PEDIATRIC ARRHYTHMIAS: ELECTROPHYSIOLOGY AND PACING

PEDIATRIC ARRHYTHMIAS: ELECTROPHYSIOLOGY AND PACING

PAUL C. GILLETTE, M.D.
Professor and Chief
Pediatric Cardiology
Medical University of South Carolina College of Medicine
Charleston, South Carolina

ARTHUR GARSON, JR., M.D.
Professor of Pediatrics and Medicine
Baylor College of Medicine;
Chief of Pediatric Cardiology
Texas Children's Hospital
Houston, Texas

1990
W.B. SAUNDERS COMPANY
Harcourt Brace Jovanovich, Inc.
Philadelphia London Toronto Montreal Sydney Tokyo

W. B. SAUNDERS COMPANY
Harcourt Brace Jovanovich, Inc.

The Curtis Center
Independence Square West
Philadelphia, PA 19106

Library of Congress Cataloging-in-Publication Data

Pediatric arrhythmias, electrophysiology, and pacing / [edited by]
Paul C. Gillette, Arthur Garson, Jr.

p. cm.

ISBN 0-7216-3201-7

1. Arrhythmia in children. I. Gillette, Paul C.
II. Garson, Arthur.
[DNLM: 1. Arrhythmia—diagnosis. 2. Arrhythmia—in infancy & childhood. 3. Arrhythmia—therapy. 4. Cardiac Pacing, Artificial—in infancy & childhood.
5. Electrophysiology—in infancy & childhood. WG 330 P371]

RJ426.A7P39 1990

618.92′128—dc20

DNLM/DLC 90-8694

Editor: W. B. Saunders Staff
Designer: W. B. Saunders Staff
Production Manager: Linda R. Turner
Manuscript Editor: Kendall Sterling
Illustration Coordinator: Ceil Kunkle
Indexer: Ella Shapiro
Cover Designer: Nina McDaid Ikeda

Pediatric Arrhythmias, Electrophysiology, and Pacing ISBN 0–7216–3201–7

Printed in the United States of America

Last digit is the print number: 9 8 7 6 5 4 3 2 1

CONTRIBUTORS

Robert H. Anderson, M.D., B.Sc., FRCPath

Professor of Paediatric Cardiac Morphology, National Heart and Lung Institute, London, U.K.; Visiting Professor, University of Pittsburgh, Pittsburgh, Pennsylvania

Embryology and Anatomy of the Normal and Abnormal Conduction System

J. Timothy Bricker, M.D.

Associate Professor of Pediatrics, Baylor College of Medicine; Director of Exercise Laboratory and Associate in Cardiology, Lillie Frank Abercrombie Section of Cardiology, Texas Children's Hospital, Houston, Texas

Arrhythmias and Sports

Henry L. Blair, C-CPT

Clinical Assistant, Medical University of South Carolina; Supervisor, Pediatric Cardiac Catheterization Laboratory, Children's Hospital, Charleston, South Carolina

Preexcitation Syndromes

David S. Buckles, Ph.D.

Instructor in Pediatrics, Division of Pediatric Cardiology, Medical University of South Carolina College of Medicine, Charleston, South Carolina

Noninvasive Diagnostic Techniques; Intracardiac Electrophysiology Studies

Christopher L. Case, D.M.D., M.D.

Assistant Professor of Pediatrics, South Carolina Children's Heart Center, Medical University of South Carolina College of Medicine, Charleston, South Carolina

Fetal Dysrhythmias

Thomas D. Christopher, M.D.

Teaching Scholar in Cardiovascular Surgery, Duke University Medical Center, Durham, North Carolina

Hemodynamic Function in Arrhythmias

Denton A. Cooley, M.D.

Clinical Professor of Surgery, University of Texas Medical School; Chief, Cardiovascular Surgery, St. Luke's Episcopal Hospital; Consultant in Cardiovascular Surgery, Texas Children's Hospital; Surgeon-in-Chief, Texas Heart Institute; Active Medical Staff, Hermann Hospital, Houston, Texas

Surgical Treatment of Tachyarrhythmias

Fred A. Crawford, M.D.

Professor of Surgery and Pediatrics; Chief of Cardiothoracic Surgery; Chairman, Department of Surgery, Medical University of South Carolina College of Medicine; Co-Director, Palmetto Heart Institute, Medical University of South Carolina Medical Center, Charleston, South Carolina
Preexcitation Syndromes; Surgical Treatment of Tachyarrhythmias

Ralph J. Damiano, Jr., M.D.

Assistant Professor of Surgery, Medical College of Virginia, Richmond, Virginia
Hemodynamic Function in Arrhythmias

David J. Driscoll, M.D.

Professor of Pediatrics, Mayo School of Medicine; Head, Section of Pediatric Cardiology, Mayo Clinic, Rochester, Minnesota
Complete Atrioventricular Block

Lesley Ewing, M.D.

Assistant Professor of Pediatrics, University of Missouri, Kansas City, Medical School; Pediatric Cardiology, Children's Mercy Hospital, Kansas City, Missouri
Bundle-Branch and Fascicular Blocks

Richard A. Friedman, M.D.

Assistant Professor of Pediatrics, Baylor College of Medicine; Associate in Pediatric Cardiology, Director of Pediatric Electrocardiography, Texas Children's Hospital, Houston, Texas
Unoperated Congenital and Acquired Heart Disease

Derek A. Fyfe, M.D., Ph.D.

Associate Professor of Pediatrics and Assistant Professor of Obstetrics and Gynecology, Medical University of South Carolina College of Medicine; Director, Pediatric Echocardiography Laboratory, Medical University of South Carolina, Charleston, South Carolina
Hemodynamic Function in Arrhythmias; Fetal Dysrhythmias

Arthur Garson, Jr., M.D.

Professor of Pediatrics and Medicine, Baylor College of Medicine; Chief of Pediatric Cardiology, Texas Children's Hospital, Houston, Texas
Systematic Interpretation of Cardiac Arrhythmias; Intracardiac Electrophysiology Studies; Supraventricular Tachycardia; Ventricular Arrhythmias; Arrhythmias and Sudden Death; Irregular Heart Beat in the Normal Child; Chronic Postoperative Arrhythmia

Paul C. Gillette, M.D.

Professor and Chief, Pediatric Cardiology, Medical University of South Carolina College of Medicine; Co-director, Palmetto Heart Institute, Charleston, South Carolina
Intracardiac Electrophysiology Studies; Preexcitation Syndromes; Catheter Ablation of Dysrhythmias; Transvenous Implantation Technique

Mark Harold, C-CPT

Electrophysiology Technologist, Children's Hospital, Medical University of South Carolina, Charleston, South Carolina
Intracardiac Electrophysiology Studies

Kenneth W. Hewett, Ph.D.

Assistant Professor of Pediatrics, Pediatric Cardiology, Medical University of South Carolina College of Medicine, Charleston, South Carolina
Developmental Cellular Electrophysiology

Siew Yen Ho, B.Sc., Ph.D.

Senior Lecturer, Paediatric Cardiac Morphology, National Heart and Lung Institute, London, U.K.
Embryology and Anatomy of the Normal and Abnormal Conduction System

John D. Kugler, M.D.

Professor of Pediatrics, Section of Cardiology, University of Nebraska Medical Center, and Children's Memorial Hospital, University of Nebraska College of Medicine, Omaha, Nebraska
Sinus Node Dysfunction

James E. Lowe, M.D.

Associate Professor of Surgery and Pathology, Duke University School of Medicine; Director, Surgical Electrophysiology Service and Attending Cardiovascular Surgeon, Duke University Medical Center, Durham, North Carolina
Hemodynamic Function in Arrhythmias

Achi Ludomirsky, M.D.

Assistant Professor of Pediatrics, Baylor College of Medicine; Associate in Pediatric Cardiology, Director of Echocardiography Research, Texas Children's Hospital, Houston, Texas
Supraventricular Tachycardia

Jeffrey P. Moak, M.D.

Assistant Professor of Pediatrics, Molecular Physiology, and Biophysics, Baylor College of Medicine; Director, Pacing and Electrophysiology and Associate in Pediatric Cardiology, Texas Children's Hospital, Houston, Texas
Pharmacology and Electrophysiology of Antiarrhythmic Drugs; Acute Nonpharmacologic Treatment of Tachyarrhythmias and Bradyarrhythmias

Martin P. O'Laughlin, M.D.

Assistant Professor of Pediatrics, Division of Pediatric Cardiology, Baylor College of Medicine, Texas Children's Hospital, Houston, Texas
Syncope

David A. Ott, M.D.

Clinical Professor, Surgery, Division of Thoracic and Cardiovascular Surgery, University of Texas; Active Staff, St. Luke's Episcopal Hospital, Texas Children's Hospital, and Hermann Hospital, Houston, Texas
Epicardial Pacemaker Implantation; Surgical Treatment of Tachyarrhythmias

James C. Perry, M.D.

Assistant Professor of Pediatrics, Baylor College of Medicine; Associate in Pediatric Cardiology, Texas Children's Hospital, Houston, Texas
Acute Pharmacologic Treatment of Cardiac Arrhythmias

William W. Pinsky, M.D.

Professor of Pediatrics, Wayne University School of Medicine; Vice Chairman of Pediatrics and Director of Pediatric Cardiology, Children's Hospital of Michigan, Detroit, Michigan
Complete Atrioventricular Block

Co-burn J. Porter, M.D.

Associate Professor of Pediatrics, Mayo Medical School; Consultant, Section of Pediatric Cardiology, Mayo Clinic and Mayo Foundation, Rochester, Minnesota
Premature Atrial Contractions and Atrial Tachyarrhythmias

Bertrand A. Ross, M.D.

Assistant Professor of Pediatrics, Eastern Virginia Medical School, Norfolk, Virginia
First and Second Degree Atrioventricular Block; Complete Atrioventricular Block; Arrhythmias and Sports

Richard T. Smith, Jr., M.D.

Director of Pediatric Electrophysiology and Pacing, The Sanger Clinic, Carolina's Medical Center, Charlotte, North Carolina
Pacemakers for Children

Henry B. Wiles, M.D.

Assistant Professor of Pediatrics and Radiology, Division of Pediatric Cardiology, Medical University of South Carolina College of Medicine, Charleston, South Carolina
Noninvasive Diagnostic Techniques

Vicki L. Zeigler, B.S.N.

Pediatric Arrhythmia Program Nurse Specialist, Division of Cardiovascular Nursing and Division of Pediatric Cardiology, Medical University of South Carolina, Charleston, South Carolina
Noninvasive Diagnostic Techniques; Transvenous Implantation Technique

PREFACE

This book is intended as a textbook of diagnosis and treatment of arrhythmias in children and young adults. To this end, it is much larger and more inclusive than our former book. The book is divided into five sections: Basic Principles (including a chapter on anatomy and pathology), Techniques, Specific Arrhythmias, Methods of Treatment, and Clinical Situations. We hope that fellows in pediatric cardiology will read the entire book. Pediatric cardiologists, adult cardiologists, and others who intermittently treat children and young adults with arrhythmias may find it useful to consult individual chapters as the specific clinical need arises.

Although we have tried to present different views of controversial points, we know that in some cases we have favored our own biases. Everything written here is not proved as fact, since there are many gaps in our knowledge. However, at present we are challenged by children with problems in these gray areas, and we must react to these problems now! We have written what we feel is most appropriate for now, the present. Although we have worked closely with most of the authors of this volume, there are areas of differing opinion among some of the chapters. To do justice to such controversy, we have tried not to eliminate areas where real differences of opinion exist.

The decade of the 1990s undoubtedly will bring improvements in the treatment of arrhythmias in children. There are still episodes of sudden death to be prevented, particularly in postoperative patients. Our goals must involve establishing definitive treatments that avoid iatrogenic complications.

The areas of fetal diagnosis and management will mature in the 1990s. We may witness the beginnings of fetal cardiac surgery. The implantation of a pacemaker might be the first fetal heart surgical procedure.

Application of nonpharmacologic arrhythmia therapy to the pediatric patient will certainly flourish in the next decade. Direct surgical treatment of arrhythmias matured in the 1980s and is currently an option for managing most arrhythmias, including its use in control of infantile, neonatal, and perhaps even fetal arrhythmias. We will probably witness major advances in catheter treatment of arrhythmias with the use of more efficacious and gentler energy sources.

Major strides have been made and will continue to be made in pediatric cardiac pacing. Transvenous implantation is now firmly established, and the predicted problems have failed to materialize. Physiologic pacing is now the standard. Antitachycardia pacing is beginning to be recognized. The 1990s should bring increased applications of all these concepts.

The past, present, and future advances outlined in this book should allow children with cardiac arrhythmias to lead normal, productive lives.

PAUL C. GILLETTE
ARTHUR GARSON, JR.

CONTENTS

SECTION I

BASIC PRINCIPLES

CHAPTER 1

EMBRYOLOGY AND ANATOMY OF THE NORMAL AND ABNORMAL CONDUCTION SYSTEM

Siew Yen Ho & Robert H. Anderson

The beginning of the twentieth century began an exciting new era for scientists interested in the rhythmic working of the heart. Discoveries of a specialized tissue network for the transmission of impulses[1] and the impulse generator itself[2] were followed swiftly by the electrical studies of Lewis,[3] which established the role of these structures. Most subsequent studies were refinements and confirmations of the original investigations, although a few contentious issues were also produced.

Investigative techniques on the physiologic aspects of cardiac conduction have progressed well ahead of anatomic and histologic methods. In recent years, investigators of the tissue and subtissue substrates are called on increasingly by their waveform-watching colleagues to find an anatomic basis for aberrations in their tracings. The pressure to "find something" is often unwarranted, because the normal system itself shows a range of anatomic variations.[4, 5] Until a large reservoir of normal material can be gathered with complete electrographic data, the correlations for most arrhythmias will remain a challenge. In the normally structured hearts, the better understood substrates are to be found in congenital heart block and some types of ventricular preexcitation. Abnormal architecture of the conduction system can also be found in some groups of congenitally malformed hearts. Awareness of anatomically abnormal systems is useful to the pediatric cardiologist. In this chapter, we provide a review of the developmental aspects of the normal conduction system and we cite instances of abnormal development.

DEVELOPMENT

Information on the early development of the cardiac conduction system in humans remains scanty. Most of our present knowledge is inferred from studies on animal species, in spite of limiting factors such as species variations. Nonetheless, phylogenetic studies have shown the presence of rings of specialized tissue separating the five components of the primitive heart tube. These rings are found at the junctions between venous sinus, primitive atrium, inlet and outlet parts of the ventricular segment, and the arterial segment. This interpretation of development is perhaps simplistic, but the approach aids in the understanding of the formation of both the normal and abnormal cardiac conduction system (Fig. 1–1). Thus it would seem that the rings form the primordium of the conduction tissues and that the ring concept can be extended to account for ectopic distributions of the conduction system in malformed hearts.[6] There is evidence that a ring of specialized tissue exists at the atrioventricular junction in human embryos[7] as described by Keith and Flack in 1907.[2] The existence of

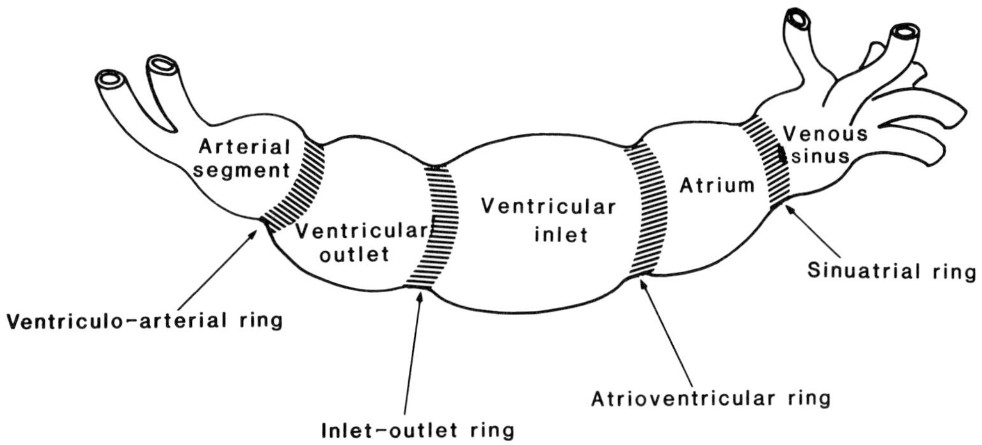

FIGURE 1–1
Diagrammatic representation of the five components of the primitive heart tube, with rings of specialized tissue at the junctions.

the other rings, however, is difficult to ascertain in the human heart after the completion of septation.

The sinus node is a recognizable structure from as early as the stage of cardiac looping.[8] The nodal primordium is situated at the junction of the superior caval vein with the right atrium. Although the nodal primordium is initially a horseshoe-shaped structure, usually only the lateral part persists. The nodal cells are histologically discrete from the adjacent myocardium in their arrangement and staining characteristics. The cells are set in a connective tissue matrix, but the volume of connective tissue appears to increase and become more evident as the fetus nears the time of birth.[8] Also, at the early stages the size of the node is largest relative to the rest of the atrial tissues.

Apart from the nodal primordium, the remainder of the sinoatrial junction is infolded to form the valves of the venous sinus. These tissues do not show any histologically specialized characteristics. As development proceeds, the valves become less cellular and more fibrous. Although they extend from the primordium of the sinus node to the developing atrioventricular junction, they cannot be shown to have any conduction properties. The ring of specialized tissue at the atrioventricular junction forms the primordium of the atrioventricular node. It is initially sandwiched between atrioventricular sulcus tissue and endocardial cushion tissue. The histologically discrete ring is recognized as soon as the heart tube is formed.

Following looping, outpouchings of the ascending and descending limbs of the ventricular loop form the trabecular components of the right ventricle and left ventricle, respectively, with the developing trabecular septum formed between the pouches (Fig. 1–2). The primordia of the bundle branches develop like a drape across the trabecular septum, reaching into the subendocardium of the trabecular pouches. Development of the inlet septum (which partitions the inlet component of the ventricular loop) carries with it a tongue of atrioventricular ring tissue that is also sandwiched by sulcus and cushion tissue. Further growth and development of the inlet septum and trabecular septum transfers the right atrioventricular orifice to the trabecular pouch of the right ventricle.[9] Consequently, the conduction tissue on the inlet and apical trabecular components of the septum are brought together to form a continuous ventricular conduction axis (Fig. 1–3). The definitive atrial septum has yet to be formed at this stage, and the ventricular conduction bundle is in contact with atrial tissues only at the posterior atrial wall. As the atrial septum forms, the atrial tissues are separated from the conduction tissue on the inlet septum by the endocardial cushions. The endocardial cushions regress gradually with increasing development, bringing the conduction bundle into direct contact with the inferior rim of the atrial septum. The atrial tissues immediately around the contact region become established as the transitional cell zone, while the end of the bundle becomes the compact atrioventricular node. Since the atrial septum grows down onto the conduction axis, the

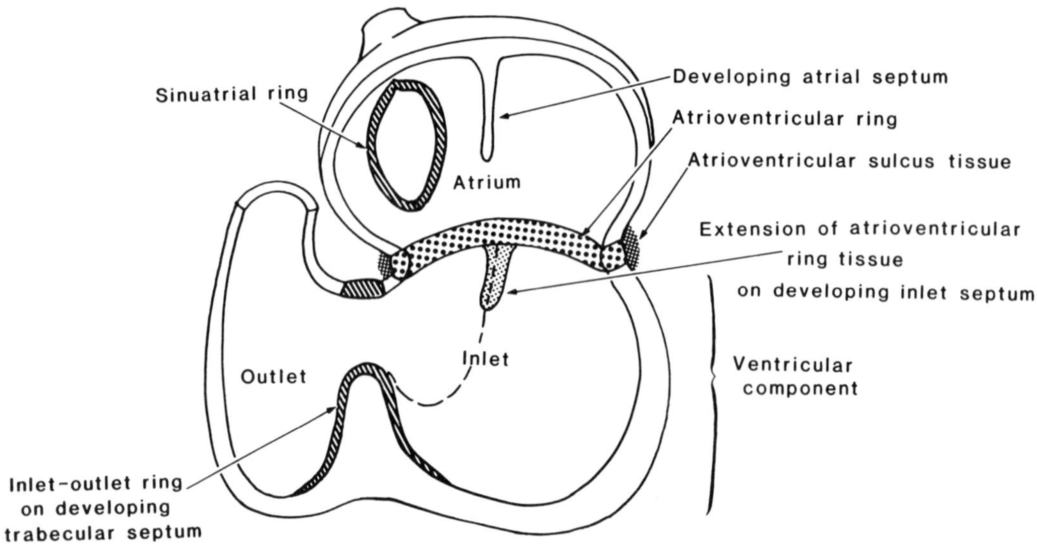

FIGURE 1–2
Diagrammatic representation of the frontal view of the heart tube after looping to show the development of the trabecular septum and the inlet septum, which carry the specialized tissue.

definitive compact node is an interatrial structure. The node becomes the penetrating bundle where the remnants of the cushions persist to separate the axis from the atrial septal tissues; sulcus tissue separates the axis from ventricular myocardium.

The primordial ventricular conduction tissues on the trabecular septum are more extensive in early than later development. The subendocardial network in the trabecular regions probably becomes the ramifications of the bundle branches. The origin of the defin-

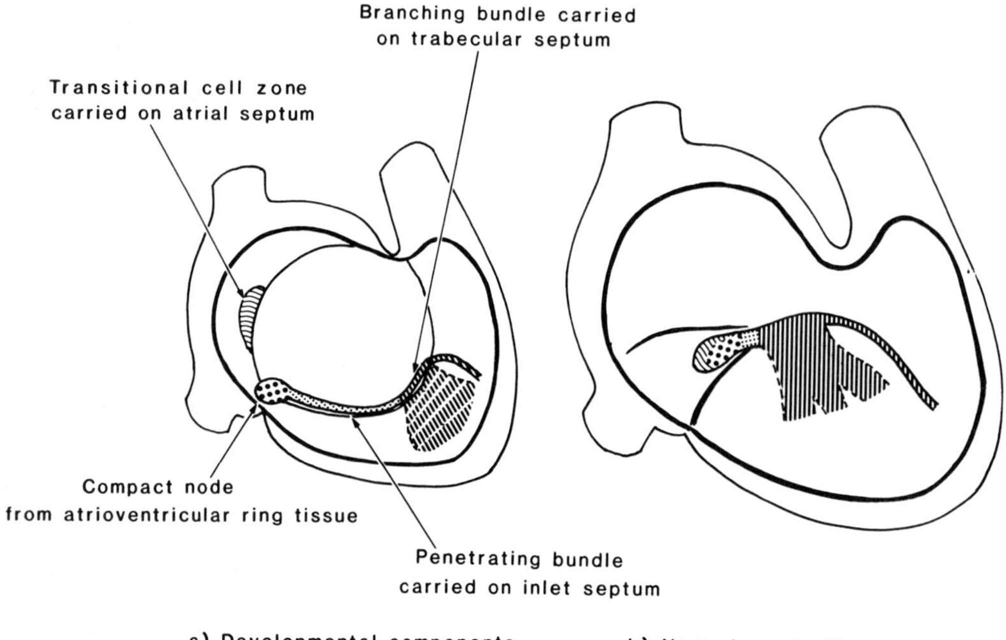

FIGURE 1–3
Diagrammatic representations of the lateral views of the heart to show the developmental components of the atrioventricular conduction axis *(left)* and the normal conduction system *(right)*.

itive cord-like right bundle branch in human hearts is still not clear. It may be a remnant of ring tissue at the ventriculoarterial junction[6] or may be formed by the contraction of a sleeve of trabecular septal tissue.[10]

The remainder of the specialized atrioventricular ring tissue largely regresses with development and with ingrowth of the atrioventricular sulcus tissue. The latter tissue contributes to the formation of the perimeter of the atrioventricular valve orifices. Ingrowing sulcus tissue eventually serves to separate the atrial from the ventricular myocardial masses. Remnants of the embryonic ring tissue occasionally persist in the margin of atrial musculature nearest the valve orifice. These areas that have histologic characteristics of conduction tissue are termed the *atrioventricular ring specialized tissue.*[11] They may persist in some congenitally malformed hearts to form abnormally positioned connecting atrioventricular nodes.

THE NORMAL SYSTEM

The atrial component of the normal system is the sinus node. The node is spindle shaped in the definitive heart and is located on the lateral margin of the junction between the superior caval vein and the right atrium. Occasionally, the node is shaped like a horseshoe draped over the crest of the right atrium. This configuration would seem to be a persistence of the embryonic form. Our studies of neonatal hearts have shown the spindle shape with a tapering tail to be the norm, rather than the horseshoe arrangement.[12, 13] The terminal groove (which is the epicardial marker for the position of the terminal crest) is also a good guide to the position of the sinus node. When viewed in cross-section, the node appears as a triangular-shaped structure in immediately subepicardial position wedged in the terminal groove (Fig. 1–4). As Truex has pointed out, the shape of the node is highly variable according to the plane of section.[14] Problems resulting from this fact can be overcome by serial section reconstructions.[12]

The nodal cells are smaller than the ordinary atrial myocytes and grouped into clusters. The feature that makes the sinus node readily recognizable under low histologic section magnifications is the fibrous tissue matrix in which the clusters of nodal cells are enmeshed. The fibrous matrix is less apparent in neonatal hearts but increases in prominence with age.[15] Another feature that aids in locating the sinus node under microscopy is the sinus node artery. The main artery supplying the node is often seen penetrating the nodal body. However, the course taken by the artery relative to the node is variable. The artery may approach the node from the medial aspect of the cavo-atrial junction or from a more lateral aspect. Furthermore, the artery may ramify within the node or adjacent to the node (Fig. 1–5). The origin of the nodal artery, too, is highly variable.[16, 17]

Detailed studies of the cellular constituents of the sinus node by both light and electron microscopy have revealed a rather homogeneous composition of nodal cells. Large pale cells described by some investigators as "Purkinje" cells or "intercalated clear cells"[18, 19] were rarely observed by us in our light microscopy studies on infant tissues or by Tranum-Jensen's ultrastructural studies using animal material.[20] From his own experience, Tranum-Jensen suggested that the "clear" cells may be artefactual. The body of the node is composed of specific nodal cells within a framework of fibrous tissue; the borders of the node show cells of intermediate form between nodal and working myocardium (the *transitional cells*). Transitional cell zones are not found uniformly around the node. In places there is a discrete junction between the tightly packed nodal cells and the individual atrial myocardial cells. In others, particularly the borders of the node facing the terminal crest, tongues of transitional cells extend into the ordinary atrial musculature (Fig. 1–6). The tail of the node, usually composed of transitional cells, penetrates intramyocardially to varying distances within the musculature of the terminal crest before merging with the surrounding myocardium.

The sinus node is richly innervated. Collections of ganglion cells are frequently seen in the epicardium in the environs of the node. Studies on human fetal tissues using histochemical techniques have also shown a rich cholinesterase-positive innervation.[7]

INTERNODAL MYOCARDIUM

As previously stated, electron microscopy has not revealed any discrete specialized tis-

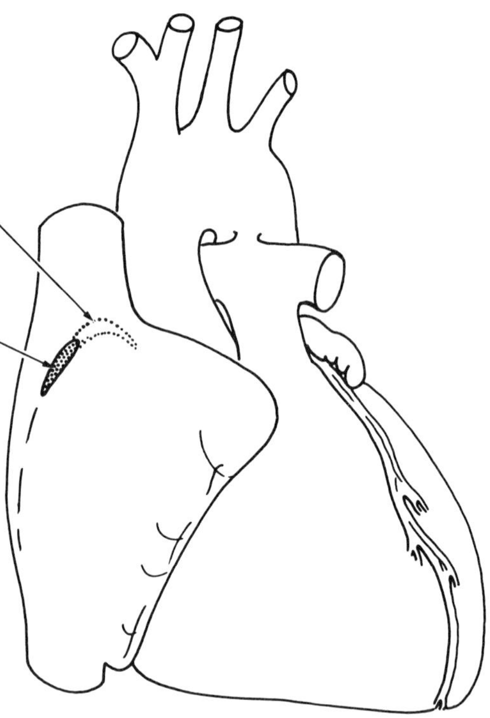

FIGURE 1–4
Diagram showing the usual spindle shape of the sinus node occupying a lateral position in the terminal groove. Occasionally, the node is horseshoe-shaped and occupies a more medial position.

sue tracts between the two cardiac nodes. Light microscopic examination of the internodal atrial myocardium in infant hearts yielded similar results (Fig. 1–7).[21] Anatomico-electrophysiologic correlative studies also were unable to demonstrate such tissue tracts.[22] Apart from the occasional extension of the tail of the sinus node into the terminal crest musculature, no histologically recognizable pathways are seen. Our anatomic findings do not discount the existence of preferential pathways for internodal conduction. Indeed, such pathways have been shown to exist.[23–25] The walls of the atrium are made up of broad bands of muscular tissue. The terminal crest and anterior rim of the oval fossa show a better degree of myocyte organization than the remaining walls. The myocardial fibers are arranged in the same direction in contrast to the lack of alignment (e.g., in the atrial appendages). The spread of excitation from sinus node to atrioventricular node has been shown to progress preferentially along these bands as broad wave fronts. The myocardium in these bands is made up of ordinary atrial myocardium, unlike the specialized conduction bundles found in the ventricles. Proponents of internodal specialized pathways have used various criteria for designating "specialization" to a cell (see Janse and Anderson 1974[23]), but none of the criteria is consistent with the generally accepted specialized characteristics shown by the sinus node or atrioventricular conduction system when viewed under a light microscope.

ATRIOVENTRICULAR SYSTEM

The atrioventricular specialized junctional area comprises the transitional cell zone, the compact atrioventricular node, the penetrating atrioventricular bundle, and the branching atrioventricular bundle (Fig. 1–8). The branching atrioventricular bundle gives origin to the ventricular bundle branches. The anatomy of this system, first described in 1906 by Tawara,[1] has been confirmed by subsequent investigators. The gross anatomic landmarks to the specialized junctional area are related to right atrial structures. It must be remembered, however, that the atrial component of the area is an interatrial structure and not exclusively a right atrial structure.[26]

The most reliable gross landmark to the position of the atrioventricular node is a triangular area in the right atrium known as the *triangle of Koch*. Koch[27] described the area

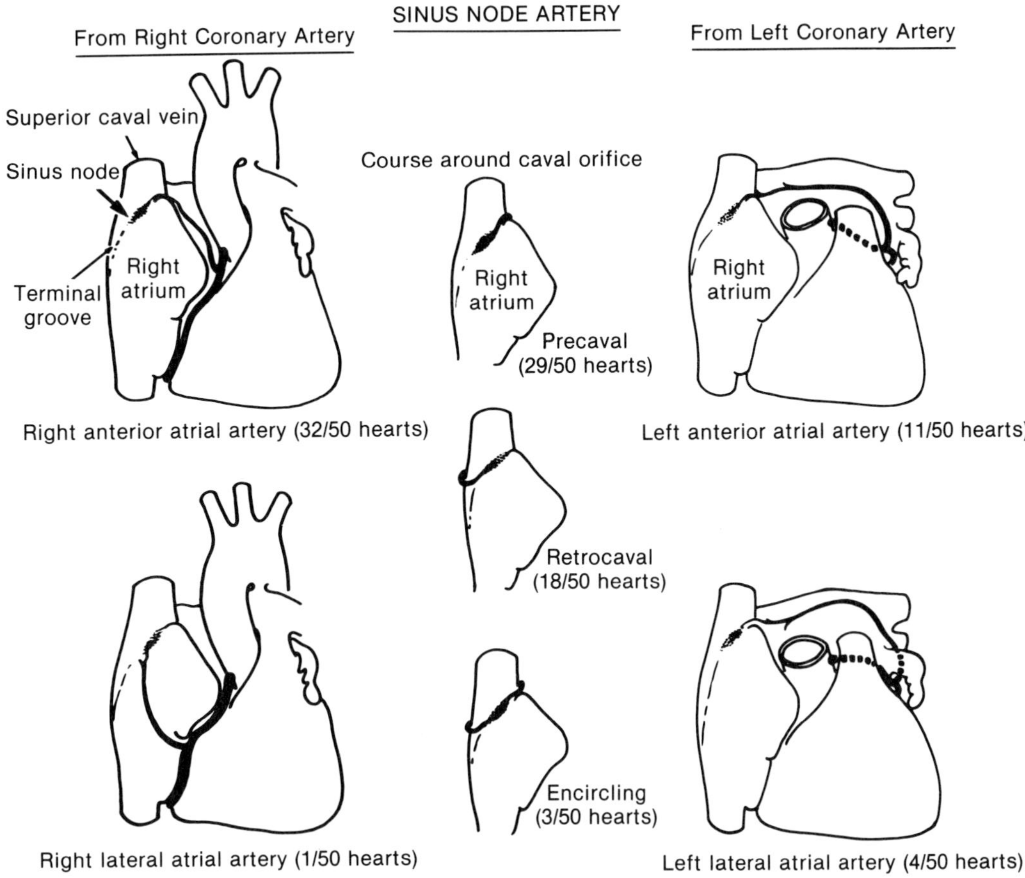

FIGURE 1–5
Diagram showing the origin and course of the sinus node artery found in 50 normal hearts. (Adapted from a study by Busquet et al: The surgical significance of the atrial branches of the coronary arteries. Int J Cardiol 6:223–224, 1984.)

as being delineated by the continuation of the eustachian valve and the annular insertion of the tricuspid valve (Fig. 1–9). The continuation of the eustachian valve and thebesian valve commissure is a tendinous structure (the tendon of Todaro) that springs forward when tension is applied on the eustachian valve. The tendon inserts into the central fibrous body, and it is at the apex of the triangle thus formed that the atrioventricular node is situated. The base of the triangle is the coronary sinus. Some investigators and surgeons continue to use the coronary sinus as a landmark, but our own observations have shown that the coronary sinus is variably distant from the node or may be absent altogether, making it a poor reference point.[28]

Since the insertion of the mitral valve is at a higher level than the tricuspid valve, anatomically there is a region of septal musculature that is atrioventricular in position, separating the right atrium from the left ventricle. The compact atrioventricular node sits against the fibrous annulus in the atrial aspect of this atrioventricular muscular septum, which is toward the apex of the triangle of Koch (Fig. 1–10). The transitional cell zone comprises fibers that extend posteriorly and superiorly, interposing between the ordinary atrial myocardium and the specialized cells of the compact node. The transitional cells are attenuated and are frequently separated by fine fibrous septa. The compact atrioventricular node is made up of interconnecting fascicles of small cells. While the nodal body is closely adherent to the fibrous annulus, two prong-like extensions usually run posteriorly to follow the curvature of the mitral and tricuspid valve rings. When viewed in cross section, the nodal body appears like a half-oval structure (Fig. 1–10), frequently with a bilaminar composition of deep and superficial layers.[29] Transitional

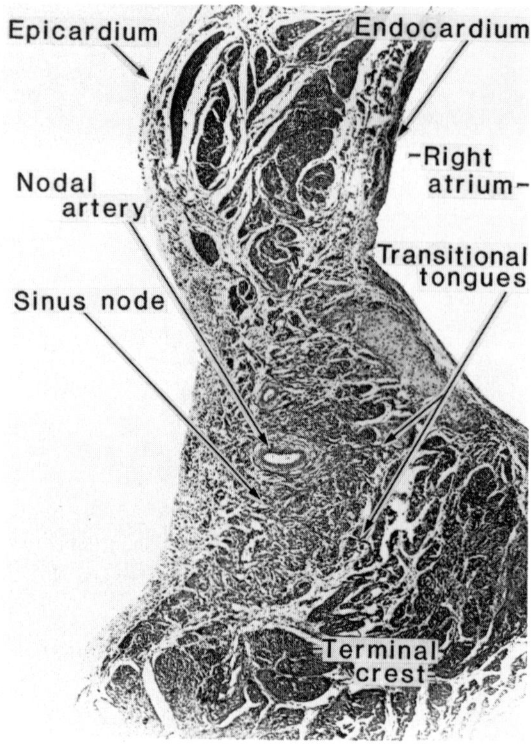

FIGURE 1–6
Photomicrograph showing the cross-section of a neonatal sinus node. Note the subepicardial position.

FIGURE 1–7
Photomicrograph of a longitudinal section through the right atrium. The cardiac nodes are distinguishable from the ordinary internodal myocardium.

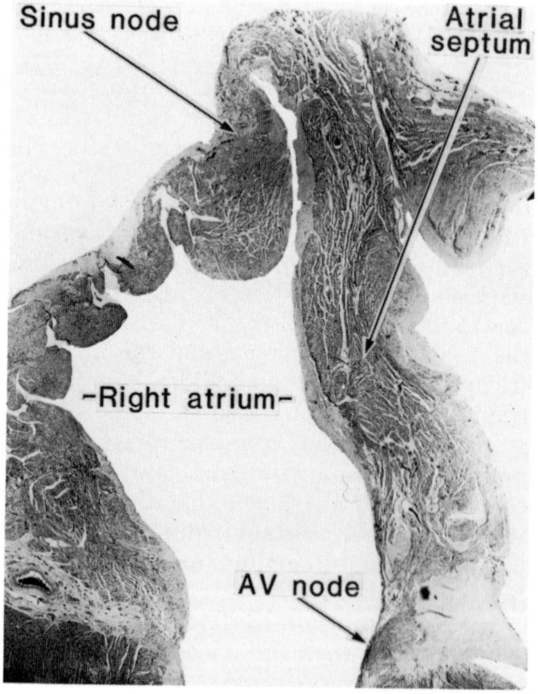

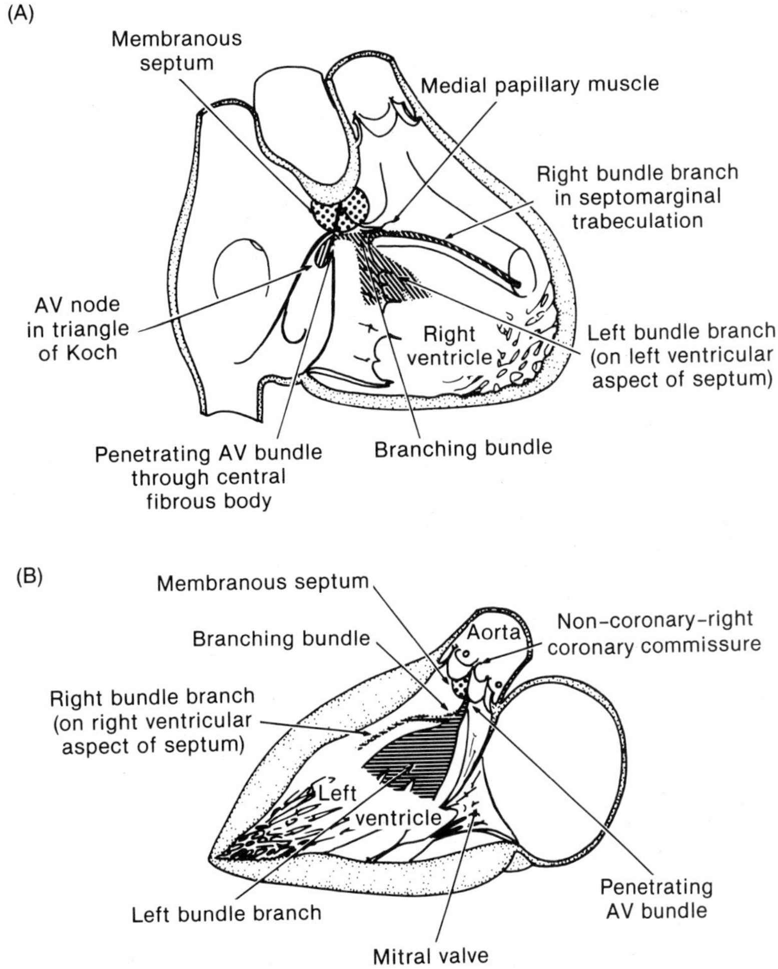

FIGURE 1–8

Diagrams showing the course of the atrioventricular conduction system as viewed from *(A)* the right side and *(B)* the left side of the heart.

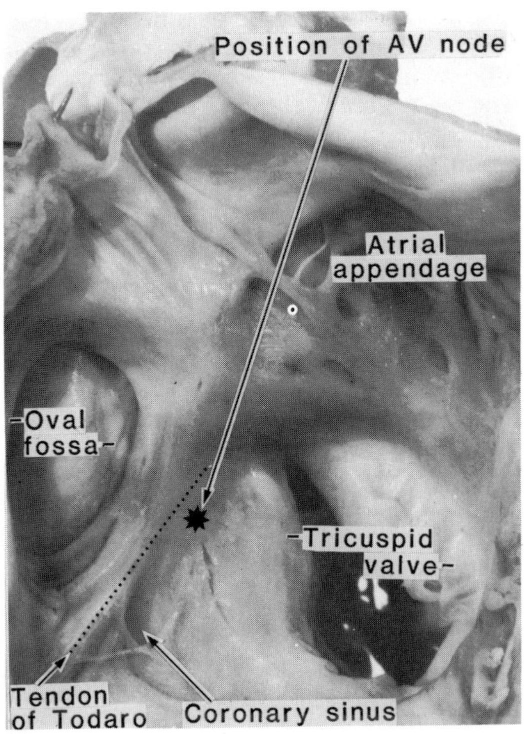

FIGURE 1–9

Right atrial view showing the boundaries of the triangle of Koch. The tendon of Todaro is represented by the dotted line.

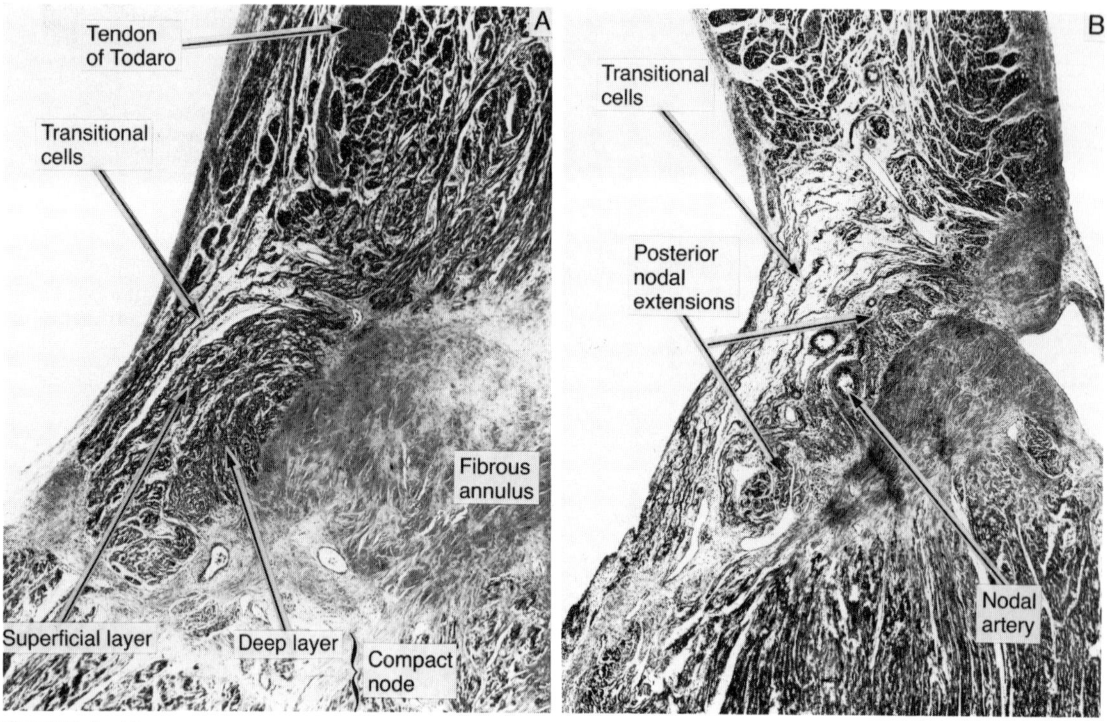

FIGURE 1–10
Histologic sections through the atrioventricular junctional area. The components of the atrioventricular node are shown in *(A)*. The posterior extensions of the node are shown in *(B)*.

cells that overlie the superficial layer give the structure a trilaminar look.

Being closely related to the fibrous annulus and the central fibrous body, the atrioventricular node seems to occupy a position in the middle of the heart. It is, in fact, an epicardial structure. This is because a tissue plane extends from the posterior atrioventricular groove tissue at the cardiac crux and runs underneath the coronary sinus into the muscular atrioventricular septum. It is in this tissue plane that the atrioventricular node artery approaches and penetrates the node (Fig. 1–11). The artery, a branch of the dominant coronary artery, is usually disproportionately large. This tissue plane is an important landmark for the surgeon attempting to destroy posterior septal accessory pathways responsible for the Wolff-Parkinson-White syndrome.

The compact node becomes the penetrating bundle at the apex of the triangle of Koch (Fig. 1–12) and enters the ventricular tissues at this point. Histologically, the transition between compact node and penetrating bundle is gradual, with imperceptible cellular distinction. When following serial histologic sections, the change from the distal portion of the node to the penetrating bundle is the point at which the axis of cells becomes completely surrounded by the fibrous annulus tissue. While the distal node is in contact with atrial myocardium, the penetrating bundle is sequestrated from both atrial and ventricular myocardium. When following the axis further into the ventricles, it can be seen that the specialized cells become aligned in a more parallel fashion but still retain their small size. The gross landmark to this portion of the axis is the membranous septum (see Fig. 1–8). As the penetrating bundle passes beneath the insertion of the tendon of Todaro into the central fibrous body, the nonbranching and branching bundles are sandwiched between the membranous septum and the muscular ventricular septum. The branching bundle may be seen astride the muscular septal crest or to the left of it (Fig. 1–13). The nonbranching component is usually very short, and the conduction axis shifts obliquely to emerge into the left ventricular outflow tract. The branching of the bundles is usually beneath the commissure between the right coronary and noncoronary leaflets of the

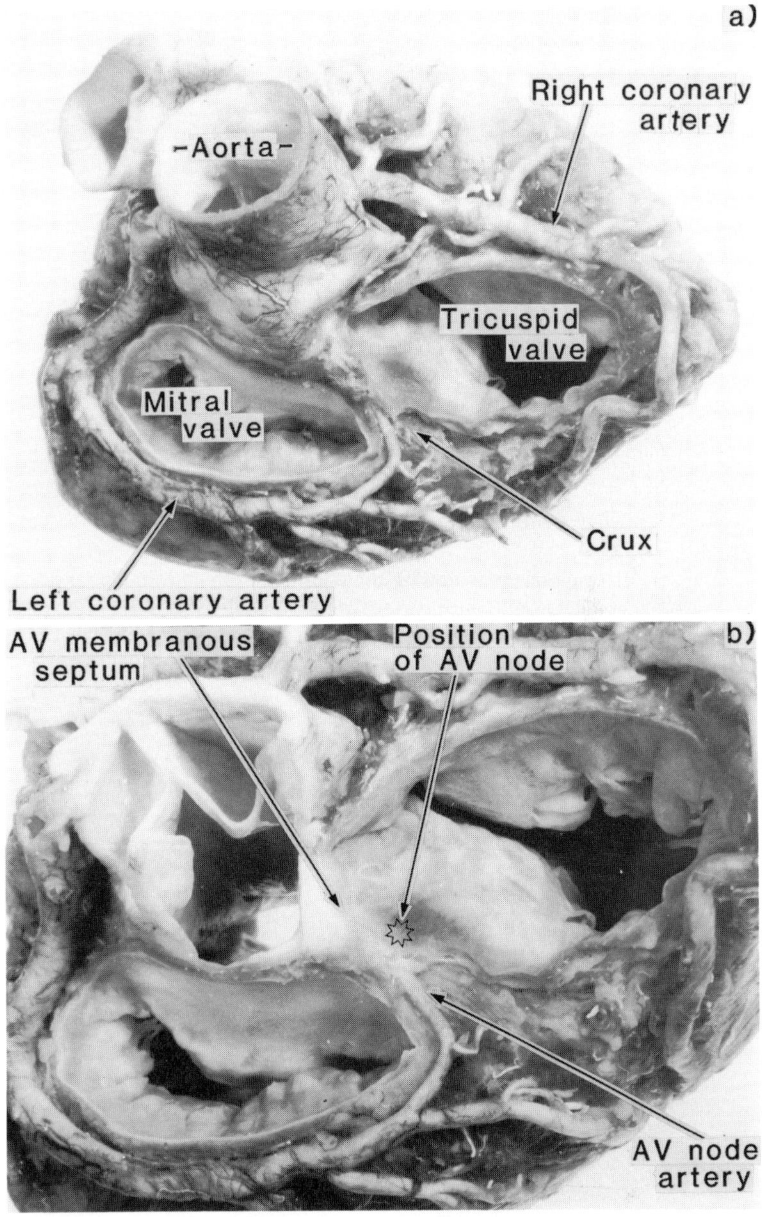

FIGURE 1–11
Dissection of a heart viewed from above to show the courses of the coronary arteries around the atrioventricular junction *(a)*. A deeper dissection *(b)* shows the origin of the atrioventricular node artery from the dominant left coronary artery at the cardiac crux.

aortic valve (see Fig. 1–8). The origin of the medial papillary muscle on the right ventricular aspect of the septum usually marks the point of descent of the right bundle branch.

The branching bundle commences at the origin of the left bundle branch. The left bundle branch is sheetlike and immediately subendocardial on the left aspect of the ventricular septum (see Fig. 1–8). Topographically, the initial fibers are within the subendocardial tissues of the aortic outflow tract. They then fan out into diverging plates of fascicles. The precise morphology of the distal division of the fascicles is controversial. Tawara's original reconstructions show the bundle radiating in fanlike fashion into three major divisions that are, in turn, interconnected distally in the left ventricle.[12] Some subsequent investigators have endorsed this arrangement,[30–33] but a bifascicular constitution has been promulgated by others, notably Rosenbaum, Elizari, and Lazzari.[34] The latter view appears to correlate well with the electrocardiographic concept of bundle branch blocks, although anatomically a trifascicular arrangement is more usual. However, be-

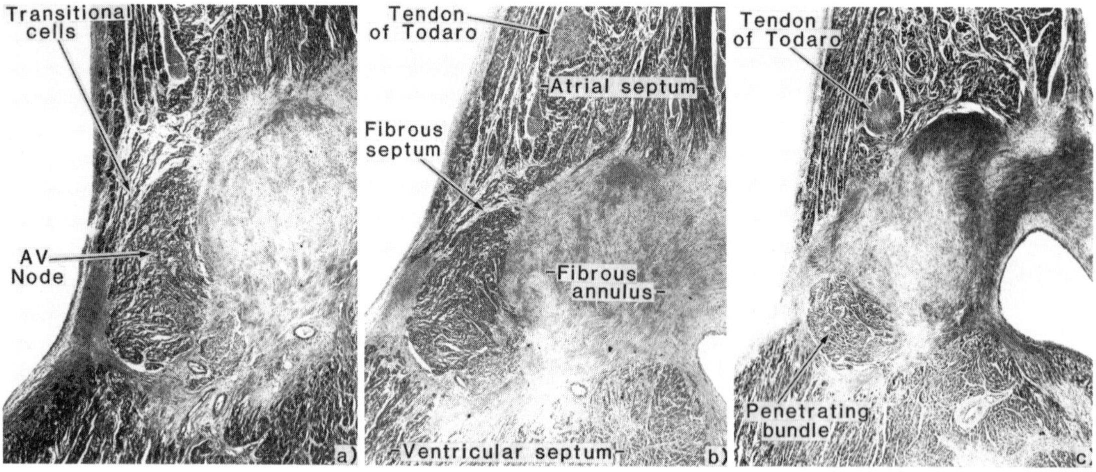

FIGURE 1–12

A series of histologic sections showing the transition from atrioventricular node to penetrating bundle. In *(a)* the nodal cells are still in contact with atrial myocardium. This contact is lost in *(b)* when a fibrous septum intervenes. The axis then becomes the penetrating bundle, although the histologic appearance is similar to that in *(a)*. The penetrating bundle is more readily recognized in *c*, where it is surrounded by a prominent fibrous collar.

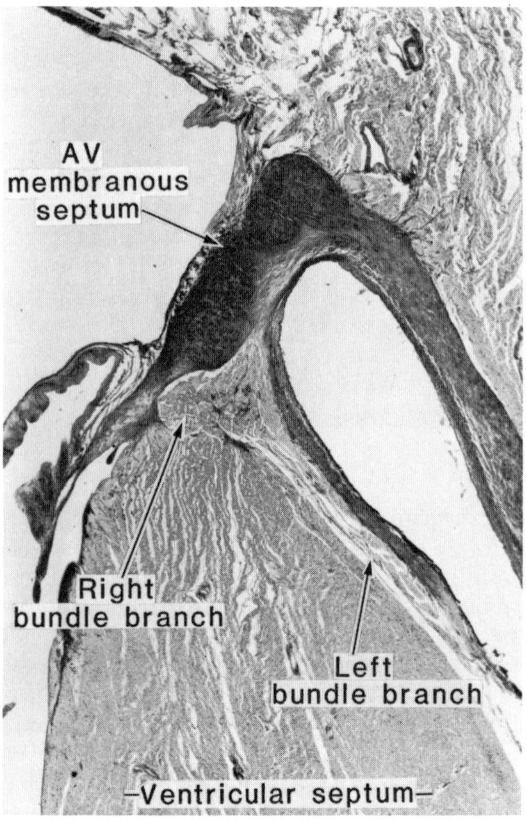

FIGURE 1–13

Histologic section showing the branching bundle offset to the left of the septal crest. (Photomicrograph courtesy of Prof. A. E. Becker)

cause the upper portion of the left bundle branch is insulated from ventricular myocardium, the manner of distal division seems less important, since the very remote ramifications are themselves interconnected in the form of a network.

The right bundle branch is morphologically very different from the left bundle branch. It is usually the direct continuation of the nodal bundle conduction axis. In some hearts it is a branch from the axis, and the axis itself continues anteriorly to terminate in the outlet musculature.[35] In terms of development, this "dead-end tract" has been considered to be a persistence of the ventriculoarterial ring tissue. The right bundle branch is characteristically a cordlike structure within a fibrous sheath (see Fig. 1–13). It penetrates intramyocardially from its branch-point origin through the substance of the septomarginal trabeculation and then passes toward the apex of the right ventricle. It then ramifies subendocardially in the apex, while the main bundle crosses the ventricular cavity within the moderator band.

The cellular makeup of the bundle branches is sometimes described as being of large, clear, "Purkinje-like" elements. Although such cells are found in ungulate hearts, our experience with infants has shown these cells to be the exception. More usually the bundle branch cells are comparable in size to ventricular myocytes, although some cells may be vacuolated. The Purkinje-like cellular appearance is more frequently encountered as fixation artefacts or in older hearts. As the bundle branches ramify, they lose their fibrous tissue sheaths and become exceedingly difficult to identify. Cells of the peripheral conduction fibers become indistinguishable from other ventricular myocytes.

The effect of aging on the conduction system is still not well known. This is probably a result of the fact that investigators tend to work either with very young patients or with only adult patients. In general, there is an increase of fibrous tissue with age.[36] In adult hearts, the bulk of the conduction tissues becomes less in relation to the cardiac mass. The globular shape of the infant atrioventricular node is not seen in adult hearts. Furthermore, older hearts often show adipose tissue deposition in the transitional cell zone. Another effect of aging that still lacks quantitative and systematic examination is the "molding" process of extensions of atrioventricular nodal fibers into the central fibrous body. These extensions, frequently seen in fetal and infant hearts, are seen with less frequency in adult hearts. It has been suggested that maturation of the central fibrous body eliminates the extensions.[37] These fiber extensions have also been implicated as a possible cause of sudden infant death syndrome,[38] but in our experience these are also not uncommonly seen in "normal" hearts.

ABNORMAL CONDUCTION SYSTEM

Congenital Heart Diseases

Both the sinus node and the atrioventricular conduction tissues can be abnormally positioned in congenitally malformed hearts, but it is convenient to describe them separately.

Sinus Node. The majority of malformed hearts have the atrial chambers in the usual position, and the sinus node in its regular position. Abnormal positions of the sinus node have been found to occur in hearts with juxtaposition of the right atrial appendage and hearts with an atrial arrangement other than the usual type.

Juxtaposition exists when the atrial appendages lie to the same side of the arterial pedicle rather than to either side at the base of the heart. Right juxtaposition, in which the left atrial appendage lies alongside the right atrial appendage to the right side of the pedicle, is uncommon. This distortion of atrial anatomy does not seem to affect the location of the sinus node. In contrast, left juxtaposition, in which the right atrial appendage is positioned alongside the left atrial appendage to the left side of the pedicle, is a more common anomaly.[39] In this malformation, the communication of the right appendage with the right atrium occupies a position between the superior caval vein and the oval fossa. Therefore, the right cavoatrial junction marked by the terminal crest is usually deviated. Our study of six patients with left juxtaposition showed a variable displacement of the node anteriorly (Fig. 1–14).[40]

Other malformations having abnormal positions of the sinus node are those that affect the arrangement of the atrial chambers.

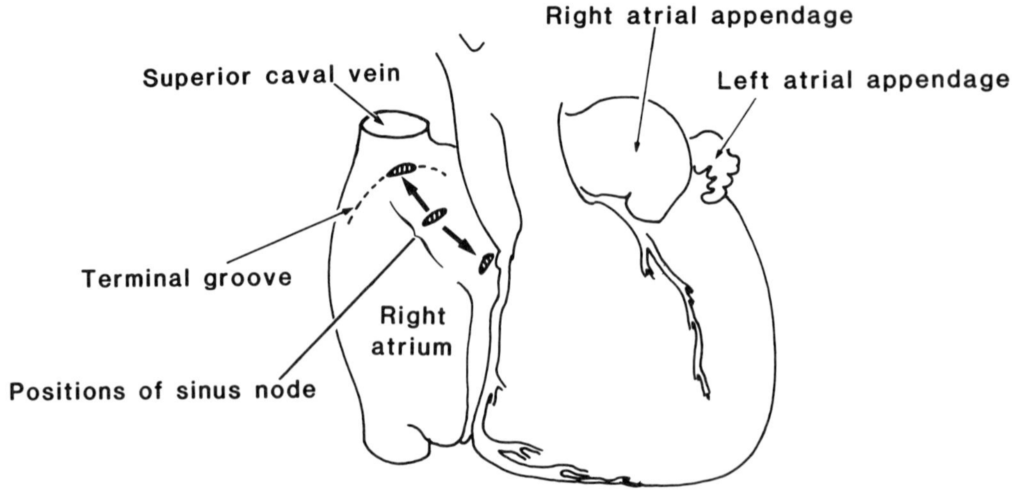

FIGURE 1–14
Diagram showing the variable locations of the sinus node in hearts with left juxtaposition of the atrial appendages.

When atrial chambers are arranged in mirror-image fashion, the morphologically right atrium (carrying the sinus node) is in left-sided position (Fig. 1–15). When there are bilateral right atrial chambers, as exists in right atrial isomerism,[41] the sinus node is duplicated and is situated in both right and left positions. When both atrial chambers are of left morphology, as in left atrial isomerism, the terminal crests are lacking.[42] Although in this group bilateral superior caval veins can be present, the sinus node is not found in its anticipated position relative to either caval vein. While in some hearts a remnant of specialized tissue is found in the posterior atrial wall near the atrioventricular junction, in other hearts such tissue cannot be identified.

Atrioventricular Conduction Tissue. As previously described, the atrioventricular conduction system is derived from several components that come together to produce a continuous conduction axis. It is not surprising that any malformation involving an absence or malalignment of any of these components will also have an abnormal disposition of the conduction axis. The most abnormal locations are produced when the inlet ventricular septum is either absent or grossly malaligned with the atrial septum. In

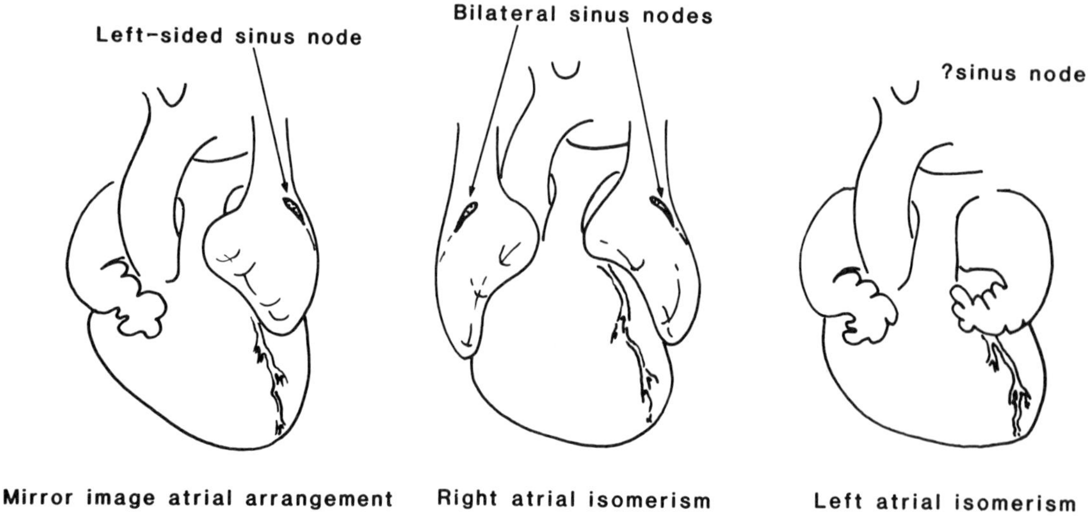

FIGURE 1–15
Diagrams showing the locations of the sinus node in three variants of atrial arrangement.

these circumstances, a malpositioned atrioventricular node is connected to the displaced axis (Fig. 1–16).

DEFECTS IN HEARTS WITH NORMALLY ALIGNED SEPTAL STRUCTURES

Most congenital heart lesions are simple holes in the cardiac septum or abnormal ventricular origins of the great arteries. These malformations have little effect on the proper alignment of atrial and ventricular septal structures, and therefore, with minor differences, a regular posteriorly situated atrioventricular conduction system is to be expected. The key prerequisite to a regular system in these hearts is concordant connection at the atrioventricular level (i.e., the morphologically right atrium connects to the morphologically right ventricle, and the morphologically left atrium connects to the morphologically left ventricle). These hearts, when associated with mirror-image arrangement of the atrial chambers (situs inversus), have mirror-image distribution of the atrioventricular conduction axis.

The more common malformations in this group are hearts with an isolated ventricular septal defect, with atrioventricular septal defect, and with tetralogy of Fallot. Except for those hearts with atrioventricular septal defect, the triangle of Koch remains a good landmark for the location of the atrioventricular node.

In terms of distribution of the atrioventricular conduction axis, hearts with tetralogy of Fallot are directly comparable to hearts with isolated ventricular septal defect, since a defect in the ventricular septum is a cardinal feature of tetralogy of Fallot. Most ventricular septal defects, whether existing in isolation or otherwise, are located in the environs of the membranous septum. These are termed *perimembranous defects,* and they have a fibrous component to their borders (Fig. 1–17). The fibrous component usually represents a remnant of the membranous septum situated in the region of fibrous continuity between the atrioventricular valves and an arterial valve. The nonbranching bundle is usually short in the normal heart, but it can be considerably longer in hearts with a ventricular septal defect. The normal leftward shift of the bundle axis brings the bundle into the left ventricular outflow tract. The penetrating and nonbranching component of the axis therefore emerges directly underneath the membranous septal remnant. Thus the posteroinferior rim of the defect is the most critical area for any surgeon contemplating a patch closure of the defect.

The disposition of the branching bundle shows a slight variation in hearts with isolated perimembranous ventricular septal defects and those associated with tetralogy of Fallot. It is frequently found astride the septal crest or, rarely, to the left side when the defect exists in isolation.[43–45] The contrary exists in hearts with tetralogy of Fallot: a minority of cases have the axis directly astride the septum.[46] This latter point is of major surgical significance.

Muscular defects situated immediately beneath both arterial valves have a relationship to the conduction axis that is similar to that of perimembranous defects. If present, a muscular posteroinferior rim provides the conduction axis with greater protection from all but the deepest sutures (see Fig. 1–17).

Defects with completely muscular borders have varying relationships with the conduction axis depending on their location within the septum (Fig. 1–18). Defects situated in the outlet part are remote from the conduction axis, while defects in the apical trabecular part are in the environs of the bundle branch ramifications. Defects in the inlet septum are particularly significant. They need to be distinguished from perimembranous defects, which have an extensive posterior extension into the inlet septum. In muscular inlet defects, the conduction axis is found at its anterosuperior quadrant. This is in stark contrast to the posteroinferior position found in the presence of perimembranous inlet defects (see Fig 1–17). When both a perimembranous defect and a muscular inlet defect exist in the same heart, the conduction axis traverses the muscular bridge separating the defects (Fig. 1–19).

In terms of conduction tissue disposition, the atrioventricular septal defect can be thought of as a perimembranous defect that has extended posteriorly to the cardiac crux. Indeed, one hypothesis suggests that the membranous septum is split into anterior and posterior components by the atrioventricular septal defect.[47] The ventricular portion of the specialized tissue axis is similar in the variants of atrioventricular septal defect having either a common atrioventricular valve

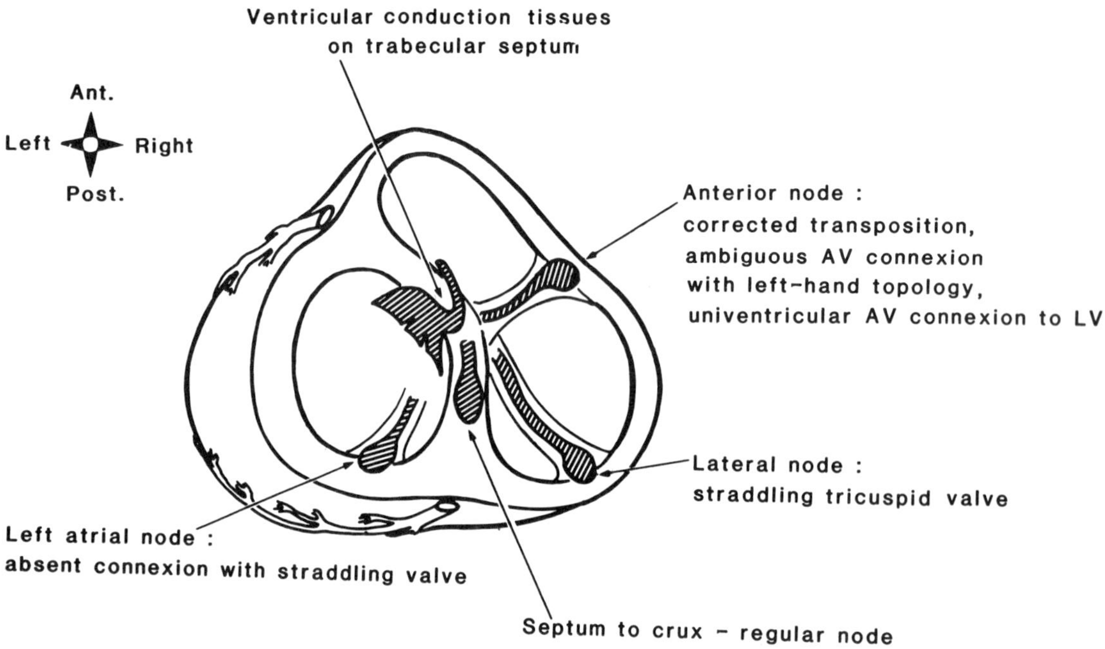

FIGURE 1–16
Diagram showing the various types of arrangement of the atrioventricular conduction system in relation to the ventricular septum.

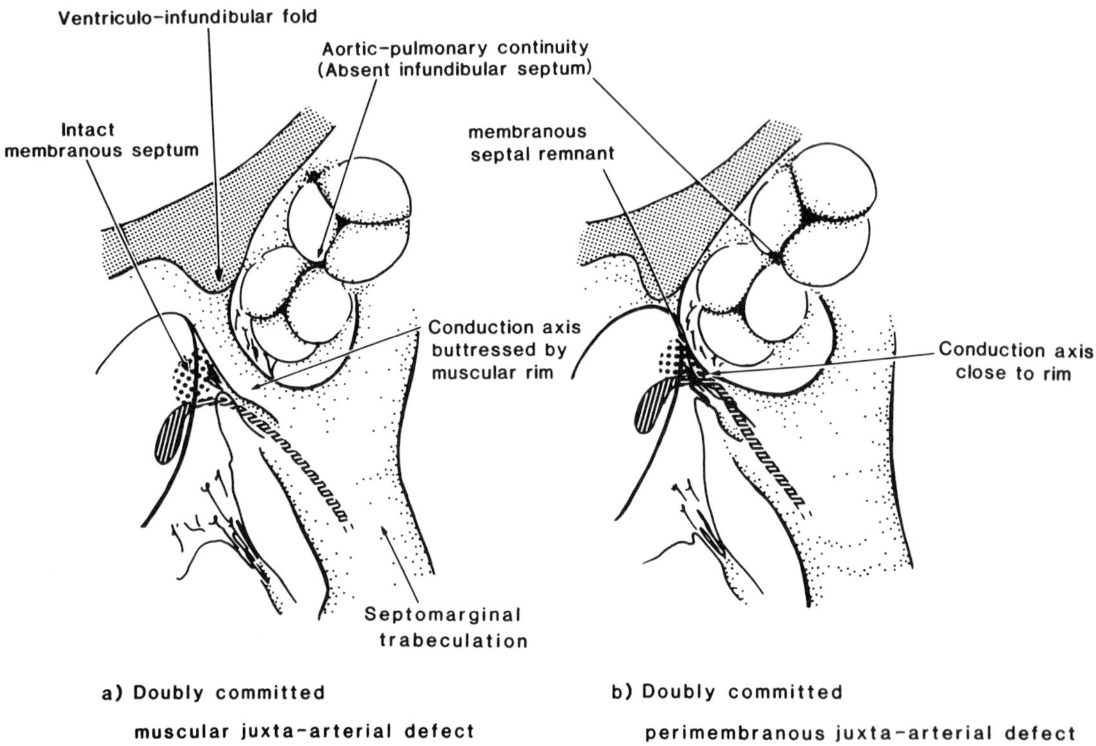

FIGURE 1–17
Diagrams showing the proximity of the conduction axis to the postero-inferior rim of the defect in muscular *(a)* and perimembranous *(b)* defects. The defect shown is of a doubly committed juxta-arterial type, but the relationship is equally relevant in those defects situated immediately underneath one arterial valve.

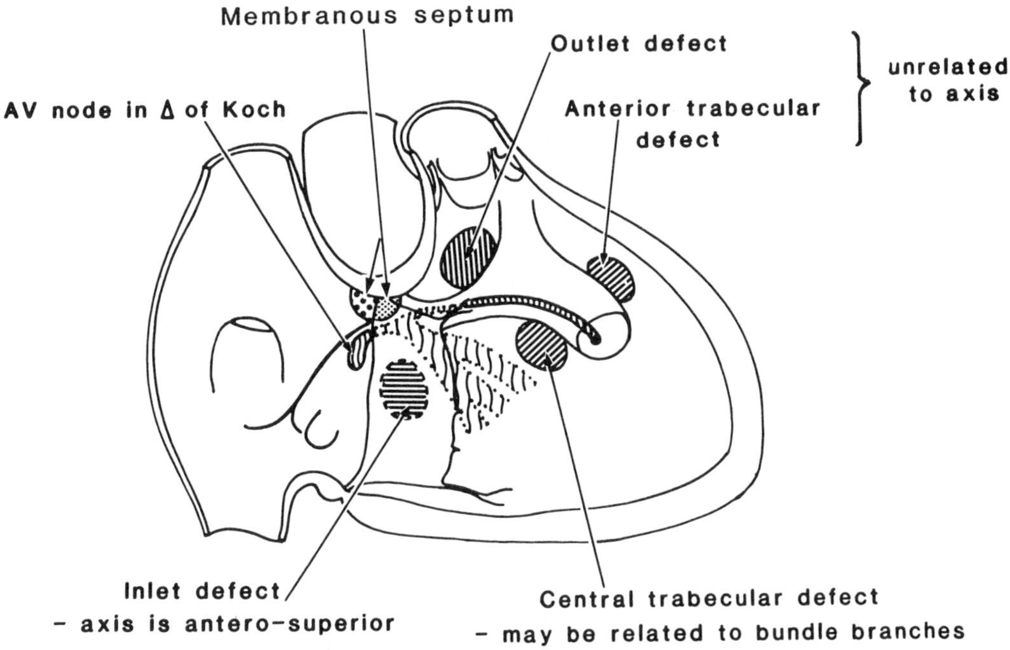

FIGURE 1–18
Diagram of the right side of the heart showing the relationship of the conduction axis to the various locations of defects that have completely muscular borders.

orifice or separate right and left atrioventricular valve orifices (ostium primum defects). The scooped-out appearance of the excavated inlet septum is present in both types to equal extent. This appearance of the ventricular septum is reminiscent of that seen in the developing heart before the fusion between atrial and ventricular components of the cardiac septum. Because of this wide separation between atrial and ventricular septal structures, the connecting atrioventricular node is not located within the limits of the triangle of Koch. Instead, the connecting node is situated more posteriorly and is found at the atrial side of the junction between the atrial and ventricular septums (Fig. 1–20). The penetrating bundle pierces the inferior part of the valve annulus at the cardiac crux.

DEFECTS IN HEARTS WITH MALALIGNMENT OF THE SEPTAL STRUCTURES

In several malformations, the atrial and ventricular septa are not in alignment. We will consider here hearts with straddling tricuspid valve, hearts with discordant atrioventricular connection in the setting of lateralized atrial arrangement, hearts with left-hand topology in the setting of atrial isomerism, and some varieties of hearts with univentricular atrioventricular connection.

The simplest hearts in this group are those with straddling tricuspid valve. The essence of this malformation is the rightward deviation of the inlet septum from the cardiac crux. As a result, the atrial septum is no longer aligned with the inlet ventricular septum. The connecting atrioventricular node is displaced to a position on the atrial wall that is nearest the point where the inlet septum ascends to meet the tricuspid valve orifice (Fig. 1–21). The penetrating bundle burrows through the valve annulus in this region. Rightward deviation of the inlet septum exists not only in hearts with discrete mitral and tricuspid valves but also in hearts with atrioventricular septal defects where a common valve exists.[48]

Hearts with usual atrial arrangement and discordant atrioventricular connection have a ventricular arrangement similar to hearts with atrial isomerism in association with left-hand ventricular topology. The conduction tissue distribution is also similar.[42, 49] In these hearts, the anterosuperior ventricular chamber is morphologically a left ventricle. The connecting atrioventricular node is situated

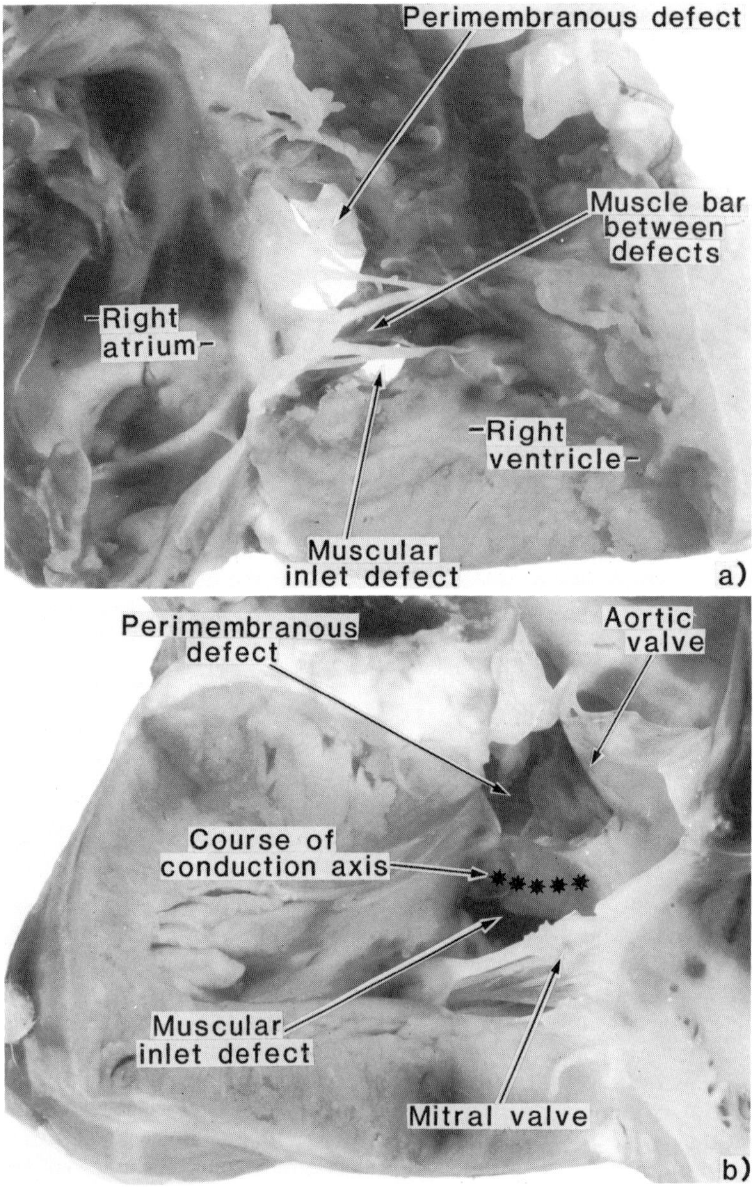

FIGURE 1–19
A heart with co-existing perimembranous inlet and muscular inlet defects. View of the right side of the heart is shown in *(a)*. Reconstructions from serial histologic sections showed the course of the axis in the muscle bar between the two defects. This course is marked in *(b)*, which shows the relationship of the defects as viewed from the left heart.

in the atrial wall that is in the anterolateral quadrant of the mitral valve. The penetrating bundle runs in the region of fibrous continuity between the mitral valve and the arterial valve of the posterior great artery. A long nonbranching bundle then courses anterior to the outflow tract of the posterior great artery before descending along the anterior margin of a ventricular septal defect (Fig. 1–22). The branching bundle gives origin to the left bundle branch, which descends down the right aspect of the ventricular septum, and the right bundle branch, which penetrates the septum to emerge in the left side of the septum. Occasionally a second atrioventricular node is present. This is the regular node located within the triangle of Koch. When the regular node also connects with the ventricular bundle branches, a conduction tissue sling is formed.[50, 51] Rarely, only the regular node may make contact with the ventricles.

Hearts with univentricular atrioventricular connection include hearts with double inlet connection and those with absence of either the right or left atrioventricular connection. Those that are significant in having an abnormal disposition of the conduction axis are

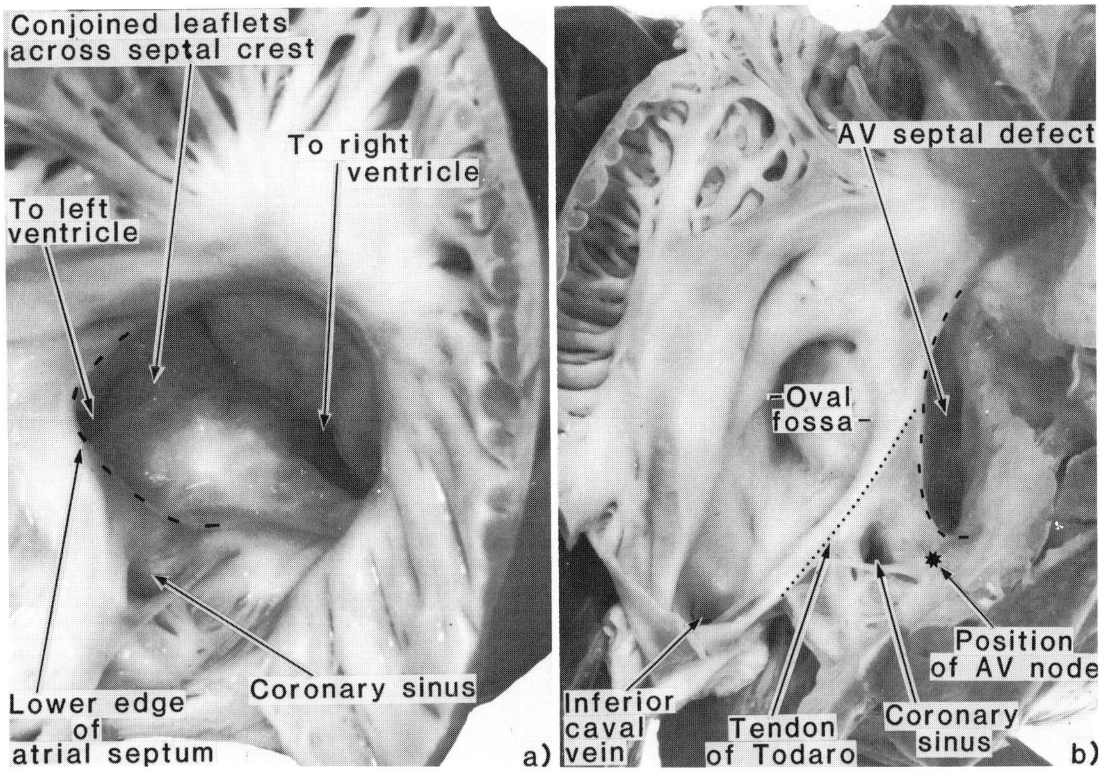

FIGURE 1–20

A heart with atrioventricular septal defect. The view from the right atrium toward the ventricular mass *(a)* shows the partition of the atrioventricular valve orifice by the conjoined leaflets. A lateral view of the right atrium *(b)* shows the posteriorly displaced position of the atrioventricular node. The angle between the tendon of Todaro (dotted line) and lower edge of the atrial septum (dashed line) does not contain the connecting node.

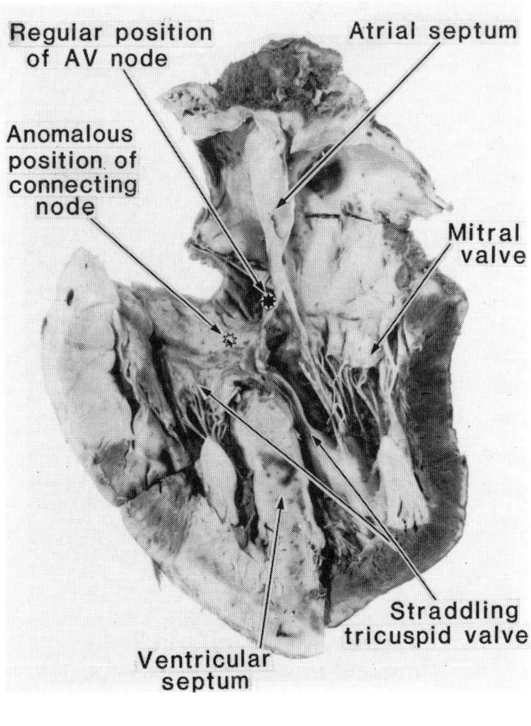

FIGURE 1–21

Four-chamber section through a heart with straddling tricuspid valve. The connecting node is deviated to the right.

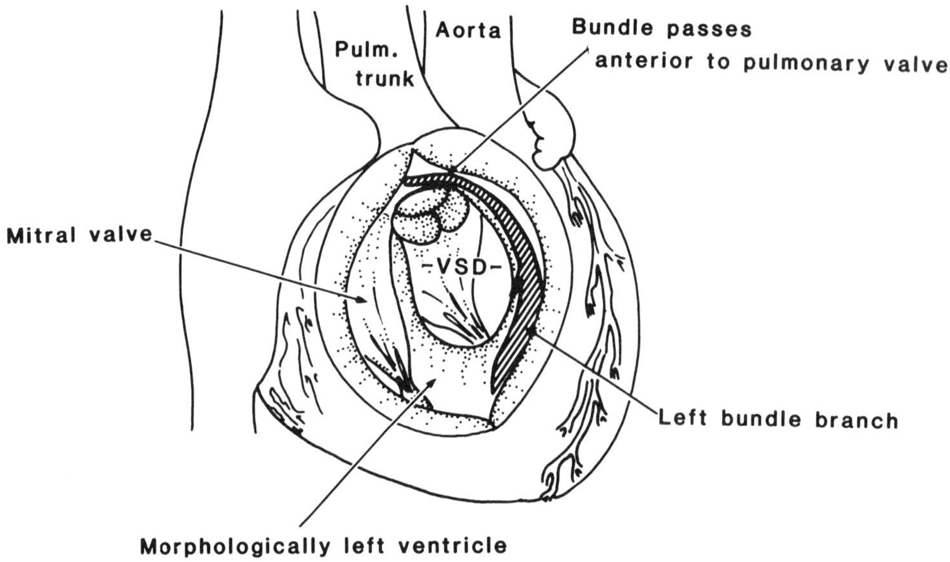

FIGURE 1–22
Diagram showing the course of the nonbranching bundle as viewed through an incision in the morphologically left ventricle in a heart with congenitally corrected transposition of the great arteries.

hearts with the atria connected to a dominant left ventricle and those with a solitary indeterminate ventricle. These diverse arrangements are detailed in Davies, Anderson, and Becker.[52] Essentially, hearts with dominant left ventricle usually have an anteriorly located ventricular septum. Those hearts with double inlet connection have a connecting atrioventricular node at the acute marginal position of the right atrioventricular orifice. From here the bundle perforates the valve annulus to enter the septum. The length of the connecting bundle depends on whether the incomplete (rudimentary) right ventricle

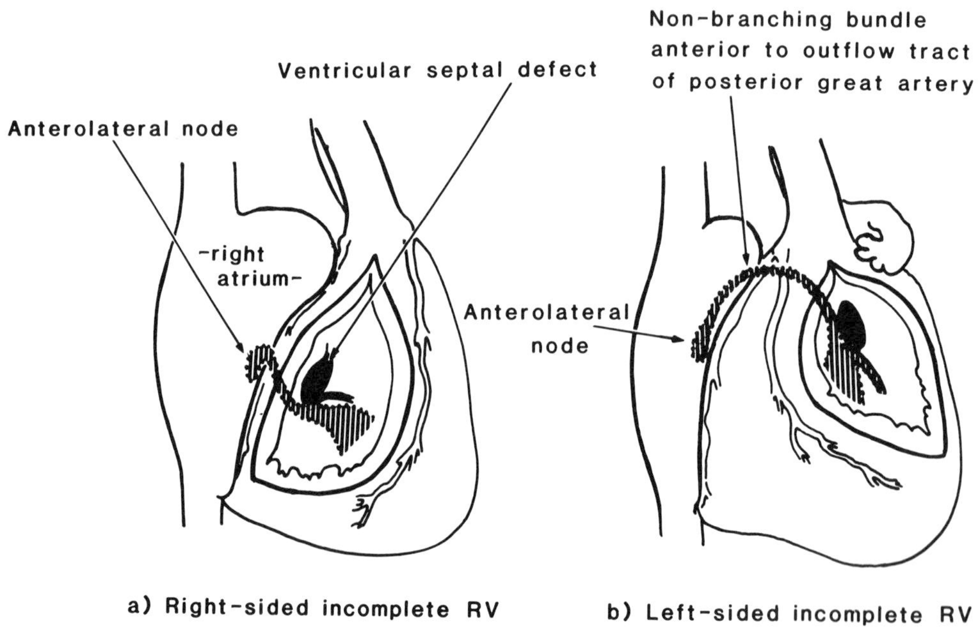

FIGURE 1–23
Diagrams showing the course of the conduction axis as viewed through incisions in the incomplete right ventricle in hearts with double inlet atrioventricular connection to a dominant left ventricle. *A*, right-sided incomplete right ventricle. *B*, left-sided incomplete right ventricle.

is right or left sided. The connecting bundle descends directly into the left ventricular aspect of the septum when the incomplete ventricle is right sided (Fig. 1–23).[53] When the incomplete right ventricle is left sided, the bundle is elongated and runs in front of the outflow tract to the posterior great artery (usually the pulmonary trunk) before reaching the septum (see Fig. 1–23). In either situation there is usually an associated septal defect. When the defect is viewed from the aspect of the incomplete right ventricle, the margin nearest the acute cardiac margin contains the descending bundle.

Most hearts with absent right atrioventricular connection have the node situated in the muscular floor of the right atrium.[54] The descent of the bundle is comparable to that previously described for double inlet connection (Fig. 1–24).

Hearts with a solitary ventricle of indeterminate morphology have been found to have an anteriorly or anterolaterally situated atrioventricular node.[55] The bundle either penetrates directly into the ventricular wall or descends through a large, free-running trabeculation to the ventricular apex. Bundle branches have not been identified.

CONGENITAL HEART BLOCK

Congenital complete heart block can occur in congenitally malformed hearts or in otherwise normal hearts.[56] Complete block associated with a cardiac defect is most frequently seen in the anomaly of congenitally corrected transposition and in some atrioventricular septal defects. Although complete block may be present at birth, it is more usual for the arrhythmia to be progressive. This may be a result of increasing fibrosis of the atrioventricular bundle, which is positioned in a particularly mobile part of the heart compared to the normal situation.[50]

When occurring in a structurally normal heart, the pattern of the cardiac conduction system can take one of three anatomic forms: atrial-axis discontinuity, nodal-ventricular discontinuity, or intraventricular discontinuity (Fig. 1–25). The last form is extremely rare.[57] In normal development, a continuous atrioventricular conduction axis is formed from the fusion of the atrial segment with the inlet and trabecular components. These different parts are themselves enveloped by loose mesenchymal tissues (the putative sulcus tissue). These tissues form the connective tissue sheaths that insulate the different components of the axis from atrial and ventricular myocardium. When the components are brought into approximation to form a continuous axis, parts of the connective tissue sheath break down. Persistence of these parts produces breaches in axis continuity.[52]

The association of congenital complete heart block with maternal connective tissue disease is well documented.[58, 59] Recent studies have pointed to the presence of anti-Ro (SS-A) antigen in maternal serum as a marker for isolated congenital heart block.[60] Our studies of hearts from eight afflicted children have shown the lack of an atrioventricular node in seven whose maternal sera were anti-Ro positive, and nodal-ventricular discontinuity in the remaining one whose maternal serum was anti-Ro negative.[61] This difference in anatomy may be etiologically significant.

ANATOMIC SUBSTRATES OF VENTRICULAR PREEXCITATION

The conduction of impulses that bypass the usual delay-producing area of the atrioventricular junction facilitates early ventricular activation. There are several potential short-circuiting pathways through which impulses may travel (Fig. 1–26). We have found it convenient to describe these according to location rather than to use eponymous terms.[62] These pathways can be described as accessory atrioventricular connections, accessory nodoventricular connections, accessory fasciculoventricular connections, accessory atriofascicular connections, and intranodal bypass tracts.

Better understanding of the mechanism underlying the Wolff-Parkinson-White syndrome has emerged from detailed histologic studies.[63–65] It is generally accepted that this syndrome is caused by accessory atrioventricular connections, which can be present at any site along either atrioventricular junction. These connections can be distinguished as left-sided, right-sided, and posterior septal types. They are particularly amenable to surgical interruption or cryoablation.[66–68] Improved understanding of the anatomy of the atrioventricular junctional area has made the notorious posterior septal connections more accessible.[69]

Accessory atrioventricular connections have been located both in structurally normal

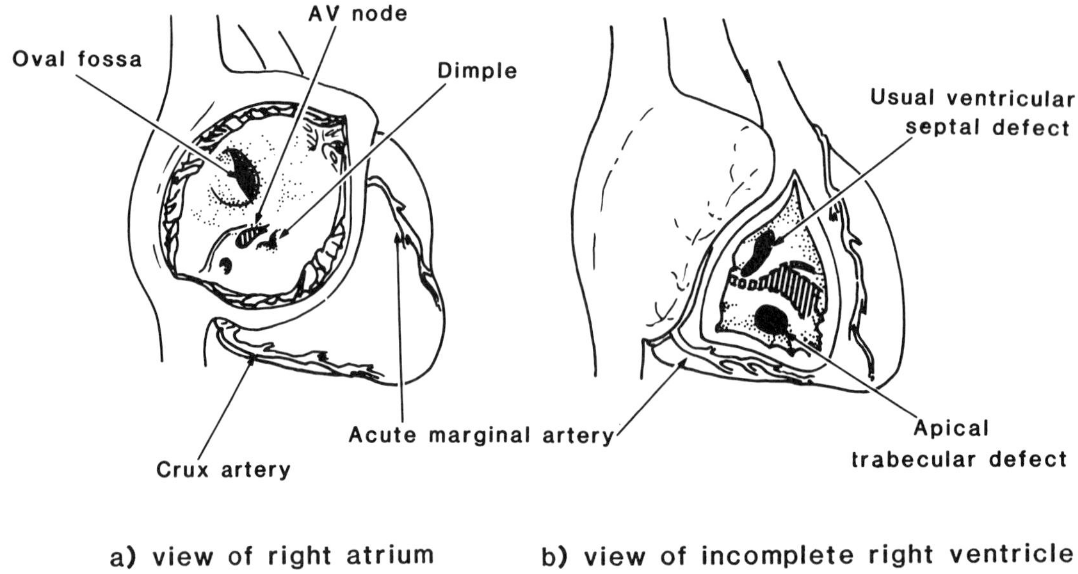

FIGURE 1–24
Diagrams showing the course of the conduction axis in a heart with absent right atrioventricular connection and dominant left ventricle. When an apical trabecular defect is present in addition to the usual defect, the axis runs in the muscle bridge between the defects. *A*, view of the right atrium. *B*, view of the incomplete right ventricle.

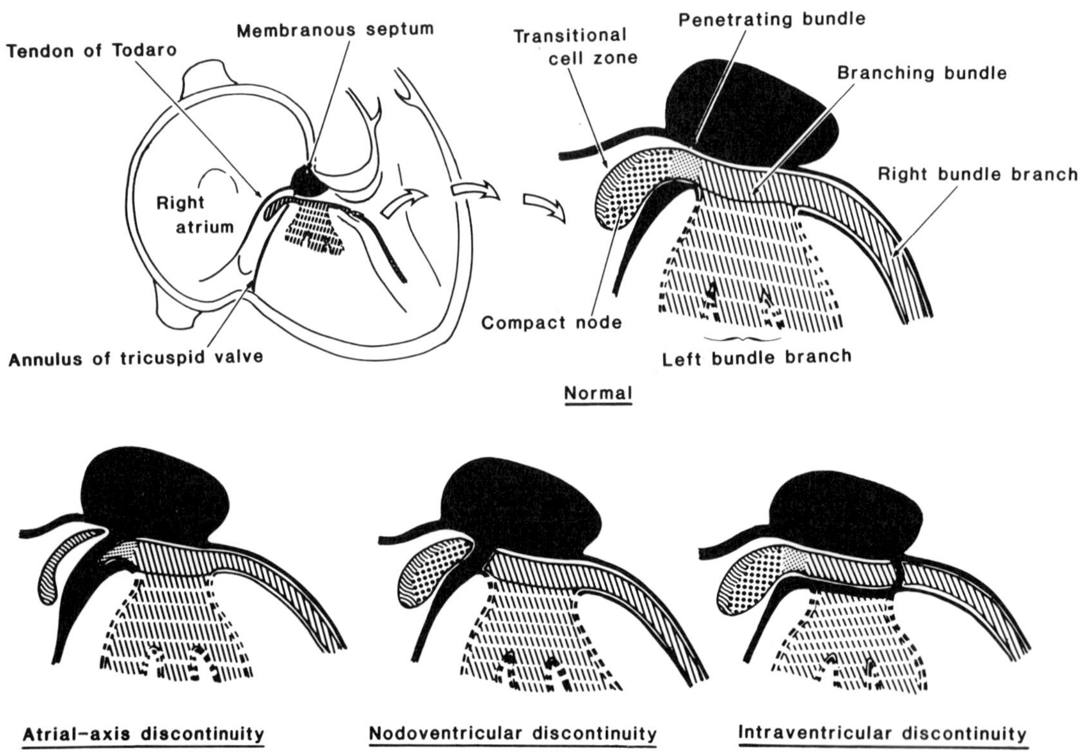

FIGURE 1–25
Diagram showing the components of the normal conduction axis and the three anatomic forms of congenitally complete heart block.

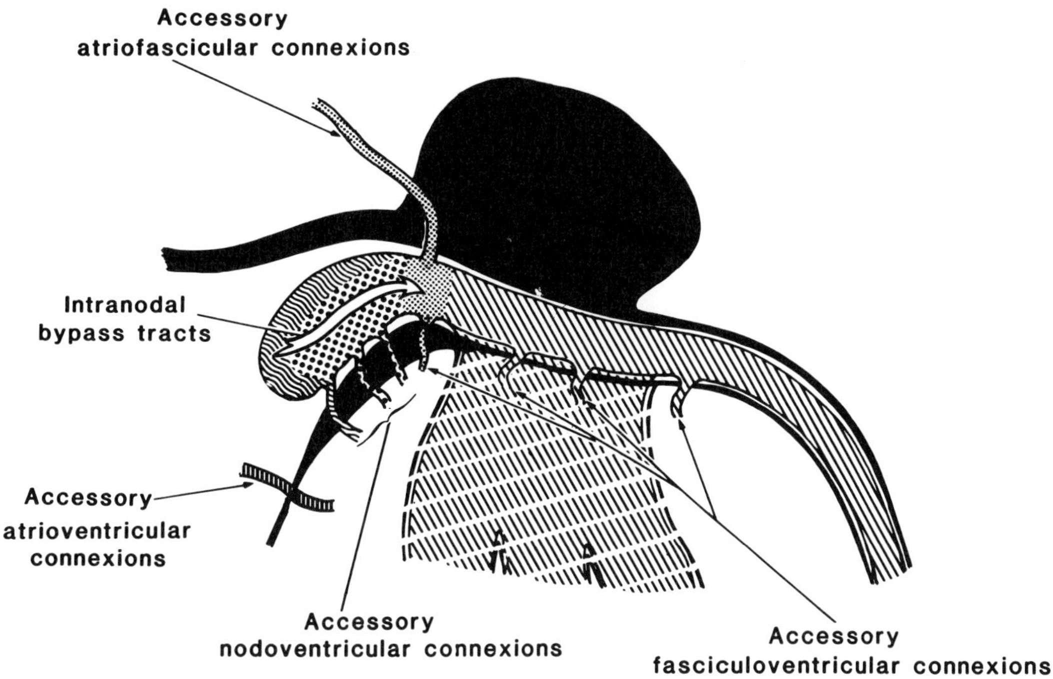

FIGURE 1–26
Diagram showing the potential anatomic substrates of ventricular pre-excitation.

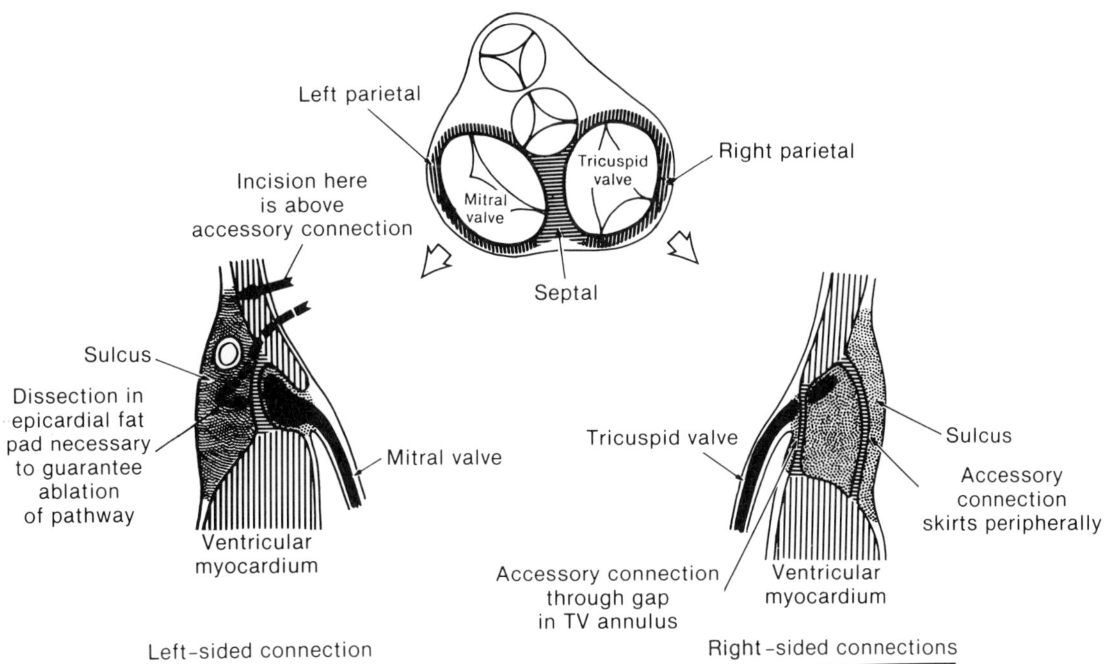

FIGURE 1–27
Diagram showing the locations of the accessory atrioventricular connections and their relationship to the mitral and tricuspid valves.

hearts and in hearts with congenital malformations (particularly Ebstein's malformation, congenitally corrected transposition, tricuspid atresia, and some forms of cardiomyopathies).[70] In most cases, the accessory connection is composed of ordinary myocardial fibers connecting the atrial and ventricular muscle masses. Occasionally the connection is composed of a bundle of specialized cells originating from a nodelike structure reminiscent of a ring-tissue remnant. The atrial origin of an accessory atrioventricular connection is in the form of a single trunk, but it frequently branches near its ventricular insertion. The diameter of the bundle is about 0.5 mm to 2 mm, and its length varies between 5 mm and 10 mm. More than one connection can exist in the same patient. Histologic studies have revealed subtle differences in the courses of right-sided and left-sided connections. Left-sided connections tend to be very close to the mitral valve annulus, whereas right-sided connections may either perforate between the poorly developed tricuspid valve annulus or else skirt near the epicardial aspect of the fat pad (Fig. 1–27).

Accessory pathways between the crest of the ventricular septum and the nodal and fascicular components of the nodal bundle axis are described as nodoventricular and fasciculoventricular connections, respectively. As mentioned previously, extensions of specialized tissue into the central fibrous body are a common feature of infant hearts. Such "archipelagoes" do not constitute accessory connections unless actual cellular contact between specialized tissues and the myocytes on the crest of the septum can be demonstrated. Systematic post mortem studies of serial histologic sections of the junctional area are required to identify these pathways.

Pathways that bypass the atrioventricular nodal delay mechanism but utilize the ventricular portion of the axis for conduction are the atriofascicular connections and intranodal bypass tracts. The atriofascicular connection consists of a bundle of atrial fibers that makes contact with the branching bundle or penetrating bundle distal to the nodal region. These atrial fibers have to be distinguished from those that normally enter the posterior region of the atrioventricular node.[71, 72]

While anatomico-electrophysiologic evidence exists in favor of the previous types of accessory connections as functioning pathways, conclusive anatomic proof of the existence of the intranodal bypass tract remains elusive. In view of the intricate structure of the atrioventricular node, it is probably impossible to identify with certainty such a tract within the nodal bundle axis by histologic means. The intranodal bypass tract must remain, for the present, an electrophysiologic entity.

CONDUCTION TISSUE AND SUDDEN INFANT DEATH

Many mechanisms have been promoted as a cause of sudden and unexpected death in infancy.[73] Not surprisingly, the heart, which works under a fine synchrony of its conduction system, is one of the favorite suspect organs. As with the other mechanisms, however, the role of the heart and its conduction tissues in this issue remains controversial.

Some of the more popularly advanced theories center on defects of the conduction system. These can be classified broadly as mechanisms of reentry, gross abnormalities of the system, and petechial hemorrhages. Anatomic abnormalities have been observed in a fair proportion of hearts in a blind series of infants dying in the first year of life.[4] A recent anatomic study pointed to the role played by accessory pathways in some cases.[74] Although stenosis of the penetrating bundle has been demonstrated in association with sudden death in a breed of dogs,[75] this has not been proven as an isolated lesion in human subjects. It is exceedingly difficult to ascertain whether hemorrhagic lesions in the cardiac nodes are the cause or effect of sudden death. Ferris and Kendeel[76] observed such lesions in infants who died from sudden infant death syndrome, but these lesions have also been found in hearts from children dying from other, known causes.[77]

Persistent fetal dispersion of the atrioventricular node was one of the earliest suggested links between instability of the conduction system and sudden infant death.[38] The loops and whorls of specialized tissue extending from the atrioventricular node into the central fibrous body are thought to be potential substrates for electrical instability. While such a possibility exists for reentry circuits that could provide a substrate for ventricular fibrillation and sudden death, the fact remains that these extensions are seen both in hearts from infants dying suddenly and in hearts from infants with known causes of death.[77–79] It would seem that these structures are part of the normal developing process and should not be implicated as a cause of death. In James' words, "Although all of us are looking at the same thing, we interpret its functional significance differently."[80] Until we are able to amass large quantities of pre- and postmortem data, anatomico-functional correlations will remain elusive.

ACKNOWLEDGMENTS

This work was supported by the Joseph Levy Foundation together with the British Heart Foundation. We thank Mrs. Rachel Marinos and Mrs. Christine Anderson for their help during the preparation of this manuscript.

References

1. Tawara S: Das Reizleitungssytem des Saugetierherzens. Jena: Gustav Fischer, 1906.
2. Keith A, Flack M: The form and nature of the muscular connections between the primary divisions of the vertebrate heart. J Anatom Physiol 41:172–189, 1907.
3. Lewis T: The mechanism and graphic registration of the heart beat. London: Shaw and Sons, 1920, p 14.
4. Anderson RH, Anderson KR, Ho SY, Becker AE: The anatomy of arrhythmias. In Godman MJ, Marquis RM (eds): Paediatric Cardiology, Volume 2. Heart Disease in the Newborn. Edinburgh: Churchill Livingstone, 1979, pp 367–386.
5. Ho SY, Mortimer G, Anderson RH, Pomerance A, Keeling JW: Conduction system defects in three perinatal patients with arrhythmia. Br Heart J 53:158–163, 1985.
6. Wenink ACG: Development of the human cardiac conducting system. J Anat 121:617–631, 1976.
7. Anderson RH, Taylor IM: Development of atrioventricular specialized tissue in the human heart. Br Heart J 34:1205–1214, 1972.
8. Anderson RH, Ho SY, Becker AE, Gosling JA: The development of the sinoatrial node. In Bonke FIM (ed): The Sinus Node. Structure, Function and Clinical Relevance. The Hague: Martinus Nijhoff, 1978, pp 166–182.
9. Anderson RH, Becker AE: Cardiac Anatomy—An Integrated Text and Colour Atlas. Edinburgh/London: Gower/Churchill Livingstone, 1980.
10. Vassall-Adams PR: The development of the atrioventricular bundle and its branches in the avian heart. J Anat 134:169–183, 1982.
11. Anderson RH, Davies MJ, Becker AE: Atrioventricular ring specialized tissue in the normal heart. Eur J Cardiol 2:219–230, 1974.
12. Anderson KR, Ho SY, Anderson RH: The location and vascular supply of the sinus node in the human heart. Br Heart J 41:28–32, 1979.
13. Hudson REB: The human pacemaker and its pathology. Br Heart J 22:153–167, 1960.
14. Truex RC: The sinuatrial node and its connections with the atrial tissues. In Wellens HJJ, Lie KI, Janse MJ (eds): The Conduction System of the Heart: Structure, Function and Clinical Implications. New York: Lea & Febiger, 1976, pp 209–226.
15. Lev M: Ageing changes in the human sinoatrial node. J Gerontol 9:1–9, 1954.
16. Busquet J, Fontan F, Anderson RH, Ho SY, Davies MJ: The surgical significance of the atrial branches of the coronary arteries. Int J Cardiol 6:223–234, 1984.
17. Nerantzis CE, Toutozas P, Avgoustakis D: The importance of the sinus node artery in the blood supply of the atrial myocardium. An anatomical study of 360 cases. Acta Cardiol 38:35–47, 1983.
18. James TN: Anatomy of the human sinus node. Anatom Rec 141:109–116, 1961.
19. James TN, Sherf L, Fine G, Morales AR: Comparative ultrastructure of the sinus node in man and dog. Circulation 34:139–163, 1966.
20. Tranum-Jensen J: The fine structure of the sinus node: a survey. In Bonke FIM (ed): The Sinus Node. The Hague: Martinus Nijhoff Medical Division, 1978, pp 149–165.
21. Anderson RH, Ho SY, Smith A, Becker AE: The internodal atrial myocardium. Anatom Rec 201:75–82, 1981.
22. Anderson RH, Becker AE, Tranum-Jensen J, Janse MJ: Anatomico-electrophysiological correlations in the conduction system—a review. Br Heart J 45:67–82, 1981.
23. Janse MJ, Anderson RH: Specialized internodal atrial pathways—fact or fiction. Eur J Cardiol 2:117–136, 1974.
24. Spach MS, King TD, Barr RC, Boaz DE, Morrow MN, Herman-Giddens S: Electrical potential distribution surrounding the atria during depolarization and repolarization in the dog. Circ Res 24:857–873, 1969.
25. Spach MS, Miller WTIII, Barr RC, Gesolowitz DB: Electrophysiology of the internodal pathways. Determining the difference between anisotropic cardiac muscle and a specialized tract system. In Little RC (ed): Physiology of Atrial Pacemakers and Connective Tissues. Mount Kisco, NY: Futura Publishing Company Inc., 1980, pp 367–380.
26. Scherf D, Cohen J: The Atrioventricular Node And Selected Cardiac Arrhythmias. New York: Grune & Stratton, 1964, pp 1–46.
27. Koch W: Weiter Mitteilungen uber den Sinusknoten der Herzens. Verh Deutsch Pathol Ges 13:85–92, 1909.
28. Chiu I-S, Hegerty AS, Anderson RH, de Leval M: The landmarks to the atrioventricular conduction system in hearts with absence or unroofing of the coronary sinus. J Thorac Cardiovasc Surg 90:297–300, 1985.
29. Truex RC, Smythe MQ: Reconstruction of the human atrioventricular node. Anatom Rec 158:11–20, 1967.
30. Demoulin JC, Kulbertus HE: Histopathological examination of concept of left hemiblock. Br Heart J 34:807–814, 1972.
31. Massing GK, James TN: Anatomical configuration of the His bundle and bundle branches in the human heart. Circulation 53:609–621, 1976.

32. Rossi L: Sistema di conduzione trifascicolare ed emiblocchi di branca sinistra. Considerazioni anatomiche ed istopatologiche. G Ital Cardiol 1:55–62, 1971.
33. Rossi L: Histopathology of conducting system in left anterior hemiblock. Br Heart J 38:1304–1311, 1976.
34. Rosenbaum MB, Elizari MV, Lazzari JO: The hemiblocks. Tampa Tracings, FL: Oldsmar, 1970.
35. Kurosawa H, Becker AE: Dead-end tract of the conduction axis. Int J Cardiol 7:13–18, 1985.
36. Erickson EE, Lev M: Ageing changes in the human AV node, bundle and bundle branches. J Gerontol 7:1–12, 1952.
37. James TN, Marshall TK: De subitaneis XVIII. Persistent fetal dispersion of the atrioventricular node and His bundle within the central fibrous body. Circulation 53:1026–1034, 1976.
38. James TN: Sudden death in babies. New observations in the heart. Am J Cardiol 22:479–506, 1968.
39. Melhuish BPP, Van Praagh R: Juxtaposition of the atrial appendages. A sign of severe cyanotic congenital heart disease. Br Heart J 30:269–284, 1968.
40. Ho SY, Monro JL, Anderson RH: The disposition of the sinus node in left-sided juxtaposition of the atrial appendage. Br Heart J 41:129–132, 1979.
41. Van Mierop LHS, Wiglesworth FW: Isomerism of the cardiac atria in the asplenia syndrome. Lab Invest 11:1303–1315, 1962.
42. Dickinson DF, Wilkinson JL, Anderson KR, Smith A, Ho SY, Anderson RH: The cardiac conduction system in situs ambiguus. Circulation 59:879–885, 1979.
43. Latham RA, Anderson RH: Anatomical variations in atrioventricular conduction system with reference to ventricular septal defects. Br Heart J 34:185–190, 1972.
44. Titus JL, Daugherty GW, Edwards JE: Anatomy of the atrioventricular conduction system in ventricular septal defect. Circulation 28:72–81, 1963.
45. Truex RC, Bishof JK: Conduction system in human hearts with interventricular septal defects. J Thorac Surg 35:421–439, 1958.
46. Anderson RH, Monro JL, Ho SY, Smith A, Deverall PB: Les voies de conduction auriculo-ventriculaires dans le tetralogie de Fallot. Coeur 8:793–807, 1977.
47. Thiene G, Wenink ACG, Frescura C, Wilkinson JL, Gallucci V, Ho SY, Anderson RH: The surgical anatomy of the conduction tissues in atrioventricular defects. J Thorac Cardiovasc Surg 82:928–937, 1981.
48. Pillai R, Ho SY, Anderson RH, Shinebourne EA, Lincoln C: Malalignment of the interventricular septum with atrioventricular septal defect. Its implications concerning conduction tissue disposition. Thorac Cardiovasc Surg 32:1–3, 1984.
49. Becker AE, Anderson RH: Conditions with discordant atrioventricular connexions—anatomy and conducting tissues. In Anderson RH, Shinebourne EA (eds): Paediatric Cardiology 1977. Edinburgh: Churchill Livingstone, 1978, pp 184–197.
50. Anderson RH, Becker AE, Arnold R, Wilkinson JL: The conducting tissues in congenitally corrected transposition. Circulation 50:911–923, 1974.
51. Symons JC, Shinebourne EA, Joseph MC, Lincoln C, Ho Y, Anderson RH: Criss-cross heart with congenitally corrected transposition. Report of a case with d-transposed aorta and ventricular preexcitation. Eur J Cardiol 5:493–505, 1977.
52. Davies MJ, Anderson RH, Becker AE: The Conduction System of the Heart. London: Butterworths, 1983.
53. Wenink ACG: The conduction tissues in primitive ventricle with outlet chamber. Two different possibilities. J Thorac Card Surg 75:747–753, 1978.
54. Dickinson DF, Wilkinson JL, Smith A, Becker AE, Anderson RH: Atrioventricular conduction tissues in univentricular hearts of left ventricular type with absent right atrioventricular connection ("tricuspid atresia"). Br Heart J 42:1–8, 1979.
55. Wilkinson JL, Anderson RH, Arnold R, Hamilton DI, Smith A: The conducting tissues in primitive ventricular hearts without an outlet chamber. Circulation 53:930–938, 1976.
56. Lev M: Pathogenesis of congenital atrioventricular block. Prog Cardiovasc Dis 15:145–157, 1972.
57. Husson GS, Blackman MS, Rogers MC, Bharati S, Lev M: Familial congenital bundle branch system disease. Am J Cardiol 32:365–369, 1973.
58. Hull D, Binns BAO, Joyce D: Congenital heart block with widespread fibrosis due to maternal lupus erythematosus. Arch Dis Child 41:688–690, 1966.
59. McCue CM, Mantakas ME, Tingelstad JB, Ruddy S: Congenital heart block in newborns of mothers with connective tissue disease. Circulation 56:82–89, 1977.
60. Scott JS, Maddison PJ, Taylor PV, Esscher E, Scott O, Skinner RD: Connective tissue disease, antibodies to ribonucleoprotein, and congenital heart block. N Engl J Med 4:209–212, 1983.
61. Ho SY, Esscher E, Anderson RH, Michaelsson M: Anatomy of congenital complete heart block and relation to maternal anti-Ro antibodies. Am J Cardiol 58:291–294, 1986.
62. Anderson RH, Becker AE, Brechenmacher C, Davies MJ, Rossi L: Ventricular preexcitation. A proposed nomenclature for its substrates. Eur J Cardiol 3:27–36, 1975.
63. Becker AE, Anderson RH, Durrer D, Wellens HJJ: The anatomical substrates of Wolff-Parkinson-White Syndrome. A clinico-pathologic correlation in seven patients. Circulation 57:870–879, 1978.
64. Frank R, Brechenmacher C, Fontaine G: Apport de l'histologie dans l'etude des syndromes de pre-excitation ventriculaire. Coeur Med Int 15:337–344, 1976.
65. Ohnell RF: Preexcitation, a cardiac abnormality. Acta Med Scand 152:79–81, 1944.
66. Gallagher J, Svenson R, Sealy WC, Wallace A: The Wolff-Parkinson-White syndrome and the pre-excitation dysrhythmias. Med Clin North Am 60:101–123, 1976.
67. Sealy WC, Gallagher JJ: The surgical approach to the septal area of the heart based on experience with 45 patients with Kent bundles. J Thorac Card Surg 79:542–551, 1980.
68. Sealy WC, Gallagher JJ, Wallace AG: The surgical treatment of the Wolff-Parkinson-White syndrome. Evolution of improved methods of identification and interruption of the Kent bundle. Ann Thorac Surg 22:443–457, 1976.
69. Cox JL, Gallagher JJ, Cain ME: Experience with 118 consecutive patients undergoing operation for the Wolff-Parkinson-White syndrome. J Thorac Cardiovasc Surg 90:440–501, 1985.
70. Wellens HJJ, Lubbers WJ, Losekoot TG: Preexcitation. In Roberts NK, Gelband H (eds): Cardiac Arrhythmias in the Neonate, Infant, and Child. New York: Appleton-Century-Crofts. 1977, pp 321–264.
71. Brechenmacher C: Atrio-His bundle tracts. Br Heart J 37:853–855, 1975.
72. James TN: Morphology of the human atrioventric-

ular node, with remarks pertinent to its electrophysiology. Am Heart J 62:756–771, 1961.
73. Guntheroth WG: Crib Death: Sudden Infant Death Syndrome. Mount Kisco, NY: Futura Publishing Company, 1982.
74. Marino TA, Kane BM: Cardiac atrioventricular junctional tissues in hearts from infants who die suddenly. J Am Coll Cardiol 5:1178–1184, 1985.
75. James TN, Drake EH: Sudden death in Doberman pinschers. Ann Intern Med 68:821–829, 1968.
76. Ferris JAJ, Kendeel SR: Sudden death in infancy. Br Med J 2:559–560, 1974.
77. Anderson RH, Bouton J, Burrow CT, Smith A: Sudden death in infancy. A study of the cardiac specialized tissue. Br Med J 2:135–139, 1974.
78. Lie JT, Rosenberg HS, Erickson EE: Histopathology of the conduction system in the sudden infant death syndrome. Circulation 53:3–8, 1976.
79. Ho SY, Anderson RH: Conduction tissue and SIDS. In Schwartz PJ, Southall DP, Valdes-Dapena M (eds): The sudden infant death syndrome. Ann NY Acad Sci 533:176–190, 1987.
80. James TN: Crib death. (Editorial) J Am Coll Cardiol 5:1185–1187, 1985.

CHAPTER 2

DEVELOPMENTAL CELLULAR ELECTROPHYSIOLOGY

Kenneth Hewett

The physiologic development of the heart has been studied for almost 100 years. In 1893, Pickering visually observed sequential contraction of the atria and ventricles (AV conduction) in the embryonic chick.[1] He also noted differences in sensitivity to autonomic agents at various stages of development. More quantitative electrocardiographic measurements were made on a midterm human fetus in vitro by Easby in 1934.[2] These recordings showed all of the electrocardiographic components of the adult at this stage of development.

A report by Fingl, Woodbury, and Hecht probably marks the beginning of developmental cellular cardiac electrophysiology.[3] In these experiments glass capillary microelectrodes were inserted into embryonic chick hearts, and the transmembrane action potentials were recorded. Definite modifications in the action potential characteristics occurred with development. The chick cardiac embryonic development has been extensively studied, because it is accessible to microelectrodes and relatively easy to maintain in vitro. Only recently has the mammalian embryologic and postnatal cellular electrophysiologic development been studied. These experiments have described age-related changes in action potentials from the early embryonic stages through early adulthood. Action potential data are an excellent source of information. By making certain assumptions about specific membrane currents, we can speculate from action potential recordings about changes in specific membrane currents during development. Drugs with relatively specific blocking action on individual currents are helpful in supporting these speculations. Ultimately, quantification of specific currents, using various voltage clamp techniques on isolated heart cells, will provide more conclusive data regarding age-related changes in cardiac currents.

A brief review and update of the major aspects of cellular cardiac electrophysiology may be helpful for some readers. At least seven currents are commonly referred to in the literature. The following description of these currents is intended only as a summary and is not an exhaustive review of the literature.

I_{Na}. The fast sodium current is the large inward current that produces the rapid upstroke of the cardiac action potential. This upstroke provided by I_{Na} is the driving force for cell-to-cell propagation of the action potential. In general, the larger the I_{Na} and the greater the velocity of the upstroke, the more rapidly this waveform will propagate through the tissue. I_{Na} activation and inactivation kinetics are highly voltage dependent. Under normal physiologic conditions in Purkinje fibers or muscle cells, I_{Na} activates in less than 1 ms and inactivates completely in 5–10 ms. There may be a second population of sodium channels that either inactivate more slowly or simply do not inactivate at all as a result of the overlap of steady-state activation and inactivation curves within the voltage range of -80 to -90 mV.[5,6] These "window current" channels serve to maintain the action potential plateau and prolong the action potential.

I_{To}. The transient outward current has been previously called the positive dynamic current (I_{qr}) or the early outward current (I_{eo}) and was originally thought to be carried by Cl^- ions. Kenyon and Gibbons in 1977 showed that K^+ was a better candidate for this current.[7] I_{To} is largely responsible for the notch in Purkinje fiber action potentials, occurring immediately after the upstroke in the earliest part of the plateau (Fig. 2–1). A similar notch is found in some myocardial cells.[8] This current is strongly frequency dependent (i.e., the current is larger at longer cycle lengths). Coraboeuf and Carmeliet have described two separate transient outward currents in sheep Purkinje fibers.[9] The faster current, which they call I_{bo}, appears to be calcium activated and has a mean inactivation time constant of 12 ms. The slower current, I_{lo}, corresponds to I_{To} in other species.

I_{si}. The slow inward current has been found to be much faster in isolated heart cells than previously seen in intact tissue preparations, reaching peak activation in 2–5 ms, and may contribute to the fast upstroke in some tissues.[10] Thus the designation I_{Ca} may be more appropriate than I_{si} for this current. I_{si} is activated at potentials positive to −50mV. I_{si} appears to be the primary inward current responsible for the action potential in central AV nodal cells, because Ca^{+2} current blockers almost completely eliminate these action potentials.[11] In normal atrial and ventricular myocardium, I_{si} provides excitation by maintaining the action potential plateau and contraction by providing the calcium trigger for activating the myofilaments. In ventricular tissue depolarized to between −40mV and −55mV, rapid, spontaneous, depolarization-induced automaticity can be produced. This automaticity is eliminated by I_{si} blockers, suggesting that "abnormal" automaticity may be produced by I_{si}.[12] Recently, Bean[38] and Nilius et al have found two separate calcium conductances in canine atrial myocytes and in guinea pig ventricular myocytes, respectively, through distinctions in their kinetics and sensitivity to organic and inorganic blockers. The physiologic significance of these conductances remains to be determined.

I_K. This current was originally described by Noble and Tsien and called I_x because the reversal potential suggested that this delayed outward plateau current was carried partially by potassium, with contributions from other ions.[13] Noble and Tsien described two components of the current, I_{x1} and I_{x2}, with distinctively different kinetics. Several other investigators have supported Noble and Tsien's findings in a variety of experiments.

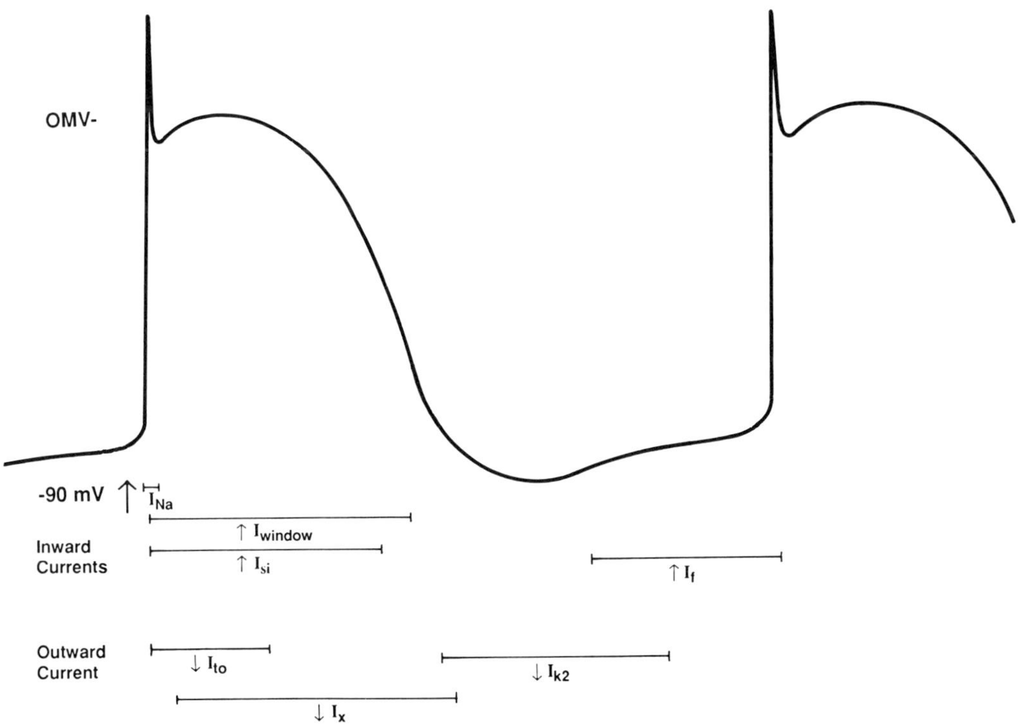

FIGURE 2–1
An idealized drawing of Purkinje fiber action potentials in a spontaneous firing preparation. At the bottom is a graphic representation of the approximate time-course of the gated conductances. These are only rough approximations at best.

However, some evidence indicates that I_{x2} is artifactually produced by ion accumulation and depletion phenomena occurring during the long voltage clamp steps required to measure I_{x2}.[14, 15] Jaeger and Gibbons have suggested that an I_x-like current may be simulated in certain experiments through effects on I_{si}.[16] If the I_K current does exist (and the preponderance of data indicates it does), the I_x current is likely to have a large influence on action potential duration, the role of which in arrhythmogenesis is well known.

I_{K1}. I_{K1} is the current that provides the resting potential in heart cells (see Fig. 2–1) and is a voltage-dependent outward current carried largely by potassium. Carmeliet has recently described a time-dependent component of I_{K1} that may contribute to the nature of the inwardly rectifying current at potentials less negative than normal resting potential.[4] A small inward leak current, carried primarily by Na^+, slightly reduces the membrane potential from the equilibrium potential for K^+ (E_K) predicted by the Nerst equation.

PACEMAKER CURRENTS

In recent years, pacemaker currents throughout the heart have undergone much scrutiny and reinterpretation. The slow diastolic depolarization of the ventricular pacemaker cells (Purkinje fiber cells) may be the product of two currents: a slowly decaying outward current and a slowly activating inward current. The biphasic nature of the diastolic depolarization often seen in spontaneously firing Purkinje fibers and illustrated in Figure 2–1 may indicate multiple currents.

I_{K2}. The original pacemaker current was described by Noble and Tsien in voltage clamp experiments using sheep Purkinje fibers.[17] They found an outward current at potentials greater than −70 mV that slowly deactivated during the diastolic interval, depolarizing the tissue.

I_f. A second pacemaker current has been described more recently. I_f is an inward current carried primarily by sodium. This current was first described by Brown, Clark, and Noble in frog sinus venosus and was termed I_f because of its "funny" behavior. I_f appeared much like I_{K2}, but it did not reverse near E_K as would be expected of a potassium current. In voltage clamp experiments, DiFrançesco found that partially blocking I_{K1} with barium ions unmasked a similar pacemaker current in Purkinje fibers.[19] The rationale for partially blocking I_{K1} is that a large potassium-depletion component will overlap the outward current during long hyperpolarizing voltage clamp steps and interfere with voltage clamp measurements. Reducing I_{K1} with barium is believed to eliminate this problem partially, thereby permitting the recording of I_f without excessive distortion.

The relative contributions of these two pacemaker currents remain to be determined and may be tissue specific. I_f may be the dominant pacemaker current at low potentials in sinus or AV nodal tissue cells with a small I_{K2} or I_{K2}-like current that is modulated by autonomic agents. On the other hand, I_{K2} may provide the majority of pacemaker current in ventricular pacemakers at potentials greater than −70 mV, while I_f may have a greater contribution at less negative potentials.

DEVELOPMENTAL ELECTROPHYSIOLOGY OF THE HEART

Developmental changes in canine Purkinje fiber action potential from early fetal stages through adulthood have been comprehensively studied. Table 2–1 contains these data acquired from several sources. As can be seen in the consistent changes from the early fetal stage through adulthood, there is an ontogenic process that increases resting potential (MDP); increases action potential amplitude (AMP) and $\dot{V}max$, and prolongs the action potential duration (APD_{50} and APD_{90}). One deviation from this pattern was observed by Escande et al, who found no difference in the MDP of human atrial myocardium taken from young patients (2 months to 22 months of age) and adults (30 years to 67 years of age).[20] Possibly, the human atrial tissue may have matured by the age of 1 to 2 years, or alternatively, adult specimens may not remain polarized in the tissue bath to the same extent as younger tissue.

Typical action potential recordings from neonatal and adult canine Purkinje fibers and ventricular myocardium are shown in Figure 2–2. As indicated in Figure 2–2 (panels A

TABLE 2–1
ACTION POTENTIAL CHARACTERISTICS OF CANINE PURKINJE FIBERS FROM EARLY FETUS TO ADULT*

	No.	MDP (−mV)	AMP (mV)	$\dot{V}_{max}$ (v/s)	APD_{50} (ms)	PD_{100} (ms)
Early Fetal†	5	−78.5 ± 0.9	115.7 ± 3.5	323 ± 21	108.5 ± 9.0	181.7 ± 22.4
Late Fetal†	6	−85.8 ± 2.1	121.7 ± 2.9	481 ± 33	132.5 ± 7.0	210.5 ± 8.2
Neonatal‡	12	−85.9 ± 4.6	125.4 ± 5.4	513 ± 85	142.4 ± 15.4	247.5 ± 27.3
Adult‡	9	−91.6 ± 8.0	130.2 ± 6.6	591 ±85	160.7 ± 23.1	281.7 ± 22.1

*All measurements were made at 37°C in Tyrode's solution, $[K^+]_o$ = 4 mm at a basic cycle length of 500 ms. †Data are mean ± SD.

‡Data from Danilo et al.[32]

‡Data from Reder et al.[24]

and B), the plateau potential is less positive in the adult Purkinje fiber action potential than in the neonate. The complete absence of a notch immediately following the upstroke is not unusual, but the degree of notching can vary from one region of a particular fiber to another. A less negative MDP with shorter action potential duration is consistently found in neonatal tissue. The differences between adult and neonatal myocardial action potentials are in some ways less striking than the Purkinje fiber action potential differences. For example, APD_{90} is 205 ms and 215 ms for adult and neonatal myocardial tissue, respectively, in the action potentials shown in Figure 2–2(C,D). Our preliminary studies indicate that there do not appear to be significant differences in $\dot{V}$max between these two age groups in canine myocardium (Lesley Ewing and Kenneth Hewett, unpublished results). Figure 2–2 does demonstrate a very consistent finding analogous to the Purkinje fiber: there is an age-related decrease in the action potential plateau potential and an increase in the notch between phases 1 and 2, which also appears to be caused by I_{To}.[8] The small notch seen in the neonatal myocardium occurs immediately after the upstroke and is not clearly evident at the paper speed used in this figure. Adult myocardium has a larger and somewhat delayed notch (Fig. 2–2[C]). The physiologic significance of these differences has not been determined.

The resting potential of heart cells is largely determined by the passive efflux of K^+ ions and the parallel influx of Na^+. The net charge on the membrane is therefore determined by the relative permeability to K^+ and Na^+ ions and the electrochemical gradient for each ion. This relationship is summarized mathematically by a modification of the Goldman equation (shown in the upper right corner of Figure 2–3, where P is the permeability coefficient of the ion). This equation assumes that chloride is passively distributed and at equilibrium. With development, embryonic chick heart cells have been shown to have decreasing permeability at resting potentials.[21] Sperelakis and Shigenobu[22] calculated the relative permeabilities of Na^+ and K^+ in 3-, 5-, and 15-day-old chick embryonic myocardium by assuming a constant intracellular potassium concentration of 150 mmol/L and an intracellular sodium concentration of 30 mmol/L (Fig. 2–3) for various concentrations of $[K^+]_o$, using the equation shown in the upper right box in Figure 2–3. The relative permeabilities (P_{Na}/P_K) decreased from 0.2 to 0.1 and .01 in the 3-, 5-, and 15-day-old tissue respectively. These results suggest that the membrane selectivity for K^+ over Na^+ increases with development of the heart and would result in higher resting potentials if intracellular ion activities remained constant. Because the cardiac membrane does behave much like a K^+ electrode, the $[K]_o$ at which zero membrane potential is produced indicates that $[K]_o$ is approximately equal to $[K]_i$. Using this indirect method, Sperelakis and Shigenobu estimated $[K]_i$ to be approximately 150 mmol/L for all age groups.[22]

More recent direct intracellular measurements with ion-selective electrodes have shown that in the embryonic chick ventricular myocardium, K^+ activity increases from 71 mmol/L at day 4 to 90 mmol/L at day 18, and that Na^+ activity decreases from 12.5 mmol/L to 7.0 mmol/L at these ages.[23] Reder et al demonstrated an increase in intracellular potassium activity from neonatal canine Purkinje fibers through adulthood; a parallel increase in MDP was also found.[24] Therefore, with development there is an overall decrease in membrane permeability, an increase in

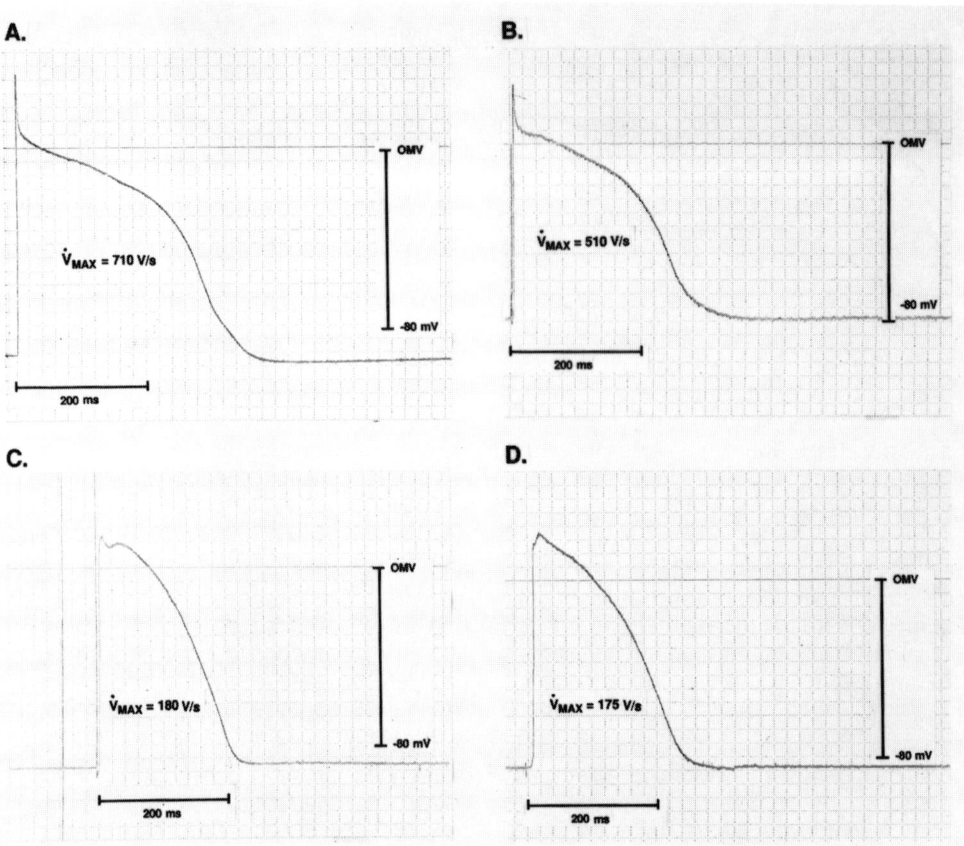

FIGURE 2–2

Representative adult and neonatal canine Purkinje fiber and papillary muscle action potentials. Panel *A:* adult canine Purkinje fiber action potential. Panel *B:* neonatal canine Purkinje fiber action potential. Panel *C:* adult papillary muscle action potential. Panel *D:* neonatal papillary muscle. These recordings were made at basic cycle length of 1000 ms, with superfusion of standard physiologic saline solution ($[K^+]_o$ = 4) and standard microelectrode recording technique. The analog data were digitized at 6–13 kHz depending on the electronic estimation of V_{max} that was monitored during the experiments. The action potential characteristics were measured automatically with a waveform detection algorithm, and $\dot{V}_{max}$ was estimated by a first difference calculation of the upstroke data.[37] These data were displayed by D/A conversion output to a Gould electrostatic recorder.

selectivity for K^+ permeability, and an increase in the electrochemical gradient of potassium, which may explain, in part, the age-related increase in resting potential.

A third developmental factor in determining resting potential may be the degree of electrogenic Na^+- and K^+-ATPase (Na^+ pump) activity. The ability of the Na^+ pump to produce net charge in the resting membrane potential has been postulated for many years and demonstrated in a variety of tissues. (For a review, see Glitsch.[25]) The embryonic or very young postnatal heart cells, being very small, have a high surface-to-volume ratio and high permeability. Both of these factors should contribute to increasing Na^+ pump activity. In fact, Marsh et al found higher Na^+- and K^+-ATPase activity in neonatal guinea pig myocardium compared with adults.[26] Therefore, the degree to which this Na^+ pump activity in immature hearts is electrogenic and contributes to the resting potential is likely to be larger in immature than in mature myocardium.

A number of experiments have shown that action potential amplitude and sensitivity to the sodium current blocker tetrodotoxin increase with development in the embryonic chick heart. Tetrodotoxin sensitivity and action potential amplitude also increase in fetal mammalian Purkinje fibers from the late embryonic stage to adulthood.[27–29] The lower resting potential found in fetal canine Purkinje fibers compared with adults does not contribute to greater sodium current inactivation or, subsequently, to the smaller action

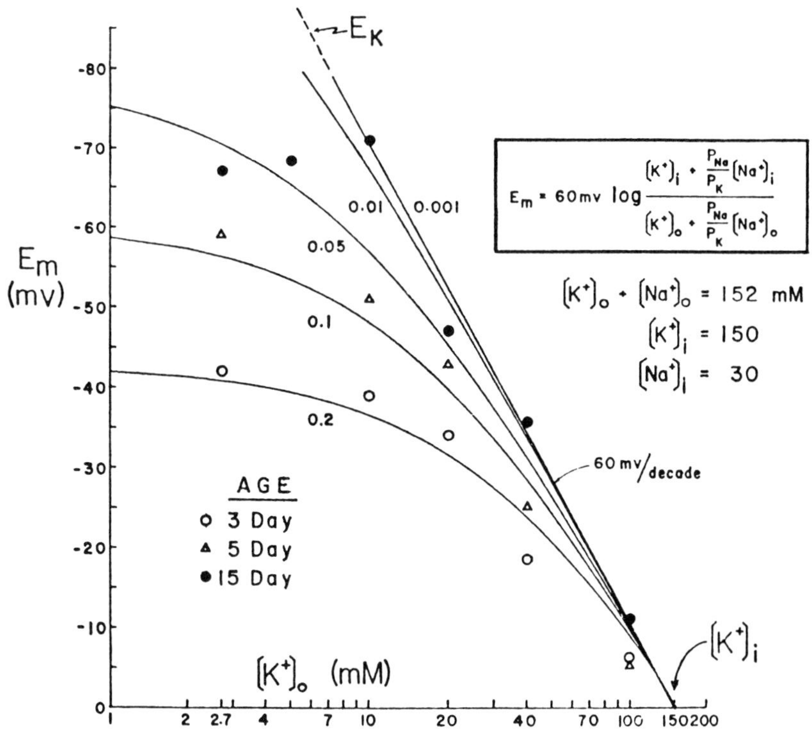

FIGURE 2–3

Resting potential (E_m) plotted as a function of $[K^+]_o$ on a logarithmic scale. $[K^+]_o$ was elevated by substitution of K^+ for equimolar amounts of Na^+. Continuous lines give theoretical calculations from the constant-field equation (shown in inset) of resting E_m as a function of $[K^+]_o$ for various assumed P_{Na}/P_K ratios of 0.001, 0.01, 0.05, 0.1, and 0.2. Calculations were made assuming a $[K^+]_i$ of 150 mmol/L, $[Na^+]_i$ of 30 mmol/L (estimated from $[Na^+]_o$ level at which excitability is lost); the sum of $[K^+]_o$ + $[Na^+]_o$ was held constant at 152 mmol/L, which was the method used to obtain the experimental data given here. As indicated by the equation, the shapes of these theoretical curves are dependent on the assumed values for $[Na^+]_i$. For a P_{Na}/P_K ratio of 0.001, the curve is linear over the entire range with a slope of 60 mV/decade (i.e., it closely follows E_K); at higher ratios, the slope continually diminishes as $[K^+]_o$ is lowered, and the curve flattens at low $[K^+]_o$ levels. Symbols give representative data obtained from embryonic chick hearts at days 3, 5, and 15. The data points for the 3-day heart follow the curve for a P_{Na}/P_K ratio of 0.2, those for the 5-day heart follow the theoretical curve for 0.1, and those for the 15-day heart follow the curve for a ratio of 0.01. The estimated intracellular K^+ activity ($[K^+]_i$) levels obtained by extrapolation to zero potential are nearly the same for a heart of any age. (From Sperelakis N, Shigenobu, K: Changes in membrane properties of chick embryonic hearts during development. J Gen Physiol 60:430–453, 1972.)

potential amplitudes and lower $\dot{V}max$ seen in the younger age group. These results suggest that the density of sodium channels may increase during development.

The shape and potential of the early plateau of the cardiac action potential is largely controlled by I_{si} and the transient outward current(s) I_{To}. Escande et al have found that there appear to be age-related differences in I_{To} of atrial myocardium recorded during cardiac bypass surgery.[17] They found that adult patients more often exhibited a pronounced notch between phases 1 and 2 of the action potential as compared with patients from 2 months to 22 months of age. Also, the plateau in the older tissue was generally at a lower potential (i.e., less positive). 4-Aminopyridine and caffeine were used to block the two transient outward currents, I_{lo} and I_{bo}, respectively,[6] producing rather similar plateaus in both age groups. These results suggest that transient outward currents increase with age and greatly affect action potential shape. Similar results have been observed in canine Purkinje fibers.[24] As can be seen in Figure 2–2(C,D), the canine ventricular myocardial action potential plateau is more positive and less notched in the neonate than in the adult.

It is interesting to note that the action potential duration was not significantly affected by I_{To} blockade in the experiments of

Escande et al.[17] APD_{90} remained greater following I_{To} blockade in adults, suggesting that developmental differences in other currents (such as I_{si}, I_K, I_{window}, or possibly I_{K1}) are responsible for age-related differences in action potential duration. A concomitant developmental change in I_{si} may also be partly responsible for these age-related changes in the action potential plateau.

Unfortunately, voltage clamp studies describing the developmental aspects of the I_{si} current are not available. It has been shown that the newborn myocardium is more dependent on extracellular Ca^{+2} than is adult tissue.[30] This dependency on extracellular Ca^{+2} may result from more myofilaments being in close proximity to the sarcolemma as a result of the high surface-to-volume ratio in neonatal cells. Another important factor may be the immaturity of the sarcoplasmic reticulum (SR), as evidenced by the low enzyme activities in the SR of neonatal heart cells.[31, 32] The I_{si} current density (a function of the number of channels per unit area of membrane and the kinetics of those channels) may also change during the maturation of heart cells. Immature heart cells appear to require a greater influx of extracellular calcium than adult cells require for the promotion of contractility. This observation would appear to explain the relative sensitivity of young individuals to the negative inotropic effects of calcium antagonists.[33]

Virtually nothing is known about the age-related changes in the delayed outward currents or the pacemaker currents. Because the I_x current probably has an important role in controlling action potential duration, it is likely that there are developmental changes in I_x that correspond to the age-related changes in action potential duration shown in Table 2–1. Developmental changes in pacemaker currents are even more difficult to interpret, because changes in autonomic innervation and in adrenergic and cholinergic agonists that accompany fetal and postnatal development have profound effects on the expression of pacemaker conductances, although the kinetics of these pacemaker currents may be unchanged.

Finally, the age-related differences in cardiac electrophysiology do relate to demonstrable differences in functional aspects of the heart. For example, the neonatal Purkinje fibers have an average maximal conduction velocity that is 33% less than that in adult fibers.[34] The degree to which age-related differences in passive membrane properties and threshold potential contribute to conduction velocity differences is not known. At least part of the slower conduction velocity, however, is attributable to significantly lower V_{max} in the neonatal fibers compared with adults (Table 2–1).

Adult canine Purkinje fibers have a relatively consistent pattern of increasing action potential duration from the proximal to distal end of the free-running segment.[35] The broadening of the action potential immediately before the Purkinje fiber inserts into the endocardium of the free wall is called the "gate." This has been postulated to act as a low-pass filter or ventricular node, giving the gates longer refractory periods and preventing some premature responses from conducting to the working myocardium. Untereker, Danilo, and Rosen[36] found that, compared with adults, the neonatal canine Purkinje fiber is much more homogeneous along its free-running segment in terms of action potential duration; there is no clear area of maximum action potential duration. This may be an indication of the progressive change in the repolarizing plateau currents from the neonatal period through adulthood.

As yet no one has demonstrated that the shorter, more homogeneous, action potential duration and slower conduction velocity predisposes the neonatal heart to reentry arrhythmias, even though these factors would tend to do so. This is because for the excitable gap necessary for reentry to exist, the following must be true:

$$\text{reentry circuit length (cm)} \geq \text{conduction velocity (cm/s)} \times \text{effective refractory period (s)}.$$

Therefore, by reducing both the effective refractory period (a function of the action potential duration) and conduction velocity, the minimum pathway length required for reentry to occur will be decreased. Given the fact that the neonatal heart is 10 to 15 times smaller than the adult heart, the potential reentry pathway is disproportionately small in the neonate. The conduction velocity is 33% less and the action potential duration 12% less in the neonate than in the adult. For this reason, severe pathologic conditions or anatomic abnormalities may be required for reentry in the very young and small heart, in spite of the normally low conduction velocity and short action potential duration.

In conclusion, in most cardiac tissues, MDP

increases during the maturation of the heart. Independent of this, the action potential amplitude and $\dot{V}max$ also increase. Action potential duration increases at a given basic cycle length. The action potential plateau generally becomes less positive with development. Conductances that might be involved in the changes in the plateau potential with development remain to be determined.

References

1. Pickering JW: Observations on the physiology of the embryonic heart. J Physiol (London) 14:383–466, 1883.
2. Easby MH: Electrocardiograms from a four and a half month old fetus. Am Heart J 10:118–119, 1934.
3. Fingl E, Woodbury LA, Hecht HH: Effects of innervation and drugs upon direct membrane potentials of embryonic myocardium. J Pharm Exp Ther 104:103–114, 1952.
4. Carmeliet E: Inward going rectification in sheep cardiac Purkinje fibers. In Paes de Carvalho A, Hoffman BF, Lieberman M (eds): Normal and Abnormal Conduction in the Heart. Mt. Kisco, NY: Futura Publishing Co., p 211–221, 1982.
5. Attwell D, Cohen I, Eisner D, Ohba M, Ojeda C: The steady-state TTX-sensitive ("window") sodium current in cardiac Purkinje fibers. Pflugers Arch 379:137–142, 1979.
6. Coraboeuf E, Deroubaix E, Coulombe A: Effects of tetrodotoxin on action potentials of the conducting system in the dog heart. Am J Physiol H:236:561–567, 1979.
7. Kenyon JL, Gibbons WR: 4-Aminopyridine and the early outward current of sheep cardiac Purkinje fibers. J Gen Physiol 73:139–157, 1979.
8. Hewett KW, Robinson RB, Hoffman BF: Evidence for a transient outward current in isolated canine ventricular myocytes. Circulation 68:III–25, 1983.
9. Coraboeuf E, Carmeliet E: Existence of two transient outward currents in sheep cardiac Purkinje fibers. Pflugers Arch 392:352–359, 1982.
10. Isenberg G: Cardiac Purkinje fibres. The slow inward current component under the influence of modified $[Ca^{2+}]_i$. Pflugers Arch 371:61–69, 1977.
11. Zipes DP, Mendez C: Action of manganese ions and tetrodotoxin on atrioventricular nodal transmembrane potentials in isolated rabbit hearts. Circ Res 32:447–454, 1973.
12. Imanishi S, McAllister RG Jr, Surawicz B: The effects of verapamil and lidocaine on the automatic depolarizations in guinea pig ventricular myocardium. J Pharm Exp Ther 207:294–303, 1978.
13. Noble D, Tsien RW: Outward membrane currents activated in the plateau range of potentials in cardiac Purkinje fibers. J Physiol 200:205–231, 1969.
14. Cohen IS, Falk RT, Kline RP: Pacemaker activity in cardiac Purkinje fibers: Voltage clamp analysis. In Paes de Carvalho A, Hoffman BF, Lieberman M (eds): Normal and Abnormal Conduction in the Heart. Mount Kisco, NY: Futura Publishing Company, pp 287–311, 1982.
15. Noble SJ: Potassium accumulation and depletion in frog atrial muscle. J Physiol (London) 258:579–613, 1976.
16. Jaeger JM, Gibbons WR: Slow inward current may produce many results attributed to I_{x1} in cardiac Purkinje fibers. Am J Physiol 249:H122–H132, 1985.
17. Noble D, Tsien RW: The kinetics and rectifier properties of slow potassium current in cardiac Purkinje fibers. J Physiol (London) 195:185–214, 1968.
18. Brown HF, Clark A, Noble SJ: Identification of the pacemaker current in frog atrium. J Physiol (London) 258:521–545, 1976.
19. DiFrancesco D: A new interpretation of the pacemaker current in calf Purkinje fibers. J Physiol (London) 314:359–376, 1981.
20. Escande D, Loisance D, Planche C, Coraboeuf E: Age-related changes of action potential plateau shape in isolated human atrial fibers. Am J Physiol 249:H843–H850, 1985.
21. Carmeliet EE, Horres CR, Lieberman M, Vereecke JS: Developmental aspects of potassium flux and permeability of the embryonic chick heart. J Physiol (London) 254:673–692, 1976.
22. Sperelakis N, Shigenobu K: Changes in membrane properties of chick embryonic hearts during development. J Gen Physiol 60:430–453, 1972.
23. Fozzard HA, Sheu SS: Intracellular potassium and sodium activities of chick ventricular muscle during embryonic development. J Physiol (London) 306:579–586, 1980.
24. Reder RF, Miura DS, Danilo P Jr, Rosen MR: The electrophysiological properties of normal neonatal and adult canine cardiac Purkinje fibers. Circ Res 48:658–668, 1981.
25. Glitsch HG: Characteristics of active Na transport in intact cardiac cells. Am J Physiol 236:H189–H199, 1979.
26. Marsh AJ, Lloyd BL, Taylor RR: Age dependence of myocardial Na^+- K^+-ATPase activity and digitalis intoxication in dog and guinea pig. Circ Res 48:329–333, 1981.
27. Shigenobu K, Sperelakis N: Development of sensitivity to tetrodotoxin of chick embryonic hearts with age. J Mol Cell Cardiol 3:271–286, 1971.
28. Marcus NC, Fozzard H: Tetrodotoxin sensitivity in the developing and adult chick heart. J Mol Cell Cardiol 13:335–340, 1981.
29. Pappano AJ: Action potentials in chick atria. Ontogentic changes in the dependence of tetrodotoxin-resistant action potentials on calcium, strontium and barium. Circ Res 39:99–105, 1976.
30. George BL, Jarmakani J: The effects of lanthanum and manganese on excitation contraction coupling in the newborn rabbit heart. Dev Pharm Ther 5:1–13, 1982.
31. Nakanishi T, Jarmakani JM: Developmental changes in myocardial mechanical function and subcellular organelles. Am J Physiol 246:H615–H625, 1984.
32. Danilo P Jr, Reder RF, Binah O, Legato MJ: Fetal canine cardiac Purkinje fibers. Electrophysiology and ultrastructure. Am J Physiol 246:H250–H260, 1984.
33. Gibson R, Driscoll D, Gillette P, Hartley C, Entman ML: The comparative electrophysiologic and hemodynamic effects of verapamil in puppies and adult dogs. Dev Pharm Ther 2:104–116, 1981.

34. Rosen MR, Legato MJ, Weiss RM: Developmental changes in impulse conduction in the canine heart. Am J Physiol 240:H546–H554, 1981.
35. Myerburg RJ, Gelband H, Hoffman BF: Functional characteristics of the gating mechanism in the canine A-V conducting system. Circ Res 28:136–147, 1971.
36. Untereker WJ, Danilo P Jr, Rosen MR: Developmental changes in action potential duration, refractoriness, and conduction in the canine ventricular conduction system. Ped Res 18:53–58, 1984.
37. Buckles DS, Hewett KW: Assessment of the maximum frequency components and digital sampling of cardiac Purkinje fiber action potentials. Comp Biomed Res 19(5):410–416, 1986.
38. Bean BP: Two kinds of calcium channels in canine atrial cells. J Gen Physiol 86:1–30, 1985.
39. Nilius B, Hess P, Lansman JB, Tsiam RW: A novel type of calcium channel in ventricular cells. Nature 316:443–446, 1985.

CHAPTER 3

PHARMACOLOGY AND ELECTROPHYSIOLOGY OF ANTIARRHYTHMIC DRUGS

Jeffrey P. Moak

Despite advances in surgical and pacemaker therapy, antiarrhythmic drugs are still the most commonly used treatment for arrhythmias. The successful use of antiarrhythmic drugs requires a thorough understanding of the disposition of these agents within the body and insight into their pharmacodynamic effects. Facility with antiarrhythmic pharmacology has multiple advantages over empiric treatment: successful drug therapy is likely to be achieved earlier; the number of agents tested is likely to be lower; and, as a result, patient acceptance and safety are more likely as well.

Two principles are well established: (1) the disposition and electrophysiologic effects of antiarrhythmic drugs differ developmentally with age, so that marked differences are not only apparent between children and adults but also exist within the pediatric age group; and (2) the pharmacologic profile of each antiarrhythmic drug is unique. Therefore, although general statements about classes of antiarrhythmic drugs can be made, each agent must also be considered individually.

This chapter will first present general information on basic pharmacologic principles (pharmacokinetics and pharmacodynamics). Subsequently, the clinical pharmacology and toxicity of the various agents useful in treating arrhythmias in children will be reviewed.

PRINCIPLES OF CLINICAL PHARMACOLOGY

The aim of antiarrhythmic therapy is elimination of the index arrhythmia. Short of this, the frequency of the index arrhythmia should be decreased. Elimination of the index arrhythmia requires the administration of a drug in an appropriate dosage that accounts for individual variations in genetic composition and disease processes.[1] The intensity of the therapeutic effect depends on the drug concentration at the site of action. Changes in drug concentration are determined by the dosage schedule, route of administration, and metabolic fate of the drug within the body.[1] Two major factors influence variability in drug response: drug disposition in the body, and sensitivity to the agent at its site of action. Drug disposition comprises distribution, absorption, biotransformation, and elimination. Drug sensitivity is examined by studying an agent's dose-response relationship to the target organ or cell.

Drug Distribution: Developmental Considerations

Several important maturational changes in body composition occur during development that influence drug distribution during childhood.[2] These changes are responsible for the increased volume of distribution of most antiarrhythmic drugs in younger patients and partially account for the higher dosage requirements for these agents. Total body water is increased in newborns and young infants compared to older children, thereby increasing the volume of the central compartment. (The central compartment consists of the serum or blood volume, together with the extracellular fluid of highly perfused tissues such as the heart, lungs, liver, kidneys, and spleen. Drugs distribute throughout this compartment within a few minutes.[3]) The peripheral compartment, normally composed of low-perfusion tissues such as fat, muscle, skin, and bone, is decreased in the younger child. In addition, several factors have been shown to decrease protein binding in the younger age group:

1. Reduced protein concentration (albumin and γ-globulins).
2. Structural and molecular alterations in fetal albumin composition that decrease its ability to bind drugs.
3. The presence of endogenous substrates (free fatty acids and bilirubin) that compete for drug binding sites.
4. Lower blood pH.
5. Decreased renal function.

Drug Absorption

Absorption is defined as the movement of a drug from the site of administration (gastrointestinal tract, respiratory system, intramuscular, or cutaneous) to the circulatory system.[4] Drug absorption is generally a "first order" kinetic process, with the rate of absorption proportional to the drug concentration remaining at the site of absorption.[5] The rate of absorption will affect both the time to and duration of the peak plasma concentration. A slow absorption rate will delay the time to peak plasma concentration and prolong the duration of its peak.

Only if a drug is administered intravenously is it fully available to reach the targeted receptor site. The systemic availability of drugs administered intramuscularly or via the gastrointestinal tract is frequently incomplete, with absorption levels ranging between 50% and 95%. *Bioavailability* is a measure of the completeness and rate of drug absorption into the central compartment after oral or intramuscular administration. Availability, in the case of oral dosaging, may be reduced either by incomplete absorption and/or drug metabolism by the intestine or liver during passage from the gut lumen to the systemic circulation. This latter effect is known as "first pass" elimination and occurs with many antiarrhythmic drugs (propranolol, lidocaine, and verapamil).

Absorption may further be attenuated by differences in biopharmaceutical formulation. Different preparations of the same drug (e.g., digoxin or phenytoin) may undergo different rates and completeness of absorption because of differences in dissolution rate. Before a drug can be absorbed after oral administration, it must first dissolve into solution (dissolution). Most antiarrhythmic drugs are formulated into solid medications to enhance stability, taste, and convenience. Thus two brands of the same drug may produce different serum concentration-time profiles and therapeutic effectiveness.

In neonates and young infants, drug absorption is known to be immature.[2] Maturational changes in gastric secretions, intestinal motility, and blood flow to the gastrointestinal tract occur throughout childhood. Gastric emptying is prolonged in newborns (6 to 8 hours) but reaches adult values by 6 to 8 months of age.[3] Slower gastric emptying delays peak plasma concentration. A relative state of gastric achlorhydria exists until 3 years of age. Neutrality of gastric secretions has the effect of diminishing absorption of antiarrhythmic drugs that are weak acids (e.g., phenytoin). Newborns also have a higher pH in the small intestine, allowing bacterial colonization. For antiarrhythmic drugs that may be recirculated enterohepatically (e.g., digoxin), bacterial colonization of the small intestine may decrease drug clearance. Irregular intestinal peristalsis delays drug absorption until the age of 4 years. In addition, as children mature, the surface area of the intestinal mucosa grows allowing for greater drug absorption. The net result of these development changes is to decrease drug absorption, with adult values not attained until the age of 4 years.

Disease states and alterations in blood flow to the gastrointestinal tract can also alter drug bioavailability. Congestive heart failure may cause intestinal mucosal edema as well as decreased blood flow, thus impairing the absorption of orally administered drugs. Malabsorption syndromes, concomitant use of other drugs (antacids), various foods, or changes in intestinal motility may similarly decrease the rate or completeness of drug absorption.

Steady-state serum concentrations are high when administered doses are large, the time interval between doses is small, when drug elimination is slow, or when the apparent volume of distribution is small. Conversely, steady-state serum concentrations are low when doses are small or infrequent, when the drug is rapidly eliminated, or when the apparent volume of distribution is large.

In practice, a steady-state serum concentration is never achieved during repeated oral administration of antiarrhythmic drugs.[6] Drug levels fluctuate about a mean during the interval between doses. At some time after each dose (determined by the rates of absorption, distribution, and elimination) serum concentration reaches a peak that is higher than the mean. During the rest of the dosage interval, serum concentration falls to and then below the mean. The longer the dosage interval, the greater the variation about the mean. The degree of fluctuation can be reduced without affecting the mean serum concentration by dosing at more frequent intervals.

INTRAVENOUS INFUSION

Because the time taken to reach a therapeutic plasma concentration may take too long during repeated oral drug administration for patients who require urgent arrhythmia suppression, an intravenous infusion may be used to rapidly achieve pharmacologic effect.[4] Intravenous drug administration can achieve high plasma concentrations almost instantaneously. Although the time taken to achieve a therapeutic plasma concentration is rapid using intravenous infusion, a steady state will only be reached when the rate of drug delivery equals the elimination rate.

Drug Elimination

The action of most drugs is terminated by metabolism, excretion, or both. Hepatic biotransformation, renal excretion, pulmonary exhalation, and fecal excretion are the usual process of drug elimination.[4] *Clearance* is a quantitative measure of the volume of blood totally cleared of drug during a unit of time. The rate of elimination is proportional to drug concentration.

Clearance is influenced by such factors as organ blood flow, degree of plasma protein binding, and organ function. Therefore, drug clearance can be anticipated to change during developmental maturation and with disease. Clearance of a drug that is highly extracted by an organ (e.g., liver or kidney) strongly depends on blood flow to that organ. A reduction in blood flow to an organ will compromise that organ's ability to eliminate drug from the blood. Because only the free fraction of drug in plasma is available for metabolism or renal excretion, the degree of protein binding can significantly affect the clearance of a drug. For drugs that are highly protein bound, only the small fraction that is unbound to plasma proteins can be cleared. Function of the organ system that eliminates a given drug from the body will modify the drug's elimination half-life. Disease-induced dysfunction of the organ system primarily responsible for the elimination of a drug will diminish its clearance.

HEPATIC METABOLISM

Biotransformation is the major mechanism for elimination of most antiarrhythmic drugs from the body.[4] Hepatic metabolism of drugs is substantially different in the newborn, infant, and adult.[2] In the neonatal period, phase I and II enzymes have reduced functional activity and are easily saturable. This is manifested clinically by decreased clearance rates and prolonged half-lives for drugs that need to be biotransformed. However, after age 6 months, the intrinsic ability for hepatic metabolism of drugs exceeds that in the adult. Thus higher dosage requirements, short dosing intervals, or both, may be necessary to maintain therapeutic drug levels in children.

A number of other factors have been shown to significantly alter enzyme activity or levels. These include enzyme induction from prior administration of the drug or another agent, enzyme inhibition from other substrates that are similarly metabolized, nutritional state, and body temperature. Disease or drugs that reduce hepatic blood flow may significantly diminish hepatic clearance. Similarly, drug metabolism may be altered by hepatocellular necrosis.

RENAL EXCRETION

In general, excretion of drugs and metabolites is primarily a renal function.[4] It is carried out by three mechanisms: glomerular filtration, tubular secretion, and tubular reabsorption. Glomerular filtration removes large molecules of high molecular weight from the plasma. Along the proximal tubule, separate mechanisms exist for secreting acids and bases from the plasma into the tubule lumen. Reabsorption is the most important factor controlling renal handling of drugs. The degree of reabsorption depends on the lipid-soluble nature of the drug, its state of ionization, and its molecular weight.

Diminished renal function is characteristic of the neonatal period and early infancy.[2] All three renal processes (tubular reabsorption, renal secretion, and glomerular filtration) are affected, and adult levels of function are attained at different ages. At birth, glomerular as well as tubular function is only 20% to 30% of that observed in the adult. Tubular reabsorption matures rapidly, with adult abilities attained at age 6 months. By about 1 month of age, the renal secretory handling of acids attains adult values. When fully matured, glomerular filtration capabilities match those of the adult kidney. Glomerular filtration matures to 70% of adult values by 6 months of age, with 100% levels not reached until age 1 year.

Drug accumulation and adverse effects may occur in neonates and young infants when doses of drugs that are cleared by the kidney are not adjusted to reflect the intrinsic excretory capability of the kidney. At any age, primary renal disease, in addition to reducing renal blood flow (low cardiac output states), may compromise the clearance capabilities of the body and result in drug accumulation if dosage is not properly adjusted. Pharmacologic therapy with antiarrhythmic drugs that are not primarily excreted unchanged by the kidney, but whose metabolites are, demand special consideration if renal failure occurs. Procainamide is one such drug.[7] *N*-acetylprocainamide prolongs action potential duration and the QTc interval and may accumulate to a greater extent than the parent drug and produce ventricular arrhythmias (torsades de pointes).

THERAPEUTIC DRUG MONITORING

The capability to measure the plasma concentration of most antiarrhythmic drugs has become widely available. However, for a drug concentration to be clinically useful, the plasma drug concentration must reflect the concentration of the drug at the receptor site, and the intensity of pharmacologic effect must correlate with receptor site drug concentration. The correlation of plasma levels with therapeutic effect is weak for drugs that exert their pharmacologic effect long after their plasma concentration disappears (e.g., amiodarone).

Much misunderstanding of drug levels pervades clinical practice. "Therapeutic" plasma concentrations encompass a range within which a large number of arrhythmias are suppressed or improved by the antiarrhythmic drug, and only a small number of patients demonstrate evidence of toxicity. When concentrations are below this range, relatively few patients receive therapeutic benefit. When the plasma concentration exceeds the therapeutic range, a large percentage of patients develop side effects. Not infrequently, however, a number of arrhythmias may be successfully controlled with antiarrhythmic blood levels within the "toxic" range, yet few patients report symptoms. Conversely, there are patients who display adverse drug effects at therapeutic blood levels. How then should plasma concentrations of antiarrhythmic drugs be used? Drugs are administered to achieve a desired therapeutic goal, and blood levels should guide the clinician in dosaging. The target of antiarrhythmic therapy should never be to achieve a desired plasma concentration.

What are the indications to measure plasma concentrations of antiarrhythmic drugs? Plasma concentration monitoring may be helpful in the evaluation of therapeutic failures. Failure to achieve arrhythmia suppression with reasonably high doses may represent a true therapeutic failure, low bioavailability, altered pharmacokinetics (high metabolic clearance), or poor patient compliance.[8] Evaluation of the plasma concentration will differentiate a true therapeutic failure from a pharmacokinetic or compliance problem. Measuring antiarrhythmic plasma concentrations may also be helpful when alterations of drug absorption, distribution, or elimination are anticipated in a patient with congestive heart failure or renal or hepatic failure. These pathophysiologic changes will alter the usual relationship between administered dose and plasma concentration. Concurrent administration of an interacting drug may confound therapy and may be resolved by measuring antiarrhythmic drug concentrations. In cases of deliberate or accidental drug overdosage, determination of plasma concentration may have important therapeutic value. Lastly, monitoring plasma concentration may elucidate whether a sign or symptom can be attributable to an adverse drug reaction or to some concurrent underlying disease.

Plasma drug levels should be interpreted in light of certain factors that modify the relationship between measured plasma concentration and cardiac effects. All antiarrhythmic drugs are variably bound to plasma proteins in the systemic circulation. However, only the unbound or free fraction can cross cell membranes and interact with the target receptor site. In almost all cases, the actual measured plasma concentration represents total (both bound and free) drug in the plasma. Interpretation of plasma concentration may therefore be complicated for antiarrhythmic drugs that exhibit concentration-dependent plasma protein binding (e.g., disopyramide and lidocaine), or if changes in protein binding occur.

Choosing the proper time to obtain a plasma drug concentration is also crucial. In general, it takes four to five drug half-lives for steady-state conditions to be attained. Sampling before steady-state conditions occur may provide misleadingly low (for orally administered drugs) or high (for intravenously administered drugs) plasma concentrations. Furthermore, levels can change significantly within a dosage interval. Because of interpatient variability in timing of the peak drug plasma concentration, it is generally recommended that blood samples be obtained near the end of the dosage interval (trough level).

Blood samples collected in containers with TRIS buffer can give falsely low plasma drug levels for drugs such as lidocaine, propranolol, and quinidine.[8] Displacement of drugs from α_1-acid glycoprotein by TRIS buffer results in an increase in unbound drug, which quickly diffuses into the red cells. Following centrifugation and removal of the red cell fraction, the resultant drug serum concentration will be spuriously low.

Differences in the analytic method for measuring plasma drug levels can produce significant discrepancies in drug concentrations. Limitations in assay capability to resolve parent drug from metabolites or other drugs may influence the quantitative accuracy of the procedure. Nonspecific assays may confound interpretation by reporting falsely elevated drug levels.

Most antiarrhythmic drugs are extensively metabolized. In some cases the metabolites are electrophysiologically active and may exert potent cardioactive effects. The time course of accumulation and elimination of drug metabolites frequently differs from the parent drug. Therefore, in evaluating the therapeutic effect of antiarrhythmic drugs that are biotransformed to active metabolites, it is important to consider the relative contribution of parent drug and metabolites (e.g., encainide and *N*-acetylprocainamide). Analytic methods to measure drug metabolites are infrequently available in clinical practice.

After a plasma drug level is obtained, the potential for therapeutic effectiveness or toxicity must be interpreted in light of certain clinical considerations. Clinical responsiveness to antiarrhythmic therapy, in the presence of an adequate drug concentration at the target receptor site, may be further influenced by the type of arrhythmia treated, amount of myocardial drug uptake, previous drug therapy, acid-base and metabolic disturbances, autonomic tone, myocardial ischemia, or cardiac pump dysfunction.

CLINICAL IMPORTANCE OF DRUG METABOLITES

The clinical importance of antiarrhythmic drug metabolites in producing unanticipated drug efficacy or toxicity has become increasingly evident. Drug metabolites may have synergistic or totally different pharmacologic actions, may accumulate and produce drug toxicity, can inhibit the electrophysiologic effect or metabolism of the parent drug, or can result in displacement of the drug from plasma protein or myocardial receptor sites.[7] Drug metabolites are of little concern unless they accumulate to a significant concentration. Metabolite accumulation is likely to occur when a major fraction of the parent drug is converted to the metabolite or when the total clearance of the metabolite is less than that of its parent. Furthermore, the plasma concentration of drug metabolites may be insignificant under ordinary circumstances but can accumulate to therapeutic or toxic levels in patients with congestive heart failure, renal failure, or hepatic insufficiency. Important pharmacologic effects of drug metabolites have been clinically demonstrated for procainamide, quinidine, lidocaine, and encainide.

DRUG INTERACTIONS

Drug interactions occur when the pharmacokinetic or pharmacodynamic effects of one drug are altered by another drug.[9] Interactions arise frequently, because patients with cardiac disease are often treated with multiple cardiovascular medications. Drug interactions may be beneficial or adverse. Beneficial drug interactions occur when two drugs are used together to achieve greater efficacy or less toxicity. All too often, however, drug interactions impair the action of one or more drugs or produce adverse side effects.

The mechanisms by which drugs interact are numerous and may be multiple. Drug interactions are best distinguished on the basis of whether they are pharmacokinetic or pharmacodynamic in origin (Table 3–1). In pharmacokinetic interactions, changes occur in the plasma concentration of one or both drugs. A change in plasma concentration of either drug is therefore expected to alter the intensity of pharmacologic action. In contrast, pharmacodynamic interactions are characterized by changes produced by one drug in the pharmacologic effects of another drug without a change in its free plasma concentration.

TABLE 3–1
MECHANISMS FOR DRUG INTERACTION

I. Pharmacokinetic
    a. Absorption
    b. Distribution
    c. Elimination
        1. Biotransformation
        2. Excretion
II. Pharmacodynamic
    a. Competitive inhibition at receptor sites
    b. Change in tissue sensitivity
    c. Effect on intermediate pathway between receptor binding and pharmacologic effect
    d. Summation or inhibition of combined drug effects

Pharmacokinetic Interactions

When several drugs are concomitantly administered orally, a change in the rate and completeness of gastrointestinal absorption of any of them may occur. Physicochemical interactions between drugs may produce insoluble complexes (tetracycline, cholestyramine resin) that retard drug dissolution and availability for absorption. Most antiarrhythmic drugs are weak acids or bases and, like most drugs, are best absorbed in the nonionized form. Alterations in gastric or intestinal pH (e.g., caused by antacids) may decrease drug bioavailability by displacing drug equilibrium to the ionized form. Drugs that depress gastrointestinal transit time may increase the bioavailability of drugs that are slowly absorbed. In contrast, agents that quicken gastrointestinal motility may reduce the completeness of absorption of drugs that are slowly absorbed.

Cardiovascular drugs that reduce cardiac output or alter regional blood flow to the gastrointestinal tract may also depress drug absorption. The reduction of cardiac output may decrease the volume of distribution of other drugs, thereby increasing their serum concentration.

All antiarrhythmic drugs are bound to plasma proteins (albumin and α_1-acid glycoprotein), although to a variable extent. Changes in plasma protein levels (secondary to either acute or chronic illness) may secondarily increase or decrease the concentration of free, unbound drug available to interact with tissue-binding sites. Alternatively, antiarrhythmic drugs may be displaced from plasma protein–binding sites by other drugs, thereby increasing the unbound drug concentration. For antiarrhythmic agents that are highly protein bound, small increases in the free, unbound concentration can intensify the pharmacologic action.

Many drugs are capable of enhancing hepatic biotransformation capabilities (e.g., microsomal enzyme induction; two such drugs are phenobarbital and phenytoin). To be effectively eliminated, most antiarrhythmic drugs require hepatic biotransformation. Increased hepatic enzyme activity will significantly enhance antiarrhythmic metabolism, thereby decreasing a drug's activity-time profile. In contrast to such drugs are those agents that inhibit metabolic transformation (e.g., cimetidine, isoniazid, and chloramphenicol). Hepatic microsomal enzyme inhibitors diminish antiarrhythmic drug clearance and increase the drug's plasma concentration level during the dosage interval.

Concomitantly administered drugs may influence the renal handling of antiarrhythmic drugs by altering renal blood flow, active tubular secretion, or passive reabsorption. Renal blood flow may be changed by cardiovascular drugs that alter cardiac output or the distribution of blood flow. Competition between antiarrhythmic drugs that are actively secreted by the renal tubules may decrease the clearance of the agent with a lower affinity for the transporter site. Changes in real tubular fluid pH may significantly affect reabsorption of antiarrhythmic agents that are predominantly excreted in the urine. The overall renal excretion of basic drugs (procainamide or quinidine) is increased by urinary acidification and decreased by alkalinization. The converse is true for acidic drugs.

Pharmacodynamic Interactions

Pharmacodynamic interaction frequently involves competition for receptor occupancy. Such interaction involves either two drugs that activate the same receptor site with different effectiveness (antiarrhythmic therapy with quinidine and mexiletine) or an active drug combined with a receptor-blocking agent (e.g., β-blockers combined with serum catecholamines). A second type of pharmacodynamic interaction results from changes in tissue sensitivity (such as increased myocardial sensitivity to digoxin after diuretic-induced hypokalemia). Not infrequently, one agent may alter the intermediate pathway by which a second drug exerts its pharmacologic effect. Most commonly, pharmacodynamic interaction results from summation or inhibition of pharmacologic action through diverse mechanisms. An example is the adverse effects of myocardial ischemia resulting from drug-induced hypotension (verapamil) combined with diuretic-induced hypokalemia.

CLASSIFICATION OF ANTIARRHYTHMIC DRUGS

Categorization of antiarrhythmic drugs into various classes is useful to the clinician treating arrhythmias. The grouping of antiarrhythmic agents with similar electrophysiologic properties provides a framework for understanding possible mechanisms of pharmacologic action. By highlighting shared effects, however, such a classification ignores the drugs' individuality. All drugs assigned to a single group do not exhibit entirely similar actions (i.e., some drugs exert more than one type of action). The classification of antiarrhythmic drugs is primarily based on their observed effects on healthy His-Purkinje tissue. Antiarrhythmic drugs may exert different effects on atrial or ventricular myocardium in different species, on depressed tissues, or when the electrolyte milieu is altered. Lastly, many antiarrhythmic agents produce their effects in vivo not by direct electrophysiologic actions on cardiac cells, but indirectly through the central or peripheral autonomic nervous system, by active metabolites, or by anti-ischemic actions.

With these reservations in mind, a clinically useful classification of antiarrhythmic agents is presented in Table 3–2. This classification will also provide the structure for the discussion that follows in the next section on individual antiarrhythmic agents.

In brief, local anesthetic agents are the

TABLE 3–2
CLASSIFICATION OF ANTIARRHYTHMIC DRUGS

I. Local anesthetic agents (primarily slow conduction)
  a. Agents that prolong refractoriness
    Quinidine, procainamide, disopyramide
  b. Agents that shorten refractoriness
    Lidocaine, phenytoin, mexiletine, ethmozine
  c. Agents producing only minor changes in refractoriness
    Encainide, flecainide, propafenone
II. β-adrenergic blockers
  Subclasses:
  a. Cardioselectivity (atenolol)
  b. Partial agonist activity
  c. Membrane stabilizing activity (propranolol)
  d. Lipid solubility
III. Agents that primarily prolong cardiac refractoriness
  Amiodarone, bretylium
IV. Calcium channel blockers
  Verapamil
V. Digitalis glycosides
  Digoxin
VI. Purinergic agonists
  Adenosine

largest in number and the most frequently used category of antiarrhythmic drugs. They exert their predominant direct electrophysiologic effect by blocking cardiac sodium channels, thereby slowing conduction within the heart. These agents are further subclassified by their associated effects (i.e., alteration of repolarization and refractoriness). The type IA agents (see Table 3–2) prolong His-Purkinje cell and ventricular muscle action potential duration (APD) and the effective refractory period (ERP). This contrasts with the type IB drugs, which shorten APD and ERP. Despite the fact that the type IC local anesthetic drugs are the most potent group as a whole in depressing cardiac conduction, they have minimal effects on myocardial refractoriness.

The second largest group of antiarrhythmic drugs are the β-blocking agents. Their predominant effect is to decrease sympathetic activity by competitively blocking the β-adrenergic receptor. While all β-blockers share this property, they can be further subclassified by cardioselectivity, partial agonist activity, membrane stabilizing activity, and lipid solubility.

Class III antiarrhythmic agents predominantly prolong APD and ERP without producing significant depression of cardiac conduction. Calcium channel blockers (class IV) primarily inhibit the slow inward calcium current and have profound effects on the sinus and atrioventricular nodes. These agents are becoming increasingly popular in use and important in arrhythmia control. Digitalis glycosides (class V) have the longest history of usage in the control of cardiac arrhythmias. Finally, the newest group of agents (class VI) to be explored for arrhythmia control are the purinergic agonists (adenosine and its analogues).

The next section will present a comprehensive discussion of the individual antiarrhythmic agents that are commonly used to treat pediatric arrhythmias.

Local Anesthetic Agents

QUINIDINE

Quinidine is the oldest of the currently used and available antiarrhythmic agents. It is derived from the dextrostereoisomer of quinine, a cinchona derivative. Although quinidine usage dates back to the mid-sixteenth century, it was not until the reports of Wenckebach (1914) and Frey (1918) that its use was popularized. Of all the available antiarrhythmic drugs, quinidine's pharmacokinetics and dynamic actions are among the best studied.

Cellular Electrophysiologic Effects

Quinidine can be characterized electrophysiologically as the prototype local anesthetic agent. By inhibiting sodium entry through its membrane channel, quinidine can markedly depress cardiac excitability, conduction, and membrane responsiveness. In healthy atrial, Purkinje, and ventricular muscle cells, quinidine depresses action potential amplitude and the maximum velocity of phase zero upstroke ($\dot{V}max$), two indices of cardiac conduction.[10, 11] Its effect on atrial or ventricular tissues depressed by hypoxia, stretch, ischemia, or hyperkalemia are more pronounced. At low concentrations, quinidine has no effect on resting membrane potential or maximum diastolic potential (MDP). Exposure to high concentrations, however, will decrease MDP.

Depression of cardiac conduction and $\dot{V}max$ (an indirect measure of sodium current) are enhanced at higher frequences of stimulation. Hondeghem and Matsubara have found that quinidine binds to the sodium channel as it activates.[12] During the action potential plateau and diastolic period, quinidine unbinds from its sodium channel receptor. The rate at which quinidine unbinds from the sodium channel is slow enough that at physiologic heart rates, not all of the bound quinidine dissociates. The result is cumulative block of the sodium channel with each successive depolarization cycle until an equilibrium is established (rate of drug unbinding equals the rate of drug binding).

Hiraoka, Sawadak, and Kawano have demonstrated that by depressing the delayed outward K^+ current, quinidine prolongs APD.[12a] Delay in recovery from sodium channel inactivation, as well as decreases in plateau currents (slow inward calcium current and delayed K^+ current), probably explains the prolongation of cardiac refractoriness induced by quinidine. Quinidine increases refractoriness to a greater extent than APD.

At therapeutic concentrations, quinidine

diminishes the slope of phase 4 depolarization in sinus node, atrial pacemaker, and His-Purkinje cells, the net effect is to prolong spontaneous cycle length.[10, 11] At higher concentrations, quinidine depresses sinus and atrioventricular nodal action potential amplitude and $\dot{V}max$. Quinidine's direct electrophysiologic effect is to prolong nodal APD.

Several investigators have demonstrated age-related changes in sensitivity to quinidine's cellular electrophysiologic effects. In a study of atrial action potentials in rats of different ages, the ability of quinidine to depress $\dot{V}max$ seemed to decrease with increasing age (i.e., more mature atria were less sensitive).[13] Morikawa and Rosen could not demonstrate development differences in tonic (resting) or use-dependent depression of $\dot{V}max$ between neonatal and adult Purkinje cells.[13a] However, the action of quinidine on His-Purkinje repolarization did demonstrate age dependence. Action potential prolongation was significantly greater in the neonatal group.

Clinical Electrophysiologic Effects

Quinidine often increases sinus heart rate indirectly through its anticholinergic actions.[10, 11] In the denervated transplanted heart, quinidine prolongs spontaneous sinus cycle length. Sinoatrial conduction time is frequently prolonged. Atrioventricular (AV) nodal conduction is similarly affected. In healthy patients, quinidine can enhance AV nodal conduction (i.e., shorten AH interval) through its vagolytic effects. However, the direct electrophysiologic action of quinidine is to depress atrioventricular nodal conduction (increase AH interval) and prolong AV nodal refractoriness. Conduction velocity in the atrium, His-Purkinje system, and ventricle is decreased by quinidine and is manifested electrophysiologically as prolongations in the PA, high right atrial–low right atrial (HRA–LRA), and His-ventricular (HV) intervals. Quinidine prolongs refractoriness in the atrium, His-Purkinje conduction system, and ventricle and has been reported to prolong the refractory period of accessory atrioventricular pathways. Dorian et al could not demonstrate any changes in defibrillation threshold following quinidine administration.[14]

Electrocardiographic Effects

Quinidine produces dose-dependent changes in the electrocardiogram.[10, 11] At therapeutic plasma concentrations, quinidine widens QRS duration and the rate-corrected QT interval. Depending on prevailing parasympathetic tone, the PR interval may remain unchanged or may lengthen. High plasma levels of quinidine can induce second or third degree AV block. Significant sinus bradycardia and long sinus pauses may occur in patients with sick sinus syndrome. Right or left bundle-branch block may develop during quinidine therapy in patients with preexisting abnormalities of the His-Purkinje conduction system.

Clinical Pharmacokinetics

Quinidine is almost always administered orally as either quinidine sulfate or quinidine gluconate. Intravenous administration is only rarely indicated (because of the frequent occurrence of hypotension and cardiovascular collapse).[15] Quinidine sulfate contains 20% more base than the gluconate preparation.[10, 11] Quinidine gluconate is more slowly absorbed, and peak plasma concentrations occur 3 to 5 hours after oral administration. In contrast, quinidine sulfate is rapidly absorbed, with peak concentrations occurring 30 to 90 minutes after ingestion. Bioavailability is high (sulfate, 80%; gluconate, 70%).[16] Systemic availability varies widely (40% to 93%) with the gluconate salt. Concurrent administration with food slows quinidine absorption but does not change the overall bioavailability.[17] Several long-acting quinidine preparations are available (e.g., quinidine polygalacturonate and extended-release quinidine sulfate); they combine quinidine alkaloid with different chemical moieties.[18] Their absorption characteristics have not been extensively studied in children.

Quinidine disposition differs markedly between children and adults. Szefler, Shen, and Gingell found the plasma clearance of quinidine higher in children (0.38 L/h/kg) than in adults (0.29 L/h/kg).[19] Elimination half-life changes with age:neonatal period, 6 h; children age 4 to 6 years, 4.7 h; adults, 6.3 h. Quinidine is highly protein bound in adults (85% to 90%). Pickoff et al have noted age- and disease-related changes in protein binding of quinidine.[20] The fraction of unbound, free quinidine decreases with maturation: newborns, 37%; infants, 21%; older children, 14%. Patients with cyanotic heart disease demonstrated a high fraction of unbound quinidine (34%), compared to age-matched controls (14%).

Several investigators have demonstrated important alterations in the pharmacokinetics of quinidine in patients with congestive heart failure. Ueda and Dzindizio found a diminished volume of distribution (68%) and total clearance (70%), but no change occurred in the half-life.[21] This accounts for the clinically documented higher plasma concentrations (43%) observed in congestive heart failure patients who were administered normal doses of quinidine. Therefore, quinidine dosage should be reduced in heart failure patients.

Quinidine is extensively biotransformed (60% to 70%) in the liver to an electrophysiologically active metabolite, 3-hydroxy-quinidine. Vozeh et al administered 3-hydroxy-quinidine to four healthy subjects; in two of them, quinidine prolonged the QT interval.[22] Wooding-Scott, Visco, and Slaughter have provided evidence to support the role of 3-hydroxy-quinidine in determining part of the pharmacologic effect of quinidine.[23] In subjects with normal quinidine clearance values, the unbound plasma concentration of 3-hydroxy-quinidine exceeds the quinidine concentration.

Less than 20% of quinidine is excreted unchanged in the urine, and renal excretion is decreased by alkalinization of the urine. Kessler et al found little need to reduce quinidine dosage in patients with renal failure.[24] However, liver disease can decrease quinidine clearance, and therefore, modification of dosage is recommended for these patients.

Quinidine blood levels of 2 to 6 μg/mL have been therapeutically effective. Levels of 7 μg/mL or higher are associated with a high incidence of toxicity. Some children may have a therapeutic response with quinidine plasma concentrations of less than 2 μg/mL. The clinician should also be aware of possible differences in plasma quinidine determinations based on the method of assay.[8] Quinidine assayed by high-performance liquid chromatographic techniques (HPLC) will give a 20% to 25% lower plasma concentration compared to spectroflurometric methods, which concurrently measure quinidine metabolites (3-hydroxy-quinidine).

Dosage

Children frequently require a larger quinidine dosage per kilogram than adults.[25, 26] A quinidine sulfate dosage of 30–60 mg/kg/d (450–900 mg/m^2) will generally prove therapeutically effective in the pediatric age group, compared to a therapeutic dosage of 10 mg/kg/d for adults. If quinidine gluconate is prescribed, a 20% higher dosage will be required (20% less quinidine base compared to sulfate).

Adverse Effects

Although quinidine is an excellent drug for treatment of arrhythmias, 30% to 40% of patients experience adverse side effects.[10] Gastrointestinal disturbances are the most common (nausea, vomiting, diarrhea, abdominal pain, and anorexia). Indications of central nervous system toxicity (cinchonism) include tinnitus, hearing loss, visual disturbances, confusion, delirium, and headache. Allergic reactions may manifest as fever or rash. Hematologic abnormalities (e.g., immune-mediated thrombocytopenia, hemolytic anemia, or agranalocytosis) may also develop during quinidine therapy.

Cardiovascular symptoms, although less common, can be more ominous. Quinidine may produce syncope in 0.5% to 2.0% of patients. Two mechanisms for quinidine-induced syncope have been described. Acquired prolonged QT syndrome with torsades de pointes is the most frequent mechanism of syncope. In a clinical review of 24 patients with quinidine-associated QT syndrome, Roden, Woosley, and Primm found the following associations: syncope usually occurred within 5 days of initiating therapy, quinidine plasma concentrations were frequently low (at or below the lower limit of therapeutic range), hypokalemia was a frequent occurrence, and marked QT prolongation was evident on the electrocardiogram.[27] Administration of an excessive quinidine dosage with toxic plasma concentrations (10 μg/ml) is the other mechanism for quinidine-induced syncope.

Quinidine, like most antiarrhythmic agents, can increase the frequency of spontaneous ventricular ectopy (proarrhythmic effect) or worsen underlying conduction abnormalities, thereby precipitating AV block. Sinus bradycardia or long sinus pauses may occur in patients with bradycardia-tachycardia syndrome.

Quinidine should be used cautiously in patients with myocardial dysfunction. The negative inotropic actions of quinidine may produce or exacerbate congestive heart failure. Hypotension is a frequent problem during intravenous administration. Peripheral vasodilation occurs with α_1- and α_2-adrenergic blockade.[28]

Drug Interactions

Several drug interactions with quinidine are clinically important. Quinidine may elevate plasma digoxin levels by 100% to 150% by decreasing its volume of distribution, clearance (renal and non-renal), and affinity for tissue receptors. Pedersen has also reported an increase in the bioavailability of digoxin.[29] Quinidine-induced elevation in plasma digoxin concentration occurs in children older than 5 years.[30] Koren and Soldin did not observe any digoxin concentration increase in infants younger than 2 months of age.[30]

Quinidine has on occasion been used concurrently with verapamil. Significant hypotension and cardiovascular collapse may result from the combined administration.[28] Two different mechanisms have been demonstrated. Verapamil may decrease the clearance of quinidine, resulting in a reduced half-life and high plasma concentration. The second mechanism is thought to be additive α-adrenergic blockade resulting in marked peripheral vasodilation.

Quinidine metabolism may be accelerated when administered with drugs that enhance hepatic microsomal enzyme activity (e.g., phenobarbital, phenytoin, and rifampin). In contrast, several agents have been observed to impair quinidine elimination (e.g., cimetidine and amiodarone). Administration of quinidine with warfarin may result in excessive prolongation of the prothrombin time.

Indications

Quinidine is a versatile antiarrhythmic drug, useful for treating both supraventricular and ventricular arrhythmias. Quinidine successfully terminates atrial flutter or atrial fibrillation in 10% to 20% of patients.[10] Chronic therapy is useful in preventing recurrence. Quinidine is an excellent drug for treating reentrant supraventricular tachycardias (AV node reentry and reciprocating AV tachycardia). In patients with Wolff-Parkinson-White syndrome, quinidine may prolong the antegrade effective refractory period of the accessory pathway and slow the ventricular response during atrial flutter or atrial fibrillation. Several investigators have reported the successful use of quinidine to treat in utero supraventricular tachycardia. Placental transfer of quinidine (24% to 94%) appears to be higher than that for other agents (0% to 25%).[31] Quinidine may provide effective long-term therapy for ventricular arrhythmias, particularly in those with "normal hearts" or cardiomyopathy.[32]

PROCAINAMIDE

The demonstration by Mautz that direct application of procaine to the myocardium elevated the threshold for stimulating ventricular muscle opened the way for the development of procainamide. Investigators during the 1930s found the antiarrhythmic effects of procaine limited by its short duration of action and prominent neurologic toxicity. Replacement of the ester linkage with an amide structure (procainamide) prolonged the duration of action of procaine and expanded its therapeutic/toxic ratio.

Cellular Electrophysiologic Effects

The cellular electrophysiologic effects of procainamide are very similar to those of quinidine.[11] The pharmacologic effects of procainamide include direct local anesthetic actions and indirect autonomic effects (parasympatholytic). In normal atrium, ventricle, and Purkinje fibers, procainamide produces a concentration-dependent depression of action potential AMP and $\dot{V}max$, as well as prolongation of APD and refractoriness. Like quinidine, procainamide prolongs the effective refractory more than it prolongs the APD (ERP/APD > 1). Compared with quinidine, procainamide produces less anticholinergic effect, but more local anesthetic effect. High concentrations of procainamide can decrease maximum diastolic potential. In therapeutic concentrations, procainamide depresses spontaneous diastolic automaticity in Purkinje fibers; however, it does not affect sinus node automaticity.

The membrane-depressant effects of procainamide are greater in diseased or infarcted tissues.[33] Studies of human atrial tissue showed that procainamide dramatically depressed action potential characteristics from cells in diseased regions. In vitro studies by Myerburg et al on cat myocardium subjected to acute and chronic myocardial infarction noted that procainamide decreased the dispersion of refractoriness between normal and infarcted tissues.[34] Procainamide prolonged action potential duration and refractoriness more in acutely ischemic cells (which had the shortest action potential duration and refractoriness) than in chronically injured cells with the longest action potential duration and refractoriness. Procainamide had intermediate effects on normal cells. Depressed fast-response action potentials in the acutely infarcted regions were very sensitive to the local anesthetic action of procainamide in concentrations that had no membrane-depressant effects on normal cells. Michelson, Spear, and Moore similarly observed that procainamide prolonged ventricular muscle refractoriness to a greater extent in regions of subacute myocardial infarction than in normal ventricular tissue;[33] however, these investigators noted that procainamide increased the difference in refractoriness between normal and infarcted regions.

Like quinidine, the local anesthetic action of procainamide is dependent on the frequency of stimulation. Slowing of conduction and inhibition of the rapid inward sodium current is greater at rapid stimulation rates. The onset and recovery from the sodium channel blocking effects of procainamide are slow and differ from those of lidocaine.[35] Procainamide has a high-affinity, short time constant for the open channel state, and a low-affinity, long time constant for the inactivated state of the sodium channel.

Procainamide has one other known antiarrhythmic mechanism: it can suppress delayed afterdepolarizations (i.e., decrease their amplitude and prolong their coupling interval), particularly at rapid stimulation rates.[36]

Neonatal canine cardiac Purkinje fiber and ventricular muscle cells have been demonstrated by Ezren et al to be less sensitive to the electrophysiologic effects of procainamide than those of adult canines.[37] Membrane-depressant effects were not evident until neonatal Purkinje cells were superfused with a five-fold higher concentration. Likewise, prolongation of APD did not result until neonatal fibers were superfused with a 500-fold higher concentration of procainamide.

Clinical Electrophysiologic Effects

Procainamide has a variable effect on sinus cycle length, frequently shortening the cycle length by an average of 7% through its vagolytic action. Goldberg et al observed a shortening of the corrected sinus node recovery time with no change in the sinoatrial conduction time in patients with normal sinus node function.[38] However, in patients with sinus node dysfunction, different results were evident. Procainamide shortened sinoatrial conduction time and lengthened the maximum corrected sinus node recovery time. In patients with abnormal sinus node function, procainamide has been reported to produce prolonged sinus pauses, sinus arrest, and sinoatrial exit block. Procainamide slows conduction in the atrium (by prolonging high right atrial to low right atrial conduction time), in the AV node (by increasing the AH interval), in the His-Purkinje system (by lengthening the HV interval) and in the ventricle (by prolonging QRS duration). Gang et al[39] and Morady et al[40] have demonstrated frequency-dependent effects of procainamide on His-Purkinje and intraventricular conduction in the human heart. Further depression of His-Purkinje conduction (an 18% increase in HV interval), as demonstrated by Scheinman et al, can occur when patients with preexisting intraventricular conduction defects are given procainamide.[41] Fortunately, complete block is rare.

As has been demonstrated in vitro, procainamide lengthens atrial, His-Purkinje, and ventricular myocardial refractoriness; AV nodal refractoriness responds differently. Josephson et al found that procainamide shortened the AV nodal effective refractory period but had little effect on the AV nodal functional refractory period.[42] In patients with the Wolff-Parkinson-White syndrome, procainamide prolongs the refractory period and slows both antegrade and retrograde conduction over the accessory atrioventricular pathway. The effect of procainamide on the refractoriness of accessory pathways is more pronounced in patients with relatively long initial refractory periods (>270 ms), and may be absent when the initial refractory period is short (<270 ms).[43] Sellers et al noted that quinidine was slightly better than procainamide in prolonging the accessory pathway functional refractory period (i.e., shortest RR interval) during atrial fibrillation.[44]

Electrocardiographic Effects

Procainamide produces dose-related increases in the PR, QRS, and QT intervals.[11] Widening of the QRS duration by more than 25% is considered a sign of toxicity and is used to limit further dosage increases. Procainamide lengthens the QT interval less than does quinidine. Rarely, in patients with preexisting conduction abnormalities, procainamide may further depress conduction so that bundle-branch block or complete atrioventricular block develops.

Clinical Pharmacokinetics

Following oral administration, procainamide is rapidly absorbed and undergoes a small amount (15% to 20%) of first-pass hepatic elimination.[45] The bioavailability of the conventional preparation (83%) and the sustained-released formulation (79%) are equivalent. Plasma levels show wide variability (up to 10 fold) when the same dose of procainamide is given to a group of patients.[46] Procainamide is rapidly distributed (distribution half-life = 10 min) following intravenous administration and is highly concentrated in the peripheral tissues, as evidenced by its large volume of distribution (children, 2.2 L/kg; adults, 1.9 L/kg).[47] The volume of distribution of procainamide is generally thought to be reduced in patients with congestive heart failure or shock. However, the recent experience of Kessler et al in myocardial infarction patients with congestive heart failure suggests this may not be globally applicable.[48] Procainamide is minimally bound to serum proteins (15% to 30%). Protein binding does not vary during acute illness, thereby keeping the free drug concentration constant.[45]

Elimination of procainamide occurs by hepatic biotransformation and renal excretion. The majority of procainamide (55% to 60%) is renally excreted unchanged in the urine.[45] Both glomerular filtration and tubular secretion contribute to its excretion. Procainamide is hepatically biotransformed by acetylation to *N*-acetylprocainamide (NAPA), which is pharmacologically active. The rate of formation of NAPA is genetically determined by the patient's acetylation phenotype (fast or slow).[49] Almost all of the NAPA metabolite (85%) is cleared in the urine. The elimination of procainamide and NAPA are reduced in the presence of renal insufficiency, and accumulation of both may occur. Therefore, dosage adjustments must be made in patients with renal failure. The rate of elimination of procainamide is not affected by chronic administration.

Significant pharmacokinetic differences exist between procainamide formulations. As previously mentioned, the overall bioavailability of the slow-release and conventional preparations does not differ. However, the elimination half-life of the slow-release preparation ($t\frac{1}{2}$ = 6 h to 7 h) is longer than that of the conventional tablets ($t\frac{1}{2}$ = 2.5 h to 4.7 h), allowing for less frequent administration.[45] In addition, variability (difference between peak and trough) in plasma procainamide levels is 32% less during dosaging with the slow-release form. The wax matrix of the sustained-release procainamide tablets is occasionally passed in the stool without affecting its absorption.

The little available data suggests that the elimination kinetics of procainamide are age dependent. Lima et al studied the disposition of procainamide in a neonate born to a mother treated chronically with procainamide.[50] They noted a markedly reduced renal clearance (0.7 mL/min) in the neonate when compared with the maternal clearance (400 mL/min) of procainamide, and a prolonged elimination half-life in the neonate (13.5 h). When procainamide was studied by Singh et al in a small group of children age 7 to 12 years, the elimination half-life was found to be shorter than that previously reported in adult patients (1.7 h vs 2.8 h).[47] This was consistent with the observation that plasma clearance was higher in children (19 mL/min/kg vs 6 mL/min/kg).

Most arrhythmias are suppressed at plasma procainamide levels of 4 to 8 μg/mL, although higher concentrations (up to 12 μg/mL) may be required in some patients. Minor adverse effects are very uncommon with procainamide levels lower than 8 μg/mL. Side effects become more frequent as plasma levels increase. When procainamide concentration exceeds 16 μg/mL, adverse electrical or hemodynamic effects usually occur.

Procainamide has been well documented to cross the placenta and have electrophysiologic effects in the fetus.[51] Neonatal plasma levels measured at birth vary between 25% and 100% of maternal concentrations. Procainamide is also known to be excreted into human breast milk.[45]

Dosage

Procainamide can be administered orally or intravenously. The recommended intravenous dose is 10–15 mg/kg (total maximum dosage = 1000 mg).[45] In order to avoid hypotension, the rate of administration should not exceed 0.5 mg/kg/min or a total of 50 mg/min. For patients with impaired myocardial function, the infusion rate should be even slower. A continuous maintenance infusion of 30–80 μg/kg/min should be instituted following completion of the loading phase if a salutory effect is observed. Chronic oral therapy with procainamide requires a total dosage between 50–100 mg/kg/d to achieve therapeutic effects. For the slow-release form, dosaging is at 6- to 8-hour intervals; for the immediate-release tablets, procainamide should be administered every 3 to 4 hours. The total daily dosage is equivalent with either formulation.

Adverse Effects

Multiple noncardiac adverse effects have been reported during procainamide therapy (Table 3–3), the most serious of which is a drug-induced lupus syndrome. Procainamide-induced systemic lupus erythematosus (SLE) is characterized by the occurrence of fever, arthralgia, pleuropericarditis (rarely, with tamponade) and hepatomegaly. Central nervous system and renal involvement are much less common than in idiopathic SLE. Procainamide-induced SLE may have an earlier onset and be more frequent in patients with a slow acetylation phenotype, although the evidence is controversial.[52] Of patients receiving procainamide, 50% to 90% develop antinuclear antibodies, but only 20% to 30% develop clinical symptoms. The clinical syndrome reverses when procainamide is stopped. Continuation of procainamide therapy in the presence of antinuclear antibodies is acceptable as long as the patient has no clinical symptoms. Procainamide less frequently produces gastrointestinal or central nervous system side effects.

Recently, attention has focused on the propensity for procainamide to produce agranulocytosis (0.6% of patients).[53] Life-threatening neutropenia occurs most frequently in patients taking the sustained-release preparation of procainamide and in patients recovering from cardiovascular surgery. The use of procainamide in patients with myasthenia gravis or hypersensitivity to procaine is contraindicated.

High plasma concentrations of procainamide can impair myocardial contractility and promote hypotension or congestive heart failure. Similar to quinidine therapy, a variety of conduction disturbances and proarrhythmia events (e.g., polymorphic ventricular tachycardia) can appear during procainamide treatment.

TABLE 3–3
CLINICAL MANIFESTATIONS OF PROCAINAMIDE TOXICITY

Noncardiac Symptoms
Gastrointestinal: anorexia, nausea, vomiting, abdominal pain, diarrhea, hepatitis
Neurologic: mental confusion, depression, insomnia, hallucinations, psychosis, headache
Skin: rash, pruritis
Hematologic: agranulocytosis, thrombocytopenia, hemolytic anemia, neutropenia
Indications of hypersensitivity: fever, drug-induced lupus syndrome, Raynaud's phenomenon
Cardiac Symptoms
Sinus bradycardia, sinus arrest
AV conduction disturbances
Ventricular arrhythmia (torsades de pointes)
Incessant supraventricular tachycardia
Hypotension, congestive heart failure

Drug Interactions

Very few drug interactions with procainamide have been described. Saal et al noted that when amiodarone was added to a stable regimen of procainamide, plasma levels of both procainamide and NAPA increased by 57% and 32%, respectively.[54] The mechanism for this drug interaction was not investigated. Cimetidine has been found to decrease by 36% the renal clearance of procainamide (by inhibiting renal tubular secretion) and to prolong its elimination half-life by 24%.[55] Weidler et al have studied the effect of propranolol on the pharmacokinetics of procainamide.[56] They demonstrated a 16% decrease in plasma clearance owing to a reduction in hepatic blood flow, a 51% increase in the volume of distribution of procainamide, and a 56% reduction in its elimination half-life. The clinical significance of these changes has yet to be documented. Procainamide has no effect on the pharmacokinetics of digoxin.

Indications

Procainamide is useful for treating a variety of atrial and ventricular arrhythmias and has a clinical spectrum of activity similar to that of quinidine. Procainamide may be used to convert acute-onset atrial fibrillation, supraventricular tachycardia, or ventricular tachycardia to sinus rhythm. For patients with supraventricular tachycardia, procainamide is most effective in AV node reentry and atrioventricular reciprocating tachycardia. It has, on rare occasion, been reported to control atrial muscle reentry or atrial ectopic tachycardia. Although it will rarely eliminate automatic supraventricular tachycardias (AET or JET), procainamide can be used to slow their rates. Procainamide is only moderately effective for treatment of ventricular arrhythmias in children with congenital heart disease.

DISOPYRAMIDE

Since its introduction in 1962, disopyramide has been demonstrated to have an antiarrhythmic efficacy comparable to that of either quinidine or procainamide. It has been used to treat a variety of supraventricular and ventricular arrhythmias. The electrophysiologic effects of disopyramide are similar to those of quinidine, with the major difference being disopyramide's greater anticholinergic effect.[57]

Cellular Electrophysiologic Effects

The cellular electrophysiologic effects of disopyramide are best interpreted in light of its direct membrane-depressant action and its indirect (anticholinergic) effects on the autonomic nervous system, particularly on supraventricular structures. Katoh et al noted that disopyramide accelerated sinus cycle length during periods of enhanced parasympathetic activity (i.e., indirect anticholinergic effect).[58] However, during cholinergic receptor blockade, disopyramide slowed sinus rate by prolonging action potential duration and decreasing the slope of phase 4 depolarization. Disopyramide did not alter maximum diastolic potential in the sinus node, sinoatrial conduction time, or sinus node response to overdrive pacing. Exposure to high concentrations of disopyramide can depress sinus node action potential amplitude and $\dot{V}max$ through inhibition of the slow inward calcium current. By using the voltage clamp technique in rabbit sinus node tissue, Kotake et al were able to demonstrate that disopyramide could decrease the delayed-onset outward potassium current responsible for repolarizing the sinus node membrane, and thereby prolong APD.[59]

The direct electrophysiologic effect of disopyramide on atrial, His-Purkinje, and ventricular muscle cells is to decrease membrane excitability, action potential amplitude, $\dot{V}max$, membrane responsiveness, and conduction velocity.[60, 61] Only during superfusion with high concentrations of disopyramide does membrane potential decrease. Using single ventricular myocytes from adult rats, Yatani and Akaike were able to show that disopyramide produced a dose-dependent depression of the fast inward sodium current and prolonged its recovery from inactivation.[62]

Disopyramide prolongs action potential duration to a greater extent than it does the effective refractory period (APD/ERP $>$ 1).[60, 61] The effect of disopyramide on His-Purkinje fiber action potential duration is to decrease the dispersion of repolarization normally present. Lengthening action potential duration is more prominent in regions with shorter action potential duration than it is at the "gate" region.

The electrophysiologic response to disopyramide can be further modified by the state of health of the tissue studied or by changes in the superfusion milieu. Similar to quinidine and procainamide, disopyramide produces a rate-dependent depression of phase 0 upstroke velocity and conduction velocity (i.e., a greater degree of $\dot{V}max$ depression at faster stimulation rates). However, this depression is less evident than with these other two agents. Sasyniuk and Kus[63] and Frame and Hoffmann[64] have demonstrated that the frequency-dependent depression of conduction was enhanced in abnormal tissues (as in myocardial infarction or hyperkalemia). The extent to which disopyramide induced depression of action potential characteristics (action potential AMP, V̇max, and membrane potential) in cells from infarcted regions was much greater than that observed in healthy, noninfarcted ventricular cells.[63] During hypoxic superfusion of Purkinje fibers, Yamada, Nishimura, and Watanabe were also able to demonstrate that the electrophysiologic effects of disopyramide were enhanced.[65] In an in vitro experimental myocardial infarction model, Sasyniuk and Kus demonstrated that, like procainamide, disopyramide reduced the difference in action potential duration between normal and infarcted tissue by lengthening APD of normal cells more than it lengthened the duration of repolarization from infarcted regions, thereby decreasing the degree of refractoriness dispersion.[63]

Stereochemical properties influence the electrophysiologic effects of disopyramide. The commercially prepared formulation of disopyramide is a racemic composite of its *d* and *l* isomers; however, their pharmacodynamic actions differ. *d*-Disopyramide prolongs canine Purkinje fiber action potential duration and corrected QT interval, whereas the *l* isomer shortens repolarization.[66] The *d* isomer exerts greater anticholinergic effects that offset some of its antiarrhythmic actions. In contrast, *l*-disopyramide has been demonstrated in a canine model to depress intraventricular conduction (i.e., prolong QRS duration) and lengthen ventricular muscle refractoriness to a greater extent than does the *d* isomer.

Studies of the developmental electrophysiologic effects of disopyramide have not been performed.

Clinical Electrophysiologic Effects

The reported clinical electrophysiologic effects of disopyramide are frequently variable and inconsistent. This can best be explained by the dual mode of action of disopyramide—direct membrane effects and vagolytic action—that counteracts its direct effects. Bexton et al were able to separate each component by investigating the clinical electrophysiologic effects of disopyramide in human cardiac transplant recipients.[57] Disopyramide shortened sinus cycle length and the sinus node recovery time of the recipient sinus node region, thus reflecting its anticholinergic action. In contrast, the sinus cycle length and the sinus node recovery time response to rapid atrial pacing were lengthened in the donor heart. Disopyramide had no effect on sinoatrial conduction. In in vitro studies, disopyramide slowed conduction throughout the atrium, His-Purkinje system, and ventricle (i.e., prolonged PA, AH, and HV intervals and Wenckebach cycle length). Although no changes in atrial, AV nodal, or ventricular muscle refractoriness were found, some investigators have demonstrated that disopyramide can lengthen the effective refractory period of these structures. Similar results were reported by Kashani et al in a study of the electrophysiologic effects of disopyramide in a group of children ranging in age from 7 months to 14 years.[67] The most consistent changes were prolongation of the atrial and AV nodal effective and functional refractory periods, in addition to prolongation of the HV interval. Disopyramide can slow conduction and prolong the refractory period of accessory atrioventricular pathways in both the antegrade and retrograde direction, making it useful for the treatment of arrhythmias in patients with Wolff-Parkinson-White syndrome.

Careful consideration should be given to the administration of disopyramide to patients with preexisting conduction system disease or sinus node dysfunction. Bergfeldt et al noted a marked (43%) prolongation of the HV interval and the frequent occurrence of second and third degree atrioventricular block (14/27) in a group of patients with bifascicular block who were given disopyramide.[68] In a group of 16 symptomatic patients with sinus node dysfunction, LaBarre et al noted the development of second degree sinoatrial exit block in two patients, and marked prolongation of the sinus node response to overdrive pacing (i.e., sinus node recovery time) in 11 patients following administration of disopyramide, thus demonstrating the marked pauses likely to occur after tachycardia termination.[69]

Electrocardiographic Effects

Increasing concentrations of disopyramide result in prolongation of the P wave duration, PR interval, QRS duration, and corrected QT interval. Lengthening of QRS duration is less marked than with quinidine.

Clinical Pharmacokinetics

Disopyramide is well absorbed following oral administration (>90%); however, first-pass hepatic metabolism decreases its systemic bioavailability to between 80% and 85%.[70] Peak plasma concentration occurs 0.5 h to 3 h after ingestion of the immediate-release formulation, and between 3.4 h and 4 h with the slow-release preparation. The overall bioavailability of both dosage forms are equivalent. Disopyramide absorption is diminished in congestive heart failure patients.

Distribution to the peripheral tissues is rapid following intravenous disopyramide administration ($t\frac{1}{2}$ = 3 min). The elimination half-life in healthy subjects varies between 4.5 h and 7.8 h. Compared with quinidine or procainamide, disopyramide does not have as extensive a volume of distribution (V_d = 0.8–1.3 L/kg). The fraction of disopyramide bound to serum proteins varies inversely with the total disopyramide plasma concentration (10% to 70%). Unlike most other antiarrhythmic drugs, protein binding of disopyramide is not linear, but dose dependent. Disopyramide is bound almost exclusively to α_1-acid glycoprotein (90% to 95%), it is minimally bound to albumin (5% to 10%).

Disopyramide is biotransformed by *N* dealkylation to an electrophysiologically active metabolite, *N*-monodealkylated disopyramide (NMD). The NMD metabolite possesses considerably more anticholinergic activity (three fold), but only 25% the antiarrhythmic activity of disopyramide.[71] Under usual circumstances, NMD does not contribute much to the antiarrhythmic effect of disopyramide, its plasma concentration being only 10% of the parent drug. However, in the presence of renal failure, it may accumulate. Fifty-two percent of a dose of disopyramide is excreted unchanged in the urine by both glomerular filtration and tubular secretion. The remaining 48% is metabolized in the liver. Of this 48%, 25% to 35% of a dose of disopyramide appears in the urine as NMD; the rest is excreted by the biliary system. Bonde et al observed an increase in the unbound fraction of disopyramide, as well as a decrease in its clearance and volume of distribution, in the presence of hepatic disease, therefore recommending a 25% reduction in disopyramide dosage.[72] Other investigators have noted a decrease in the volume of distribution and clearance of disopyramide during renal failure, indicating the need to similarly decrease disopyramide dosage during renal insufficiency.

The pharmacokinetics of disopyramide are altered in patients with cardiac disease. Landmark et al have demonstrated a reduction in the distribution half-life, volume of distribution, and clearance of disopyramide, as well as moderate prolongation of its elimination half-life, in patients with significant organic heart disease.[73] Absorption was slowed, decreasing the peak concentration of disopyramide. Based on their results, Landmark et al suggested increasing the time interval between doses of disopyramide.

Few data are available on the pharmacokinetics of disopyramide in children. Protein binding of disopyramide seems to increase with age (neonate, 37%; infants, 56%; children, 66%; adults, 66%). Although studied in only two patients, the elimination half-life found by Hordoff et al in children ($t\frac{1}{2}$ = 4.8 h) is shorter than that reported for adult patients with cardiac disease.[74] Further suggestive evidence for enhanced clearance or a larger volume of distribution of disopyramide in children has been provided by Holt et al.[75] These investigators noted marked elevation of the oral dosage of disopyramide required to produce plasma concentrations comparable to those in adults, whether the dosage was calculated on the basis of body weight or surface area.

Disopyramide can be transferred across the human placenta. Fetal cord blood levels have been shown to approximate maternal plasma levels by 39%.[70] Secretion of disopyramide into human breast milk has also been described, approximating 50% of maternal plasma concentrations.[70,76] However, Hoppu, Neuvonen, and Korte have calculated the maximum amount of disopyramide ingested by the nursing infant to be 2 mg/d.[76] They could detect only a trace of drug in the nursing infant's blood.

The therapeutic range for plasma levels of disopyramide is frequently referenced between 2 and 5 μg/mL; however, there are considerable problems with correlating total plasma drug levels of disopyramide and antiarrhythmic efficacy. As previously described, disopyramide is equally composed of a *d* and *l* enantiomer, each exhibiting different pharmacokinetic properties. The free or unbound fraction of an antiarrhythmic drug is thought to represent the therapeutically important fraction (concentration) of agent at the receptor site. Differences in protein binding (the *d* isomer is more highly protein bound at similar total plasma concentration, and therefore has a lower free, unbound fraction), clearance (higher for the *d* isomer), volume of distribution (greater for the *d* isomer), and elimination half-life (shorter for the *d* isomer) influence the relative concentration (unbound) of each isomer at the cardiac receptor site.[66, 71] The relationship between antiarrhythmic efficacy and plasma concentration is further complicated by stereoselective differences in pharmacodynamic action of the two enantiomers.

Dosage

Disopyramide is available for oral usage only. Holt et al have reported the largest experience with disopyramide usage in children.[75] The total average daily dosage required to achieve satisfactory arrhythmia control (or a plasma concentration of 2–5 μg/mL) varied with age: less than 2 years old, 30 (23–33) mg/kg; 2 to 10 years old, 20 (9–24) mg/kg; 11 to 14 years, 8 (5–13) mg/kg. Hordoff et al used a similar dosage of disopyramide (6–14 mg/kg/d) to treat older children with atrial and ventricular arrhythmias, a dosage not markedly different from that recommended for adult subjects.[74] The maximum total daily dose should not exceed 1200 mg. Disopyramide may be administered on every 6 hours (immediate-release formulation) or every 12 hours (sustained-release preparation).

Adverse Effects

The therapeutic efficacy of disopyramide therapy is not infrequently dampened by adverse effects.[77] Anticholinergic side effects are the most frequent (70% of patients) and include xerostomia, urinary retention, hesitancy, constipation, and blurred vision. Myasthenia gravis and glaucoma are contraindications for the use of disopyramide. Gastrointestinal symptoms, although less common than during quinidine therapy, may occur and include anorexia, nausea, vomiting, and diarrhea. Adverse cardiovascular effects are the most serious and may result in cardiac death (hypotension, congestive heart failure, complete AV block, sinus node dysfunction). Disopyramide has been reported to produce ventricular tachyarrhythmias, presumably by causing marked QT prolongation. Depression of cardiac automaticity and exacerbation of conduction disturbances are particularly prevalent in patients receiving disopyramide in combination with other local anesthetic agents (e.g., lidocaine, procainamide, or phenytoin). Rare side effects include cholestatic jaundice, agranulocytosis, acute psychosis, and fasting hypoglycemia.

Drug Interactions

Unlike quinidine, disopyramide has not been observed to alter the pharmacokinetics of digoxin. However, several antiarrhythmic agents have been reported to alter the metabolism and elimination of disopyramide. Bonde et al have documented that atenolol (a β-blocker) can decrease the clearance of disopyramide from 1.9 to 1.6 mL/kg/min.[78] They further observed that combined administration markedly reduced cardiac output, making combined therapy precarious. Phenytoin has been reported by Matos, Fisher, and Kim to increase the metabolism of disopyramide, thereby decreasing its plasma concentration by 54%.[79]

Indications

The spectrum of clinical arrhythmias responsive to disopyramide is similar to those responsive to quinidine and procainamide and includes paroxysmal supraventricular tachycardia (AV node reentry, reciprocating AV tachycardia), atrial fibrillation, atrial flutter, and ventricular arrhythmias (simple and complex forms).

LIDOCAINE

Lidocaine, synthesized in 1946, was first used as an antiarrhythmic agent in 1950. Its rapid onset and limited toxicity has made it the most widely used drug for the emergency treatment of ventricular arrhythmias. In addition, lidocaine has favorable pharmacokinetic characteristics (rapid metabolism and excretion) that make it especially easy to administer as a continuous intravenous infusion.

Cellular Electrophysiologic Effects

Similar to other local anesthetic antiarrhythmic agents, the basic electrophysiologic action of lidocaine is to block transmembrane passage of sodium ions through the fast inward sodium channel.[80] By this mechanism lidocaine has important depressant effects on cardiac excitability, conduction, and automaticity. The effects of lidocaine on calcium channels are minor in comparison.[81]

At therapeutic plasma concentrations, lidocaine has little effect on the membrane action potential characteristics of sinus node, atrial, or AV nodal cells.[82] High concentrations of lidocaine (clinical toxicity range) have been observed to diminish sinoatrial automaticity (by only 14%) and to decrease action potential AMP and V̇max slightly. When tissues were exposed to toxic concentrations of lidocaine, Mandel and Bigger noted prolongation of atrial APD and refractoriness.[82] They also noted that lidocaine could abolish ectopic atrial rhythms in vitro.

In contrast to the relative insensitivity of the atrium, the specialized conduction system and ventricular muscle are markedly affected by lidocaine.[83–85] The electrophysiologic response to lidocaine is dependent on a number of factors: external potassium concentration, spontaneous or paced cycle length, and the state of health of the tissue studied. Lidocaine accelerates repolarization of healthy Purkinje fibers exposed to low concentrations (5 mg/L).[83–85] Only at moderate concentrations (50 mg/L) does lidocaine decrease MDP, action potential amplitude, and V̇max, as well as shift membrane responsiveness (demonstrated by a curve relating rate of rise of premature responses to level of membrane potential) in the hyperpolarized direction. Shortening of repolarization preferentially occurs in regions with the longest action potential durations (e.g., the gate region). Therapeutic concentrations of lidocaine have little effect on ventricular muscle APD. However, high concentrations prolong ventricular muscle repolarization and refractoriness. Lidocaine decreases phase 4 depolarization and automaticity of normal Purkinje fibers, in addition to decreasing excitability.

The action of lidocaine is highly selective for depressed myocardial tissue.[86] At low concentrations in experimental myocardial infarction preparations, lidocaine markedly decreased action potential amplitude, V̇max, and conduction, and prolonged ventricular muscle refractoriness. The local anesthetic effects of lidocaine are similarly enhanced under conditions of hyperkalemia ($[K]_o \geq 6.0$ mmol/L).

Lidocaine-induced depression of sodium channel activity (measured by changes in V̇max or conduction velocity) is sensitive to cardiac rate.[12, 35, 40, 87] At low frequencies of stimulation in healthy Purkinje fibers, lidocaine has little effect on V̇max. However, at rapid frequencies of stimulation, moderate depression of V̇max occurs. Lidocaine binds with sodium channel receptor sites during their open and inactivated states. Unbinding from local anesthetic receptor sites occurs during the resting state and is rapid when compared with that produced by quinidine or flecainide therapy. This observation accounts for the absence of tonic block (depression of V̇max) of sodium channel activity at low stimulation rates.

Tissues from neonatal hearts have different sensitivity to the effects of lidocaine than those of adults. Roberts and Goldberg have found that the same concentration of lidocaine has a greater effect on rat atria from older animals.[13] In studies of canine Purkinje fibers, Mary-Rabine and Rosen found that the depressant effect of lidocaine on membrane action potentials in the neonatal age group was less than that observed in adult fibers.[88] Morikawa and Rosen studied age-related changes in use dependence of lidocaine in canine Purkinje fibers.[89] With the onset of rapid stimulation, V̇max decreased to steady state more rapidly in adult fibers (1 beat) than in the younger age group (3 beats). In contrast, however, recovery from sodium channel blockade was faster in the neonatal group.

Clinical Electrophysiologic Effects

Lidocaine has little effect on normal sinus node function, intraatrial conduction, or AV node function.[90, 91] In patients with sinoatrial dysfunction, lidocaine has been reported to prolong sinoatrial conduction time. Rarely, sinus arrest may occur following lidocaine administration. At therapeutic concentrations, lidocaine shortens the effective and relative refractory periods of the His-Purkinje system. Prolongation of the HV interval may occur in patients with preexisting conduction abnormalities.[92] Inconsistent effects on ventricular muscle refractoriness have been reported.[93] Lidocaine significantly increases the ventricular fibrillation threshold as well as the defibrillation threshold.[94] No significant effects of lidocaine on the refractory periods of the atrium, AV node, or right ventricle could be demonstrated in a group of young children studied by Shakibi and Aryanpur.[95]

Electrocardiographic Effects

Lidocaine has little effect on heart rate, PR interval, or QRS duration.[80] Slight shortening of the QT interval has been reported. Lidocaine-induced sinus node depression and AV block have been described in patients with conduction system disease.[92]

Clinical Pharmacokinetics

Since lidocaine undergoes extensive first-pass elimination (70% to 80% of the dose), effective plasma levels are seldom achieved with oral administration.[80] Plasma clearance of lidocaine following intravenous injection occurs as a biexponential process. The initial distribution phase has an average half-life of 5–10 min. In adults, the second phase of elimination has an average half-life of 80–110 min.

Lidocaine is metabolized by the liver to two pharmacologically active metabolites, methylglycinexylide (MEGX) and glycinexylide (GX).[80] Accumulation of these two metabolites may further block sodium channel activity and depress cardiac conduction enough to produce toxicity. Lidocaine clearance is greatly altered by changes in liver blood flow and cardiac output and by the presence of liver disease.[96] In patients with heart failure, clearance is reduced to 60% of normal (probably the result of reduced liver blood flow), and therefore the administered dosage should be reduced. A similar reduction of dosage is required for patients with liver disease. Less than 10% of the drug is excreted unchanged in the urine, and therefore dosage adjustment is not required in the presence of renal disease.

Lidocaine is excreted in breast milk (40% of maternal plasma levels) and crosses the placenta to produce moderate fetal plasma concentrations (fetal/maternal plasma ratio approximates 0.5).[97, 98]

Lidocaine, although not highly bound to plasma proteins (25% to 50%), exhibits concentration-dependent binding. As the total plasma concentration of lidocaine is increased, the free fraction simultaneously increases.

Clinical pharmacokinetic study of lidocaine distribution and metabolism in infants and children has been limited but suggests some important differences when compared with adults, particularly in the neonatal age group. Studies by Mihaly et al of lidocaine pharmacokinetics in neonates have demonstrated an increased volume of distribution (neonate, 2.8 L/kg; adult, 1.1 L/kg) and prolonged elimination half-life (neonate, $t^1\!/\!_2$ = 3.2 h; adult, $t^1\!/\!_2$ = 1.8 h).[99] These investigators could find no significant differences in total plasma clearance. The neonates did seem to excrete a greater fraction of lidocaine unchanged in the urine, implying that hepatic metabolism was limited. Tucker et al found that protein binding of lidocaine was decreased in the neonatal age group by 20%.[100] Lidocaine pharmacokinetics in children ages 6 months to 3 years, as studied by Finholt et al, were comparable to adult values.[101]

Most ventricular arrhythmias respond to plasma lidocaine concentrations between 1.5 and 5 μg/mL. Toxic effects occur at concentrations greater than 6 μg/mL.

Dosage

Intravenously, lidocaine is given as a bolus of 1 mg/kg at a rate not to exceed 50 mg/min.[80] If, after 5 to 10 minutes, no improvement of the arrhythmia is evident, a second bolus (1 mg/kg) may be infused. If the arrhythmia does not improve after 3 mg/kg of lidocaine it is possible that the rhythm may respond to more lidocaine, but the likelihood of toxicity will significantly increase. If bolus infusions of lidocaine improve the rhythm, a continuous intravenous infusion should be started at a rate of 20–50 μg/kg/min. If the arrhythmia recurs within the first several hours after initiating the continuous infusion, it is likely that rapid distribution and metabolism have caused the blood level to fall below the therapeutic concentration. In this situation it is recommended that a 0.5-mg/kg lidocaine bolus be administered to increase the plasma concentration.

Modification of lidocaine dosage is important under several different circumstances.[96] Prolonged infusions (>24 h) reduce lidocaine clearance and require a 50% reduction in the infusion rate. In the presence of low cardiac output, congestive heart failure, or shock, the volume of distribution of lidocaine will be diminished, thereby requiring 50% dosage reduction during the loading phase. Henry et al recommended a dosage reduction for lidocaine loading in cardiac patients with right-to-left shunts, based on their studies using a canine model of right-to-left intracardiac shunting.[102]

Adverse Effects

Central nervous system toxicity is the earliest and most frequent sign of lidocaine toxicity.[80] When plasma concentration exceeds 5 μg/mL, vertigo, paresthesias, and slurring of speech may occur. Obtundation, seizures, or respiratory arrest can occur when levels exceed 6 μg/mL. Sinus node depression and His-Purkinje block have been reported in patients with preexisting electrical conduction system disease.[92] On rare occasions, lidocaine may accelerate the ventricular rate when administered during atrial flutter or atrial fibrillation.[103] In the presence of depressed myocardial contractility, lidocaine may precipitate congestive heart failure or produce hypotension. Similar to other local anesthetic agents, lidocaine can aggravate ventricular arrhythmias.

Drug Interactions

Alterations in hepatic blood flow may have important interactive effects on lidocaine clearance (hepatic biotransformation). Drugs that lower hepatic blood flow (propranolol or cimetidine) diminish hepatic clearance of lidocaine and subsequently increase its plasma concentration.[104] Lidocaine clearance may be increased by drugs that increase hepatic blood flow (isoproterenol) or enhance microsomal enzyme activity (phenobarbital or phenytoin).

Indications

Lidocaine is primarily used for the acute emergency treatment of life-threatening ventricular arrhythmias. Although lidocaine has been demonstrated to decrease the ventricular response in patients with atrial fibrillation and Wolff-Parkinson-White syndrome, several reports have observed that lidocaine may shorten the accessory pathway effective refractory period and accelerate the ventricular response. Lidocaine rarely converts orthodromic reciprocating atrioventricular tachycardia to sinus rhythm (15% of patients). Although it rarely converts automatic atrial or junctional tachycardias to sinus rhythm, lidocaine may be used to slow their rates, allowing better hemodynamic tolerance.

PHENYTOIN

Phenytoin was originally introduced into clinical medicine by Merritt and Putnam in 1938 as an anticonvulsant agent. However, it was not until 1950, when Harris and Kokernot found phenytoin effective against the cardiac arrhythmias of myocardial infarction, that phenytoin's role as an effective antiarrhythmic drug was appreciated.[105] The electrophysiologic effects of phenytoin are not unlike those of lidocaine. However, it is effective when orally administered and has a long duration of action. The therapeutic effects of phenytoin are probably mediated through a combination of direct actions on the heart and effects exerted through the sympathetic nervous system.

Cellular Electrophysiologic Effects

The cellular electrophysiologic actions of phenytoin are more pronounced in the His-Purkinje system and ventricular myocardium than in atrial tissue.[105–109] The effects of phenytoin vary depending on its concentration, on the extracellular potassium concentration, and more importantly, on the condition of the tissue studied.[105–112] When external potassium concentration is low (<3 mmol/L), low concentrations of phenytoin (1–3 μg/mL) may increase the resting membrane potential, action potential AMP, $\dot{V}max$, and conduction velocity of His-Purkinje and ventricular myocardial cells.[108] Membrane responsiveness may also be increased, indicating an increase in $\dot{V}max$ at all levels of membrane potential at which an action potential can be elicited. All these effects are pronounced in cells from depressed tissues. When the external potassium concentration is low, high concentrations of phenytoin (10–20 μg/mL) cause little alteration in action potential characteristics.[108]

Therapeutic concentrations of phenytoin in the presence of a normal superfusate potassium concentration (>4.0 mmol/L) exert local anesthetic effects. Action potential AMP, V̇max, conduction velocity, and membrane responsiveness are depressed.[105, 106] Similar to lidocaine, phenytoin produces a concentration-dependent shortening of APD and the effective refractory period. APD is abbreviated more than is the effective refractory period; thus the ratio of the effective refractory period to APD is increased. Using single isolated rat ventricular myocytes, Sanchez-Chapula and Josephson were able to demonstrate that the sodium channel blockade induced by phenytoin was both voltage and frequency dependent.[113] These observations provide an explanation for two important aspects of the local anesthetic action of phenytoin: (1) in cells from depolarized tissue, phenytoin depresses action potential characteristics and conduction further; and (2) the ability of phenytoin to slow conduction is enhanced at rapid stimulation rates. Like lidocaine, phenytoin binds preferentially to sodium channels in the inactivated state. Reactivation of the sodium current is also slowed, thus providing insight into the experimental findings of El-Sherif and Lazzara, who noted slowing of conduction and prolonged refractoriness in regions of myocardial infarction exposed to phenytoin.[112]

Low concentrations of phenytoin have little effect on sinus node automaticity or action potential characteristics.[109, 110] High concentrations can decrease phase 4 depolarization (slow sinus rate), membrane potential, action potential AMP, and V̇max of sinus node cells. In the case of atrial cells, low concentrations of phenytoin increase membrane potential, action potential AMP, and V̇max. Low concentrations of phenytoin in the presence of a low superfusate potassium concentration may shorten atrial APD. In contrast, slight prolongation of APD occurs at high superfusate concentrations, as does a decrease in action potential AMP, V̇max, and membrane responsiveness. Yatani, Hamilton, and Brown have been able to show that phenytoin blocks cardiac calcium channels, thus accounting for its effects on the sinus node.[114]

Phenytoin decreases automaticity of Purkinje fibers (whether normal or depressed) as well as specialized atrial fibers at therapeutic concentrations.[105–110] In normal fibers, this negative chronotropic effect results from a decrease in phase 4 depolarization and in depressed fibers, from a combination of a decrease in phase 4 depolarization and an increase in membrane potential. In addition, phenytoin depresses delayed afterdepolarization amplitude and triggered activity induced by digitalis glycosides.[115]

No age-related differences in sensitivity to the electrophysiologic actions of phenytoin could be demonstrated by Spinelli and Rosen.[116] Using a canine cardiac Purkinje fiber model, they noted similar responses of neonatal and adult fibers to phenytoin, whether healthy sodium dependent action potentials or slow responses were studied.

Phenytoin is known to exert antiarrhythmic effects through the central nervous system.[117, 118] In situations in which increased cardiac sympathetic discharge enhances arrhythmias (digitalis toxicity), phenytoin has been shown to decrease nerve traffic in cardiac sympathetic nerves. When injected into the cerebrospinal fluid, phenytoin delays the onset and suppresses the occurrence of digitalis-induced ventricular arrhythmias. Phenytoin has no peripheral cholinergic or β-adrenergic blocking effects.

Clinical Electrophysiologic Effects

Phenytoin has a variable electrophysiologic effect on the human sinus node, depending on its state of function.[119] In normal subjects, phenytoin causes little change in the spontaneous sinus cycle length, sinoatrial conduction time, or the maximum corrected sinus node recovery time. In contrast, marked suppression of sinus node automaticity (prolongation of spontaneous cycle length and maximum corrected sinus node recovery time) has been demonstrated in individuals with sinus node dysfunction. Sinus arrest with AV junctional escape rhythms has been reported. Phenytoin does not slow conduction or prolong refractoriness in the atrium.[120, 121] Therapeutic concentrations of phenytoin accelerate AV nodal conduction (i.e., shorten the AH interval and Wenckebach cycle length) and decrease its functional and effective refractory period, although these effects are not invariable. The effects of phenytoin on human AV nodal conduction when it has been depressed by drugs or disease is not known; however, it is likely to further impair AV nodal conduction and cause AV block. Phenytoin has no effect on conduction in the His-Purkinje system or ventricle; therefore, no changes occur in the HV interval or QRS duration.[120, 121] The effective and functional refractory periods of the specialized conduction system are shortened, both in the antegrade and retrograde direction, thereby facilitating the rapid conduction of early premature beats. Phenytoin can shorten ventricular muscle refractoriness.

Electrocardiographic Effects

Phenytoin has only a slight effect on the surface electrocardiogram. Shortening of the corrected QT interval may be the only significant change.[105, 106] No alterations of spontaneous heart rate, PR interval, or QRS duration are usually evident.

Clinical Pharmacokinetics

Although phenytoin is well absorbed from the gastrointestinal tract (primarily the duodenum), its absorption is delayed; peak plasma concentrations occur 4–12 h after an oral dose.[105, 106] For most preparations, the systemic bioavailability ranges between 65% and 97%. Phenytoin absorption may be impaired by the concomitant ingestion of certain drugs (Table 3–4). Food intake can have clinically important effects on phenytoin absorption. Nasogastric tube feedings and ingestion of pudding have been reported to impair the absorption of phenytoin. In contrast, meals enriched with protein or fat facilitate phenytoin absorption. Diseases of the gastrointestinal system may also diminish the absorption of phenytoin. Finally, the relative oral bioavailability of phenytoin increases with age (0 to 5 years, 65%; 6 to 10 years, 74%; 11 years–adulthood, 78%).[122]

TABLE 3–4
DRUG INTERACTIONS WITH PHENYTOIN

1. Inhibitors of gastrointestinal absorption:
   - Antacids
   - Charcoal
   - Sucralfate
2. Inhibitors of phenytoin metabolism:
   - Bishydroxycoumarin
   - Chloramphenicol
   - Isoniazid
   - Chlorpromazine
   - Phenylbutazone
   - Prochlorperazine
   - Chlordiazepoxide
   - Diazepam
   - Methylphenidate
   - Disulfiram
3. Stimulators of phenytoin metabolism:
   - Phenobarbital
   - Carbamazepine

Phenytoin is not as widely distributed throughout the body as other antiarrhythmic agents (apparent V_d = 0.8 L/kg). Few age-related differences in the apparent V_d of phenytoin exist (premature infants, 0.8 L/kg; full-term infants, 0.8 L/kg; older infants, 0.7 L/kg).[123–125] The high degree of protein binding (predominantly to albumin) is primarily responsible for phenytoin's limited distribution. The plasma protein binding of phenytoin is diminished in the neonate and does not attain adult values until 3 months of age (newborn, 80%; 3 months to 2 years, 85%; adults, 87%).[123–125] The protein binding of phenytoin is further altered by a number of disease states and by various agents. Decreased plasma protein binding has been observed during renal failure, nephrotic syndrome, hypoalbuminemia, hyperbilirubinemia, and hepatic disease and following surgical procedures. Phenytoin can also be displaced from its binding sites by thyroxine, acetylsalicylic acid, phenylbutazone, penicillin, acetazolamide, valproic acid, and sulfisoxazole.

Phenytoin is almost completely hydroxylated in the liver to metabolites with less activity, the major metabolite being *p*-hydroxyphenytoin.[105, 106] Less than 5% of an oral dose of phenytoin is excreted unchanged in the urine. The glucuronide conjugate of *p*-hydroxyphenytoin and the other biotransformation products are eliminated by the kidneys and may accumulate during renal insufficiency. Dosage reduction is therefore recommended for patients with renal failure or hepatic dysfunction. The hepatic biotransformation of phenytoin can be importantly modified by patient age, concomitant administration of other drugs, and genetic influences. Young infants exhibit a greater capacity to biotransform phenytoin than either newborns or adult subjects.[123–125] The early increase in phenytoin metabolism in the newborn to young infant age group reflects a rapid maturation in drug oxidative metabolism. The higher ratio of liver weight (enzyme mass) to surface area in young infants may account for their enhanced capacity to eliminate phenytoin in comparison to adults. Although young infants and children rapidly eliminate phenytoin, the pattern of urinary metabolites does not differ significantly from that in adults, suggesting similar metabolic pathways. Coadministration of phenytoin with a number of drugs can increase or decrease the metabolism of phenytoin (see Table 3–4). Rarely, some families may exhibit genetic factors that alter phenytoin metabolism. A small number of patients cannot metabolize more than 1–2 mg/kg/d; others have a higher-than-usual hydroxylation capacity, resulting in low plasma phenytoin levels. Leppik et al have reported altered phenytoin metabolism during febrile illnesses, when phenytoin plasma levels may be decreased by as much as 40%.[126]

The elimination half-life of phenytoin in premature and full-term newborns is prolonged (premature, 75±64 h; full-term, 21±12 h) and demonstrates wide interpatient variability.[123–125] A rapid increase in phenytoin metabolism shortens its elimination half-life to 8±4 h in infants older than 1 month. In contrast, the elimination half-life of phenytoin in adults averages 22 hours (7–40 h).

The hepatic metabolism of phenytoin is unique among antiarrhythmic agents; its metabolism can be saturated at high dosages.[105, 106] The amount of hydroxylated phenytoin increases linearly with dosage (first-order kinetics) until a critical drug concentration occurs at the enzyme site. Most patients can metabolize a daily dosage of phenytoin of up to 10 mg/kg. However, in some individuals, the dosage of phenytoin necessary to produce a concentration that saturates the enzyme system may be less within what is considered the therapeutic range. Once the enzyme system becomes saturated, any further increase in phenytoin dosage will precipitously elevate plasma levels (i.e., drug metabolism becomes fixed at a maximum value; zero-order kinetics). Therefore, when phenytoin plasma levels are high, relatively small increases in daily dosage may produce large increases in plasma levels and result in toxicity.

Phenytoin has been demonstrated to easily cross the human placenta.[123] Because of its high degree of teratogenicity, therapy with phenytoin during pregnancy is contraindicated. Secretion of phenytoin into human breast milk has been reported.

Dosage

Conventional oral dosaging produces steady-state plasma concentrations only after 5 to 13 days. To expedite therapeutic effectiveness, a loading regimen of phenytoin must be administered (either intravenously or orally). For rapid arrhythmia control, phenytoin may be safely administered intravenously according to the protocol of Garson and Gillette.[127] One-thirteenth of the total loading dose (10–15 mg/kg, maximum total dose = 1000 mg) is injected every 5 minutes and flushed with normal saline in order to avoid precipitation in glucose-containing solutions with an acid pH. Despite the slow rate of this loading regimen, hypotension was experienced by 3 of 19 patients treated by Garson and Gillette. Phenytoin loading is better tolerated orally. An effective regimen established by Garson et al was to administer phenytoin (15 mg/kg) orally in four divided doses on day 1, and 7.5 mg/kg in four divided doses on day 2.[128] Depending on the level of arrhythmia control and plasma concentration on day 3, another half-loading dose (7.5 mg/kg/d) may be needed before maintenance dosaging is instituted. Recommended maintenance dosages for phenytoin vary according to age: newborn, 4–8 mg/kg/d divided every 12 h; infants older than 2 weeks, 8–12 mg/kg/d divided every 8 h; children, 5–6 mg/kg/d divided every 12 h; adults, 4–5 mg/kg/d divided every 12 h. Plasma phenytoin concentrations between 10 and 25 μg/mL are frequently required for arrhythmia control.

Adverse Effects

Although side effects during phenytoin therapy are common, fortunately the most frequent ones are relatively minor. Serious adverse effects are rare (Table 3–5). The most common adverse reactions involve the central nervous system (nystagmus, ataxia, drowsiness and stupor, and coma). Neurologic symptoms occur frequently when plasma phenytoin levels exceed 20 μg/mL. Skin rashes usually disappear with termination of treatment. Proper dental hygiene can limit gingival hyperplasia. Rapid intravenous phenytoin administration may produce bradycardia and hypotension, particularly in patients with borderline cardiac hemodynamics. Oral phenytoin therapy rarely exacer-

TABLE 3–5
PHENYTOIN-INDUCED ADVERSE EFFECTS

1. Central Nervous System
   - Nystagmus, diplopia
   - Ataxia
   - Drowsiness, stupor, coma
   - Movement disorders (choreoathetosis, hemiballismus)
   - Peripheral neuropathy
2. Cutaneous
   - Rashes
   - Erythema multiforme
   - Steven-Johnson syndrome
3. Gastrointestinal
   - Anorexia
   - Nausea
   - Abdominal pain
   - Hepatitis, hepatic necrosis
4. Oral
   - Gingival hyperplasia
5. Hematologic
   - Aplastic anemia
   - Pure red cell aplasia
   - Megaloblastic anemia
   - Agranulocytosis
6. Immunologic
   - Malignant lymphoma
   - Lymph node hyperplasia
7. Collagen-Vascular Disorders
   - Drug-induced SLE syndrome
8. Metabolic
   - Hyperglycemia
   - Hypocalcemia
   - Rickets
   - Hypothyroidism
9. Cardiovascular
   - Hypotension
   - Congestive heart failure
10. Teratogenicity
    - Fetal hydantoin syndrome

bates compensated congestive heart failure. Ventricular proarrhythmia has rarely been observed in our experience.

One potential untoward effect must be highlighted: the teratogenic potential of phenytoin. Fetal hydantoin syndrome, a constellation of fetal anomalies including craniofacial defects (cleft lip, cleft palate, hypertelorism, low nasal bridge), growth deficiency (small for gestational dates), mental retardation (microcephaly), hypoplasia of the fingers and nails, and congenital heart disease occurs in 11% of infants exposed to phenytoin in utero.[129] A higher percentage (31%) of exposed fetuses show lesser degrees of impairment of mental performance, growth, and morphogenesis. For these reasons, phenytoin therapy of adolescent and young adult females must be avoided.

Drug Interactions

In addition to the pharmacokinetic interactions enumerated previously, several other important antiarrhythmic drug interactions with phenytoin should be mentioned. Concomitant antiarrhythmic treatment with phenytoin and amiodarone has been shown by Gore, Haffajee, and Alpert to elevate plasma phenytoin levels, the mechanism of which was not studied.[130] Rameis observed that phenytoin can shorten the elimination half-life of digoxin by 29% by increasing its nonrenal clearance.[131] Further investigation is needed to determine whether this interaction is of clinical importance. Phenytoin has also been demonstrated to augment the anticoagulant action of coumadin. Lastly, phenytoin may enhance the electrophysiologic effects of verapamil by increasing its unbound concentration (i.e., displacing it from plasma proteins).

Indications

Phenytoin is very effective in the treatment of digitalis-induced atrial, junctional, and ventricular tachyarrhythmias. However, phenytoin cannot be recommended for treatment of digitalis-induced bradycardia or conduction disturbances. In addition to digitalis-induced arrhythmias, phenytoin is highly successful in controlling ventricular arrhythmias in patients with congenital heart disease and abnormal hemodynamics. Otherwise, phenytoin is rarely useful in the management of cardiac arrhythmias (supraventricular tachycardia, atrial flutter, or atrial fibrillation).

MEXILETINE

Mexiletine, originally synthesized in the 1960s as an anorectic agent, was quickly noticed during clinical investigation to exhibit anticonvulsant and antiarrhythmic actions.[132] Early in vitro studies demonstrated that mexiletine had local anesthetic effects, and subsequent clinical trials confirmed that mexiletine was an effective antiarrhythmic drug for ventricular arrhythmias. Structurally, mexiletine resembles the amine structure of lidocaine, and many of the electrophysiologic effects of mexiletine also resemble those of lidocaine. However, enough important differences exist between the two that mexiletine should not be considered an orally active form of lidocaine.

Cellular Electrophysiologic Effects

Like lidocaine and phenytoin, the cellular electrophysiologic effects of mexiletine depend on the nature of the tissue studied, extracellular concentration of potassium, and most importantly, on the state of health of the tissue.[132, 133] The electrophysiologic actions of mexiletine on the His-Purkinje system and ventricular myocardium are more pronounced than those in atrial tissue.[133, 134] Mexiletine blocks the fast inward sodium current thereby slowing conduction, decreasing excitability and spontaneous automaticity.[133–135] Low concentrations of mexiletine decrease action potential AMP, $\dot{V}$max, membrane responsiveness, APD, and the effective refractory period of His-Purkinje fibers when studied with extracellular potassium concentrations >4.0 mmol/L. However, low concentrations of mexiletine exert no electrophysiologic effects on healthy Purkinje fibers studied at an external potassium concentration of 2.7 mmol/L, implying that the membrane-depressant effects of mexiletine are voltage dependent (MDP is more negative when the external potassium concentration = 2.7 mmol/L). High concentrations of mexiletine further depress action potential AMP, $\dot{V}$max, membrane responsiveness, and conduction velocity, and shorten APD. The effective refractory period, in contrast, can increase, suggesting delayed reactivation of the sodium current.[135] (In contrast, high concentrations of lidocaine shorten both APD and the effective refractory period.) Mexiletine-induced shortening of APD is uniform throughout the specialized conduction system, showing no preferential action on the gate region (i.e., region of longest APD). Restitution of action potential duration during premature stimulation may be altered. Mexiletine inhibits the normal shortening of APD (and, presumably, refractoriness) during early premature beats, thereby antagonizing the "peeling back" of refractoriness that may be important for ventricular tachycardia initiation.[136]

Several investigators have shown that the ability of mexiletine to decrease $\dot{V}$max or the fast inward sodium current was amplified at rapid stimulation frequencies.[137, 138] Both the onset and recovery from sodium channel blockade is rapid, similar to lidocaine and phenytoin. Like these other agents, mexiletine blocks inactivated sodium channels as well as channels in the open state. Frame, Gitant, and Hoffman demonstrated that recovery from the use-dependent effects of mexiletine is five times slower than from lidocaine.[138] At similar concentrations, mexiletine has a greater effect on $\dot{V}$max than does lidocaine.

In ventricular myocardium, mexiletine decreases conduction velocity, action potential AMP, $\dot{V}$max, and membrane responsiveness.[132, 133] However, unlike its effect in Purkinje fibers, mexiletine prolongs the effective refractory period with little to no change in APD.[139]

The electrophysiologic action of mexiletine is enhanced in diseased or depressed tissues (e.g., in acidosis, hyperkalemia, hypoxia, or ischemia). When studied under hypoxia conditions, Burke and Berman noted pronounced local anesthetic effects and marked slowing of conduction in Purkinje fibers at concentrations of mexiletine that had little effect during normoxia.[140] Yoon and Han have also discovered that in ischemic hearts, the effect of mexiletine on the diastolic excitability threshold, refractoriness, and conduction is exaggerated.[141]

Mexiletine can be effective in suppressing certain types of automatic rhythms. It can decrease phase 4 depolarization in normal and partially depolarized Purkinje fibers. In addition, Amerini et al have demonstrated the ability of mexiletine to reduce digitalis-induced delayed afterdepolarization amplitude and triggered activity.[142] Mexiletine is surprisingly effective in terminating triggered activity arising from early afterdepolarizations.

At therapeutic concentrations, mexiletine exerts trivial depressant effects on sinus node automaticity (spontaneous cycle length, sinoatrial conduction time, or response to overdrive atrial pacing).[134] However, superfusion with high concentrations of mexiletine slows the spontaneous sinus rate, prolongs sinoatrial conduction, and decreases action potential AMP and $\dot{V}$max. Action potential duration is also prolonged. Using the voltage clamp technique, Igawa, Kotake, and Mushiba observed that mexiletine could depress the slow inward calcium and pacemaker currents in sinus node tissue, thereby explaining the electrophysiologic effects of mexiletine.[134] Similarly, only at relatively high concentrations does mexiletine alter atrial action potential characteristics and slow conduction within the atrium.[143] Atrial action potential duration and refractoriness exhibit little change. No studies have yet reported the in vitro pharmacologic effects of mexiletine on the AV node.

Mexiletine may exert additional antiarrhythmic effects by modifying autonomic nervous system activity. Mexiletine has been demonstrated by Kitagawa, Takeda, and Kohei to inhibit norepinephrine release from sympathetic nerves.[144] They were able to demonstrate that through sympathetic antagonism, mexiletine increased the dose of ouabain necessary to produce digitalis toxicity. Evidence exists to suggest that mexiletine may also be vagolytic.

The developmental pharmacology of mexiletine has received little attention, and only one report is available. Using isolated rat ventricular myocytes, Hering, Bodewei, and Wollenberger noted that neonatal cells were more sensitive to mexiletine.[135] The concentration of mexiletine required to achieve 70% block of the sodium current in adult myocytes was 50 mmol/L, whereas a much smaller concentration (15 mmol/L) produced 65% block in neonatal ventricular cells. This data must be considered preliminary. For all other local anesthetic agents studied to date, cardiac tissues from immature animals have either been less sensitive or have not differed.

Clinical Electrophysiologic Effects

The clinical electrophysiologic effects of mexiletine have been studied in normal individuals and in patients with sinus node dysfunction or conduction abnormalities.[145] Mexiletine has little effect on normal sinus node function (sinus node recovery time or sinoatrial conduction time). No change in spontaneous sinus cycle length has been observed in adult subjects. However, Shakibi and Moezzi have found that mexiletine reduced sinus cycle length in children, probably through a vagolytic mechanism.[146] Results in patients with sinus node dysfunction differ. Mexiletine produces a significant increase in sinus cycle length and sinus node recovery time and impairs sinoatrial conduction. Sinoatrial arrest, as well as sinoatrial exit block, have been observed. Published data on the effects of mexiletine on the AV node have been variable. McComish et al reported that mexiletine had no effect on AV nodal conduction time or refractory periods, but other investigators have shown an increase in the AV nodal functional refractory period as well as an increase in the AH interval and Wenckebach cycle length.[147]

Conduction within the atrium and ventricle, as well as refractoriness in these structures, remains unchanged after administration of mexiletine.[132, 145, 146] The relative refractory period of the His-Purkinje conduction system is decreased in normal subjects, but mexiletine usually increases the effective and relative refractory periods of the His-Purkinje system in patients with preexisting conduction abnormalities. Similarly, mexiletine has little effect on His-ventricular conduction time in normal individuals, but may further increase conduction delay in patients with His-Purkinje disease. Rarely, second or third degree infra-Hisian block may complicate mexiletine administration.

The reported electrophysiologic effects of mexiletine on atrioventricular bypass pathways have also been variable.[132, 145] In one reported series, mexiletine produced a significant increase in both the antegrade and retrograde refractory periods of the accessory connection; however, all the studied patients had relatively long refractory periods during the basal state. Other investigators have found that mexiletine did not produce changes in either the conduction properties or refractoriness of accessory pathways in patients with Wolff-Parkinson-White syndrome.

Electrocardiographic Effects

Mexiletine causes no significant change in the PR interval, QRS duration, or corrected QT interval.[132] Heart rate changes depend on patient age and whether sinus node dysfunction exists. Rarely, mexiletine may produce prolongation of QRS duration in patients with diffuse organic heart disease, or AV block in patients with conduction system abnormalities.

Clinical Pharmacokinetics

Orally administered, mexiletine is rapidly and well absorbed from the small intestine, with peak plasma concentrations occurring 1 to 3 hours after a dose.[132, 148] Unlike lidocaine, mexiletine has a high systemic bioavailability (79% to 88%). Absorption can be delayed in patients concomitantly taking cimetidine, antacids, or narcotic analgesics, and in patients suffering from recent myocardial infarction.

Mexiletine has a large apparent volume of distribution (5–9 L/kg) because of avid tissue binding. Only 61% to 75% of the mexiletine in the blood is bound to serum proteins. The nature of the plasma protein to which mexiletine binds is unknown. The disposition kinetics of mexiletine are most consistent with a three-compartment model, representing fast and slow distribution phases and a much slower elimination phase.[132, 148]

Mexiletine is extensively metabolized in the liver by oxidation and by reduction and conjugation reactions; eight metabolites have been identified. Unlike phenytoin metabolism, mexiletine metabolism is not saturable. None of the metabolites of mexiletine have so far been shown to possess pharmacologic activity. Less than 15% of an administered dose is excreted unchanged in the urine. Mexiletine has a relatively long plasma elimination half-life, varying between 6.3 and 11.8 hours. The half-life is prolonged in patients with acute myocardial infarction (17 h) and functional class III or IV congestive heart failure (15.4 h), largely because of reduced hepatic blood flow, suggesting the need to reduce mexiletine dosage in these patients.

Hepatic dysfunction can affect the pharmacokinetics of mexiletine. Several observers have identified a reduced elimination rate in patients with liver disease (e.g., cirrhosis). Pentikainen et al noted no change in the volume of distribution or protein binding of mexiletine, but clearance was reduced (26% of normal), and the elimination half-life was markedly prolonged (28.7 h) in these patients. These investigators therefore recommended that the maintenance dosage of mexiletine be reduced by 25% to 33%.

Urinary excretion of mexiletine is facilitated by acidification.[133] Urinary excretion at a urine pH of 5.0 can account for 30% to 55% of the dose administered, compared to 10% at normal pH. The elimination half-life can thus be decreased from a normal value of 9 hours to 4.5 hours with urinary acidification. El Allaf et al have studied the elimination kinetics of mexiletine during renal failure.[150] Their results indicated that dosage reduction was not necessary unless the creatinine clearance was ≤10 mL/min.

Mexiletine readily crosses the human placenta, and levels in maternal and cord blood are equal.[148] No teratogenicity has been reported in fetuses delivered to mothers who were chronically administered mexiletine throughout pregnancy. Mexiletine is also excreted into human breast milk, with levels in breast milk approximating those in maternal plasma. The total quantity ingested by the nursing infant is insufficient to produce detectable plasma levels.

The reported range of therapeutic plasma concentrations for mexiletine is between 0.8 and 2.0 μg/mL. However, our experience and that of several other investigators has failed to reveal a correlation between therapeutic efficacy, adverse effects, and plasma levels.

Mexiletine is marketed as a racemic mixture of equal parts of the *d* and *l* enantiomer. Grech-Belanger, Turgcon, and Gilbert have shown differences in the pharmacokinetics of the two enantiomers.[151] The *d* enantiomer exhibits greater plasma concentration over time, suggesting higher bioavailability or decreased clearance. However, there are no reports as yet regarding differences in pharmacologic effects, making the significance of these pharmacokinetic differences uncertain.

Mexiletine pharmacokinetics have been relatively unexplored in children. Holt et al have made the only pertinent observations.[75] They noticed that in treating two young infants (one age 2 weeks and one age 20 months), the dose of mexiletine required (15–25 mg/kg/d) to produce plasma levels comparable to adults was much larger. The mechanism(s) for the higher daily dosage of mexiletine in these young infants was not delineated.

Dosage

For treatment of arrhythmias in children, the oral dosage of mexiletine we found effective ranged between 1.4 and 5.1 mg/kg (median = 3.3 mg/kg) administered every 8 hours. Higher dosages (up to 8 mg/kg) may be required in infants. The total daily dosage recommended for treatment of arrhythmias in adults varies between 450 mg and 1200 mg (average = 600 mg). Loading doses should be avoided because of the high incidence of adverse effects.

Adverse Effects

Side effects occur not infrequently during mexiletine treatment (20% to 70% of patients). Fortunately they are minor and can be abated with reduction in dosage. The two most common adverse reactions observed with mexiletine are gastrointestinal and neurologic. Gastrointestinal side effects consist of nausea, vomiting, abdominal pain, and epigastric distress. Rarely, liver function tests may show elevated levels or hepatitis may occur. Adverse effects involving the gastrointestinal tract result from a direct irritant effect of mexiletine on the stomach; it may be prevented by administering mexiletine with food, antacids, or cimetidine.[133] Neurologic side effects include tremor, nystagmus, diplopia, dizziness, dysarthria, paresthesias, ataxia, headache, confusion, personality changes, and in rare instances, seizures. Cardiovascular complications, specifically hypotension, worsening of congestive heart failure, and aggravation of arrhythmias, are extremely uncommon. Skin rash, thrombocytopenia, agranulocytosis, and a positive antinuclear antibody test have also been reported.

Drug Interactions

Concurrent treatment with antacids, cimetidine, and narcotic analgesics can slow the absorption of mexiletine. Hepatic enzyme inducers such as phenytoin and rifampin have been shown to increase the clearance of mexiletine and shorten its elimination half-life, thus requiring increased mexiletine dosage in patients needing such medications.[132, 133, 148] No evidence exists to suggest an interaction between mexiletine and digoxin or between mexiletine and coumadin.

Indications

Mexiletine is most effective in treating ventricular arrhythmias that occur in the setting of associated congenital heart disease. Mexiletine is less efficacious in patients with cardiomyopathy or normal hearts. Mexiletine has been reported to suppress ventricular arrhythmias resulting from digitalis toxicity. Because it has little effect on atrial or atrioventricular junctional tissue, mexiletine is rarely effective for therapy of supraventricular tachycardia (Wolff-Parkinson-White syndrome), atrial flutter, or atrial fibrillation.

ETHMOZINE

Ethmozine, the ethyl ester hydrochloride of 10-(3-morpholinopropionyl) phenothiazine-2-carbamic acid, was synthesized and initially studied in the Soviet Union during the 1960s.[152] Ethmozine, a phenothiazine chemical derivative, was noted by early investigators to share similar antiarrhythmic properties in common with other phenothiazines (i.e., local anesthetic effects). Numerous clinical investigative trials have reported ethmozine to be a safe and effective agent for control of atrial and ventricular arrhythmias.

Cellular Electrophysiologic Effects

The cellular electrophysiologic effects of ethmozine have been studied almost exclusively in Purkinje tissue and ventricular myocardium.[153, 154] Few studies report the pharmacologic action of ethmozine on atrial myocardium or in the sinus or AV nodes.[155] In His-Purkinje cells, low concentrations of ethmozine (0.05 μg/mL) depress $\dot{V}max$ without having a significant effect on other action potential parameters. Higher concentrations (0.2 μg/mL) further reduce $\dot{V}max$; depress action potential AMP, overshoot, and membrane responsiveness; and shorten APD. Only at extremely toxic concentrations (1 μg/mL) does membrane potential decrease. Although ethmozine shortens the effective refractory period and APD, the degree of shortening of the effective refractory period is smaller than that of APD ($\Delta ERP/APD > 1$). The net result of these changes is a relative prolongation of the effective refractory period. Furthermore, the takeoff potential of the earliest propagated premature response becomes more negative, in addition to an increase in $\dot{V}max$, after ethmozine superfusion. The effect of these changes is faster conduction of early premature beats, thereby lessening the probability of re-entrant excitation. Ventricular diastolic excitability has been demonstrated by Ruffy et al to increase in the canine ventricle after exposure to ethmozine.[153]

Similar to lidocaine and the other type Ib local anesthetic agents, the electrophysiologic response to ethmozine is enhanced in depressed or unhealthy tissue.[156] Ruffy et al were the first to observe that ethmozine markedly depressed conduction in ischemic regions of the left ventricle in comparison to its effects on conduction in healthy ventricular myocardium.[153] Supportive observations were later made by Tsuji et al, who investigated the membrane actions of ethmozine on hypoxic depressed canine Purkinje fibers.[156] They noted that the local anesthetic action of ethmozine was exaggerated at concentrations that produced minimal effects on normoxic Purkinje fibers. During superfusion with similar concentrations, ethmozine decreased maximum diastolic potential 2.4% in the presence of normoxia and 4.9% during hypoxia. Similarly, ethmozine produced a 27% decrease of $\dot{V}max$ in the presence of normoxia and a 34% decrease during hypoxic superfusion.

Several reports have demonstrated that the local anesthetic effect of ethmozine results from blockade of the fast inward sodium current.[157, 158] Early investigators thought that ethmozine did not delay the reactivation kinetics of the sodium channel and thus demonstrated no use dependence. However, experimental studies in nerve fibers and recent work by Schubert et al on isolated rat ventricular myocytes have shown that ethmozine delays recovery from the inactivated state and augments sodium channel block at rapid stimulation rates.[159] Thus, in cardiac muscle, the local anesthetic effects of ethmozine are both frequency dependent and voltage dependent.

When its effects were studied on slow response action potentials in depolarized Purkinje cells (high K^+ + isoproterenol), ethmozine produced no appreciable changes in $\dot{V}max$ or APD. Furthermore, ethmozine injected directly into the canine sinus node artery or the AV nodal artery had no detectable direct chronotropic or dromotropic effects in the studies either by Ruffy et al or by Urthaler et al.[153, 160] Therefore the data (although indirect and limited) suggests that ethmozine has little or no inhibitory action on the slow calcium channel current.

Microelectrode studies of the electrophysiologic effects of ethmozine on atrial structures has been restricted to the work by Yuryavichus et al.[155] These investigators noted a decrease in frog atrium in $\dot{V}max$ following ethmozine exposure. No changes in APD were evident.

Ethmozine exhibits interesting effects on spontaneous automatic rhythms. In normally automatic Purkinje fibers (MDP ≥ -80 mV), ethmozine decreases the spontaneous rate by shifting the threshold potential in the depolarized direction instead of reducing phase 4 depolarization (as lidocaine does).[154] Ethmozine is very effective in decreasing the rate of diastolic depolarization and terminating abnormal automaticity (i.e., automaticity occurring from membrane potentials between -68 mV and -38 mV).[154] (In contrast, lidocaine may prolong the cycle length of abnormally automatic rhythms but never terminates them.) Finally, ethmozine can depress the amplitude of delayed afterdepolarizations and abort triggered activity that has been induced by either barium chloride, myocardial infarction, or digitalis toxicity in Purkinje fibers.

Similar to the other type Ib antiarrhythmic agents, ethmozine can depress sympathetic nerve conduction and thereby diminish sympathetic activity to the heart. The studies by Urthaler et al have demonstrated that ethmozine significantly diminishes the sinus node and AV junctional responses to stellate ganglion stimulation.[161] Careful experiments have eliminated a direct post-synaptic sympathetic blocking action, but additional effects on the autonomic nervous system were detected. Urthaler et al found that ethmozine had vagolytic effects (although minor and variable in magnitude) at both the sinus node and AV junctional levels.[161] How and if changes in autonomic activity contribute to the antiarrhythmic effects of ethmozine needs further investigation.

No developmental studies of the electrophysiologic actions of ethmozine have been reported to date.

Clinical Electrophysiologic Effects

When injected intravenously, ethmozine slows conduction throughout the human heart. Chazov, Shugushev, and Rosenshtraukh observed significant slowing of conduction within the atrium (increase in PA interval), the AV node (prolongation of AH interval), the His-Purkinje system (lengthening of HV interval), and the ventricle (increase in QRS duration).[152] No changes occurred in atrial, AV nodal, or ventricular refractoriness.

Ethmozine can produce complete conduction block or prolong the effective refractory period of accessory atrioventricular pathways in patients with Wolff-Parkinson-White syndrome. Following ethmozine administration, Chazov, Shugushev, and Rosenshtraukh noted complete antegrade accessory pathway conduction block in six of 10 patients and prolongation of the effective refractory period in three others.[152] Retrograde accessory pathway conduction was similarly altered (complete conduction block in two of 16 patients) and prolongation of the retrograde effective refractory period was noted in 9 of 9 patients.

The effects of ethmozine on the sinus node depend on whether there is preexistent sinus node dysfunction.[162] In patients with normal sinus node function, ethmozine may shorten the spontaneous cycle length (i.e., anticholinergic action). Ethmozine usually has little effect on either the response to overdrive atrial pacing or the sinoatrial conduction time. In contrast, ethmozine usually increases the maximum corrected sinus node recovery time and sinoatrial conduction time in subjects with symptomatic sinus node dysfunction. Shugushev et al noted the development of sinoatrial exit block in four of nine patients administered ethmozine.[162] In these individuals, ethmozine usually did not alter the spontaneous sinus heart rate.

Fox, Hoffman, and Rosen were unable to demonstrate any changes in the ventricular fibrillation threshold following ethmozine administration to dogs.[163] Ethmozine, however, did seem to elevate the defibrillation threshold. In animal studies, ethmozine appears to raise the ventricular diastolic excitability threshold.

Electrocardiographic Effects

Ethmozine usually produces modest prolongation of the PR interval and QRS duration on the surface electrocardiogram; these effects are dose related.[164] No significant changes occur in the corrected QT interval.

Clinical Pharmacokinetics

The clinical pharmacokinetics of ethmozine have had only limited evaluation in adult subjects, and no data exist for infants and young children.[165–167] Ethmozine is well absorbed from the gastrointestinal tract, and peak plasma levels occur 1 to 3 hours after oral doses. Once absorbed, ethmozine is extensively distributed in the body (V_d = 11.1 ± 3.1 L/kg). Ethmozine is extensively bound to plasma proteins (90% to 95%). The nature of the plasma protein(s) has not been investigated.

Biotransformation is thought to be the predominant route of elimination (99%). Over 30 metabolites have been identified, and their electrophysiologic activity has not been studied in any significant detail. Less than 1% of ethmozine is excreted unchanged in the urine. Radiolabeled studies indicate that ethmozine metabolites are excreted in the feces (60%) and urine (40%). In healthy subjects the elimination half-life ranges from 3 to 6 hours after a single dose and approximates 8 hours during chronic dosing. Ethmozine appears to have a longer elimination half-life in patients with heart disease (6.4 to 13.1 h) and renal insufficiency (47 h). Morganroth reported that despite the relatively short plasma half-life (mean = 4 h), the biologic half-life of ethmozine exceeds 48 hours, raising questions concerning the pharmacologic importance of ethmozine metabolites.[168] Plasma ethmozine levels correlate poorly with therapeutic efficacy or toxicity.

Dosage

Oral therapy with ethmozine should be instituted at a starting dosage of 200 mg/m²/d (5 mg/kg/d), divided into 8-hour doses, and slowly increased (as necessary) to a maximum dosage of 600 mg/m²/d (15 mg/kg/d).

Adverse Effects

Side effects are relatively uncommon (25% to 30% of patients) and are most likely to occur at high dosages (15 mg/kg/d).[169] The most frequent adverse effects are neurologic and include vertigo, dizziness, blurred vision, tinnitus, headache, paresthesias, euphoria, perioral tingling, and muscle twitches. Symptoms involving the gastrointestinal tract are the next most common and include nausea, vomiting, diarrhea, epigastric distress, and constipation. Cardiovascular side effects are the most serious and include hypotension, exacerbation of congestive heart failure, and arrhythmia aggravation. Only at high doses has ethmozine been noted to depress ventricular function, and only in patients with significant preexisting compromised function. Proarrhythmia effects (either incessant supraventricular or ventricular tachycardia) are relatively uncommon (less than 10% of patients). Prolonged sinus pauses and His-Purkinje conduction disturbances (bundle-branch block) have also been reported in patients with organic heart disease. Rare symptoms include rash, pruritis, and the malignant neuroleptic syndrome (fever, stupor, and dystonia). Slit lamp examination has revealed no ophthalmologic abnormalities, as has been observed with other phenothiazine-derived drugs.

Drug Interactions

Few important drug interactions with ethmozine have been described. Data exist suggesting that calcium may interfere with the oral absorption of ethmozine. Biollaz, Shaheen, and Wood have studied the effect of cimetidine on the pharmacokinetics of ethmozine.[167] Cimetidine reduced the clearance of ethmozine (19.7 ± 4.2 mg/kg/min vs 38.2 ± 10.7 mg/kg/min) and prolonged its elimination half-life (4.6 ± 1.6 h vs 3.3 ± 1.6 h). However, Biollaz et al could not demonstrate any additional electrocardiographic changes, implying little pharmacodynamic interaction. Kennedy et al noted no changes in the pharmacokinetics of digoxin following ethmozine administration.[170]

Indications

Ethmozine promises to be a useful agent for the management of both supraventricular and ventricular arrhythmias. Chazov, Shugushev, and Rosenshtraukh have reported it effective in the treatment of Wolff-Parkinson-White syndrome and AV nodal reentry tachycardia.[152] In our own experience, ethmozine has been effective in suppressing atrial ectopic tachycardia.[171] Several investigators have found ethmozine moderately successful in controlling ventricular arrhythmias (PVCs, couplets, and nonsustained ventricular tachycardia). Pratt et al reported that ethmozine was highly effective for suppressing ventricular arrhythmias in patients with mitral valve prolapse.[164] On the other hand, ethmozine has not been found useful in atrial flutter or atrial fibrillation.

FLECAINIDE

Flecainide acetate is a new antiarrhythmic drug belonging to a unique series of trifluoroethoxybenzamides.[172] Its primary action is to depress membrane responsiveness by inhibiting the rapid transmembrane influx of sodium through its ion channel. Flecainide is several times more potent than procainamide, quinidine, or lidocaine in depressing cardiac conduction. Because of its marked negative dromotropic effect in association with minor changes in repolarization, flecainide has been classified as a type IC local anesthetic agent. Clinical studies have shown it to be of value in the treatment of a broad spectrum of atrial, junctional, and ventricular arrhythmias.

Cellular Electrophysiologic Effects

Flecainide was the first of a new subclass of local anesthetic drugs to be studied. The type IC agents are distinguished by their ability to bind to previously activated sodium channels (channels that exist in the inactivated state) and markedly retard their recovery to the rested state. By this effect, the type IC antiarrhythmic agents diminish the availability of sodium channels to depolarize the cell membrane during the subsequent action potential. During electrical diastole, inactivated sodium channels generally recover to the rested state, allowing for maximum membrane depolarization during the next propagated impulse. Local anesthetic agents dissociate from their binding sites on sodium channels during diastole with different rate constants. Flecainide and the other type IC agents unbind from the sodium channel with a long time constant (10 to 30 s), thereby markedly slowing recovery from inactivation. Delayed recovery from inactivation is manifested as a decrease in $\dot{V}max$ and depression of cardiac conduction.

Flecainide exerts electrophysiologic effects primarily on working myocardium (atrial and ventricular) and on the specialized conduction system.[173] When superfused with concentrations of flecainide in the therapeutic range, only minor effects are observed on the sinus and AV nodes.[174] Flecainide can decrease sinus node automaticity and decrease AV nodal conduction velocity. In general, flecainide depresses slow response action potentials only when studied at high concentrations (10 μg/mL). Singh et al observed flecainide to depress atrial action potential AMP and $\dot{V}max$ at clinically relevant concentrations.[174] Flecainide was noted to have little effect on MDP, APD, or ERP in atrial tissue. Similar to its effects on atrial cells, flecainide has been reported by Ikeda et al to decrease action potential AMP and $\dot{V}$max in ventricular muscle and His-Purkinje fibers.[173]

Several studies have noted that flecainide altered repolarization and refractoriness.[175] At low concentrations (0.1–1.0 mg/mL), flecainide shortens Purkinje fiber APD and ERP and inhibits spontaneous automaticity and membrane responsiveness. Flecainide has the opposite effect on ventricular repolarization: APD is prolonged in a dose-dependent manner.

The acute cellular electrophysiologic effects of flecainide on adult and neonatal Purkinje and ventricular cardiac tissues have been reported by Yabek et al.[176] These investigators noted diminished sensitivity to flecainide (a response similar to that to other local anesthetic agents) in the neonatal age group. In neonatal ventricular myocardium, the ability of flecainide to prolong repolarization and to depress $\dot{V}$max were significantly attenuated. Flecainide had no effect on action potential AMP and only minor effects on neonatal Purkinje fiber APD. The use-dependent blocking effect of flecainide on sodium channel activity was also less marked in neonatal tissues.

Clinical Electrophysiologic Effects

The electrophysiologic effects of flecainide in the intact human heart can be anticipated from its in vitro cellular effects. Sinus cycle length has been reported to change variably (either no change or a decrease).[177] In patients with sick sinus syndrome, flecainide administration may cause significant sinus dysfunction (bradycardia), requiring pacemaker implantation. Flecainide inhibits conduction throughout the heart. In the atrium, this is manifested by an increase in the PA interval. Flecainide can depress AV nodal conduction, as demonstrated by prolongation of the AH interval and the Wenckebach cycle length. As in other atrial tissues, flecainide does not alter AV nodal refractoriness. Flecainide usually prolongs the HV interval and therefore should be administered cautiously to patients with preexisting abnormalities of the His-Purkinje conduction system. Prolonged ventricular refractoriness and increased pacing threshold have been observed during flecainide therapy. Flecainide also prolongs refractoriness and slows conduction (frequently producing block) in accessory atrioventricular pathways. The effects of flecainide are different from those of other local anesthetic agents in that it can significantly prolong the refractoriness of accessory pathways with short baseline ERPs (ERP < 270 ms). Flecainide can produce profound depression of retrograde conduction in accessory pathways.

Electrocardiographic Effects

Several electrocardiographic changes have been noted following flecainide administration.[177] Flecainide will prolong the PR, QRS, and QTc intervals. The prolongation of the QTc interval is largely a result of marked QRS prolongation. Some reports have suggested a relationship between the degree of QRS prolongation and serum concentrations. However, no investigator has been able to demonstrate a relationship between the degree of QRS lengthening and the proarrhythmic effects of flecainide. Slowing of interatrial conduction is manifested electrocardiographically as a prolongation of P wave duration. Flecainide can decrease the degree of preexcitation evident on the ECG in patients with Wolff-Parkinson-White syndrome.

Clinical Pharmacokinetics

Flecainide is well absorbed from the gastrointestinal tract (70% to 100% of an orally administered dose).[177, 178] Peak plasma concentrations occur 2 to 3 hours following administration. The rate and extent of flecainide absorption are not affected by food or antacids. Bioavailability studies have not indicated any important presystemic hepatic metabolism. Following intravenous administration (2 mg/kg), flecainide has a rapid-onset effect (1.5–10 min, average = 5 min). Flecainide has a large apparent volume of distribution (range 5–13.4 L/kg, average = 8.7 L/kg).

Flecainide and its metabolites are primarily excreted in the urine (86%); only 27% is excreted unchanged.[178] A small amount (5%) is eliminated through the gastrointestinal tract, suggesting that biliary excretion does not contribute importantly to the elimination of flecainide. However, flecainide is biotransformed by the liver to two electrophysiologically active metabolites: meta-*O*-dealkylated flecainide and the meta-*O*-dealkylated lactam of flecainide. The plasma concentration of flecainide metabolites are considerably lower than that of the parent drug, thereby making it unlikely that the metabolites contribute substantially to the effects of flecainide. Flecainide is not extensively bound to plasma proteins (40%).

In normal healthy adults, the elimination half-life of flecainide averages 13 hours (range 7–19 h).[177, 178] Till et al reported a slightly shorter $t\frac{1}{2}$ in seven children aged 1 month to 13.7 years (mean, 8.7 h; range, 7–12 h).[179] The clearance of flecainide is decreased in patients with congestive heart failure and moderate renal failure, thereby making it important to make appropriate dosage adjustments in these patients.[180] In patients with congestive heart failure, total clearance is generally reduced 20% and the elimination half-life is prolonged (average, 19 h; range, 14–26 h). More marked changes in the clearance of flecainide are apparent during renal failure (40% decrease in total clearance).

Therapeutic effects have been reported with serum concentrations between 0.2 and 1.0 μg/mL. Many investigators have noted an increasing incidence of proarrhythmic effects and toxicity when trough serum concentrations exceed 1.0 μg/ml. Preliminary data suggest that serum concentrations of flecainide can increase during chronic therapy, making it important to serially follow levels.

Dosage

Wren and Campbell reported the successful treatment of 12 children with varied arrhythmias using an oral flecainide dosage of 3–6 mg/kg/d. The equivalent dosage calculated by the body surface area method would be 115–230 mg/m.[2, 181] The total daily dose should never exceed 400 mg.[177] Flecainide can be administered by twice-daily dosing, but in patients with side effects and in young children, antiarrhythmic efficacy frequently improves with three doses per day. In order to avoid drug accumulation and toxicity, Morganroth, Anderson, and Gentzkow have recommended not increasing the dosage more often than every 4 days.[182]

Adverse Effects

Adverse effects have been reported to be common (30% to 40% of patients) during flecainide therapy but are frequently self-limited and disappear with a decrease in dosage or by altering the frequency of administration from twice daily to three times daily.[177] Transient central nervous system symptoms are the most frequent and include blurred vision, focusing difficulties, drowsiness, dizziness, oral paresthesias, and headache. Unlike the type IA agents, gastrointestinal side effects (nausea, obstipation) are rare.

The provocation of serious ventricular arrhythmias is of more concern.[182] When used at high dosages during early clinical investigation, flecainide therapy was not infrequently complicated by induction of sustained ventricular tachycardia or ventricular fibrillation, often resistant to DC cardioversion and pacing. Since recognition of the importance of limiting the maximum dosage, proarrhythmic effects are much less frequent. Morganroth, Anderson, and Gentzkow have extensively studied this problem and observed ventricular proarrhythmia to be related to arrhythmia classification on treatment entry (most common in patients being treated for sustained ventricular tachycardia), the presence of structural heart disease, and preexisting sinus node dysfunction.[182] As mentioned previously, flecainide therapy should be initiated carefully in patients with abnormalities in His-Purkinje conduction. New-onset bundle-branch block and infranodal conduction block have been reported. Flecainide has also been documented to facilitate incessant supraventricular tachycardia. Precipitation or exacerbation of congestive heart failure may occur in patients with diminished cardiac contractile function.

Drug Interactions

Little data are available on drug interactions with flecainide. Tjandra-Maga et al have noted a 24% ± 35% rise in digoxin serum concentration in normal volunteers treated jointly with digoxin and flecainide.[178] Propranolol and flecainide each appear to raise the other's plasma concentration and to exert additive negative inotropic effects.[183] Shea et al have reported elevated flecainide concentrations during concomitant amiodarone therapy.[184] Lastly, Tjandra-Maga et al have noted that cimetidine decreases the nonrenal clearance of flecainide and prolongs its elimination half-life.[185]

Indications

Flecainide has been reported to treat effectively a wide variety of both supraventricular and ventricular arrhythmias.[177] Flecainide appears to be very successful in treating supraventricular tachycardias secondary to atrioventricular nodal reentry and reciprocating tachycardias incorporating an accessory atrioventricular pathway. Satisfactory arrhythmia control has been documented for automatic supraventricular tachycardias (e.g., atrial automatic tachycardia and junctional ectopic tachycardia). Flecainide has also been used for chemical conversion of atrial fibrillation. However, experience in the clinical usage of flecainide is most extensive in the treatment of ventricular arrhythmias. Flecainide provides better antiarrhythmic suppression of simple and complex ventricular ectopy in adult subjects than does quinidine or disopyramide. Our preliminary data suggest that flecainide is moderately effective in suppressing ventricular tachycardia in children.

ENCAINIDE

Encainide hydrochloride is a benzanilide derivative synthesized in 1969.[186] Despite the fact that its chemical structure does not resemble any of the known antiarrhythmic agents, the major electrophysiologic action of encainide is to block cardiac sodium channels.[187] Encainide is a class IC antiarrhythmic drug whose cellular pharmacologic effects cause marked slowing of conduction, with little alteration of cardiac refractoriness.[187] Clinical experience with encainide suggests that it is very effective in treating a wide spectrum of atrial and ventricular arrhythmias.

Cellular Electrophysiologic Effects

Encainide is a local anesthetic antiarrhythmic agent with no β-blocking or calcium channel blocking properties. The cellular electrophysiologic effects of encainide have been best studied in fibers from the His-Purkinje conduction system and ventricular myocardium.[188–190] Gibson, Somani, and Bassett were the first to demonstrate a concentration-dependent reduction in $\dot{V}max$ of canine Purkinje fibers by encainide.[188] Superfusion with high concentrations of encainide ($>10^{-6}$ mol/L) reduced action potential AMP, conduction velocity, APD, and excitability. Membrane responsiveness is similarly depressed. Although APD is shortened, Gibson, Somani, and Bassett observed that the effective refractory period increased, with the ratio of the change in the effective refractory period to APD being greater than 1.[188] Carmeliet has demonstrated similar effects, with the exception of the changes in APD, in atrial and ventricular myocardium.[190] Action potential duration was observed to increase in rabbit and guinea pig ventricular tissues and in guinea pig atrial tissues.

The depressant effects of encainide on conduction are enhanced in diseased tissues and during rapid stimulation. Wong et al showed that the electrophysiologic effects of encainide were more marked and occurred at a lower drug concentration in ischemic rabbit ventricular myocardium.[191] In a canine model of myocardial infarction investigated by Ro, Gillon, and Kupersmith, encainide caused more marked increases in ventricular refractoriness and more slowing of conduction in infarcted tissue than in normal tissue.[192] King and Man demonstrated marked use dependence of encainide during superfusion of infarcted subendocardial Purkinje fibers.[193] At rapid stimulation frequencies, encainide induced marked depression of $\dot{V}max$, whereas in the absence of drug, the cycle length of stimulation did not affect $\dot{V}max$. Campbell noted an extremely long (20 s) time constant of recovery from use-dependent block, compared with that of mexiletine (0.5 s) or disopyramide (12 s).[194] The slow time course of recovery from cardiac sodium channel blockage in relation to the relatively brief diastolic period at physiologic heart rate accounts for the reduced His-Purkinje and ventricular conduction seen clinically. The exact nature of the interaction of encainide with the sodium channel (whether open or inactivated) is still unexplored.

Several investigators have evaluated the electrophysiologic effects of encainide on automatic rhythms. Gibson, Somani, and Bassett noted the suppressant effects of encainide on spontaneous automaticity occurring in normally polarized Purkinje fibers.[188] Carmeliet found that encainide could slow depolarization-induced abnormal automaticity and terminate delayed afterdepolarization-induced triggered activity.[190] The enhanced abnormal automaticity that commonly develops in the first 24 hours following myocardial infarction was shown by King and Man to slow in a dose-dependent fashion after exposure to encainide.[193]

Microelectrode studies of the cellular electrophysiologic effects of encainide on the sinus and AV nodes have not been reported. In addition, little understanding exists of the developmental electrophysiology of encainide.

Encainide is extensively metabolized, and all three of its known metabolites are electrophysiologically active.[187] The metabolites vary in potency and in their pharmacologic action. The metabolites *O*-demethylencainide (ODE) and 3-methoxy-*O*-demethylencainide (MODE) produce changes qualitatively similar to those of encainide on the action potential characteristics of canine Purkinje fibers and ventricular muscle cells. On a concentration basis, ODE was found by Elharrar and Zipes to be nine times more potent in reducing $\dot{V}max$ than either MODE or encainide.[189] In isolated Langendorff perfused heart preparation and in vivo, encainide slows impulse conduction in the His-Purkinje system and ventricle and increases the atrial effective refractory period. Encainide does not alter AV nodal conduction or ventricular refractoriness. His bundle observations in dogs given ODE have shown depression of atrial, AV nodal, His-Purkinje, and intraventricular conduction, and its effects on either atrial or ventricular refractoriness are variable (either no change or prolongation). In an in vivo model, Davy et al noted the electrophysiologic effects of ODE to be more potent than those of encainide in reducing both His-Purkinje conduction (4.7 times) and intraventricular conduction (7.2 times).[195] In the same animal model, MODE was demonstrated to be 10 times more potent in depressing atrial conduction and 2.5 times more potent in depressing intraventricular conduction, as well as four times more potent in prolonging atrial refractoriness, in comparison to encainide. Unlike either encainide or ODE, MODE could prolong ventricular refractoriness. The third metabolite of encainide, *N*-dimethylencainide (NDE), has similar potency to encainide, but it can prolong atrial or ventricular refractoriness. Encainide metabolites assume importance during chronic therapy, because they accumulate to concentrations that exceed those of the parent drug, and thus importantly contribute to the clinical electrophysiologic actions of encainide.

Encainide has been shown to produce little or no alteration in the autonomic nervous system. When investigated at high concentrations, no adrenergic (α- or β-), cholinergic agonist, or antagonist activity could be demonstrated.

Clinical Electrophysiologic Effects

The most evident clinical electrophysiologic action of encainide is to markedly slow conduction throughout the heart. Only modest changes in refractory periods are observed. In subjects with normal sinus node function, encainide does not usually alter the spontaneous cycle length, maximum corrected sinus node recovery time, or sinoatrial conduction time.[187] However, encainide can slow sinus node automaticity following autonomic blockade. The effects of encainide in patients with sinus node dysfunction differ; prolonged sinus pauses and dramatic increases in overdrive suppression of sinus node automaticity have been reported. Encainide slows conduction through the AV node as manifested by prolongation of the AH interval and Wenckebach cycle length. Slowed conduction in the atrium (prolongation of the PA interval), in the His-Purkinje system (increase in the HV interval), and in the ventricle (lengthening of the QRS duration) are readily evident. Encainide can markedly prolong His-Purkinje conduction time (HV interval) in subjects with preexisting abnormalities. The development of new-onset bundle-branch block or infra-Hisian block has been described. In addition, encainide prolongs atrial, AV nodal, and ventricular refractoriness.[187]

The electrophysiologic effects of encainide on accessory pathways in patients with Wolff-Parkinson-White syndrome are quite interesting. Encainide causes complete antegrade conduction block in approximately 50% of patients; its effects on retrograde conduction are more variable.[196] Encainide is a unique antiarrhythmic agent in that it can prolong refractoriness in accessory pathways that have short antegrade effective refractory periods (<270 ms), unlike other local anesthetic agents.

Encainide alters excitability in the human heart. Increases in the ventricular diastolic threshold have been reported, and this may be of importance in pacemaker-dependent patients with marginal ventricular capture thresholds.[187] Fain et al have observed that both encainide and ODE greatly increase the energy requirements for successful defibrillation.[197] In animal studies, Dawson et al found that ODE could lower the ventricular fibrillation threshold, possibly explaining some of the proarrhythmic effects of encainide.[198]

Electrocardiographic Effects

On the surface electrocardiogram, encainide typically prolongs the PR interval and QRS duration, but prolongation of the corrected QT interval is minimal. Most of the QT prolongation is secondary to lengthening of the QRS duration. Encainide usually does not alter the resting heart rate, except in individuals with sick sinus syndrome.

Clinical Pharmacokinetics

Encainide is well absorbed after oral administration, and peak plasma concentrations occur 1 to 2 hours after dosing.[187, 199–202] Plasma levels of encainide and its metabolites are highly variable as a result of differences in intersubject ability to oxidatively metabolize encainide in the liver. McAllister et al have characterized two distinct populations of subjects with pronounced differences in the disposition pharmacokinetics of encainide (extensive metabolizers and poor metabolizers).[200] The capacity to oxidatively metabolize encainide appears linked with the metabolic pathway for hydroxylation of debrisoquine, a genetic autosomal recessive defect. In extensive metabolizers (90% to 92% of patients), the oral bioavailability of encainide is relatively low (25% to 30%) because of first-pass metabolism. After multiple oral doses, the elimination half-life of encainide is 2.5 hours. Encainide is extensively distributed in adult patients (376 ± 48 L). Its protein binding is moderate (70%). During chronic therapy in extensive metabolizers, ODE and MODE accumulate to plasma concentrations in excess of those of encainide. The metabolites are eliminated much more slowly than encainide itself (ODE, 11.4 ± 9.6 h; MODE, >24 h), accounting for the long biologic half-life of encainide. Encainide and its metabolites are primarily excreted in the urine.

In poor metabolizers (8% to 10% of patients), systemic bioavailability is much higher (83% to 88%), and the elimination half-life of encainide is longer (8–11 h).[200] The apparent volume of distribution of encainide in poor metabolizers is smaller (172 ± 13 L), possibly related to higher protein binding (78%) and less extensive accumulation of metabolites. Encainide concentrates in plasma 10 to 20 times greater in the poor metabolizer group than in the extensive metabolizer group. However, plasma concentrations of ODE are only one-fifth those of encainide, and no MODE levels are detectable. NDE, not present in extensive metabolizers, has been measured at significant concentrations in the poor metabolizer group. In this group, encainide is primarily excreted unchanged in the urine (>40%). The clinical importance of differences in the ability of individual patients to metabolize encainide in determining its antiarrhythmic efficacy is still undetermined, as are the pharmacokinetics of encainide in infants and young children. Based on the pharmacokinetics of encainide, however, it is recommended that the total daily dosage not be increased more frequently than every 2 to 3 days.

Encainide pharmacokinetics have been studied during renal failure (creatinine clearance <40 mL/min).[202] The results indicated a three-fold decrease in clearance of encainide and its metabolites, and an increase in the degree of protein binding (70% to 81%). In patients with renal failure there is significant accumulation of both ODE and MODE to levels identical to those in normal subjects receiving twice the dosage of encainide. It is therefore recommended that major adjustments be made in encainide dosage during renal insufficiency in order to prevent adverse reactions.

Alteration of the pharmacokinetics of encainide have been observed during advanced hepatic cirrhosis.[202, 203] In patients with cirrhosis, bioavailability rose three fold (from 26% to 76%), and the elimination half-life has been noted to be prolonged (3.6 h). Although mean encainide plasma concentrations are elevated in patients with cirrhosis, no increases are appreciated in plasma levels of either ODE or MODE. More importantly, the pharmacologic effect of encainide as measured by the degree of QRS prolongation is comparable between patients with cirrhosis and normal subjects. No major adjustments in encainide dosage during hepatic disease have therefore been recommended.[203]

Data on encainide disposition in congestive

heart failure patients are not yet available. The role of plasma levels of encainide or its metabolites in guiding antiarrhythmic therapy is currently under investigation and appears to be quite complex.

Dosage

Based on our experience in the use of encainide to treat supraventricular tachycardia in children, we recommend an oral encainide dosage of 60–120 mg/m²/d, divided into 8-hour doses.[204] In infants and young children, we have occasionally needed to administer encainide more frequently (every 6 hours). The total daily dosage should not exceed 225 mg. Furthermore, dosage increases should be stopped if the PR interval exceeds 0.28 s or the QRS duration exceeds 0.16 s (or more than 100% of the pre-encainide QRS duration). Increases in dosage should not be made more frequently than every 2 to 3 days.

Adverse Effects

Side effects can occur in up to 60% of adult patients administered encainide, but such effects are less common in children (26%).[187, 199, 204] The most frequent drug-related adverse effects are neurologic (dizziness, lightheadedness, headache, tremor, sleep disturbances, paresthesias, visual disturbances, nystagmus, photophobia, ataxia, and lip numbness). Gastrointestinal complaints are the next most frequent and include nausea, constipation, metallic taste, and vomiting. Transient elevation of liver transaminases has been reported in 2% to 3% of adult patients; drug-induced hepatitis is extremely rare. Laboratory studies have not shown changes in renal function or hematologic parameters. Most of these side effects are dose related and can be eliminated by decreasing the dosage of encainide.

Cardiovascular complications (hypotension, exacerbation of congestive heart failure, and proarrhythmia) are more serious. The proarrhythmic effects of encainide are not related to the degree of QRS or QT prolongation but seem to occur in patients with a history of sustained ventricular tachycardia and depressed cardiac function. Some evidence exists to suggest that it may relate to high ODE plasma concentrations (>300 ngm/mL).[199] Encainide is extremely well tolerated from a hemodynamic point of view. Rare are instances of new-onset congestive heart failure or exacerbations of compensated congestive heart failure. Other adverse cardiac effects include drug-induced conduction disturbances and sinus bradycardia with prolonged sinus pauses.

Drug Interactions

Very few clinically important drug interactions with encainide have been reported.[205] Cimetidine, a known inhibitor of the cytochrome $P\text{-}_{450}$ system, has been demonstrated to significantly elevate plasma levels of encainide, ODE, and MODE. The relevance of this interaction, however, is unknown. Several investigators have validated the lack of interaction between encainide and digoxin and between encainide and anticoagulants.

Indications

The antiarrhythmic efficacy of encainide in the treatment of supraventricular tachyarrhythmias has been well documented, particularly for AV nodal reentry tachycardia, reciprocating atrioventricular tachycardia, the permanent form of junctional reciprocating tachycardia, and atrial ectopic tachycardia. Encainide rarely controls atrial fibrillation. Investigative clinical trials in adults have shown that encainide is effective in the treatment of isolated ventricular premature beats, couplets, and nonsustained ventricular tachycardia. Suppression of sustained ventricular tachycardia, especially in patients with marked compromise of ventricular function, is less successful.

PROPAFENONE

Propafenone, synthesized in 1970, is still under clinical investigation as an antiarrhythmic agent.[206] Although its chemical structure resembles a β-blocking agent, the predominant electrophysiologic effect of propafenone is to interfere with sodium conductance. The antiarrhythmic action of propafenone is a composite of its local anesthetic activity, β-adrenergic blockade and slow inward current inhibition. Clinically, propafenone has been used successfully to treat a variety of supraventricular and ventricular tachyarrhythmias. Our experience with the use of this agent has been limited to the treatment of postoperative junctional ectopic tachycardia.[207]

Cellular Electrophysiologic Effects

As already mentioned, the overwhelming electrophysiologic action of propafenone is to block the fast inward sodium current, thereby slowing conduction and spontaneous automaticity.[208] In Purkinje fibers and ventricular muscle, propafenone decreases action potential amplitude, $\dot{V}$max, membrane responsiveness, excitability, and conduction velocity in a concentration-dependent manner.[209, 210] High concentrations of propafenone can depress maximum diastolic potential. The effect of propafenone on APD and refractoriness in Purkinje fibers and ventricular myocytes is discordant: it decreases APD and the effective refractory period in Purkinje fibers, but lengthens both parameters in ventricular myocardial cells. However, the effect of propafenone is to increase the effective refractory period/APD ratio in Purkinje fibers and ventricular myocardium. The effect of propafenone on atrial tissue is similar to that on ventricular myocardium.[210]

Propafenone produces tonic and use-dependent block of $\dot{V}$max in Purkinje cells and ventricular myocardium. Kohlhardt and Seifert studied the recovery from use-dependent block induced by propafenone and found that the time constant of recovery was slow (15.5 s), as with other IC agents.[209] The effect of propafenone on $\dot{V}$max was also demonstrated to be voltage sensitive, explaining the enhanced action of propafenone in depressed myocardial tissue (such as is seen in myocardial infarct preparations).

Satoh and Hashimoto studied the effect of propafenone on sinoatrial tissue from rabbit hearts.[211] Propafenone depressed spontaneous automaticity, action potential AMP, $\dot{V}$max, and MDP and prolonged APD. Voltage clamp analysis revealed inhibition of the slow inward calcium (I_{ca}), pacemaker (I_f), and delayed outward potassium (I_k) currents. Slow response action potentials in Purkinje fibers have been observed by Delgado, Tamargo, and Tejerina to be similarly sensitive to the depressant effects of propafenone.[210]

Propafenone is effective in suppressing many different forms of automaticity. The spontaneous automaticity that occurs in Purkinje fibers at normal levels of membrane potential is easily inhibited by propafenone.[210] Tamargo, Delgado, and Tejerina showed that propafenone was effective in suppressing abnormal automaticity induced in ventricular myocardium by barium chloride.[212, 213] Similar observations were noted during ouabain-induced delayed afterdepolarizations and triggered activity.[213]

Propafenone exerts several important effects on the autonomic nervous system that either facilitate or oppose its direct depressant effects.[206] In vitro electrophysiologic studies as well as radioligand binding assays have demonstrated the ability of propafenone to block β-adrenergic receptors (propafenone exhibits 1/40th the β-blocking potency of propranolol). The effect of propafenone on β_2 receptors surpasses that on β_1 receptors. Propafenone also inhibits isoproterenol-stimulated increases in adenylate cyclase activity. Following intravenous propafenone administration to conscious dogs, Li et al observed an elevation of resting rate.[214] Pharmacologic studies suggested a vagolytic mechanism for the positive chronotropic action of propafenone.

During elimination, propafenone is metabolized to an electrophysiologically active metabolite, 5-hydroxypropafenone.[206] The overall cellular electrophysiologic effects of 5-hydroxypropafenone resemble those of its parent drug.[215] However, the two differ in relative magnitude of effect on the sodium and calcium channels, as well as in their β-blocking actions. Philipsborn et al have demonstrated that the antagonistic effect of 5-hydroxypropafenone on cardiac conduction and calcium activity was more marked than that of propafenone.[215] Despite this difference, the antiadrenergic effects of propafenone were observed to exceed those of 5-hydroxyproprafenone.

Clinical Electrophysiologic Effects

Similar to the other type IC local anesthetic agents, propafenone slows conduction throughout the heart—atrium, AV node, His-Purkinje system, and ventricular myocardium.[216] His bundle electrophysiologic investigations have noted increases in the HRA-LRA conduction time, AH and HV intervals, and QRS duration. Shortly following intravenous administration, sinus heart rate may be observed to increase (a vagolytic effect). In individuals with normal sinus node function, propafenone has a variable effect on the sinus node response to rapid atrial pacing (either no change or an increase in the maximum corrected sinus node recovery time). Sinoatrial conduction time is usually increased. In subjects with sinus node dysfunction, propafenone usually decreases the spontaneous heart rate and prolongs both the corrected sinus node recovery time and sinoatrial conduction time.[217] Propafenone has been reported to produce sinoatrial exit block and long sinus pauses in patients with sick sinus syndrome. Propafenone slows conduction through the AV node and prolongs the Wenckebach cycle length. The development of bundle-branch block has been described in patients with preexisting His-Purkinje conduction abnormalities. Although the major electrophysiologic effect of propafenone is to slow cardiac conduction, Alboni et al have noted that propafenone can prolong atrial, AV nodal, and ventricular refractoriness.[217]

Several investigators have noted important effects of propafenone on accessory atrioventricular pathways. Breithardt et al observed complete antegrade conduction block in seven of 15 patients with Wolff-Parkinson-White syndrome who were administered propafenone.[218] In those individuals in whom propafenone failed to produce conduction block (usually patients whose accessory pathway ERP $<$ 270 ms), propafenone was still able to significantly prolong the accessory pathway refractoriness. Propafenone is also effective in slowing retrograde accessory pathway conduction and prolonging its refractoriness. Rudolph et al made similar observations in a group of Wolff-Parkinson-White syndrome patients with recurrent supraventricular tachycardia treated with propafenone. They observed complete conduction block in eight of 10 patients with antegrade accessory pathway conduction.[219] Garcia-Civera et al showed that propafenone was very effective in depressing retrograde fast pathway conduction in patients with dual AV nodal pathways.[220]

The reported clinical electrophysiologic effects of propafenone in children and young animals are similar to those described in adults and in cardiac tissues from mature animals.[221, 222] No study to date has made a quantitative developmental comparison. Musto et al investigated the clinical electrophysiologic effects of propafenone in 20 children whose mean age was 9.8 years.[221] They noted that propafenone slowed conduction throughout the heart and prolonged atrial, AV nodal, and ventricular refractoriness. Propafenone was shown to slow spontaneous sinus cycle length. Similar observations were made by Villafane et al during investigation of the electrophysiologic effects of propafenone in young dogs (age 5–11 days).[222]

Electrocardiographic Effects

Electrocardiographic changes are common following propafenone administration. Blood level–related prolongations of the PR interval and QRS duration are the most frequently observed changes.[206] Alterations of the QTc are more variable (either no change or a prolongation). Conduction disturbances and sinus pauses may be noted in subjects with abnormal hearts.

Clinical Pharmacokinetics

Following its oral administration, propafenone is well absorbed (>95%); its maximum plasma concentration occurs 2 to 3 hours after a dose.[206, 223–225] Systemic bioavailability is modest (12% to 50%) and is dose dependent. Propafenone undergoes extensive presystemic clearance. As a result, increases in oral dosage produce nonlinear elevations in maximum plasma concentration. Connolly et al reported that a threefold increase in total daily dosage resulted in a 10-fold increase in peak plasma concentration. They also noted that the overall bioavailability of propafenone increased during chronic oral therapy.[225]

After an intravenous dose, drug effect occurs within 5 minutes, is maintained for 20 minutes, and dissipates after 45 minutes. The half-life of distribution following intravenous administration is 4 minutes. Propafenone is highly protein bound (97%) and has a large apparent volume of distribution (1.9–3.3L/kg).

Propafenone is dependent on hepatic metabolism for its elimination. Less than 1% is excreted unchanged in the urine. Like debrosoquine and encainide, the oxidative metabolism of propafenone is bimodally distributed.[226] Extensive metabolizers are able to oxidatively metabolize propafenone to two metabolites: 5-hydroxypropafenone and a hydroxymethoxy metabolite. The metabolites are further conjugated with glucuronide and sulfate and are then in turn excreted in the stool and urine. The elimination half-life of propafenone is relatively short in extensive metabolizers ($t½ = 4.7 \pm 1.3$ h), and because it does not follow a linear pattern, Kates, Yee, and Winkle could not determine the elimination half-life of 5-hydroxyproprafenone.[227] In contrast, the elimination half-life of propafenone is much longer in subjects who are slow metabolizers ($t½ = 16.8 \pm 10.6$ h). In both groups, the elimination half-life lengthens during chronic treatment.

The clinical importance of 5-hydroxypropafenone in mediating the antiarrhythmic actions of propafenone is unknown but may partially explain the wide variability in plasma concentrations noted to be clinically useful in arrhythmia control.[225] No therapeutic range of plasma concentrations for propafenone has been established to date. Understanding of the clinical pharmacokinetics of propafenone in children is limited.

Dosage

Our experience with propafenone has been restricted to the intravenous preparation. The protocol we have found effective for propafenone loading is to administer 0.2 mg/kg boluses every 10 minutes to a maximum dose of 2 mg/kg. During the loading period, because of the negative inotropic effect of propafenone, 10 mg/kg of colloid solution is usually infused to maintain a stable blood pressure. The usual loading dose required ranges from 1.6 mg/kg to 1.8 mg/kg. Following achievement of a satisfactory response, propafenone loading is suspended, and a continuous infusion of 0.004–0.007 mg/kg/min is instituted.

Dressler et al reported the results of a multicenter European study using chronic oral propafenone therapy to treat a variety of arrhythmias in children.[228] Using a mean dosage of 300 mg/m^2/d, they achieved arrhythmia control in 30 of 35 patients (86%). Propafenone was administered every 8 hours. Musto et al reported a slightly higher arrhythmia control rate (92%) using a mean oral propafenone dosage of 411 ± 84 mg/m^2/d in a group of 20 children.[221]

Adverse Effects

Side effects during oral propafenone treatment are relatively uncommon, particularly in children.[206, 221, 225, 228] The most commonly reported adverse effects involve the central nervous system (blurred vision, weakness, paresthesias, dizziness, and tremor). Gastrointestinal effects include vomiting, abdominal pain, nausea, constipation, bitter taste, and cholestatic hepatitis. Although rare, propafenone can produce a drug-induced SLE syndrome. Cardiovascular side effects are more serious and include congestive heart failure, hypotension, sinus pauses, conduction abnormalities, AV block, and (rarely) exacerbation of ventricular arrhythmias. Often cardiovascular toxicity is unpredictable and not related to plasma drug levels.

Drug Interactions

Two important drug interactions have been reported during propafenone treatment. Propafenone may produce a variable (40% to 100%) elevation of plasma digoxin levels. Cardaioli et al noted no changes in renal clearance of digoxin and proposed that an increase in digoxin bioavailability was the probable mechanism for the increase in plasma digoxin levels.[229] Propafenone may aggravate ventricular arrhythmias in patients being concomitantly treated with amiodarone. The occurrence of torsades de pointes in patients treated with a combination of amiodarone and propafenone has been reported.

Indications

Propafenone has been successfully used in patients with supraventricular and ventricular arrhythmias. Successfully treated supraventricular arrhythmias include atrial flutter, atrial fibrillation, supraventricular tachycardia that utilizes an accessory atrioventricular connection or AV nodal reentry, and postoperative junctional ectopic tachycardia. Propafenone has also been reported to be effective in suppressing simple and complex ventricular ectopy. The role that propafenone may play in the treatment of any specific arrhythmia, particularly in pediatric patients, is still under clinical investigation.

β-Adrenoreceptor Blocking Agents

The past decade has witnessed an explosion in the availability of new β-adrenergic blocking agents. All of these drugs act by antagonizing the actions of the endogenous adrenergic agonists (epinephrine and norepinephrine) at the β-adrenergic receptor. The result of this competitive inhibition of receptor sites is that higher concentrations of endogenous agonists are required in order to induce the same β-adrenergic receptor–mediated response. Although unified as one broad group of agents by their mechanism of action, these drugs are distinguished by important pharmacodynamic differences: adrenoceptor selectivity, membrane stabilizing activity, and intrinsic sympathomimetic activity.

Ahlquist initially classified the adrenergic receptor into two types (α and β) according to the potency of different sympathomimetic amines.[230] Subsequent studies by Lands et al further suggested two types of β-adrenergic receptors.[231] Stimulation of β_1-adrenergic receptors produces inotropic and chronotropic effects on the heart, whereas β_2-adrenergic stimulation causes smooth muscle relaxation along with dilation of the bronchi and of certain vascular beds. Much research has gone into the development of cardioselective β-blockers, but selectivity is concentration dependent. At low doses, cardioselective β-blockers preferentially bind and block β_1-adrenergic receptors more than β_2-adrenergic receptors (Table 3–6). Selective binding to β_1-adrenergic receptor sites, however, disappears at high concentrations. In contrast, the nonselective β-blockers inhibit both β_1- and β_2-adrenergic receptors at similar concentrations.

Early in vitro studies suggested that at concentrations of propranolol above those associated with β-blockade, additional electrophysiologic effects (not β-adrenergic receptor–mediated) were evident. High concentrations of propranolol (also recently observed with several of the newer β-blocking agents) have been noted to decrease action potential $\dot{V}max$ without having any effect on membrane potential.[232–234] This local anesthetic effect (i.e., membrane stabilizing activity) results from a reduction in sodium influx through its membrane channel, thereby decreasing cardiac excitability and conduction. Recent data suggest that membrane stabilizing activity may be an important mechanism by which β-blockers exert their antiarrhythmic effects in certain patients.[235]

TABLE 3–6
PHARMACODYNAMIC PROPERTIES OF BETA BLOCKERS*

	SELECTIVITY FOR β_1-RECEPTORS	MEMBRANE STABILIZING ACTIVITY	ISA
Atenonol	+	0	0
Metoprolol	+	0	0
Nadolol	0	0	0
Propranolol	0	+	0

* + = present; 0 = absent; ISA = intrinsic sympathomimetic activity.

Intrinsic sympathomimetic activity (ISA) refers to the ability of certain β-blocking drugs (see Table 3–6) not only to combine with the β-adrenoceptor site to inhibit the action of endogenous agonists (when present in high concentration), but also to stimulate the receptor activation site when endogenous agonist concentration is low.[236] Under conditions of low sympathetic activity, β-blockers with ISA bind with the β-adrenergic receptor and stimulate its activity, therefore acting as a partial agonist. However, they are unable to stimulate receptor activity to the same extent as full agonists. Intrinsic sympathomimetic activity appears to balance the direct negative pharmacologic actions of β-blocking agents on cardiac rate and contractility.

Since its introduction in 1964, propranolol remains the most widely prescribed β-blocking agent in the treatment of arrhythmias. However, recent reports of central nervous system side effects and compliance problems with frequent administration of propranolol have popularized the use of atenolol and nadolol. This section will detail the pharmacology of propranolol and highlight certain facets of the pharmacokinetics and pharmacodynamics by which atenolol and nadolol differ from propranolol (Table 3–7). Because of its recent clinical availability and unexplored use in children, the new ultrashort-acting β-blocking agent, esmolol, will only be briefly discussed.

PROPRANOLOL

Cellular Electrophysiologic Effects

Propranolol modifies cellular electrophysiologic properties through two different

TABLE 3–7
PHARMACOKINETIC PROPERTIES OF β-BLOCKERS

	ABSORPTION (%)	BIOAVAIL-ABILITY (%)	PROTEIN BINDING (%)	HALF-LIFE (hrs)	METABOLISM	URINARY EXCRETION UNCHANGED (%)
Atenolol	45–60	55	<55	6–7	Minimal	85–100
Metoprolol	>.95	50	12	3–4	Extensive	<5
Nadolol	15–25	20	25–30	12–24	Minimal	70
Propranolol	100	33	90	4–6	Extensive	<1

mechanisms.[232–234] At low concentrations (<100 ng/mL), the electrophysiologic action of propranolol is to competitively inhibit catecholamine binding at β_1- and β_2- (nonselective) adrenoreceptor sites, an effect almost entirely the result of its levorotatary stereoisomer. At high concentrations (3000 ng/mL) propranolol can decrease action potential amplitude, $\dot{V}$max, and membrane responsiveness. Propranolol significantly alters sinus and AV nodal electrophysiology.[232] Propranolol usually decreases the slope of phase 4 depolarization and subsequently the spontaneous cycle length of sinus node automaticity. Through its weak calcium channel blocking properties, propranolol at high concentrations may depress sinus and AV nodal action potential amplitude and $\dot{V}$max, thereby slowing sinoatrial and AV nodal conduction. AV nodal refractoriness becomes prolonged. Propranolol has little effect on healthy atrial cells.

In Purkinje fibers displaying fast response action potentials, low concentrations of propranolol decrease APD and automatic rate with no significant effect on other membrane parameters.[232–234] Acceleration of repolarization is most marked in areas of the ventricular conduction system in which action potential duration is the longest. The reduction in refractory period is not as great as the reduction in APD (ERP/APD >1). Through its sodium channel blocking effects, propranolol at high concentrations will decrease action potential AMP and $\dot{V}$max. In ventricular myocardium, propranolol has little effect in low concentrations, but exposure to high concentrations decreases action potential AMP, $\dot{V}$max, and membrane potential and shortens APD slightly. Long-term administration of propranolol lengthens APD.[237]

In depressed, partially depolarized cardiac tissues, the actions of propranolol are enhanced.[232–234] Depressed fast response action potentials are more sensitive to the membrane-depressant effects of propranolol, especially if catecholamines are facilitating inward membrane currents. Spinelli et al have demonstrated significant age-related changes in sensitivity of Purkinje fiber automaticity to propranolol.[238] In both adult and neonatal Purkinje fibers, propranolol produced a dose-dependent decrease in spontaneous automaticity; however, neonatal Purkinje fiber automaticity exhibited a five-fold greater sensitivity to propranolol.

Clinical Electrophysiologic Effects

Propranolol slows sinus heart rate in a dose-dependent manner.[239, 240] Severe sinus bradycardia may result if the heart is particularly dependent on sympathetic tone or if sinus node dysfunction is present. Yabek, Berman, and Dillon observed that propranolol increased the maximum corrected sinus node recovery time and had little effect on sinoatrial conduction in children.[239] In contrast, studies by Vasquez et al in adult patients with normal sinus node function showed that propranolol can prolong both the corrected sinus node recovery time and the sinoatrial conduction time.[240] Propranolol will also slow AV nodal conduction and prolong its refractoriness, as evidenced by prolongation of the AH interval, the AV nodal Wenckebach cycle length, and the AV nodal effective refractory period.[241] Propranolol has little effect on atrial, His-Purkinje, or ventricular muscle conduction or refractoriness. Denes et al could not demonstrate any effect of propranolol on accessory atrioventricular pathways.[242] β-blockers have also been shown to raise the ventricular fibrillation threshold.[243]

Electrocardiographic Effects

Treatment with propranolol usually alters the surface electrocardiogram.[232–234] Depression of sinus heart rate and prolongation of the PR interval are the most common changes. Shortening of the corrected QT interval may also be noted.

Clinical Pharmacokinetics

Bioavailability of orally administered propranolol is limited because of its high degree of hepatic extraction and clearance.[244–247] Consequently, larger oral doses must be given to achieve a plasma concentration equivalent to that attained by intravenous dosing. During the attainment of a steady state after multiple oral doses, bioavailability increases secondary to a 65% reduction in hepatic extraction. Saturation of hepatic tissue receptor sites is thought to explain the changes in systemic availability (see Tables 3–6 and 3–7).

Propranolol is almost entirely metabolized by the liver to a pharmacologically active metabolite (4-hydroxypropranolol).[244] Reduction in hepatic blood flow (such as occurs in congestive heart failure, low cardiac output, or liver disease) decreases hepatic extraction of propranolol. Riopel and Walle demonstrated a relationship between hemoglobin concentration (i.e., degree of polycythemia) and plasma propranolol levels in a group of children with cyanotic congenital heart disease.[247] Hyperviscosity and reduced hepatic blood flow were suggested as the mechanisms for reduced clearance (prolonged half-life). Less than 1% of propranolol is excreted unchanged in the urine. However, during renal failure, significant alterations in propranolol pharmacokinetics occur, requiring dosage adjustment. Drug metabolites accumulate, and higher plasma propranolol levels are observed (decreased first-pass elimination effect).

A wide variation in plasma levels (as much as a 20-fold difference) has been observed in patients given the same oral dose of propranolol.[244] The high degree of hepatic extraction undoubtedly is one cause. The therapeutic range of propranolol concentrations in the treatment of arrhythmias has not been clearly defined. Plasma levels of 25–150 ng/mL are required for physiologic β-receptor blockade. However, Woosley et al found that 40% of patients who responded to treatment with propranolol for ventricular arrhythmias required plasma levels between 150 ng/mL and 1000 ng/mL.[248] Differences in pharmacologic response to high plasma propranolol concentrations have similarly been noted by Duff, Mitchell, and Wyse.[235]

Propranolol is highly protein bound (90% to 95%) and is widely distributed (3.6 L/kg).[244] Its distribution half-life following intravenous administration is 10 minutes. The elimination half-life is longer following oral administration (3.2 h) than following intravenous injection (2.3 h). The elimination half-life of 4-hydroxypropranolol (the major metabolite) is longer than the parent compound (5.2–7.5 h). Under normal circumstances, propranolol is completely eliminated within 36–48 hours.

Few data are available on the pharmacokinetics of propranolol during childhood. During the neonatal period, protein binding is diminished (68%, compared to 90% to 95% in adults). The volume of distribution of propranolol is increased in this age group, as is its elimination half-life. In contrast, Riopel and Walle found that the elimination half-life of propranolol in a group of children aged 9 months to 6 years did not significantly differ from that reported in adults.[247]

Propranolol easily crosses the human placenta.[249] Cord blood levels approximate maternal plasma concentrations, thereby explaining recent reports of adverse fetal effects. Propranolol is also excreted into breast milk.[250] Peak concentrations occur 2–3 hours after an oral dose. Since levels in breast milk are only 64% of maternal plasma concentrations, the nursing infant is unlikely to be administered quantities of propranolol significant enough to have a pharmacologic effect.

Wilson, Atwood, and Shand have studied the bioavailability of two different pharmaceutical formulations of propranolol (oral solution and tablet) in children.[251] Both had similar bioavailability and produced similar peak plasma concentrations. As expected, peak plasma concentrations occurred earlier with the oral solution (2 h) compared with the tablet preparation (3 h). Propranolol is also available in a long-acting formulation. Kubik, Gill, and Dawes found the long-acting preparation as effective as the conventional formulation in suppressing ventricular arrhythmias in adult patients.[252] Both produced similar plasma concentrations, suggesting that, by improving patient compliance, the long-acting formulation may be more therapeutically useful.

Dosage

The currently recommended starting dosage of propranolol is 2 mg/kg/d, divided into four doses. Shand, Nuckolls, and Oates, as well as Riopel and Walle, found administration of propranolol in a dosage ≤1.8 mg/kg/d produced very low propranolol plasma levels (<25 ng/mL).[246, 247] In contrast, high propranolol blood levels may be required for arrhythmia suppression in some children. Both Gillette et al and Pickoff et al have cautiously administered propranolol in dosages of up to 14 mg/kg/d in selected patients resistant to therapy at lower dosages.[253, 254] Because of the high incidence of adverse effects, we generally recommend alternative therapy if dosages of 5 mg/kg/d are ineffective. Long-acting formulations of propranolol may provide effective therapy for some children. Although these preparations have not been studied, we anticipate that they would have to be administered twice daily in children because of the enhanced hepatic biotransforming capacity in this age group.

Adverse Effects

Adverse effects from propranolol therapy are usually cardiovascular in origin and include hypotension, bradycardia, and congestive heart failure. Bradycardia may be caused by sinus bradycardia or AV block. Propranolol may precipitate congestive heart failure in patients with compromised cardiac function.

Several noncardiac side effects are also significant. Propranolol may increase the risk of hypoglycemia in insulin-dependent patients or in normal patients during fasting. Bronchospasm may be induced, particularly in asthmatic patients. Propranolol has also been reported to produce significant central nervous system side effects (fatigue; disturbing, vivid dreams; insomnia; depression; proximal muscle myopathy; and impaired psychomotor performance).[255]

Drug Interactions

Concurrent administration of propranolol with several other drugs has been demonstrated to significantly alter the pharmacokinetics of propranolol.[9, 244] Cimetidine has been reported to increase propranolol blood levels through a reduction in the clearance of propranolol. Cimetidine has been shown to decrease hepatic blood flow, thus prolonging the clearance of a number of agents that are primarily biotransformed in the liver. By reducing extracellular fluid, simultaneous administration of propranolol with furosemide results in elevated plasma concentrations of propranolol and augmentation of its β-adrenergic blocking actions. Concurrent treatment with propranolol and a calcium channel antagonist is contraindicated, because of synergism in their negative inotropic effects on myocardial contractility. Their combined use frequently results in hypotension and cardiovascular collapse.

Indications

As an antiarrhythmic drug, propranolol is effective in the treatment of many supraventricular and ventricular arrhythmias. Propranolol may be employed to decrease the rate of persistent sinus tachycardia that results from thyrotoxicosis or pheochromocytoma. Propranolol usually does not convert atrial flutter or atrial fibrillation to sinus rhythm, but it may be used to decrease the ventricular rate during these arrhythmias. For reentrant supraventricular tachycardias that use the AV node as one of the reentrant pathways (AV node reentry or reciprocating AV tachycardia), propranolol may acutely terminate the tachycardia and provide long-term prophylaxis against arrhythmia recurrence. Propranolol may be effective in other atrial arrhythmias such as sinus node reentry tachycardia and digitalis-induced paroxysmal atrial tachycardia. Propranolol can also be used successfully to treat ventricular arrhythmias. It is particularly effective in patients with mitral valve prolapse, congenital prolonged QT interval syndrome, and catecholamine-sensitive ventricular arrhythmias.

ATENOLOL

Atenolol is a cardioselective β-blocker with favorable pharmacokinetic properties; it may be administered once daily. It differs pharmacodynamically from propranolol in its relative selectivity in blocking β_1-adrenergic receptors, thereby lessening the risk of bronchospasm in susceptible patients and avoiding blood glucose control problems in insulin-dependent diabetics, and hypotension caused by its vascular spacing effects. Atenolol lacks any intrinsic sympathomimetic activity and membrane stabilizing activity (see Table 3–6).[256]

Cellular Electrophysiologic Effects

Similar to propranolol at low concentrations, atenolol competitively inhibits catecholamine-mediated effects. At high concentrations, atenolol lacks any local anesthetic actions or the ability to depress action potential amplitude and V̇max.

Clinical Electrophysiologic Effects

Subtle differences in the clinical electrophysiologic effects of propranolol and atenolol are apparent.[257] When the two are given in equipotent β-blocking doses, depression of sinus heart rate is less during atenolol administration than during propranolol administration. Shimotori, Kobayashi, and Chiba thought this reflected atenolol's lack of membrane stabilizing activity.[258] Atenolol impairs sinus and AV nodal function to a greater extent than do β-adrenergic blocking agents that exhibit partial agonist activity (ISA). Atenolol can prolong atrial refractoriness and, like propranolol, has no effect on His-Purkinje conduction.

Clinical Pharmacokinetics

Atenolol is rapidly absorbed from the gastrointestinal tract, with peak levels appearing between 2 and 3 hours.[259] Bioavailability varies from 45% to 55%. Unlike propranolol, atenolol undergoes little hepatic extraction (<10%) and is widely distributed in the body. Less than 5% is bound to serum proteins. Most of the absorbed fraction of atenolol is excreted unchanged in the urine. The half-life of atenolol varies from 5–9 hours in normal subjects but is markedly increased during renal failure. Accumulation occurs in patients with impaired renal function, suggesting the need for dosage adjustment during renal failure.[260] Excretion in healthy subjects is complete approximately 48 hours after administration of the last dose. Metabolism of atenolol is minimal, and there are no pharmacologically active metabolites. Little correlation exists between plasma levels and the pharmacologic action of atenolol (see Tables 3–6 and 3–7).

Atenolol readily crosses the placenta.[261] At birth, cord blood and maternal plasma concentrations are equal. Elimination of atenolol is markedly decreased in the neonate (half-life in the neonate, 16 h; half-life in adults, 6–9 h). Atenolol is also excreted into breast milk. No data is currently available regarding the pharmacokinetics of atenolol in older children.

Dosage

Atenolol is as effective as propanolol in its β-blocking effects. However, few data are available from which to make dosage recommendations. We initiate therapy with 1 mg/kg/d; if ineffective, the dosage is increased to 2 mg/kg/d. Once-daily administration is generally effective, but on rare occasions we have administered atenolol in two divided doses.

Adverse Effects

The cardiovascular adverse effects are not unlike those of propranolol. Atenolol differs significantly from propranolol in its lower incidence of respiratory complications (bronchoconstriction) and central nervous system side effects. Of all currently marketed β-blockers, atenolol has the lowest concentration in human brain tissue.[262]

Drug Interactions

Unlike propranolol, atenolol does not decrease hepatic metabolism of lidocaine.

NADOLOL

Nadolol, like propranolol, is a nonselective β-adrenergic blocking agent. However, it has several pharmacokinetic advantages over propranolol. It may be administered once daily (similar to atenolol) and causes fewer central nervous system side effects. Like atenolol, nadolol lacks partial agonist activity (ISA) and membrane stabilizing effects.[263]

Cellular and Clinical Electrophysiologic Effects

The cellular and clinical pharmacologic actions of nadolol mimic atenolol, with the exception of its cardioselectivity. Nadolol exhibits no preferential effect on either of the β-adrenergic receptor subtypes. Chronic nadolol administration, like chronic propranolol administration, results in prolongation of atrial and ventricular muscle action potential duration and refractoriness. From a developmental perspective, neonatal animals appear to be more sensitive to the β-blocking effects of nadolol, not unlike studies using propranolol.[264]

Clinical Pharmacokinetics

Nadolol is poorly absorbed from the gastrointestinal tract (30%), but to its advantage, it is not metabolized prior to systemic availability (first-pass effect).[244] Peak levels occur 3–4 hours after oral administration. Concurrent ingestion with food does not affect the rate or extent of absorption. Only 20% to 30% is bound to serum proteins. Nadolol is primarily eliminated by renal excretion; less than 30% is metabolized. As a result, no pharmacologically active metabolites have been identified. The elimination half-life of nadolol ranges from 20 to 24 hours, and thus it can be administered once daily. Dosage adjustment is required during compromised renal function (see Tables 3–6 and 3–7).

Dosage

In its β-blocking effects, nadolol is approximately 50% less potent than propranolol. However, clinical studies by Escoubet et al have suggested that nadolol may be as much as 10 times more potent than propranolol when assessed by its effects on resting spontaneous sinus heart rate.[257] We therefore recommend initiating therapy with 1.0–2.0 mg/kg/d. When a steady state has been achieved (approximately 5 days), the dosage can be adjusted upward or downward as clinically indicated.

Adverse Effects

Like atenolol, only minimal amounts of nadolol gain access to the brain, thereby making the incidence of central nervous system side effects low.

ESMOLOL

Recently released for clinical usage, the ultrashort-acting β-blocker, esmolol, is effective in the acute management of tachyarrhythmias. For the emergency treatment of a hemodynamically compromising arrhythmia, an ideal β-blocking agent should have a rapid onset of effect, an easily titratable dosing regimen, and a short duration of action to allow prompt recovery from adverse effects.

Cellular Electrophysiologic Effects

Esmolol is a cardioselective β_1-adrenergic blocker that has minimal partial agonist activity and membrane stabilizing effects (only at high concentrations ($\geq 10^{-4}$ mol/L).[265]

Clinical Electrophysiologic Effects

The major pharmacologic action of esmolol is on sinus and AV nodal function.[265] Esmolol can prolong the spontaneous sinus cycle length and corrected sinus node recovery time. Depression of AV nodal conduction (prolongation of the AH interval and Wenckebach cycle length) is its most prominent effect. No effects are evident on atrial, His-Purkinje, or ventricular muscle conduction and refractoriness.

Clinical Pharmacokinetics

For clinical usage, esmolol is administered intravenously. It has a rapid distribution half-life (2 minutes) and an elimination half-life of 9 minutes.[266] Metabolism is predominantly blood based, chiefly by erythrocyte esterases. The hydrolysis of esmolol results in the formation of an acid metabolite that is only 0.003% as potent. Less than 2% is excreted unchanged in the urine. Unlike propranolol, alteration of hepatic blood flow does not change the metabolism of esmolol. Esmolol is moderately protein bound (55%). Blood levels of esmolol are not detectable 30 minutes after discontinuation of an infusion. No data regarding its pharmacokinetics in children exist (see Tables 3–6 and 3–7).

Dosage

Esmolol is best administered as a series of progressive titration steps, with each step including a 1-minute loading infusion.[267] Therapy is initiated with a loading dose of 500 μg/kg/min for 1 minute, followed by a maintenance infusion of 50 μg/kg/min. If arrhythmia control is unsatisfactory after 4 minutes, a second loading dose is administered, and the maintenance infusion rate is increased to 100 μg/kg/min. This sequence of administering a loading infusion (500 μg/kg/min for 1 minute) and then increasing the maintenance infusion rate is repeated until either the arrhythmia is controlled or the maintenance infusion rate equals 200 μg/kg/min.

Adverse Effects

A transient decrease in systemic blood pressure is the most frequent side effect (up to 44% of patients) of esmolol therapy.[267] Central nervous system side effects (somnolence, agitation, headache, dizziness, and confusion) are the next most common. Nausea and vomiting occur in 16% of patients. Respiratory tract symptoms, suggestive of bronchoconstriction, are rare.

Drug Interactions

Digoxin, morphine, and warfarin each produce well-documented interactions with esmolol when administered concomitantly.[266] Esmolol may increase plasma digoxin levels by 10% to 19%. Both morphine and warfarin have been demonstrated to increase plasma esmolol levels, suggesting the need to administer esmolol at a lower maintenance infusion rate for patients requiring a combination of these drugs.

Indications

Esmolol is very effective in acute reduction of ventricular rate during atrial tachyarrhythmias (atrial fibrillation, atrial flutter, or automatic atrial tachycardia). The one notable exception is atrial fibrillation associated with Wolff-Parkinson-White syndrome; esmolol has no effect on accessory pathway conduction or refractory properties.

Agents That Primarily Prolong Cardiac Refractoriness

AMIODARONE

Amiodarone, a benzofuran derivative, was initially developed and marketed as an antianginal agent.[268] More recently, it has been employed successfully as an antiarrhythmic drug to treat both supraventricular and ventricular tachyarrhythmias. Based on in vitro studies, it has been categorized as a class III agent; its major action is to prolong action potential duration and cardiac refractoriness.

Cellular Electrophysiologic Effects

Amiodarone exerts several electrophysiologic effects. It was originally thought that the pharmacologic action of amiodarone was solely to prolong repolarization and refractoriness in all cardiac tissues (sinus node, atrium, AV node, His-Purkinje system, and ventricle). However, recent studies have demonstrated that amiodarone can block sodium channels, thereby depressing cardiac conduction in atrial and ventricular myocardium, as well as in the specialized His-Purkinje conduction fibers.[269, 270] Slowing of conduction is more marked at rapid rates of stimulation.[271]

In the sinus node, amiodarone predominantly decreases the slope of phase 4 depolarization and prolongs action potential duration, thus slowing spontaneous automaticity.[272] Action potential amplitude and $\dot{V}max$ are also decreased, probably through inhibition of calcium channel currents. Studies by Nishimura et al have demonstrated that amiodarone can block the calcium current in isolated guinea pig ventricular muscle cells.[273] Amiodarone prolongs AV nodal repolarization and refractoriness, in addition to slowing conduction through the AV node. Talajic, DeRoode, and Nattel found that amiodarone depressed AV nodal conduction most at fast rates of stimulation.[274]

Refractoriness is significantly lengthened

by amiodarone.[275] Neliat et al observed that amiodarone could inhibit the delayed outward potassium current as well as delay reactivation of the fast sodium current.[276] These actions probably underlie the ability of amiodarone to prolong repolarization and refractoriness. As in the sinus node, amiodarone will decrease His-Purkinje fiber automaticity. At slow rates of stimulation, amiodarone has no effect on membrane potential, action potential amplitude, or $\dot{V}max$.[270] However, at rapid stimulation frequencies, amiodarone will decrease $\dot{V}max$ and slow cardiac conduction. Detailed investigation by Mason, Hondegheim, and Katzung has revealed that amiodarone blocks cardiac sodium channels that are in an inactivated state (i.e., during phase 2 and part of phase 3 of the action potential).[269] Thus amiodarone depresses cardiac conduction more in depolarized tissue (more sodium channels exist in the inactivated state), in tissue with a brief diastolic period (as during tachycardia), and in tissue with long action potential durations (e.g., Purkinje fibers). Amiodarone has only minor effects on cardiac conduction during bradycardia, in fully polarized tissue, and in muscle with short action potential durations (atrial myocardium).

Amiodarone exerts several other important antiarrhythmic actions. It has been shown to block noncompetitively both α- and β-adrenergic receptors.[268] Amiodarone also inhibits the release of neurotransmitters from presynaptic adrenergic neurons. Ohta et al found that amiodarone is effective in decreasing delayed afterdepolarization amplitude and suppressing triggered automaticity.[277]

Significant age-related pharmacodynamic differences in response to amiodarone have been noted. Yabek, Kato, and Singh studied the acute electrophysiologic effects of amiodarone on neonatal and adult Purkinje and ventricular muscle cells.[270] Amiodarone had no effect on canine neonatal ventricular cells at concentrations that prolonged APD and refractoriness in ventricular muscle from adult dogs. Acute exposure to amiodarone shortened APD in Purkinje fibers from both adult and neonatal animals, with the effect being greater in the immature age group. Using an intact canine model, Pickoff et al also evaluated age-related differences in electrophysiologic responsiveness to amiodarone.[278] Amiodarone depressed sinus node automaticity and prolonged atrial refractoriness to a much greater extent in the younger age group. However, the opposite was true for the AV node. When administered in a similar dosage, amiodarone prolonged AV nodal conduction time (AH interval) and Wenckebach cycle length significantly more in the adult age group. Collectively, these results suggest that different regions of the heart have variable developmental sensitivity to the pharmacologic action of amiodarone.

Clinical Electrophysiologic Effects

Most of the electrophysiologic effects of amiodarone identified in vitro have been demonstrated clinically.[268, 271, 275] Following long-term administration, amiodarone has been found to depress spontaneous sinus node automaticity and prolong both the sinus node recovery time response to rapid pacing and the sinoatrial conduction time. Marked sinus bradycardia can occur in individuals with sinus node dysfunction. Conduction in the atrium is slowed (i.e., prolonged HRA-LRA conduction time). Amiodarone increases the AH interval and paced cycle length maintaining 1:1 AV nodal conduction, and prolongs AV nodal refractoriness. Prolongation of the HV interval is usually minor, but may be marked in patients with preexisting conduction system disease. Infra-Hissian block has been observed on rare occasions. Wellens et al found that amiodarone prolonged refractoriness in accessory AV pathways in the antegrade direction in virtually all patients with Wolff-Parkinson-White syndrome, whereas the effective refractory period in the retrograde direction was lengthened in only 50% of patients.[279]

Amiodarone has an antifibrillatory effect when studied using models of myocardial ischemia.[280] It can also elevate the defibrillation threshold and make cardioversion/defibrillation more difficult. Little change occurs in atrial or ventricular pacing thresholds.

The development of the electrophysiologic effects of amiodarone are time- and cardiac tissue-dependent. Following acute intravenous administration, slowing of AV nodal conduction and prolongation of refractoriness are the only evident changes. Several days to several weeks of administration are required before atrial and ventricular refractoriness lengthen.[281] Singh and Vaugh Williams studied the evolution of the cellular electrophysiologic changes that occur in rabbits in response to intraperitoneal administration of amiodarone.[282] After 1 week of treatment, ventricular muscle action potential duration increased 11%; after 3 weeks, it lengthened 23%; and after 6 weeks, APD was prolonged 30%. A similar time course has been observed in the clinical setting. Tuna et al examined the temporal onset of electrophysiologic effects following chronic oral administration of amiodarone in a canine model. The maximum effect of amiodarone on refractoriness occurred earlier in the right atrium than in the right ventricle (3 days vs 12 days).[283]

Electrocardiographic Effects

Electrocardiographic effects of amiodarone include reduction in heart rate and prolongation of the PR, QRS, and corrected QT intervals.[268] T wave amplitude may decrease, and prominent U waves may develop.

Clinical Pharmacokinetics

Despite its high lipid solubility, oral absorption of amiodarone is slow and variable (22% to 95%).[268, 284, 285] Peak plasma concentrations occur 3 to 7 hours after a dose. Erratic absorption is thought to result from either gastrointestinal or hepatic metabolism. Once absorbed, amiodarone has a large volume of distribution (0.9–148 L/kg) and accumulates extensively in muscle, liver, subcutaneous fat, lung, and skin tissues. Unlike most other antiarrhythmic drugs, the distribution and elimination of amiodarone can best be characterized by a three-compartment model: a central compartment, a peripheral compartment formed by well perfused organs, and a deep compartment of poorly perfused tissues with a high affinity for lipid-soluble compounds (equilibration is reached within several weeks to months).

Amiodarone is predominantly metabolized in the liver to its major metabolite, desethylamiodarone.[285] Desethylamiodarone can accumulate to a greater extent than its parent compound and has significant electrophysiologic effects. The electrophysiologic effects of desethylamiodarone on cardiac conduction and refractoriness may be substantially greater than those of amiodarone, although this is controversial. In vitro, Yabek, Kato, and Singh found desethylamiodarone to have less effect than amiodarone on $\dot{V}max$ and ventricular refractoriness.[270] However, Talajic, DeRoode, and Nattel demonstrated in anesthetized dogs that desethylamiodarone produced larger increases in QRS duration and in atrial and ventricular refractoriness than did amiodarone.[274] Significant amounts of amiodarone can be found in bile. Renal elimination of both amiodarone and desethylamiodarone is negligible. In plasma, amiodarone is highly protein bound (96%).

After long-term therapy, amiodarone persists in the body, with the terminal elimination half-life estimated to be from 8 to 107 days. During drug withdrawal, elimination from the plasma is biphasic. In the first 10 days after cessation of therapy, plasma concentrations are halved. However, 12 to 21 days after termination of therapy, plasma concentrations rebound. Measurable plasma levels of amiodarone and desethylamiodarone may be detected for as long as 9 months after cessation of therapy.

The effects of liver disease, renal failure, or congestive heart failure on the pharmacokinetics of amiodarone have not been studied. Data applicable to children are scant. Observations by Coumel and Fidelle suggest that the onset of amiodarone effect in children may occur within a few hours of oral administration.[286] Full effect occurs after 4 days of therapy, in contrast to the 7- to 10-day period observed in adult patients. Following withdrawal of treatment, arrhythmias relapse earlier in children than in adults (3 weeks vs several months).

The lower limit of the therapeutic range has been estimated, on the basis of symptomatic arrhythmia recurrence after amiodarone withdrawal, to be 1.0 μg/mL.[268] Establishment of a safe upper limit has been more difficult. Many investigators have been unable to find an association between plasma levels and therapeutic effectiveness. Adverse reactions are more common when plasma concentrations exceed 2.5 μg/mL. Nademanee et al have found the monitoring of reverse T_3 levels helpful in guiding dosage.[287] Serious adverse effects occurred with marked elevations of reverse T_3 levels (>110 ng/mL). In our experience, reverse T_3 levels exceeding 90 ng/mL are frequently related to symptomatic side effects.[288]

Intravenous administration of amiodarone results in a rapid onset effect (1–30 min) that persists for 1 to 3 hours. Antiarrhythmic efficacy is delayed with oral usage. Loading doses are therefore required to quicken antiarrhythmic activity.

Amiodarone has been demonstrated to cross the human placenta.[289] Fetal cord blood levels are 10% to 25% of maternal plasma levels. Amiodarone is also excreted into breast milk, where its concentration exceeds maternal plasma levels. Because the total amount ingested is low (1.5 mg/kg/d) breast feeding is not contraindicated.

Dosage

Amiodarone is initially given in a loading dosage of 10 mg/kg/d (5 mg/kg twice daily) for 10 days. The dose is subsequently decreased to 5 mg/kg once per day and continued for 1 to 2 months. If there is no arrhythmia recurrence, dosage can be decreased every 4 to 6 months to a minimal dosage of 2.5 mg/kg/d. If the arrhythmia recurs, or if it did not respond during the initial 10-day loading period, the long-term dose may be increased to 10–15 mg/kg/d. Some investigators have used initial loading doses of up to 60 mg/kg/d for shorter time periods (3 to 5 days).

Intravenous amiodarone has been used on occasion in the management of refractory life-threatening ventricular tachyarrhythmias. Marked hypotension and depression of cardiac contractility can occur following too rapid intravenous administration, particularly in patients with preexisting abnormalities in cardiac function. Intravenous amiodarone should be given in a dosage of 5 mg/kg over a 15- to 30-minute period. This dosage can be repeated 15 minutes later if satisfactory arrhythmia control has not been achieved. After the loading dose has been given, a maintenance infusion can be started (10–20 mg/kg/d).

Adverse Effects

Side effects are very common in adult patients treated with amiodarone (Table 3–8).[268, 284] The reported overall incidence of side effects has been as high as 93%, with serious side effects occurring in up to 26% of patients. Our experience to date suggests that adverse effects are less common in children and young adults (30%).[288] None of our patients younger than 10 years of age have had side effects. Amiodarone-induced corneal microdeposits is the most common side effect (18%), but usually causes no symptoms. Dermatologic side effects, the next most common, have included skin rash and slate gray pigmentation in sun-exposed areas. Headache, nausea, and paresthesias have only rarely been reported by our patients. Biochemical changes in thyroid function tests have been common, but treatment for hypo- or hyperthyroidism is rare. No pulmonary toxicity has occurred (see Table 3–8).

TABLE 3–8
AMIODARONE-INDUCED SIDE EFFECTS

Ocular	*Endocrine*
Corneal microdeposits	Hypo- and hyperthyroidism
Halo vision	Parotid swelling
Xerophthalmia	
Photophobia	
Macular degeneration	*Cutaneous*
	Rash
Gastrointestinal	Photosensitivity
Nausea	Hyperkeratosis
Constipation	Pruritis
Anorexia	Hair loss
Ageusia	Erythema nodosum
Elevated transaminases	
	Pulmonary
Neurologic	Interstitial pneumonitis
Sleep disturbances	Chronic cough
Tremor	
Paresthesias	*Renal*
Myopathy	Renal dysfunction
Neuropathy	
Headache	*Cardiovascular*
Vertigo	Hypotension
Ataxia	Worsening CHF
Myoclonus	Bradycardia
Depression	AV block
Fatigue	Proarrhythmia
Restless legs syndrome	
	Miscellaneous
	Epididymitis

In a collective review of 215 children treated with amiodarone, Dick and Scott found a 16% overall incidence of adverse effects.[290] Amiodarone-induced keratopathy was the most frequent side effect (6.5%), followed by skin rash (3%). Amiodarone-induced hepatic failure has been reported (0.5%). Neurologic symptoms (alterations in behavior, nightmares, personality changes, or suicide attempts) have occurred in 3% of patients. Hypothyroidism requiring treatment occurred in 2% of the patients, most commonly in younger children (3 months to 41 months old) who were given high doses of amiodarone.

Like other antiarrhythmic drugs, amiodarone may produce sinus bradycardia or long pauses in patients with sinus node dysfunction. Atrioventricular block may occur in those with conduction system abnormalities (0.7%). Rarely, amiodarone may be proarrhythmic (i.e., may induce torsades de pointes or increase the frequency of supraventricular tachycardia).

Other symptoms, reported to occur in adults but not yet noted in children, are numerous. Both total daily dosage and duration of therapy have been correlated with the frequency of adverse effects in adult patients, suggesting the importance of cumulative dosage in producing side effects. Therefore, to minimize adverse effects, we feel that amiodarone should be used only for refractory arrhythmias, at the lowest effective dosage, and for the shortest period of time possible. With reduction of dosage or cessation of treatment, side effects eventually disappear.

Drug Interactions

Amiodarone has a marked effect on the pharmacokinetics of many commonly used cardiovascular drugs.[291] The most frequent interaction, and one of the best studied, occurs between amiodarone and digoxin. In patients on a stable dosage of digoxin, concurrent therapy with amiodarone will elevate plasma digoxin levels 69% to 100%, usually starting within 24 hours of combined treatment. This interaction with digoxin appears to result from a decrease in its renal and nonrenal clearance, a decrease in volume of distribution, and perhaps from displacement from tissue-binding sites. It is generally recommended that digoxin dosage be decreased by 50% prior to initiating simultaneous therapy with amiodarone. Amiodarone has been demonstrated to interact with other antiarrhythmic drugs, specifically quinidine, procainamide, phenytoin, and flecainide. Plasma levels of these agents usually begin to increase (32% to 100%) within 1 to 5 days of concurrent treatment. The pharmacokinetic bases for these interactions have been less extensively evaluated than those for digoxin. When amiodarone therapy is given concurrently with one of these agents, their dosage should be reduced 30% to 50%.

The interaction of amiodarone with warfarin is also well documented. Patients have been noted to have dramatic increases (78%) in prothrombin times and occasionally to develop bleeding complications. Almong et al have noted a 55% decrease in warfarin clearance.[292] Potentiation of the anticoagulation effect of warfarin begins as early as 4 days after initiating amiodarone therapy. Most investigators suggest a 35% to 65% reduction in warfarin dosage when administered concurrently with amiodarone.

Amiodarone should be used cautiously in combination with β-blockers or calcium channel blockers. A few reports suggest that concurrent treatment may synergistically depress sinus node function or atrioventricular conduction.

Indications

Amiodarone has a broad antiarrhythmic spectrum, making it effective in both automatic and reentry arrhythmias. Amiodarone has been used successfully to treat refractory paroxysmal atrial fibrillation (71% success rate), atrial flutter (95% success rate), ectopic atrial tachycardia, supraventricular tachycardia from either AV nodal reentry or AV reciprocation (78% success rate), and ectopic junctional tachycardia.[268, 288, 290] Furthermore, amiodarone is very effective in controlling ventricular tachycardia resistant to other antiarrhythmic drugs (86% success rate).[284, 288, 290]

BRETYLIUM TOSYLATE

Bretylium tosylate, a quaternary ammonium compound with potent antiarrhythmic and adrenergic blocking actions was developed in the 1950s for the treatment of hypertension.[293] Because of poor absorption and the development of tolerance to its hypotensive action, it proved unsatisfactory for this purpose. Leveque was the first to report on the antiarrhythmic properties of bretylium.[294] A number of subsequent studies have established its role in the treatment of refractory and recurrent ventricular arrhythmias, particularly ventricular fibrillation.

Cellular Electrophysiologic Effects

Bretylium has significant autonomic nervous system effects as well as direct myocardial effects.[293] Bretylium is preferentially taken up by sympathetic ganglia and their postganglionic nerve terminals, where it has a biphasic effect. Although it initially causes norepinephrine release, bretylium prevents further norepinephrine release during sympathetic nerve stimulation without altering the ultrastructural integrity of the adrenergic neuronal vesicles, depressing preganglionic or postganglionic sympathetic nerve transmission, impairing sympathetic ganglionic transmission, depleting the adrenergic terminal of norepinephrine, or diminishing the responsiveness of adrenergic receptors to agonists. Additionally, bretylium impairs the uptake of norepinephrine into the adrenergic nerve terminals and thus potentiates the effect of infused norepinephrine on the adrenergic receptors. The effects of bretylium on the autonomic nervous system are not limited to adrenergic blockade. Schreiber, Friedman, and Sokolovsky have reported that bretylium can competitively inhibit cardiac muscarinic receptors, thereby exerting anticholinergic activity.[295]

The direct electrophysiologic effects of bretylium on isolated cardiac tissues differ from those of the local anesthetic or β-blocking agents previously discussed. In Purkinje fiber and ventricular muscle tissues, bretylium prolongs action potential duration and the effective refractory period without affecting their ratio, similar to the electrophysiologic action of amiodarone.[296, 297] In healthy tissue, therapeutic concentrations of bretylium have no effect on MDP, action potential AMP, $\dot{V}$max, membrane responsiveness, or diastolic excitability. Soon after bretylium exposure, MDP, action potential AMP, $\dot{V}$max, conduction velocity, and spontaneous automaticity may increase, particularly in partially depolarized tissues.[297] These changes may be associated with shortened action potential duration and refractoriness, but these are transient and short-lived. The effect of bretylium on atrial myocardium is more variable.[296, 298] Action potential duration and atrial refractoriness have been reported either to increase or not to change significantly when exposed to bretylium. DeAzevedo, Watanabe, and Dreifus demonstrated in rabbits that bretylium slowed conduction through the atrioventricular node and prolonged nodal refractoriness.[299]

The direct electrophysiologic effects of bretylium on depressed or diseased tissues differ from those just described. Microelectrode studies performed on infarcted canine hearts indicate that bretylium lengthens APD most in Purkinje cells located in the proximal portion of the specialized conduction system of normal myocardium and least in cells located within the infarct region, where APD was already lengthened.[300, 301] This differential effect reduced the disparity in repolarization and refractoriness between normal and infarcted regions. Bretylium had no other significant action on normal fibers, but it improved phase 0 action potential characteristics (action potential AMP, $\dot{V}$max, and conduction velocity) of infarcted Purkinje cells. Fujimoto et al demonstrated that bretylium could significantly alter the conduction of premature ventricular beats in ischemic ventricular myocardium.[300] By delaying conduction of premature impulses into the ischemic region and shortening the conduction delay of impulses out of the ischemic region, bretylium decreased the conduction differences in the ischemic border zone, thus lessening the possibility for unidirectional conduction block. In a Purkinje fiber model of ischemia (superfusion with hypoxic Tyrode's solution), Nishimura and Watanabe reported that bretylium restored action potential characteristics (previously depressed during exposure to hypoxia) to control values.[301]

No reports are currently available assessing age-related influences on the direct in vitro electrophysiologic actions of bretylium.

Clinical Electrophysiologic Effects

Following intravenous administration in humans, the clinical electrophysiologic effects of bretylium resemble those of sympathetic stimulation, suggesting that the indirect electrophysiologic effects of bretylium are predominant.[302] Anderson et al serially studied the clinical electrophysiologic effects of bretylium in a group of patients for a 90-minute period following intravenous administration of bretylium (5 mg/kg).[302] Spontaneous sinus cycle length was observed to shorten. No significant changes were demonstrated in the corrected sinus node recovery time; PA, AH, or HV intervals; or Wenckebach cycle length. Bretylium did, however, shorten the right atrial, AV nodal, and right ventricular effective refractory periods.

Bretylium increases the ventricular fibrillation threshold, probably through its action on sympathetic neurons. Frame and Wang observed in a canine model that when access of bretylium to the adrenergic neuron was prevented (either by antagonism of the presynaptic amine transport pump or by chemical sympathectomy), the antifibrillatory effect of bretylium was absent.[303] Furthermore, when blockade of adrenergic neurotransmission by bretylium was reversed by the administration of *d*-amphetamine, the ventricular fibrillation threshold decreased. Unlike many other antiarrhythmic agents such as lidocaine, bretylium does not increase the energy requirement for defibrillating the heart.[304]

Electrocardiographic Effects

Bretylium usually has little effect on the surface electrocardiogram.[302] Sinus heart rate may be transiently elevated, but no changes in the PR interval, QRS duration, or corrected QT interval are observed.

Clinical Pharmacokinetics

Bretylium is absorbed poorly and erratically from the gastrointestinal tract; peak plasma concentration occurs 1 to 9 hours after a dose.[305–308] Systemic bioavailability ranges between 18% and 27%. Unlike most other antiarrhythmic drugs, the distribution and elimination of bretylium is best demonstrated by a three-compartment model (see discussion on the clinical pharmacokinetics of amiodarone). Bretylium is widely distributed and concentrates in the tissues (V_d = 3.4–8.6 L/kg). The half-life of distribution is rapid, averaging 25 minutes. In the plasma, protein binding is negligible (1% to 8%) and is not concentration dependent.

Bretylium is predominantly eliminated in the urine as unchanged drug (75% to 85% of a dose).[306] Renal excretion occurs by both glomerular filtration and tubular secretion. The renal clearance of bretylium decreases during renal insufficiency, particularly when creatinine clearance is depressed below 30 mL/min/1.73 m^2.[308] Bretylium's half-life of elimination in normal patients and in patients with arrhythmias ranges between 6.3 hours and 13.6 hours. The pharmacokinetics of bretylium in normal subjects does not differ from those in patients with ventricular arrhythmias. During renal failure, the half-life of elimination can be prolonged up to 87.4 hours; therefore the dosage should be reduced in patients with renal insufficiency.[308] Bretylium is insignificantly metabolized, and no clinically active metabolites have been recognized.

Following the intravenous administration of bretylium, electrical cardioversion is facilitated within minutes, but antiarrhythmic effects are often delayed (30 minutes to 2 hours). Monitoring plasma concentration is not helpful during acute treatment (i.e., a therapeutic range has not been defined). The experimental findings of Anderson et al can best explain these two observations. Using a canine model, Anderson et al noted that the direct electrophysiologic and antifibrillatory effects of bretylium paralleled myocardial drug levels and not plasma concentration.[309] They showed that the myocardial concentration of bretylium was slow to increase, peaking 1.5 to 6 hours after intravenous administration. Peak myocardial concentrations occurred at a time when plasma concentrations were low and decreasing.

The risk of the use of bretylium during pregnancy has not been studied, and little is understood of its transplacental passage or excretion in breast milk. In addition, the clinical pharmacokinetics of bretylium in children has not been explored.

Dosage

Bretylium should be given by parenteral administration only. The recommended intravenous dosage is 5–10 mg/kg. During ventricular fibrillation or unstable ventricular tachycardia, bretylium should be infused rapidly. However, to avoid toxicity (hypotension, nausea and vomiting) in patients with stable ventricular tachycardia, bretylium should be diluted in 5% dextrose water and infused slowly over a 10- to 20-minute period. Bretylium dosaging can be repeated 30 minutes to 2 hours later if the arrhythmia persists. The total daily dose should not exceed 30 mg/kg. If a salutary antiarrhythmic effect is observed, bretylium can be continued as a continuous infusion (15–30 μg/kg/min) or by intermittent boluses (5–10 mg/kg every 6 to 8 hours).

Adverse Effects

The major undesirable side effect of parenteral bretylium administration is hypotension secondary to adrenergic blockade, which reduces peripheral vascular resistance.[306] Postural hypotension occurs in 50% to 75% of patients, but hypotension of variable severity may occur even in supine patients. Supine hypotension may be treated with plasma volume expansion or catecholamine infusion. The initial release of norepinephrine caused by bretylium may transiently increase blood pressure, produce symptoms related to catecholamine release (anxiety, excitement, flushing, chest pain, headache), or exacerbate the baseline level of ventricular ectopy (10% to 15% of patients). The rapid intravenous administration of bretylium may cause nausea, vomiting, or diarrhea. Long-term administration has been reported to produce parotitis, nasal stuffiness, and conjunctional suffusion and is not recommended.

Drug Interactions

Three drug interactions should be considered when administering bretylium to treat arrhythmias. Available data suggest an important interaction between quinidine and bretylium. DeAzevido, Watanabe, and Dreifus were the first to demonstrate in vitro that bretylium could reverse the local anesthetic effects of quinidine on atrial and His-Purkinje conduction.[299] Bretylium has been used clinically to effectively terminate quinidine-induced torsades de pointes. However, these two agents can have a synergistic effect in depressing atrioventricular nodal conduction and when administered together can produce a high degree of atrioventricular block.

Bretylium is contraindicated for the treatment of digitalis-induced ventricular arrhythmias. The early transient release of norepinephrine from sympathetic nerve terminals has been experimentally demonstrated to worsen such arrhythmias (see section on digoxin).[293]

Bretylium-induced postural hypotension results from bretylium's neuronal blocking action and subsequent peripheral vasodilatation. Tricyclic antidepressant drugs can be used to block the presynaptic amine transport pump, thereby inhibiting the intracellular transport of bretylium and its ability to cause adrenergic blockade. Protripyline is the tricyclic antidepressant agent most frequently used for this indication.[307]

Indications

Bretylium is recommended for the treatment of ventricular fibrillation and ventricular tachycardia resistant to lidocaine and other antiarrhythmic drugs. Bretylium has been demonstrated to be equally as effective as lidocaine in facilitating an organized rhythm during ventricular fibrillation. However, in the treatment of ventricular tachycardia, it must be considered a second choice. A wide spectrum of arrhythmias has proved responsive to bretylium, including those occurring as a result of ischemic heart disease, primary myocardial disease, valvular heart disease, and possibly the prolonged QT interval syndromes; those occurring following cardiac surgery; and those occurring during cardiopulmonary resuscitation.[305] Bretylium has been demonstrated to be ineffective in suppressing simple ventricular ectopy (isolated PVCs). The use of bretylium to treat atrial tachyarrhythmias is relatively unexplored.

Calcium Channel Blockers

VERAPAMIL

Verapamil, a papaverine derivative, was initially introduced as a coronary vasodilator in 1962.[310] Subsequent studies found that it exerted antiarrhythmic effects, but these effects were different from other antiarrhythmic agents. The therapeutic action of verapamil and other calcium channel blockers arises from their ability to directly inhibit the influx of calcium ions across the plasma membrane of excitable cells. By decreasing the inward flux of calcium ions during excitation, calcium channel antagonists diminish the net current available to depolarize the cell membrane. In cardiac cells that have sodium-dependent action potentials, calcium channel inhibition has only minor electrophysiologic effects. However, in cardiac cells that are dependent on calcium ion flux for membrane depolarization (e.g., sinus and AV nodal cells) calcium channel blockers can markedly suppress membrane excitability and conduction. Of the currently marketed calcium channel blocking agents, verapamil has enjoyed the greatest clinical usage as an antiarrhythmic agent. Three other calcium channel antagonists (diltiazem, bepredil, and lidoflazine) are currently undergoing evaluation for their antiarrhythmic potential.

Cellular Electrophysiologic Effects

In therapeutic concentrations, verapamil exerts its electrophysiologic effects on slow response action potentials (i.e., those dependent on calcium ions crossing the sarcolemma through slow cardiac channels).[310] The time-dependent transitions in the sarcolemmic calcium channel state (channel opening, inactivation, and reactivation) are much slower than those of the fast sodium channels responsible for the inward depolarizing current in atrial, His-Purkinje, and ventricular myocardial cells. As a result, verapamil decreases the slope of diastolic depolarization, action potential amplitude, and V̇max in sinus node cells.[311] Little to no change occurs in the maximum diastolic potential. Verapamil also depresses action potential amplitude and V̇max in upper AV nodal cells, with much less effect evident in the lower node (NH region).[311] Verapamil preferentially binds to the calcium channel in the inactivated state.[312] By slowing channel recovery from the inactivated state, verapamil can prolong AV nodal refractoriness and depress conduction. The blocking effects of verapamil are more apparent at faster rates of stimulation.

Low concentrations of verapamil (1 mg/L) have little effect on atrial, His-Purkinje, or ventricular muscle cells.[313] Wit and Cranfield found some decrease in action potential plateau voltage and shortening of early repolarization.[311] Otherwise, no alterations in MDP, action potential AMP, V̇max, or action potential duration at full repolarization were noted. Rosen et al observed that high concentrations of verapamil (>1 mg/L) could decrease MDP and action potential amplitude and depress membrane responsiveness of His-Purkinje cells.[313] When high concentrations of verapamil were administered, APD and refractoriness were prolonged.

The local anesthetic effects of verapamil result from its racemic nature; it is composed of equal parts of the *d* and *l* isomers. Much evidence exists to suggest stereospecific differences in electrophysiologic effects. Bayer, Kaufmann, and Mannhold, using cat papillary muscles, demonstrated that *d*-verapamil has quite specific inhibitory effects on the fast inward sodium current.[314] By contrast, the *l*-isomer had a more potent negative inotropic effect on papillary muscle contraction and depressed upstroke velocity in cat sinus node action potentials to a greater extent. Satoh, Yanagisawa, and Taira, by injecting various concentrations of each isomer into the AV nodal artery, have shown that the *l* isomer is six times more potent than the *d* isomer in depressing AV nodal conduction.[315] It therefore appears that the *l* isomer predominantly inhibits slow channel current, whereas the *d* isomer can block either the fast or slow channel.

Verapamil may exert several other important antiarrhythmic effects. Verapamil can depress membrane excitability in atrial or ventricular action potentials previously affected by disease.[310] By decreasing action potential amplitude and V̇max, verapamil may slow or block conduction into these depressed regions. Verapamil is also effective in inhibiting four types of automaticity: the spontaneous automaticity inherent to normally polarized Purkinje cells; the membrane current responsible for delayed afterdepolarizations (transient inward current); the calcium current important in generating early afterdepolarizations; and spontaneous automaticity occurring at depolarized membrane potentials.[310] Verapamil is a potent α-adrenergic blocking agent and can delay the onset and attenuate the electrophysiologic effects of myocardial ischemia.[28, 316]

Age-related changes in sensitivity of slow response action potentials to verapamil have been observed. In studying calcium-dependent slow response action potentials in canine Purkinje fibers superfused with a sodium-free, calcium-rich solution, Reder et al found that low concentrations of verapamil could significantly decrease action potential AMP in adult (but not in neonatal) Purkinje fibers.[317] Ezrin, Bassett, and Gelband noted that verapamil prolonged the APD of adult rabbit Purkinje fibers at concentrations ≥0.5 mg/L.[318] In contrast, verapamil shortened action potential duration in neonatal fibers. Arnold, Vallner, and Tackett were able to demonstrate that, at blood levels that prolonged atrioventricular conduction in adult dogs, verapamil had no effect on the PR interval in newborn puppies.[319]

Clinical Electrophysiologic Effects

The predominant clinical pharmacologic action of verapamil is to prolong conduction time through the AV node (AH interval and Wenckebach cycle length) and lengthen its functional refractory periods without affecting intra-atrial (PA interval) or His-Purkinje conduction (HV interval).[320] The spontaneous sinus heart rate may decrease slightly; more commonly, it does not change significantly, especially in adults. Verapamil usually does not affect the sinus node recovery time response to rapid atrial pacing or the sinoatrial conduction time in patients with normal sinus node function. In those with sinus node dysfunction, however, verapamil can increase sinus node recovery time or produce sinus arrest.

Age-related changes in sensitivity to the clinical electrophysiologic effects of verapamil have been demonstrated. In adults, verapamil does not alter the refractory periods of the atrium, His-Purkinje system, or ventricle. However, Shakibi et al found a 12% increase in the atrial effective refractory period in children aged 50 days to 12 years.[321] Pickoff et al noted similar observations in a canine developmental study of the electrophysiologic effects of verapamil.[322] Verapamil had no effect on atrial refractoriness in adult dogs, but significantly increased (by 32%) the effective refractory period in newborn puppies. Observations from both human and animal studies suggest developmental differences in response of the sinus node to verapamil. Pickoff et al and Gibson et al both noted a decrease in spontaneous heart rate in young animals following verapamil administration.[322, 323] Similar findings were reported by Shakibi et al in children.[321] As previously mentioned, sinus heart rate changes very little in adults, but may increase from reflex sympathetic stimulation secondary to peripheral vasodilation. Verapamil is also more effective in depressing retrograde AV nodal conduction in children than in adults.[324]

The electrophysiologic changes in accessory atrioventricular pathway refractoriness vary following verapamil administration. Most frequently, verapamil does not alter accessory pathway refractoriness. Rarely, it has been documented to shorten it, particularly in cases of atrial fibrillation (either from reflex sympathetic stimulation or by decreasing concealed retrograde conduction).[325]

Electrocardiographic Effects

The predominant electrocardiographic effect of verapamil is to prolong the PR interval.[310] Decreases in P wave amplitude and sinus heart rate may accompany depression of atrioventricular conduction. No significant effect on the QRS duration or corrected QT interval are apparent.

Clinical Pharmacokinetics

Verapamil is readily absorbed following oral administration (80% to 90%).[310, 326–328] Because of extensive first-pass biotransformation, systemic bioavailability is reduced (10% to 35%), and plasma levels may vary by more than a factor of 10 following administration of the same oral dose to different patients. Maximum plasma levels are attained 2.2 hours after oral ingestion. Therapeutic effects begin within 30 minutes after oral administration and persist for up to 6 hours.

Following absorption, verapamil is widely distributed (5 L/kg) and is highly bound to plasma proteins (83% to 92%).[326, 327] Its clearance varies from 0.71 L/kg/h to 0.83 L/kg/h in adults, with an elimination half-life of 2.8 to 6.3 hours. During long-term oral administration, drug accumulation occurs with reduced clearance and a two-fold prolongation of the elimination half-life. Dosage adjustment should not be undertaken until steady-state plasma concentrations are achieved, usually 4 to 5 days after drug initiation.

Metabolism of verapamil occurs largely in the liver.[326, 327] Of the various metabolites produced, only the *N*-demethylated form (norverapamil) has significant activity, which is about 20% of that of the parent drug. Seventy-four to eighty percent of a given dose is excreted as metabolites in the bile. Less than 5% is excreted unchanged by the kidney.

In patients with hepatic disease, first-pass effects are diminished, bioavailability is enhanced (52%), clearance is decreased (50%), and plasma half-life is prolonged (fourfold).[326, 327] Verapamil may accumulate to toxic levels if the dosage is not appropriately decreased; oral doses should be decreased to one-fourth the usual dose, and intravenous doses decreased to one-half the usual dose. No dosage alterations are necessary in patients with renal failure. Although little data are available on the pharmacokinetics of verapamil in cardiac patients, its clearance is probably decreased in the presence of congestive heart failure.

Therapeutic effects of verapamil begin shortly after intravenous administration.[326, 327] Verapamil has a distribution half-life of 49 minutes. The elimination half-life after intravenous administration is similar to that after oral administration. The plasma level–effect relationship for verapamil is complex. After intravenous drug administration, a linear relationship between drug levels and effects on atrioventricular conduction can be demonstrated. However, to achieve similar clinical effects following oral administration, much higher plasma levels are required (two- to three-fold). Hoon et al have suggested that this is a result of preferential first-pass extraction of the relatively more active *l*-isomer during oral administration.[329] Therefore no therapeutic concentration range has been defined to date.

Verapamil is excreted into human breast milk, with concentrations varying between 23% and 100% of maternal plasma levels. Verapamil could not be detected in the plasma of a breast-fed infant, suggesting the safety of administration of verapamil during lactation. Transplacental passage of verapamil has also been demonstrated.[31, 326] Fetal cord blood concentrations vary between 15% and 50% of maternal plasma levels.

Information regarding the clinical pharmacokinetics of verapamil in children is scant. Epstein et al studied the elimination half-life and pattern of hepatic biotransformation of verapamil in five infants ranging in age from 4 days to 9 months.[331] Their results showed that infants metabolized verapamil differently (i.e., produced less norverapamil) but cleared verapamil in a manner similar to adults ($t½$ varied between 4 and 7 hours). DeVonderweid et al observed a slightly shortened half-life (2.1 h and 3.1 h) in the two infants (aged 15 days and 4 months, respectively) they studied.[332] In older children (7 to 19 years old), Wagner, Rocchini, and Vasiliades found that verapamil had a slower clearance (0.5 L/min, compared with 0.58–1.6 L/min in adults) and a prolonged elimination half-life (9.2 h).[333]

A sustained-release preparation of verapamil has recently been marketed. Unlike conventional formulations, it has a high bioavailability (90 ± 30%) and produces more stable plasma levels over a 12-hour period.[328] With conventional formulations, plasma levels can vary as much as 412% between trough and peak plasma concentrations, but a significantly lower (130%) difference was observed with the sustained-release preparation.

Dosage

Intravenously, verapamil is administered slowly over a 1- to 2-minute period in a dosage ranging from 0.075 mg/kg to 0.150 mg/kg (maximum dose, 10 mg). A second injection may be given 15 minutes later if arrhythmia control is unsatisfactory. The initial effect achieved with bolus injection (e.g., slowing the ventricular response during atrial fibrillation) may be maintained by a continuous infusion at a rate of 0.005 mg/kg/min. We do not recommend the use of intravenous verapamil to treat supraventricular tachycardia in infants younger than 12 months.[334] For chronic oral administration, a dosage of 4–17 mg/kg/d has been shown to be effective in arrhythmia suppression.[335] The most efficacious dosage schedule in children is to administer verapamil three times daily.

Adverse Effects

Major side effects forcing discontinuation of verapamil are rare in children (8%); however, minor side effects occurred in 44% of children chronically administered verapamil and retrospectively reviewed by Hesslein et al (Table 3–9).[336] Most adverse effects are an extension of the pharmacologic action of verapamil. Cardiovascular complications are most frequent (15%) and include hypotension, sinus bradycardia, AV block, asystole, and congestive heart failure. Bradycardia and conduction disturbances occur frequently in patients with preexisting sinus or AV nodal abnormalities or in those receiving β-adrenergic blocking agents.

Contraindications to the use of verapamil include the presence of advanced congestive heart failure, second or third degree AV block, significant sinus node dysfunction, and

TABLE 3–9 VERAPAMIL-INDUCED SIDE EFFECTS

Cardiovascular	*Gastrointestinal*
Hypotension	Constipation
Sinus bradycardia—asystole	Hepatitis
AV block	Nausea, vomiting
Congestive heart failure	*Endocrine*
Fluid retention-peripheral edema	Hyperglycemia
Polymorphic ventricular tachycardia	*Cutaneous*
	"Allergic" vasculitis
Respiratory	Rash
Pulmonary edema	Pruritis
Asthma	
Central Nervous System	
Headache	
Dizziness, vertigo	
Perceptual disorders	
Behavior changes	

hypotensive states; it should not be administered intravenously to children younger than 12 months. Both experimental and clinical experience suggest that the negative inotropic effects of verapamil are exaggerated in young patients; numerous reports suggest the frequent occurrence of cardiovascular collapse (hypotension or asystole) following intravenous verapamil administration to infants less than 12 months of age.[334] Chronic oral administration of verapamil results in a more balanced and well tolerated hemodynamic state and is therefore safe to use in young infants.

Drug Interactions

A number of drug interactions with verapamil have been described.[9] Although the concomitant administration of β-adrenergic blockers and the oral form of verapamil has been safely used in adult patients with mildly impaired cardiac function, we do not recommend their combined usage in children. Both are negatively inotropic and depress sinus automaticity and atrioventricular conduction. The concurrent use of propranolol with verapamil has been associated with a high risk of hypotension, bradycardia, and asystole. Under all circumstances, the intravenous administration of verapamil to patients taking β-blockers is definitely contraindicated.

When verapamil is added to a therapeutic regimen that includes digoxin, plasma glycoside concentrations increase 40% to 75%. Pedersen has demonstrated that verapamil can decrease the renal tubular secretion of digoxin and probably its nonrenal clearance as well.[29] No changes in the volume of distribution or tissue binding of digoxin were evident. The increase in plasma digoxin levels is dependent on the dose of verapamil; most investigators of this interaction recommend a 50% reduction of the digoxin dosage.

Cimetidine, which has pronounced effects on both liver blood flow and drug metabolizing enzyme systems, might be expected to alter the elimination kinetics of verapamil. Some authors have found that hypercalcemia can antagonize the electrophysiologic effects of verapamil on AV nodal conduction. Thus the co-administration of calcium and verapamil may reduce verapamil's therapeutic efficacy. Matsuda et al studied the combined electrophysiologic effects of disopyramide and verapamil in patients with Wolff-Parkinson-White syndrome.[337] When administered together, the anticholinergic action of disopyramide blocked the antiarrhythmic effect of verapamil on AV nodal conduction. Combined administration of verapamil with quinidine is contraindicated (see the section on quinidine).[28]

Indications

Intravenous verapamil is very effective (80% to 97%) in terminating acute episodes of supraventricular tachycardia, bearing in mind the age limitations in its use.[338] Verapamil is most effective in treating supraventricular tachycardias that incorporate the AV node in the tachycardia circuit (AV node reentry and atrioventricular reciprocating tachycardia). Gomes et al have demonstrated that verapamil may also be therapeutically efficacious in sinus node reentry tachycardia.[339] In the multicenter study reported on by Hesslein et al, chronic oral verapamil therapy was effective in controlling supraventricular tachycardia in 82% of the children enrolled in this study.[336] Verapamil is less effective (22%) for atrial ectopic tachycardia and may accelerate the rate of junctional ectopic tachycardia. In contrast, multifocal atrial tachycardia appears quite sensitive to the antiarrhythmic effects of verapamil, especially in cases of pulmonary disease and theophylline toxicity.

Verapamil slows the ventricular response over the AV node in the presence of atrial fibrillation or atrial flutter.[340] It may convert a small number of episodes (10%) to sinus rhythm, particularly if the atrial flutter or atrial fibrillation is of recent onset. Some patients with atrial flutter may develop atrial fibrillation following verapamil administration. In patients with atrial fibrillation associated with Wolff-Parkinson-White syndrome, verapamil may accelerate the ventricular response and is therefore contraindicated.[325]

In general, verapamil is rarely effective in treating patients who have recurrent ventricular tachycardia. However, there are three subsets of ventricular tachycardia that may be responsive to verapamil: (1) ventricular tachycardia with right bundle-branch block and left axis deviation occurring in the absence of organic heart disease; (2) ventricular tachycardia that can be induced by rapid atrial and ventricular pacing or atrial premature extrastimuli but not by programmed ventricular extrastimulus testing; and (3) exercise-induced ventricular tachycardia (either right or left bundle-branch block morphology).[341, 342]

Digitalis Glycosides

DIGITALIS

Since William Withering's report, "An Account of the Foxglove and Some of Its Medicinal Uses," digitalis has become the most frequently prescribed and studied antiarrhythmic and inotropic agent.[343] Withering recognized in 1785 that optimal use of digitalis glycosides required considerable skill and knowledge on the part of the physician because of their unusually narrow therapeutic/toxic dose ratio. Most of the antiarrhythmic effects of digitalis glycosides result from their action on the atria and atrioventricular junction.

Cellular Electrophysiologic Effects

The electrophysiologic effects of digitalis glycosides are the net result of direct effects on myocardial cells and indirect effects mediated via the autonomic nervous system.[344, 345] The direct electrophysiologic effects of digitalis glycosides are thought to occur through inhibition of the sacrolemmic Na^+ pump.[344] Binding of digitalis to the Na^+- and K^+-activated transport enzyme complex known as Na^+-K^+-ATPase blocks the active outward transport of sodium ions across the myocardial cell membrane, leading to increased intracellular sodium activity. Intracellular sodium accumulation enhances Na^+-Ca^{++} exchange, which consequently increases the intracellular calcium concentration. Digitalis binding to the sodium pump is dependent on Na^+ and K^+ concentrations, with low extracellular K^+ and high intracellular Na^+ enhancing binding.

In therapeutic concentrations, digitalis glycosides appear to have no direct effect on sinus node action potential characteristics.[346] They slow the sinus rate primarily by enhancing vagal discharge. In addition, digitalis slows sinus heart rate by increasing the sensitivity of sinus node cells to acetylcholine and decreasing sensitivity to β-adrenergic catecholamines.[345]

The effect of digitalis on atrial action potential characteristics and conduction are variable and depend on concentration.[346, 347] At low concentrations, atrial cells hyperpolarize (an effect mediated through the parasympathetic nervous system), action potential AMP and $\dot{V}$max increase, and conduction is accelerated. Associated changes include a decrease in action potential duration and a shortening of the atrial effective refractory period. Membrane hyperpolarization decreases phase 4 depolarization (if present) and increases membrane responsiveness. High digitalis concentrations partially depolarize atrial cells and decrease action potential AMP and $\dot{V}$max, thereby slowing atrial conduction.[347] When exposed to high concentrations of digitalis, atrial APD and the effective refractory period are prolonged.

In the AV node, digitalis (at low concentrations) slows conduction and prolongs nodal refractoriness through its cholinergic and antiadrenergic effects. At high concentrations, digitalis primarily decreases MDP, action potential AMP, and $\dot{V}$max.[347] These actions are associated with impaired AV nodal conduction and, on occasion, block of atrioventricular transmission.

Digitalis in therapeutic concentrations has little effect on His-Purkinje or ventricular muscle cells.[348] At low concentrations, the only direct effect is a small, somewhat variable prolongation of APD and refractoriness. With prolonged superfusion or exposure to higher digitalis concentrations, APD and refractoriness are shortened. Other effects noted at high concentrations include decreases in MDP, action potential AMP, $\dot{V}$max, membrane responsiveness, and conduction velocity. Toxic concentrations of digitalis can increase the rate of spontaneous depolarization, thereby increasing automaticity.[349] In addition, digitalis may induce delayed afterdepolarizations that can lead to triggered arrhythmias. By decreasing membrane potential, high concentrations of digitalis increase Purkinje cell excitability.

Age-related changes in Purkinje fiber and ventricular muscle sensitivity to the direct toxic electrophysiologic effects of digitalis have been well demonstrated. Rosen et al. has shown that neonatal canine cardiac Purkinje fiber action potentials are more resistant to the toxic effects of digitalis (membrane depolarization, depression of conduction, and enhancement of automaticity) than are those of adult Purkinje fibers.[348] Kelliher and Roberts have similarly demonstrated that the dose of digitalis required to produce ventricular tachyarrhythmias and death in immature rabbits was larger than that required in developmentally mature rabbits.[350] These experimental findings are consistent with the clinical observation that infants and young children tolerate higher plasma and myocardial concentrations of digitalis than do adults.

Experimental evidence suggests that the greater tolerance of the young to the toxic electrophysiologic effects of digitalis may partially relate to differences in end-organ responsiveness. Marsh, Lloyd, and Taylor have shown that young dogs and guinea pigs exhibit higher myocardial Na^+-K^+-ATPase activity and total ouabain binding, when compared with adults of the same species.[351] Kearin, Kelly, and O'Malley studied digoxin binding to human erythrocytes from both newborn and adult subjects, and noted twice as many digoxin-binding sites in erythrocytes obtained from neonates.[352] The same investigators noted, however, that the dissociation constant of digoxin in the neonate was twice as large (i.e., lower binding affinity) as that in the adult erythrocytes. They hypothesized that if the occupation of a critical number of binding sites was necessary to obtain a therapeutic effect, an increased number of binding sites having a lower affinity for digoxin would require higher digoxin concentrations for a therapeutic response. Consistent with these observations are those of Ng, Akera, and Brody, who examined the developmental abundance of the two molecular forms of Na^+-K^+-ATPase activity during postnatal maturation in ferret cardiac tissue.[353] They found a relative deficiency of high affinity α^+-binding sites in neonatal hearts and diminished sensitivity to ouabain inhibition of Na^+-K-ATPase activity.

Neurally Mediated Effects. On the basis of both animal and clinical studies, it is known that one important mechanism by which digitalis glycosides exert their electrophysiologic effects is through the parasympathetic nervous system.[345, 346] Various studies have shown that digitalis increases vagal activity by acting on several components of the parasympathetic nervous system. Digitalis can activate reflexogenic areas of the cardiovascular system (e.g., arterial baroreceptors, chemoreceptors, and other afferent nerve fibers in the nodose ganglion and the heart). Digitalis also acts on efferent pathways to augment parasympathetic tone. Effects have been demonstrated on autonomic ganglia as well as on efferent parasympathetic nerves. Digitalis can potentiate end-organ responsiveness to acetylcholine, particularly in the sinoatrial and atrioventricular nodes. Lastly, augmented parasympathetic tone can modulate sympathetic activity by inhibiting norepinephrine release from sympathetic terminals.

Digitalis glycosides alter sympathetic activity at multiple levels, but probably only at higher (toxic) concentrations than those required to produce parasympathetic effects.[345] Several studies have shown that high concentrations of digitalis glycosides in the brain increase efferent sympathetic neural activity. At high concentrations, digitalis glycosides can induce the release of catecholamines and prevent catecholamine re-uptake, both of which result in cardiac stimulation.

Clinical Electrophysiologic Effects

Dhingra et al have studied the clinical electrophysiologic effects of ouabain on adult atrium and sinus node.[354] They found that ouabain had little effect on spontaneous sinus heart rate but prolonged the maximum corrected sinus node recovery time and sinoatrial conduction time. In addition, ouabain prolonged atrial refractoriness (atrial ERP and FRP) and slowed intra-atrial conduction (prolonged the PA interval). Engel and Gonzalez have also demonstrated that digitalis can protect against atrial fibrillation and atrial flutter in adults by prolonging atrial refractoriness and curtailing the duration of the vulnerable period.[355] These results differ from those reported by Kugler, Garson, and Gillette in a group of young children in which the only electrophysiologic effect of ouabain was to prolong the sinoatrial conduction time.[356] Ouabain had no effect on atrial refractoriness or conduction. Whether these results reflect pharmacokinetic or developmental differences in electrophysiologic sensitivity to digitalis will need future exploration. In patients with sinus node dysfunction, digitalis, even in therapeutic concentrations, may markedly depress sinus automaticity and conduction, resulting in prolonged sinus pauses, sinoatrial exit block, or sinus arrest.

Therapeutic concentrations of digoxin have been demonstrated by Przybyla et al to slow AV nodal conduction (increase AH interval) and prolong its effective and functional refractory periods.[357] In contrast, Gomes et al could not demonstrate any effect of ouabain on His-Purkinje refractoriness or conduction.[358] Digitalis has been consistently observed to shorten ventricular muscle refractoriness.[359]

Electrocardiographic Effects

The effects of digitalis glycosides administration on the surface electrocardiogram include a decrease in sinus heart rate, prolongation of the PR interval, shortening of the QT interval, depression of the ST segment, and flattening of the T wave.[346]

DIGOXIN

Clinical Pharmacokinetics

Digoxin has become the digitalis preparation predominantly used, principally because of its flexibility in administration and its intermediate duration of action. Following oral administration, the systemic bioavailability of digoxin in children and adults is equivalent and depends on the formulation assessed (tablet, 75%; elixir, 80%; encapsulated gel, 95%).[360–364] Onset of pharmacologic action begins 15 to 30 minutes following absorption; peak plasma concentration occurs 30 to 90 minutes after an oral dose. Absorption can be affected by malabsorption states, disorders of gastrointestinal motility, drugs, or food. Meals delay the absorption peak but do not affect the total amount absorbed. Drugs that depress gastrointestinal motility increase digoxin bioavailability. On the other hand, cathartics or drugs that increase gastrointestinal transit time can render digoxin absorption less complete. Co-administration of digoxin with drugs that interact with it physiochemically (e.g., antacids, antidiarrheals, charcoal, or cholestyramine) may make digoxin unabsorbable.[9]

Once absorbed, digoxin is rapidly distributed to the tissues, with a distribution half-life ranging from 20 to 60 minutes.[360–364] Digoxin is not highly bound to plasma proteins (34±4%); its protein binding does not change between infancy and adulthood. In contrast, digoxin is highly bound to tissue proteins, giving it a large apparent volume of distribution, particularly in infants and young children. The volume of distribution of digoxin changes with age (premature neonates, 5 L/kg; full-term neonates, 7.5 L/kg; adults, 5 L/kg). The greater apparent volume of distribution for digoxin in infants and young children is reflected in higher myocardial digoxin concentrations compared with adults. The ratio of digoxin content in the right atrial appendage to that in serum was 149:1 in infants, 78:1 in children, and 28:1 in adults.

Digoxin is excreted primarily by the kidneys, with 60% to 80% excreted unchanged in the urine.[360–364] Nonrenal elimination is higher in pediatric patients (32%) compared with adults (25%). The renal elimination of digoxin occurs predominantly through glomerular filtration but also involves tubular secretion. The tubular secretion of digoxin is more pronounced in children and may account for the enhanced clearance in this age group. The renal clearance of digoxin is low in low-birth-weight premature neonates (53 mL/kg/h) and steadily increases until 1 year of age (253 mL/kg/h), when it attains its maximum value. Renal clearance subsequently declines with age until adulthood (149 mL/kg/h). The age-related changes in renal elimination of digoxin are reflected by changes in the elimination half-life (premature neonates 61 h; full-term neonates, 35 h; infants, 18 h; children, 37 h; and adults, 35–48 h). Renal excretion of digoxin is proportional to glomerular filtration, suggesting the need to alter the dosage in patients with renal failure.

Digoxin is known to cross the placenta.[365] Fetal cord plasma levels are similar to maternal plasma concentrations. Digoxin is also secreted into human breast milk at a concentration similar to steady-state maternal plasma concentration. However, the total daily excretion of digoxin in lactating mothers usually does not exceed 1–2 μg, an amount unlikely to be of pharmacologic significance to the nursing infant.

The use of plasma levels to guide pharmacologic therapy with digoxin remains controversial.[360, 361] It is generally agreed that digoxin levels between 0.7 and 2.0 ng/mL augment cardiac contractile function. Positive inotropic effects do not appear to be greater at higher plasma levels (>2 ng/mL), but less is understood about the electrophysiologic effects of digoxin, which usually occur at higher concentrations than its inotropic action. Plasma digoxin levels exceeding 2 ng/

mL may be associated with digitalis toxicity in children and adults. In contrast, high plasma concentrations of digoxin (up to 3.5 ng/mL) are tolerated by infants and young children, who appear to be less prone to the direct arrhythmogenic effects of digoxin. The upper limit of the therapeutic range for antiarrhythmic effects has yet to be established. Furthermore, measurement of plasma digoxin concentration may be complicated by the presence of an endogenous digoxin-like immunoreactive substance that cross-reacts with the immunoassay antibody to digoxin, particularly in infants less than 6 months of age or in older patients with renal failure. To measure plasma digoxin concentration, blood levels should be obtained at least 6 hours after a dose or, preferably, immediately before the next dose (i.e., 12 hours after a dose). Loes et al, as well as Henion et al, have proposed the usefulness of red blood cell electrolytes as a sensitive indicator of the toxic effects of digoxin.[366, 367] Red blood cell (RBC) sodium concentration and the RBC Na^+/K^+ ratio were significantly greater in patients who demonstrated toxicity than in patients who did not. However, this assay is restricted to research applications and is generally not available to the clinician.

Dosage

Recommendations for digoxin dosage should be based on pharmacokinetic data and generally aim for a plasma concentration of 1.1–1.7 ng/mL.[361] A loading dose is given to shorten the time to onset of desired effect (Table 3–10). The daily maintenance dose is 25% of the loading dose and is given in two divided doses to minimize the possibility of toxic peak levels and subtherapeutic trough levels. When used intravenously, the dosage should be reduced 20% to 25% because only 75% to 80% of an orally administered dose is absorbed.

Adverse Effects

Digitalis toxicity persists as one of the most prevalent adverse drug reactions encountered in clinical practice.[346, 347, 349] The noncardiac manifestations of digitalis toxicity include gastrointestinal, central nervous system, and visual symptoms (Table 3–11). Although the noncardiac symptoms are the earliest manifestation of digitalis toxicity, these symptoms are nonspecific and difficult to evaluate in infants and children. Therefore the diagnosis of digitalis toxicity in children frequently rests on electrocardiographic abnormalities. Cardiac toxicity manifested by arrhythmias can simulate every known rhythm disturbance (see Table 3–11). The electrocardiographic signs of digitalis toxicity differ between children and adults. Infants are more likely to develop profound sinus bradycardia and AV conduction disturbances than tachyarrhythmias. Arrhythmias as warning signs of toxicity are relatively late in appearance. A number of factors are known to influence individual sensitivity to digitalis and predisposition to adverse effects (Table 3–12).[368]

Drug Interactions

A myriad of drug interactions with digoxin have been documented for a number of agents, some of which have been discussed in previous sections of this chapter (Table 3–13).[9, 369, 370] Spironolactone has been demonstrated to inhibit renal tubular secretion of digoxin, thereby decreasing its renal clearance. Moreover, spironolactone has been found to interfere with the digoxin radioimmunoassy, leading to spuriously high results. Diuretics may produce renal insufficiency and reduce the volume of distribution of digoxin, raising its concentration accordingly. Diuretic-induced hypokalemia may also predispose to digitalis toxicity. Digoxin is metab-

TABLE 3–10 RECOMMEND ORAL DIGOXIN DOSAGE

	LOADING DOSAGE (μg/kg/d)	MAINTENANCE DOSAGE (μg/kg/d)
Premature Infant	20	5
Full-Term Neonate (up to age 2 mo)	30	8–10
Infants < 2 yrs old	40–50	10–12
Children > 2 yrs old	30–40	8–10
Adults	1.25–1.50 mg total dosage	0.25 mg/d total dosage

TABLE 3–11
CLINICAL MANIFESTATIONS OF DIGITALIS TOXICITY

Noncardiac
- Gastrointestinal: nausea, vomiting, anorexia
- Neurologic: lethargy, weakness, headache, disorientation, confusion, seizures
- Visual: scotomas, halos, flickering, changes in color perception
- Breast: gynecomastia
- Skin: allergic rash

Cardiac
- Profound sinus bradycardia or sinoatrial exit block
- AV junctional escape rhythm
- AV conduction disturbances (second or third degree block)
- Isolated atrial, junctional, or ventricular ectopic beats (unifocal or multifocal)
- Atrial, junctional, or ventricular tachycardia
- Ventricular fibrillation

olized by the gastrointestinal flora in about 10% of the population; in these patients, antibiotics (e.g., erythromycin or tetracycline) may inhibit bacterial growth and result in as much as a two-fold increase in plasma digoxin concentrations. When indomethacin is used for pharmacologic closure of a patent ductus arteriosus in premature infants, it may impair renal function. Thus indomethacin may inhibit elimination of digoxin and result in a 50% elevation in plasma concentration. Patients with congestive heart failure often have reduced renal blood flow; vasodilator therapy may acutely improve renal hemodynamics and thereby increase digoxin clearance.

TABLE 3–12
FACTORS PREDISPOSING TO DIGITALIS TOXICITY

1. *High plasma digoxin levels*
   - Decreased renal excretion of digoxin (premature and full-term neonates and patients with renal failure)
   - High dose requirements (used for treatment of arrhythmias)
   - Hypothyroidism
   - Drug interactions
   - Obstruction hepatic disease
2. *Increased sensitivity of myocardium (with normal plasma digoxin concentration)*
   - Myocardial factors
     - Myocardial ischemia
     - Myocarditis (rheumatic, viral)
   - Systemic changes
     - Electrolyte abnormalities (hypokalemia, hypomagnesemia, hypercalcemia)
     - Hypoxemia
     - Alkalosis
     - Catecholamine and sympathetic drug administration
     - Anesthesia
   - Electric shock (cardioversion)
   - Autonomic Nervous System tone
3. *Open Heart Surgery (Immediate Post-Operative Period)*
4. *Allergy and Hypersensitivity to Digitalis*

Indications

Digitalis is one of the most frequently used antiarrhythmic drugs to control paroxysmal supraventricular tachycardia, atrial fibrillation, and atrial flutter. Recent electrophysiologic studies have demonstrated that digoxin can decrease the refractory period (effective and functional) of accessory atrioventricular connections in patients with Wolff-Parkinson-White syndrome. The use of digitalis in patients with Wolff-Parkinson-White syndrome and atrial flutter or atrial fibrillation is contraindicated because of its potential to increase the ventricular response rate and predispose to ventricular fibrillation.[371]

Purinergic Agonists

ADENOSINE

Adenosine, an endogenous purine nucleoside important as an intermediate metabolite in many biochemical pathways, is also known to have potent antiarrhythmic effects.[372] The electrophysiologic effects of adenosine were first described by Drury and Szent-Gyorgi in 1929.[373] These investigators demonstrated that intravenous administration of adenosine slowed sinus heart rate and produced transient atrioventricular block, but only during the past several years have the electrophysiologic effects of adenosine been further defined and its role as an antiarrhythmic agent useful for treating episodes of supraventricular tachycardia been established.

Cellular Electrophysiologic Effects

The electrophysiologic effects of adenosine predominate in the atrium. West and Belardinelli have studied the cellular electrophysiologic effects of adenosine on the rabbit sinus node.[374] Adenosine decreased the slope of phase 4 depolarization, action potential amplitude, and action potential duration. Following hyperpolarization of maximum diastolic potential, $\dot{V}max$ increased. In the guinea pig atrioventricular node, adenosine

TABLE 3–13
PHARMACOKINETIC DRUG INTERACTIONS WITH DIGOXIN

INTERACTIVE SUBSTANCE	MECHANISM OF INTERACTION*	MEAN MAGNITUDE OF INTERACTION
Cholestyramine (colestipol)	↓ absorption	↓ 25%
Antacids	↓ absorption	↓ 25%
Kaolin-pectate	↓ absorption	?
Bran	↓ absorption	↓ 20%
Neomycin	↓ absorption	↓ 28%
Erythromycin Tetracycline	↓ bioavailability by ↑ intestinal metabolism of digoxin	↑ 43% to 116%
Quinidine	↓ volume of distribution, ↓ renal and nonrenal clearance	↑ 100%
Amiodarone	↓ renal and nonrenal clearance	↑ 70% to 100%
Verapamil	↓ renal and nonrenal clearance	↑ 70% to 100%
Spironolactone	↓ renal and nonrenal clearance	↑ 30%
Triamterene	↓ renal clearance	↑ 20%
Indomethacin	↓ renal clearance	↑ 50%

*↓ = decreased; ↑ = increased; ? = unknown.

was similarly observed to impair atrioventricular conduction and depress action potential amplitude and $\dot{V}max$. Belardinelli and Isenberg have demonstrated in isolated atrial myocytes that adenosine increases membrane potential, action potential amplitude, and $\dot{V}max$, and shortens action potential duration and refractoriness.[375]

In contrast, adenosine has little or no direct effect on ventricular myocardium. However, adenosine can indirectly antagonize the electrophysiologic effects of β-adrenergic stimulation (shortening of ventricular refractoriness).[376] In the His-Purkinje system, several investigators have demonstrated that adenosine will decrease the rate of phase 4 depolarization and slow the spontaneous automatic rate.[377, 378] Wesley and Belardinelli noted a concomitant shortening of action potential duration, but this effect has not been observed by other investigators.[378]

The electrophysiologic effects of adenosine are thought to be mediated through extracellular A_1-purinoceptors coupled to adenylate cyclase and sarcolemmic potassium channels. Voltage clamp and flux studies have demonstrated that adenosine depresses the slow inward calcium current.[379] However, the shortening of action potential duration and membrane hyperpolarization produced by adenosine are probably secondary to augmentation of potassium currents during repolarization, brought about through an increase in potassium channel conductance.[375]

Clinical Electrophysiologic Effects

In the clinical electrophysiologic laboratory, adenosine exerts negative chronotropic and dromotropic effects; spontaneous sinus cycle length, the AH interval, and Wenckebach cycle length all increase.[380] No change in the HV interval has been observed. Perrot, Clozel, and Faivre have noted some interesting observations in patients with Wolff-Parkinson-White syndrome.[381] While adenosine had no effect on the antegrade conduction characteristics of the accessory connection, in 15 of 22 patients the degree of preexcitation became more apparent as the contribution to ventricular activation from conduction through the atrioventricular node was diminished. In the remaining seven patients (all with accessory pathways that had either prolonged refractory periods or Mahaim fibers), adenosine abolished the preexcitation pattern. DiMarco et al have similarly observed the ability of adenosine to prolong refractoriness and suppress conduction in the accessory pathway associated with the permanent form of junctional reciprocating tachycardia.[382]

Electrocardiographic Effects

Following administration, adenosine slows the spontaneous heart rate and prolongs the PR interval.[380] Transient complete atrioventricular block has been reported to occur with the use of high dosages.[380]

Clinical Pharmacokinetics

The onset of adenosine effect is rapid (17 ± 3 s).[382] Similarly, its electrophysiologic

TABLE 3–14
CELLULAR ELECTROPHYSIOLOGIC ACTION OF ANTIARRHYTHMIC DRUGS*
(HIS-PURKINJE OR VENTRICULAR MYOCARDIUM)

DRUG	MDP	AMP	$\dot{V}max$	MEMBRANE RESPONSIVENESS	APD	ERP	SPONTANEOUS AUTOMATICITY	ET
Class I								
Quinidine	0	↑	↑	↑	↑	↑	↓	↑
Procainamide	0	↓	↓	↓	↑	↑	↓	↑
Disopyramide	0	↓	↓	↓	↑	↑	↓	↑
Lidocaine	0	0	0↓	0↓	↓	↓	↓	↑
Phenytoin	0	0↓	0↓	0↓	↓	↓	↓	↑
Mexiletine	0	↓	↓	↓	↓	↓	↓	↑
Ethmozine	0	↓	↓	↓	↓	↓	↓	↑
Encainide	0	↓	↓	↓	↓	↑	↓	↑
Flecainide	0	↓	↓	↓	↓0↑	↑	↓	↑
Propafenone	0	↓	↓	↓	↓0↑	↑	↓	↑
Class II								
Propranolol	0	0↓	0↓	0	↓	↓	↓	0↑
Atenolol	0	0	0	0	↓	↓	↓	0
Class III								
Amiodarone	0	↓	↓	↓	↑	↑	↓	↑
Bretylium	0↑	0↑	0↑	0↑	↑	↑	↑	↓
Class IV								
Verapamil	0	0	0	0	0	0	↓	0
Class V								
Digoxin	0↓	0↓	0↓	0↓	↓0↑	↓0↑	0↓	↓0↑
Class VI								
Adenosine	0	0	0	0	0	0	0	0

*AMP = action potential amplitude; APD = action potential duration; ERP = effective refractory period; ET = excitability threshold; MDP = maximum diastolic potential; $\dot{V}max$ = maximum velocity of phase 0 upstroke; 0 = no charge; ↑ = increase; ↓ = decrease.

action quickly dissipates. The half-life of adenosine in human blood was found to be 9.3 seconds when studied by Klabunde.[383] Therefore, the duration of its pharmacologic action is short. Adenosine is taken up by circulating blood elements (erythrocytes) and endothelial cells. Once cellular uptake occurs, adenosine is preferentially metabolized to inosine and hypoxanthine-xanthine by adenosine deaminase. In an alternative route of metabolism, adenosine is phosphorylated by adenosine kinase for reincorporation into nucleotides. The intracellular transport of adenosine can be diminished by dipyridamole and diazepam.[383] By inhibiting cellular uptake of adenosine and, subsequently, its metabolism, these agents indirectly increase the extracellular concentration of adenosine and intensify its action. Aminophylline has been reported to antagonize the effects of adenosine.[376] Furthermore, the potency of adenosine is influenced by the site and rate of administration. The effects of adenosine are greater if delivered centrally, particularly as a bolus, in contrast to either a peripheral infusion or administration at a slow rate. Patients born with congenital adenosine deaminase deficiency may be extremely sensitive to exogenous adenosine.

In addition to its electrophysiologic effects, adenosine produces vasodilation of the coronary and system vascular beds. Hypotension may therefore occur at higher dosages.

Dosage

A wide range of adenosine dosage has been reported to be effective in supraventricular tachycardia termination. This partially reflects differences in the site of administration (either peripheral or intracardiac). The mean effective dosage reported by DiMarco et al required to terminate supraventricular tachycardia was 83±35 μg/kg.[382] The patients treated by Watt et al required a slightly higher dosage (135 μg/kg).[384] Both investigators used a similar administration protocol. The initial injection consisted of a dosage equal to 30–40 μg/kg. If no effect was observed within 60 seconds, a second injection of 60–80 μg/kg was administered. The dosage of adenosine was progressively increased by 30–40 μg/kg increments until either tachy-

TABLE 3–15
CLINICAL ELECTROPHYSIOLOGIC EFFECTS OF ANTIARRHYTHMIC DRUGS*

DRUG	AH	HV	ERP A	ERP AVN	ERP HPS	ERP V
Class I						
Quinidine	↓0↓	0↓		↑	↓0↑	↑
Procainamide	0↑	0↑	↑	0↓	↑	↑
Disopyramide	0↑	0↑	↑	0↑	↑	↑
Lidocaine	0↓	0↑	0	0↓	0↓	0↓
Phenytoin	0↓	0↑	0	0↓	↓	0↓
Mexiletine	0↑	0↑	0	0↑	0↓	0
Ethmozine	0↑	0↑	0	0	0↓	0
Encainide	↑	↑	↑	↑	↑	↑
Flecainide	↑	↑	↑	0	↓	↑
Propafenone	↑	↑	↑	↑	↓	↑
Class II						
Propranolol	0↑	0	0	↑	0	0
Atenolol	0↑	0	0	↑	0	0
Class III						
Amiodarone	↑	0↑	↑	↑	↑	↑
Bretylium	0↓	0	↓0↑	↓0↑	↓0↑	↓0↑
Class IV						
Verapamil	↑	0	0↑	↑	0	0
Class V						
Digoxin	↑	0	↓0↑	↑	0	0↓
Class VI						
Adenosine	↑	0	↓	↑	0	0

*A = atrium; AH = low septal right atrium to His bundle activation interval; AVN = atrioventricular node; ERP = effective refractory period; HPS = His-Purkinje system; HV = His bundle to ventricular activation interval; V = ventricle; 0 = no change; ↑ = increase; ↓ = decrease.

TABLE 3–16
ALTERATION OF ELECTROCARDIOGRAPHIC INTERVALS BY ANTIARRHYTHMIC DRUGS*

DRUG	SINUS RATE	PR	QRS	QT
Class I				
Quinidine	↓0↑	0↑	↑	↑
Procainamide	↓0↑	↑	↑	↑
Disopyramide	↓0↑	0↑	↑	↑
Lidocaine	0	0	0	0↓
Phenytoin	0	0	0	0↓
Mexiletine	0↓	0	0	0
Ethmozine	0↑	0↑	0↑	0
Encainide	0↓	↑	↑	0↑
Flecainide	0↓	↑	↑	↑
Propafenone	↓0↑	↑	↑	0↑
Class II				
Propranolol	↓	↑	0	↓
Atenolol	↓	↑	0	↓
Class III				
Amiodarone	↓	↑	↑	↑
Bretylium	0↑	0↑	0	0
Class IV				
Verapamil	↓0↑	↑	0	0
Class V				
Digoxin	0↓	↑	0	↓
Class VI				
Adenosine	↓	↑	0	0

*0 = no change; ↑ = increase; ↓ = decrease.

TABLE 3–17
DOSAGE REGIMEN FOR ANTIARRHYTHMIC DRUGS*

DRUG	INTRAVENOUS ADMINISTRATION Loading (mg/kg)†	Maintenance (μg/kg/min)†	ORAL ADMINISTRATION (mg/kg/d)†
Class I			
Quinidine	Not recommended		30–60
Procainamide	10–15 (max = 1000 mg)	30–80	50–100
Disopyramide	N.A.		<2 years of age: 20–33 2–10 years of age: 10–24 >10 years of age: 6–14
Lidocaine	1–3	30–50	N.A.
Phenytoin	10–15		Day 1: 15 Day 2: 7.5 Maintenance: 4–8
Mexiletine	N.A.		4.2–15
Ethmozine	N.A.		5–15
Encainide	N.A.		60–120 mg/m²/day
Flecainide	N.A		3–6
Propafenone	1–2	0.004–0.007 mg/kg/min	N.A.
Class II			
Propranolol	0.01–0.15		2–5
Atenolol	N.A.		1–2
Class III			
Amiodarone	5		10–15 for 1–2 weeks; Maintenance: 5–10
Bretylium	5–15	15–30	Not recommended
Class IV			
Verapamil	0.075–0.15	0.005 mg/kg/min	4–17
Class V			
Digoxin		See Table 3–10	
Class VI			
Adenosine	30–250 μg/kg		Not recommended

*N.A. = not available.
†Unless otherwise noted.

cardia terminated or AV block ensued. Clarke et al administered 50–250 μg/kg of adenosine to four pediatric patients to terminate supraventricular tachycardia.[385]

Adverse Effects

Side effects, although short-lived, are not infrequent following adenosine administration, and can be either cardiovascular, pulmonary, or neurologic. Sinus bradycardia and atrioventricular block occur following administration of high doses of adenosine. Long sinus pauses (75 seconds) may ensue after termination of supraventricular tachycardia in patients with sick sinus syndrome.[382, 384] Adenosine administration during supraventricular tachycardia has on rare occasions induced atrial fibrillation.[386] Pulmonary symptoms include dyspnea and coughing. Adenosine has also been reported to produce bronchoconstriction and wheezing in patients predisposed to asthma. Neurologic side effects such as flushing and headache may develop secondary to vasodilatation. Agitation, vomiting, and (rarely) seizure activity have also been observed.

Drug Interactions

Meszaros et al have documented several important drug interactions with adenosine in vitro using guinea pig atrial tissue.[387] These investigators found that quinidine will antagonize the effects of adenosine (shortening of repolarization and hyperpolarization of membrane potential). BMA, an antiarrhythmic drug with class III effects, will similarly suppress the effect of adenosine on atrial action potential duration. In contrast, Meszaros et al noted a synergistic effect between verapamil and adenosine. Superfusion of guinea pig atrial tissue with the combination of adenosine and verapamil markedly shortened action potential duration. Drug interactions with dipyridamole have been previously discussed.

Despite these in vitro observations, it is still relatively unknown if important antiarrhythmic drug interactions occur in the clinical setting. DiMarco et al did not observe any such interactions in 11 patients who received adenosine in combination with another antiarrhythmic drug to terminate supraventricular tachycardia.[382]

Indications

Adenosine administration provides a rapid and effective method for terminating acute episodes of supraventricular tachycardia that incorporate the atrioventricular node in the reentrant circuit (AV node reentry, AV reciprocating tachycardia, and the permanent form of junctional reciprocating tachycardia (PJRT). Because of its very short half-life, adenosine is not effective for long-term management of recurrent paroxysms of supraventricular tachycardia. Adenosine may be diagnostically helpful in demonstrating the mechanism of supraventricular arrhythmias that fail to terminate following its administration (e.g., atrial flutter, sinus node reentry tachycardias, or primary atrial tachycardias). Preliminary data suggest that adenosine may be effective in terminating ventricular tachycardia in the small subset of patients with normal hearts and exercise-induced ventricular tachycardia.[388]

The use of adenosine to terminate supraventricular tachycardia has one major advantage over other antiarrhythmic drugs: its short half-life. After bolus administration, the effects of adenosine dissipate within 60 seconds. This allows the clinician to administer progressively larger doses until therapeutic effect is achieved, without reaching a toxic effect resulting from drug accumulation.

SUMMARY

The cellular and clinical electrophysiologic effects, electrocardiographic effects, and dosage information for the drugs discussed in this chapter are summarized in Tables 3–14 through 3–17, pages 102 to 104.

References

1. Woosley RL, Shand DG: Pharmacokinetics of drugs. Am J Cardiol 41:986–995, 1978.
2. Maxwell GM: Principles of Pediatric Pharmacology. New York, Oxford University Press, 1984.
3. Evans ME, Bhat R, Vidyasagar D: Factors modulating drug therapy and pharmacokinetics. In Yeh TF (ed): Drug Therapy in the Neonate and Small Infant. Chicago, Year Book Medical Publishers, 1985, pp 3–18.
4. Rowland M, Tozer TN: Clinical Pharmacokinetics: Concepts and Applications. Philadelphia, Lea and Febiger, 1980.
5. Greenblatt DJ, Koch-Weser J: Clinical pharmacokinetics. I. N Engl J Med 293:702–705, 1975.
6. Greenblatt DJ, Koch-Weser J: Clinical pharmacokinetics. II. N Engl J Med 293:964–970, 1975.
7. Kates RE, Woosley RL, Harrison DC. Clinical importance of metabolites of antiarrhythmic drugs. Am J Cardiol 53:248–251, 1984.
8. Friedman H, Greenblatt DJ: Rational therapeutic monitoring. JAMA 256:2227–2233, 1986.
9. Koch-Weser J: Drug interactions in cardiovascular therapy. Am Heart J 90:93–116, 1975.
10. Mason JW, Hondeghem LM. Quinidine. Ann NY Acad Sci 432:162–176, 1984.
11. Hoffman BF, Rosen MR, Wit AL: Electrophysiology and pharmacology of cardiac arrhythmias. VII. Cardiac effects of quinidine and procainamide. Am Heart J 90:117–122, 1975.
12. Hondeghem LM, Matsubara T: Quinidine and lidocaine: Activation and inactivation block. Proc West Pharmacol Soc 27:19–21, 1984.

12a. Hiraoka M, Sawadak, Kawano S: Effects of quinidine on plateau currents of guinea-pig ventricular myocytes. J Mol Cell Cardiol 18:1097–1106, 1986.

13. Roberts J, Goldberg P: Changes in responsiveness of the heart to drugs during aging. Fed Proc 38:1927–1932, 1979.

13a. Morikawa Y, Rosen MR. Effects of quinidine on the transmembrane potential of young and adult canine Purkinje fibers. J Pharm Exp Ther 236:832–837, 1986.

14. Dorian P, Fain ES, Davy JM, et al: Effects of quinidine and bretylium on defibrillation energy requirements. Am Heart J 112:19–25, 1986.
15. Woo E, Greenblatt DJ: A reevaluation of intravenous quinidine. Am Heart J 96:829–832, 1978.
16. Covinsky JO, Russo J, Kelly KL, et al: Relative bioavailability of quinidine gluconate and quinidine sulfate in healthy volunteers. J Clin Pharmacol 19:261–269, 1979.
17. Woo E, Greenblatt DJ: Effect of food on enteral absorption of quinidine. Clin Pharmacol Ther 27:188–193, 1980.
18. Morganroth J, Hunter H: Comparative efficacy and safety of short acting and sustained release quinidine in the treatment of patients with ventricular arrhythmias. Am Heart J 110:1176–1181, 1985.
19. Szefler SJ, Shen D, Gingell RL: Quinidine elimination in pediatric patients. Pediatr Res 14(suppl 1):473, 1980.
20. Pickoff AS, Kessler KM, Singh S, et al: Age related differences in the protein binding of quinidine. Dev Pharmacol Ther 3:108–115, 1981.
21. Ueda CT, Dzindizio BS. Quinidine kinetics in

congestive heart failure. Clin Pharmacol Ther 23:158–164, 1978.
22. Vozeh S, Uematsu T, Guentert TW, et al: Kinetics and electrocardiographic changes after oral 3-OH-quinidine in healthy subjects. Clin Pharmacol Ther 37:575–581, 1985.
23. Wooding-Scott RA, Visco J, Slaughter RL: Total and unbound concentrations of quinidine and 3-hydroxyquinidine at steady state. Am Heart J 113:302–306, 1987.
24. Kessler KM, Lisker B, Conde C, et al: Abnormal quinidine binding in survivors of pre-hospital cardiac arrest. Am Heart J 107:665–669, 1984.
25. Burkart GJ, Marin-Garcia J: Quinidine dosage in children using population estimates. Pediatr Cardiol 6:269–273, 1986.
26. Newton G, Crawford EJ: A study of quinidine dosage in infants and children. J Pediatr 47:700–715, 1955.
27. Roden DM, Woosley RL, Primm RK: Incidence and clinical features of the quinidine associated long QT syndrome: Implications for patient care. Am Heart J 111:1088–1093, 1986.
28. Maisel AS, Motulsky HJ, Insel PA: Hypotension after quinidine plus verapamil. Possible addictive competition at alpha-adrenergic receptors. N Engl J Med 312:167–170, 1985.
29. Pedersen KE: Digoxin interactions. The influence of quinidine and verapamil on the pharmacokinetics and receptor binding of digitalis glycosides. Acta Medica Scand 697:1–40, 1985.
30. Koren G, Soldin SJ: Cardiac glycosides. Clin Lab Med 7:587–606, 1987.
31. Guntherroth WG, Cyr DR, Mack LA, et al: Hydrops from reciprocating atrioventricular tachycardia in a 27 week fetus requiring quinidine for conversion. Obstet Gynecol 66(suppl 3):29S–33S, 1985.
32. Krongrad E, Hordof AJ: Tachycardias in children. In Surawicz B, Reddy CP, Prystowsky EN (eds): Tachycardias. Boston, Martinus Nijhoff, 1984, pp 319–354.
33. Michelson EL, Spear JF, Moore EN: Effects of procainamide on strength-interval relations in normal and chronically infarcted canine myocardium. Am J Cardiol 47:1223–1232, 1981.
34. Myerburg RJ, Bassett AL, Epstein K, et al: Electrophysiological effects of procainamide in acute and healed experimental ischemic injury of cat myocardium. Circ Res 50:386–393, 1982.
35. Ehring GR, Hondeghem LM: Structural similarities and cardiac electrophysiological differences between lidocaine and procainamide. Proc West Pharmacol Soc 23:163–166, 1980.
36. Hewett K, Gessman L, Rosen MR: Effects of procainamide, quinidine and ethmozine on delayed afterdepolarizations. Eur J Pharmacol 96:21–28, 1983.
37. Ezrin AM, Epstein K, Bassett AL, et al: Effects of procaine amide on cellular electrophysiology of neonatal and adult dog myocardium. Dev Pharmacol Ther 1:352–363, 1980.
38. Goldberg D, Reiffel JA, Davis JC, et al: Electrophysiologic effects of procainamide on sinus node function in patients with and without sinus node disease. Am Heart J 103:75–79, 1982.
39. Gang ES, Denton TA, Oseran DS, et al: Rate-dependent effects of procainamide on His-Purkinje conduction in man. Am J Cardiol 55:1525–1529, 1985.
40. Morady F, DiCarlo LA, Baerman JM, et al: Rate dependent effects of intravenous lidocaine, procainamide and amiodarone on intraventricular conduction. J Am Coll Cardiol 6:179–185, 1985.
41. Scheinman MM, Weiss AN, Shafton E, et al: Electrophysiologic effects of procainamide in patients with intraventricular conduction delay. Circulation 49:522–529, 1974.
42. Josephson ME, Caracta AR, Ricciutti MA, et al: Electrophysiologic properties of procainamide in man. Am J Cardiol 33:596–603, 1974.
43. Wellens HJJ, Braat S, Brugada P, et al: Use of procainamide in patients with the Wolff-Parkinson-White syndrome to disclose a short refractory period of the accessory pathway. Am J Cardiol 50:1087–1089, 1982.
44. Sellers TD, Campbell RWF, Bashore TM, et al: Effects of procainamide and quinidine sulfate in the Wolff-Parkinson-White syndrome. Circulation 55:15–22, 1977.
45. Anderson JL: Conventional and sustained release procainamide: Update on pharmacology and clinical use. Clin Ther 7:618–640, 1985.
46. Koch-Weser J, Klein SW: Procainamide dosage schedules, plasma concentrations and clinical effects. JAMA 215:1454–1460, 1971.
47. Singh S, Gelband H, Mehta A, et al: Procainamide elimination kinetics in pediatric patients. Pediatr Res 15:472, 1981.
48. Kessler KM, Kayden DS, Estes DM, et al: Procainamide pharmacokinetics in patients with acute myocardial infarction or congestive heart failure. J Am Coll Cardiol 5:1131–1139, 1986.
49. Ylitalo P, Ruosteenoja R, Leskinen O, et al: Significance of acetylator phenotype in pharmacokinetics and adverse effects of procainamide. Eur J Clin Pharmacol 25:791–795, 1983.
50. Lima JJ, Kuritzky PM, Schentag JJ, et al: Fetal uptake and neonatal disposition of procainamide and its acetylated metabolite: A case report. Pediatrics 61:491–493, 1978.
51. Given BD, Phillipe M, Sanders SP, et al: Procainamide cardioversion of fetal supraventricular tachyarrhythmia. Am J Cardiol 53:1460–1461, 1984.
52. Woosley RL, Drayer DE, Reidenberg MM, et al: Effect of acetylator phenotype on the rate at which procainamide induces antinuclear antibodies and the lupus syndrome. N Engl J Med 298:1157–1159, 1978.
53. Meyers DG, Gonzalez ER, Peters LL, et al: Severe neutropenia associated with procainamide: Comparison of sustained release and conventional preparations. Am Heart J 109:1393–1395, 1985.
54. Saal AK, Werner JA, Greene HL, et al: Effect of amiodarone on serum quinidine and procainamide levels. Am J Cardiol 53:1264–1267, 1984.
55. Christian CD, Meredith CG, Spery KV: Cimetidine inhibits renal procainamide clearance. Clin Pharmacol Ther 36:221–227, 1984.
56. Weidler DJ, Gary DC, Jallad NJ, et al: The effect of long term propranolol administration on the pharmacokinetics of procainamide in humans. Clin Pharmacol Ther 29:289, 1981.
57. Bexton RS, Hellestrand KJ, Cory-Pearce R, et al: The direct electrophysiologic effects of disopyramide phosphate in the transplanted human heart. Circulation 67:38–45, 1983.
58. Katoh T, Karaguezian HS, Jordan J, et al: The cellular electrophysiologic mechanism of the dual

actions of disopyramide on rabbit sinus node function. Circulation 66:1216–1224, 1982.
59. Kotake H, Hasagawa J, Hata T, et al: Electrophysiological effect of disopyramide on rabbit sinus node cells. J Electrocardiol 18:377–384, 1985.
60. Kus T, Sasyniuk BI: Electrophysiological actions of disopyramide phosphate on canine ventricular muscle and Purkinje fibers. Circ Res 37:844–854, 1975.
61. Danilo P, Hordof A, Rosen MR: Effects of disopyramide on electrophysiological properties of canine cardiac Purkinje fibers. J Pharm Exp Ther 201:701–710, 1977.
62. Yatani A, Akaike N: Blockade of the sodium current in isolated single cells from rat ventricle with mexiletine and disopyramide. J Mol Cell Cardiol 17:467–476, 1985.
63. Sasyniuk BI, Kus T: Cellular electrophysiologic changes induced by disopyramide phosphate in normal and infarcted hearts. J Int Med Res 4(suppl 1):20–25, 1976.
64. Frame LH, Hoffman BF: Disopyramide's effects are enhanced by fast pacing rates in depolarized tissues. Circulation 64(suppl 4):272, 1981.
65. Yamada S, Nishimura M, Watanabe Y: Electrophysiologic effects of disopyramide studied in a hypoxic canine Purkinje fiber model. J Electrocardiol 15:31–40, 1982.
66. Giacomini KM, Nelson WL, Pershe RA, et al: In vivo interaction of the enantiomers of disopyramide in human subjects. J Pharmacokinet Biopharm 14:335–356, 1986.
67. Kashani IA, Shakibi JG, Siassi B: Electrophysiologic effects of disopyramide in children. Jpn Heart J 21:491–496, 1980.
68. Bergfeldt L, Rosenqvist M, Vallin H, et al: Disopyramide induced second and third degree atrioventricular block in patients with bifascicular block: An acute stress test to predict atrioventricular block progression. Br Heart J 53:328–334, 1985.
69. La Barre A, Strauss HC, Scheinman MM, et al: Electrophysiologic effects of disopyramide phosphate on sinus node function in patients with sinus node dysfunction. Circulation 59:226–235, 1979.
70. Siddoway LA, Woosley RL: Clinical pharmacokinetics of disopyramide. Clin Pharmacokinet 11:214–222, 1986.
71. Chiang WT, Von Bahr C, Calissendorff B, et al: Kinetics and dynamics of disopyramide and its dealkylated metabolite in healthy subjects. Clin Pharmacol Ther 38:37–44, 1985.
72. Bonde J, Graudal NA, Pedersen LE, et al: Kinetics of disopyramide in decreased hepatic function. Eur J Clin Pharmacol 31:73–77, 1986.
73. Landmark K, Bredesen JE, Thaulow E, et al: Pharmacokinetics of disopyramide in patients with imminent to moderate cardiac failure. Eur J Clin Pharmacol 19:187–192, 1981.
74. Hordoff A, Moak J, Steeg C, et al: Treatment of cardiac arrhythmias with disopyramide (Norpace). Pediatr Res 15:465, 1981.
75. Holt DW, Walsh AC, Curry PV, et al: Pediatric use of mexiletine and disopyramide. Br Med J 2:1476–1477, 1979.
76. Hoppu K, Neuvonen PJ, Korte T: Disopyramide and breast feeding. Br J Clin Pharmacol 21:553, 1986.
77. Taylor EH, Pappas AA: Disopyramide: Clinical indications, pharmacokinetics and laboratory assessment. Ann Clin Lab Sci 16:289–295, 1986.
78. Bonde J, Bodtkar S, Angelo HR, et al: Atenolol inhibits the elimination of disopyramide. Eur J Clin Pharmacol 28:41–43, 1985.
79. Matos JA, Fisher JD, Kim SG: Disopyramide-phenytoin interaction. Circulation 64(suppl 4):264, 1981.
80. Rosen MR, Hoffman BF, Wit AL: Electrophysiology and pharmacology of cardiac arrhythmias. V. Cardiac antiarrhythmic effects of lidocaine. Am Heart J 89:526–536, 1975.
81. Ono K, Kigosue T, Arita M: Comparison of the inhibitory effects of mexiletine and lidocaine on the calcium current of single ventricular cells. Life Sci 39:1465–1470, 1986.
82. Mandel WJ, Bigger JT: Electrophysiologic effects of lidocaine on isolated canine and rabbit atrial tissue. J Pharm Exp Ther 178:81–93, 1971.
83. Davis LD, Tempte JV: Electrophysiological actions of lidocaine on canine ventricular muscle and Purkinje fibers. Circ Res 24:639–655, 1969.
84. Bigger JT, Mandel WJ: Effect of lidocaine on the electrophysiological properties of ventricular muscle and Purkinje fibers. J Clin Invest 49:63–77, 1970.
85. Wittig J, Harrison LA, Wallace AG: Electrophysiological effects of lidocaine on distal Purkinje fibers of canine heart. Am Heart J 86:69–78, 1973.
86. El-Sherif N, Scherlag BJ, Lazzara R, et al: Reentrant ventricular arrhythmias in the late myocardial infarction period. 4. Mechanism of action of lidocaine. Circulation 56:395–402, 1977.
87. Davis J, Matsubara T, Scheinman MM, et al: Use-dependent effects of lidocaine on conduction in canine myocardium: Application of the modulated receptor hypothesis in vivo. Circulation 74:205–214, 1986.
88. Mary-Rabine L, Rosen MR: Lidocaine effects on action potentials of Purkinje fibers from neonatal and adult dogs. J Pharm Exp Ther 205:204–211, 1978.
89. Morikawa Y, Rosen MR: Developmental changes in the effects of lidocaine on the electrophysiological properties of canine Purkinje fibers. Circ Res 55:633–641, 1984.
90. Dhingra RC, Deedwania PC, Cummings JM, et al: Electrophysiologic effects of lidocaine on sinus node and atrium in patients with and without sinoatrial dysfunction. Circulation 57:448–454, 1978.
91. Rosen KM, Lau SH, Weiss MB, et al: The effect of lidocaine on atrioventricular and intraventricular conduction in man. Am J Cardiol 25:1–5, 1970.
92. Roos J, Dunning AJ: Effects of lidocaine on impulse formation and conduction defects in man. Am Heart J 89:686–699, 1975.
93. Josephson ME, Caracta AR, Lau SH, et al: Effects of lidocaine on refractory periods in man. Am Heart J 84:778–786, 1972.
94. Chow MSS, Kluger J, DiPersion DM, et al: Antifibrillatory effects of lidocaine and bretylium immediately postcardiopulmonary resuscitation. Am Heart J 110:938–943, 1985.
95. Shakibi JG, Aryanpur I: Electrophysiologic effects of lidocaine in children. Jpn Heart J 20:271–276, 1979.
96. Wyman MG, Slaughter RL, Farolino DA, et al: Multiple bolus technique for lidocaine administration in acute ischemic heart disease. II. Treatment of refractory ventricular arrhythmias and the pharmacokinetic significance of severe left ventricular failure. J Am Coll Cardiol 2:764–769, 1983.

97. Zeisler JA, Gaarder TD, De Mesquita SA: Lidocaine excretion in breast milk. Drug Intell Clin Pharmacol 20:691–693, 1986.
98. Sakuma S, Oka T, Okuno A, et al: Placental transfer of lidocaine and elimination from newborns following obstetrical epidural and pudendal anesthesia. Pediatr Pharmacol 5:107–115, 1985.
99. Mihaly GW, Moore G, Thomas J, et al: The pharmacokinetics and metabolism of the anilide local anesthetics in neonates. Eur J Clin Pharmacol 13:143–152, 1978.
100. Tucker GT, Boyes RN, Bridenbaugh PO, et al: Binding of anilide type local anesthetics in human plasma. I. Relationship between binding, physiochemical properties and anesthetic activity. Anesthesiology 33:287–303, 1970.
101. Finholt DA, Stirt JA, DiFazio CA, et al: Lidocaine pharmacokinetics in children during general anesthesia. Anesth Analg 65:279–282, 1986.
102. Henry W, Casto D, Keagy B, et al: The effect of right to left intracardiac shunting on arterial lidocaine levels in a canine model. Pediatr Res 19(suppl 1):128, 1985.
103. Dunahy DT, Aronow WS: Lidocaine-induced cardiac rate changes in atrial fibrillation and atrial flutter. Am Heart J 95:474–482, 1978.
104. Bauer LA, Edwards WAD, Randolph FP, et al: Cimetidine-induced decrease in lidocaine clearance. Am Heart J 108:413–415, 1984.
105. Wit AL, Rosen MR, Hoffman BF: Electrophysiology and pharmacology of cardiac arrhythmias. VIII. Cardiac effects of diphenylhydantoin, A. Am Heart J 90:265–272, 1975.
106. Wit AL, Rosen MR, Hoffman BF: Electrophysiology and pharmacology of cardiac arrhythmias. VIII. Cardiac effects of diphenylhydantoin, B. Am Heart J 90:397–404, 1975.
107. Bigger JT, Bassett AL, Hoffman BF: Electrophysiological effects of diphenylhydantoin on canine Purkinje fibers. Circ Res 22:221–236, 1968.
108. Rosen MR, Danilo P, Alonso MB, et al: Effects of therapeutic concentrations of diphenylhydantoin on transmembrane potentials of normal and depressed Purkinje fibers. J Pharm Exp Ther 197:594–603, 1976.
109. Strauss HC, Bigger JT, Bassett AL, et al: Actions of diphenylhydantoin on the electrical properties of isolated rabbit and canine atria. Circ Res 23:463–477, 1968.
110. Singh BN, Vaughn-Williams EM: Effect of altering potassium concentration on the action of lidocaine and diphenylhydantoin on rabbit atrial and ventricular muscle. Circ Res 24:286–295, 1971.
111. Hondeghem LM, Grant AO, Jensen RA: Antiarrhythmic drug action: Selective depression of hypoxic cardiac cells. Am Heart J 87:602–605, 1974.
112. El-Sherif N, Lazzara R: Reentrant ventricular arrhythmias in the late myocardial infarction period. 5. Mechanisms of action of diphenylhydantoin. Circulation 57:465–472, 1978.
113. Sanchez-Chapula J, Josephson IR: Effect of phenytoin on the sodium current in isolated rat ventricular cells. J Mol Cell Cardiol 15:515–522, 1983.
114. Yatani A, Hamilton S, Brown AM: Diphenylhydantoin blocks cardiac calcium channels and binds to the dihydropyridine receptor. Circ Res 59:356–361, 1986.
115. Wasserstrom JA, Ferrier GR: Effects of phenytoin and quinidine on digitalis induced oscillatory afterpotentials, aftercontractions, and inotropy in canine ventricular tissues. J Mol Cell Cardiol 14:725–736, 1982.
116. Spinelli W, Rosen MR: Frequency dependent actions of phenytoin in adult and young canine Purkinje fibers. J Pharm Exp Ther 238:794–801, 1986.
117. Garan H, Ruskin JN, Powell WJ: Centrally mediated effect of phenytoin on digoxin-induced ventricular arrhythmias. Am J Physiol 241:H67–72, 1981.
118. Gillis RA, McClellan JR, Sauer TS, et al: Depression of cardiac sympathetic nerve activity by diphenylhydantoin. J Pharm Exp Ther 173:599–610, 1971.
119. Tsuchioka Y, Yamoaka K, Hashimoto M, et al: Electrophysiological effects of diphenylhydantoin in patients with sinus node dysfunction. Jpn Heart J 27:159–166, 1986.
120. Caracta AR, Damato AN, Josephson ME, et al: Electrophysiologic properties of diphenylhydantoin. Circulation 47:1234–1241, 1973.
121. Damato AN, Berkowitz WD, Patton RD, et al: The effect of diphenylhydantoin on atrioventricular and intraventricular conduction in man. Am Heart J 79:51–56, 1970.
122. Matsukura M, Ikeda T, Higashi A, et al: Relative bioavailability of two different phenytoin preparations: Evidence for an age dependency. Dev Pharmacol Ther 7:160–168, 1984.
123. Shah Y, Miller RK: The pharmacokinetics of phenytoin in perfused human placenta. Pediatr Pharmacol 5:165–179, 1985.
124. Loughnan PM, Greenwald A, Purton WW, et al: Pharmacokinetic observations of phenytoin disposition in the newborn and young infant. Arch Dis Child 52:302–309, 1977.
125. Leff R, Fischer LJ, Roberts RJ: Phenytoin metabolism in infants following intravenous and oral administration. Dev Pharmacol Ther 9:217–223, 1986.
126. Leppik IE, Fischer J, Kriel R, et al: Altered phenytoin clearance with febrile illness. Neurology 33:173–178, 1983.
127. Garson A, Gillette PC: Intravenous dilantin protocol for ventricular dysrhythmias in children. Pediatr Res 15:463, 1981.
128. Garson A, Kugler JD, Gillette PC, et al: Control of late postoperative ventricular arrhythmias with phenytoin in young patients. Am J Cardiol 46:290–294, 1980.
129. Hanson JW, Smith DW: The fetal hydantoin syndrome. J Pediatr 87:285–290, 1975.
130. Gore JM, Haffajee CI, Alpert JS: Interaction of amiodarone and diphenylhydantoin. Am J Cardiol 54:1145, 1984.
131. Rameis H: On the interaction between phenytoin and digoxin. Eur J Clin Pharmacol 29:49–53, 1985.
132. Campbell RWF: Mexiletine. N Engl J Med 316:29–34, 1987.
133. Woosley RL, Wang T, Stone W, et al: Pharmacology, electrophysiology and pharmacokinetics of mexiletine. Am Heart J 107:1058–1065, 1984.
134. Igawa O, Kotake H, Mushiba H: Electrophysiological actions of mexiletine on rabbit sinoatrial node cells. Eur J Pharmacol 122:11–17, 1986.
135. Hering S, Bodewei R, Wollenberger A: Sodium current in freshly isolated and in cultured single rat myocardial cells: Frequency and voltage dependent block by mexiletine. J Mol Cell Cardiol 15:431–444, 1983.

136. Matsuo S, Kishida H, Munakata K, et al: The effects of mexiletine on action potential duration and its restitution in guinea pig ventricular muscle. Jpn Heart J 26:271–287, 1985.
137. Campbell TJ: Resting and rate dependent depression of maximum rate of depolarization ($\dot{V}$ max) in guinea pig ventricular action potentials by mexiletine, disopyramide, and encainide. J Cardiovasc Pharmacol 5:291–296, 1983.
138. Frame L, Gitant G, Hoffman BF: Mexiletine and tocainide differ from lidocaine in their use-dependent kinetics. Circulation (suppl 2)66:292, 1982.
139. Arita M, Gato M, Nagamoto Y, et al: Electrophysiological actions of mexiletine (Ko 1173) on canine Purkinje fibers and ventricular muscle. Br J Pharmacol 67:143–152, 1979.
140. Burke G, Berman ND: Differential electrophysiologic effects of mexiletine on normal and hypoxic canine Purkinje fibers. J Cardiovasc Pharmacol 7:1096–1100, 1985.
141. Yoon MS, Han J: Electrophysiologic effects of mexiletine on normal and ischemic ventricles. J Electrocardiol 15:109–114, 1982.
142. Amerini S, Carboni P, Cerbai E, et al: Electrophysiological mechanisms for the antiarrhythmic action of mexiletine on digitalis-, reperfusion-, and reoxygenation-induced arrhythmias. Br J Pharmacol 86:805–815, 1985.
143. Singh BN, Vaughn-Williams EM: Investigations of the mode of action of a new antidysrhythmic drug, Ko 1173. Br J Pharmacol 44:1–9, 1972.
144. Kitagawa H, Takeda F, Kohei H: Inhibition of sympathetic nervous system by mexiletine, an antiarrhythmic agent, and its antagonism by oubain. Arzneim-Forsch 35:356–359, 1985.
145. Saksena S, Craelius W: The electropharmacology and therapeutic role of mexiletine. Clin Prog Electrophysiol Pacing 1:122–141, 1983.
146. Shakibi JG, Moezzi B: Electrophysiologic effects of mexiletine in children. Jpn Heart J 23:733–738, 1982.
147. McComish M, Kitson D, Robinson C, et al: Clinical electrophysiological effects of mexiletine. Postgrad Med J 53(suppl 1):85–91, 1977.
148. Grech-Belanger O: Clinical pharmacokinetics of mexiletine. Clin Prog Electrophysiol Pacing 4:553–560, 1986.
149. Pentikainen PJ, Hietakorp S, Halinen MO, et al: Cirrhosis of the liver markedly impairs the elimination of mexiletine. Eur J Clin Pharmacol 30:83–88, 1986.
150. El Allaf D, Henrard L, Crochelet L, et al: Pharmacokinetics of mexiletine in renal insufficiency. Br J Clin Pharmacol 14:431–435, 1982.
151. Grech-Belanger O, Turgcon J, Gilbert M: Stereoselective disposition of mexiletine in man. Br J Clin Pharmacol 21:481–487, 1986.
152. Chazov EI, Shugushev KK, Rosenshtraukh LV: Ethmozine. I. Effects of intravenous drug administration on paroxysmal supraventricular tachycardia in the ventricular preexcitation syndrome. Am Heart J 108:475–482, 1984.
153. Ruffy R, Rosenshtraukh LV, Elharrar V, et al: Electrophysiological effects of ethmozine on canine myocardium. Cardiovasc Res 13:354–363, 1979.
154. Dangman KH, Hoffman BF: Antiarrhythmic effects of ethmozine in cardiac Purkinje fibers: Suppression of automaticity and abolition of triggering. J Pharm Exp Ther 227:578–586, 1983.
155. Yuryavichus IA, Rosenshtraukh LV, Undrovinas AI, et al: The effect of ethmozine, a new antiarrhythmic agent, on the force of contraction, transmembrane potential and rapid incoming sodium flow of the frog atrial muscle. Kardiologiia 18:118–125, 1978.
156. Tsuji Y, Nishimara M, Osada M, et al: Membrane action of ethmozine on normoxic and hypoxic canine Purkinje fibers. J Cardiovasc Pharmacol 5:961–967, 1983.
157. Rvenko SV, Bolotina VM, Khodorov BI: Tonic and frequency dependent block of Na channels by ethmozine. J Mol Cell Cardiol 12(suppl 1):135, 1980.
158. Undrovinas AI, Yushmanova AV, Rosenshtraukh LV: Effects of ethmozine and lidocaine on sodium currents in single internally perfused myocardial cells. J Mol Cell Cardiol 12(suppl 1):171, 1980.
159. Schubert B, Hering S, Bodewei R, et al: Use- and voltage-dependent depression by ethmozine (moricizine) on the rapid inward sodium current in single rat ventricular muscle cells. J Cardiovasc Pharmacol 8:358–366, 1986.
160. Urthaler F, Rosenshtraukh LV, Walker AA, et al: Differential inotropic actions of ethmozine and ethacizin. Am Heart J 111:462–465, 1986.
161. Urthaler F, Rosenshtraukh LV, Hageman GR, et al: Differential modulation of autonomic activity by ethmozine and ethacizin (analog of ethmozine) on the canine sinus node and atrioventricular junction. J Am Coll Cardiol 8:86A–94A, 1986.
162. Shugushev KK, Rosenshtraukh LV, Smetnev AS: Electrophysiologic effects of ethmozine on sinus node function in patients with and without sinus node dysfunction. Clin Cardiol 9:443–448, 1986.
163. Fox S, Hoffman BF, Rosen MR: Effects of ethmozine and lidocaine on ventricular fibrillation and defibrillation in anesthetized dogs. Am J Cardiol 45:474, 1980.
164. Pratt CM, Young JB, Wierman AM, et al: Complex ventricular arrhythmias with the mitral valve prolapse syndrome. Effectiveness of moricizine (ethmozine) in patients resistant to conventional antiarrhythmics. Am J Med 80:826–832, 1986.
165. Piotrovsky VK, Merkulova IN, Romina MN, et al: Pharmacokinetics of ethmozine after a single intravenous injection. Kardiologiia 22:75–80, 1982.
166. MacFarland RT, Moeller VR, Pieniaszek HJ, et al: Assessment of the potential pharmacokinetic interaction between digoxin and ethmozine. J Clin Pharmacol 25:138–143, 1985.
167. Biollaz J, Shaheen O, Wood AJJ: Cimetidine inhibition of ethmozine metabolism. Clin Pharmacol Ther 37:665–668, 1985.
168. Morganroth J: Safety and efficacy of a twice daily dosing regimen for moricizine (ethmozine). Am Heart J 110:1188–1192, 1985.
169. Pratt CM, Wierman A, Seals AA, et al: Efficacy and safety of moricizine in patients with ventricular tachycardia: Results of a placebo controlled prospective long term clinical trial. Circulation 73:718–726, 1986.
170. Kennedy HL, Sprague MK, Redd RM, et al: Serum digoxin concentrations during ethmozine antiarrhythmic therapy. Am Heart J 111:667–672, 1986.
171. Evans V, Garson A, Smith RT, et al: Ethmozine: A promising drug for "automatic" atrial ectopic focus tachycardia. Circulation 72(suppl 3):173, 1985.
172. Guehler J, Gornick CC, Tobler HG, et al: Electrophysiologic effects of flecainide acetate and its

major metabolites in the canine heart. Am J Cardiol 55:807–812, 1985.
173. Ikeda N, Singh BN, Davis LD, et al: Effects of flecainide on the electrophysiologic properties of isolated canine and rabbit myocardial fibers. J Am Coll Cardiol 5:303–310, 1985.
174. Singh BN, Nademaneek, Josephson MA, et al: The electrophysiology and pharmacology of verapamil, flecainide and amiodarone: Correlations with clinical effects and antiarrhythmic actions. Ann NY Acad Sci 432:210–235, 1984.
175. Estes NAM, Garan H, Ruskin JN: Electrophysiologic properties of flecainide acetate. Am J Cardiol 53:26B–29B, 1984.
176. Yabek SM, Kato R, Ikeda N, et al: Effects of flecainide on the cellular electrophysiology of neonatal and adult cardiac fibers. Am Heart J 113:70–76, 1987.
177. Roden DM, Woosley RL: Flecainide. New Engl J Med 315:36–41, 1986.
178. Tjandra-Maga TB, Verbesselt R, Van Hecken A, et al: Flecainide: Single and multiple oral dose kinetics, absolute bioavailability and effect on food and antacid in man. Br J Clin Pharmacol 22:309–316, 1986.
179. Till J, Holt D, Shinebourne EA, et al: Efficacy and pharmacokinetics of flecainide acetate in the treatment of supraventricular tachycardia in children. J Am Coll Cardiol 9:129A, 1987.
180. Woosley RL, Echt DS, Roden DM: Effects of congestive heart failure on the pharmacokinetics and pharmacodynamics of antiarrhythmic drugs. Am J Cardiol 57:25B–33B, 1986.
181. Wren C, Campbell RWF: The response of paediatric arrhythmias to intravenous and oral flecainide. Br Heart J 57:171–175, 1987.
182. Morganroth J, Anderson JL, Gentzkow GD: Classification by type of ventricular arrhythmia predicts frequency of adverse cardiac events from flecainide. J Am Coll Cardiol 8:607–615, 1986.
183. Lewis GP, Holtzman JL: Interaction of flecainide with digoxin and propranolol. Am J Cardiol 52B–57B, 1984.
184. Shea P, Lal R, Kim SS, et al: Flecainide and amiodarone interaction. J Am Coll Cardiol 7:1127–1130, 1986.
185. Tjandra-Maga TB, Verbesselt R, Van Hecken A, et al: Oral flecainide elimination kinetics: Effects of cimetidine. Circulation 68(suppl 3):416, 1983.
186. Sami M, Mason JW, Peters F, et al: Clinical electrophysiologic effects of encainide, a newly developed antiarrhythmic agent. Am J Cardiol 44:526–532, 1979.
187. Naccarelli GV, Rinkenberger RL, Dougherty AH, et al: Encainide: A review of its electrophysiology, pharmacology and clinical efficacy. Clin Prog Electrophysiol Pacing 3:268–291, 1985.
188. Gibson JK, Somani P, Bassett AL: Electrophysiologic effects of encainide (MJ 9067) on canine Purkinje fibers. Eur J Pharmacol 52:161–169, 1978.
189. Elharrar V, Zipes DP: Effects of encainide and metabolites (MJ 14030 and MJ 9444) on canine cardiac Purkinje and ventricular fibers. J Pharm Exp Ther 220:440–447, 1982.
190. Carmeliet E: Electrophysiological effects of encainide on isolated cardiac muscle and Purkinje fibers and on the Langendorff-perfused guinea pig heart. Eur J Pharmacol 61:247–262, 1980.
191. Wong SS, Myerburg RJ, Ezrin AM, et al: Electrophysiologic effects of encainide on acutely ischemic rabbit myocardial cells. Eur J Pharmacol 80:323–329, 1982.
192. Ro JH, Gillon J, Kupersmith J: Electrophysiologic effects of encainide following acute coronary occlusion in dogs. J Cardiovasc Pharmacol 3:532–540, 1981.
193. King BW, Man RYK: Electrophysiological effects of encainide (MJ 9067) on canine subendocardial Purkinje fibers surviving infarction. J Cardiovasc Pharmacol 6:547–554, 1984.
194. Campbell TJ: Resting and rate dependent depression of maximum rate of depolarization ($\dot{V}$ max) in guinea pig ventricular action potentials by mexiletine, disopyramide, and encainide. J Cardiovasc Pharmacol 5:291–296, 1983.
195. Davy JM, Dorian P, Kantelip JP, et al: Qualitative and quantitative comparison of the cardiac effects of encainide and its major metabolites. J Pharm Exp Ther 237:907–911, 1986.
196. Prystowsky EN, Klein GJ, Rikenberger RL, et al: Clinical efficacy and electrophysiologic effects of encainide in patients with Wolff-Parkinson-White syndrome. Circulation 69:278–287, 1984.
197. Fain ES, Dorian P, Davy JM, et al: Effects of encainide and its metabolites on energy requirements for defibrillation. Circulation 73:1334–1341, 1986.
198. Dawson AK, Roden DM, Duff HJ, et al: Differential effects of O-demethyl encainide on induced and spontaneous arrhythmias in the conscious dog. Am J Cardiol 54:654–658, 1984.
199. Roden DM, Woosley RL: Clinical pharmacology of the new antiarrhythmic encainide. Clin Prog Electrophysiol Pacing 2:112–119, 1984.
200. McAllister CB, Wolfenden HT, Aslanian WS, et al: Oxidative metabolism of encainide: Polymorphism, pharmacokinetics and clinical considerations. Xenobiotica 16:483–490, 1986.
201. Wehmeyer AE, Thomas RL: Encainide: A new antiarrhythmic agent. Drug Intell Clin Pharmacol 20:9–13, 1986.
202. Roden DM, Wood AJJ, Wilkinson GR, et al: Disposition kinetics of encainide and metabolites. Am J Cardiol 58:4C–9C, 1986.
203. Bergstrand RH, Wang T, Roden DM, et al: Encainide disposition in patient with chronic cirrhosis. Clin Pharmacol Ther 40:148–154, 1986.
204. Strasburger JF, Moak JP, Smith RT, et al: Encainide for refractory supraventricular tachycardia in children. Am J Cardiol 58:49C–54C, 1986.
205. Quart BD, Gallo DG, Sami MH, et al: Drug interaction studies and encainide use in renal and hepatic impairment. Am J Cardiol 104C–113C, 1986.
206. Siddoway LA, Roden DM, Woosley RL: Clinical pharmacology of propafenone: Pharmacokinetics, metabolism, and concentration-response relations. Am J Cardiol 54:9D–12D, 1984.
207. Garson A, Moak JP, Smith RT, et al: Control of post-operative junctional ectopic tachycardia with propafenone. Am J Cardiol 59:1422–1424, 1987.
208. Kohlhardt M: Block of sodium channels by antiarrhythmic agents: Analysis of the electrophysiologic effects of propafenone in heart muscle. Am J Cardiol 54:13D–19D, 1984.
209. Kohlhardt M, Seifert C: Inhibition of $\dot{V}$ max of the action potential by propafenone and its voltage time and pH dependence in mammalian ventricular myocardium. Naunyn Schmiedebergs Arch Pharmacol 315:55–62, 1980.

210. Delgado C, Tamargo J, Tejerina T: Electrophysiological effects of propafenone in untreated and propafenone-pretreated guinea-pig atrial and ventricular muscle fibers. Br J Pharmacol 86:765–775, 1985.
211. Satoh H, Hashimoto K: Effect of propafenone on the membrane currents of rabbit sinoatrial node cells. Eur J Pharmacol 118:331–340, 1985.
212. Tamargo J, Delgado C, Tejerina T: Effect of propafenone on ventricular automaticity. Eur Heart J 5(suppl 1):131, 1984.
213. Tamargo J, Delgado C: Electrophysiologic effects of propafenone on isolated guinea pig ventricular muscle and sheep Purkinje fibers. Eur J Pharmacol 118:331–340, 1985.
214. Li JH, Boucher M, Carpentier A, et al: Propafenone in the conscious dog with chronic atrioventricular block: Mechanisms of chronotropic cardiac effects and plasma concentration-response relationships. J Cardiovasc Pharmacol 8:885–891, 1986.
215. Philipsborn G, Gries J, Hoffman HP, et al: Pharmacological studies on propafenone and its main metabolite 5-hydroxy-propafenone. Arzheim-Forsch 34:1489–1497, 1984.
216. Prystowsky EN, Heger JJ, Chilson DA, et al: Antiarrhythmic and electrophysiologic effects of oral propafenone. Am J Cardiol 54:26D–28D, 1984.
217. Albini P, Fillippi L, Pirani R, et al: Electrophysiologic effects of propafenone in patients with sinus node dysfunction. G Ital Cardiol 14:297–303, 1984.
218. Breithardt G, Borggrefe M, Wiebringhaus E, et al: Effect of propafenone in the Wolff-Parkinson-White syndrome: Electrophysiologic findings and long term follow up. Am J Cardiol 54:29D–39D, 1984.
219. Rudolph W, Petri H, Kafka W, et al: Effects of propafenone on the accessory pathway (AP) in patients with WPW syndrome. Am J Cardiol 43:430, 1979.
220. Garcia-Civera R, Sanjuan R, Morell S, et al: Effects of propafenone on induction and maintenance of atrioventricular nodal reentrant tachycardia. PACE 7:649–655, 1984.
221. Musto B, D'onofrio A, Musto A, et al: Electrophysiologic effects and clinical efficacy of propafenone in patients in pediatric age with recurrent supraventricular tachycardia. G Ital Cardiol 16:336–343, 1986.
222. Villafane J, Gelband H, Xu H, et al: The electrophysiologic effects of propafenone hydrochloride in the neonatal canine. Pediatr Res 22:50–54, 1987.
223. Hollman M, Brode E, Hotz D, et al: Investigation of the pharmacokinetics of propafenone in man. Arzheim-Forsch 33:763–770, 1983.
224. Connolly S, Lebsack CS, Winkle RA, et al: Propafenone disposition kinetics in cardiac arrhythmias. Clin Pharmacol Ther 36:163–168, 1984.
225. Connolly S, Kates RE, Lebsack CS, et al: Clinical pharmacology of propafenone. Circulation 68:589–596, 1983.
226. Siddoway LA, McAllister CB, Wang T, et al: Polymorphic oxidative metabolism of propafenone in man. Circulation 68(suppl 3):64, 1983.
227. Kates RE, Yee YG, Winkle RA: Metabolite cumulation during chronic propafenone dosing in arrhythmia. Clin Pharmacol Ther 37:610–614, 1985.
228. Dressler F, Gravinghoff L, Grutte E, et al: Antiarrhythmic drug therapy with propafenone in infants and children—results of a multicenter study. Monatsschr Kinderheilkd 133:154–157, 1985.
229. Cardaioli P, Compostella L, De Domenico R, et al: Changes induced by propafenone on digoxin kinetics: Study on healthy volunteers. G Ital Cardiol 16:237–240, 1986.
230. Ahlquist RP: A study of the adrenotropic receptors. Am J Physiol 153:586–600, 1948.
231. Lands AM, Arnold A, McAwliff JP, et al: Differentiation of receptor systems activated by sympathomimetic amines. Nature 214:597–598, 1967.
232. Wit AL, Hoffman BF, Rosen MR: Electrophysiology and pharmacology of cardiac arrhythmias. IX. Cardiac electrophysiologic effects of beta adrenergic receptor stimulation and blockade, part A. Am Heart J 90:521–533, 1975.
233. Wit AL, Hoffman BF, Rosen MR: Electrophysiology and pharmacology of cardiac arrhythmias. IX. Cardiac electrophysiologic effects of beta adrenergic receptor stimulation and blockade, part B. Am Heart J 90:665–675, 1975.
234. Wit AL, Hoffman BF, Rosen MR: Electrophysiology and pharmacology of cardiac arrhythmias. IX. Cardiac electrophysiologic effects of beta adrenergic receptor stimulation and blockade, part C. Am Heart J 90:795–803, 1975.
235. Duff HJ, Mitchell LB, Wyse G: Antiarrhythmic efficacy of propranolol: Comparison of low and high serum concentrations. J Am Coll Cardiol 4:959–965, 1986.
236. Taylor SH: Intrinsic sympathomimetic activity: Clinical fact or fiction? Am J Cardiol 52:16D–26D, 1983.
237. Vaughn-Williams EM, Dennis PD, Garnham C: Circadian rhythm of heart rate in the rabbit: Prolongation of action potential duration by sustained beta adrenoceptor blockade is not due to associated bradycardia. Cardiovasc Res 20:528–535, 1986.
238. Spinelli W, Danilo P, Buchthal S, et al: Developmental changes in the effects of beta adrenergic blocking concentrations of propranolol on canine Purkinje fibers. Dev Pharmacol Ther 9:412–426, 1986.
239. Yabek S, Berman W, Dillon T: Electrophysiologic effects of propranolol on sinus node function in children. Am Heart J 104:612–616, 1982.
240. Vasquez M, Chuquimia R, Shantha N, et al: Clinical electrophysiological effects of propranolol on normal sinus node function. Br Heart J 41:709–715, 1979.
241. Berkowitz WD, Wit AL, Lau SH, et al: The effects of propranolol on cardiac conduction. Circulation 40:855–862, 1969.
242. Denes P, Cummings JM, Simpson R, et al: Effects of propranolol on anomalous pathway refractoriness and circus movement tachycardias in patients with preexcitation. Am J Cardiol 41:1061–1067, 1978.
243. Coram WM: Comparative effects of β-blockers on ventricular fibrillation threshold. Primary Cardiol 1:11–12, 1986.
244. Johnson G, Regardh CG: Clinical pharmacokinetics of β-adrenoreceptor blocking drugs. Clin Pharmacokinet 1:233–263, 1976.
245. Bharadwaja K, Promisloff R: Clinical pharmacology of propranolol. Drug Ther 7:22–37, 1977.
246. Shand DG, Nuckolls EM, Oates JA: Plasma propranolol levels in adults, with observations in four children. Clin Pharmacol Ther 11:112–120, 1970.
247. Riopel DA, Walle T: Kinetic and clinical observa-

tions in cyanotic children on propranolol therapy. Clin Pharmacol Ther 28:743–750, 1980.
248. Woosley RL, Kornhauser DK, Smith RL, et al: Suppression of chronic ventricular arrhythmias with propranolol. Circulation 60:819–827, 1979.
249. Cottrill CM, McAllister RG, Gettes L, et al: Propranolol therapy during pregnancy, labor and delivery: Evidence for transplacental drug transfer and impaired neonatal drug disposition. J Pediatr 91:812–814, 1977.
250. Bauer JH, Pape B, Zajicek J, et al: Propranolol in human plasma and breast milk. Am J Cardiol 43:860–862, 1979.
251. Wilson JT, Atwood GF, Shand DG: Disposition of propoxyphene and propranolol in children. Clin Pharmacol Ther 19:264–270, 1976.
252. Kubik MM, Gill B, Dawes PM: Propranolol in cardiac arrhythmias: A comparative study of the conventional and long acting formulations. Cur Med Res Opin 10:215–220, 1986.
253. Gillette P, Garson A, Eterovic E, et al: Oral propranolol treatment in infants and children. J Pediatr 92:141–144, 1978.
254. Pickoff A, Zies L, Ferrer PL, et al: High dose propranolol therapy in the management of supraventricular tachycardia. J Pediatr 94:144–146, 1979.
255. Kotis JB, Rosen RC: Central nervous system effects of β-adrenergic-blocking drugs: The role of ancillary properties. Circulation 75:204–212, 1987.
256. Shand DG: State of the art: Comparative pharmacology of the beta adrenoceptor blocking drugs. Drug 25(suppl 2):92–99, 1983.
257. Escoubet B, LeClerq JF, Maison-Blanche P, et al: Comparison of four beta-blockers as assessed by 24 hour ECG recording. Clin Pharmacol Ther 39:361–368, 1986.
258. Shimatori M, Kobayashi M, Chiba S: Comparative study of four beta-adrenoceptor blocking agents on sinoatrial conduction time in isolated blood perfused canine atria. Arch Int Pharmacodyn 274:240–252, 1985.
259. Fitzgerald JD, Ruffin R, Smedstad KG, et al: Studies on the pharmacokinetics and pharmacodynamics of atenolol in man. Eur J Clin Pharmacol 13:81–89, 1983.
260. Campese VM, Feinstein EI, Gura V, et al: Pharmacokinetics of atenolol in patients treated with chronic hemodialysis or peritoneal dialysis. J Clin Pharmacol 25:393–395, 1985.
261. Rubin PC, Butters L, Reynolds B, et al: Atenolol elimination in the neonate. Br J Clin Pharmacol 16:659–662, 1983.
262. Cruickshank JM, Neil-Dwyer G, Bartlett J, et al: Beta blockers and the blood brain barrier. Primary Cardiol 6(suppl 1):34–37, 1980.
263. Wood AJJ: Pharmacologic differences between beta blockers. Am Heart J 108:1070–1077, 1984.
264. Hamra M, Danilo P, Rosen M: Developmental changes in the cardiac electrophysiologic and beta blocking effects of nadolol. Fed Proc 45:781, 1986.
265. Gorczynski RJ: Basic pharmacology of esmolol. Am J Cardiol 56:3F–11F, 1985.
266. Lowenthal DT, Porter S, Saris SD, et al: Clinical pharmacology, pharmacodynamics and interactions with esmolol. Am J Cardiol 56:14F–17F, 1985.
267. Esmolol Research Group: Intravenous esmolol for the treatment of supraventricular tachyarrhythmia: Results of a multicenter, baseline controlled safety and efficacy study in 160 patients. Am Heart J 112:498–505, 1986.
268. Naccarelli GV, Rinkenberger RL, Dougherty AH, et al: Amiodarone: Pharmacology and antiarrhythmic and adverse effects. Pharmacotherapy 5:298–313, 1985.
269. Mason JW, Hondeghem LM, Katzung BG: Amiodarone blocks inactivated cardiac sodium channels. Pflugers Arch 396:79–81, 1983.
270. Yabek SM, Kato R, Singh BN: Acute effects of amiodarone on the electrophysiologic properties of isolated neonatal and adult cardiac fibers. J Am Coll Cardiol 5:1109–1115, 1985.
271. Morady F, DiCarlo LA, Krol RB, et al: Acute and chronic effects of amiodarone on ventricular refractoriness, intraventricular conduction and ventricular tachycardia induction. J Am Coll Cardiol 7:148–157, 1986.
272. Goupil N, Lenfant J: The effects of amiodarone on the sinus node activity of the rabbit heart. Eur J Pharmacol 39:23–31, 1976.
273. Nishimura M, Follmer CH, Cigan AL, et al: Amiodarone blocks Ca^{++} current in guinea pig ventricular myocytes. Circulation 74(suppl 2):169, 1986.
274. Talajic M, DeRoode MR, Nattel S: Comparative electrophysiologic effects of intravenous amiodarone and desethylamiodarone in dogs: Evidence for clinically relevant activity of the metabolic. Circulation 75:265–271, 1987.
275. Ikeda N, Nademanee K, Kannan R, et al: Electrophysiologic effects of amiodarone: Experimental and clinical observation relative to serum and tissue drug concentrations. Am Heart J 108:890–898, 1984.
276. Neliat G, Moreau M, Ducouret P, et al: Electrophysiological effects of butoprozine on isolated heart preparations: Comparison with amiodarone and verapamil. Arch Int Pharmacodyn 255:220–236, 1982.
277. Ohta M, Karagueuzian HS, Mandel WJ, et al: Acute and chronic effects of amiodarone on delayed afterdepolarization and triggered automaticity in rabbit ventricular myocardium. Am Heart J 113:289–296, 1987.
278. Pickoff AS, Singh S, Flinn CJ, et al: Dose dependent electrophysiologic effects of amiodarone in the immature canine heart. Am J Cardiol 52:621–625, 1983.
279. Wellens HJJ, Lie KI, Bar FW, et al: Effect of amiodarone in the Wolff-Parkinson-White syndrome. Am J Cardiol 38:189–194, 1976.
280. Patterson E, Eller BT, Abrams GD, et al: Ventricular fibrillation in a conscious canine preparation of sudden coronary cardiac death—prevention by short and long term amiodarone administration. Circulation 68:857–864, 1983.
281. Kennedy EE, Rosenfeld LE, McPherson CA, et al: Evaluation by serial electrophysiologic studies of an abbreviated oral loading regimen of amiodarone. Am J Cardiol 56:867–871, 1985.
282. Singh BN, Vaugh-Williams EM: The effect of amiodarone, a new anti-anginal drug, on cardiac muscle. Br J Pharmacol 39:657–667, 1970.
283. Tuna IC, Qi A, Gornick C, et al: Kinetics of electrophysiologic changes during oral loading of amiodarone and after withdrawal of amiodarone in the unsedated dog. Circulation 72:1380–1385, 1985.
284. Mason JW: Amiodarone. N Engl J Med 316:455–466, 1987.

285. Latini R, Toynoni G, Kates RE: Clinical pharmacokinetics of amiodarone. Clin Pharmacokinet 9:136–154, 1984.
286. Coumel P, Fidelle J: Amiodarone in the treatment of cardiac arrhythmias: One hundred thirty-five cases. Am Heart J 100:1063–1069, 1980.
287. Nademanee K, Singh BN, Hendrickson JA, et al: Pharmacokinetic significance of serum reverse T_3 levels during amiodarone treatment: A potential method for monitoring chronic drug therapy. Circulation 66:202–212, 1982.
288. Garson A, Gillette PC, McVey P, et al: Amiodarone treatment of critical arrhythmias in children and young adults. J Am Coll Cardiol 4:749–755, 1984.
289. Arnoux P, Seyral P, Llurens M, et al: Amiodarone and digoxin for refractory fetal tachycardia. Am J Cardiol 59:166–167, 1987.
290. Dick M, Scott WA: Amiodarone in pediatric patients. Clin Prog Electrophysiol Pacing 4:522–527, 1986.
291. Greene HL, Saal AK: Interaction of amiodarone with other drugs. Clin Prog Electrophysiol Pacing 4:419–425, 1986.
292. Almong S, Shafran N, Halkin H, et al: Mechanism of warfarin potentiation by amiodarone: Dose and concentration dependent inhibition of warfarin elimination. Eur J Clin Pharmacol 28:257–261, 1985.
293. Heissenbuttel RH, Bigger JT: Bretylium tosylate: A newly available antiarrhythmic drug for ventricular arrhythmias. Ann Int Med 91:229–238, 1979.
294. Leveque PE: Antiarrhythmic action of bretylium. Nature 207:203–204, 1965.
295. Schreiber G, Friedman M, Sokolovsky M: Interaction of bretylium tosylate with rat cardiac mascarinie receptors: Possible pharmacological relevance to antiarrhythmic action. Circ Res 55:653–659, 1984.
296. Papp JG, Vaughn-Williams EM: The effect of bretylium on intracellular cardiac action potentials in relation to its antiarrhythmic and local anesthetic activity. Br J Pharmacol 37:380–390, 1969.
297. Wit AL, Steiner C, Damato AN: Electrophysiologic effects of bretylium tosylate on single fibers of the canine specialized conducting system and ventricle. J Pharm Exp Ther 173:344–356, 1970.
298. Mirro MJ, Webel RR, Kelly KJ, et al: Electrophysiologic properties of bretyllium tosylate on atrial myocardium. J Cardiovasc Pharmacol 3:1312–1320, 1981.
299. DeAzevedo IM, Watanabe Y, Dreifus L: Electrophysiologic antagonism of quinidine and bretylium tosylate. Am J Cardiol 33:633–638, 1974.
300. Fujimoto T, Hamamoto H, Peter T, et al: Electrophysiologic effects of bretylium on canine ventricular muscle during acute ischemia and reperfusion. Am Heart J 105:966–972, 1983.
301. Nishimura M, Watanabe Y: Membrane action and catecholamine release action of bretylium tosylate in normoxic and hypoxic canine Purkinje fibers. J Am Coll Cardiol 2:287–295, 1983.
302. Anderson JL, Brodine WN, Patterson E, et al: Serial electrophysiologic effects of bretylium in man and their correlation with plasma concentration. J Cardiovasc Pharmacol 4:871–882, 1982.
303. Frame VB, Wang HH: Importance of interaction with adrenergic neurons for antifibrillatory action of bretyllium in the dog. J Cardiovasc Pharmacol 8:336–345, 1986.
304. Kerber RE, Pandian NG, Jensen SR, et al: Effect of lidocaine and bretylium on energy requirements for transthoracic defibrillation: Experimental studies. J Am Coll Cardiol 7:397–405, 1986.
305. Koch-Weser J: Bretylium. N Engl J Med 300:473–477, 1979.
306. Rapeport WG: Clinical pharmacokinetics of bretylium. Clin Pharmacokinet 10:248–256, 1985.
307. Benditt DG, Tobler G, Benson DW, et al: Antiarrhythmic actions of bretylium, bethanidine and related compounds. Clin Prog Electrophysiol Pacing 1:349–362, 1983.
308. Josselson J, Narang PK, Adir J, et al: Bretylium kinetics in renal insufficiency. Clin Pharmacol Ther 33:144–150, 1983.
309. Anderson JL, Patterson E, Conlon M, et al: Kinetics of antifibrillatory effects of bretylium: Correlation with myocardial drug concentrations. Am J Cardiol 46:583–592, 1980.
310. Rosen MR, Wit AL, Hoffman BF: Electrophysiology and pharmacology of cardiac arrhythmias. VI. Cardiac effects of verapamil. Am Heart J 89:665–673, 1975.
311. Wit AL, Cranfield PF: Effect of verapamil on the sinoatrial and atrioventricular nodes of the rabbit and the mechanism by which it arrests reentrant atrioventricular nodal tachycardia. Circ Res 35:413–425, 1974.
312. Woods JP, West TC: Frequency dependence of $\dot{V}$ max in K-depolarized guinea pig ventricle: Effects of nifedipine and verapamil. J Cardiovasc Pharmacol 7:197–204, 1985.
313. Rosen MR, Ilvento JP, Gelband H, et al: Effects of verapamil on electrophysiologic properties of canine cardiac Purkinje fibers. J Pharm Exp Ther 189:414–422, 1974.
314. Bayer R, Kaufmann R, Mannhold R: Inotropic and electrophysiological actions of verapamil and D600 in mammalian myocardium. III. Effects of the optical isomers on transmembrane potentials. Naunyn Schmiedeberg's Arch Pharmacol 290:81–97, 1975.
315. Satoh K, Yanagisawa T, Taira N: Effects of atrioventricular conduction and blood flow of enantiomers of verapamil and of tetrodotoxin injected into the posterior and the arterior septal artery of the atrioventricular node preparation of the dog. Naunyn Schmiedeberg's Arch Pharmacol 308:89–98, 1979.
316. Temesy-Armos PN, Legenza M, Southworth SR, et al: Effects of verapamil and lidocaine in a canine model of sudden coronary death. J Am Coll Cardiol 6:674–681, 1985.
317. Reder RF, Miura DS, Danilo P, et al: The electrophysiological properties of normal neonatal and adult canine Purkinje fibers. Circ Res 48:658–668, 1981.
318. Ezrin AM, Bassett AL, Gelband H: Cellular electrophysiology in the developing mammalian heart: Modification by antiarrhythmic agents. In Roberts NK, Gelband H (eds): Cardiac Arrhythmias in the Neonate, Infant and Child. East Norwalk, Connecticut, Appleton-Century-Crofts, pp 37–58, 1983.
319. Arnold TH, Vallner JJ, Tackett RL: Age related changes in the pharmacodynamics of verapamil. Am Heart J 110:981–985, 1985.
320. Singh BN, Nademanee K, Baky SH: Calcium antagonists: Clinical use in the treatment of arrhythmias. Drugs 25:125–153, 1983.
321. Shakibi JG, Kashani IA, Mehranpur M, et al:

Electrophysiologic effects of verapamil in children. Jpn Heart J 20:789–801, 1979.
322. Pickoff AS, Flinn CJ, Singh S, et al: The effects of verapamil on the electrophysiology of the intact immature mammalian heart. J Cardiovasc Pharmacol 7:125–130, 1985.
323. Gibson R, Driscoll D, Gillette P, et al: The comparative electrophysiologic and hemodynamic effects of verapamil in puppies and adult dogs. Dev Pharmacol Ther 2:104–116, 1981.
324. Kashani IA, Shakibi JG, Siassi B: Effect of verapamil on retrograde ventriculo-atrial conduction in children. Jpn Heart J 21:485–490, 1980.
325. Gulamhusein S, Ko P, Klein GJ: Ventricular fibrillation following verapamil in the Wolff-Parkinson-White syndrome. Am Heart J 106:145–147, 1983.
326. McAllister RG: Clinical pharmacokinetics of calcium channel antagonists. J Cardiovasc Pharmacol 4:S340–S345, 1982.
327. Follath F, Ha HR, Schutz E, et al: Pharmacokinetics of conventional and slow release verapamil. Br J Clin Pharmacol 21:149S–153S, 1986.
328. Follath F, Schutz E, Ha HR, et al: Serum drug levels on slow release verapamil. Clin Pharmacol Ther 33:205, 1983.
329. Hoon TJ, Bauman JL, Rodvold KA, et al: The pharmacodynamic and pharmacokinetic differences of the d- and l- isomers of verapamil: Implications in the treatment of paroxysmal supraventricular tachycardia. Am Heart J 112:396–403, 1986.
330. Miller MR, Withers R, Bhamra R, et al: Verapamil and breast feeding. Eur J Clin Pharmacol 30:125–126, 1986.
331. Epstein ML, Seibel MA, Hill MR, et al: Pharmacokinetics of chronic oral verapamil therapy in infants. Circulation 74(suppl 2):77, 1986.
332. DeVonderweid U, Benettoni A, Piovan D, et al: Use of oral verapamil in long term treatment of neonatal, paroxysmal supraventricular tachycardia: A pharmacokinetic study. Int J Cardiol 6:581–584, 1984.
333. Wagner JG, Rocchini AP, Vasiliades J: Prediction of steady state verapamil plasma concentrations in children and adults. Clin Pharmacol Ther 32:172–181, 1982.
334. Epstein ML, Kiel EA, Victorica BE: Cardiac decompensation following verapamil therapy in infants with supraventricular tachycardia. Pediatrics 75:737–740, 1985.
335. Porter CJ, Gillette PC, Garson A, et al: Effects of verapamil in supraventricular tachycardia in children. Am J Cardiol 48:487–491, 1981.
336. Hesslein PS, Finlay CD, Garson A, et al: Chronic oral verapamil: Pediatric experience. Circulation 74(suppl 2):176, 1986.
337. Matsuda H, Konishi T, Matsuyama E, et al: Combined effect of verapamil and disopyramide on induction of circus movement tachycardia in patients with pre-excitation. Jpn Circ J 45:1138–1146, 1981.
338. Soler-Soler J, Sagrista-Sauleda J, Cabrerra A, et al: Effect of verapamil in infants with paroxysmal supraventricular tachycardia. Circulation 59:876–879, 1979.
339. Gomes JA, Harriman RJ, Kang PS, et al: Sustained symptomatic sinus node reentrant tachycardia: Incidence, clinical significance, electrophysiologic observations and the effects of antiarrhythmic agents. J Am Coll Cardiol 5:45–47, 1985.
340. Schwartz J: Verapamil in atrial fibrillation: The expected, the unexpected and the unknown. Am Heart J 106:173–175, 1983.
341. Woelfel A, Foster JR, McAllister RG, et al: Efficacy of verapamil in exercise-induced ventricular tachycardia. Am J Cardiol 56:292–297, 1985.
342. Sang RJ, Shapiro WA, Shen EN, et al: Effects of verapamil on ventricular tachycardias possibly caused by reentry, automaticity, and triggered activity. J Clin Invest 72:350–360, 1983.
343. Fisch C: William Withering: an account of the foxglove and some of its medical uses 1785–1985. J Am Coll Cardiol 5:1A–2A, 1985.
344. Fozzard HA, Sheets MF: Cellular mechanisms of action of cardiac glycosides. J Am Coll Cardiol 5:10A–15A, 1985.
345. Watanabe AM: Digitalis and the autonomic nervous system. J Am Coll Cardiol 5:35A–42A, 1985.
346. Smith TW, Haber E: Digitalis, part 1. N Engl J Med 289:945–951, 1973.
347. Rosen MR, Wit AL, Hoffman BF: Electrophysiology and pharmacology of cardiac arrhythmias. IV. Cardiac antiarrhythmic and toxic effects of digitalis. Am Heart J 89:391–399, 1975.
348. Rosen MR, Hordof AJ, Hodess AB, et al: Ouabain induced changes in the electrophysiologic properties of neonatal, young and adult canine cardiac Purkinje fibers. J Pharm Exp Ther 194:255–263, 1975.
349. Rosen MR: Cellular electrophysiology of digitalis toxicity. J Am Coll Cardiol 5:22A–34A, 1985.
350. Kelliher GJ, Roberts J: Effect of age on the cardiotoxic action of digitalis. J Pharm Exp Ther 197:10–18, 1976.
351. Marsh AJ, Lloyd BL, Taylor RR: Age dependence of myocardial Na^+-K^+ ATPase activity and digitalis intoxication in the dog and guinea pig. Circ Res 48:329–333, 1981.
352. Kearin M, Kelly JG, O'Malley K: Digoxin receptors in neonates: An explanation of less sensitivity to digoxin than in adults. Clin Pharmacol Ther 28:346–349, 1980.
353. Ng YC, Akera T, Brody TM: Developmental changes in digitalis sensitivity and relative abundance of two molecular forms of Na^+-K^+ ATPase in the ferret heart. Fed Proc 46:560, 1987.
354. Dhingra RC, Amat-Y-Leon F, Wyndham C, et al: The electrophysiological effects of ouabain on sinus node and atrium in man. J Clin Invest 56:555–562, 1975.
355. Engel TR, Gonzalez ADC: Effects of digitalis on atrial vulnerability. Am J Cardiol 42:570–576, 1978.
356. Kugler JD, Garson A, Gillette PC: Electrophysiologic effects of digitalis on sinoatrial nodal function in children. Am J Cardiol 44:1344–1348, 1979.
357. Przybyla AC, Paulay KL, Stein E, et al: Effects of digoxin on atrioventricular conduction patterns in man. Am J Cardiol 33:344–350, 1974.
358. Gomes JAC, Damato AN, Bobb GA, et al: The effect of digitalis on refractoriness of the intact canine His-Purkinje system. Circulation 58:284–294, 1978.
359. Bissett JK, DeSoyza NDB, Kane JJ, et al: Effect of digitalis on human ventricular refractoriness. Cardiovasc Res 12:288–293, 1978.
360. Smith TW: Pharmacokinetics, bioavailability and serum levels of cardiac glycosides. J Am Coll Cardiol 5:43A–50A, 1985.
361. Park MK: Use of digoxin in infants and children,

with special emphasis on dosage. J Pediatr 108:871–878, 1986.
362. Wettrell G: Digoxin therapy in infants: A clinical pharmacokinetic study. Acta Pediatr Scand 257:7–28, 1976.
363. Collins-Nakai RL, Schiff D, Ng PK: Multiple dose kinetics of digoxin in neonates. Pediatr Pharmacol 5:117–122, 1985.
364. Morselli PL, Assuel BM, Gomeni R, et al: Digoxin pharmacokinetics during human development. In Morselli PL, Garattini S, Sereni F (eds): Basic and Therapeutic Aspects of Perinatal Pharmacology. New York, River Press, 1975, pp 377–392.
365. Nagushima M, Asai T, Suzuki C, et al: Intrauterine supraventricular tachyarrhythmias and transplacental digitalisation. Arch Dis Child 61:996–1000, 1986.
366. Loes MW, Singh S, Lock JE, et al: Relation between plasma and red cell electrolyte concentrations and digoxin levels in children. N Engl J Med 299:501–504, 1978.
367. Henion WA, Montondo D, Hilal A, et al: Changes in red blood cell electrolyte concentrations in digitalis intoxication. Am Heart J 106:14–20, 1983.
368. Surawicz B: Factors affecting tolerance to digitalis. J Am Coll Cardiol 5:69A–81A, 1985.
369. Koren G: Interaction between digoxin and commonly coadministered drugs in children. Pediatrics 75:1032–1037, 1985.
370. Marcus FI: Pharmacokinetic interactions between digoxin and other drugs. J Am Coll Cardiol 5:82A–90A, 1985.
371. Byrum C, Wahl RA, Behrendt DM, et al: Ventricular fibrillation associated with the use of digitalis in a newborn infant with Wolff-Parkinson-White syndrome. J Pediatr 101:400–403, 1982.
372. Sparks HV, Bardenheuer H: Regulation of adenosine formation by the heart. Circ Res 58:193–201, 1986.
373. Drury AN, Szent-Gyorgyi A: The physiologic activity of adenine compounds with special reference to their action upon the mammalian heart. J Physiol 68:213–237, 1929.
374. West GA, Belardinelli L: Sinus slowing and pacemaker shift caused by adenosine in rabbit SA node. Pflugers Arch 403:66–74, 1985.
375. Belardinelli L, Isenberg G: Isolated atrial myocytes: Adenosine and acetylcholine increase potassium conductance. Am J Physiol 224:H734–H737, 1983.
376. Pelleg A: Cardiac cellular electrophysiologic actions of adenosine and adenosine triphosphate. Am Heart J 110:688–693, 1985.
377. Rosen MR, Danilo P, Weiss RM: Actions of adenosine on normal and abnormal impulse initiation in canine ventricle. Am J Physiol 244:H715–H721, 1983.
378. Wesley RC, Belardinelli L: Role of adenosine on ventricular overdrive suppression in isolated guinea pig hearts and Purkinje fibers. Circ Res 57:517–531, 1985.
379. Goto M, Yatani A, Tsuda Y: Stabilizing effects of adenosine on the membrane currents and tension components of the bullfrog atrium. Jpn J Physiol 28:611–625, 1978.
380. DiMarco JP, Sellers TD, Berne RM, et al: Adenosine: Electrophysiologic effects and therapeutic use for terminating paroxysmal supraventricular tachycardia. Circulation 68:1254–1263, 1983.
381. Perrot B, Clozel JP, Faivre G: Effect of adenosine triphosphate on the accessory pathway. Eur Heart J 5:382–393, 1984.
382. DiMarco JP, Sellers TD, Lerman BB, et al: Diagnostic and therapeutic use of adenosine in patients with supraventricular tachyarrhythmias. J Am Coll Cardiol 6:417–425, 1985.
383. Klabunde RE: Dipyridamole inhibition of adenosine metabolism in human blood. Eur J Pharmacol 98:21–26, 1983.
384. Watt AH, Bernard MS, Webster J, et al: Intravenous adenosine in the treatment of supraventricular tachycardia: A dose-ranging study and interaction with dipyridamole. Br J Clin Pharmacol 21:227–230, 1986.
385. Clarke B, Rowland E, Barness PJ, et al: Rapid and safe termination of supraventricular tachycardia in children by adenosine. Lancet 1:299–301, 1987.
386. Belhassen B, Pelley A, Shoshani D, et al: Atrial fibrillation induced by adenosine triphosphate. Am J Cardiol 53:1405–1406, 1984.
387. Meszaros J, Klemen K, Kecskemeti V, et al: Antagonism between adenosine and bromobenzoylmethyladamantylamine, a K^+ channel blocker in atrial myocardium of guinea pigs. Eur J Pharmacol 98:265–268, 1984.
388. Lerman BB, Belardinelli L, West GA, et al: Adenosine-sensitive ventricular tachycardia: Evidence suggesting cyclic AMP-mediated triggered activity. Circulation 74:270–280, 1986.

SECTION II
TECHNIQUES

CHAPTER 4

SYSTEMATIC INTERPRETATION OF CARDIAC ARRHYTHMIAS

Arthur Garson, Jr.

Certain principles are helpful in the analysis of cardiac rhythm in children. We have developed a step-by-step method of diagnosis that, though it does not include every possible arrhythmia, will place most rhythm disturbances in a single category.

This method differs from most others in that it begins with the QRS complex. The QRS is the most obvious feature of the electrocardiogram, and in actual practice, the first determination made is usually the regularity of the QRS complexes. We have used hand-drawn electrocardiographic tracings in the teaching of this method; this has two advantages. First, it allows us to vary one part of the electrocardiogram at a time, while keeping all other parts constant; for example, keeping the QRS rate and P rate exactly the same while varying only the P mean vector. Therefore, focus is directed at the important teaching point rather than the unimportant slight change in rate or QRS morphology. The second advantage is that the tracings are easy to read, without wandering baselines or electrical interference.

The use of this method requires no expertise with the electrophysiologic principles that underlie the electrocardiogram. It is a stepwise deductive method used by pediatric cardiologists and can be learned by anyone who knows the basics of the electrocardiogram in adults or children (morphology, rate, mean vector, and duration of both the P wave and QRS complex). Once learned, this method can be easily and quickly reviewed by those who encounter arrhythmias infrequently in children.

In analyzing the electrocardiogram, certain questions must be answered sequentially (Fig. 4–1). When these questions are answered, the arrhythmia(s) will be identified.

VENTRICULAR RATE

The first step is to decide if the ventricular rate (RR interval) is regular. We consider a rhythm to be regular if the RR intervals in the electrocardiogram vary by less than 0.08 seconds (Figs. 4–2 and 4–3). The examples shown in the figures are idealized drawings taken from the electrocardiograms of different 4-year-old patients. For patients in the 3- to 4-year age range, the normal QRS rate ranges from 70/min to 140/min, the normal PR interval is 0.09–0.16 s, and the normal QRS duration is 0.04–0.10 s.

If the ventricular rate is regular, the answers to three additional questions will categorize the rhythm. The first question is whether the ventricular rate is decreased, normal, or increased for a child of the patient's age (Fig. 4–4). For example, Figure 4–5 shows three sample electrocardiograms, each taken from a 4-year-old patient. The ventricular rates are 50/min, 85/min, and 180/min. For a 4-year-old child, a ventricular rate of 50/min is bradycardia, and 180/min is tachycardia.

QRS DURATION

The second question to be answered is whether the QRS duration is normal or prolonged (Fig. 4–6). If the QRS duration is prolonged, the specific morphology must be determined. In a 4-year-old, the upper limit of normal for QRS duration is 0.08 s. Any QRS complex longer than 0.08 s is prolonged. An abnormally long QRS complex may have one of four distinct morphologies

Text continued on page 125

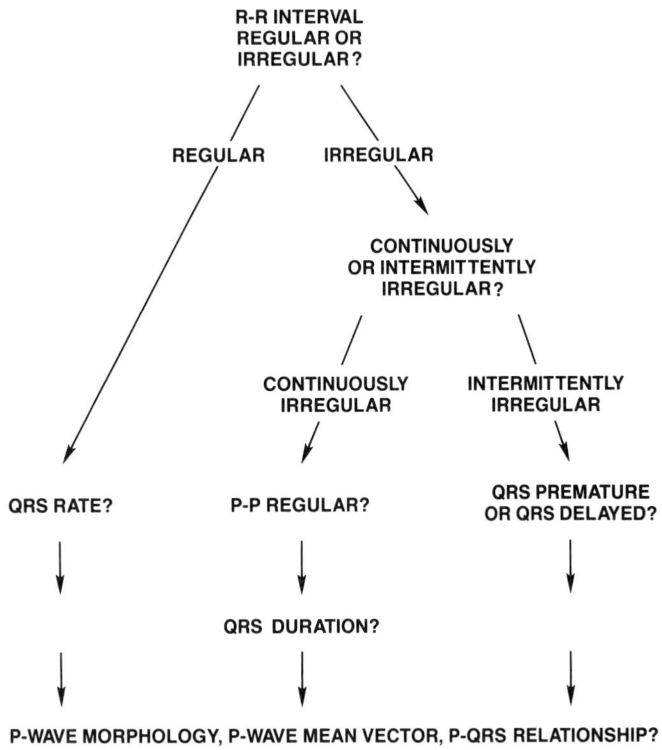

FIGURE 4–1
Schema for interpretation of arrhythmias.

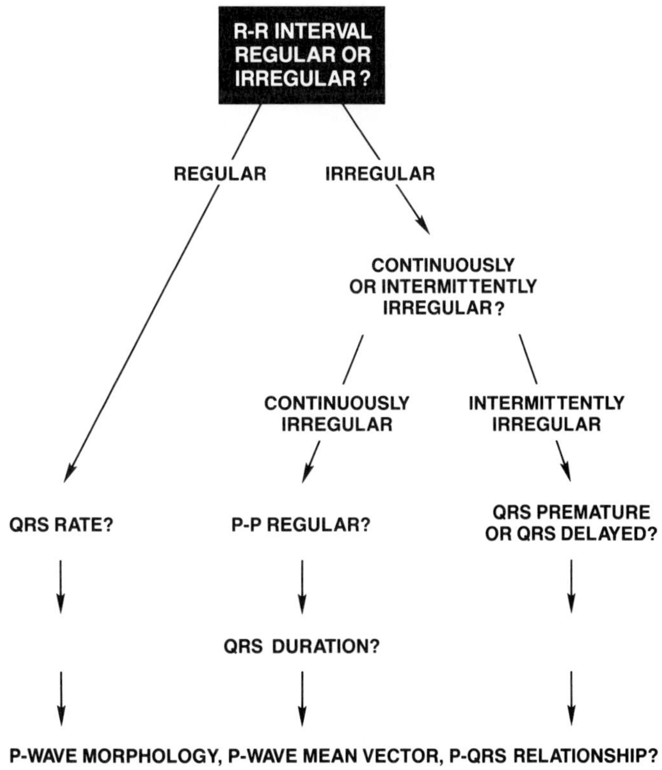

FIGURE 4–2
Regular versus irregular RR interval.

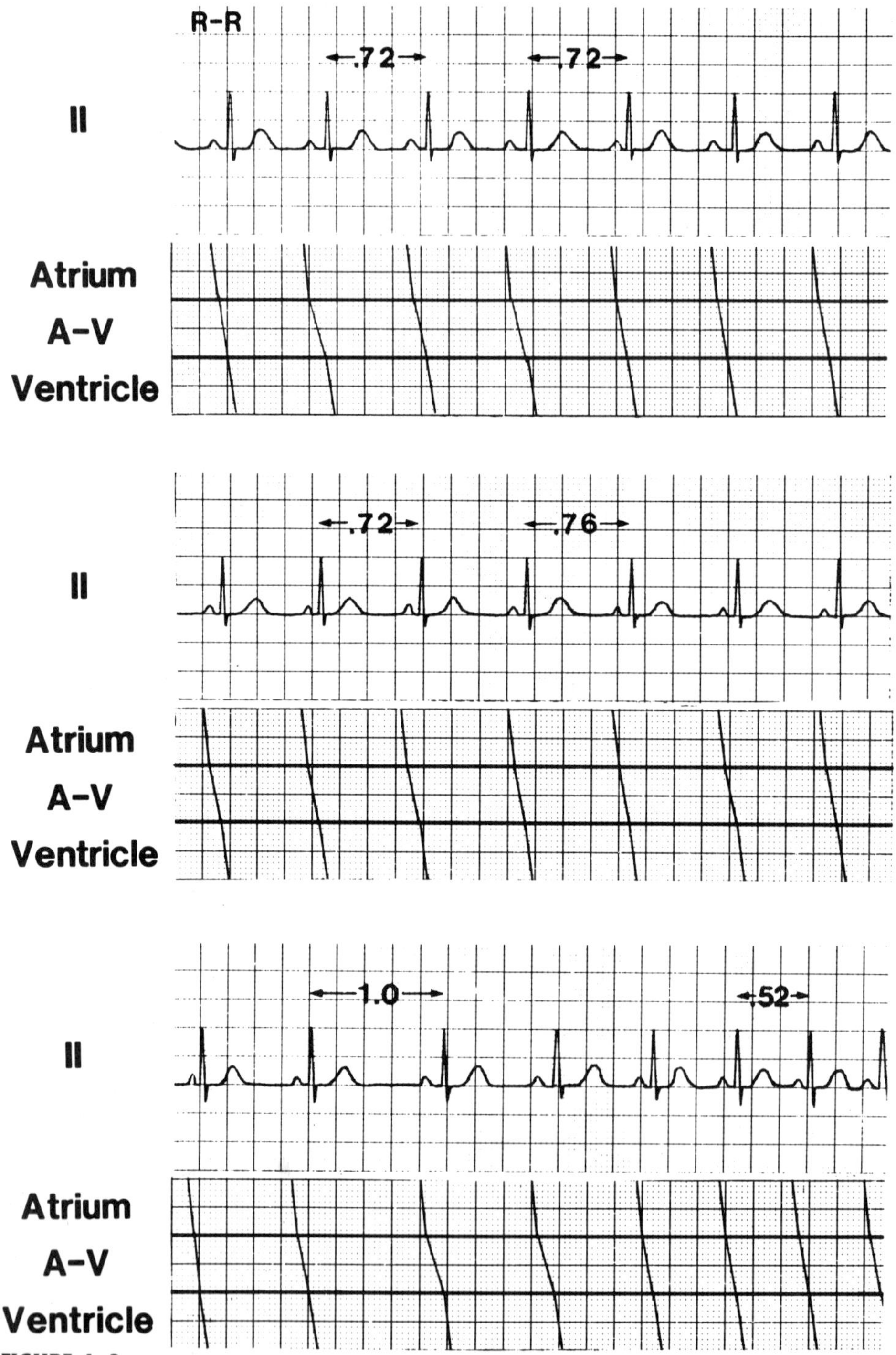

FIGURE 4–3
REGULAR vs IRREGULAR RHYTHM

Top tracing: Sinus rhythm; absolutely regular RR interval of 0.72 s (QRS rate = 85 bpm).

Middle tracing: Sinus rhythm; first three RR intervals are 0.72 s, followed by three RR intervals of 0.76 s. Since the RR intervals vary by 0.08 s or less, this is considered to be a regular rhythm.

Bottom tracing: Sinus arrhythmia; the RR intervals vary from 0.52 to 1.0 s. This is a markedly irregular rhythm.

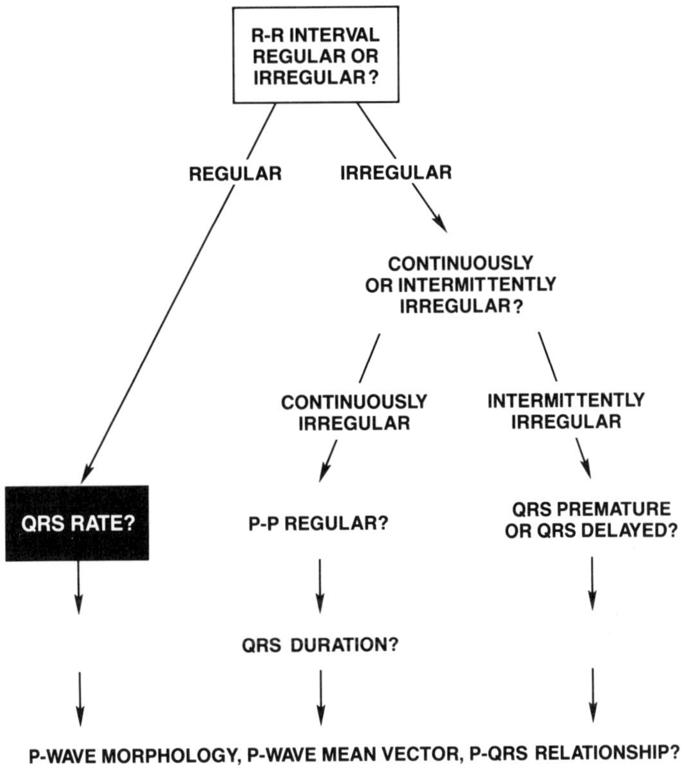

FIGURE 4–4
Regular RR interval: variation in QRS rate.

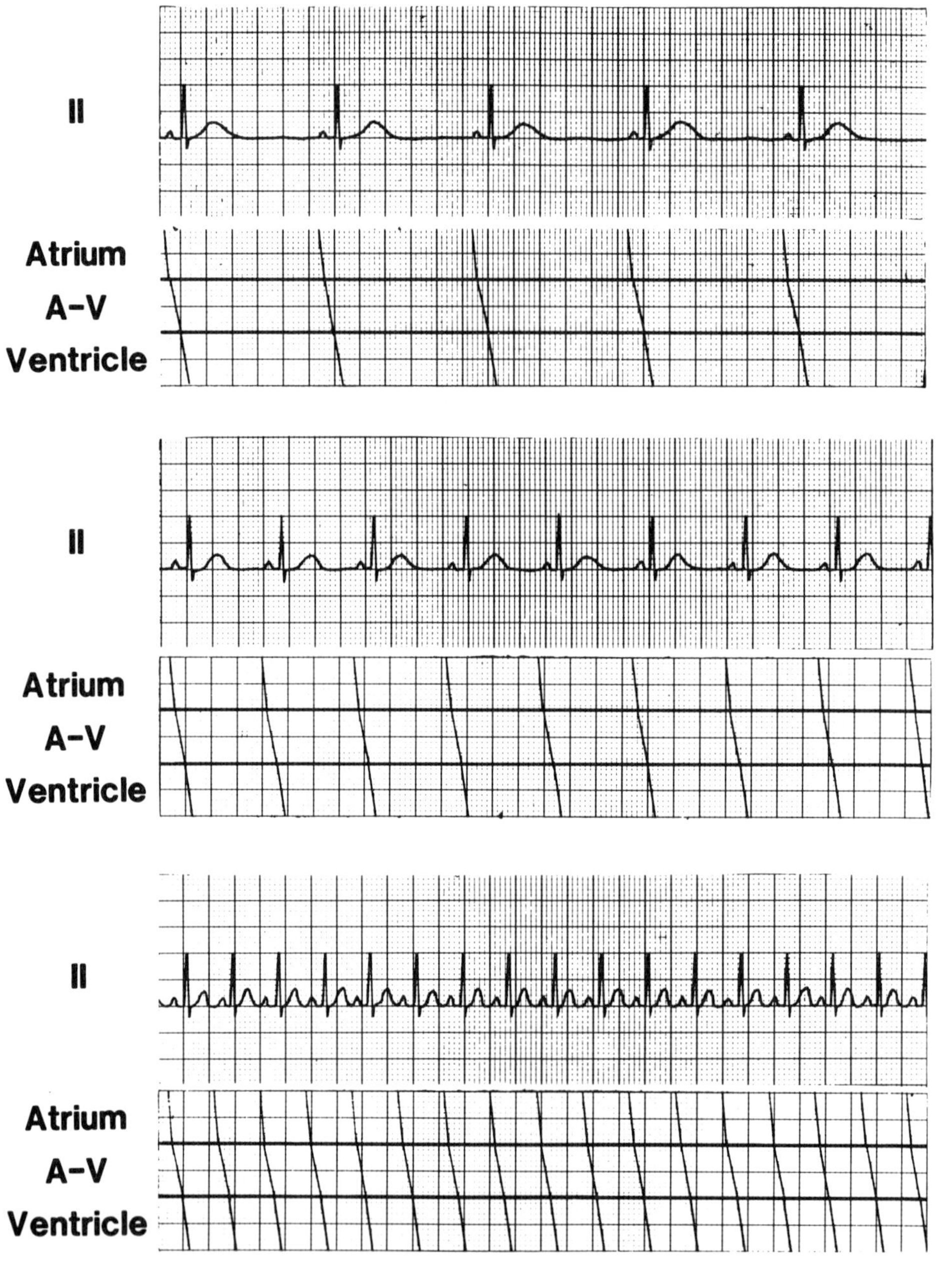

FIGURE 4–5
VARIATION IN QRS RATE

Top tracing:	Sinus bradycardia; QRS rate is 50/min.
Middle tracing:	Sinus rhythm; QRS rate is 85/min.
Bottom tracing:	Sinus tachycardia; QRS rate is 180/min.

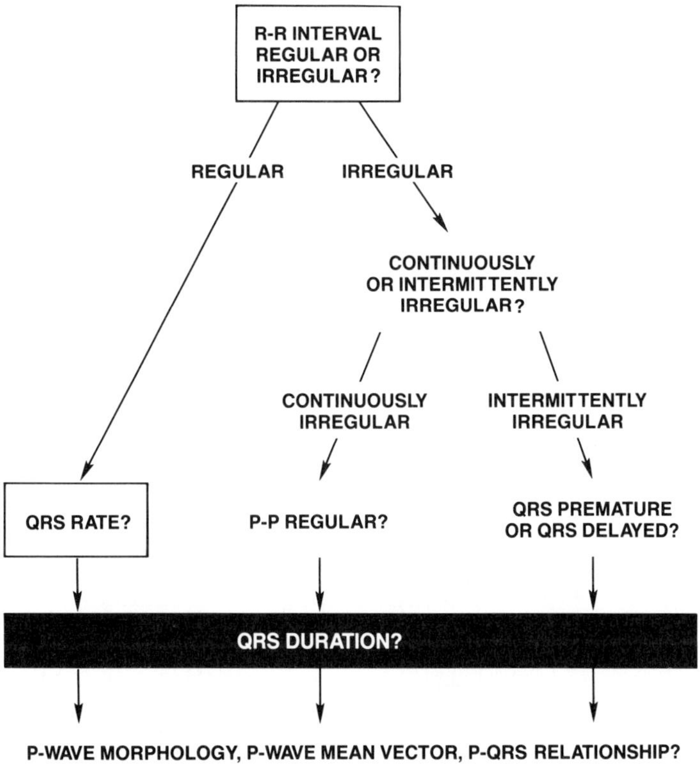

FIGURE 4–6
Regular RR interval: QRS duration.

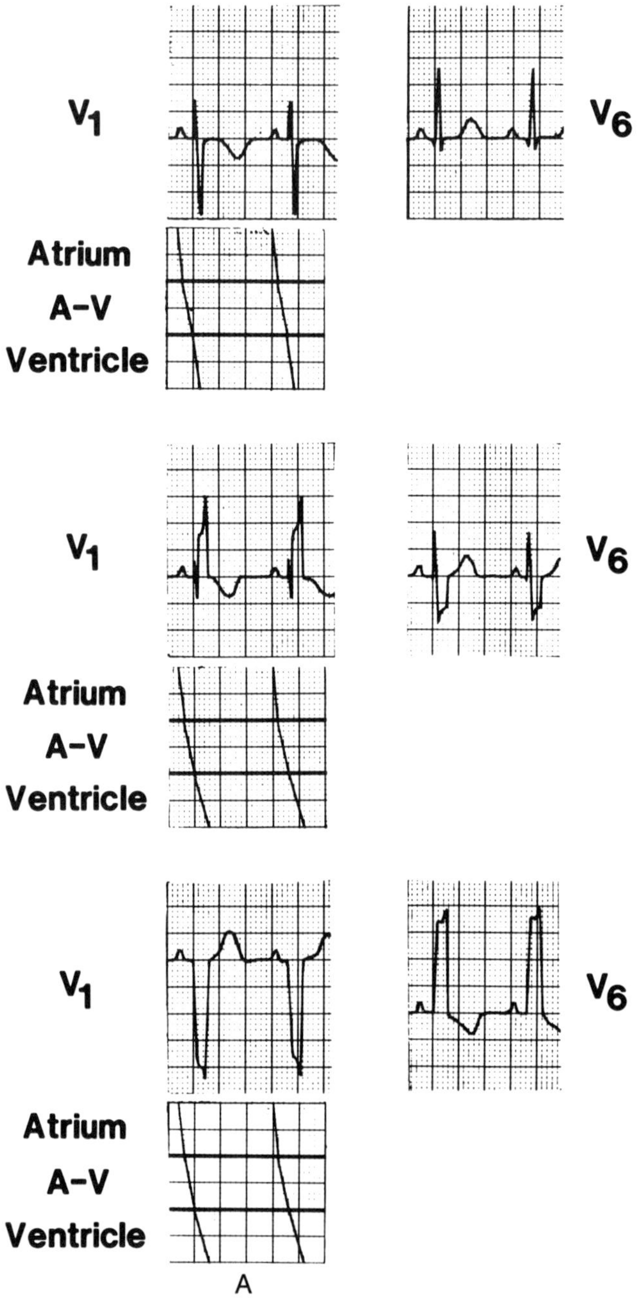

FIGURE 4–7A

TYPES OF VENTRICULAR ABERRATION

Top tracing: Normal duration (0.08 s) QRS complex.

Middle tracing: Prolonged duration (0.12 s) QRS complex with complete right bundle branch block morphology. Note the terminal slowing which is positive in V_1.

Bottom tracing: Prolonged duration (0.12 s) QRS complex with complete left bundle branch block morphology. Note the M-shaped complex with an absent Q wave in V_6.

(Figs. 4–7A and 4–7B). It is most helpful to distinguish among these different morphologies by looking at leads V_1 and V_6. In complete right bundle-branch block, the initial 0.04 s shows a rapid, normal deflection, and the terminal forces are inscribed slowly (wide QRS). These terminal forces are directed anteriorly and to the right (positive in V_1 and negative in V_6), because the right ventricle has delayed activation. Therefore, in complete right bundle-branch block, the complex in V_1 is mainly positive with an RSR′ morphology. In complete left bundle-branch block, the delayed terminal forces are directed posteriorly and to the left, because the left ventricle has delayed activation; in complete left bundle-branch block, the complex in V_1 is mainly negative, and in V_6 it is mainly positive with an RR′ morphology (Fig. 4–7A).

In Wolff-Parkinson-White syndrome, the PR interval is short, and the abnormally prolonged QRS complex is inscribed slowly in the initial 0.02–0.04 s. This slow initial deflection is called the "delta" wave. The remainder of the QRS complex is inscribed rapidly and normally.

The QRS complex of diffuse intraventricular conduction delay found in quinidine toxicity, myocarditis, hypoglycemia, myocardial ischemia, and hyperkalemia involves delay in all phases of depolarization, and the inscription of the entire QRS complex is prolonged (Fig. 4–7B).

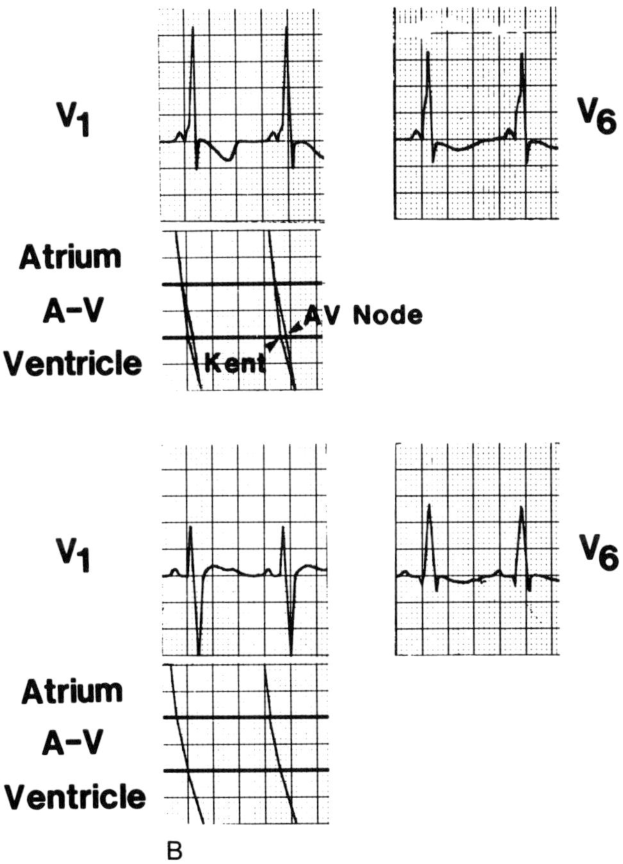

FIGURE 4–7B
TYPES OF VENTRICULAR ABERRATION *(continued)*

Top tracing: Prolonged duration (0.12 s) QRS complex with Wolff-Parkinson-White morphology. The PR interval is short (0.08 s). The initial 0.04 s of the QRS has a slurred upstroke: the "delta" wave. The latter part of the QRS is normal.

Bottom tracing: Prolonged duration (0.12 s) QRS complex with morphology of diffuse intraventricular conduction delay. This is a wide QRS complex without the specific morphologies of complete right bundle branch block, complete left bundle branch block, or Wolff-Parkinson-White.

ATRIAL ACTIVITY

The third question to be answered concerns atrial activity (Fig. 4–8). When the atria depolarize, one of three patterns is observed in the electrocardiogram (Fig. 4–9):

1. *P waves.* Distinct depolarizations, normally 0.03–0.08 s in duration and more pointed than T waves.
2. *Flutter waves.* These are 0.09–0.18 s in duration and occur in succession, giving the impression of a "sawtooth" baseline. Flutter waves may not be visible in all electrocardiographic leads; the most likely leads to show flutter waves are II, III, aV_F, and V_1.
3. *Fibrillation.* Coarse or fine irregular oscillations of the baseline without other demonstrable atrial activity.

If P waves are visible, the P wave axis must be determined (Fig. 4–10). See Figures 4–11A and 4–11B.

Text continued on page 131

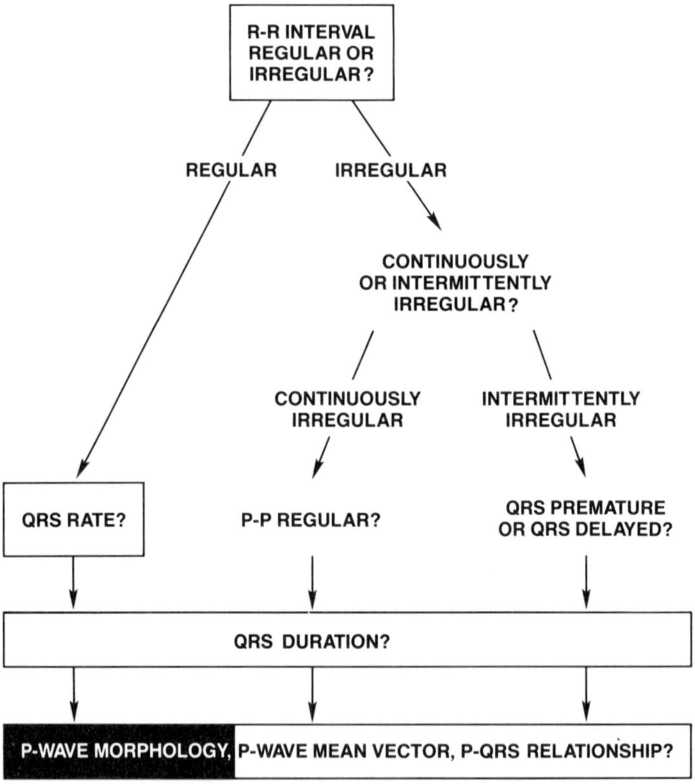

FIGURE 4–8
Regular RR interval: P wave morphology.

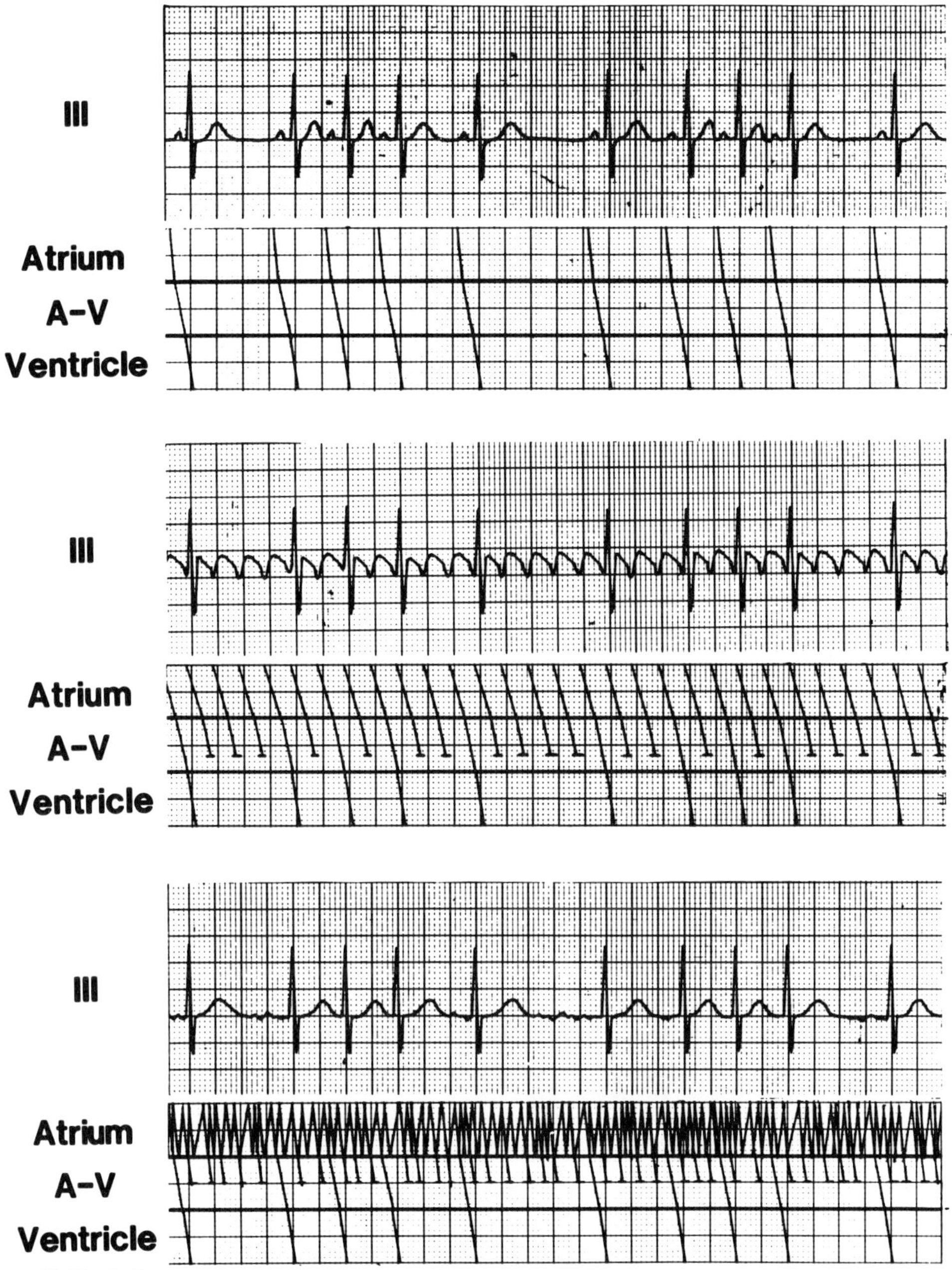

FIGURE 4–9
MORPHOLOGY OF ATRIAL DEPOLARIZATION

Top tracing: Sinus arrhythmia; a P wave precedes each QRS complex.

Middle tracing: Atrial flutter with varying type II second degree AV block; flutter waves are visible throughout the tracing.

Bottom tracing: Atrial fibrillation; note the fine oscillations in the baseline.

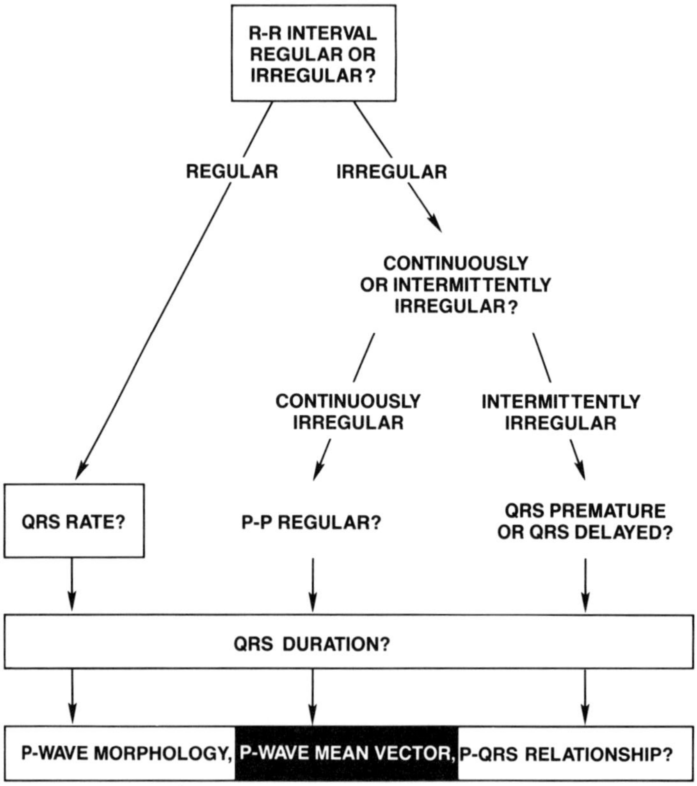

FIGURE 4–10
Regular RR interval: P wave mean vector.

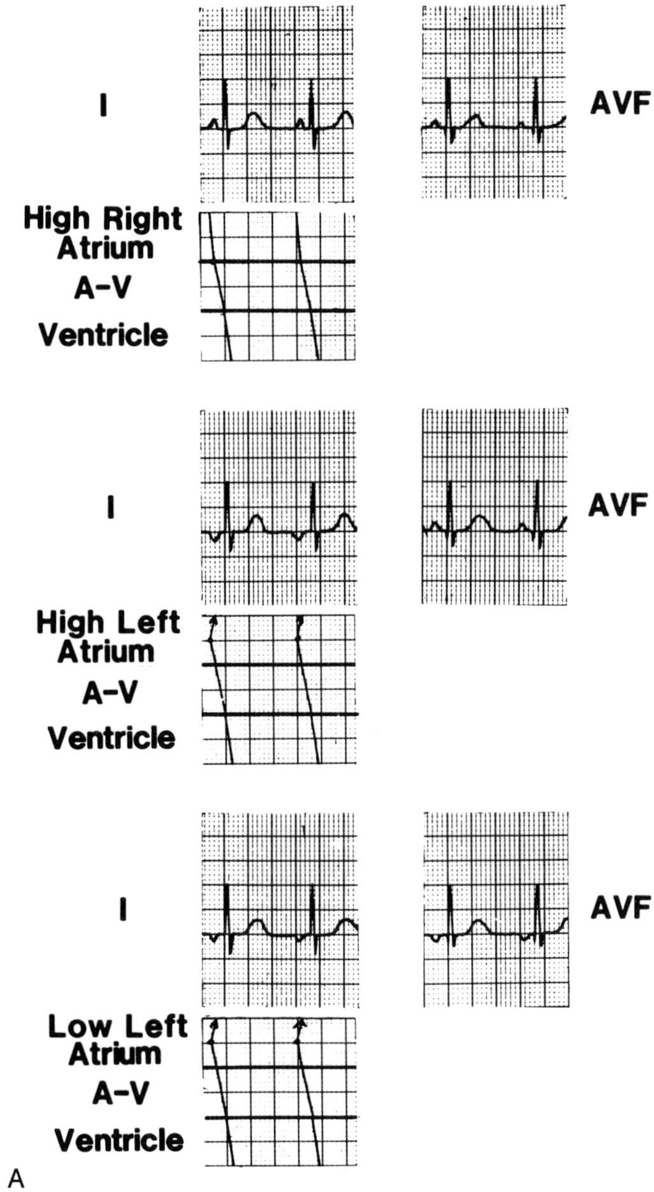

FIGURE 4–11A
P WAVE MEAN VECTOR
Top tracing: Sinus rhythm; P wave mean vector 0° to +90°.
Middle tracing: High left atrial rhythm; P wave mean vector +91° to 180°.
Bottom tracing: Low left atrial rhythm; P wave mean vector −179° to −91°.

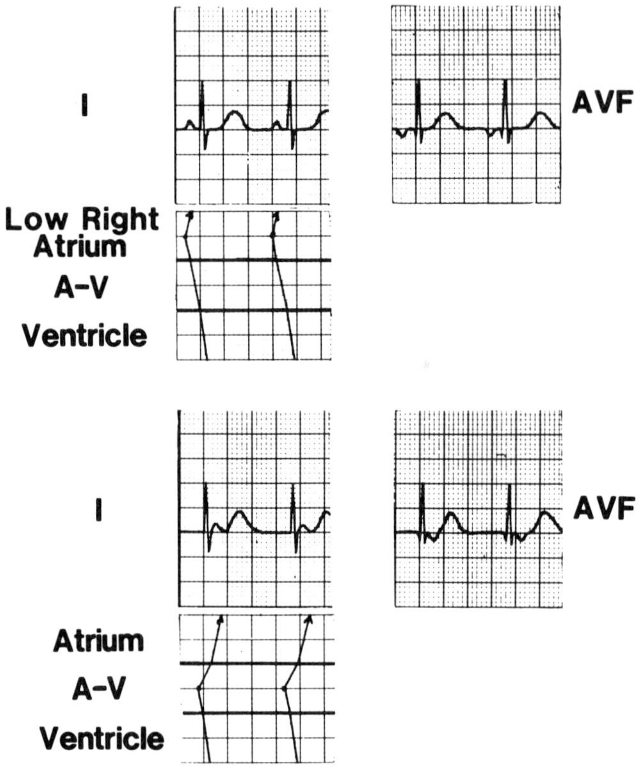

B

FIGURE 4–11B

P WAVE MEAN VECTOR *(continued)*

Top tracing: Low right atrial rhythm; P wave mean vector −1° to −90°.

Bottom tracing: Junctional rhythm; P wave mean vector −1° to −90° with P wave following QRS complex.

RELATIONSHIP OF ATRIAL DEPOLARIZATIONS TO QRS COMPLEXES

Finally, the relationship of the atrial depolarizations to the QRS complexes must be determined (Fig. 4–12). The atrial depolarizations are either related in a regular way to the QRS complexes or are unrelated to the QRS complexes (atrioventricular dissociation). If an atrial depolarization precedes each QRS complex with a constant PR interval, we assume that the atrial depolarization conducted through the His bundle and caused the ventricular depolarization (Fig. 4–13); this is known as isochronic dissociation. If an atrial depolarization follows each QRS complex with a constant RP interval (and a mean vector of −1° to −90°), we assume that the AV junction or ventricle initiated the depolarization, and the impulse conducted retrogradely through the AV node and depolarized the atrium. One other type of P–QRS relationship occurs if there are more P waves than QRS complexes; if the RR interval is regular and the PP interval (atrial rate) is a constant multiple of the ventricular rate (i.e., every second, third, or fourth atrial depolarization is followed by a QRS complex), the diagnosis is second degree AV block. In this case, each ventricular depolarization is caused by an atrial depolarization.

Atrioventricular Dissociation. If the atrial and ventricular depolarizations are unrelated, the diagnosis is atrioventricular (AV) dissociation. AV dissociation occurs in several arrhythmias of entirely different mechanisms. Therefore, AV dissociation should never be the only diagnosis in the interpretation of an electrocardiogram. There are three major causes for AV dissociation (Figs. 4–14A and 4–14B):

1. Slowing of sinus or atrial rhythm with junctional rhythm occurring at a normal junctional rate. If retrograde conduction to

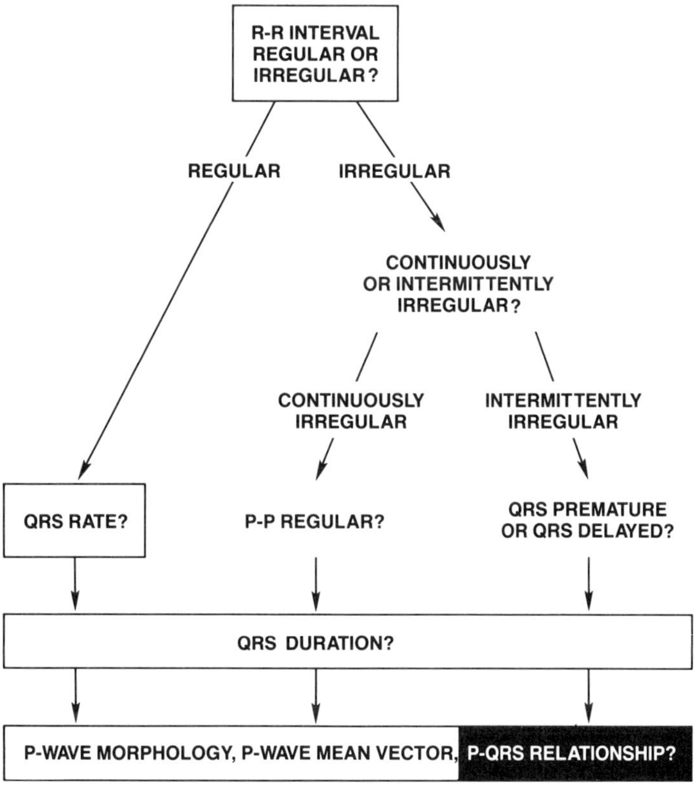

FIGURE 4–12
Regular RR interval: P-QRS relationship.

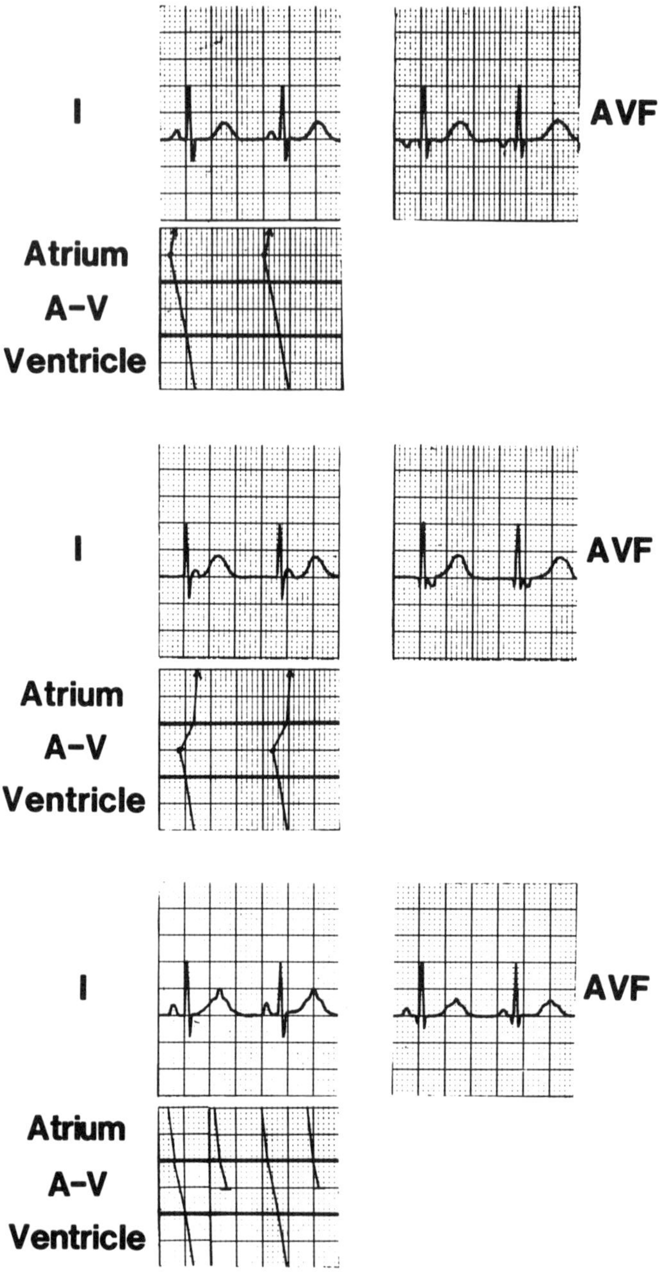

FIGURE 4–13

P-QRS RELATIONSHIP

Top tracing: Low right atrial rhythm; P wave precedes each QRS complex.

Middle tracing: Junctional rhythm; P wave follows each QRS complex.

Bottom tracing: Sinus tachycardia with fixed type II second degree AV block; a QRS complex follows every other P wave; QRS rate is 85/min, and P rate is 170/min.

the atria does not occur during junctional rhythm, AV dissociation may occur, with the slow sinus beats continuing to depolarize the atria while the impulses arising in the junction depolarize the ventricles (Fig. 4–14A).

2. An accelerated junctional rhythm or a ventricular rhythm without retrograde conduction. This results in an abnormally rapid ventricular rate with a normal sinus rate (Fig. 4–14A).

3. Complete AV block. This is the best example of AV dissociation because, by definition, the atria and ventricles are unrelated (Fig. 4–14B).

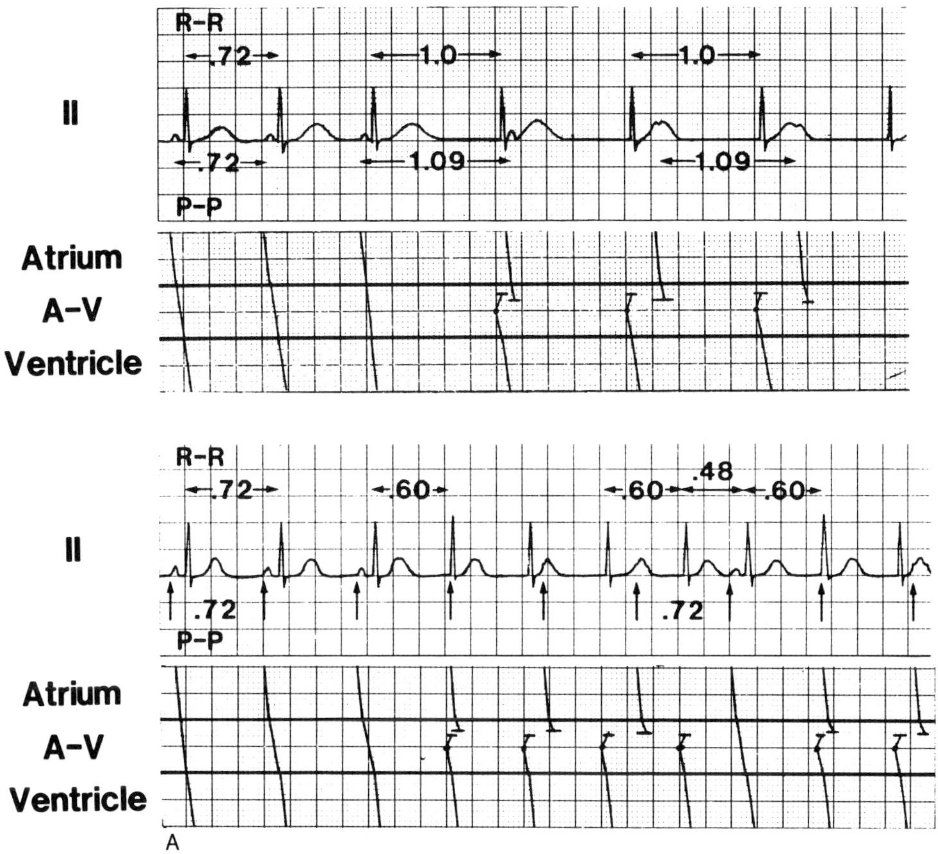

FIGURE 4–14A
AV DISSOCIATION

Top tracing: Sinus rhythm followed by junctional rhythm with AV dissociation; the first three complexes are sinus rhythm at a rate of 85/min. The sinus rate then slows to 55/min (PP interval = 1.09 s). The patient's normal junctional rate of 60/min (RR interval = 0.72 s) is usually suppressed by the faster sinus rate. However, at this time, the junctional rate is faster than the sinus rate, and the junction assumes the function of the pacemaker. The sinus P waves continue dissociated through the tracing because in this patient there is no retrograde conduction to the atrium from the junction, so sinus rhythm is not disturbed.

Bottom tracing: Sinus rhythm followed by accelerated junctional rhythm with AV dissociation. The first three complexes are sinus rhythm at a rate of 85 bpm. The sinus rate remains at 85/min (sinus P waves marked by arrows every 0.72 s), but the AV junction develops an abnormally rapid rate of 100/min (RR interval = 0.60 s) and assumes the pacemaker function. The P waves and QRS complexes are dissociated because there is no retrograde conduction from the junction to the atria; however, conduction is intact from atria to ventricles. A short RR interval (0.48 s) is found when a sinus P wave occurs a sufficient time after the preceding QRS complex such that the AV node is not refractory and AV conduction can occur. This is a sinus "capture" beat; accelerated junctional rhythm resumes after the capture beat.

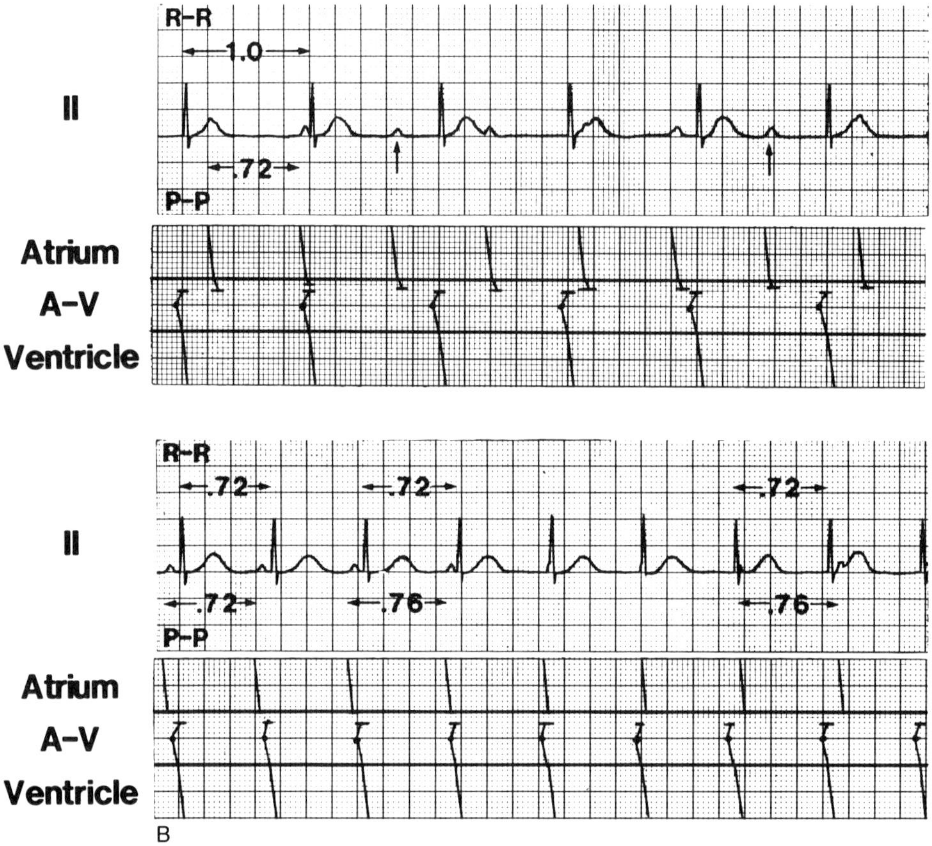

FIGURE 4–14B

AV DISSOCIATION *(continued)*

Top tracing: Complete AV block; junctional rate is 60/min (RR interval = 1.0 s); atrial rate is 85/min (PP interval = 0.72 s); the P waves and QRS complexes are dissociated because there is no conduction through the AV node in either antegrade or retrograde direction. If antegrade conduction was intact, two P waves (arrows) should have changed the RR interval (see Fig. 4–14*A*, bottom). The RR interval was not influenced by the intervening P waves, and therefore the P waves probably did not conduct to the ventricles.

Bottom tracing: Complete AV block with isochronic dissociation; the RR intervals remain absolutely constant at 0.72 s; the PP intervals begin at 0.72 s. However, the PP intervals lengthen to 0.76 s, with a shortening PR interval, and the RR interval is unaffected. The change in atrial rate without a corresponding change in ventricular rate is the clue that the first three P waves most likely were not conducted to the ventricles, but only appeared to be conducted because the atria and ventricles were beating independently at exactly the same rate (isochronic dissociation).

Isochronic Dissociation. It is possible to have the atria and ventricles beating at exactly the same rate and have a constant PR interval with no conduction from atria to ventricles. This is called "isochronic" or "isorhythmic" dissociation (Fig. 4–14B). The only way to prove the existence of isochronic dissociation is to find, in a long rhythm strip, that one of the two rates (atrial or ventricular) changes and the other stays the same. For example, if the PP interval lengthens and the RR interval remains constant, AV dissociation will then become evident.

Irregular RR Intervals. If the RR intervals are irregular, they can either be irregular continuously or there can be a basic, regular RR interval into which an irregular RR interval is intermittently introduced (Figs. 4–15 and 4–16).

If the RR interval varies continuously, the next question to be answered is whether the PP intervals are regular. Next the QRS duration should be ascertained, and finally, if the QRS is continuously irregular, the P wave mean vector, P morphology, and P-QRS relationship should be determined (Figs. 4–17 and 4–18). In pediatrics, if the PP intervals vary, generally the atrial and ventricular depolarizations are related, and therefore the RR interval will also vary. The two most common causes of irregular PP and RR intervals are sinus arrhythmia and wandering pacemaker. In sinus arrhythmia, the P wave mean vector varies between 0° and +90°. In wandering pacemaker, P waves are not always present; when P waves are present in wandering pacemaker, the P wave mean vector may vary throughout the four quadrants. Of course, atrial fibrillation is "irregularly irregular" (no two RR intervals the same) and falls into the category of irregular RR intervals.

If the RR interval is irregular but the PP interval is regular, the most likely diagnosis is second degree AV block. In typical type I second degree AV block (Wenckebach), the PR intervals progressively lengthen and the RR intervals progressively shorten until an atrial depolarization occurs without a following QRS complex, and the cycle begins again.

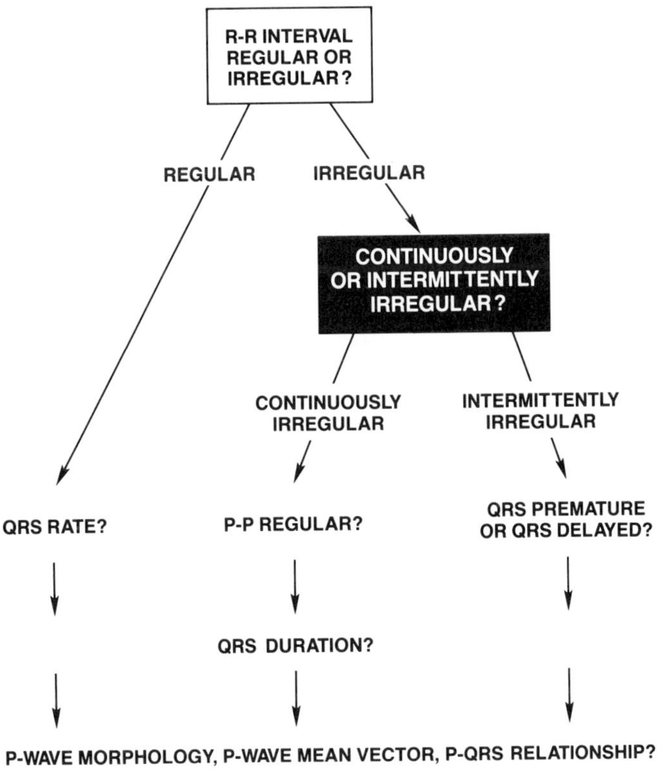

FIGURE 4–15
Irregular RR interval: Continuously versus intermittently irregular.

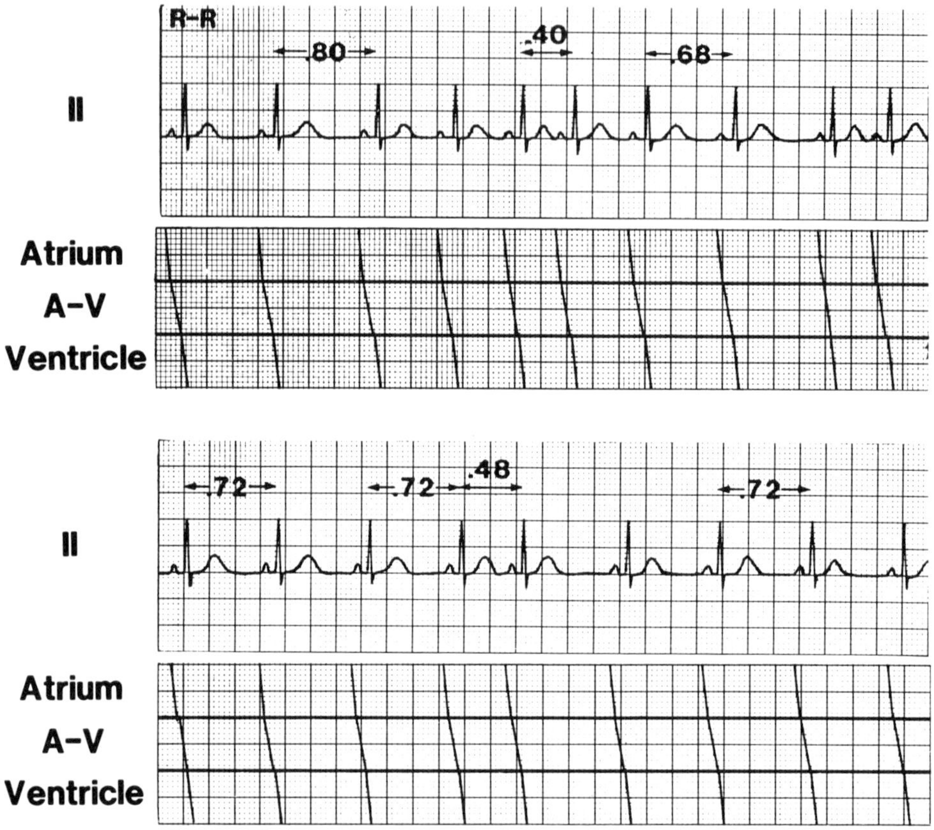

FIGURE 4–16
CONTINUOUSLY IRREGULAR vs INTERMITTENTLY IRREGULAR

Top tracing: Sinus arrhythmia; the RR intervals vary throughout the tracing; this is continuously irregular.

Bottom tracing: Sinus rhythm with premature atrial contraction; the RR intervals are basically constant but are interrupted by an irregular RR interval; this is intermittently irregular.

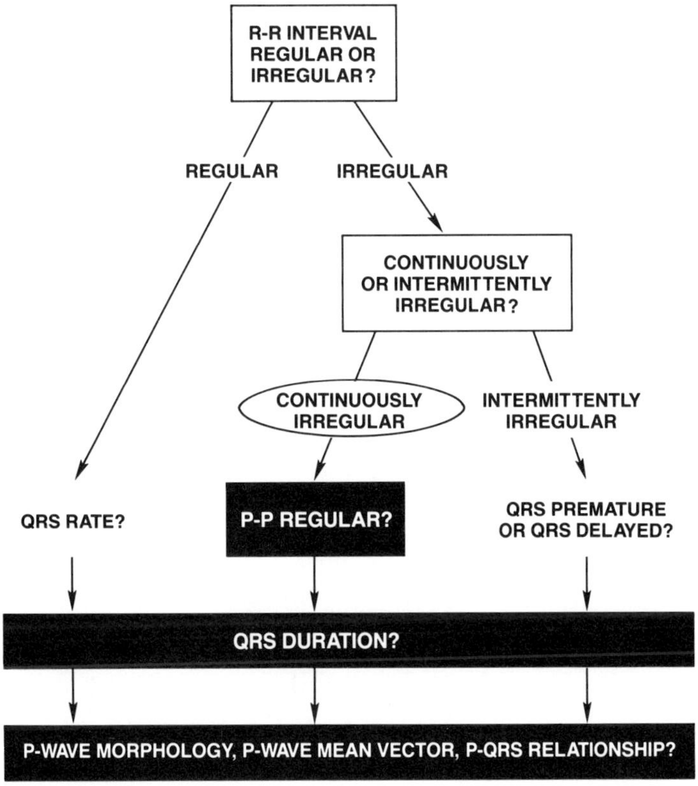

FIGURE 4–17
Continuously irregular: PP interval, QRS duration, atrial activity.

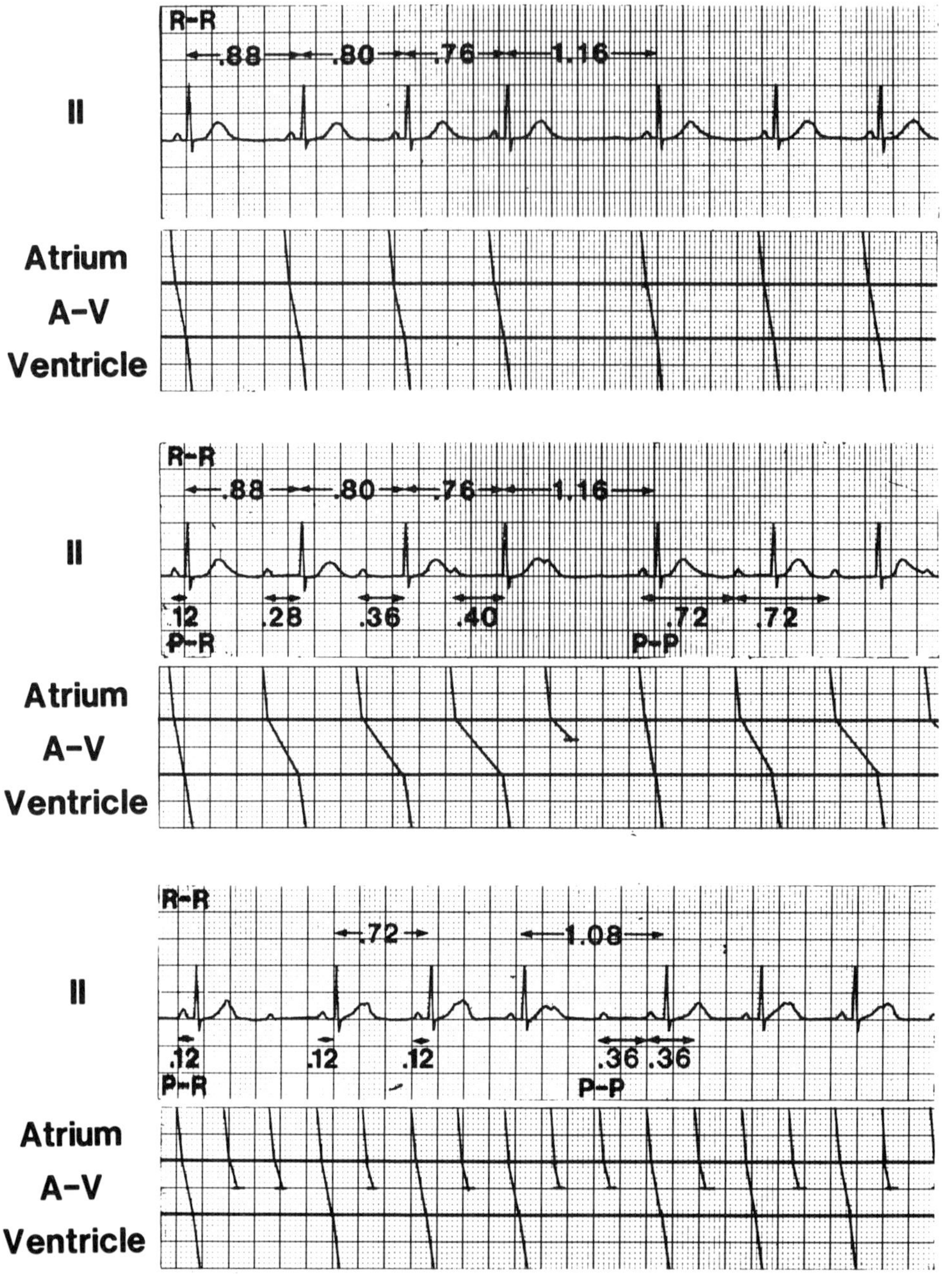

FIGURE 4–18
CONTINUOUSLY IRREGULAR RHYTHMS

Top tracing: Sinus arrhythmia: RR intervals vary from 0.76 to 1.16 s; each QRS complex is preceded by a P wave with a constant PR interval.

Middle tracing: Sinus rhythm with type I second degree AV block (Wenckebach); the RR intervals are identical to those in the top tracing; the PR interval lengthens until a P wave is not followed by a QRS (arrow).

Bottom tracing: Sinus tachycardia with varying type II second degree AV block; the atrial rate is 167 bpm (PP interval = 0.36 s); the RR interval varies from 0.72 with 2:1 block to 1.08 with 4:1 block.

In type II second degree AV block, the PR intervals remain constant, but the RR intervals may vary if the number of atrial depolarizations that are conducted to the ventricles vary (Fig. 4–18). Each type of AV block can occur with any type of supraventricular rhythm: either sinus or ectopic atrial rhythm, supraventricular tachycardia, or atrial flutter.

If there is a basic, regular RR interval that is interrupted intermittently, the initial question to be answered is whether the first irregular RR interval is shorter or longer than the basic, regular RR interval (Figs. 4–19 and 4–20). In order to be considered irregular, the RR interval must vary from the basic RR interval by 0.04 s or more.

QRS Complex. If the QRS is premature (by at least 0.04 s), the RR interval that follows the premature QRS may be prolonged (Fig. 4–21). The degree of prolongation has been used to distinguish among types of premature beats. In children, any type of premature beat may be followed by a "compensatory pause," and so the degree of prolongation is of little value.

The QRS duration is determined next. If the QRS duration is normal, the premature QRS can have one of three causes:

1. Intermittent conduction of a sinus beat. In the presence of atrial or junctional rhythm, the sinus node continues to depolarize. If the early QRS is preceded by a P wave with a normal mean vector (0° to +90°), the sinus node depolarization has conducted to the atria, causing the P wave, and the atrial impulse has conducted to the ventricles (so-called "sinus capture").
2. Premature atrial contraction. In sinus, atrial, or junctional rhythm, if the early QRS is preceded by a premature P wave, this is a premature atrial contraction.
3. Premature junctional contraction. If the QRS is not preceded by a premature P wave, this is a premature junctional contraction (Fig. 4–22).

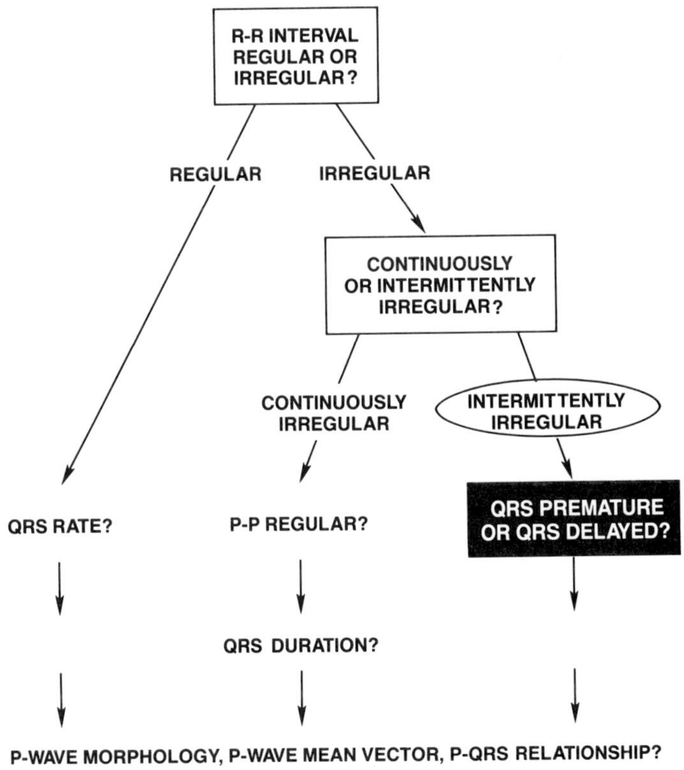

FIGURE 4–19
Intermittently irregular: Premature versus delayed QRS.

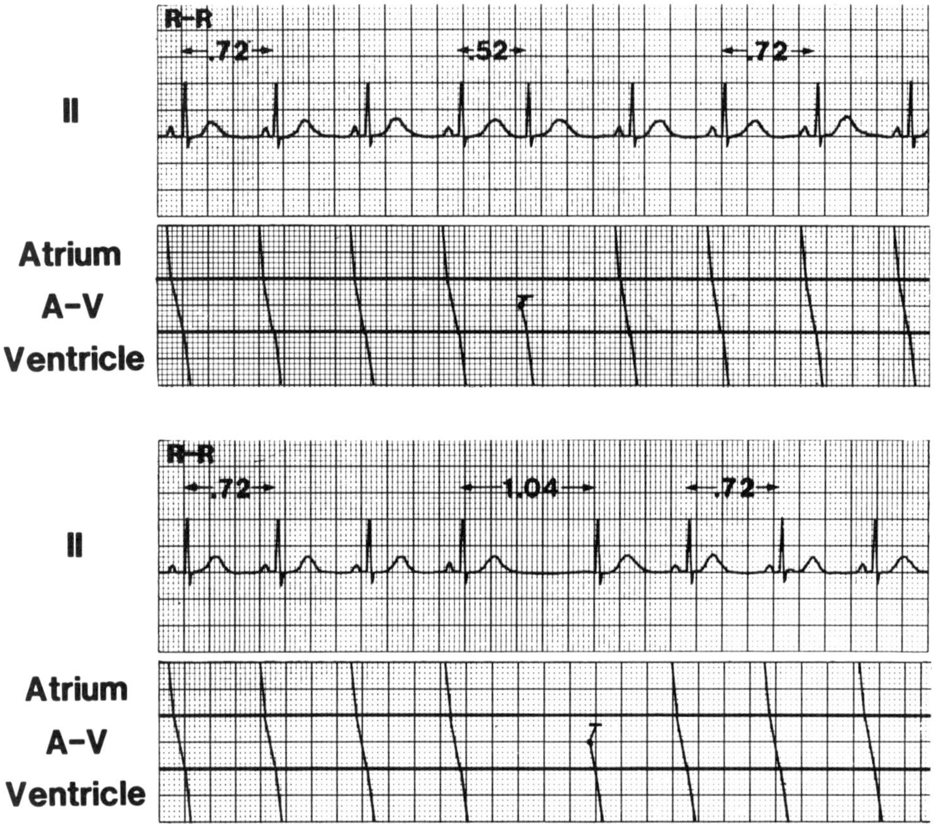

FIGURE 4–20
INTERMITTENTLY IRREGULAR; PREMATURE vs DELAYED QRS

Top tracing: Sinus rhythm with premature junctional contraction; basic RR interval is regular at 0.72 s; it is interrupted by a premature QRS with an RR interval of 0.52 s.

Bottom tracing: Sinus rhythm with sinus pause and junctional escape beat; basic RR interval is regular at 0.72 s; it is interrupted by a delayed QRS with an RR interval of 1.04 s.

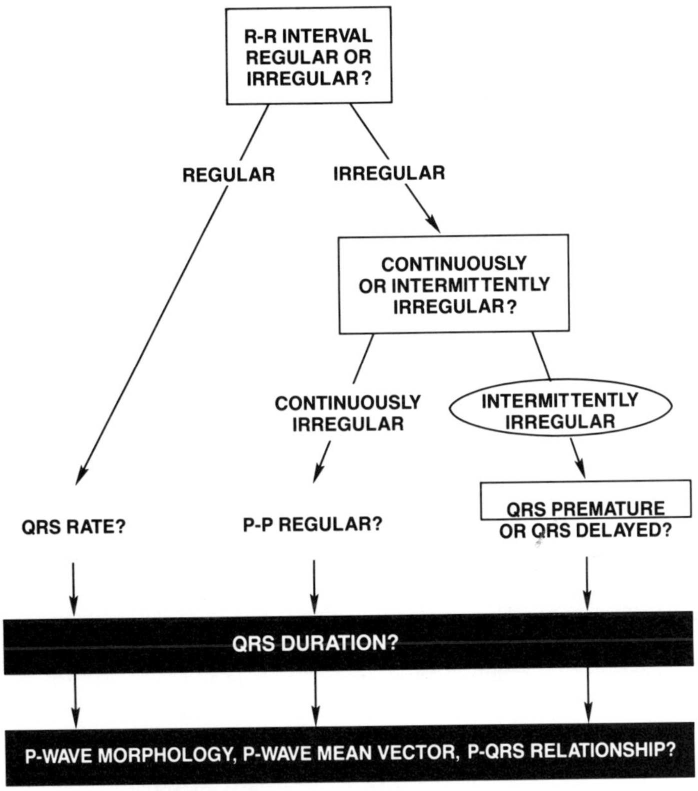

FIGURE 4–21
Premature normal duration QRS: atrial activity.

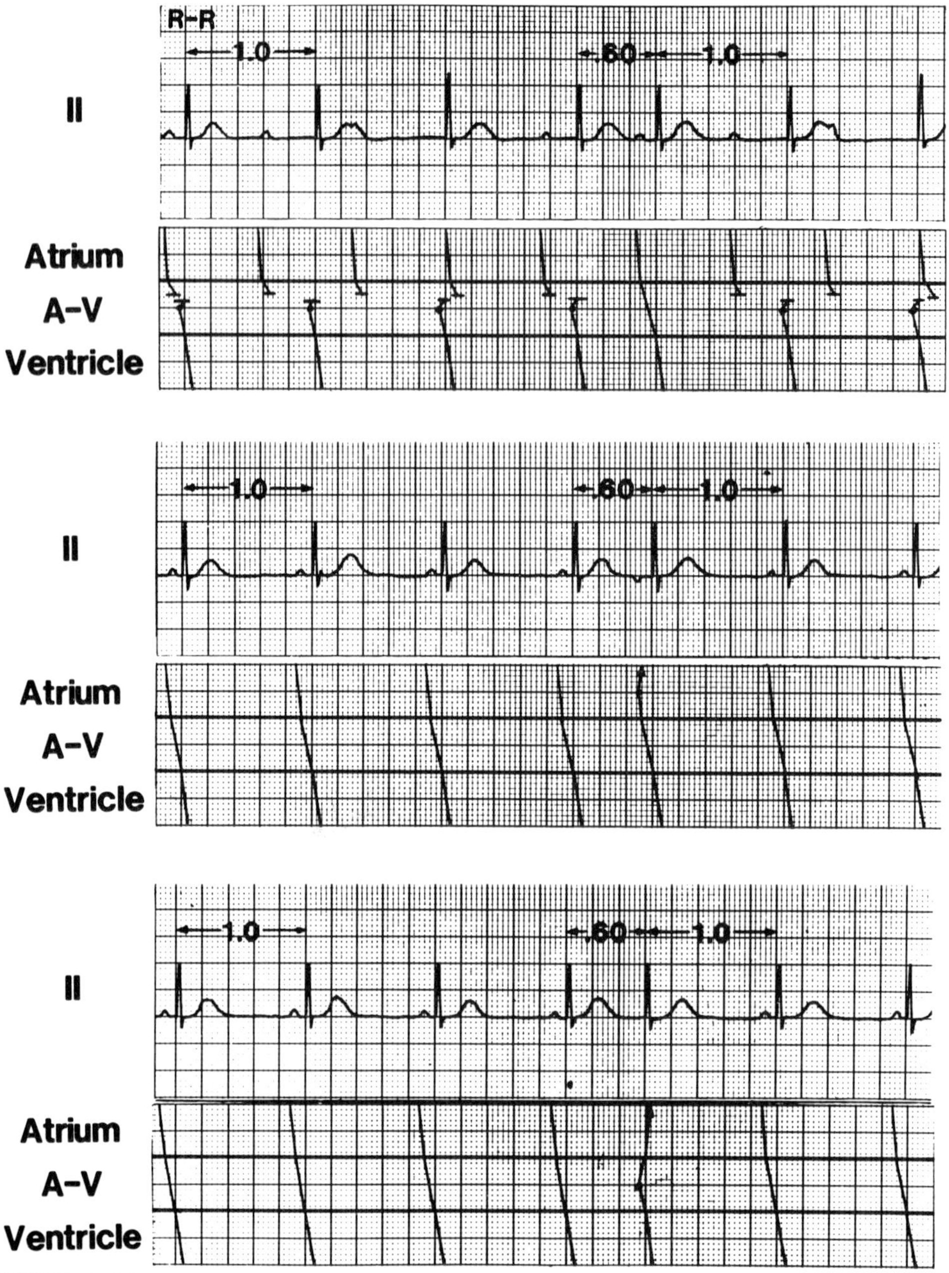

FIGURE 4–22
INTERMITTENTLY IRREGULAR: PREMATURE QRS

Top tracing: Sinus rhythm with advanced second degree AV block and junctional escape rhythm; the basic RR interval is 1.0 s (junctional rhythm at 60/min). The premature QRS is caused by a sinus "capture" beat (see Fig. 4–14*A*). This is the only P wave that conducts; all the other P waves are blocked. This is advanced second degree AV block.

Middle tracing: Sinus rhythm with premature atrial contraction; the basic RR interval is 1.0 s (sinus rhythm at 60/min). The premature QRS is preceded by a P wave that is negative in lead II; this is a premature atrial contraction originating from an inferior location in the atria.

Bottom tracing: Sinus rhythm with premature junctional contraction; the basic RR interval is 1.0 s (sinus rhythm at 60/min). The premature QRS is not preceded by a P wave; this is a premature junctional contraction.

If the premature QRS has a prolonged duration (Fig. 4–23), there are three possible causes similar to those for a normal duration QRS:

1. Sinus capture with aberration.
2. Premature atrial contraction with aberration.
3. Premature ventricular contraction.

It is possible to have a premature QRS complex without a preceding P wave as a result of a premature junctional contraction with aberration; however, it is impossible to distinguish on the surface electrocardiogram in children a premature junctional contraction with aberration from a premature ventricular contraction (Fig. 4–24). Therefore, we have chosen to classify all QRS complexes that are premature and have a prolonged duration without preceding P waves as premature ventricular contractions.

If the QRS is not premature, but rather is delayed by 0.04 s or more, the QRS duration should be determined (Fig. 4–25). If the QRS duration is normal, the answers to three questions will classify the rhythm. The first refers to the basic supraventricular rhythm. In second degree AV block, the supraventricular rhythm continues uninterrupted; in a nonconducted premature atrial contraction, a different morphology P wave is introduced prematurely; with a "pause" in the supraventricular rhythm, no atrial activity is observed (Figs. 4–26A and 4–26B).

Second, what is the RR interval from the delayed QRS complex back to the immediately preceding QRS? In type II second degree AV block, the RR interval is twice the basic RR interval; in a nonconducted premature atrial contraction, the RR interval is less than twice the basic RR interval. While most premature atrial contractions can be followed by either a compensatory or a noncompensatory pause, virtually all nonconducted premature atrial contractions have less than a fully compensatory pause. Therefore, both the PP and RR intervals should be less than twice the basic RR interval. In a

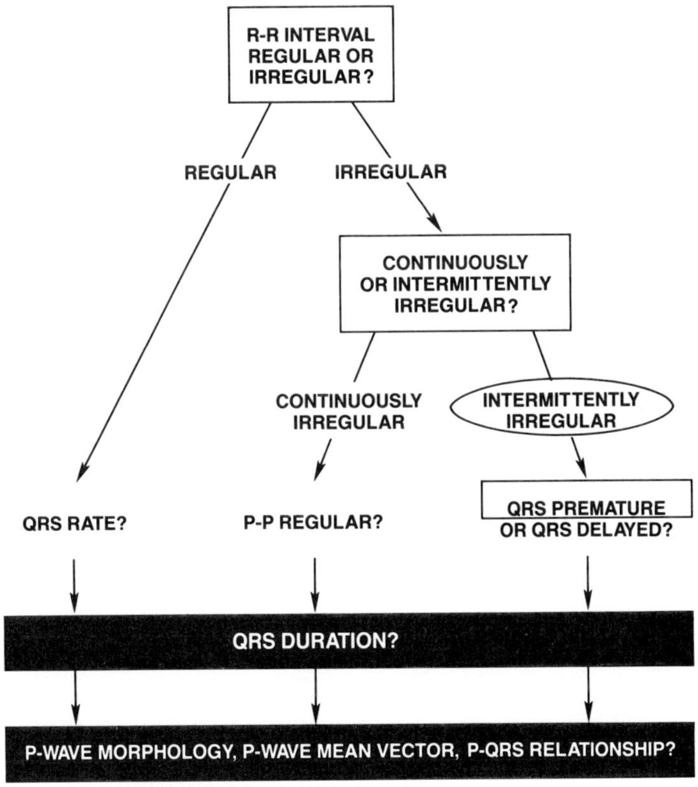

FIGURE 4–23
Premature prolonged duration QRS: atrial activity.

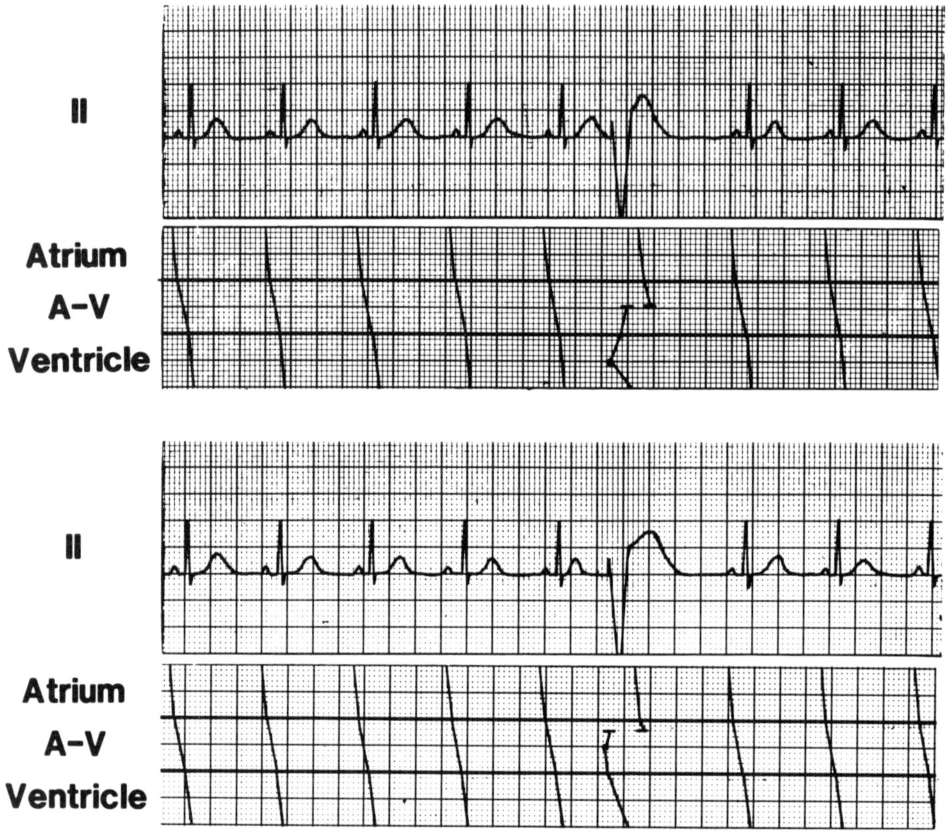

FIGURE 4–24
PREMATURE VENTRICULAR CONTRACTION vs PREMATURE JUNCTIONAL CONTRACTION WITH ABERRATION

Top tracing: Sinus rhythm and premature ventricular contraction; basic RR interval interrupted by a premature QRS with prolonged duration.

Bottom tracing: Sinus rhythm and premature junctional contraction with aberration; basic RR interval interrupted by a premature QRS with prolonged duration. These two arrhythmias are indistinguishable on the surface electrocardiogram.

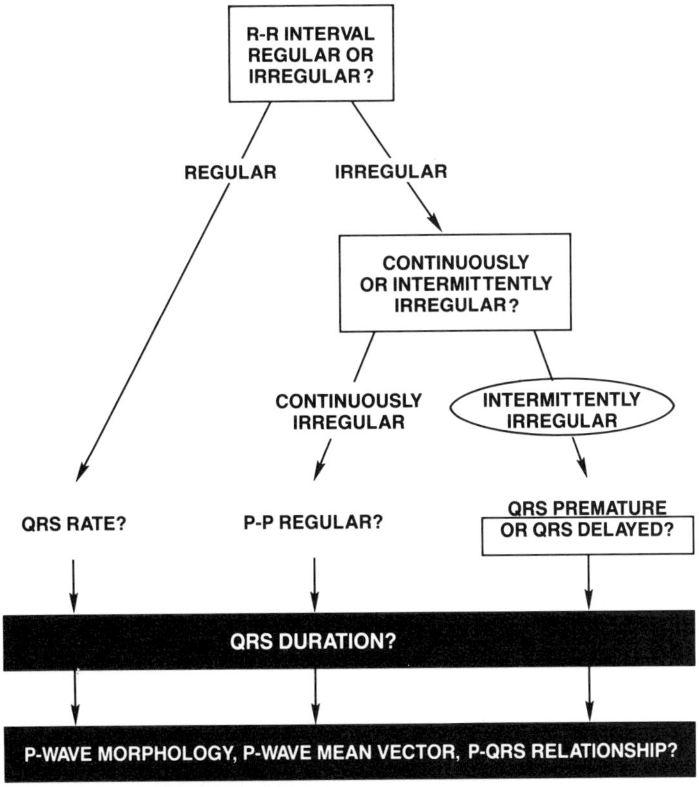

FIGURE 4–25
Delayed QRS: QRS duration, atrial activity.

"pause," the RR interval can be of any duration, but is always longer than the basic RR interval (Fig. 4–26A,B).

The third question concerns the atrial activity immediately preceding the delayed QRS complex. In AV block, the delayed QRS is preceded by a supraventricular P wave that is identical to that seen in the basic rhythm. In a nonconducted premature atrial contraction, the delayed QRS is also preceded by a supraventricular P wave that is identical to that seen in the basic supraventricular rhythm. In a pause with atrial escape, the delayed QRS is preceded by a P wave with a different mean vector and morphology from the basic P wave. In a pause with junctional escape, the delayed QRS is not preceded by a P wave.

If the QRS complex is delayed and the QRS duration is prolonged, the most common rhythm is a pause with ventricular escape (Fig. 4–26B).

With this background, the major common cardiac rhythm disturbances in children can be better understood. The arrhythmias will be discussed in 14 categories. Assignment into a category depends on:

1. Regularity of the RR interval.
2. QRS rate.
3. QRS duration.

In the following discussion, arrhythmia categories are grouped by whether the RR interval is regular (categories 1–6, Table 4–1), continuously irregular (categories 7–10, Table 4–2), or intermittently irregular (categories 11–14, Table 4–3). Each category is then discussed separately, with criteria provided for each of the arrhythmias in the category. Sample hand-drawn electrocardiographic tracings are also included with each category to facilitate comparison between arrhythmias.

Text continued on page 151

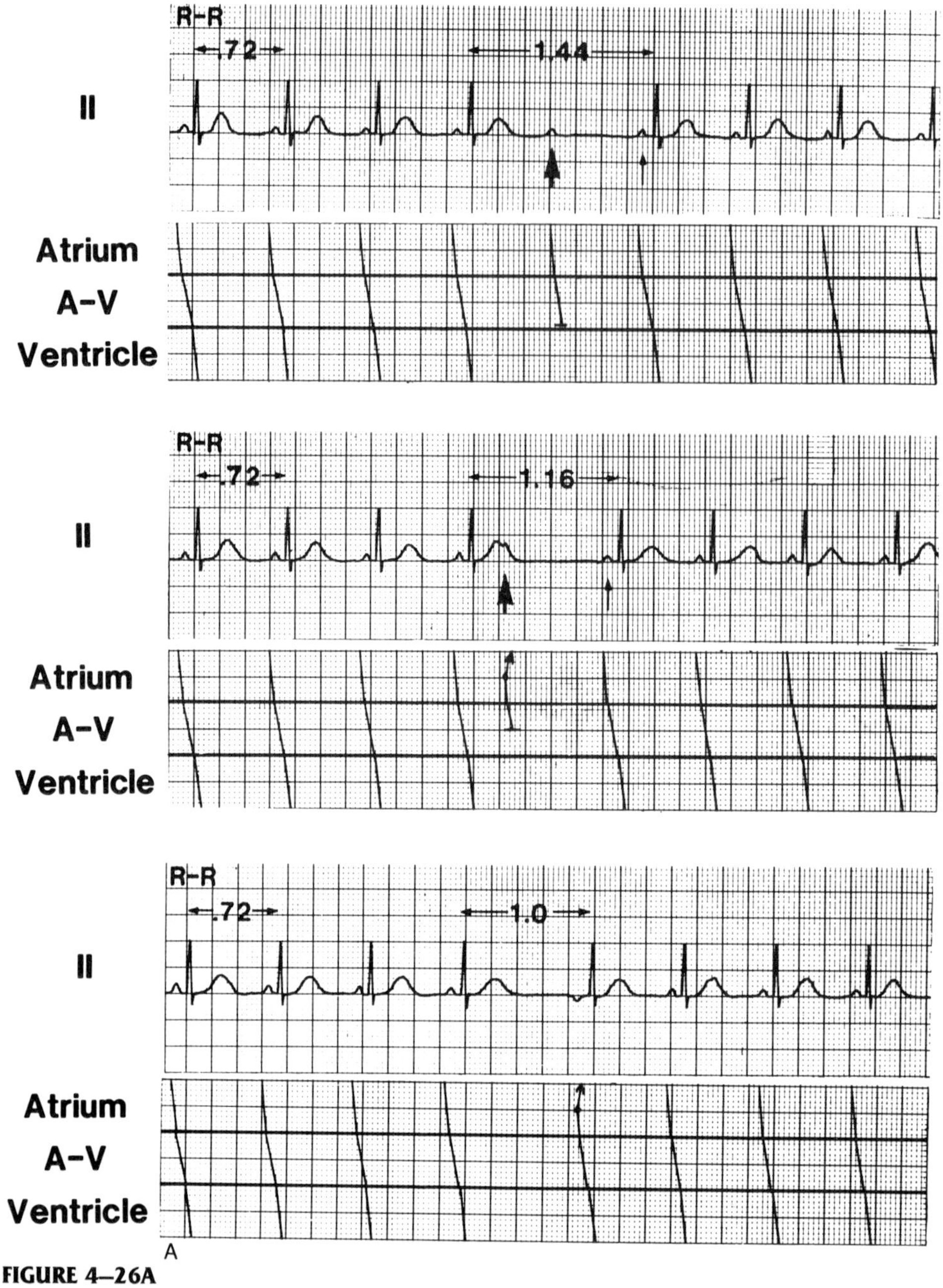

FIGURE 4–26A

INTERMITTENTLY IRREGULAR: DELAYED QRS

Top tracing: Sinus rhythm with type II second degree AV block; the basic RR interval is interrupted by an irregular RR interval that is exactly twice the basic RR interval. Sinus rhythm continues after the last regular QRS (large arrow); sinus rhythm initiates the QRS, which is delayed (small arrow).

Middle tracing: Sinus rhythm with nonconducted premature atrial contraction; the basic RR interval is interrupted by an irregular RR interval that is less than twice the basic RR interval. The last regular QRS complex is followed by a premature P wave (large arrow); sinus rhythm initiates the QRS, which is delayed (small arrow).

Bottom tracing: Sinus rhythm with sinus pause and low atrial escape beat; the basic RR interval is interrupted by an irregular RR interval that is greater than the basic RR interval. The last regular QRS complex is not followed by a P wave. An inverted P wave (small arrow) precedes the delayed QRS, indicating that this is a low atrial escape beat.

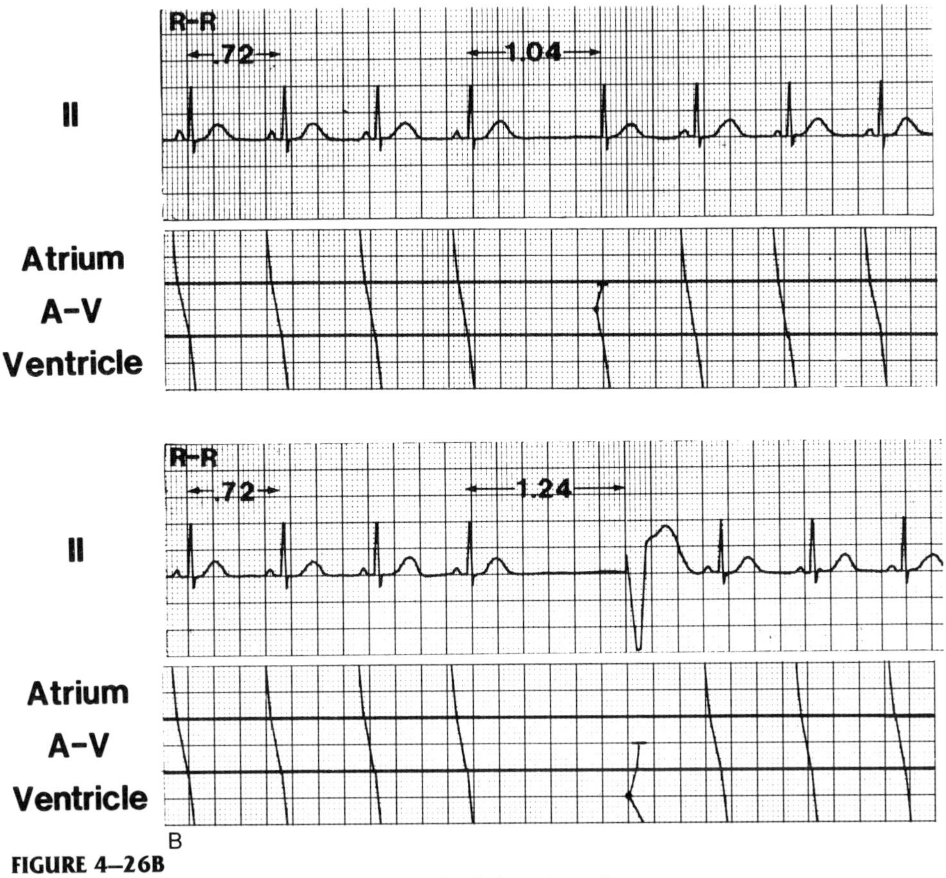

FIGURE 4–26B

INTERMITTENTLY IRREGULAR; DELAYED QRS *(continued)*

Top tracing: Sinus rhythm with sinus pause and junctional escape beat; the basic RR interval is interrupted by an irregular RR interval that is greater than the basic RR interval and also greater than the RR interval in low atrial escape (see Fig. 4–26A, bottom). This is because the junctional escape rate is slower than the atrial escape rate; the last regular QRS complex is not followed by a P wave; no P wave precedes the delayed QRS, indicating that this is a junctional escape beat.

Bottom tracing: Sinus rhythm with sinus pause and ventricular escape beat; the basic RR interval is interrupted by an irregular RR interval that is greater than the basic RR interval and also greater than the RR interval in either low atrial or junctional escape. The last regular QRS complex is not followed by a P wave. No P wave precedes the delayed QRS, which has prolonged duration, indicating that this is a ventricular escape beat. Strictly speaking, a ventricular escape beat should occur only at intervals longer than 1.5 s. Therefore, this is an accelerated ventricular escape beat, since it occurs at 1.24 s after the preceding QRS complex.

TABLE 4–1
ARRHYTHMIAS WITH A REGULAR RR INTERVAL*

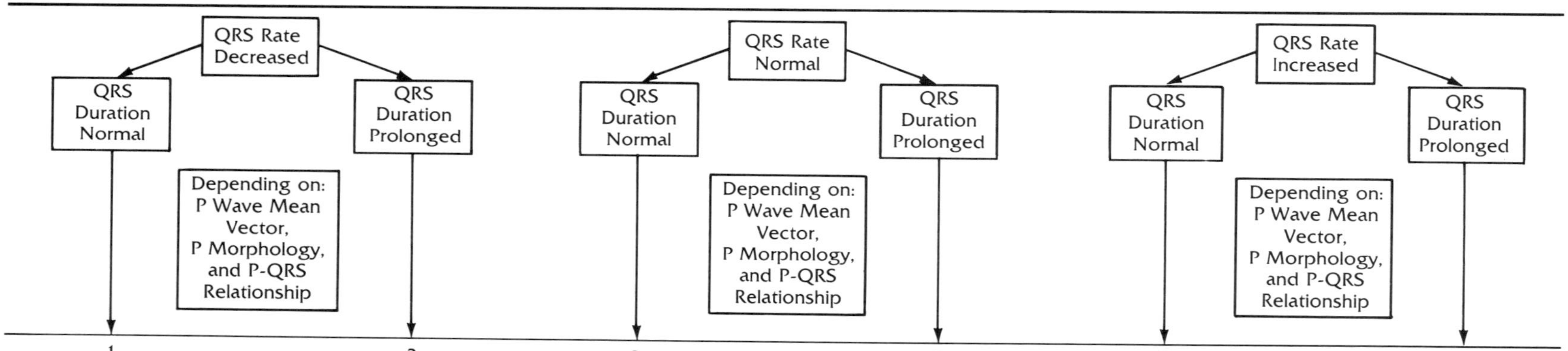

1	2	3	4	5	6
a. Sinus bradycardia	a. Sinus bradycardia with aberration	a. Sinus rhythm	a. Sinus rhythm with aberration	a. Sinus tachycardia (1:1 conduction)	a. Sinus tachycardia (1:1 conduction) with aberration
b. Ectopic atrial bradycardia	b. Ectopic atrial bradycardia with aberration	b. Ectopic atrial rhythm	b. Ectopic atrial rhythm with aberration	b. Ectopic atrial tachycardia (1:1 conduction)	b. Ectopic atrial tachycardia (1:1 conduction) with aberration
c. Junctional rhythm	c. Junctional rhythm with aberration or idioventricular rhythm	c. Accelerated junctional rhythm	c. Accelerated junctional rhythm with aberration or ventricular tachycardia	c. Supraventricular tachycardia (1:1 conduction)	c. Supraventricular tachycardia with aberration or ventricular tachycardia
d. Supraventricular rhythm with type II second degree AVB (SVT, sinus rhythm, atrial rhythm, sinus tachycardia, atrial flutter)	d. Supraventricular rhythm with aberration and fixed type II second degree AVB	d. Supraventricular rhythm with fixed type II second degree AVB	d. Supraventricular rhythm with aberration and fixed type II second degree AVB	d. Supraventricular tachycardia with fixed type II second degree AVB	d. Supraventricular tachycardia with aberration and fixed type II second degree AVB
e. Third degree AVB with junctional rhythm	e. Third degree AVB with ventricular rhythm			e. Atrial flutter with fixed type II second degree AVB	e. Atrial flutter with aberration and fixed type II second degree AVB

*Numbers and letters refer to categories that follow in the text.

TABLE 4–2
ARRHYTHMIAS WITH A CONTINUOUSLY IRREGULAR RR INTERVAL*

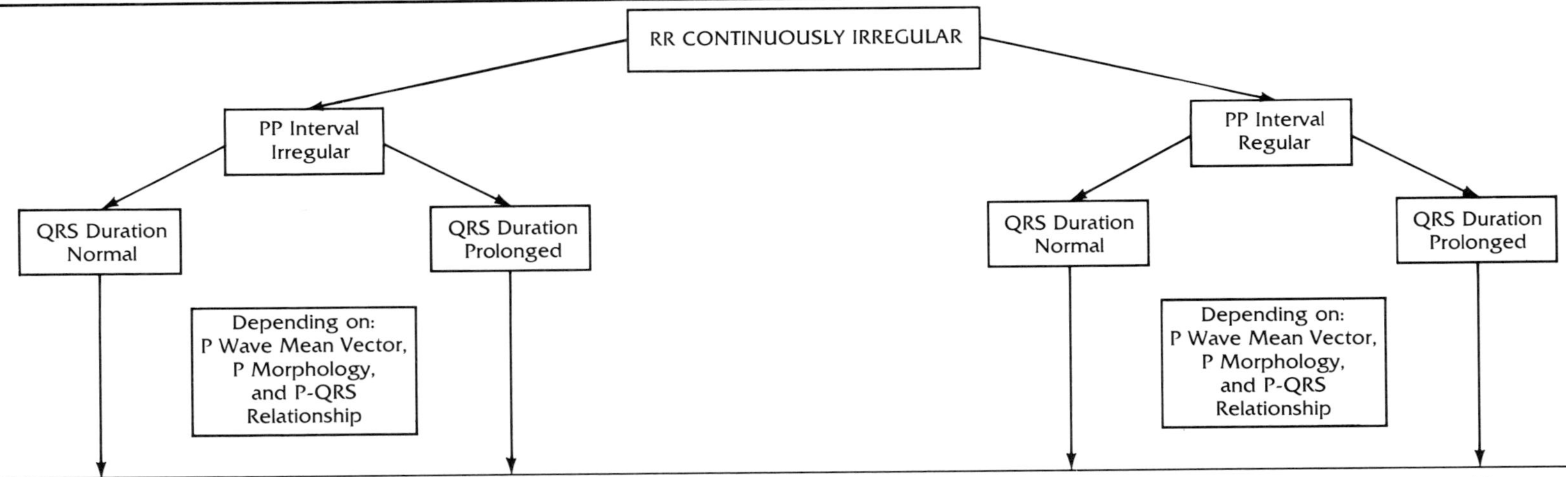

7	8	9	10
a. Sinus arrhythmia	a. Sinus arrhythmia with aberration	a. Supraventricular rhythm with varying type II second degree AVB	a. Supraventricular rhythm with aberration and varying type II second degree AVB
b. Wandering pacemaker	b. Wandering pacemaker with aberration	b. Supraventricular rhythm with type I second degree AVB (Wenckebach)	b. Supraventricular rhythm with aberration and type I second degree AVB (Wenckebach)
c. Atrial fibrillation	c. Atrial fibrillation with aberration		

*Numbers and letters refer to categories that follow in the text.

TABLE 4–3
ARRHYTHMIAS WITH AN INTERMITTENTLY IRREGULAR RR INTERVAL*

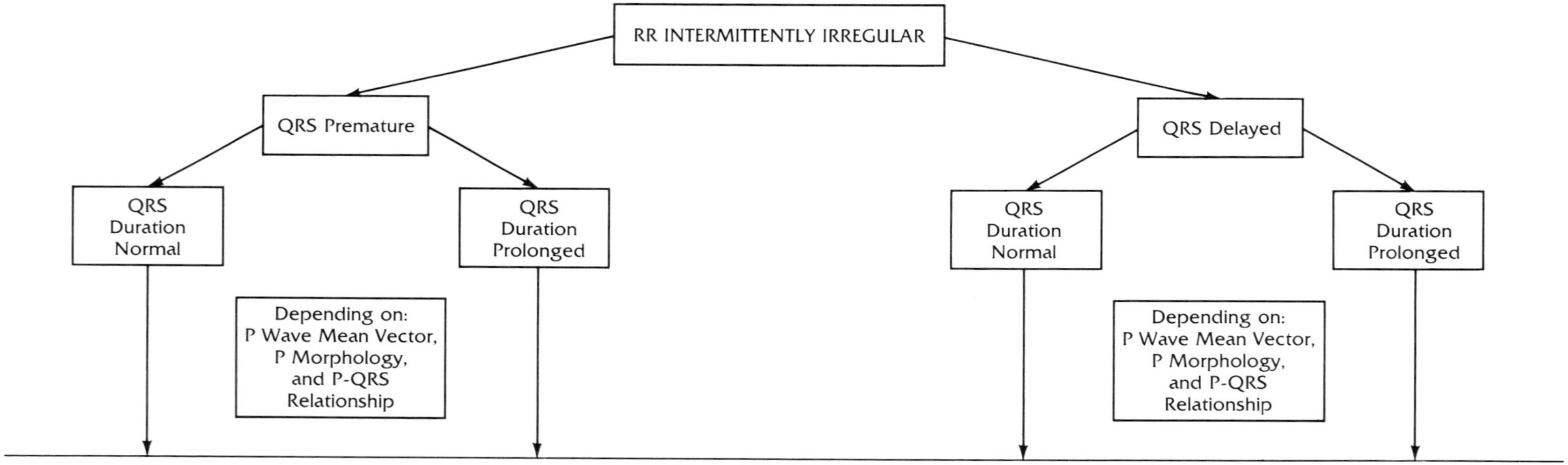

11	12	13	14
a. Ectopic atrial or junctional rhythm with sinus capture	a. Ectopic atrial or junctional rhythm with sinus capture and aberration	a. Supraventricular rhythm with intermittent type II second degree AVB	a. Pause in supraventricular rhythm with ventricular escape
b. Sinus, ectopic atrial, or junctional rhythm with premature atrial contraction	b. Sinus, ectopic atrial, or junctional rhythm with premature atrial contraction and aberration	b. Supraventricular rhythm with nonconducted premature atrial contraction	
c. Sinus, ectopic atrial, or junctional rhythm with premature junctional contraction	c. Sinus, ectopic atrial, or junctional rhythm with premature ventricular contraction	c. Pause in supraventricular rhythm with ectopic atrial escape	
		d. Pause in supraventricular rhythm with junctional escape	

*Numbers and letters refer to categories that follow in the text.

1. RR INTERVAL – REGULAR QRS RATE – DECREASED QRS DURATION – NORMAL

(See Figures 4–27A, 4–27B, and 4–27C)

a. Sinus Bradycardia
P wave precedes each QRS complex with normal P wave mean vector (0° to 90°).

b. Ectopic Atrial Bradycardia
P wave precedes each QRS complex with abnormal P wave mean vector (−1° to +91°).

c. Junctional Rhythm
1. Sinus P rate less than QRS rate with AV dissociation; or
2. "Retrograde" P wave (mean vector −1° to −90°) follows some or all QRS complexes.

d. Supraventricular Rhythm With Fixed Type II Second Degree AV Block
P rate a multiple of QRS rate with fixed relationship of P waves to QRS complexes (every second, third, or fourth P wave precedes a QRS complex with the same PR interval). The supraventricular rhythm that is blocked must then be ascertained:
1. Sinus Rhythm With AV Block
P mean vector and P rate are normal for age.
2. *Atrial Rhythm With AV Block*
P mean vector is abnormal and P rate is normal.
3. *Sinus Tachycardia With AV Block*
P mean vector is normal and P rate is increased (≤230/min).
4. *Supraventricular Tachycardia With AV Block*
P mean vector is abnormal and P rate is increased, or
P mean vector is normal and P rate is >230 min.
5. *Atrial Flutter With AV Block*
P waves have flutter morphology with fixed relationship of flutter waves to QRS complexes.

NOTE: In any rhythm with fixed type II second degree AV block, it is important to obtain long rhythm strips that demonstrate that, as the supraventricular rhythm changes, so does the ventricular response. If the ventricular response remains unchanged with a change in the supraventricular rhythm, this may be complete AV block with isochronic dissociation.

e. Complete AV Block With Junctional Rhythm
Sinus P rate equal to or greater than QRS rate with AV dissociation.

FIGURE 4–27A

1. RR INTERVAL – REGULAR QRS RATE – DECREASED QRS DURATION – NORMAL

Top tracing: Sinus bradycardia. Ventricular rate = 50/min; atrial rate = 50/min.
Second tracing: Ectopic atrial bradycardia. Ventricular rate = 50/min; atrial rate = 50/min.
Third tracing: Junctional rhythm with AV dissociation. Ventricular rate = 50/min; atrial rate = 48/min. Conduction does not occur from ventricles to atria.
Bottom tracing: Junctional rhythm. Ventricular rate = 50/min; atrial rate = 50/min. Retrograde conduction is intact with inverted P waves following each QRS complex.

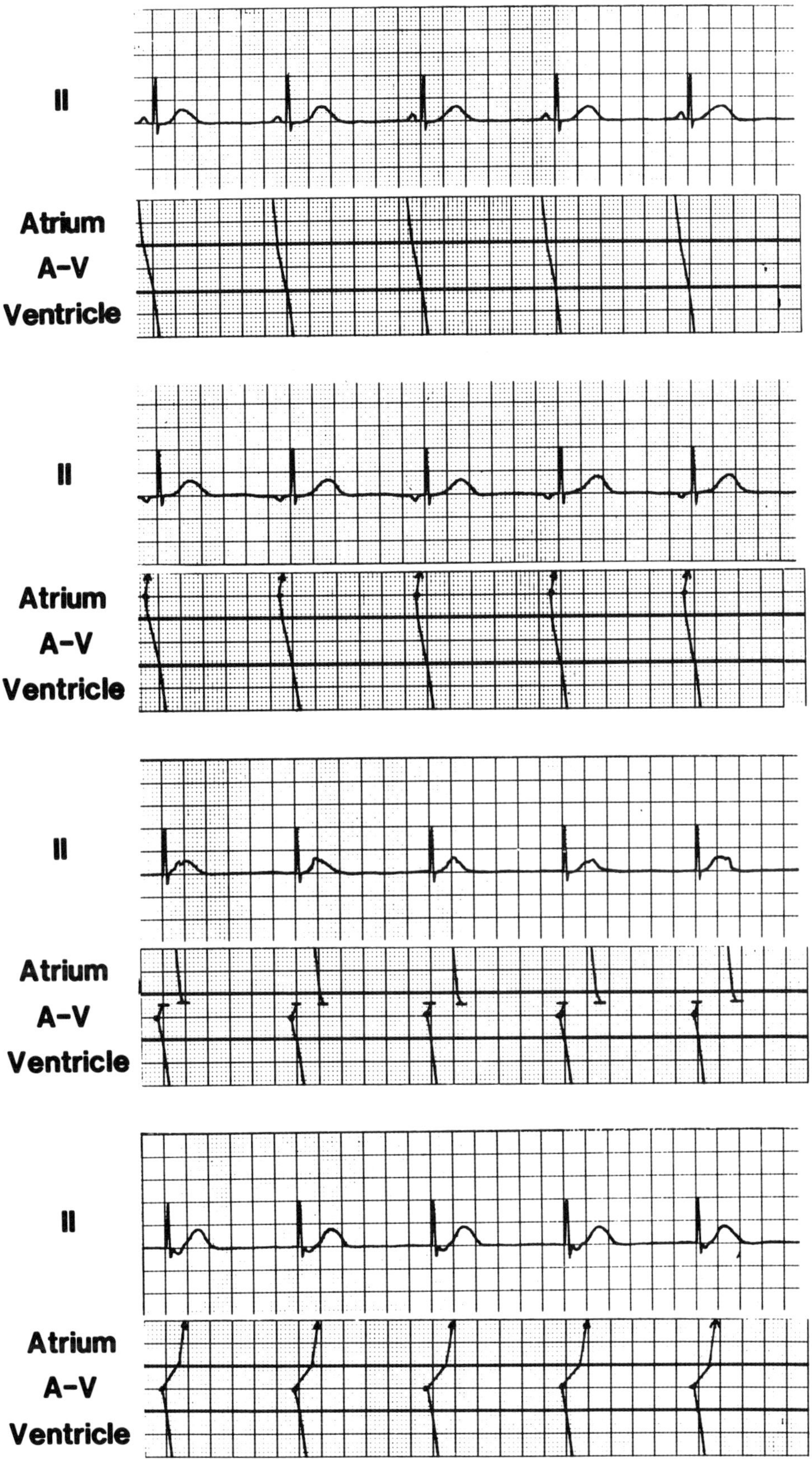
II
Atrium
A-V
Ventricle
II
Atrium
A-V
Ventricle
II
Atrium
A-V
Ventricle
II
Atrium
A-V
Ventricle
A

FIGURE 4–27B *(continued)*

1. RR INTERVAL – REGULAR
QRS RATE – DECREASED
QRS DURATION – NORMAL

Top tracing: Sinus rhythm with second degree AV block (2:1). Ventricular rate = 50/min; atrial rate = 100/min. Every other P wave is followed by a QRS complex; when AV block is 2:1, it is not possible to determine if this is type I or type II second degree AV block.

Second tracing: Atrial rhythm with second degree AV block (2:1). Ventricular rate = 50/min; atrial rate = 100/min.

Third tracing: Sinus rhythm (rapid rate) with fixed type II second degree AV block (3:1). Ventricular rate = 50/min; atrial rate = 150/min.

Bottom tracing: Supraventricular tachycardia with fixed type II second degree AV block (5:1). Ventricular rate = 50/min; atrial rate = 250/min.

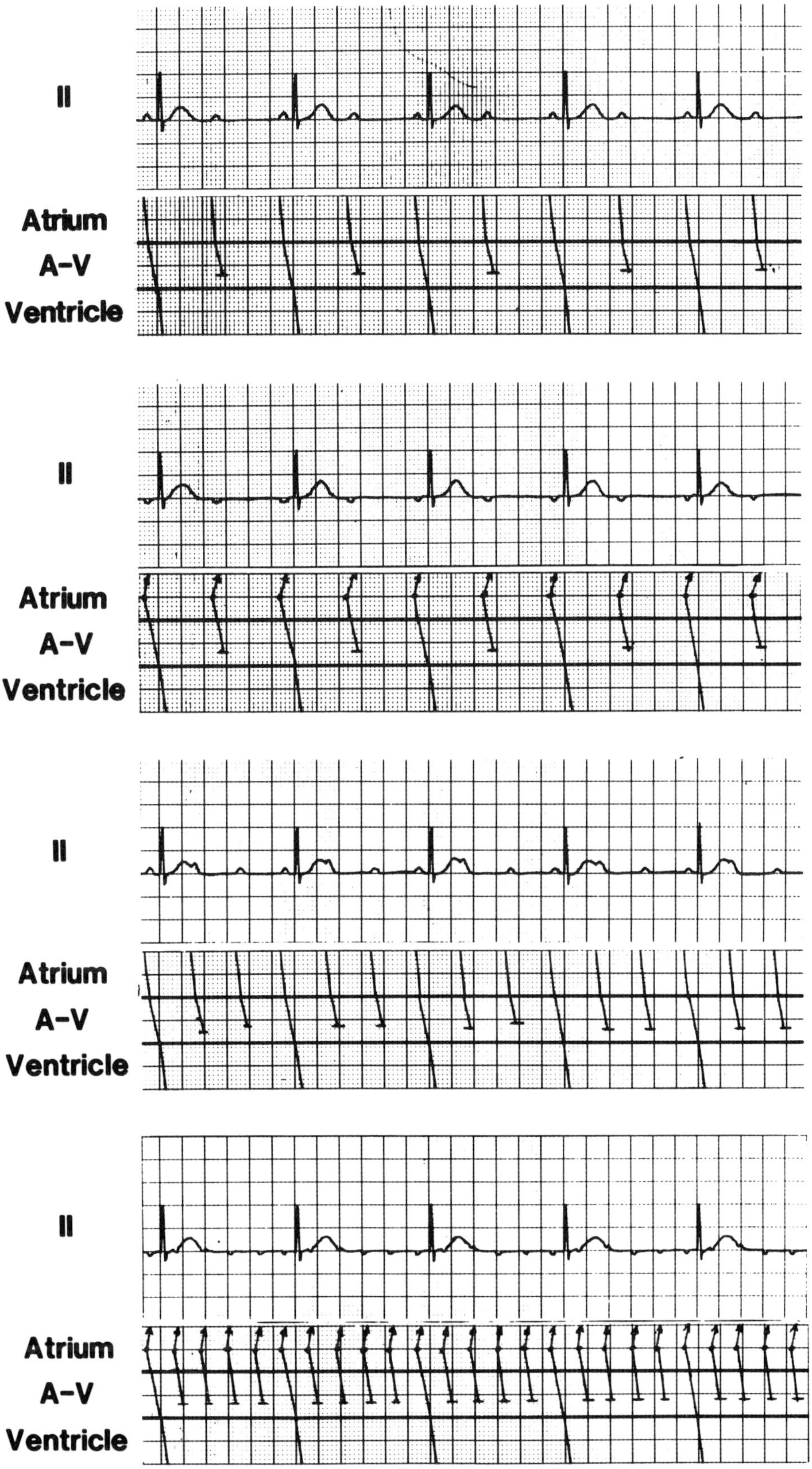
II
Atrium
A-V
Ventricle
II
Atrium
A-V
Ventricle
II
Atrium
A-V
Ventricle
II
Atrium
A-V
Ventricle

B

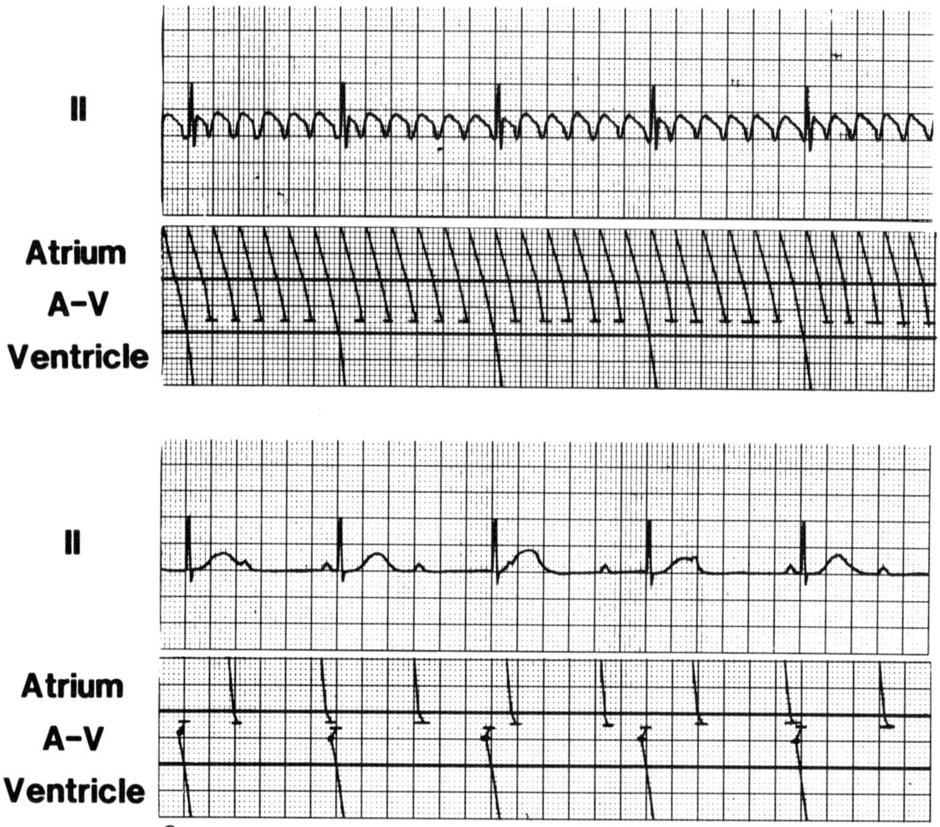

C

FIGURE 4–27C *(continued)*

---

1. RR INTERVAL – REGULAR
QRS RATE – DECREASED
QRS DURATION – NORMAL

Top tracing: Atrial flutter with fixed type II second degree AV block (6:1). Ventricular rate = 50/min; atrial rate = 300/min.

Bottom tracing: Complete AV block with AV dissociation and junctional rhythm. Ventricular rate = 50/min; atrial rate = 85/min.

2. RR INTERVAL – REGULAR
QRS RATE – DECREASED
QRS DURATION – PROLONGED

(See Figures 4–28A, 4–28B, and 4–28C)

a. Sinus Bradycardia With Aberration
P wave precedes each QRS complex with normal P wave mean vector.

b. Ectopic Atrial Bradycardia With Aberration
P wave precedes each QRS complex with abnormal P wave mean vector.

c. Junctional Rhythm With Aberration or Idioventricular Rhythm
1. P rate less than QRS rate with AV dissociation; or
2. "Retrograde" P wave follows some or all QRS complexes.

d. Supraventricular Rhythm With Fixed Type II Second Degree AV Block and Aberration
P rate a multiple of QRS rate with fixed relationship of P waves to QRS complexes (see 1*d*).

e. Complete AV Block With Ventricular Rhythm
P rate equal to or greater than QRS rate with AV dissociation.

FIGURE 4–28A

2. RR INTERVAL – REGULAR QRS RATE – DECREASED QRS DURATION – PROLONGED

Top tracing: Sinus bradycardia with complete right bundle branch block. Ventricular rate = 50/min; atrial rate = 50/min.

Second tracing: Ectopic atrial bradycardia with complete right bundle branch block. Ventricular rate = 50/min; atrial rate = 50/min.

Third tracing: Junctional rhythm with complete right bundle branch block or idioventricular rhythm with AV dissociation (it is impossible to distinguish between these on a surface electrocardiogram); a ladder diagram for each is shown. Ventricular rate = 50/min; atrial rate = 48/min. Conduction does not occur from ventricles to atria.

Bottom tracing: Junctional rhythm with complete right bundle branch block or idioventricular rhythm (inverted P waves following each QRS complex); a ladder diagram for each is shown. Ventricular rate = 50/min; atrial rate = 50/min. Retrograde conduction is intact with inverted P waves following each QRS complex.

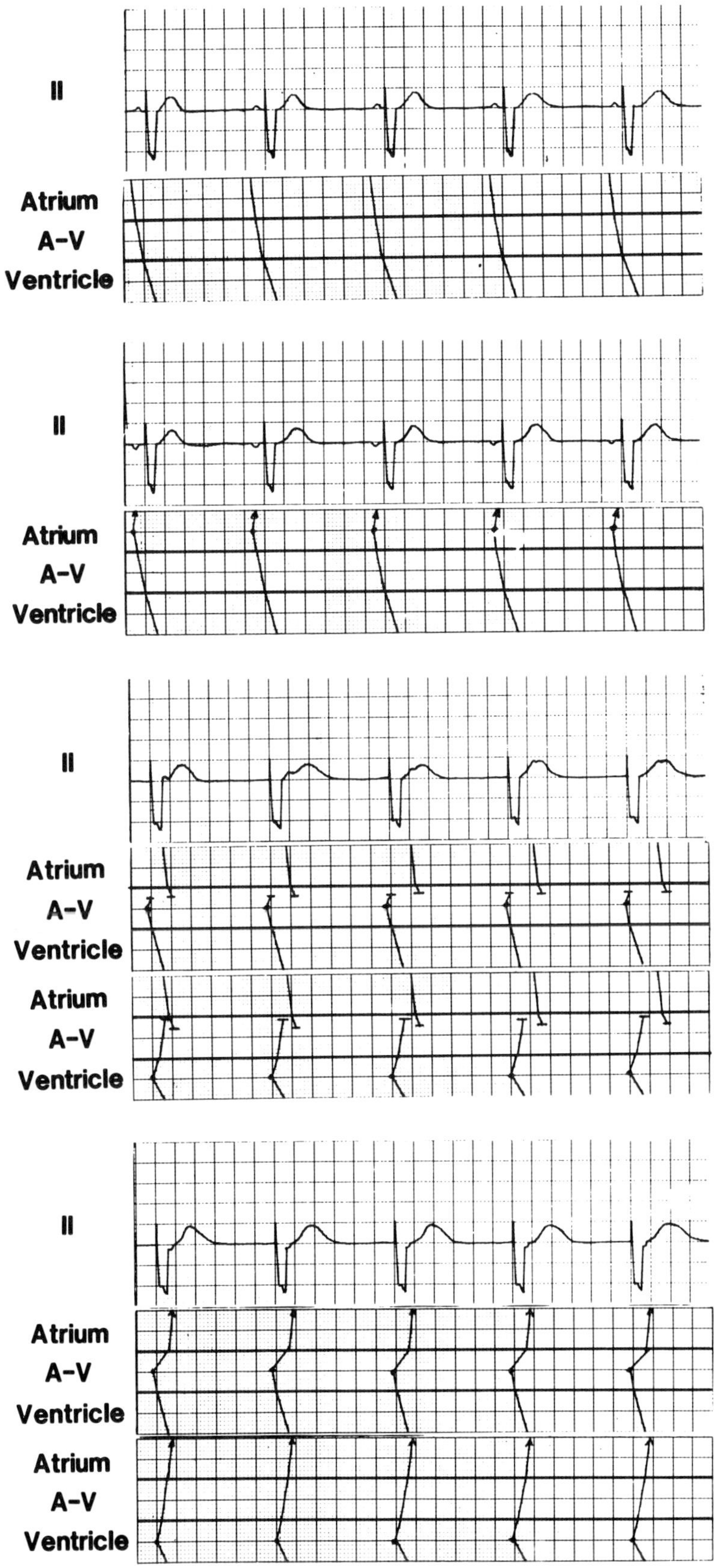
II
Atrium
A-V
Ventricle
II
Atrium
A-V
Ventricle
II
Atrium
A-V
Ventricle
Atrium
A-V
Ventricle
II
Atrium
A-V
Ventricle
Atrium
A-V
Ventricle

A

FIGURE 4–28B ***(continued)***

2. RR INTERVAL – REGULAR QRS RATE – DECREASED QRS DURATION – PROLONGED

Top tracing: Sinus rhythm with second degree AV block (2:1) and complete right bundle branch block. Ventricular rate = 50/min; atrial rate = 100/min. Every other P wave is followed by a QRS complex; when AV block is 2:1, it is not possible to determine if this is type I or type II second degree AV block.

Second tracing: Atrial rhythm with second degree AV block (2:1) and complete right bundle branch block. Ventricular rate = 50/min; atrial rate = 100/min.

Third tracing: Sinus rhythm (rapid rate) with fixed type II second degree AV block (3:1) and complete right bundle branch block. Ventricular rate = 50/min; atrial rate = 150/min.

Bottom tracing: Supraventricular tachycardia with fixed type II second degree AV block (5:1) and complete right bundle branch block. Ventricular rate = 50/min; atrial rate = 250/min.

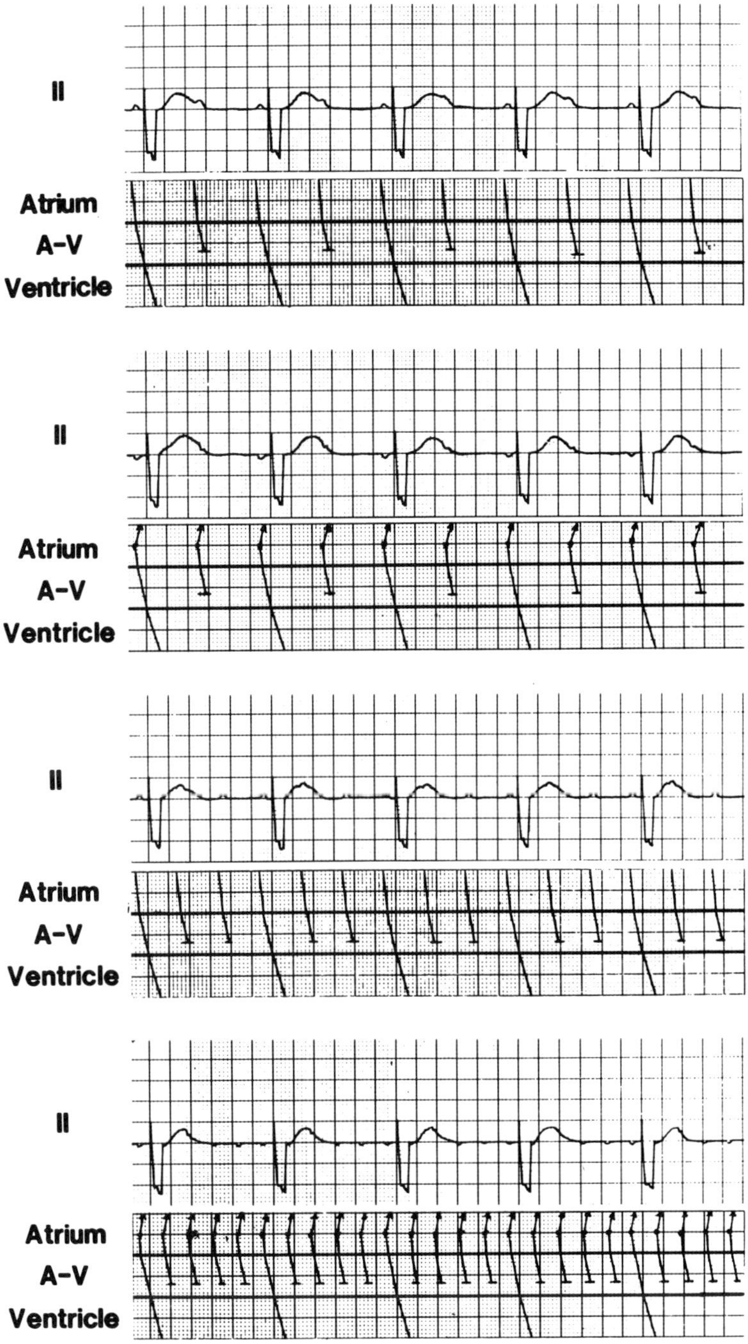
II
Atrium
A-V
Ventricle
II
Atrium
A-V
Ventricle
II
Atrium
A-V
Ventricle
II
Atrium
A-V
Ventricle
B

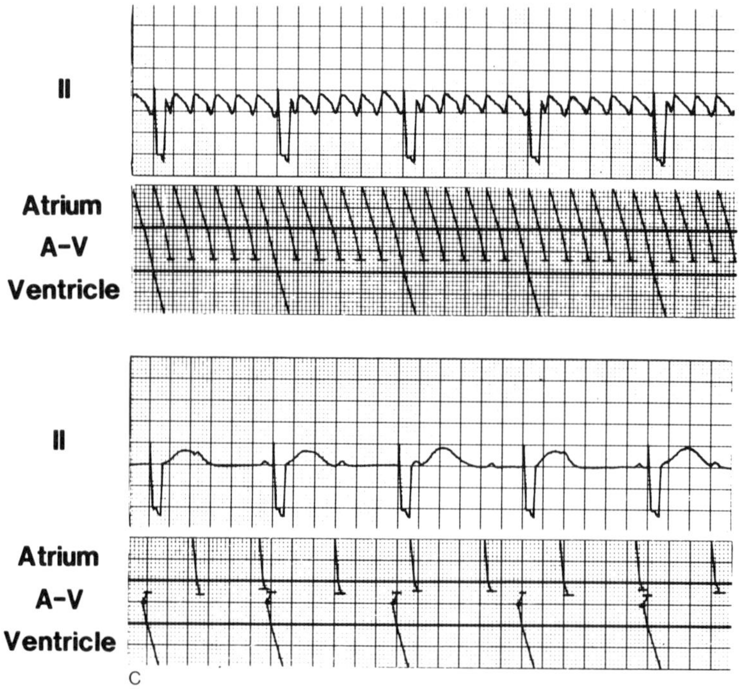

FIGURE 4–28C *(continued)*

2. RR INTERVAL – REGULAR QRS RATE – DECREASED QRS DURATION – PROLONGED

Top tracing: Atrial flutter with fixed type II second degree AV block (6:1) and complete right bundle branch block. Ventricular rate = 50/min; atrial rate = 300/min.

Bottom tracing: Complete AV block with AV dissociation and junctional rhythm with complete right bundle branch block or idioventricular rhythm. Ventricular rate = 50/min; atrial rate = 85/min.

3. RR INTERVAL – REGULAR QRS RATE – NORMAL QRS DURATION – NORMAL

(See Figures 4–29A, 4–29B, and 4–29C)

a. Sinus Rhythm
P wave precedes each QRS complex with normal P wave mean vector.

b. Ectopic Atrial Rhythm
P wave precedes each QRS complex with abnormal P wave mean vector.

c. Accelerated Junctional Rhythm
1. Sinus P rate less than QRS rate with AV dissociation; or
2. No P waves visible; or
3. Retrograde P wave follows some or all QRS complexes.

d. Supraventricular Rhythm With Fixed Type II Second Degree AV Block
P rate a multiple of QRS rate with fixed relationship of P waves to QRS complexes (see 1*d*).

FIGURE 4–29A

3. RR INTERVAL – REGULAR
QRS RATE – NORMAL
QRS DURATION – NORMAL

Top tracing:	Sinus rhythm. Ventricular rate = 75/min; atrial rate = 75/min.
Second tracing:	Ectopic atrial rhythm. Ventricular rate = 75/min; atrial rate = 75/min.
Third tracing:	Accelerated junctional rhythm with AV dissociation. Ventricular rate = 75/min; atrial rate = 71/min. Conduction does not occur from ventricles to atria.
Bottom tracing:	Accelerated junctional rhythm. Ventricular rate = 75/min; atrial rate = 75/min. Retrograde conduction is intact, with inverted P waves following each QRS complex.

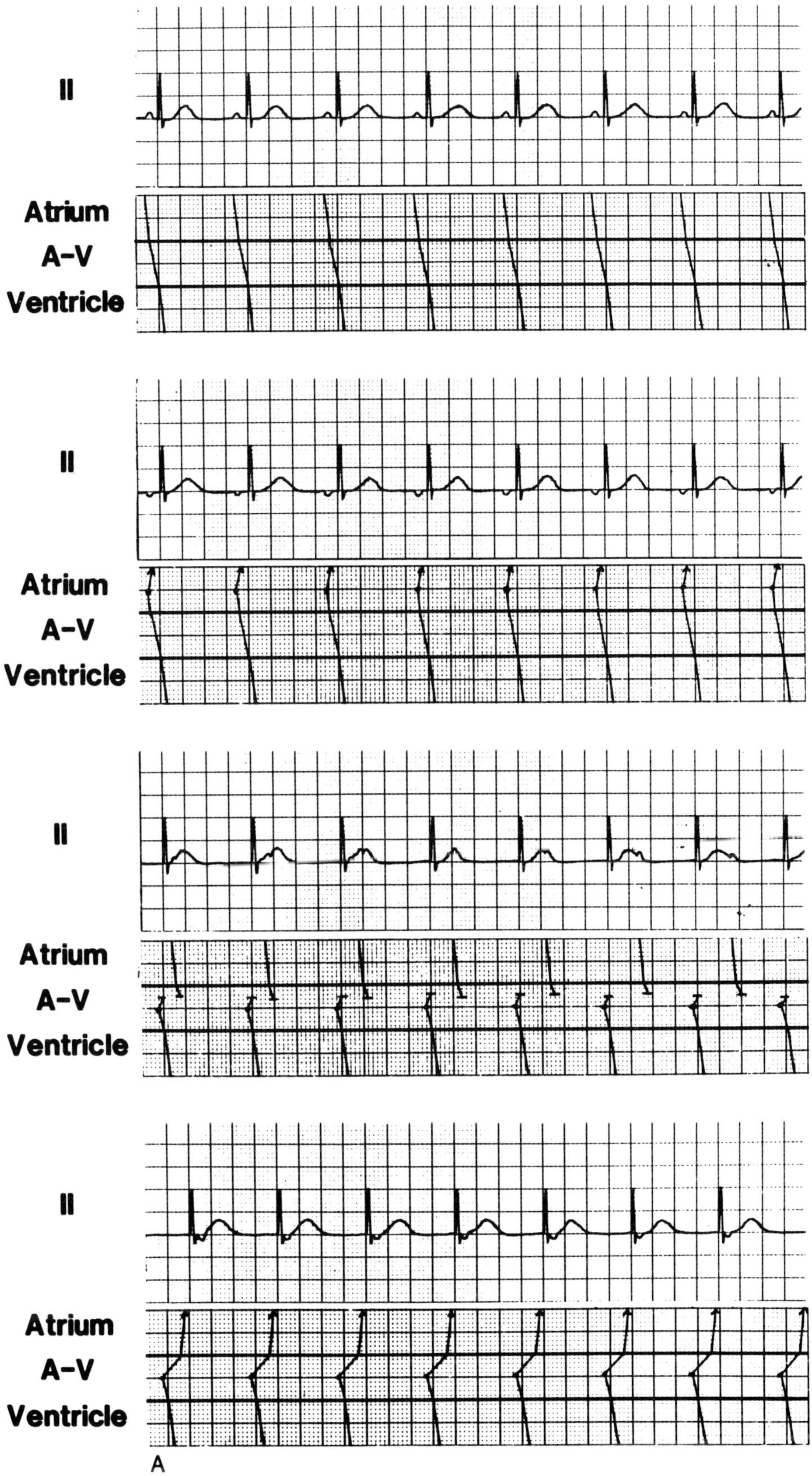
II
Atrium
A-V
Ventricle
II
Atrium
A-V
Ventricle
II
Atrium
A-V
Ventricle
II
Atrium
A-V
Ventricle
A

FIGURE 4–29B ***(continued)***

3. RR INTERVAL – REGULAR
QRS RATE – NORMAL
QRS DURATION – NORMAL

Top tracing: Sinus rhythm with second degree AV block (2:1). Ventricular rate = 75/min; atrial rate = 150/min. Every other P wave is followed by a QRS complex; when AV block is 2:1, it is not possible to determine if this is type I or type II second degree AV block.

Second tracing: Atrial rhythm with second degree AV block (2:1). Ventricular rate = 75/min; atrial rate = 150/min.

Third tracing: Sinus tachycardia with fixed type II second degree AV block (3:1). Ventricular rate = 75/min; atrial rate = 225/min.

Bottom tracing: Supraventricular tachycardia with fixed type II second degree AV block (4:1). Ventricular rate = 75/min; atrial rate = 300/min.

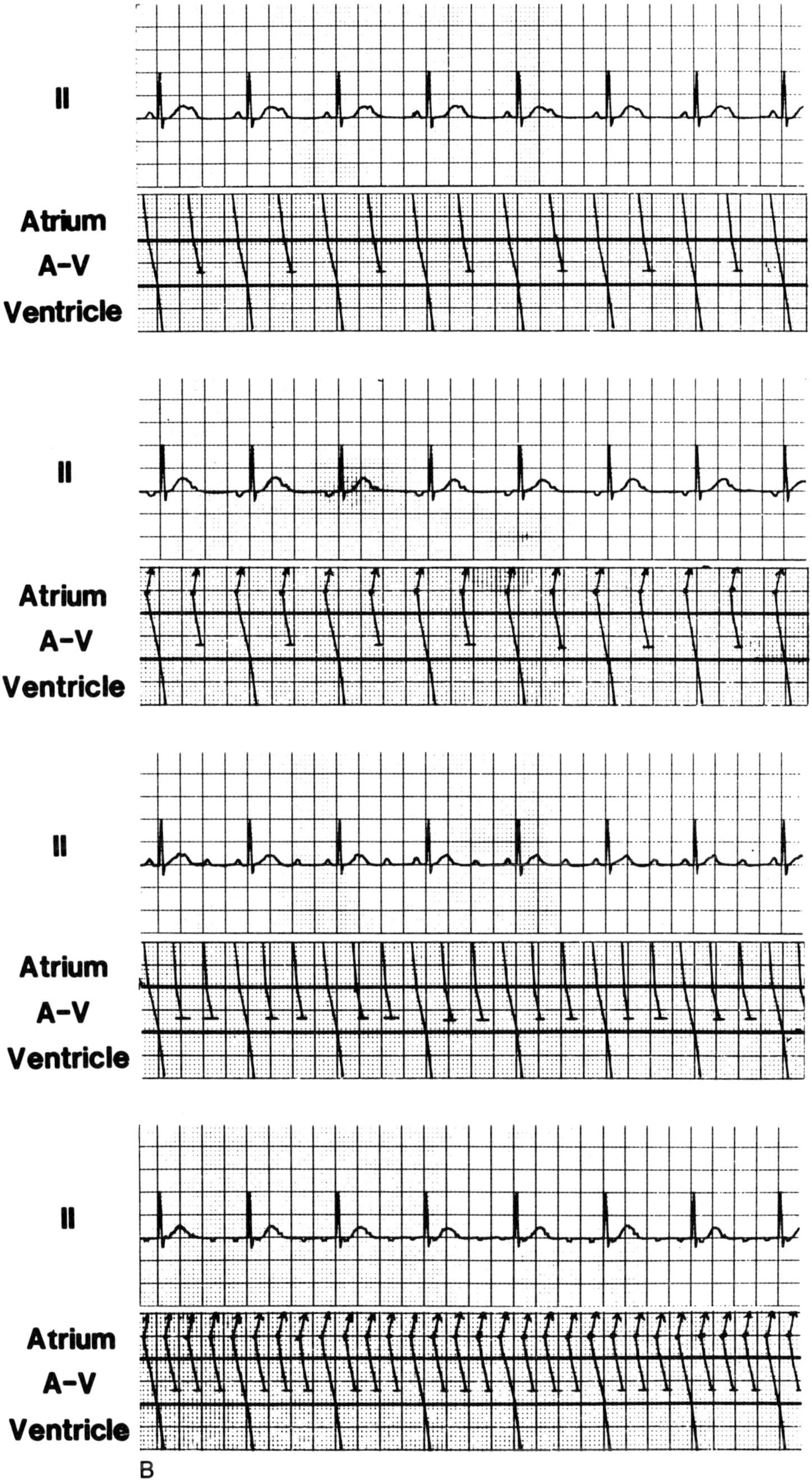
II
Atrium
A-V
Ventricle
II
Atrium
A-V
Ventricle
II
Atrium
A-V
Ventricle
II
Atrium
A-V
Ventricle
B

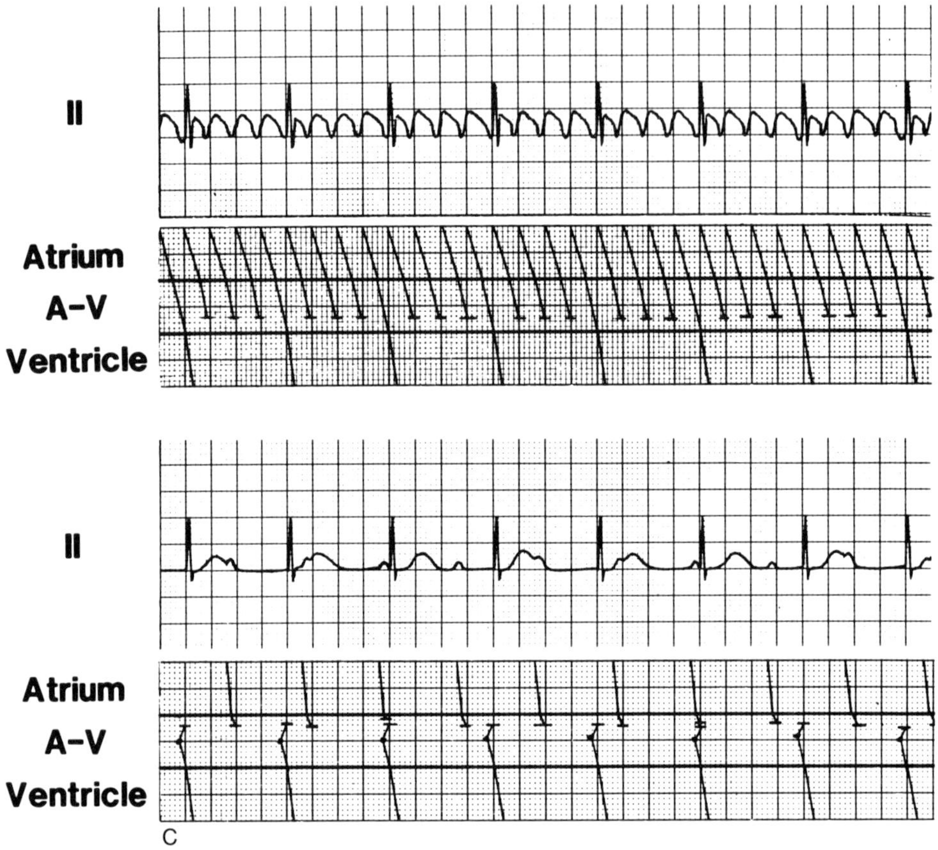

FIGURE 4–29C *(continued)*

---

3. RR INTERVAL – REGULAR
QRS RATE – NORMAL
QRS DURATION – NORMAL

Top tracing: Atrial flutter with fixed type II second degree AV block (4:1). Ventricular rate = 75/min; atrial rate = 300/min.

Bottom tracing: Complete AV block with AV dissociation and accelerated junctional rhythm. Ventricular rate = 75/min; atrial rate = 100/min.

4. RR INTERVAL – REGULAR
QRS RATE – NORMAL
QRS DURATION – PROLONGED

(See Figures 4–30A, 4–30B, and 4–30C)

a. Sinus Rhythm With Aberration
P wave precedes each QRS complex with normal P wave mean vector.

b. Ectopic Atrial Rhythm With Aberration
P wave precedes each QRS complex with abnormal P wave mean vector.

c. Accelerated Junctional Rhythm With Aberration or Ventricular Tachycardia
1. Sinus P rate less than QRS rate with AV dissociation; or
2. No P wave visible; or
3. Retrograde P wave follows some or all QRS complexes.

d. Supraventricular Rhythm With Aberration and Fixed Type II Second Degree AV Block
P rate a multiple of QRS rate with fixed relationship of P waves to QRS complexes (see 1*d*).

FIGURE 4–30A

4. RR INTERVAL – REGULAR QRS RATE – NORMAL QRS DURATION – PROLONGED

Top tracing: Sinus rhythm with complete right bundle branch block. Ventricular rate = 85/min; atrial rate = 85/min.

Second tracing: Ectopic atrial rhythm with complete right bundle branch block. Ventricular rate = 85/min; atrial rate = 85/min.

Third tracing: Accelerated junctional rhythm with complete right bundle branch block or ventricular tachycardia with AV dissociation (it is impossible to distinguish between these on a surface electrocardiogram). Ventricular rate = 85/min; atrial rate = 80/min. Conduction does not occur from ventricles to atria.

Bottom tracing: Accelerated junctional rhythm with complete right bundle branch block or ventricular tachycardia. Ventricular rate = 85/min; atrial rate = 85/min. Retrograde conduction is intact, with inverted P waves following each QRS complex.

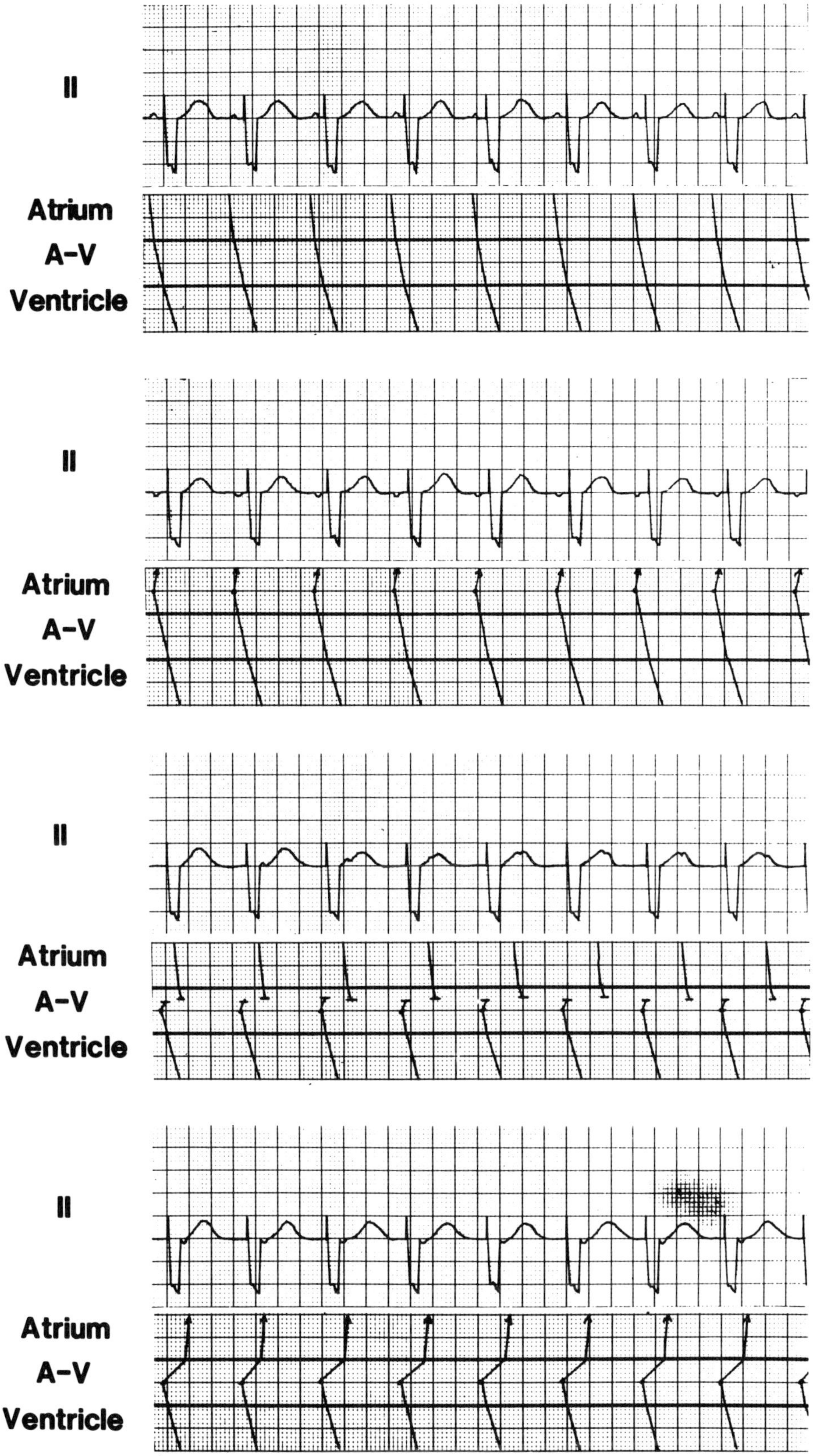
II
Atrium
A-V
Ventricle
II
Atrium
A-V
Ventricle
II
Atrium
A-V
Ventricle
II
Atrium
A-V
Ventricle

A

FIGURE 4–30B ***(continued)***

4. RR INTERVAL – REGULAR
QRS RATE – NORMAL
QRS DURATION – PROLONGED

Top tracing: Sinus rhythm with second degree AV block (2:1) and complete right bundle branch block. Ventricular rate = 75/min; atrial rate = 150/min. Every other P wave is followed by a QRS complex; when AV block is 2:1, it is not possible to determine if this is type I or type II second degree AV block.

Second tracing: Atrial rhythm with second degree AV block (2:1) and complete right bundle branch block. Ventricular rate = 75/min; atrial rate = 150/min.

Third tracing: Sinus tachycardia with fixed type II second degree AV block (3:1) and complete right bundle branch block. Ventricular rate = 75/min; atrial rate = 225/min.

Bottom tracing: Supraventricular tachycardia with fixed type II second degree AV block (4:1) and complete right bundle branch block. Ventricular rate = 75/min; atrial rate = 300/min.

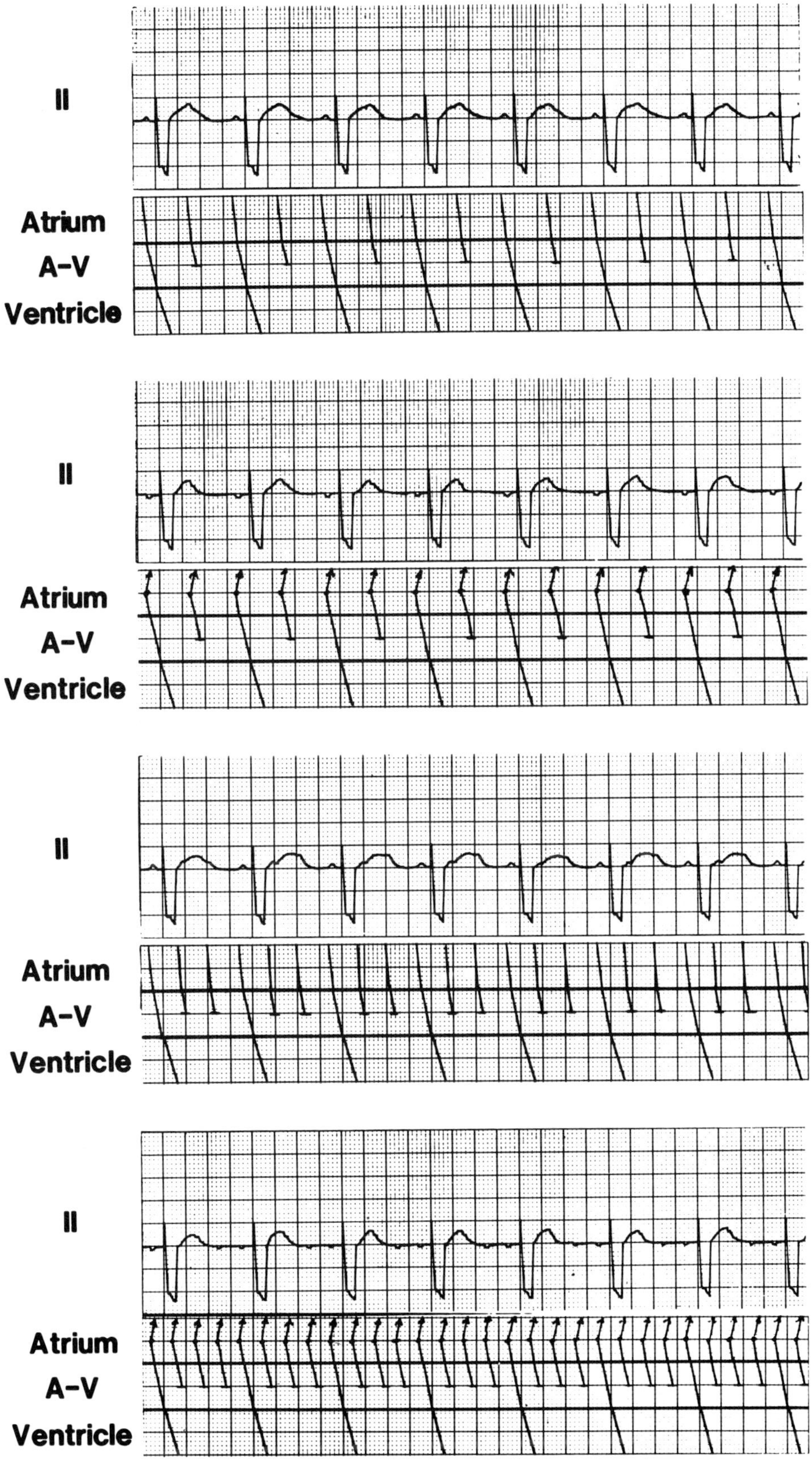
II
Atrium
A-V
Ventricle
II
Atrium
A-V
Ventricle
II
Atrium
A-V
Ventricle
II
Atrium
A-V
Ventricle

B

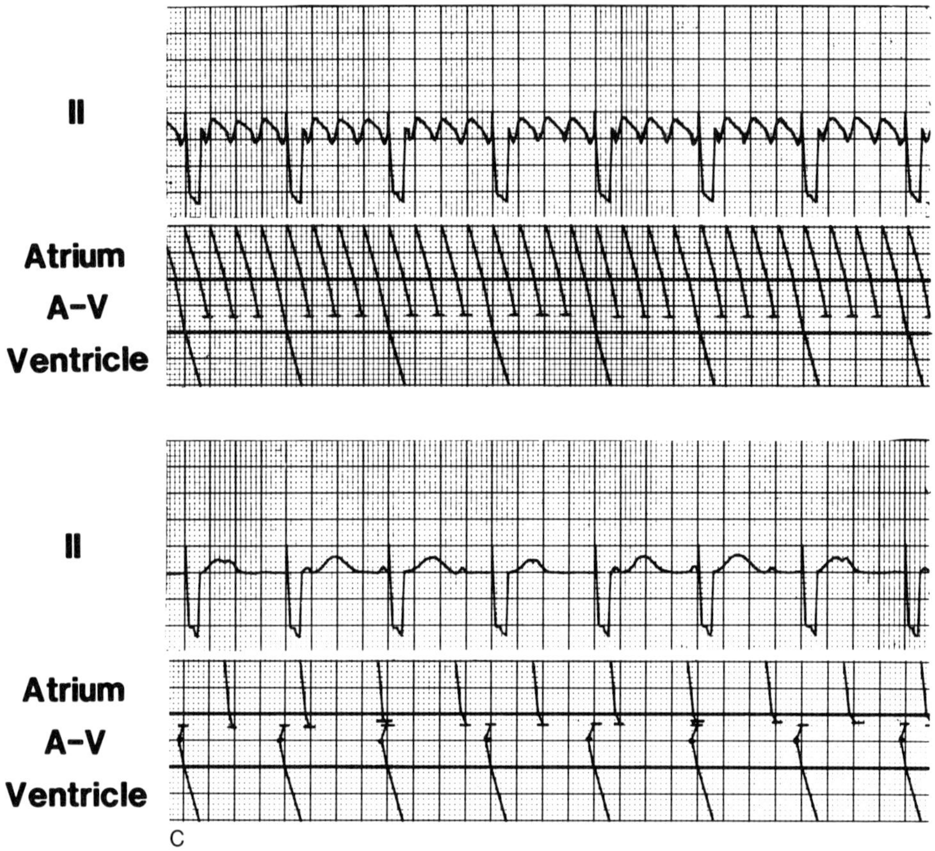

FIGURE 4–30C *(continued)*

4. RR INTERVAL – REGULAR
QRS RATE – NORMAL
QRS DURATION – PROLONGED

Top tracing: Atrial flutter with fixed type II second degree AV block (4:1) and complete right bundle branch block. Ventricular rate = 75/min; atrial rate = 300/min.

Bottom tracing: Complete AV block with AV dissociation and accelerated junctional rhythm with complete right bundle branch block or ventricular tachycardia. Ventricular rate = 75/min; atrial rate = 100/min.

5. RR INTERVAL – REGULAR
QRS RATE – INCREASED
QRS DURATION – NORMAL

(See Figures 4–31A, 4–31B, and 4–31C)

a. Sinus Tachycardia (1:1 Conduction)
P wave precedes each QRS complex with normal P wave mean vector and P rate ≤230/min.

b. Ectopic Atrial Tachycardia (1:1 Conduction)
P wave precedes each QRS complex with abnormal P wave mean vector.

c. Supraventricular Tachycardia (1:1 Conduction)
1. P wave visible between some or all QRS complexes with constant PR interval; or
2. No P wave visible; or
3. Sinus P rate less than QRS rate with AV dissociation.

d. Supraventricular Tachycardia With Fixed Type II Second Degree AV Block
P rate a multiple of QRS rate with fixed relationship of P waves to QRS complexes.

e. Atrial Flutter With Fixed Type II Second Degree AV Block
P waves have flutter morphology with fixed relationship of flutter waves to QRS complexes.

FIGURE 4–31A

5. RR INTERVAL – REGULAR QRS RATE – INCREASED QRS DURATION – NORMAL

Top tracing: Sinus tachycardia. Ventricular rate = 160/min; atrial rate = 160/min; P axis 0° to 90°; PR interval 0.12 s.

Second tracing: Ectopic atrial tachycardia. (This is a type of SVT. In SVT, P waves may be present or absent, and the PR interval may be normal or prolonged. In this and the next five tracings, some of the various morphologies of SVT are presented.) Ventricular rate = 160/min; atrial rate = 160/min; P axis = 270° to 359°; PR interval 0.12 s.

Third tracing: Supraventricular tachycardia. Ventricular rate = 160/min; atrial rate = 160/min; P axis = 270° to 359°; PR interval 0.20 s.

Bottom tracing: Supraventricular tachycardia. Ventricular rate = 160/min; no P waves are visible.

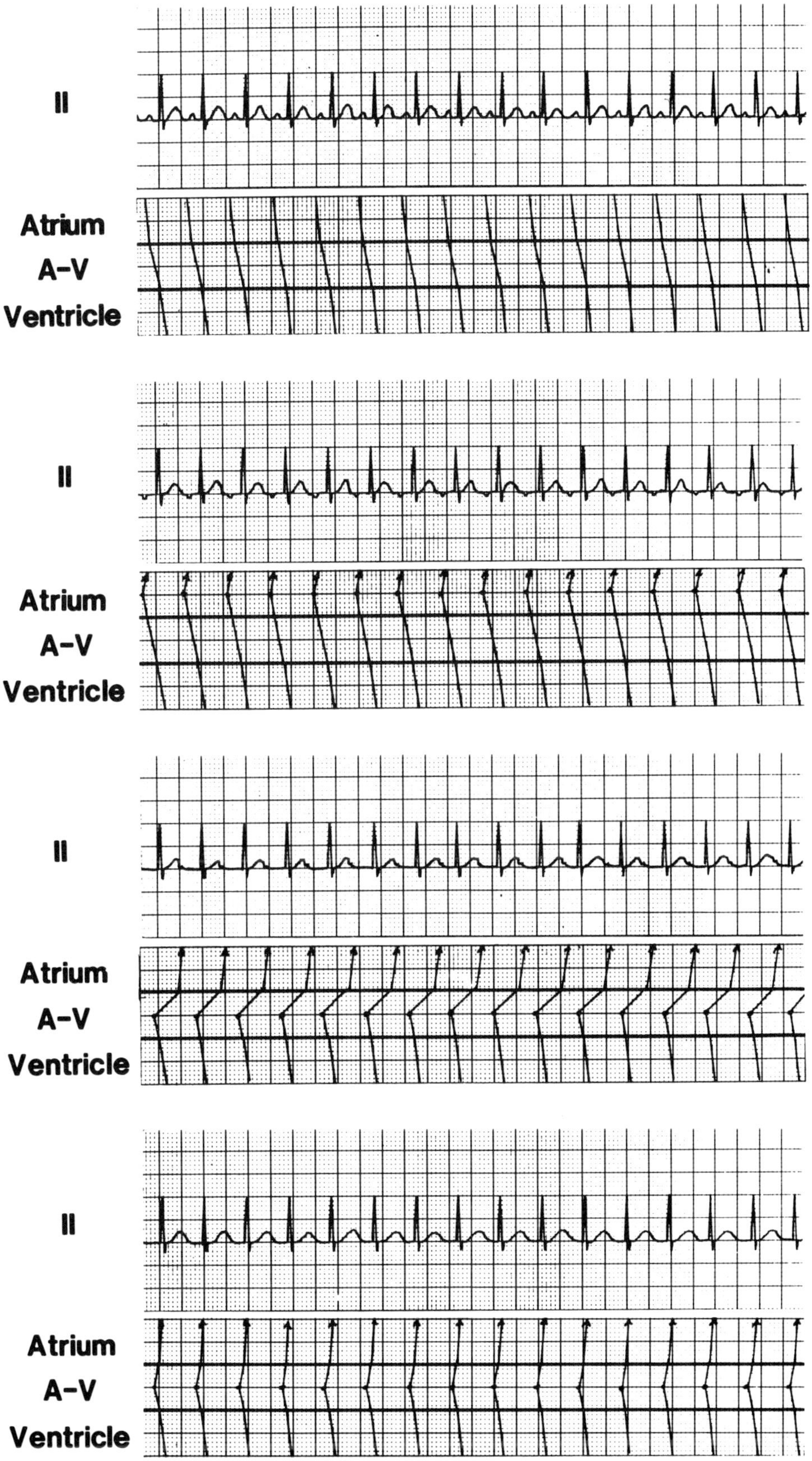
II
Atrium
A–V
Ventricle
II
Atrium
A–V
Ventricle
II
Atrium
A–V
Ventricle
II
Atrium
A–V
Ventricle

A

FIGURE 4–31B *(continued)*

5. RR INTERVAL – REGULAR QRS RATE – INCREASED QRS DURATION – NORMAL

Top tracing: Supraventricular tachycardia with AV dissociation. Ventricular rate = 160/min; atrial rate = 100/min; P mean vector, 0° to +90°; PR interval variable. The P waves are from the sinus node depolarizing the atria, and the QRS complexes are from the AV junction depolarizing the ventricles.

Middle tracing: Supraventricular tachycardia with second degree AV block (2:1). Ventricular rate = 160/min; atrial rate = 320/min; P mean vector, −1° to −90°. There are two PR intervals: 0.12 s and 0.33 s. From the surface electrocardiogram it is not possible to determine which P wave causes the QRS.

Bottom tracing: Supraventricular tachycardia. This is the same example shown in the middle tracing, but with 1:1 conduction. Ventricular rate = 320/min; atrial rate = 320/min; P mean vector, −1° to −90°; PR interval, 0.14 s. Inverted P waves immediately follow each QRS.

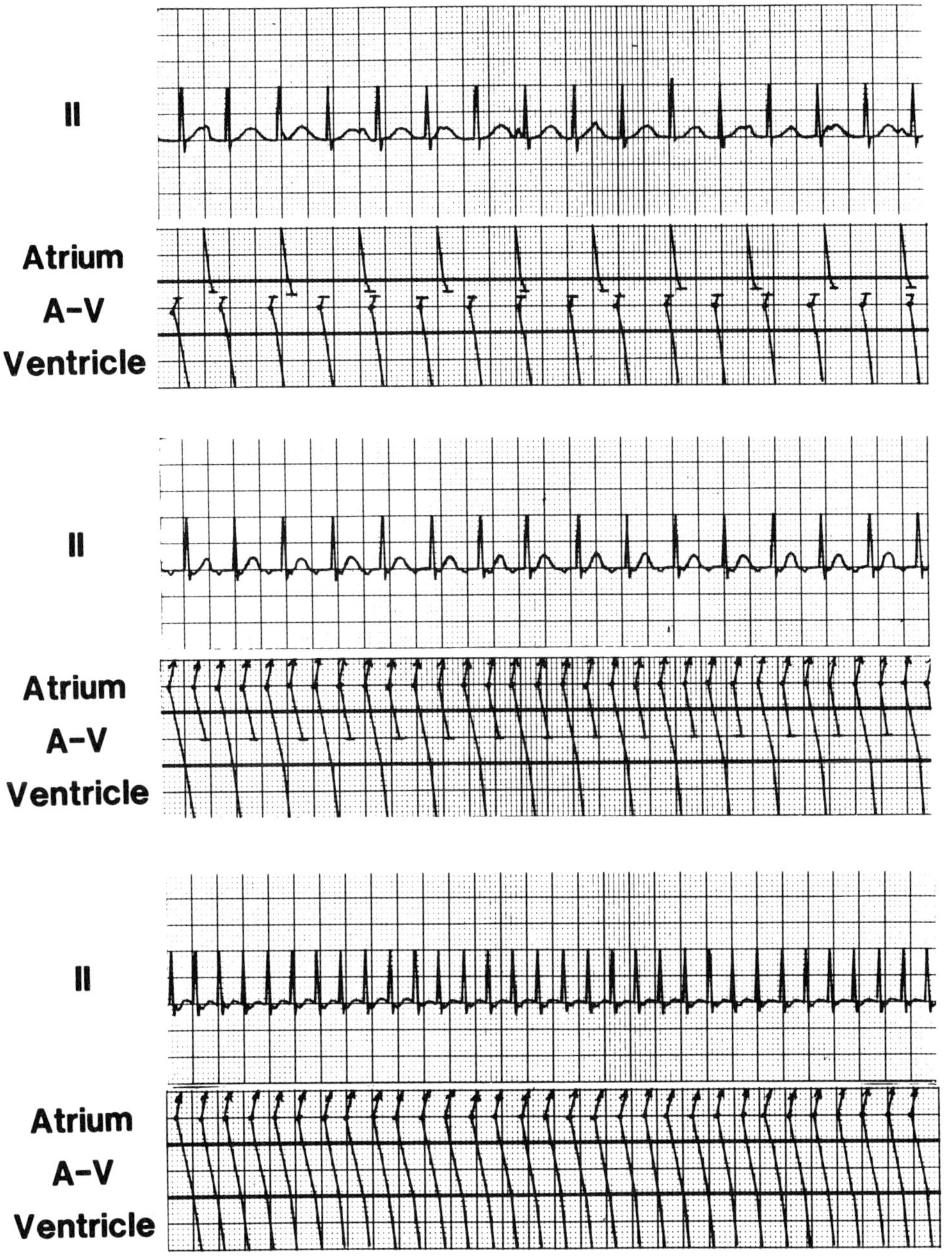
II
Atrium
A-V
Ventricle
II
Atrium
A-V
Ventricle
II
Atrium
A-V
Ventricle

B

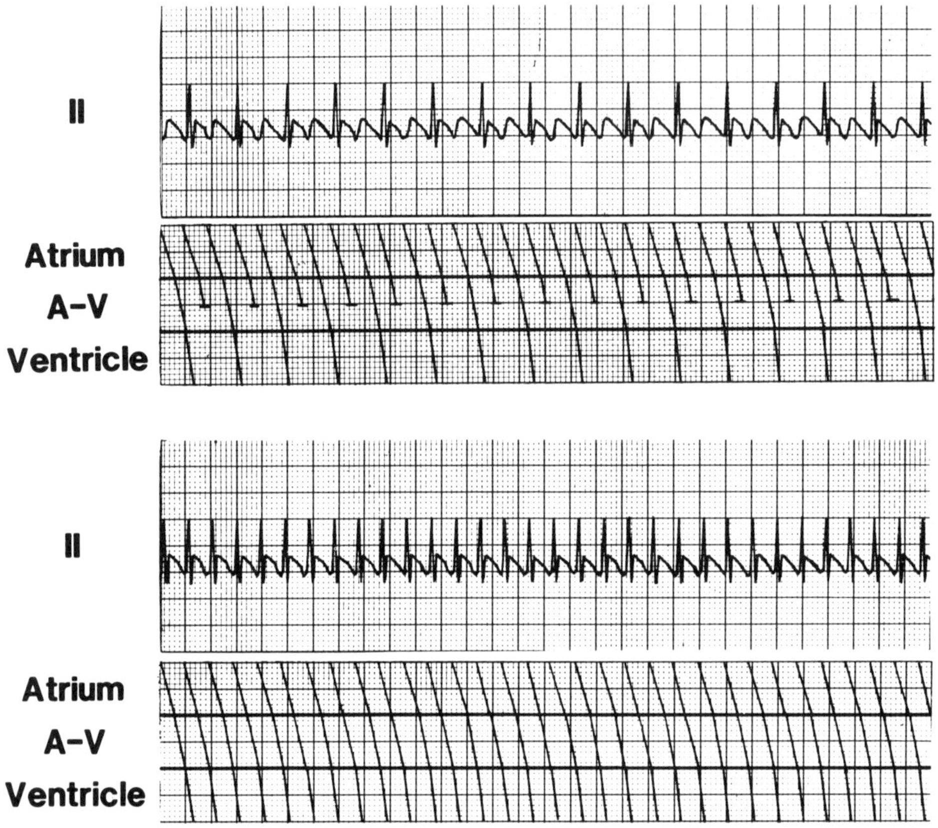

C

FIGURE 4–31C *(continued)*

5. RR INTERVAL – REGULAR
QRS RATE – INCREASED
QRS DURATION – NORMAL

Top tracing: Atrial flutter with second degree AV block (2:1). Ventricular rate = 160/min; atrial rate = 320/min.

Bottom tracing: Atrial flutter. This is the same example shown in the top tracing, but with 1:1 conduction. Ventricular rate = 320/min; atrial rate = 320/min.

6. RR INTERVAL – REGULAR
QRS RATE – INCREASED
QRS DURATION – PROLONGED

(See Figures 4–32A, 4–32B, 4–32C, and 4–32D)

a. Sinus Tachycardia (1:1 Conduction) With Aberration
P wave precedes each QRS complex with normal P wave mean vector.

b. Ectopic Atrial Tachycardia (1:1 Conduction) With Aberration
P wave precedes each QRS complex with abnormal P wave mean vector.

c. Supraventricular Tachycardia (1:1 Conduction) With Aberration or Ventricular Tachycardia

1. P wave visible between some or all QRS complexes with constant PR interval; or

2. No P wave visible; or

3. Sinus P rate less than QRS rate with AV dissociation.

d. Supraventricular Tachycardia With Aberration and Fixed Type II Second Degree AV Block
P rate a multiple of QRS rate with fixed relationship of P waves to QRS complexes.

e. Atrial Flutter With Aberration and Fixed Type II Second Degree AV Block
P waves have flutter morphology with fixed relationship of flutter waves to QRS complexes.

FIGURE 4–32A

6. RR INTERVAL – REGULAR QRS RATE – INCREASED QRS DURATION – PROLONGED

Top tracing: Sinus tachycardia with complete right bundle branch block. Ventricular rate = 160/min; atrial rate = 160/min; P mean vector, 0° to +90°; PR interval, 0.12 s.

Second tracing: Sinus tachycardia with complete right bundle branch block. This tracing is the same as the top tracing, except that the T waves have greater amplitude, and the P waves are on the downslope of the T waves. Ventricular rate = 160/min; atrial rate = 160/min; P mean vector, 0° to +90°; PR interval, 0.12 s. This is unlikely to be ventricular tachycardia, because the P waves are related to the QRS complexes, and the P wave mean vector is normal.

Third tracing: Ectopic atrial tachycardia with complete right bundle branch block or ventricular tachycardia with 1:1 retrograde conduction to the atria; a ladder diagram of each is shown below the fourth tracing. Ventricular rate = 160/min; atrial rate = 160/min; P mean vector, −1° to −90°; PR interval, 0.12 s. The P waves could either originate in the low atrium (from ectopic supraventricular tachycardia) and conduct to the ventricles or could be conducted retrogradely from ventricular tachycardia. It is impossible to distinguish between the two on a surface electrocardiogram. However, in children, supraventricular tachycardia with aberration is much less common than ventricular tachycardia.

Bottom tracing: Ectopic atrial tachycardia with complete right bundle branch block or ventricular tachycardia; a ladder diagram of each is shown below the fourth tracing. This tracing is the same as the third tracing, except that the T waves have greater amplitude, and the P waves are on the downslope of the T waves. Ventricular rate = 160/min; atrial rate = 160/min; P mean vector, −1° to −90°; PR interval, 0.12 s.

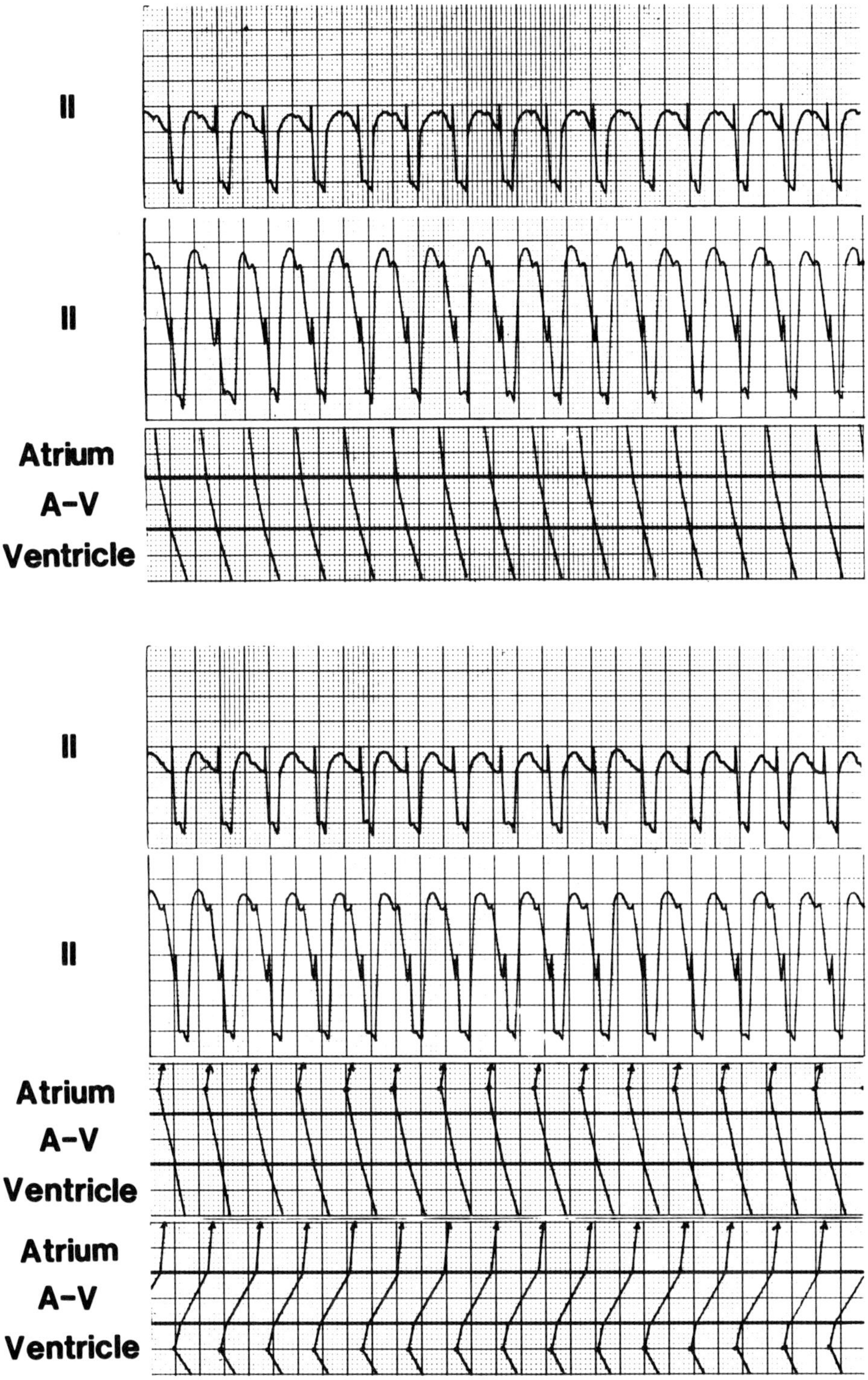
II
II
Atrium
A-V
Ventricle
II
II
Atrium
A-V
Ventricle
Atrium
A-V
Ventricle

A

FIGURE 4–32B *(continued)*

6. RR INTERVAL – REGULAR QRS RATE – INCREASED QRS DURATION – PROLONGED

Top tracing: Supraventricular tachycardia with complete right bundle branch block or ventricular tachycardia; a ladder diagram of each is shown below the top tracing. Ventricular rate = 160/min; atrial rate = 160/min; P mean vector, −1 to −90°; PR interval, 0.24 s. Inverted P waves are visible on the upstroke of the T waves.

Second tracing: Supraventricular tachycardia with complete right bundle branch block or ventricular tachycardia. Ventricular rate = 160/min. P waves are not visible consistently; no ladder diagram is shown because atrial activity cannot be discerned.

Bottom tracing: Supraventricular tachycardia with complete right bundle branch block or ventricular tachycardia; a ladder diagram of each is shown below the bottom tracing. There is complete AV dissociation. Ventricular rate = 160/min; atrial rate = 100/min; P mean vector, 0° to +90° (sinus P waves); PR interval, variable.

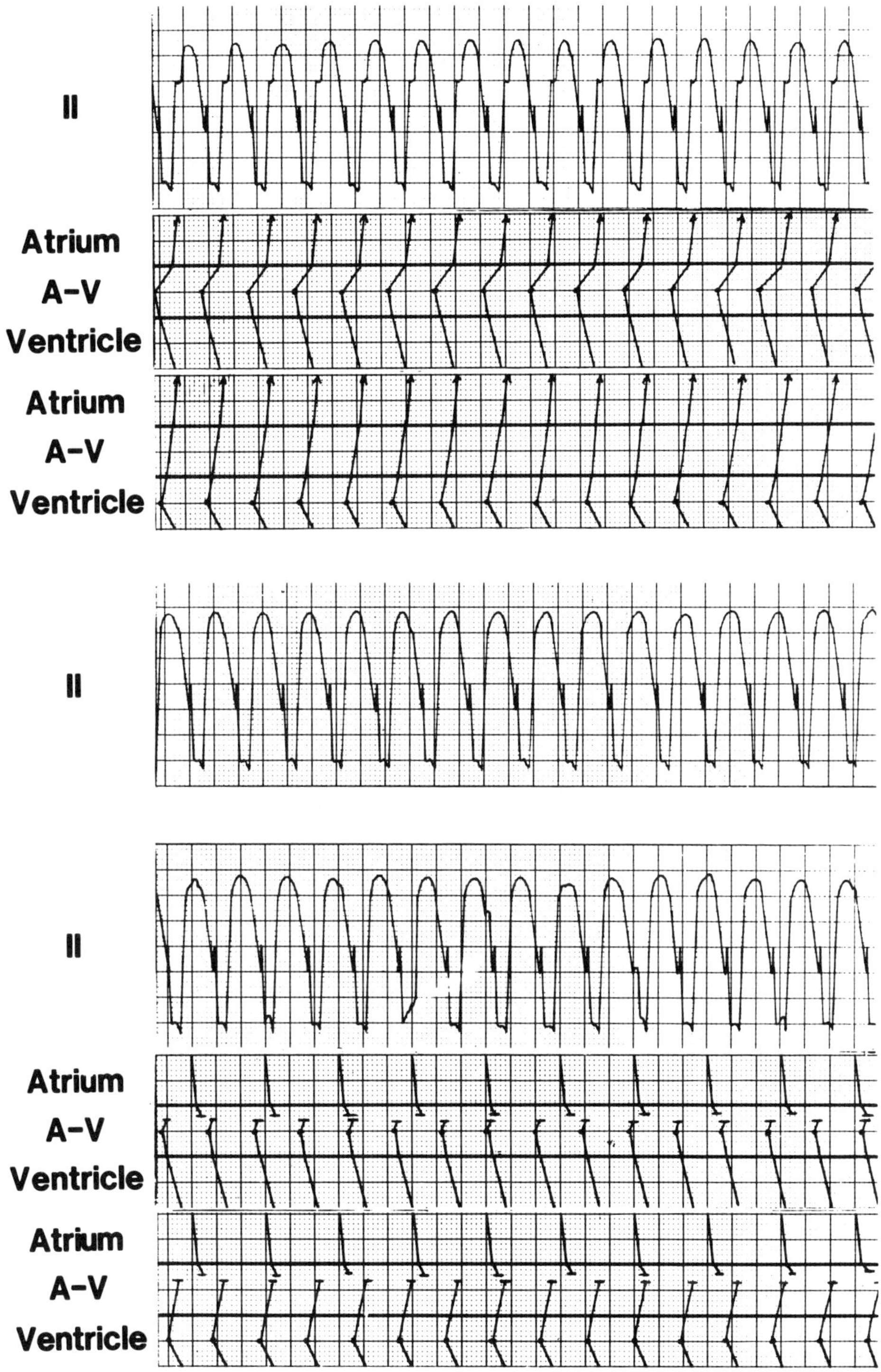
II
Atrium
A-V
Ventricle
Atrium
A-V
Ventricle
II
II
Atrium
A-V
Ventricle
Atrium
A-V
Ventricle

B

FIGURE 4–32C ***(continued)***

6. RR INTERVAL – REGULAR QRS RATE – INCREASED QRS DURATION – PROLONGED

Top tracing: Supraventricular tachycardia with complete right bundle branch block and second degree AV block (2:1). Ventricular rate = 160/min; atrial rate = 320/min; P mean vector, −1° to −90°. There are two PR intervals: 0.12 s and 0.32 s (the P wave with the PR interval of 0.32 s is concealed in the S wave of the bundle branch block pattern; compare Fig. 4–31B). Ventricular tachycardia would be an unlikely diagnosis, because the P waves and QRS complexes are related, with two P waves for each QRS complex.

Bottom tracing: Supraventricular tachycardia with complete right bundle branch block or ventricular tachycardia; a ladder diagram of each is shown. This is the same example as the top tracing, except with 1:1 conduction. Ventricular rate = 320/min; atrial rate = 320/min; P mean vector, −1° to −90°; PR interval, 0.32 s. It is impossible to distinguish between the two on a surface electrocardiogram, except that this is an uncommonly high rate for ventricular tachycardia.

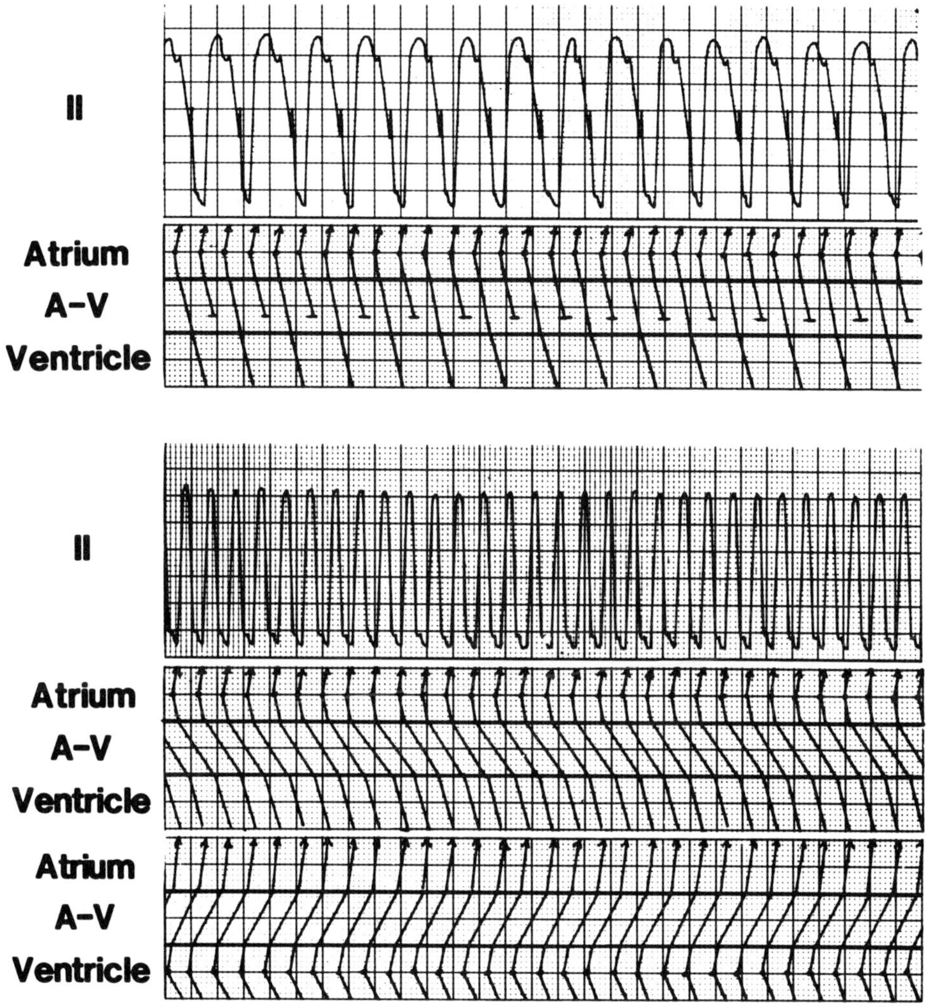
II
Atrium
A–V
Ventricle
II
Atrium
A–V
Ventricle
Atrium
A–V
Ventricle

C

FIGURE 4–32D *(continued)*

6. RR INTERVAL – REGULAR QRS RATE – INCREASED QRS DURATION – PROLONGED

Top tracing: Atrial flutter with second degree AV block (2:1) and complete right bundle branch block. Ventricular rate = 160/min; atrial rate = 320/min; P mean vector, −1° to −90°. The sawtooth baseline is partially concealed. This could be mistaken for supraventricular tachycardia with complete right bundle branch block or for ventricular tachycardia.

Middle tracing: Atrial flutter with second degree AV block (2:1) and complete right bundle branch block. This is the same example as the top tracing, except that the T waves have greater amplitude. Ventricular rate = 160/min; atrial rate = 320/min. The sawtooth baseline is concealed. This could be mistaken for supraventricular tachycardia with complete right bundle branch block or ventricular tachycardia. An esophageal lead showing two atrial depolarizations for each QRS complex would help with the diagnosis.

Bottom tracing: Atrial flutter with complete right bundle branch block or ventricular tachycardia. This is the same example as the top and middle tracings, except with 1:1 conduction. Ventricular rate = 320/min; atrial rate = 320/min. The sawtooth appearance is apparent between QRS complexes, but this could be mistaken for ventricular tachycardia. This is a very common rate for atrial flutter, and an uncommon rate for ventricular tachycardia.

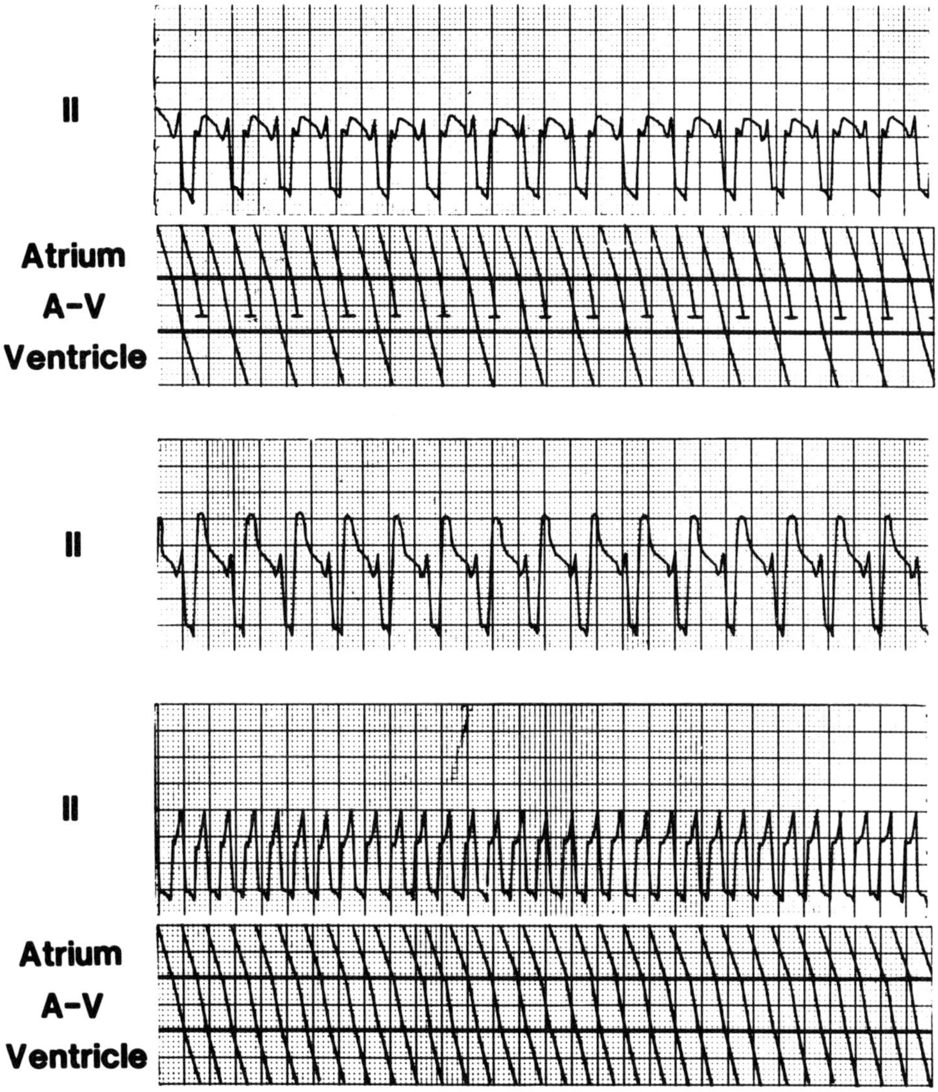

D

7. RR INTERVAL – IRREGULAR
RR INTERVAL – VARIES CONTINUOUSLY
PP INTERVAL – IRREGULAR
QRS DURATION – NORMAL

(See Figure 4–33)

a. Sinus Arrhythmia

1. P wave mean vector may vary between 0° and +90°.
2. P wave precedes each QRS complex with variation in PR interval ≤0.02 s.
3. RR interval prolongs and shortens cyclically with respiration. (Sinus, atrial, and junctional pacemakers are all under vagal influence, and so the rate of rhythms originating from all these sites can vary cyclically. Therefore, sinus, atrial, and junctional rhythm can all have "sinus arrhythmias.")

b. Wandering Pacemaker

1. P wave mean vector continually changes—sinus, atrial, junctional.
2. QRS complexes related to all P waves—P wave either precedes QRS (sinus, atrial origin of P wave) or follows QRS (junctional origin of P wave); P waves may not be visible following junctional beats.

c. Atrial Fibrillation

1. Atrial depolarizations have fibrillation morphology.
2. "Irregularly irregular"—RR intervals are all usually different.

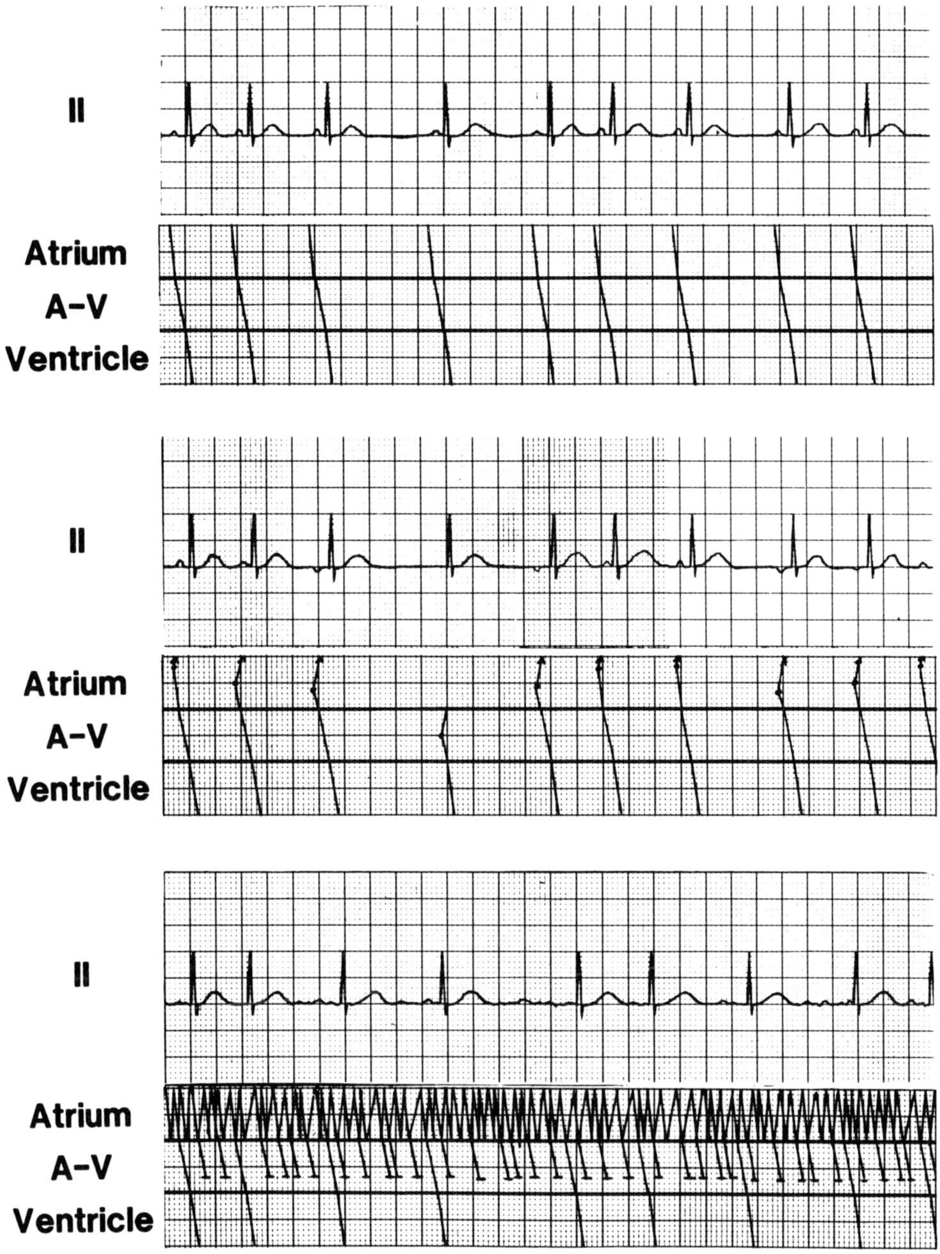

FIGURE 4–33

7. RR INTERVAL – IRREGULAR
RR INTERVAL – VARIES CONTINUOUSLY
PP INTERVAL – IRREGULAR
QRS DURATION – NORMAL

Top tracing: Sinus arrhythmia. Ventricular rate: variable (RR interval = 0.48–0.92 s). Atrial rate: variable (PP interval = 0.50–0.88 s). P mean vector: slight variation (+45° to +90°). PR interval: slight variation (0.10–0.12 s). Inspiration began at the left side of the tracing and the patient breathed approximately every 3 s (20/min).

Middle tracing: Wandering pacemaker. Ventricular rate: variable (RR interval = 0.48–0.92 s). Atrial rate: variable (PP interval = 0.45–1.72 s). P mean vector: variable, when P wave present. PR interval: slight variation, when P wave present (0.10–0.12 s).

Bottom tracing: Atrial fibrillation. Ventricular rate: variable (RR interval = 0.44–1.06 s). No two RR intervals are the same. Atrial rate: fibrillation.

8. RR INTERVAL – IRREGULAR
RR INTERVAL – VARIES CONTINUOUSLY
PP INTERVAL – IRREGULAR
QRS DURATION – PROLONGED

(See Figure 4–34)

a. Sinus Arrhythmia With Aberration

1. P wave mean vector may vary between 0° and +90°.
2. P wave precedes each QRS complex with variation in PR interval <0.02 s.
3. RR interval prolongs and shortens cyclically with respiration. (Sinus, atrial, and junctional pacemakers are all under vagal influence, and so the rate of rhythms originating from all these sites can vary cyclically. Therefore, sinus, atrial, and junctional rhythm can all have "sinus arrhythmias.")

b. Wandering Pacemaker With Aberration

1. P wave mean vector continually changes—sinus, atrial, junctional.
2. QRS complexes related to all P waves—P wave either precedes QRS (sinus, atrial origin of P wave) or follows QRS (junctional origin of P wave).

c. Atrial Fibrillation With Aberration

1. Atrial depolarizations have fibrillation morphology.
2. "Irregularly irregular"—RR intervals are all usually different.

FIGURE 4–34

8. RR INTERVAL – IRREGULAR
RR INTERVAL – VARIES CONTINUOUSLY
PP INTERVAL – IRREGULAR
QRS DURATION – PROLONGED

Top tracing: Sinus arrhythmia with complete right bundle branch block. Ventricular rate: variable (RR interval = 0.48–0.92 s). Atrial rate: variable (PP interval = 0.50–0.88 s). P mean vector: slight variation (+45° to +90°). PR interval: slight variation (0.10–0.12 s). Inspiration began at the left side of the tracing and the patient breathed approximately every 3 s (20/min).

Middle tracing: Wandering pacemaker with complete right bundle branch block. Ventricular rate: variable (RR interval = 0.48–0.92 s). Atrial rate: variable (PP interval = 0.45–1.72 s). P mean vector: variable, when P wave present. PR interval: slight variation, when P wave present (0.10–0.12 s).

Bottom tracing: Atrial fibrillation with complete right bundle branch block. Ventricular rate: variable (RR interval = 0.44–1.06 s). No two RR intervals are the same. Atrial rate: fibrillation.

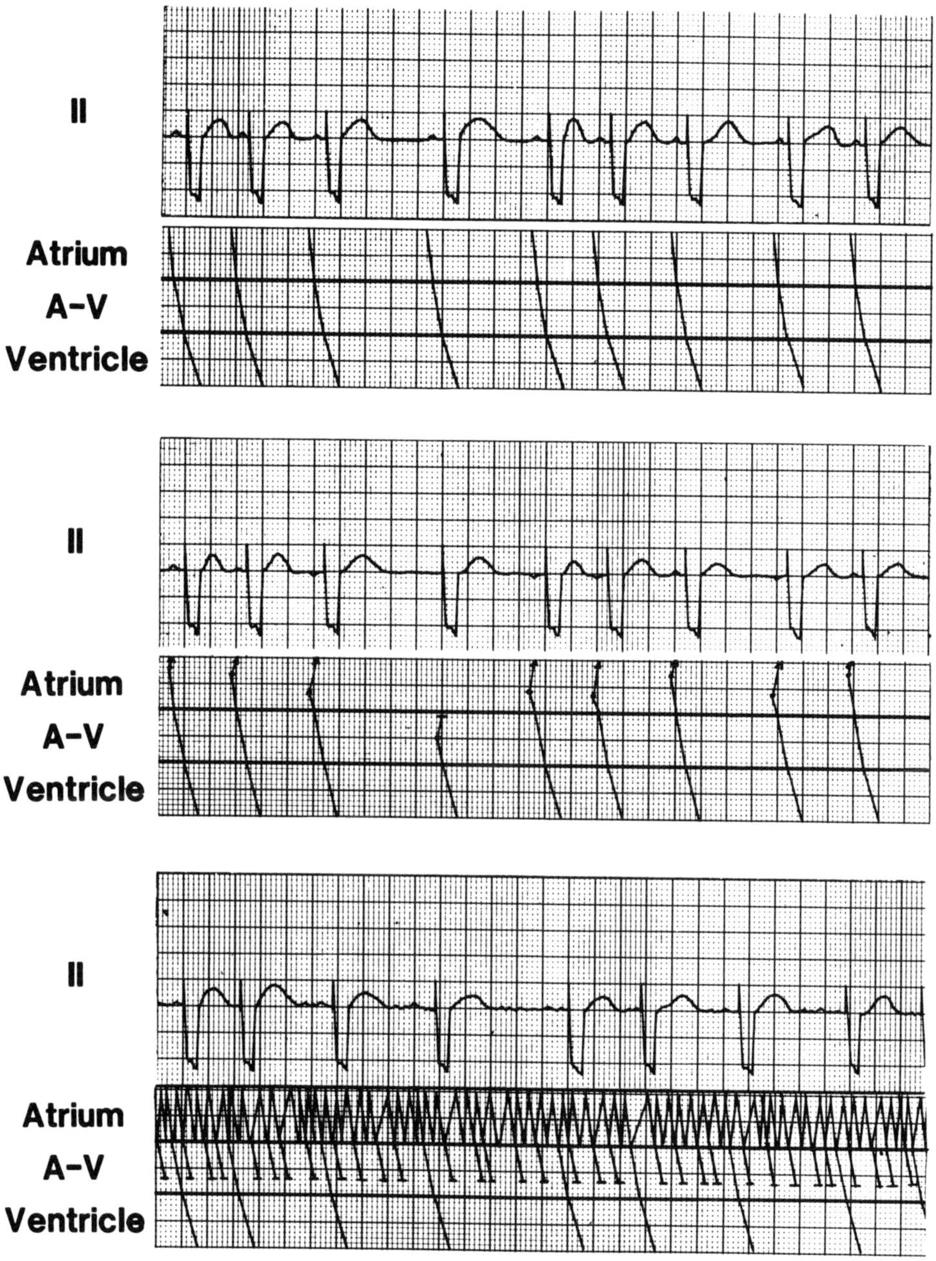
II
Atrium
A-V
Ventricle
II
Atrium
A-V
Ventricle
II
Atrium
A-V
Ventricle

9. RR INTERVAL – IRREGULAR
PP INTERVAL –VARIES CONTINUOUSLY
RR INTERVAL – REGULAR
QRS DURATION – NORMAL

(See Figure 4–35)

a. Supraventricular Rhythm (see 1d) With Varying Type II Second Degree AV Block
1. RR interval varying multiple of PP interval.
2. All R waves preceded by P wave with same PR interval.

b. Supraventricular Rhythm (see 1d) With Type I Second Degree AV Block (Wenckebach)
1. RR interval progressively shortens.
2. PR interval progressively lengthens until single P wave is not followed by QRS complex.

FIGURE 4–35

9. RR INTERVAL – IRREGULAR
RR INTERVAL – VARIES CONTINUOUSLY
PP INTERVAL – REGULAR
QRS DURATION – NORMAL

Top tracing: Sinus tachycardia with varying type II second degree AV block (3:1, 2:1, 1:1 conduction). Ventricular rate: variable (RR interval = 0.28–0.88 s); atrial rate = 214/min; P mean vector, 0° to +90°; PR interval = 0.12 s on conducted beats.

Second tracing: Atrial flutter with varying type II second degree AV block (3:1, 2:1, 1:1 conduction). Ventricular rate: variable (RR interval = 0.20–0.80 s); atrial rate = 300/min.

Third tracing: Sinus tachycardia with type I second degree AV block (5:4 Wenckebach). Ventricular rate: variable. (RR intervals progressively shorten within a group of four QRS complexes; from beginning of tracing—0.48, 0.40, 0.38 s—then the blocked P wave causes a pause of 0.74 s, and then the cycle begins again.) Atrial rate = 167/min; P mean vector, 0° to +90°; PR interval: variable. (PR intervals progressively lengthen within a group of four QRS complexes; from beginning of tracing—0.12, 0.24, 0.28, 0.30 s—then a P wave without a following QRS complex, and the cycle begins again.)

Bottom tracing: Atrial flutter with type I second degree AV block (5:4 Wenckebach). Ventricular rate: variable. (RR intervals progressively shorten within a group of four QRS complexes; from beginning of tracing—0.32, 0.24, 0.22 s. The blocked flutter wave causes a pause of 0.22 s, and the cycle begins again.) Atrial rate = 300/min; flutter-R interval: variable. (Flutter-R intervals progressively lengthen within a group of four QRS complexes; from beginning of tracing—0.12, 0.24, 0.28, 0.30 s—then a flutter wave without a following QRS complex, and the cycle begins again. Flutter waves begin on each dark line every 0.20 s.) *Note:* All supraventricular rhythms can have second degree AV block (see 1d), although only sinus tachycardia and atrial flutter are shown here.

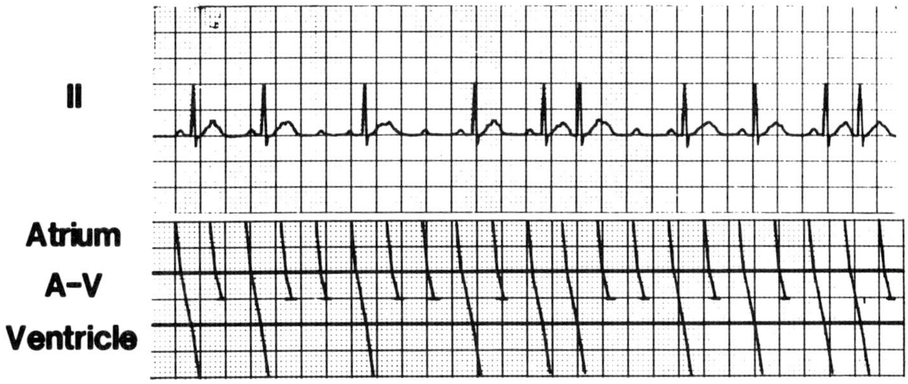
II
Atrium
A-V
Ventricle

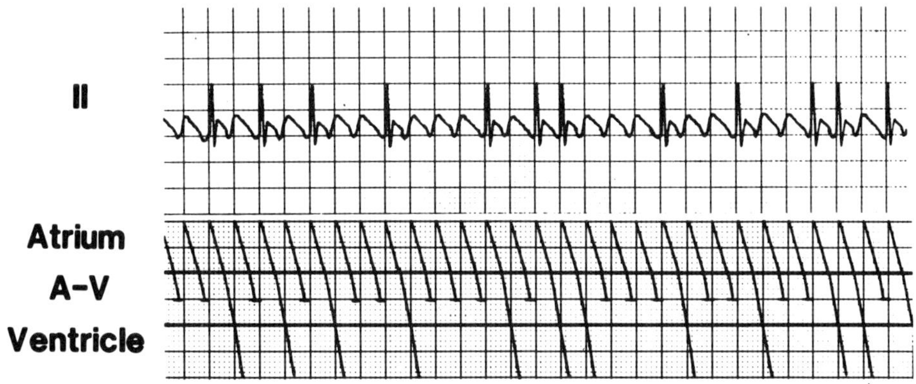
II
Atrium
A-V
Ventricle

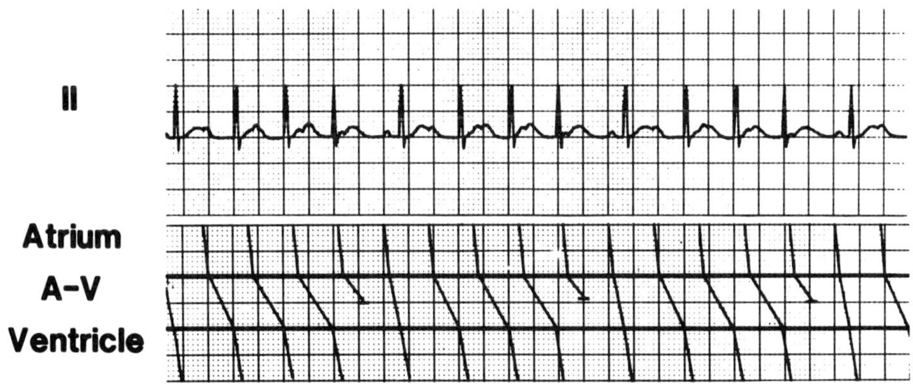
II
Atrium
A-V
Ventricle

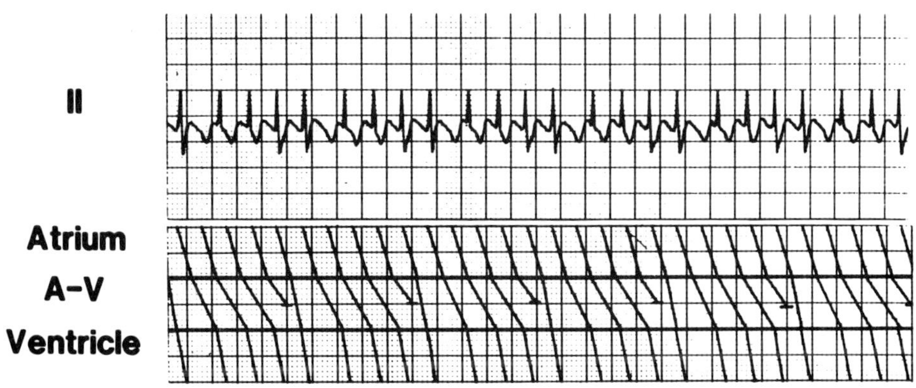
II
Atrium
A-V
Ventricle

10. RR INTERVAL – IRREGULAR
RR INTERVAL – VARIES CONTINUOUSLY
PP INTERVAL – REGULAR
QRS DURATION – PROLONGED

(See Figure 4–36)

a. Supraventricular Rhythm (see 1d) With Aberration and Varying Type II Second Degree AV Block

1. RR interval varying multiple of PP interval.
2. All R waves preceded by P wave with same PR interval.

b. Supraventricular Rhythm (see 1d) With Aberration and Type I Second Degree AV Block (Wenckebach)

1. RR interval progressively shortens.
2. PR interval progressively lengthens until single P wave is not followed by QRS complex.

FIGURE 4–36

10. RR INTERVAL – IRREGULAR
RR INTERVAL – VARIES CONTINUOUSLY
PP INTERVAL – REGULAR
QRS DURATION – PROLONGED

Top tracing: Sinus tachycardia with varying type II second degree AV block (3:1, 2:1, 1:1 conduction) and complete right bundle branch block. Ventricular rate: variable (RR interval = 0.28–0.88 s). Atrial rate = 214/min; P mean vector, 0° to +90°; PR interval = 0.12 s on conducted beats (P waves are on the upstroke of all T waves).

Second tracing: Atrial flutter with varying type II second degree AV block (3:1, 2:1, 1:1 conduction) and complete right bundle branch block. Ventricular rate: variable (RR interval = 0.20–0.80 s); atrial rate = 300/min.

Third tracing: Sinus tachycardia with type I second degree AV block (5:4 Wenckebach) and complete right bundle branch block. Ventricular rate: variable. (RR intervals progressively shorten within a group of four QRS complexes; from beginning of tracing—0.48, 0.40, 0.38 s—then the blocked P wave causes a pause of 0.74 s, and then the cycle begins again.) Atrial rate = 167/min; P mean vector, 0° to +90°; PR interval: variable. (PR intervals progressively lengthen within a group of four QRS complexes; from beginning of tracing—0.12, 0.24, 0.28, 0.30 s—then a P wave without a following QRS complex and the cycle begins again.) The P waves cause the various irregularities in the QRS complexes and T waves.

Bottom tracing: Atrial flutter with type I second degree AV block (5:4 Wenckebach) and complete right bundle branch block. Ventricular rate: variable. (RR intervals progressively shorten within a group of four QRS complexes; from beginning of tracing—0.32, 0.24, 0.22 s. The blocked flutter wave causes a pause of 0.22 s, and the cycle begins again.) Flutter waves are not visible, but the diagnosis may be inferred from the rate and pattern of the QRS complexes. The atrial rate is inferred to be 300/min. *Note:* All supraventricular rhythms can have second degree AV block (see 1d), although only sinus tachycardia and atrial flutter are shown here.

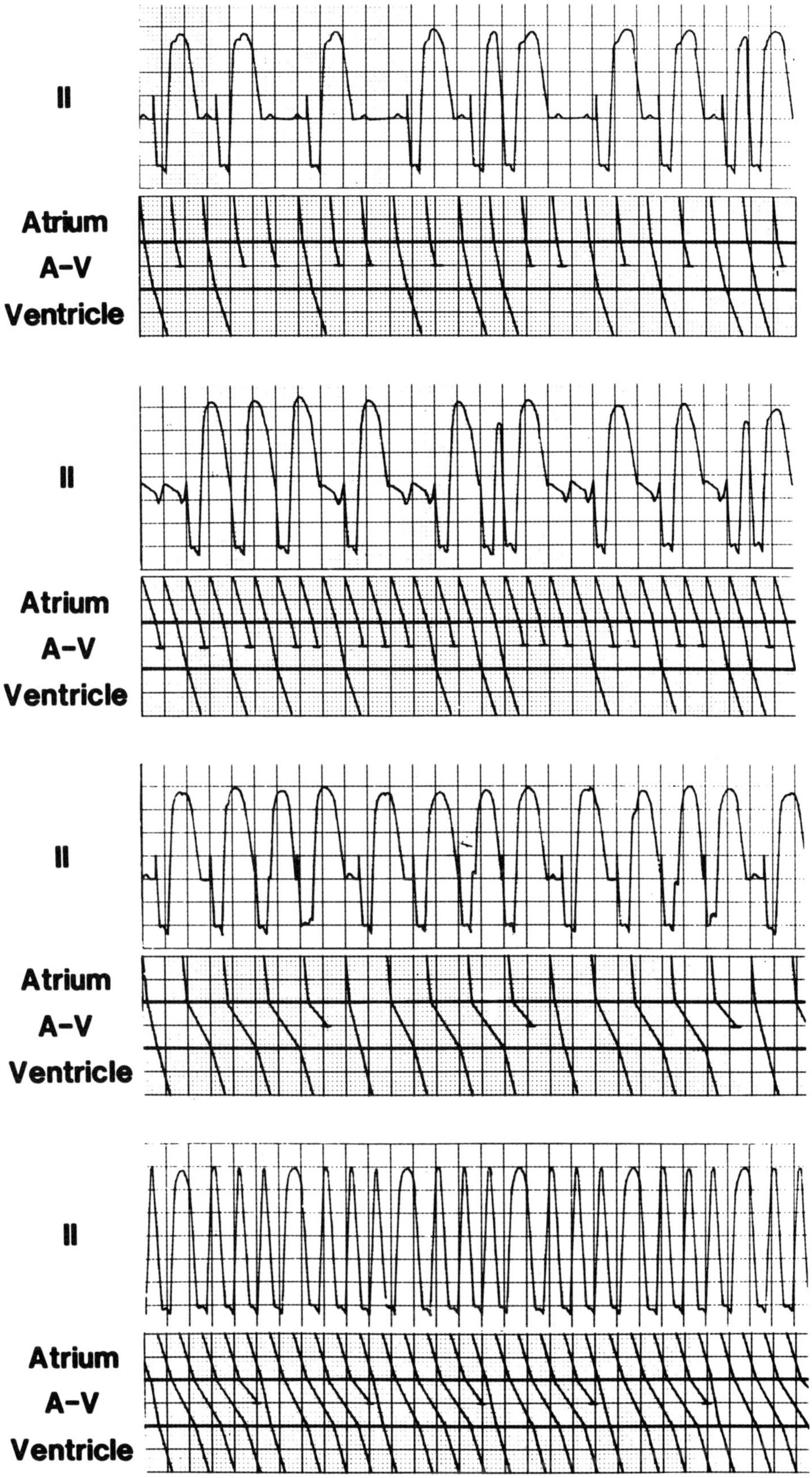
II
Atrium
A–V
Ventricle
II
Atrium
A–V
Ventricle
II
Atrium
A–V
Ventricle
II
Atrium
A–V
Ventricle

11. BASIC RR INTERVAL – REGULAR, BUT INTERRUPTED INTERMITTENTLY IRREGULAR RR INTERVAL – SHORT (PREMATURE QRS) QRS DURATION OF EARLY COMPLEX – NORMAL

(See Figure 4–37)

a. Atrial or Junctional Rhythm (see 1d) With Sinus Capture
Early QRS preceded by P wave with normal P mean vector.

b. Sinus, Atrial, or Junctional Rhythm (see 1d) With Premature Atrial Contraction
Early QRS preceded by P wave with abnormal P mean vector.

c. Sinus, Atrial, or Junctional Rhythm (see 1d) With Premature Junctional Contraction
Early QRS not preceded by P wave.

FIGURE 4–37

11. BASIC RR INTERVAL – REGULAR, BUT INTERRUPTED INTERMITTENTLY IRREGULAR RR INTERVAL – SHORT (PREMATURE QRS) QRS DURATION OF EARLY COMPLEX – NORMAL

Top tracing: Junctional rhythm with intermittent sinus capture beats. Atrial rate = 60/min (PP interval is constant at 1.0 sec). Sinus bradycardia is present also. Basic RR interval regular at 0.80 s—junctional rhythm. There are two short RR intervals (0.60 s) when the third and sixth sinus P waves in the tracing occur at an appropriate time and the AV node is not refractory. Then AV conduction occurs, and the P waves are followed closely by QRS complexes. The RR interval after the fourth QRS is 0.80 s, because the junctional rhythm begins again from the time of the last QRS complex.

Middle tracing: Sinus rhythm with premature atrial contractions. Basic ventricular and atrial rates = 75/min (RR and PP intervals = 0.80 s). The two short RR intervals (0.60 s) occur when a premature P wave (PP interval = 0.60 s) with a different P axis conducts to the ventricles. The PR interval of the premature atrial contraction is 0.18 s, which is longer than the 0.12 s found in sinus rhythm. The PR interval is longer because the AV node is still relatively refractory when the premature atrial contraction occurs. The RR interval after the fourth QRS is 0.80 s (less than compensatory pause) because the premature P wave reset the sinus node.

Bottom tracing: Sinus rhythm with premature junctional contractions. Basic ventricular and atrial rates = 75/min (RR and PP intervals = 0.80 s). The two short RR intervals (0.60 s) are caused by identical premature QRS complexes without a preceding P wave, indicating that these are premature junctional contractions. The RR interval after the fourth QRS is 0.80 s (less than compensatory pause) because the premature QRS caused the atria to be activated prematurely (retrograde P wave) and reset the sinus node.

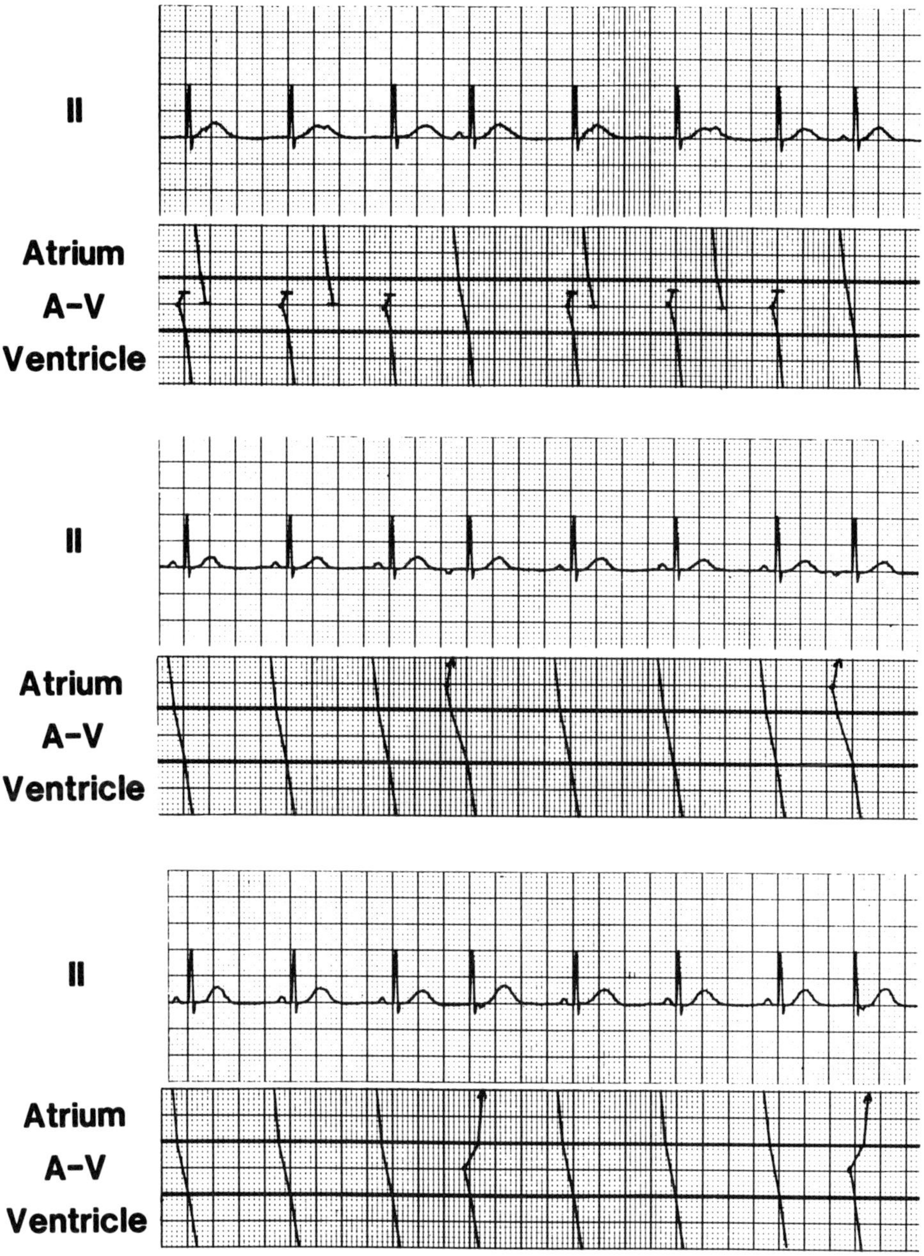
II
Atrium
A-V
Ventricle
II
Atrium
A-V
Ventricle
II
Atrium
A-V
Ventricle

12. BASIC RR INTERVAL – REGULAR, BUT INTERRUPTED INTERMITTENTLY IRREGULAR RR INTERVAL – SHORT (PREMATURE QRS) QRS DURATION OF EARLY COMPLEX – PROLONGED

(See Figure 4–38)

a. *Ectopic Atrial or Junctional Rhythm (see 1d) With Sinus Capture and Aberration*
QRS preceded by P wave with normal P mean vector.

b. *Sinus, Ectopic Atrial, or Junctional Rhythm (see 1d) With Premature Atrial Contraction and Aberration*
QRS preceded by ectopic P wave with abnormal P mean vector.

c. *Sinus, Atrial, or Junctional Rhythm (see 1d) With Premature Ventricular Contraction*
QRS not preceded by P wave.

FIGURE 4–38

12. BASIC RR INTERVAL – REGULAR, BUT INTERRUPTED INTERMITTENTLY IRREGULAR RR INTERVAL – SHORT (PREMATURE QRS) QRS DURATION OF EARLY COMPLEX – PROLONGED

Top tracing: Junctional rhythm with intermittent sinus capture beats with complete right bundle branch block. Atrial rate = 60/min (PP interval is constant at 1.0 s). Sinus bradycardia is present also. Basic RR interval regular at 0.80 s—junctional rhythm. There are two short RR intervals (0.60 s) when the third and sixth sinus P waves in the tracing occur at an appropriate time and the AV node is not refractory. Then AV conduction occurs, and the P waves are followed closely by QRS complexes. The RR interval after the fourth QRS is 0.80 s, because the junctional rhythm begins again from the time of the last QRS complex.

Middle tracing: Sinus rhythm with premature atrial contractions and complete right bundle branch block. Basic ventricular and atrial rates = 75/min (RR and PP intervals = 0.80 s). The two short RR intervals (0.60 s) occur when a premature P wave (PP interval = 0.60 s) with a different P axis conducts to the ventricles. The PR interval of the premature atrial contraction is 0.18 s, which is longer than the 0.12 s found in sinus rhythm. The PR interval is longer because the AV node is still relatively refractory when the premature atrial contraction occurs. The RR interval after the fourth QRS is 0.80 s (less than compensatory pause) because the premature P wave reset the sinus node.

Bottom tracing: Sinus rhythm with premature ventricular contractions. Basic ventricular and atrial rates = 75/min (RR and PP intervals = 0.80 s). The two short RR intervals (0.60 s) are caused by premature QRS complexes with prolonged duration without a preceding P wave, indicating that these are premature ventricular contractions. There are retrograde P waves on the upstroke of the T waves. The RR interval after the fourth QRS is 0.80 s (less than compensatory pause) because the premature QRS caused the atria to be activated prematurely (retrograde P wave) and reset the sinus node.

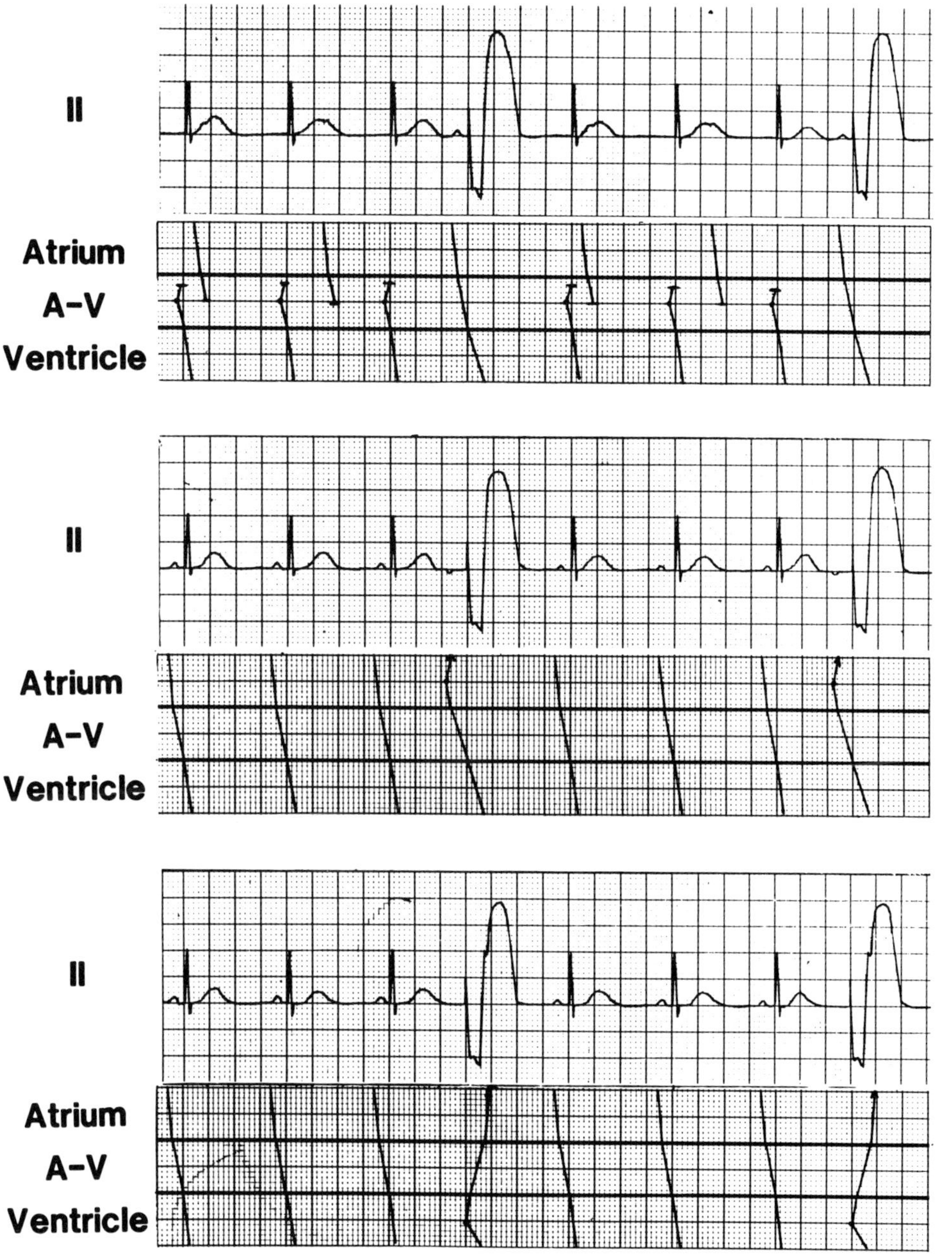
II
Atrium
A-V
Ventricle
II
Atrium
A-V
Ventricle
II
Atrium
A-V
Ventricle

13. BASIC RR INTERVAL – REGULAR, BUT INTERRUPTED INTERMITTENTLY IRREGULAR RR INTERVAL – LONG (DELAYED QRS) QRS DURATION OF DELAYED COMPLEX – NORMAL

(See Figure 4–39)

a. Supraventricular Rhythm (see 1d) With Intermittent Type II Second Degree AV Block
  1. Supraventricular P wave occurs at regular PP interval.
  2. "Delayed" QRS occurs at twice preceding RR interval.
  3. "Delayed" QRS preceded by supraventricular P wave.

b. Supraventricular Rhythm (see 1d) With Nonconducted Premature Atrial Contraction
  1. P wave with different mean vector or morphology than supraventricular P wave occurs prematurely.
  2. "Delayed" QRS complex occurs at less than twice preceding RR interval.
  3. "Delayed" QRS preceded by supraventricular P wave.

c. Pause in Supraventricular Rhythm With Ectopic Atrial Escape
  1. No supraventricular P wave occurs.
  2. "Delayed" QRS occurs at more than regular RR interval.
  3. "Delayed" QRS preceded by P wave with different mean vector or morphology than supraventricular P wave.

d. Pause in Supraventricular Rhythm With Junctional Escape
  1. No supraventricular P wave occurs.
  2. "Delayed" QRS occurs at more than regular RR interval.
  3. "Delayed" QRS not preceded by P wave.

FIGURE 4–39

13. BASIC RR INTERVAL – REGULAR, BUT INTERRUPTED INTERMITTENTLY IRREGULAR RR INTERVAL – LONG (DELAYED QRS) QRS DURATION OF DELAYED COMPLEX – NORMAL

Top tracing: Sinus rhythm with intermittent type II second degree AV block. Basic ventricular and atrial rates = 100/min (RR and PP intervals = 0.60 s). The long RR interval is 1.20 s—exactly twice the basic RR interval—because sinus rhythm continues uninterrupted, despite the blocked P wave.

Second tracing: Sinus rhythm with nonconducted premature atrial contraction. Basic ventricular and atrial rates = 100/min (RR and PP intervals = 0.60 s). The long RR interval is 1.0 s—less than twice the basic RR interval. The QRS complex preceding the pause is followed by a P wave that occurs at a time when the AV node is refractory and is not conducted to the ventricles. This premature atrial contraction resets the sinus node, and sinus rhythm begins again. There is a less than fully compensatory pause following the premature atrial contraction.

Third tracing: Sinus rhythm with sinus pause and low atrial escape beat. Basic ventricular and atrial rates = 100/min (RR and PP interval = 0.60 s). The long RR interval is 0.80 s—longer than the basic RR interval. The QRS complex preceding the delayed QRS is not followed by a sinus P wave ("pause" in sinus rhythm). The pause is ended by an identical QRS complex, which is preceded by a P wave with an axis of $-1°$ to $-90°$, which is a low atrial escape beat.

Bottom tracing: Sinus rhythm with sinus pause and junctional escape beat. Basic ventricular and atrial rates = 100/min (RR and PP intervals = 0.60 s). The long RR interval is 1.0 s—longer than the basic RR interval. The pause is longer with a junctional escape beat than with an atrial escape beat, because basic junctional rhythm (which determines the escape interval) is slower than atrial rhythm. The QRS complex preceding the delayed QRS is not followed by a sinus P wave ("pause" in sinus rhythm). The pause is ended by an identical QRS complex without a preceding P wave—a junctional escape beat.

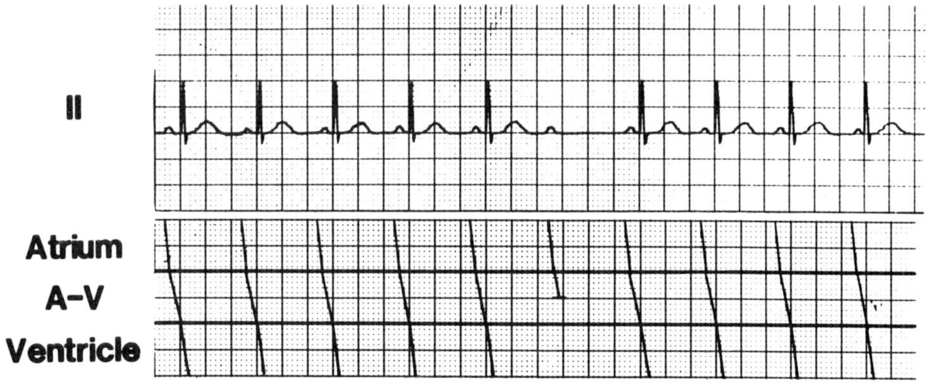
II
Atrium
A-V
Ventricle

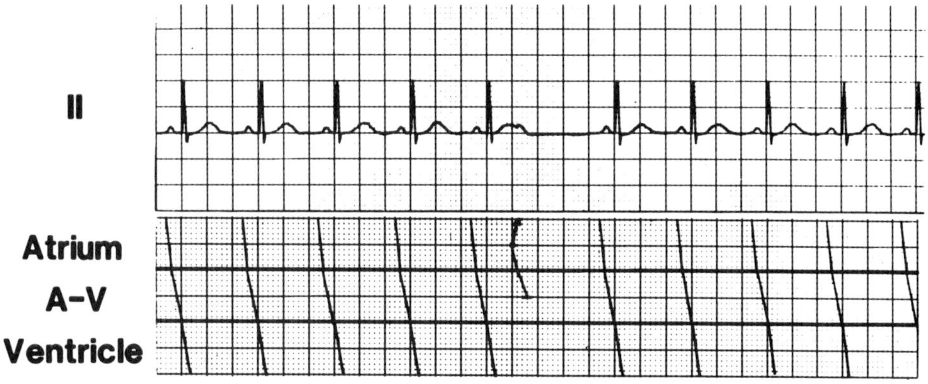
II
Atrium
A-V
Ventricle

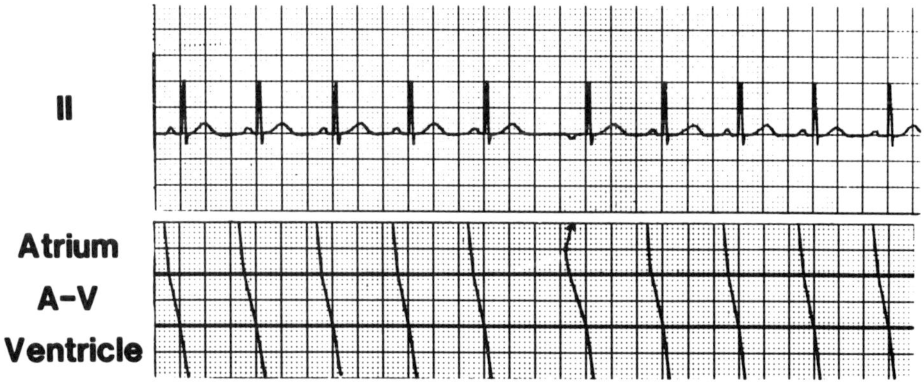
II
Atrium
A-V
Ventricle

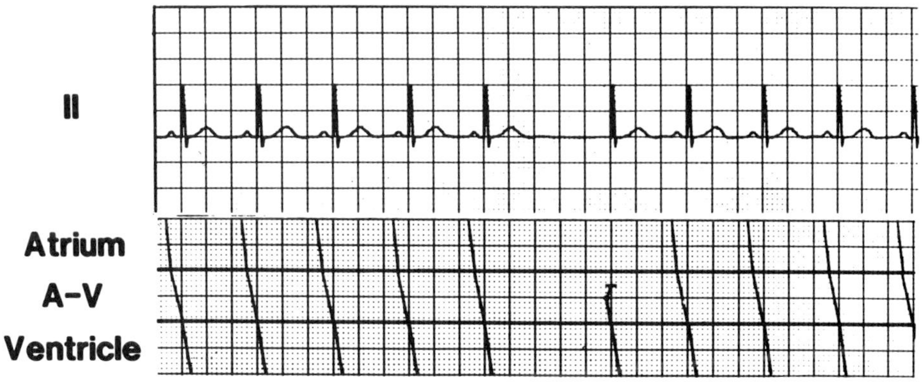
II
Atrium
A-V
Ventricle

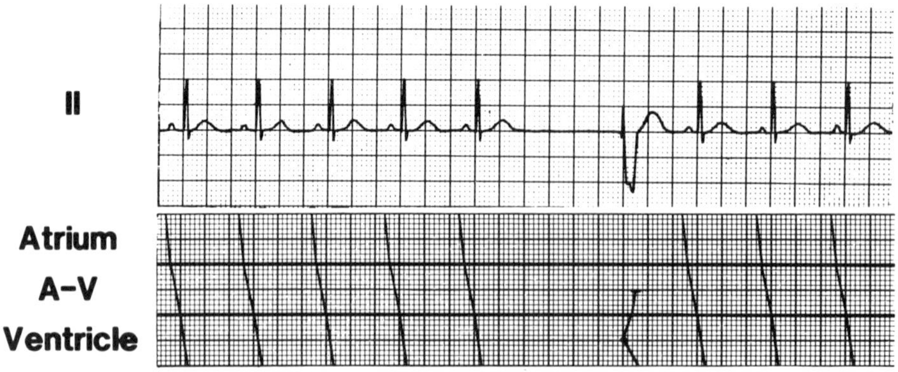

FIGURE 4–40

14. BASIC RR INTERVAL – REGULAR, BUT INTERRUPTED INTERMITTENTLY
IRREGULAR RR INTERVAL – LONG (DELAYED QRS)
QRS DURATION OF DELAYED COMPLEX – PROLONGED

Sinus rhythm with sinus pause and ventricular escape beat. Basic ventricular and atrial rates = 100/min (RR and PP intervals = 0.60 s). The long RR interval is 1.20 s—longer than the basic RR interval. The pause is longest with a ventricular escape beat, because idioventricular rhythm is the slowest in the heart. This is actually an accelerated ventricular escape beat, because for a 4-year-old child, a normal ventricular escape beat would occur at a cycle length greater than 1.5 s. The QRS complex preceding the delayed QRS is not followed by a sinus P wave ("pause" in sinus rhythm). The pause is ended by a QRS complex with prolonged duration without a preceding P wave—a ventricular escape beat.

14. BASIC RR INTERVAL – REGULAR, BUT INTERRUPTED INTERMITTENTLY
IRREGULAR RR INTERVAL – LONG (DELAYED QRS)
QRS DURATION OF DELAYED COMPLEX – PROLONGED

(See Figure 4–40)

a. Pause in Supraventricular Rhythm With Ventricular Escape

1. No supraventricular P wave follows preceding R wave.
2. "Delayed" QRS occurs at more than regular RR interval.
3. "Delayed" QRS not preceded by P wave.

Acknowledgments

This research was supported in part by grants HL24916, HL07190, and RR00188 from the National Institutes of Health, Bethesda, Maryland, and by a grant from the J. S. Abercrombie Foundation.

CHAPTER 5

NONINVASIVE DIAGNOSTIC TECHNIQUES

Henry B. Wiles, David S. Buckles & Vicki L. Zeigler

Disturbance of cardiac rhythm is an important aspect of pediatric cardiovascular medicine. Arrhythmias are seemingly increasing in frequency as a result of longer survival after "corrective" cardiac surgery and more frequent recognition by primary physicians of an arrhythmia in the child with an anatomically normal heart.[1, 2] The complication of rhythm disturbance after surgery is well documented for repair of tetralogy of Fallot,[3–6] d-transposition of the great arteries,[7–10] the Fontan procedure,[11, 12] and even simple atrial septal defect repair. Noninvasive testing beyond the standard resting 12-lead electrocardiogram (ECG) is necessary for the documentation, diagnosis, and management of arrhythmias. The resting electrocardiogram records cardiac rhythm for only a brief moment and only while the child is quiet and still. Continuous or instantaneous recording of cardiac rhythm during normal activity or during induced physiologic changes (such as exercise stress) requires the specialized techniques of 24-hour ambulatory electrocardiography, transtelephonic transmission of cardiac rhythm, telemetric transmission within the hospital setting, treadmill or bicycle exercise electrocardiography, signal-averaged electrocardiography, and nuclear cardiology evaluation of activation sequence.

AMBULATORY ELECTROCARDIOGRAPHY

The 24-hour continuous ambulatory electrocardiogram (cardioscan) has proven itself invaluable in the diagnosis and management of arrhythmias since it was first introduced by Holter.[13] Cardiac rhythm, conduction, and rate are continuously monitored while the patient is asleep and awake.[14] Current tape recorders are small and easily worn by infants and children, and adolescents can place the recorder under outer clothing so that it is less conspicuous. Many commercial systems are available with minor variations in features.

The greatest recent advancement in technology is the use of computer programs to analyze the tape recordings. Previously a trained technician reviewed the entire tape at accelerated playback speed. This was time consuming, tedious, and subject to human error. Current computer analysis allows greater speed and efficiency, with the ability to graphically represent changes in variables such as heart rate, frequency of premature beats, and ST segment depression. Computer storage of cardioscans eliminates the considerable space required to store hardcopy reports. However, accurate assessment of rhythm requires that rhythm strips be printed at 25 mm/s paper speed.

Romano et al[15] published cardioscan values for heart rate, PR interval, and QT interval in 32 normal children. They found that the range of normal heart rates and PR intervals recorded during the cardioscan was greater than that recorded during the resting electrocardiogram. We are conservative in using the cardioscan for the evaluation of QT interval and ST segment in children, since lead placement is not always accurately known. In addition, the quality of the tracing is often not as clear as with a 12-lead electrocardiogram.

Indications

Suspected Arrhythmia. The child who complains of palpitations, dizziness, or syncope deserves a 24-hour cardioscan to document the long-term baseline rhythm. By correlating symptoms with simultaneously recorded rhythm, the relationship of symptoms to heart rhythm can be shown. Porter, Gillette, and McNamara reported that 84% of cardioscans obtained in a population of children with known or suspected rhythm disturbance documented an arrhythmia, and that 48% of these cardioscans showed an arrhythmia that was not present on a previous 12-lead electrocardiogram.[16] They also found that symptoms recorded by the patient in a diary did not correlate well with timing of an arrhythmia. Since symptoms may occur only infrequently, even the 24-hour recording period may not capture the supposed arrhythmia. We often use transtelephonic recordings (discussed in a later section) in conjunction with the cardioscan to document a suspected arrhythmia.

Premature Ventricular Contraction. Benign premature ventricular contractions (PVCs) of childhood do not generally require treatment.[17] The 24-hour cardioscan is quite useful in confirming the diagnosis of benign PVCs and will define the frequency (number per hour), the timing (single, bigeminy, or couplet), and the morphology (uniform or multiform). Benign PVCs are single and uniform, while coupled and multiform PVCs require further evaluation (Fig. 5–1).

Congenital Complete Atrioventricular (AV) Block. Knowledge of the baseline heart rate during all daily activities in patients with congenital complete AV block is essential for the management of these patients. Dewey, Capeless, and Levy found a high incidence of significant symptoms in patients with a mean daytime heart rate below 50 beats per minute on a 24-hour cardioscan.[18] Permanent pacemaker implantation is indicated in children with a daytime heart rate below 45 beats per minute.[19]

Sinus Node and Atrioventricular Node Dysfunction. Sinus bradycardia, sick sinus syndrome, and atrioventricular node block (second or third degree) may occur with or without symptoms. The 24-hour cardioscan may provide the information necessary to decide whether further investigation, such as invasive electrophysiology testing, or institution of medical therapy is needed. First degree block and Wenckebach rhythm are not considered abnormal. Mobitz type II second degree block and third degree block found on 24-hour cardioscan warrant further noninvasive and invasive testing.

Cardiomyopathy. The presence of ventricular arrhythmia is a poor prognostic sign in both dilated and hypertrophic cardiomyopathy. Holmes et al found a striking direct relationship between complex ventricular ectopy recorded on the cardioscan and survival in patients with ischemic or idiopathic dilated cardiomyopathy.[20] Arrhythmias are frequently present in patients with hypertrophic cardiomyopathy and are believed to be responsible for sudden death in these patients.[21] We aggressively treat ventricular ectopy in patients with a cardiomyopathy. The cardioscan is the best way to document these arrhythmias, since they often produce no symptoms.

Postoperative Evaluation. Many corrective operations for congenital heart malformations have cardiac arrhythmia as a subsequent

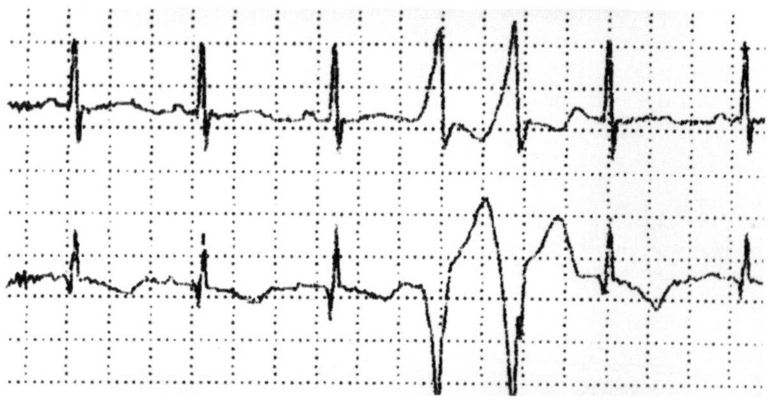

FIGURE 5–1
This 24-hour cardioscan from an asymptomatic 11-year-old girl shows a ventricular couplet. She also had a rare ventricular triplet and persistent PVCs during exercise. An invasive electrophysiology catheterization demonstrated atrial flutter and atrioventricular node reentry tachycardia. She was started on β-blockade therapy with improvement in her ventricular ectopy.

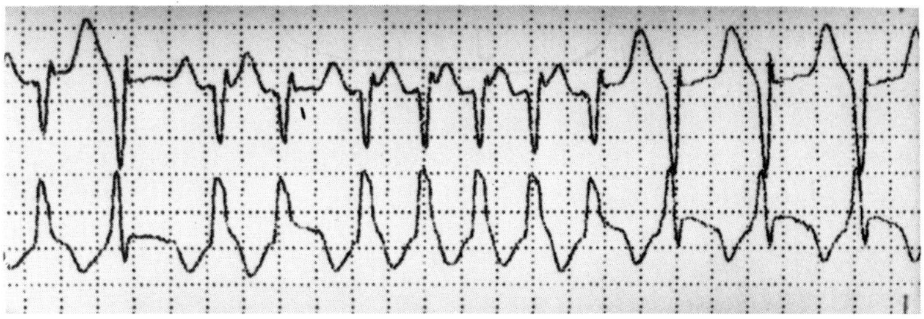

FIGURE 5–2
This 24-hour cardioscan tracing from a patient following tetralogy of Fallot repair shows ventricular tachycardia in the postoperative recovery period. Notice that he has bundle-branch block during sinus rhythm. He required treatment with phenytoin, which suppressed his ventricular ectopy.

complication (Fig. 5–2). The risk of sudden death in postoperative tetralogy of Fallot with PVCs is high enough to warrant initiation of drug therapy, such as phenytoin. Documentation of atrial and ventricular ectopy, sinus node dysfunction, and atrioventricular node dysfunction after the Senning or Mustard repair and the Fontan repair requires periodic cardioscan monitoring. The incidence of these findings is as high as 30%.[11]

Monitoring Drug Therapy. The effectiveness of antiarrhythmic drug therapy can be followed with serial cardioscans. The total number and type of conduction disturbances can be evaluated as therapy is initiated and adjusted. Many antiarrhythmic drugs have pro-arrhythmic side effects when first administered. Monitoring with telemetry and cardioscans is likely to detect these adverse reactions, and we routinely do this when starting therapy with flecainide, quinidine, mixiletine, and amiodarone. The criteria for determining a drug's effectiveness are not uniform and must be individualized with each patient and condition.

TRANSTELEPHONIC ELECTROCARDIOGRAPHY

Transtelephonic electrocardiographic monitoring was initially used for the follow-up of permanently implanted pacemakers. More recently, because of "hard-to-document" arrhythmias, it has become an important at-home diagnostic tool for arrhythmia detection.[22] Transtelephonic monitoring may also be used to evaluate the efficacy of antiarrhythmic drugs. The advantages of this type of arrhythmia documentation are (1) cost (the price of the transmitter is much less than that of a 24-hour ambulatory monitor); (2) decreased hospitalization time, which may be prolonged as a result of the inability to document an arrhythmia on 24-hour or telemetric monitoring; and (3) rapid interpretation (after documentation it takes very little time, less than that for cardioscan interpretation, to have the single-channel ECG interpreted). There are also disadvantages: (1) the patient must have or be near a telephone; (2) the onset of symptoms and the short nature of some of the arrhythmias may be too brief to allow recording; and (3) occurrences during the patient's sleep cycle may go undocumented.

Several systems for transmitting single- or multiple-channel recordings exist and can be used with any standard local or long-distance telephone system. We believe only single-channel ECGs are necessary for interpretation of basic heart rhythm and rate. We employ a simple plastic box powered by a single 9-volt battery that has four metal electrodes or "feet" on the back. It is similar in size and weight to a pocket transistor radio. The receiving center is a 15-pound, 11″ × 6″ device designed to receive transmissions via a direct telephone line connection or through an external telephone coupler. A pacemaker data module that prints out pacemaker pulse rate, atrial and ventricular pulse widths, and AV intervals on the paced patient can also be used with this system. The transmitter is purchased by the patient, who is subsequently charged for each ECG interpretation.

Our receiver unit is used with a telephone answering machine so that ECGs may be transmitted at any time during the day or night (Fig. 5–3). The messages are replayed each morning and demodulated into a standard one-channel ECG strip. Patients and parents are personally instructed in the use of the device by trained personnel. They are given written instructions and are asked to give a return demonstration prior to discharge from the hospital or outpatient clinic; this is done to obtain a baseline ECG on the single-channel machine and to evaluate the accuracy of the patient's technique (Fig. 5–4). This also helps to allay fear and anxiety somewhat, since it will have been performed once before the real event actually occurs.

Before transmission of an ECG, patients are instructed to give their name, telephone number, and description of any symptoms. They then place the monitor on the upper middle half of the chest and listen for a "beating" tone. They then place the mouthpiece of the phone over the transmitter for approximately 30 seconds. This entire process takes only 2 to 3 minutes and is easily accomplished with good teaching in a relaxed setting. Parents and patients are told that if the ECG strip is normal, there will be no contact from the arrhythmia center; however, if the ECG was not performed correctly or an arrhythmia was documented, they will be promptly informed.

Indications

Pacemakers. Transtelephonic electrocardiographic monitoring has proven valuable, informative, and reliable as a follow-up technique for those patients with permanent pacemakers.[23] Families are encouraged to call in both routinely and whenever they are concerned that the pacemaker may be malfunctioning. From January to December of 1988, a total of 247 ECGs were received from paced patients; of these, 24 (10%) were abnormal and indicated the need for patient evaluation. As elective pacemaker replacement nears, patients are encouraged to transmit more frequently (i.e., monthly or even weekly) in order for gradual rate decreases and pulse width extensions to be detected early. Another valuable technique in the pacemaker patient is that of receiving transtelephonic real-time telemetry measurements. A specific transmitter is required to obtain this information and a person trained to use the decoder must be present at the time of the call to obtain the information. Lead impedance and battery voltage are two of the most valuable pieces of information obtained in this way and may indicate either lead problems or elective replacement parameters.

Tachycardia. From January through December of 1988, 157 ECG strips were obtained from patients who did not have pacemakers. Of these 157, 24 (15%) were abnormal. Because of the transient and unpredictable nature of these arrhythmias, 24-hour ambula-

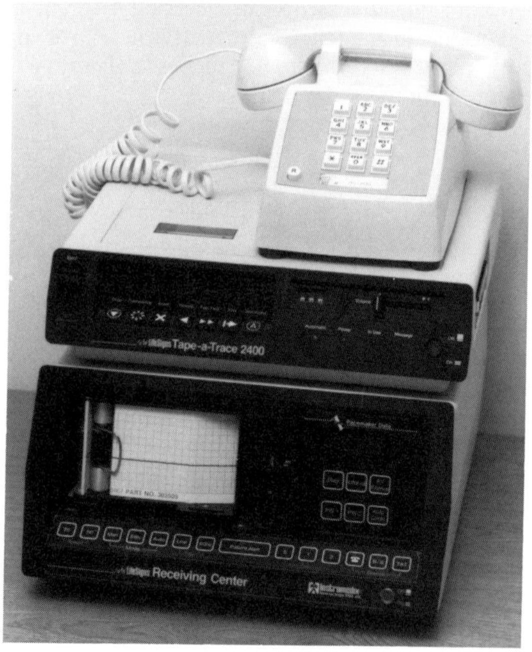

FIGURE 5–3
Transtelephonic electrocardiography requires a telephone (top), a tape recorder (middle), and a receiving center/demodulator (bottom).

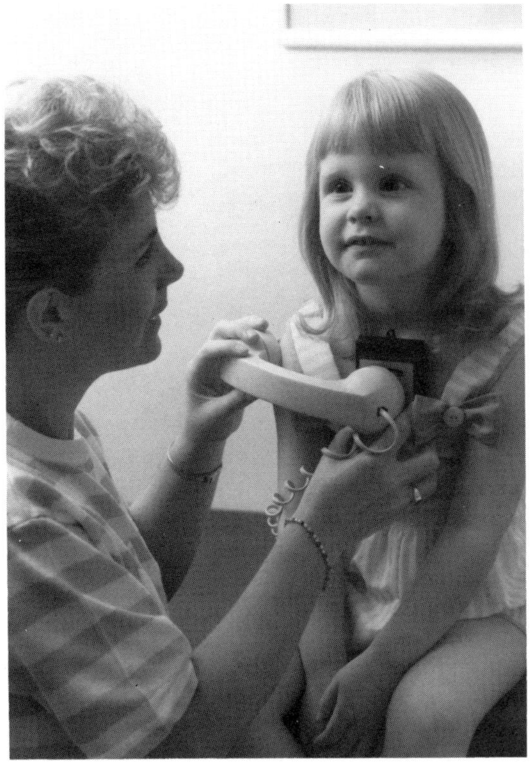

FIGURE 5–4
The telephone transmitter is easily placed over the heart, even in small children. With proper training the patient or parent can determine when the recorder is properly positioned by listening to the tones emitted from the transmitter.

tory monitoring had failed to detect any of them (Fig. 5–5). In one patient a medication change was indicated, and in 12 patients a previously undocumented supraventricular tachycardia was recorded. The remaining 11 abnormal strips were from patients whose surgical or medical treatment had failed.

For patients who have extremely short bursts of undocumented tachycardia, an event recorder may be a useful diagnostic

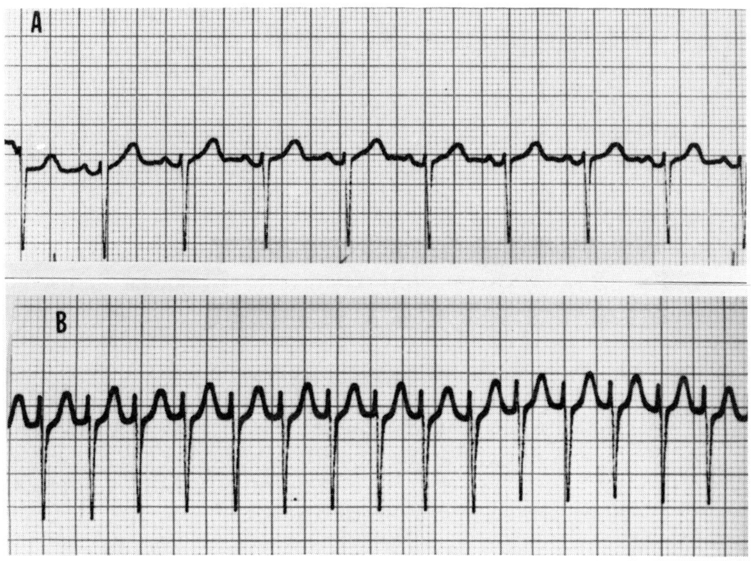

FIGURE 5–5
(*A*) This transtelephonic recording shows sinus rhythm during an episode of chest pain and shortness of breath in a 15-year-old girl. This documents that these symptoms are not a result of tachycardia. (*B*) This recording shows supraventricular tachycardia at 214 bpm in the same patient. Her only symptom at this time was the sensation of palpitations. Transtelephonic ECGs helped differentiate two types of episodes in this patient: one related to an arrhythmia and one not related to a rhythm disturbance.

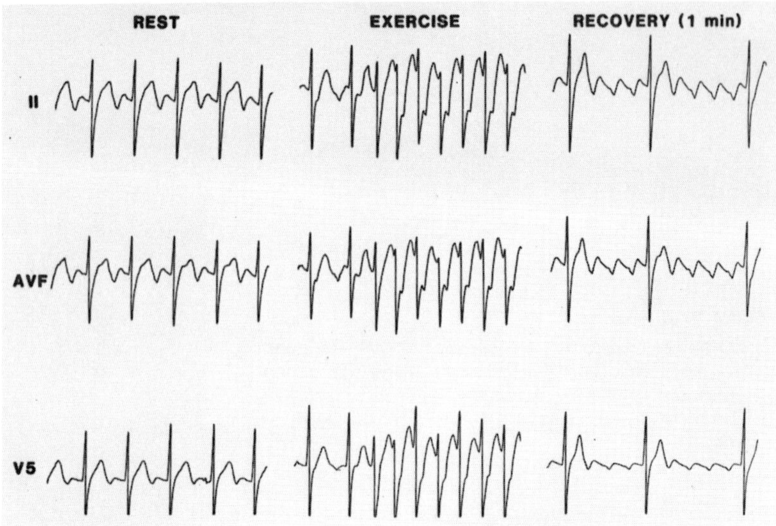

FIGURE 5–6
This exercise ECG shows wide QRS tachycardia during exercise. The recovery ECG clearly shows atrial flutter with variable conduction. The rest ECG probably represents atrial flutter with 2:1 conduction rather than sinus rhythm. Exercise testing helped establish this atrial arrhythmia.

tool. It is very similar to the conventional monitor, but slightly larger in size. It records the event as it happens but allows playback to be done at a later time.

Transtelephonic electrocardiograpic monitoring has become a very useful tool in the detection of transient arrhythmias and in permanent pacemaker follow-up. The variety of monitors available allow considerable choice in determining the appropriate device for each individual patient.

EXERCISE STRESS ELECTROCARDIOGRAPHY

The physiologic changes that occur during exercise stress can be extremely helpful in the noninvasive evaluation of cardiac arrhythmias in children. The adrenergic tone in the body during and after exercise is believed to either suppress or provoke cardiac ectopy. Benign rhythm disturbances are usually suppressed, while serious disturbances may be provoked or exacerbated by exercise (Fig. 5–6). Exercise stress is an easy noninvasive study to perform in children, even those as young as 4 years of age.

The principles of safe and effective exercise stress are well reported.[24–27] Treadmill exercise and upright bicycle exercise are both adequate techniques for maximum stress testing; we generally use treadmill exercise because it produces higher maximum oxygen consumption. Commonly used exercise protocols are the modified Bruce protocol[26] for treadmill testing and the James protocol[25] for bicycle exercise. Exercise testing in children for evaluation of rhythm disturbance uses the same techniques and safety procedures as those used for routine exercise testing.

Indications

Sinus Node Function. The sinus node has a clear and rapid response to the stress of exercise. This reproducible response is useful in differentiating sinus node dysfunction from normal sinus node variation. The patient with insignificant sinus bradycardia will have the expected rapid sinus node response, while the patient with sick sinus syndrome may not.

Supraventricular Tachycardia. Exercise stress rarely brings out supraventricular tachycardia, but patients with SVT may have ventricular ectopy or limited cardiac reserve, with reduced exercise endurance.[28] The prognostic implication of losing the delta wave during exercise in patients with Wolff-Parkinson-White syndrome is unclear, but some evidence indicates that this phenomenon is correlated with a long antegrade effective refractory period of the accessory connection.[29] We do not rely on this phenomenon for diagnosis, however, and recommend invasive electrophysiologic testing to confirm the antegrade effective refractory period.

Cardiomyopathy. Patients with either dilated or hypertrophic cardiomyopathy are at risk for complications from arrhythmias.[21, 30] Exercise testing in conjunction with 24-hour ambulatory monitoring is useful in defining the prognosis of these patients.

Ventricular Ectopy. We perform an exercise test on any patient with frequent PVCs, multiform PVCs, couplets, or ventricular tachycardia. Benign PVCs in children are generally suppressed during exercise.[17] Ventricular ectopy that worsens during exercise is not normal, and further noninvasive and invasive testing is indicated.

Patients who have undergone ventriculotomy for correction of a congenital malformation are appropriate candidates for exercise testing in an attempt to provoke ventricular ectopy. An earlier study of patients after repair of tetralogy of Fallot showed a correlation between exercise-induced ventricular ectopy and poor hemodynamic results, which is believed to be a marker for sudden death.[31] A more recent study of 70 patients after tetralogy of Fallot repair showed no correlation between exercise ECG changes and induced ventricular ectopy during electrophysiologic investigation (unpublished data of Ewing, Gillette, Buckles et al). We believe any postoperative patient with ventricular ectopy as indicated by resting ECG, 24-hour monitoring, exercise testing, or invasive studies should receive antiarrhythmic medical therapy.

Despite the reproducibility of certain parameters on sequential exercise tests, the role of exercise testing in the evaluation of drug therapy for ventricular ectopy is not well established. We are encouraged by a subsequent exercise test without ventricular ectopy following drug therapy, but do not rely on this as adequate documentation of the effectiveness of drug therapy.

TELEMETRIC ELECTROCARDIOGRAPHY

Continuous radio transmission of cardiac rhythm in hospitalized children has added significantly to the management of known, suspected, or potential rhythm disturbances. Telemetry monitors allow multiple ECG recordings to be continuously monitored at a central station. These systems use battery operated radio transmitter boxes that are attached to the patient with standard ECG electrodes. The receiving unit uses an antenna to capture the incoming signal. The ECG is displayed on an oscilloscope for continuous monitoring. Various limits and parameters, such as minimum and maximum heart rate, are set for automatic warning by an alarm system. Rhythm strips of arrhythmia, tachycardia, or bradycardia are automatically printed at 25 mm/s.

Telemetric monitoring adds great versatility to the care of postoperative patients who are at risk for rhythm disturbance. A patient may have continuous ECG monitoring while staying in a private room instead of requiring bedside monitoring in an intensive care unit (Fig. 5–7). Children with suspected arrhythmia may be monitored for documentation of any rhythm disturbance while enjoying freedom of movement within the hospital. Management of known arhythmias is facilitated by constant monitoring of the effects of antiarrhythmic drugs. Children without primary cardiac conduction disturbances, such as apnea and bradycardia, may also be monitored closely for symptoms. The disadvantage of telemetric monitoring is that rhythm disturbances may not be recognized and permanently recorded. The range of radio transmission is also limited, and monitoring cannot occur outside of this range.

SIGNAL-AVERAGED ELECTROCARDIOGRAPHY

Among the newest of the noninvasive diagnostic techniques, signal-averaged electrocardiography (SAECG) is being considered for use in cases of ventricular arrhythmias and depolarization abnormalities. A modified form of vectorcardiography, SAECG was first espoused in its present form in 1981 by Simson.[32] Recordings from 3 to 5 minutes in duration are taken simultaneously from three sets of orthogonal pairs of electrodes arranged in X, Y, and Z axes (Fig. 5–8). After the recorded signals are digitized by a computer, the QRS complexes are extracted

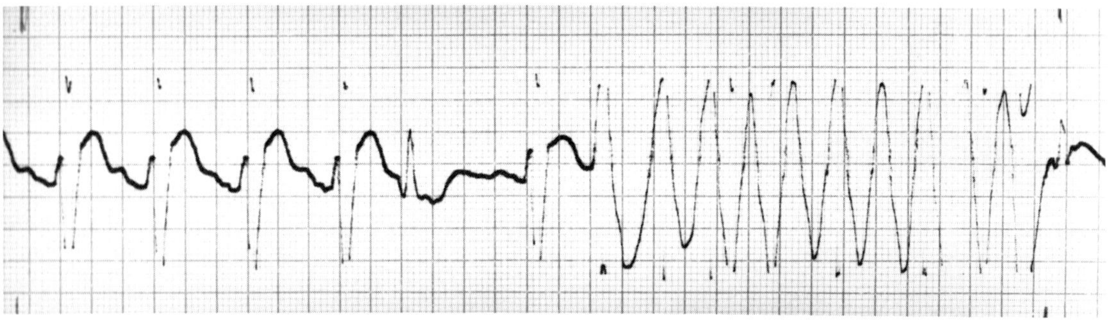

FIGURE 5–7
This telemetric ECG shows ventricular tachycardia that produced syncope in this 17-year-old boy with tricuspid atresia and transposed great arteries. His rhythm was monitored during drug therapy trials while staying in a private room. He ultimately required six simultaneous antiarrhythmic medications to control his ventricular and atrial ectopy.

using a matching template. For each of the three axes, the QRS complexes are superimposed and averaged to reduce the noise level to <2 microvolts. A vector sum is calculated from the three averaged QRS complexes, and the summed complex is filtered to remove the relatively slowly changing QRS waveform. The remaining signal contains very detailed information on ventricular depolarization characteristics in the range of microvolts.

A normal QRS complex derived from an SAECG recording is characterized by an abrupt onset, well-defined waveform variations, and abrupt cessation of electrical activity (Fig. 5–9). However, in some patients, delays in depolarization that are undetectable on the standard surface ECG appear in the final filtered QRS complex as electrical activity of very low amplitude, continuing after the normal end point of the QRS. This low-level, delayed activity has been termed "late potentials," and has been shown to be highly correlated with the presence of ventricular tachycardia in adults.[33, 34] SAECG is also used to assess vulnerability to development of malignant ventricular arrhythmias in patients following surgical repair of tetralogy of Fallot.[35] An example of an abnormal SAECG complex is presented in Figure 5–10, a recording taken from a 22-year-old patient following complete repair of tetralogy of Fal-

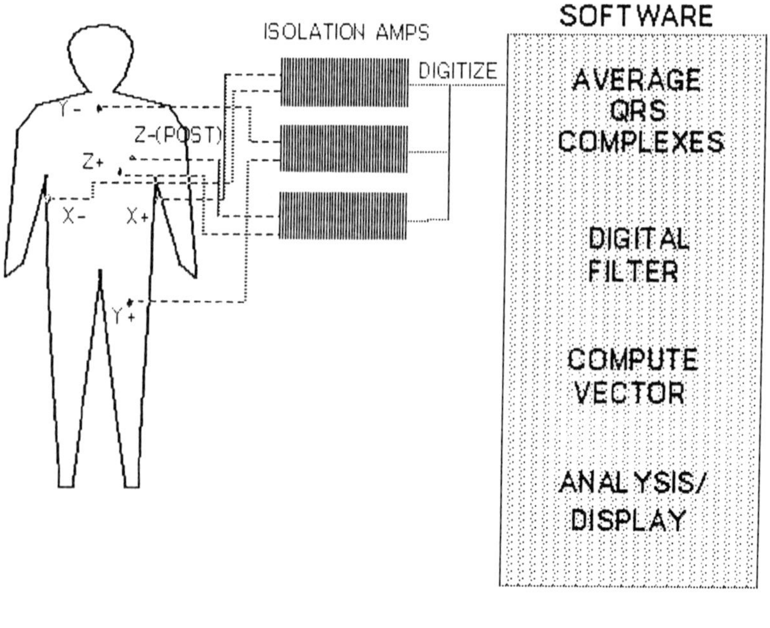

FIGURE 5–8
This schematic drawing shows the component parts necessary for signal averaged electrocardiography. POST = posterior.

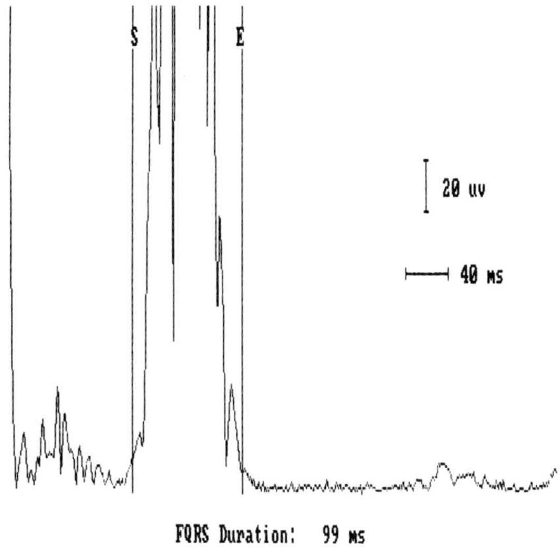

FIGURE 5–9
This signal-averaged ECG is normal and shows well-defined, abrupt changes in the waveform. S = start; E = end; F = filtered.

lot. This patient demonstrated very poor ventricular function and had numerous episodes of ventricular ectopy.

Antiarrhythmic agents that affect myocardial depolarization (such as flecainide, encainide and amiodarone) may also produce changes that are revealed by SAECG analysis. Figure 5–11 shows a set of recordings taken from a 9-year-old patient undergoing treatment with encainide for premature ventricular complexes. The two recordings were made just prior to, and 4 hours after, a regularly scheduled administration of oral encainide.

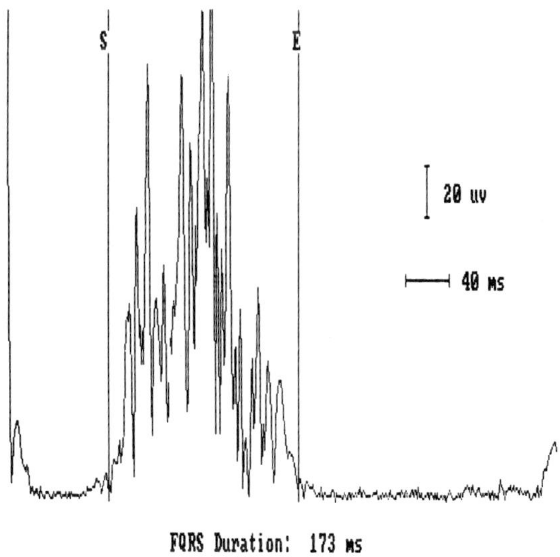

FIGURE 5–10
This signal-averaged ECG from a patient following tetralogy of Fallot repair shows abnormal prolongation of the filtered QRS with multiple fractionated waves at the upstroke and downstroke. S = start; E = end.

The advantages of signal-averaged electrocardiography include high-resolution analysis of myocardial depolarization characteristics (normally obtainable only with invasive electrode catheters), relatively short recording time, and minimal risk and discomfort to the patient. Disadvantages include the complexity and cost of the equipment and the lack of well-established guidelines for interpretation of results. Considerable research is in progress to establish standard procedures (including optimal electrode placement), to explore the various clinical situations that may benefit from the technique, and to formulate guidelines that will enhance and standardize the applications of the technique.

NUCLEAR CARDIOLOGY PHASE ANALYSIS

A relatively new technique for the noninvasive evaluation of rhythm disturbance is the phase analysis of a technetium 99m equilibrium gated nuclear cardiology study. This technique can localize the area of earliest activation in conditions of preexcitation such as Wolff-Parkinson-White syndrome[36] or ventricular tachycardia.[37] The theory of this technique is that the area in the ventricular cavity that ejects blood first must be associ-

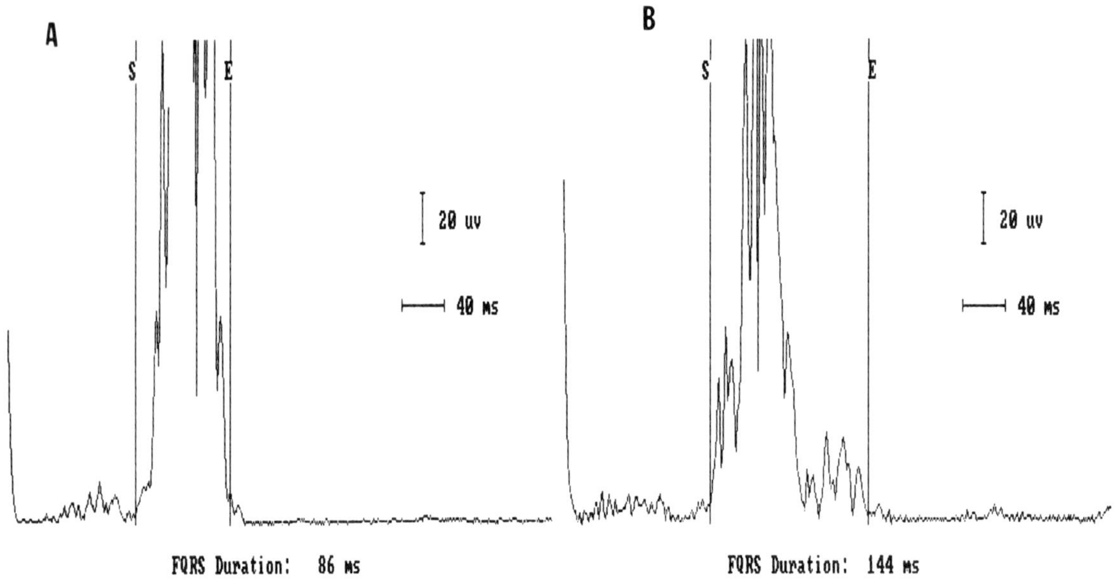

FIGURE 5–11
(*A*) This signal-averaged ECG recorded before encainide therapy shows a normal tracing. (*B*) Four hours after an oral dose of encainide, the signal-averaged ECG shows a prolonged QRS and multiple late potentials. S = start; E = end.

ated with the area that has the earliest electrical activity. Fourier analysis of the ejection of the radioactive tracer technetium 99m from the ventricular cavity gives a regional pixel-by-pixel ejection sequence. The phase of pixel-by-pixel ejection is graphically displayed for analysis and identification of earliest activation.

Johnson et al[36] showed that phase images could localize bypass tracts in both free wall and septal/paraseptal locations. They proposed that this technique may be useful in the preoperative patient with Wolff-Parkinson-White syndrome. This technique has even greater use, however, in the immediate postoperative period when a persistent bypass tract is present. Localization of the persistent or previously concealed tract can be accomplished noninvasively in the recovery area. Other studies have shown the patterns of phase mapping with bundle-branch block[38] and preexcitation through Mahaim fibers.[39] Patients with sustained ventricular tachycardia also show a phase map that localizes earliest activation in close correlation with intracardiac electrophysiologic studies.[40]

References

1. Yabek SM, Dillon T, Berman W Jr, et al: Symptomatic sinus node dysfunction in children without structural heart disease. Pediatrics 69:590–593, 1982.
2. Yabek SM, Swensson RE, Jarmakani JM: Electrocardiographic recognition of sinus node dysfunction in children and young adults. Circulation 56:235–239, 1977.
3. Gillette PC, Yeoman MA, Mullins CE, et al: Sudden death after repair of tetralogy of Fallot: Electrocardiographic and electrophysiologic abnormalities. Circulation 56:566–571, 1977.
4. Dunningan A, Pritzker MR, Benditt DG, et al: Life threatening ventricular tachycardias in late survivors of surgically corrected tetralogy of Fallot. Br Heart J 52:198–206, 1984.
5. Walsh EP, Rockenmacher S, Keane JF, et al: Late results in patients with tetralogy of Fallot repaired during infancy. Circulation 77:1062–1067, 1988.
6. Deal BJ, Scagliotti D, Miller SM, et al: Electrophysiology drug testing in symptomatic ventricular arrhythmias after repair of tetralogy of Fallot. Am J Cardiol 59:1380–1385, 1987.
7. Trusler GA, Williams WG, Duncan KF, et al: Results with the Mustard operation in simple transposition of the great arteries: 1963–1985. Ann Surg 206:251–260, 1987.
8. Musewe NN, Reisman J, Benson LN, et al: Cardiopulmonary adaptation at rest and during exercise 10 years after Mustard atrial repair for transposition of the great arteries. Circulation 77:1055–1061, 1988.
9. Flinn CJ, Wolff GS, Dick M, et al: Cardiac rhythm after the Mustard operation for complete transposition of the great arteries. N Engl J Med 310:1635–1638, 1984.
10. Vetter VL, Tanner CS, Horowitz LN: Electrophysiologic consequences of the Mustard repair of d-transposition of the great arteries. J Am Coll Cardiol 10:1265–1273, 1987.

11. Porter CJ, Battiste CE, Humes RA, et al: Risk factors for supraventricular tachyarrhythmias after Fontan procedure for tricuspid atresia. Am Heart J 112:645, 1986. Abstract.
12. Girod DA, Fontan F, Deville C, et al: Long-term results after the Fontan operation for tricuspid atresia. Circulation 75:605–610, 1987.
13. Holter NJ: New method for heart studies. Science 134:1214–1220, 1961.
14. Rees AH, Solinger R, Elbl F: Holder monitoring in the management of cardiac arrhythmias in children. Compr Ther 11:11–16, 1985.
15. Romano M, Clarizia M, Onofrio E, et al: Heart rate, PR, and QR intervals in normal children: A 24-hour Holter monitoring study. Clin Cardiol 11:839–842, 1988.
16. Porter CJ, Gillette PC, McNamara DG: 24-hour ambulatory ECGs in the detection and management of cardiac dysrhythmias in infants and children. Pediatr Cardiol 1:203–208, 1980.
17. Jacobsen JR, Garson A Jr, Gillette PC, et al: Premature ventricular contractions in normal children. J Pediatr 92:36–38, 1978.
18. Dewey RC, Capeless MA, Levy AM: Use of ambulatory electrocardiographic monitoring to identify high-risk patients with congenital complete heart block. N Engl J Med 316:835–839, 1987.
19. Frye RL, Collins JJ, DeSanctis RW, et al: Guidelines for permanent pacemaker implantation, May 1984. Circulation 70:331A–339A, 1984.
20. Holmes J, Kubo SH, Cody RJ, et al: Arrhythmias in ischemic and nonischemic dilated cardiomyopathy: Prediction of mortality by ambulatory electrocardiography. Am J Cardiol 55:146–151, 1985.
21. McKenna WJ, Chetty S, Oakley CM, et al: Arrhythmia in hypertrophic cardiomyopathy: Exercise and 48 hour ambulatory electrocardiographic assessment with and without beta adrenergic blocking therapy. Am J Cardiol 45:1–5, 1980.
22. Fyfe DA, Homes DR, Newbauer SA, et al: Transtelephonic monitoring in pediatric patients with clinically suspected arrhythmias. Clin Pediatr 23:139–143, 1984.
23. Shannon CE: Pacing system follow-up. In Gillette PC, Griffin JC (eds): Practical Cardiac Pacing. Baltimore, Williams and Wilkins, 1986, pp 137–160.
24. James FW, Blomqvist CG, Freed MD, et al: Standards for exercise testing in the pediatric age group. Circulation 66:1377A–1397A, 1982.
25. James FW, Kaplan S, Glueck CJ, et al: Responses of normal children and young adults to controlled bicycle exercise. Circulation 61:902–912, 1980.
26. Cumming GR, Everatt D, Hastman L: Bruce treadmill test in children: Normal values in a clinic population. Am J Cardiol 41:69–75, 1978.
27. Gutgesell HP, Gessner IH, Vetter VL, et al: Recreational and occupational recommendations for young patients with heart disease. A statement for physicians by the Committee of Congenital Cardiac Defects of the Council on Cardiovascular Disease in the Young, American Heart Association. Circulation 74:1195A–1198A, 1986.
28. Strasberg B, Ashley WW, Wyndham CRC, et al: Treadmill exercise testing in the Wolff-Parkinson-White syndrome. Am J Cardiol 45:742–748, 1980.
29. Bricker JT, Porter CJ, Garson A Jr, et al: Exercise testing in children with Wolff-Parkinson-White syndrome. Am J Cardiol 55:1001–1004, 1985.
30. Hofmann T, Meinertz T, Kasper W, et al: Mode of death in idiopathic dilated cardiomyopathy: A multivariate analysis of prognostic determinants. Am Heart J 116:1455–1463, 1988.
31. Garson A Jr, Gillette PC, Gutgesell HP: Stress-induced ventricular arrhythmia after repair of tetralogy of Fallot. Am J Cardiol 46:1006–1012, 1980.
32. Simson MB: Use of signals in the terminal QRS complex to identify patients with ventricular tachycardia after myocardial infarction. Circulation 64:235–242, 1981.
33. Breithardt G, Borggrefe M, Karhenn U, et al: Prevalence of late potentials in patients with and without ventricular tachycardia: Correlation with angiographic findings. Am J Cardiol 49:1932–1937, 1982.
34. Cain ME, Ambos HD, Witkowski FX, et al: Fast-Fourier transform analysis of signal averaged electrocardiograms for identification of patients prone to sustained ventricular tachycardia. Circulation 69:711–720, 1984.
35. Zimmermann M, Friedli B, Adamec R, et al: Frequency of ventricular late potentials and fractionated right ventricular electrograms after operative repair of tetralogy of Fallot. Am J Cardiol 59:448–453, 1987.
36. Johnson LL, Seldin DW, Yeh H-L, et al: Phase analysis of gated blood pool scintigraphic images to localize bypass tracts in Wolff-Parkinson-White syndrome. J Am Coll Cardiol 8:67–75, 1986.
37. Botvinick EH, Frais MA, Shosa DW, et al: An accurate means of detecting and characterizing abnormal patterns of ventricular activation by phase image analysis. Am J Cardiol 50:289–298, 1982.
38. Frais MA, Botvinick EH, Shosa DW, et al: Phase image characterization of ventricular contraction in left and right bundle branch block. Am J Cardiol 50:95–105, 1982.
39. Schechtmann N, Botvinick EH, Dae M, et al: The scintigraphic characteristics of ventricular pre-excitation through Mahaim fibers with the use of phase analysis. J Am Coll Cardiol 13:882–891, 1989.
40. Swiryn S, Pavel D, Byrom E, et al: Sequential regional phase mapping of radionuclide gated biventriculograms in patients with sustained ventricular tachycardia: Close correlation with electrophysiologic characteristics. Am Heart J 103:319–332, 1982.

CHAPTER 6

INTRACARDIAC ELECTROPHYSIOLOGY STUDIES

Paul C. Gillette, David Buckles, Mark Harold, & Arthur Garson, Jr.

Recording of the His bundle depolarization and the depolarization of several parts of the atria and ventricles together with programmed electrical stimulation of the heart has enabled the clinical electrophysiologist to verify the mechanism of cardiac dysrhythmias in humans.[1,2] Intracardiac electrophysiologic study (EPS) can also document the anatomic site of the origin of normal and abnormal rhythms and blocks. These techniques have been in use for approximately 20 years, and during this period we have learned a great deal about the mechanisms of dysrhythmias in children. Clinical electrophysiology provides the bridge between microelectrode studies in isolated tissue and the surface electrocardiograms (ECGs). We have learned enough from EPS in some groups of patients that EPS need not be performed in all cases. In other clinical situations, intracardiac recordings and stimulation are a vital tool in the study of each patient.

In this chapter we will describe the equipment, techniques, and interpretation of clinical EPS as currently used in our laboratories. We will also give examples of the use of these studies in common types of clinical dysrhythmias.

The technique for recording the His bundle depolarization in humans was first reported by Scherlag et al in 1969, and the method has been modified only minimally for use in children.[1–8] In 1970 the techniques of programmed stimulation of the heart were incorporated with His bundle recording.[8–11]

PREPARATION FOR THE ELECTROPHYSIOLOGY STUDY

Sedation

Sedation is required to perform an electrophysiology study on an infant or child. Each sedative drug has electrophysiologic effects. It is necessary to understand these effects and standardize the types and dosages of sedation used in each pediatric electrophysiology laboratory if data are to be compared among different laboratories. A mixture of meperidine and promethazine is most commonly used for sedation in pediatric cardiac catheterizations. The addition of chlorpromazine causes marked shortening of sinus node recovery times.[12] It is likely that other sedative drugs also have electrophysiologic effects, but we cannot assume that these effects are similar to those of the meperidine, chlorpromazine, and promethazine mixture. Our current procedure is to use meperidine (2 mg/kg body weight) and promethazine (1 mg/kg body weight) intramuscularly 45 minutes before the beginning of the study. If extra sedation is needed during the study, meperidine and promethazine may be given at doses of 0.5 mg/kg each. Thus the number of drugs affecting the study is minimized. Ketamine (1 mg/kg intravenously) has also been used for additional sedation. It increases heart rate and blood pressure through a sympathomimetic effect. We attempt to keep the patient lightly asleep throughout the study to maintain a steady state.

Equipment

The essential items for an EPS are a multipurpose recorder, a programmable stimulator, and electrode catheters. A storage oscilloscope and a physiologic tape recorder are useful additions. The multipurpose recorder should be capable of recording at least six (and preferably 18) electrical channels at paper speeds of 100–500 mm/s on photographic paper. At least three (preferably 13) channels must be capable of recording intracardiac electrograms; that is, they should be completely isolated from all sources of current leakage and should have the capacity to filter all waveforms below 30–50 Hz and above 250–500 Hz. Two to four additional channels are necessary for recording surface ECGs, with filter settings of dc for the lower limit and 200 Hz for the upper limit. The ECG channels must also be isolated. For optimal recordings the room should be free of 60 Hz interference and radiofrequency interference. With today's photographic recorders, the paper may be developed instantly at speeds of up to 150 mm/s, but for speeds of 200–500 mm/s, the paper must be stored in a cassette and developed by a wet process in the darkroom. Other recorders are available that use a xerographic process capable of recording at speeds up to 500 mm/s. If the recorder does not generate time lines accurately, then a separate time line generator should be used to calibrate the intervals properly. The multipurpose recorder also should have at least one blood pressure channel so that femoral artery pressure can be monitored continuously and displayed throughout the study. We consider this essential, because the child's heart can be stimulated rapidly enough to cause severe hypotension.

A junction box is necessary to connect the catheters to the recorder and select each bipolar or unipolar recording. Several commercially available junction boxes can carry up to 12 channels of data simultaneously. A junction box can also be built by most electronics laboratories. Most modern junction boxes also allow selection of pacing sites from any of the recorded sites.

A programmable stimulator is the second major piece of equipment necessary for the electrophysiologic laboratory. This stimulator should either be battery powered or, if wall current is used, be used with an optical isolation device so that there is no possibility for current to leak into the patient through the catheters. The programmable pacemaker should be capable of stimulating with pulses of 1- or 2-ms duration, 0.5–20 mA in output. Several pacing modes are necessary: continuous pacing rates of 50–600 beats per minute (bpm); pacing for 8 to 10 beats at a basic drive cycle length, followed by introduction of one to eight premature stimuli at separately controllable cycle lengths; and sensing of a spontaneous rhythm with introduction of single and multiple premature beats at separately controllable cycle lengths. If the pacemaker generates a separate isolated output of the pacemaker impulse, this may be recorded on the paper. Also, a separate output of the next-to-last sensed or paced beat before the premature beat may be used to trigger other instruments, such as the storage oscilloscope and recorder. There are several commercially available programmable stimulators that meet these specifications.

We now use a custom-designed digital computer (Compaq 386) to perform stimulation protocols, measure intervals, and prepare the report.

Specially built electrode catheters are necessary for pediatric EPS. The catheter used to record the His bundle depolarization should be 5 or 6 French diameter, usually with three electrodes. The first 1 mm ring electrode is positioned at the tip of the catheter; the second 1 mm ring electrode is 1 mm to 10 mm proximal to the first electrode; the third electrode is 10 mm proximal to the second. These catheters are available from several catheter companies and need not be custom made. For recording and stimulating other parts of the heart, a 4 or 5 French quadripolar catheter with 1 mm ring electrodes spaced 2 mm to 5 mm apart has proved the most useful. If the electrodes are placed closer than 5 mm to each other, the stimulus artifact will cause an offset on the recording from the other two electrodes on the same catheter. Multipolar catheters with up to 12 electrodes are useful for mapping the coronary sinus.

An eight-channel storage oscilloscope that allows "stop-action" visualization of the recordings is a useful addition to the laboratory. This oscilloscope is connected in series to the recorder with its isolation amplifiers; thus the amplifiers of the storage oscilloscope do not have to be isolated, and a standard electronics laboratory oscilloscope may be used—a significant financial savings. If an accurate time base is incorporated, direct on-line measurements of intervals will be accurate.

A physiologic tape recorder with a frequency response adequate to record the His bundle depolarization is useful in several respects. It serves as a backup in case the paper recordings do not develop properly, and it also allows capture of spontaneous transient electrophysiologic events that might occur when the recorder would not normally be turned on. We now use an 8-channel digital audiotape recorder that records 8 channels of data for 3 hours on a DAT cassette (Sony).

Catheter Insertion

Catheters are inserted by a percutaneous technique similar to that used by pediatric cardiologists for hemodynamic catheterization. After preparation and draping of the groin, a short bevel needle is introduced into the femoral vein and a soft, coiled guide wire is passed through the needle. It is important not to enter the heart with the wire in arrhythmia patients since they are likely to have their arrhythmia induced. The needle is withdrawn, and a small skin incision is made with a no. 11 scalpel blade in order to facilitate the introduction of the dilator and sheath. It is often effective to dilate the skin and the vein with a plastic cannula before using the sheath and dilator. Many commercial sheath and dilator sets are satisfactory for EPS. We usually use two sheaths with a sidearm that is one size larger than the catheter so we can infuse medications and sedation without having to remove an electrode catheter. A slow, continuous flush must be maintained through the sheath to prevent clotting.

It is both possible and safe to insert two catheters percutaneously into the same femoral vein in infants as young as 6 months of age. When the first sheath is in position, it is elevated to approximately a 60° angle with skin, and the needle is inserted approximately 5 mm distal to the first sheath for placement of the second sheath. In older children, 3 or 4 sheaths may be placed in one vein.

Care must be taken to aspirate when removing the sheaths, because the catheter has been left in the same position for a long time, and clots may have formed between the catheter and sheath. We have not used routine systemic heparinization in our pediatric patients, and we have noted no problems with embolization. In patients with a right-to-left shunt, we heparinize with 70 U/kg at the beginning of the procedure.

The technique for inserting a sheath percutaneously into an antecubital vein is similar to that used in the groin, except the needle and wire are introduced before local anesthesia is infiltrated into the skin.[13] In our experience it has frequently been impossible to locate and enter the vein after local anesthesia has been introduced. We generally use a 21 gauge butterfly needle with a 0.018-inch diameter guide wire. In infants and young children we insert one sheath into a femoral vein and then give an additional dose of sedative drugs before attempting to place a catheter in the antecubital vein. Local anesthesia is infiltrated after the wire has been passed into the vein but before the sheath and dilator are inserted. We have been routinely successful in introducing a 5 French sheath into the antecubital vein of children as young as 12 months.

A plastic cannula for continuous monitoring of arterial pressure is inserted into a femoral artery in every patient undergoing EPS. Pulse oximetry is a useful additional monitoring modality.

Catheter Positioning

Catheters are positioned under fluoroscopic control while the electrographic recordings are observed. The catheter for recording the His bundle potential should have a 70°–90° bend, but never more (Fig. 6–1). The distance from the tip to the bend depends on the size of the patient's heart. The length of the curved tip should allow the

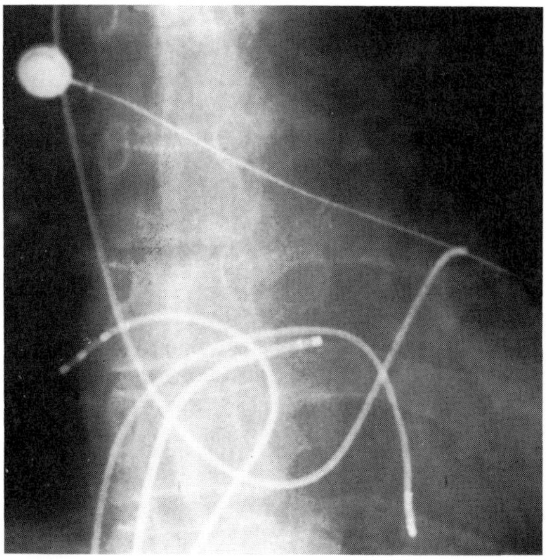

FIGURE 6–1
Anteroposterior roentgenogram showing the positioning of electrode catheters for the electrophysiologic study of a patient with supraventricular tachycardia. A surface ECG electrode and wire are superimposed. Four catheters are positioned in the heart. One passes from the superior vena cava to the right atrium, the coronary sinus, and to the left heart border for recording the distal and proximal coronary sinus electrograms. The catheter positioned against the high lateral wall of the right atrium has four electrodes: the distal two for stimulating and the proximal two for recording the high right atrial electrogram. The third catheter is positioned across the septal leaflet of the tricuspid valve and has three electrodes for recording the His bundle depolarization. The fourth catheter, positioned in the apex of the right ventricle via the inferior vena cava, has four electrodes: the distal two for stimulating and the proximal two for recording the right ventricular electrogram.

catheter to be placed with the electrodes just across the septal leaflet of the tricuspid valve when the catheter has been inserted from the femoral vein. The tip of the catheter should be pointing toward the left axilla in the posteroanterior projection (see Fig. 6–1). It should not be pointing caudad, as this would tend to record a right bundle-branch potential. Clockwise rotation of the catheter will position it against the septum, and a His bundle potential will be recorded. The catheter should be positioned across the tricuspid valve at the top (or cephalad) extent of the annulus. When the catheter is in a position thought likely to record a His bundle potential, the electrograms are observed (Fig. 6–2). If only a ventricular electrogram is recorded, then the catheter is too far into the ventricle; it should be withdrawn with clockwise rotation while the electrogram is watched on the oscilloscope. Often a very discrete appearing electrogram will be seen with slight withdrawal, but no atrial electrogram (or only a small one) will be seen. This is probably the right bundle-branch potential, and the catheter should be withdrawn further until the atrial and ventricular electrograms are of almost the same magnitude, with a discrete biphasic or triphasic potential between them. This will likely be the His bundle electrogram. His bundle pacing can be carried out by unplugging the electrodes from the junction box and plugging them into the pacemaker to determine if pacing and capture can be achieved with a stimulus to V interval the same as the potential to V interval that was previously recorded, but without causing aberration of the ventricular depolarization. Although His bundle pacing specifically confirms that the His bundle electrogram is being recorded, it is often not feasible because pacing of the adjacent ventricular myocardium can occur even though a His bundle potential is being recorded. Our experience indicates that adequate verification of recording of the His bundle potential is achieved by noting the nearly equal size of the atrial and ventricular depolarization. Once a His bundle potential is being recorded, the catheter will frequently stay in the same position for several hours. The size and morphology of the His bundle potential may vary with the respiratory cycle.

It is frequently useful to record a separate high right atrial electrogram to measure the internodal conduction time from the high right atrium to the low right atrium. The catheter should be positioned against the high lateral border of the right atrium; frequently it is possible to put a bend in the catheter to keep it positioned against the atrial wall. This also gives a separate atrial electrogram when the atrial and ventricular rhythms are dissociated, making it easier to define the atrial rhythm. The same catheter position can be used for right atrial pacing and for introducing premature atrial stimuli. A quadripolar electrode catheter should be used.

When the retrograde atrial activation sequence is needed, as in a study for supraventricular tachycardia (SVT), it is useful to record depolarization of the coronary sinus to delineate left atrial activation (see Fig. 6–1). Although it is often possible in pediatric patients to position a catheter in the left atrium through a patent foramen ovale, the coronary sinus offers several advantages. It

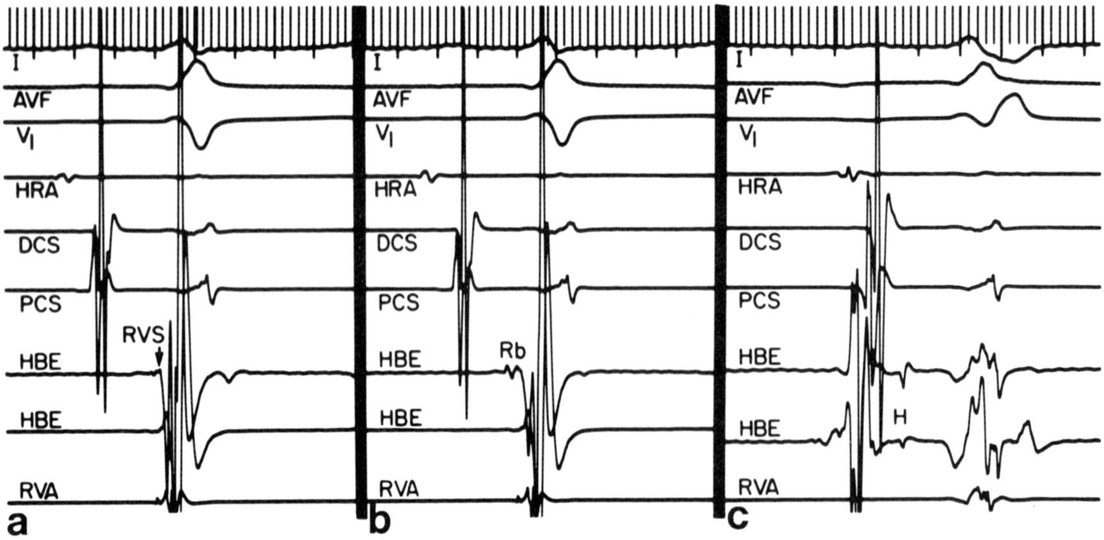

FIGURE 6–2

Three panels of intracardiac recordings showing the method of finding the His bundle depolarization. From top to bottom are 10-ms time lines, surface leads I, aVF, and V_1, high right atrium (HRA), distal coronary sinus (DCS), proximal coronary sinus (PCS), two His bundle leads (HBE), and right ventricular apex (RVA) electrograms. In panel *a* the His bundle catheter is positioned far into the right ventricle, with only ventricular depolarization (RVS) recorded. Note that no atrial or specialized conduction system potentials are recorded with this catheter position. In panel *b* the His bundle catheter has been withdrawn slightly with clockwise rotation, and a potential is recorded just before the ventricular depolarization. This is a right bundle branch potential (Rb). Still no atrial depolarization is seen. In panel *c* the catheter has been withdrawn further with continuing clockwise rotation. Now there is a large atrial depolarization on each HBE recording. There is also a His bundle depolarization (H) on each HBE recording. The potential-to-ventricle interval is considerably longer than the right bundle branch–to-ventricle interval.

is a reproducible and stable location for recording the left atrium, recording only the base of the left atrium close to the AV groove. When the catheter is introduced through a patent foramen ovale, several different parts of the left atrium may be recorded. The coronary sinus, although it records left atrial electrical activity, is not in the arterial system and does not present the problem of arterial embolization of clot material should it form on the catheter. The coronary sinus may be entered most easily by a left antecubital vein approach. A multipolar (10 to 14 electrodes) electrode catheter should be used with bipolar electrodes close together. Biplane fluoroscopy is a great help in positioning the catheter in the coronary sinus. The catheter is advanced pointing toward the spine in both the posteroanterior and the lateral projections (leftward and posterior). If only single plane fluoroscopy is available, counterclockwise rotation of a catheter in the left arm will move the catheter posteriorly. When using single plane fluoroscopy, the right anterior oblique projection is helpful. The coronary sinus catheter may also be positioned from the leg by aiming it in the same direction. It will likely be in the coronary sinus when it begins a vigorous vertical motion. This catheter also should have a 90° bend with the same distance from tip to bend as the His bundle catheter. The catheter will usually engage the mouth of the coronary sinus easily and with minimal rotation can be advanced to the left heart border. Care must be taken not to advance the catheter too vigorously, since the coronary sinus is a very thin-walled structure.

It is frequently useful to have a catheter positioned in the right ventricular apex for recording the right ventricular activation sequence and inducing single or multiple premature beats into the right ventricle. Again, a quadripolar electrode catheter is used. Ventricular stimulation is useful not only in the study of ventricular dysrhythmias but also in delineating concealed accessory AV connections that conduct only in the retrograde direction.

Generally, the high right atrial catheter and right ventricular catheter are used for both recording and stimulation. The distal two electrodes are used for stimulation, and the proximal two are used for recording. For the coronary sinus catheter, usually all electrodes are used for recording.

THE ELECTROPHYSIOLOGIC STUDY

Measurement of Intervals

Intervals should be measured only from records with stable baselines and discrete electrograms. Measuring poor quality tracings will result in serious errors and may lead to errors in patient management. The basic principle in measuring electrograms is to measure the first variation of the baseline greater than 45° from the beginning of each depolarization to the beginning of the next (Fig. 6–3). The high right atrial electrogram is measured from the beginning of the first visible depolarization recorded in the high right atrial lead. The low septal right atrial depolarization is measured on the same intracardiac lead as the His bundle electrograms. The His bundle potential is measured from the beginning of the first depolarization of the His bundle potential; it is usually separate from the atrial depolarization by at least a short isoelectric line. An exception to this is in the Lown-Ganong-Levine syndrome, in which the PR interval and the atrium to His (AH) interval are extremely short. In this instance it is sometimes difficult to separate the His bundle potential from the low right atrial potential.

The ventricular electrogram is measured at the beginning of ventricular depolarization. Usually, the earliest depolarization is found in the QRS complex on the four surface ECG leads. It is best to record leads I, aVF, V_1, and V_6 because one of these leads is likely to show the earliest ventricular activation. The ventricular activation on the His bundle electrogram has been used in the past as the beginning of the ventricular depolarization, but the right ventricular septal surface is often activated 20 ms to 60 ms later than the left ventricular septal surface (recorded by the Q wave on the ECG), which may lead to errors in measurement.

Other intra-atrial conduction intervals may also be measured (for instance, high right atrium and left atrium, from the beginning of the high right atrial depolarization to the beginning of the electrogram on the coronary sinus catheter). All parts of the atrium may be mapped in this manner. The ventricle to right ventricular apex (V-RVA) interval is measured from the beginning of ventricular depolarization on the surface ECG to the beginning of the ventricular electrogram recorded with the catheter positioned in the right ventricular apex.

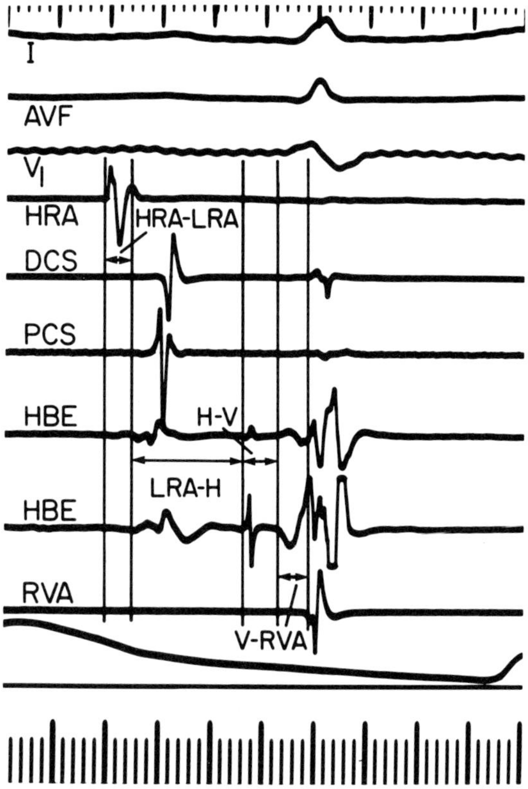

FIGURE 6–3

Measurements of intracardiac recordings. Shown are 10-ms time lines, surface leads I, aVF, and V_1, high right atrium (HRA), distal coronary sinus (DCS), proximal coronary sinus (PCS), two His bundle electrograms (HBE), and the right ventricular apex depolarization (RVA). The most frequently measured intervals are documented on this recording. The high right atrium to low right atrium interval (HRA–LRA) is measured from the beginning of the HRA depolarization to beginning of the LRA depolarization on the HBE. The LRA-His interval (LRA-H)—that is, the AV node conduction time—is measured from the beginning of the LRA depolarization to the beginning of the HBE depolarization. The His-ventricle interval (H-V)—that is, the His-Purkinje conduction time—is measured from the beginning of the HBE depolarization to the beginning of the ventricular depolarization on the surface ECG. The ventricle-to-right ventricular apex (V-RVA) conduction time is measured from the beginning of the ventricular depolarization on the surface ECG to the beginning of the right ventricular apical depolarization.

The high right atrium to low septal right atrium interval measures conduction from the sinus node to the AV node. The low septal right atrium to His interval is thought to measure AV node conduction time. The His to ventricle (HV) interval measures conduction from the proximal bundle of His to the ventricular myocardium. The V-RVA interval accurately reflects the conduction time of the right bundle branch. These intervals can also be measured by microcomputers during the electrophysiology study. Table 6–1 gives the normal values from our laboratory for the resting intervals derived from patients with no significant hemodynamic or electrophysiologic abnormalities.

Evaluation of Sinus Node Function

Evaluation of sinus node function is described in detail in Chapter 7 and will be reviewed only briefly here. Sinus node function is evaluated in the electrophysiology laboratory by recording the patient's resting sinus cycle length, noting the response of the sinus node to overdrive atrial pacing, and determining the sinoatrial conduction time.[14] Techniques are being developed for direct recording of the extracellular sinus node potential, which will allow the direct measurement of sinoatrial conduction time.[15] Intrinsic sinus node function measured after propranolol and atropine administration is also useful.

Evaluation of AV Node Function

AV node conduction time is represented on the intracardiac electrograms as the low septal right atrial to His bundle (LSRA-H) interval. The AV node also conducts in a retrograde fashion in most patients. It is generally not possible to measure the retrograde AV node conduction time (H-LSRA). Patients with marked abnormalities of AV node conduction will be found to have prolonged LSRA-H intervals on intracardiac recordings. Lesser degrees of AV node dysfunction may be detected by stressing the AV node with either continuous rapid atrial pacing or the introduction of single premature atrial extrastimuli. Rapid atrial pacing with determination of the rate at which second degree AV block occurs within the AV node (an atrial depoloarization not followed by a His bundle depolarization) is a useful method of evaluating AV node function. In children sedated by our method, 1:1 AV conduction should be maintained up to at least 180 bpm and is often maintained at rates greater than 200 bpm. The LSRA-H interval increases with increasing paced heart rate. The HV interval usually does not change with incremental rapid atrial pacing. It is mandatory to monitor the arterial blood pressure carefully during rapid atrial pacing because significant hypotension often develops with 1:1 conduction of rates above 200 bpm. In virtually every case the second degree AV block that occurs in response to rapid atrial pacing is of the Wenckebach or type I variety; i.e., there is progressive prolongation of the LSRA-H interval followed by a dropped beat. The Wenckebach sequence usually begins with a rather long cycle: 6:5 or 5:4 conduction. As the atrial pacing rate is increased, the Wenckebach sequences become shorter and shorter until eventually 2:1 AV block occurs. A 2:1 block without a preceding Wenckebach may indicate that the AV conduction is occurring in tissue other than the AV node (James fiber or Kent bundle). Block rarely occurs below the AV node ("block below the His") during incremental stimulation (Fig. 6–4).

Another method of evaluating AV node function is determination of the AV node effective and functional refractory periods by the extrastimulus technique. The clinically

TABLE 6–1
NORMAL CONDUCTION INTERVALS (n = 70)

AGE GROUP (Years)	CONDUCTION INTERVALS (MEAN ± 2 SD) (ms)*				
	Cycle Length	*HRA-V (PR)*	*HRA-LRA*	*LRA-H*	*HV*
<2	284–660	87–147	0–32	40–96	15–55
2–5	370–690	101–169	6–38	45–101	27–59
6–10	361–797	108–172	9–41	40–124	28–52
11–15	441–885	108–172	10–38	46–106	25–57
>15	504–1040	103–187	3–47	43–135	20–48

*The normal V-RVA conduction interval is 5–30 ms.

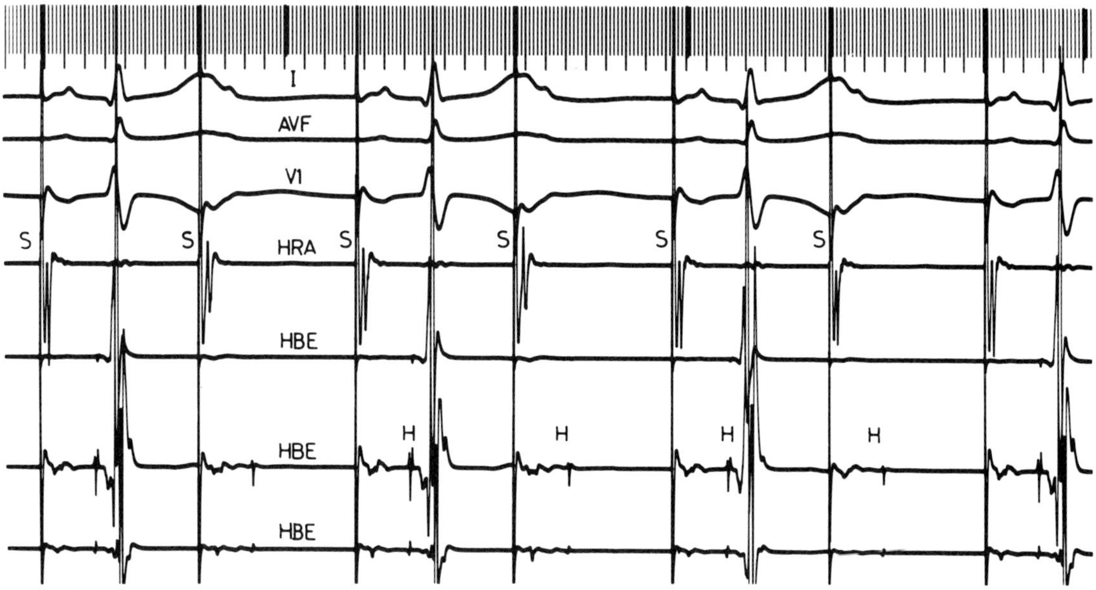

FIGURE 6–4

Electrogram documenting a 2:1 block below the bundle of His during atrial pacing at a cycle length of 400 ms, or a heart rate of approximately 150 bpm. Shown are 10-ms time lines and surface leads I, and V_1 recorded simultaneously with high right atrium (HRA) and three bipolar electrograms from a His bundle catheter (HBE). This catheter has four electrodes. The first HBE recording is from a distal pair of electrodes, the next is from the middle pair of electrodes, and the bottom recording is from the most proximal pair of electrodes. Thus the first recording is likely from the right bundle branch. There are two atrial depolarizations for each ventricular depolarization (H), and the PR interval of the second atrial depolarization is constant. The low right atrium to His interval is also constant for each beat, but there is no right bundle branch or ventricular depolarization recorded after alternate atrial paced beats (S), indicating 2:1 block below the His bundle. This is definitely an abnormal response at this cycle length.

determined refractory periods do not correlate exactly with the refractory periods measured in the microelectrode laboratory described in Chapter 2. The effective refractory period in the clinical electrophysiology laboratory is similar to the absolute refractory period measured in the microelectrode laboratory. The AV node refractory periods are determined by introducing single premature atrial depolarization into either a sinus rhythm or a basic paced rhythm. A minimum of eight beats of sinus or paced rhythm are allowed to occur between each premature beat. The first premature beat is given at a cycle length 20 ms shorter than the paced or sinus rhythm. The cycle length of the premature beat is then decreased in decrements of 10–20 ms. The last two paced or sinus beats, the premature beat, and two recovery beats are recorded for each premature atrial extrastimulus. The storage oscilloscope is very helpful at this point in determining if the electrograms recorded are of sufficient quality to determine the refractory periods. It is necessary to ensure that the His bundle potential does not decrease in amplitude to such a degree that the depolarization cannot be detected, which happens frequently with premature stimulation. If it does, the catheter must be repositioned so that a detectable His bundle depolarization is recorded both during the basic rhythm and with the premature stimulus. As the degree of prematurity is increased, the LSRA-H interval usually lengthens (Fig. 6–5). If the LSRA-H interval does not increase, a bypass tract through the James fiber or Kent bundle should be suspected.

The effective refractory period of the AV node is defined as the longest prematurity interval ($LSRA_1$-$LSRA_2$) that fails to result in a His bundle depolarization. Similarly, in any structure of the heart the effective refractory period is determined by premature stimulation and is reached when the premature stimulus fails to excite that structure. The functional refractory period can be thought of in terms of, "How close together can two impulses be and still be conducted by that structure?" It is thus defined by the shortest interval of structures stimulated distal to the point in question. The functional refractory period of the AV node is defined as the shortest H_1H_2 interval in response to a pre-

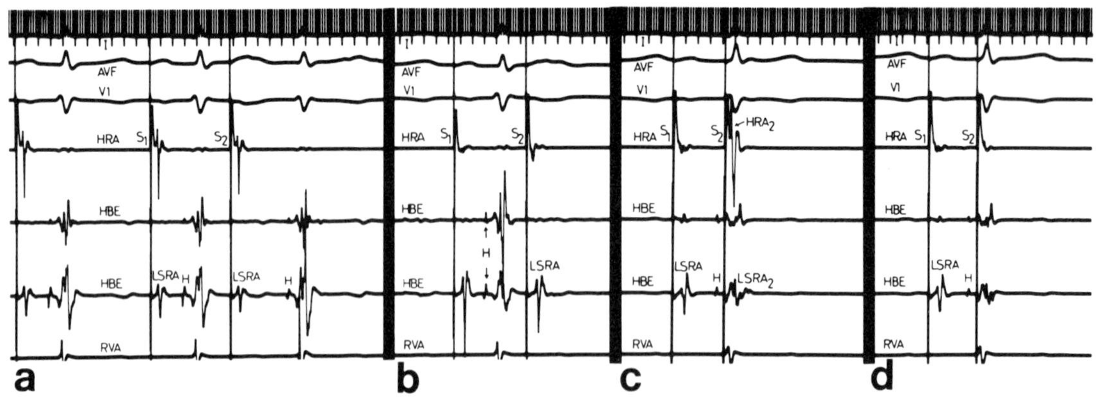

FIGURE 6–5
Demonstration of the mechanism for determining the AV node refractory periods. The four panels show 10-ms time lines, surface leads I, aVF, and V_1, high right atrium (HRA), two His bundle electrograms (HBE), and a right ventricular apical electrogram. The atrium is being paced at a steady cycle length, and progressively more premature atrial extrastimuli (S_2) are being introduced. In panel *a* a prolonged low septal right atrium to His (LSRA-H) interval has resulted from the S_2 stimulation, but conduction has occurred through the AV node to the bundle of His and the ventricle. In panel *b* the degree of prematurity has been shortened by 10 ms. The atrium is still captured and conduction occurs to the LSRA, but no conduction occurs to the bundle of His or the ventricles. Thus the AV node effective refractory period has been exceeded. In panel *c* the degree of prematurity has been shortened further. The atrium and the LSRA are still captured and conduction still does not occur to the His bundle or the ventricle. In panel *d* the degree of prematurity is 10 ms shorter than in the third panel. The HRA is no longer captured, and thus the atrial effective refractory period has been exceeded.

mature atrial stimulus (i.e., how close together the AV node transmits impulses to the His bundle). This concept can be clarified further by considering that in atrial fibrillation the functional refractory period of the AV node can be defined as the shortest two RR intervals found from the surface ECG. Since the earlier premature atrial extrastimuli result in greater degrees of AV node delay, the effective and functional refractory periods of the AV node do not occur at the same cycle length. The functional refractory period is always longer than the effective refractory period, sometimes to a large degree. In 15% to 20% of patients, the atrial effective refractory period occurs before the AV node effective refractory period (i.e., there is failure to capture the right atrium at a degree of prematurity that still allows AV node conduction). In these patients the effective refractory period of the AV node cannot be determined. The functional refractory period of the AV node can be determined in some of the them, however, because if the H_1H_2 has begun to get longer (i.e., has reached its lowest value) the functional refractory period has already been determined.

The refractory periods of all cardiac structures are cycle length dependent; therefore it is often useful to determine the refractory periods at sinus cycle length and at one or two additional faster-paced cycle lengths. At faster pacing rates, the AV node effective and functional refractory periods are prolonged, but the atrial and ventricular effective refractory periods are shortened. Thus if the atrial muscle limits refractoriness during sinus rhythm, pacing at a faster cycle length may unmask the AV node refractory period. The AV node functional refractory period has been shown to have a good correlation with the atrial paced rate at which second degree AV block occurs, whereas the AV node effective refractory period does not correlate as well with this value. The AV node functional refractory period was also found to be markedly prolonged in three patients with severe first degree AV block and an otherwise normal heart. It appears that the AV node functional refractory period has the best correlation with the actual clinical status of the AV node.

Refractory Periods of the His-Purkinje System

In only 10% to 20% of patients is it possible to measure the refractory period of the structures between the proximal bundle of His and the ventricular myocardium. Since the AV node or atrial muscle frequently has a

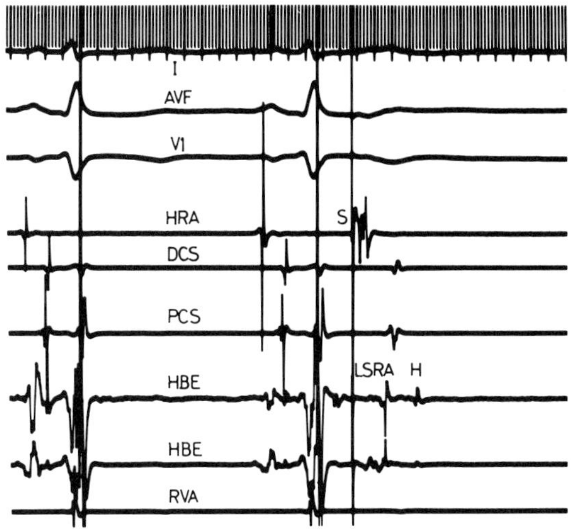

FIGURE 6–6
Demonstration of determination of the effective refractory period of the distal His-Purkinje system. Shown are surface leads I, aVF, and V_1, high right atrium (HRA), distal coronary sinus (DCS), proximal coronary sinus (PCS), two His bundle electrograms (HBE), and right ventricular apex (RVA) electrogram. Two sinus beats are shown, followed by a premature atrial extrastimulus (S). The S captures the HRA, conducts to the low septal right atrium (LSRA) and left atrium, and conducts to the bundle of His (H) with a small delay in the AV node. The His bundle depolarization is not followed by ventricular depolarization, indicating block below the His bundle and documenting the effective refractory period of the His-Purkinje system.

longer refractory period than does the His-Purkinje system, the AV node refractory period or the atrial muscle refractory period is reached before the refractory period of the His-Purkinje system; i.e., the only way to determine the refractory period of the His-Purkinje system is if "block below the His" occurs. The effective refractory period of the His-Punkinje system is defined as the longest H_1H_2 interval that fails to conduct to the ventricle (Fig. 6–6). Therefore in response to a premature atrial stimulus, the atrium and the His bundle would depolarize, but there would be no resulting ventricular depolarization. The functional refractory period of the His-Purkinje system is the shortest V_1V_2 interval obtainable by premature stimulation of the atrium.

The refractory periods of the individual bundle branches can be measured in a small number of patients (Fig. 6–7). This happens when conduction occurs to the AV node, the bundle of His, and the ventricle in response to a premature atrial stimulus, but results in a bundle-branch block pattern on the surface ECG. The effective refractory period of the bundle branch is the longest H_1H_2 interval that fails to conduct through that bundle branch as determined by the pattern on the surface ECG.

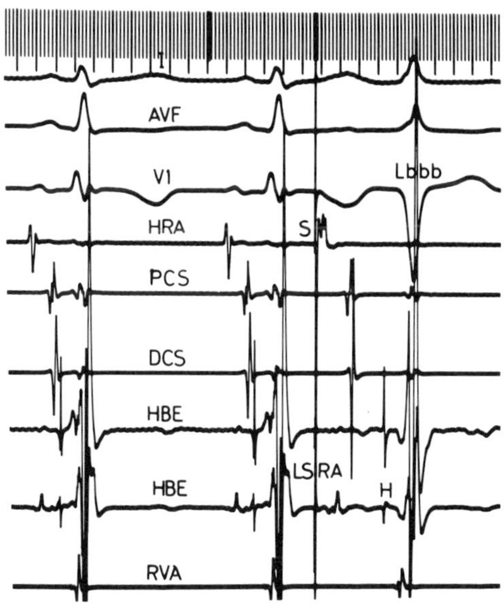

FIGURE 6–7
Demonstration of determination of the left bundle branch refractory period. Shown are surface leads I, aVF, and V_1, high right atrium (HRA), proximal and distal coronary sinus (PCS and DCS), two His bundle electrograms (HBE), and right ventricular apex (RVA) electrogram. Two sinus beats are followed by a premature atrial extrastimulus (S). A small delay in conduction is noted between the low septal right atrium (LSRA) and the His bundle depolarization (H). The H is followed at a normal interval by ventricular depolarization, but a left bundle branch block (LBBB) pattern is detected on the surface ECG, indicating that the left bundle branch effective refractory period has been exceeded.

Refractory Period of the Atrial and Ventricular Muscle and Accessory Connection

Refractory periods of the atrial and ventricular muscle may also be determined by the extrastimulus technique. The refractory period of these tissues is defined as the longest stimulus-to-stimulus interval that fails to capture the particular structure being stimulated. The functional refractory periods of the atrial and ventricular myocardium are determined as the shortest intervals that can be achieved by stimulating each structure. Thus if the high right atrium is being stimulated, the functional refractory period is the shortest $LSRA_1$-$LSRA_2$ in response to stimulation. As with the AV node, the functional refractory period is always longer than the effective refractory period, but the difference between the two is not as great. The antegrade refractory period of an accessory connection (AC) is defined by the longest interval between two atrial stimuli that fails to conduct through the AC. For example, the effective refractory period of a Kent bundle is the longest A_1A_2 that fails to conduct with a delta wave.

Retrograde Refractory Periods

The retrograde refractory period of the AV specialized conduction system (AV node, bundle of His, and bundle branches) is not usually the same as the antegrade refractory period. Therefore if it is necessary to know the function in both directions (e.g., to determine drug effect in SVT), the period must be tested separately in each direction. The technique for testing the retrograde refractory period of the AV conduction system is basically the same as for testing it in the antegrade direction, except that the pacing is carried out in the ventricle, usually the right ventricular apex (Fig. 6–8). Recording is made in the His bundle area so that clear atrial, His bundle, and ventricular deflections can be seen during sinus rhythm. During ventricular pacing the His bundle potential is usually not seen, but in some cases it may be seen between a ventricular pacing spike and the ventricular depolarization on the His bundle electrogram. With moderate degrees of prematurity of the ventricular extrastimulus, the retrograde His reflection occurs later than the end of ventricular depolarization in some patients. With further increases in prematurity, in most patients a degree of prematurity will be found at which the ventricle is captured, but there is no retrograde conduction to the atrium. If the retrograde His depolarization has been visible, it can be determined where this block has occurred; otherwise it must be stated that block occurred in the AV specialized conduction system.

The retrograde AV node conduction time is represented by the retrograde His deflection to low septal right atrial depolarization during ventricular pacing. It is not always possible to measure this interval, since the retrograde His deflection is often obscured by the ventricular muscle depolarization. In 15% to 20% of adult patients with intact antegrade conduction, there is no retrograde conduction from ventricle to atrium. This can be determined by continuous ventricular pacing and noting that the atrial cycle length continues the same as the preceding sinus cycle length while the ventricular pacing rate is faster (AV dissociation). In an additional 15% of adult patients, retrograde conduction appears to take place over some structure other than the AV node, probably either a retrograde Kent bundle that does not function in the antegrade direction or a retrograde bypass fiber from the bundle of His directly into the atrium. This can be determined by the fact that the ventricle to atrium (VA) interval remains short and constant at all cycle lengths of ventricular stimulation. The refractory period of this AC may be longer or shorter than that of the ventricular muscle, so that block may occur in the retrograde conduction before the ventricular muscle refractory period is reached; or, in many of these cases, the ventricular muscle refractory period is reached before block occurs in the retrograde conduction.

The presence of a retrograde AC can also be documented by recording a discontinuous ventriculoatrial conduction curve. For example, a VA interval that remains constant for one-half or two-thirds of the cycle lengths of ventricular extrastimulation, then suddenly increases, and then gradually increases further with a concomitant change in atrial activation sequence is indicative of conduction over an AC with a longer refractory period than the retrograde refractory period of the AV node. If a retrograde Wenckebach periodicity can be demonstrated in VA conduction during continuous ventricular pacing, the conduction is most likely through the AV node (Fig. 6–9).

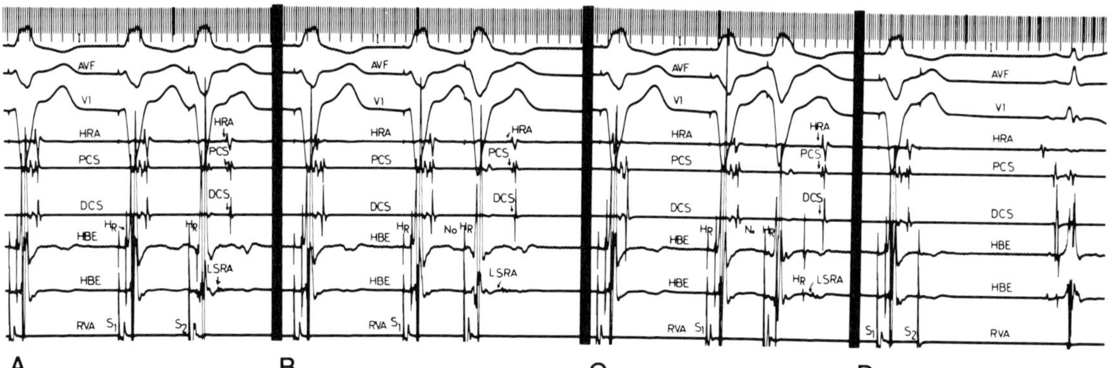

FIGURE 6–8

Determination of retrograde effective refractory periods. Shown are simultaneously recorded surface leads I, aVF, and V_1, high right atrium (HRA), proximal coronary sinus (PCS), distal coronary sinus (DCS), His bundle lead (HBE), and right ventricular apex (RVA) electrograms during ventricular pacing with ventricular premature stimulation (S). In panel *A* are shown two ventricular paced beats followed by a ventricular premature beat, each of which is given in the RVA. During both the basic ventricular drive beats and the premature beat, a retrograde His bundle depolarization (H_R) can be seen between the pacemaker spike and the ventricular depolarization, indicating that rapid conduction has occurred retrograde in the right bundle branch to depolarize the bundle of His. A retrograde atrial depolarization is seen after each ventricular depolarization, and the retrograde activation sequence is normal: low septal right atrium (LSRA) before PCS, PCS before DCS and HRA. In panel *B,* the degree of prematurity has been shortened, and no retrograde His bundle depolarization can be seen. Delay has occurred somewhere between the ventricular pacing site and the atrium, as documented by the increase in ventriculoatrial conduction time when compared with panel *A.* In panel *C* the degree of prematurity has been shortened further. The retrograde His bundle depolarization is now seen following the ventricular depolarization, and the retrograde AV node conduction time can be determined from the H-LSRA depolarization. In panel *D,* the ventricular muscle refractory period has been exceeded, and the S_2 stimulus fails to capture the ventricle. Thus in this patient it was not possible to record the retrograde refractory period of either the AV node or the distal specialized conduction system, because the ventricular muscle refractory period was longer than that of these structures.

Interpretation of Electrophysiologic Studies

In order to determine if resting function of the conduction system is normal, the measured intervals are compared to normal intervals established for similar conditions. Since methods of sedation vary markedly, each laboratory must establish its own normal limits. We have determined normal limits for sedation with meperidine, chlorpromazine, and promethazine; these determinations were made before angiography was performed in the patient. The subjects were children with suspected congenital heart lesions who were later documented to be normal, children with an insignificant cardiac lesion (such as pulmonary stenosis with 10–20 mmHg gradient or a bicuspid aortic valve), or children with pulmonary vascular abnormalities who were undergoing pulmonary angiography (see Table 6–1).

Normal values have also been established for sinus node recovery time and sinoatrial conduction time for the evaluation of sinus node function; these are given in Chapter 7. The effects of sedation are more marked on sinus node function than on AV node function; thus it is particularly important to use normal values reflecting the conditions of the study. The AV refractory period measurements are age related. Normal values have been established by Dubrow et al for AV refractory periods in three age groups of children.[16] Our normal values (Table 6–2) basically agree with those of Dubrow et al. By comparing each measurement or calculation for a particular patient with established normal values, it is possible to determine whether each index of function is normal or abnormal. The degree of abnormality may also be determined. Each study must be individualized to the needs of the particular patient, but the evaluation of each patient should be as complete as possible. We have found concealed ACs in several patients evaluated for other problems, such as apparently isolated sinus node dysfunction.

Anatomic Site of Dysrhythmia

In some types of dysrhythmias, such as second or third degree AV block, the ana-

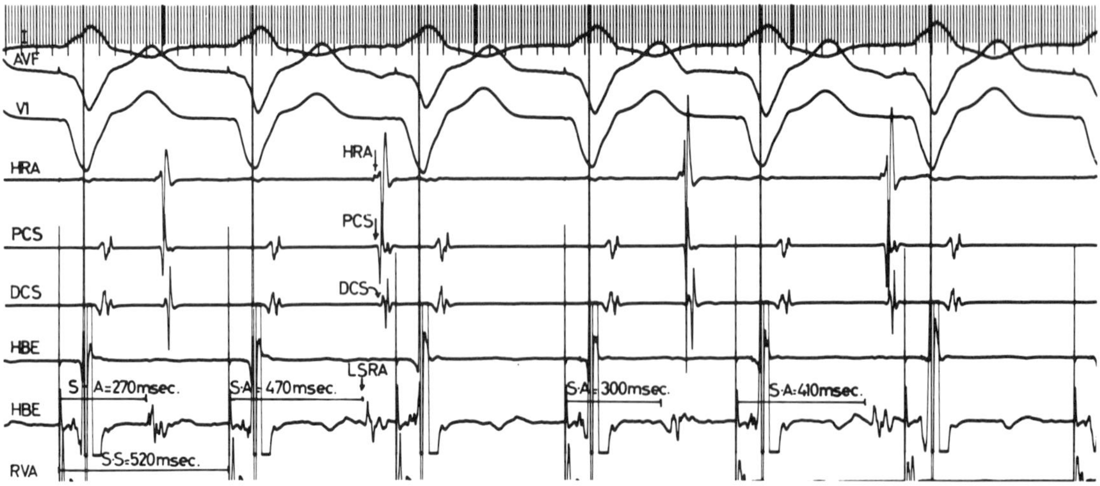

FIGURE 6–9
Demonstration of retrograde Wenckebach type I AV block. Shown are surface ECG leads I, aVF, and V_1, high right atrium (HRA), proximal and distal coronary sinus (PCS and DCS), His bundle (HBE), and right ventricular apex (RVA) electrograms. The ventricles are being paced at a steady cycle length (S-S) of 520 ms. The ventricle to atrium conduction time (S–A) increases from 270 ms to 470 ms between the first and second ventricular depolarizations. The third ventricular depolarization is not followed by an atrial depolarization. The sequence is then repeated with different retrograde conduction times. These are retrograde conducted beats, documented by the normal retrograde atrial activation sequence.

tomic location of the block may be of more prognostic significance than the mechanism. In the past great emphasis was placed on differentiating Mobitz I from Mobitz II second degree AV block because the mechanism suggested the site of block. Now the anatomic location of the block can frequently be determined by EPS, and the mechanism appears to be less important.[17, 18] For instance, in a patient with complete AV block, if His bundle depolarization is found preceding each ventricular depolarization but is not found following each atrial depolarization, the block can be said to be in the AV node (Fig. 6–10). On the other hand, if a His bundle depolarization follows each atrial depolarization and also precedes each ventricular depolarization, the block can be said to be within the bundle of His. Block within the His bundle frequently shows a normal QRS complex and thus cannot be distinguished on the surface

TABLE 6–2
NORMAL VALUES FOR AV NODE EFFECTIVE AND FUNCTIONAL REFRACTORY PERIODS (MEAN ± 2 SD) (ms) (n = 31)

CYCLE LENGTH GROUP	CYCLE LENGTH	EFFECTIVE REFRACTORY PERIOD	FUNCTIONAL REFRACTORY PERIOD
>600	353–1137	148–395	285–501
450–599	441–605	135–295	204–452
<450	252–468	126–238	195–359

ECG from AV node block, which also has a normal QRS complex.[17] Block below the His bundle, characterized by a His bundle depolarization following each atrial depolarization, is almost universally associated with a wide QRS complex on the surface ECG.

The anatomic location of a right bundle-branch block can be localized by measuring the ventricle to right ventricular apex (RVA) conduction time.[19] A prolonged V-RVA conduction time indicates a proximal right bundle-branch block.

The site of origin of premature beats is also easily determined from an intracardiac electrophysiologic recording. Premature atrial beats have both an atrial and a His bundle depolarization preceding the ventricular depolarization. Ventricular premature depolarizations have neither an atrial nor a His bundle depolarization preceding them. The only sure way to differentiate aberrantly conducted premature junctional beats from premature ventricular beats is by His bundle recording (Fig. 6–11).

Tachydysrhythmia

The mechanism of a patient's tachydysrhythmia and the anatomic site are equally important, and both may be determined dur-

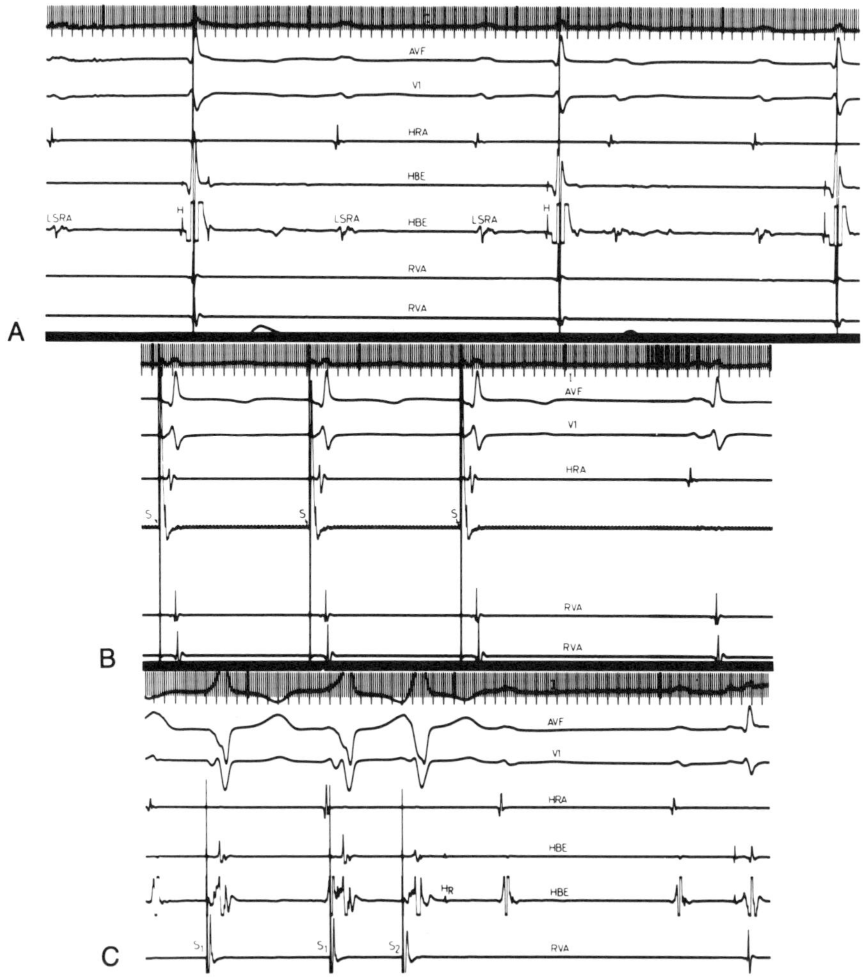

FIGURE 6–10

Demonstration of complete AV block in the AV node. Panel *A* shows leads I, aVF, and V_1, high atrium (HRA), two His bundle electrograms (HBE), and two right ventricular apex (RVA) electrograms. There is complete AV dissociation with a constant RR interval and a different constant PP interval. There are no His bundle depolarizations following the low septal right atrium (LSRA) depolarizations, but there is a His bundle depolarization (H) with a normal HV interval preceding each ventricular depolarization. His bundle pacing is shown in panel *B*. The His bundle leads have been disconnected from the recorder and connected to the pacemaker. Pacing is being carried out at a rate faster than the inherent junctional escape rate. The stimulus (S) to ventricle interval is the same as the previously recorded His to ventricle interval. The QRS complexes have not been changed by the His bundle pacing. In panel *C* ventricular pacing with premature ventricular stimulation has been carried out. A retrograde His bundle depolarization (H_R) can be seen following the ventricular premature stimulation.

ing EPS. The principles used in interpreting clinical EPS are founded in the basic electrophysiologic principles outlined in Chapter 2. There are three mechanisms for tachydysrhythmias: reentry, abnormal automaticity, and triggered dysrhythmia.

Reentry. When a single impulse enters a closed circuit through which it conducts more than once, the mechanism is termed *reentry*. In order for an impulse to reenter, one of the circuits must have different electrophysiologic properties. Generally, a reentry circuit is depicted as a diamond (Fig. 6–12), and two legs of the diamond (or "pathways") have different properties. One of these properties is the absolute refractory period. Once a cell is depolarized, a certain period of time is necessary for that cell to recover before it can again depolarize. This length of time is called the absolute refractory period. If the absolute refractory period of one side of the reentry circuit is longer than that of the other side, and if an impulse arrives at such a time that one side is in the refractory period and the other side is not, then the impulse will conduct through one side and not through

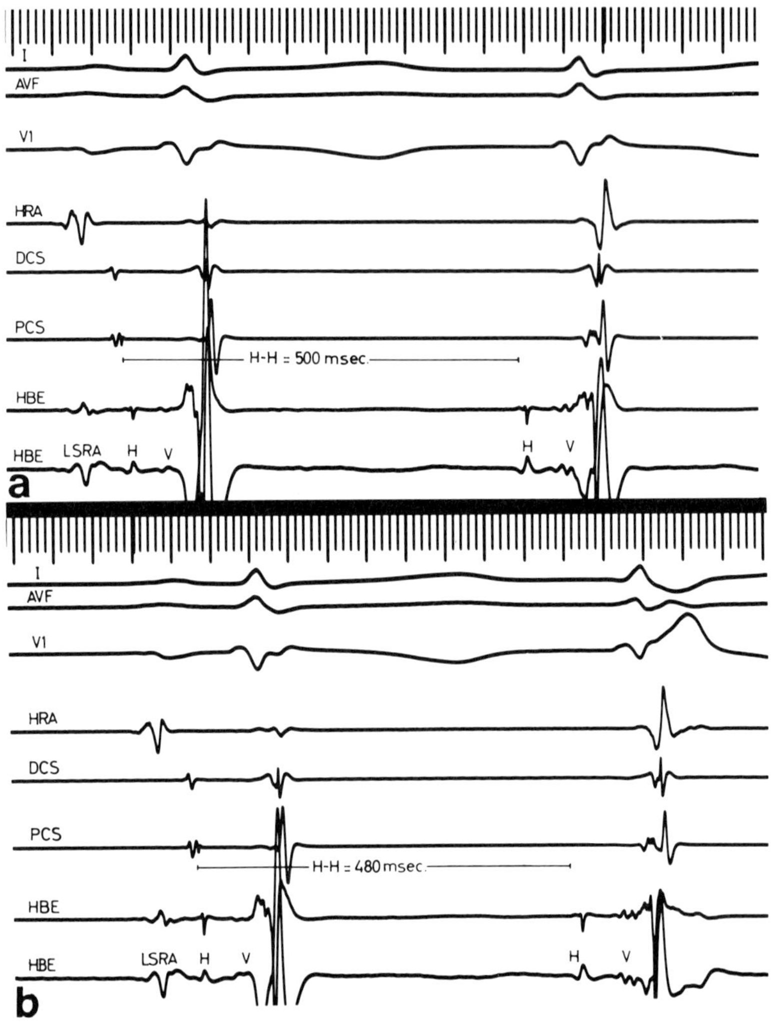

FIGURE 6–11
Demonstration of His bundle premature depolarizations (junctional premature depolarizations). In panel *a* surface leads I, aVF, and V_1, high right atrium (HRA), distal coronary sinus (DCS), proximal coronary sinus (PCS), and two His bundle electrograms (HBE) are recorded. The first beat is a sinus beat with normal activation sequence and conduction times from the HRA to the ventricle (V). The second beat occurs with an H_1H_2 interval of 500 ms. This is a premature His bundle (H) extrasystole, demonstrated by the H preceding the QRS with no atrial depolarization preceding the QRS. The morphology of the QRS depolarization is unchanged from the sinus beat. in panel *b* the same electrograms are recorded; again the first beat is a sinus beat. The second beat, with an H_1H_2 interval of 480 ms, is again a His bundle depolarization, because the H precedes the V and the HV interval is normal. Right bundle branch block aberration has occurred because this degree of prematurity apparently exceeded the right bundle branch refractory period. Intracardiac electrophysiology is the only method of determining whether such complexes as seen on the surface ECG are premature ventricular depolarizations or junctional with aberration.

the other (Fig. 6–12). This block alone does not allow reentry; slow conduction must also exist. If the impulse is slowed in the antegrade conducting limb sufficiently to delay its arrival at the distal end of the blocked limb beyond the absolute refractory period of the blocked limb, then retrograde conduction can occur through the previously blocked limb and reentry can occur (see Fig. 6–12[D]). This is the phenomenon of "unidirectional block" and implies that an impulse may not conduct in an antegrade direction in a fiber, but if the impulse arrives at the other end of the fiber with sufficient delay, the fiber may conduct in a retrograde direction.

A reentry circuit in SVT may be small and consist of a few atrial cells, or it may be large and involve the AV node and an accessory connection. The interface between the sinus node and atrial muscle provides such an area and may result in sinus node reentry SVT. The AV node has been shown in certain patients to react as if it consisted of two parallel columns of cells with separate electrophysiologic properties, one with a shorter refractory period and slow conduction (the so-called "alpha" pathway) and the other with a longer refractory period and rapid conduction (the so-called "beta" pathway).[20] The most common type of AV node reentry SVT occurs using the alpha pathway in an antegrade direction and the beta pathway in the retrograde direction. Similar differences in properties can exist in the normal bundle of His and in atrial muscle. Fibrosis resulting from either prior cardiac surgery, myocarditis, or stretch and hypertrophy may increase the difference in properties and, along with this difference, the likelihood of reentry.

Reentry involving normal anatomic structures of the heart (sinus node, atrial muscle,

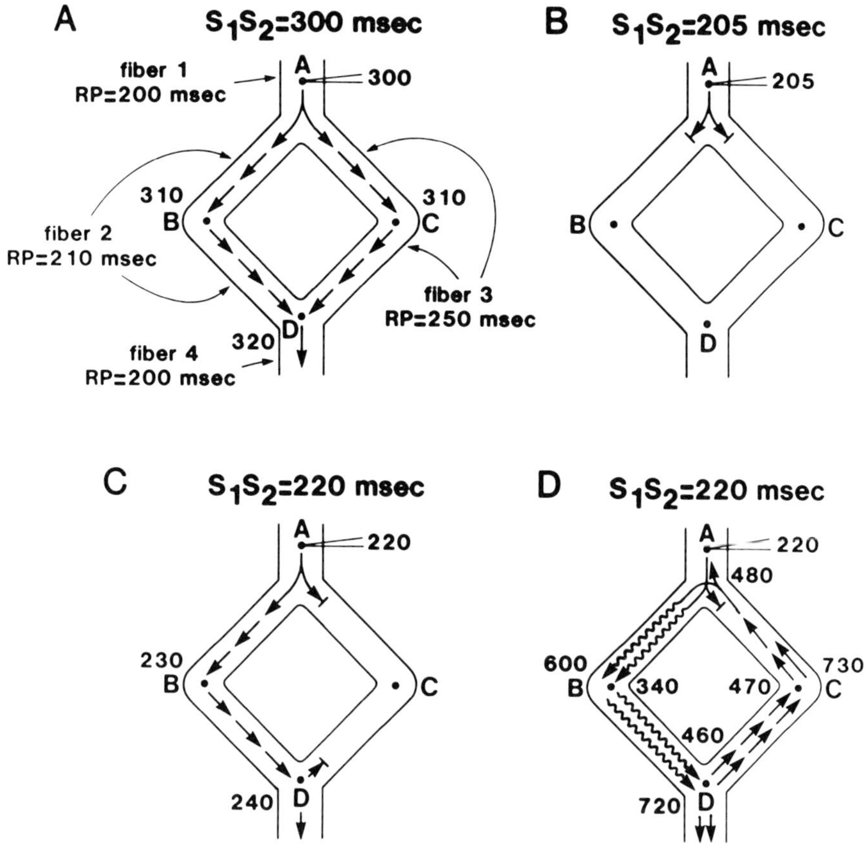

FIGURE 6–12
Electrophysiologic mechanism of reentry. Assume that four muscle fibers are located in the atrium and that these fibers may have different properties. Fiber 1 and fiber 4 have absolute refractory periods (RPs) of 200 ms. In between these fibers are two other fibers, fiber 2 with an RP of 210 ms and fiber 3 with an RP of 250 ms. In panel *A* a premature stimulus is delivered 300 ms after a basic drive stimulus (S_1S_2 = 300 ms). The RPs of both fibers 2 and 3 are less than 300 ms; thus the impulse arrives at point B in fiber 2 310 ms after the last drive stimulus (10 ms after S_2) and, with the same conduction velocity in fiber 3, arrives at point C at the same time. Fiber 4 is excited 10 ms later. in panel *B*, the S_1S_2 interval is 205 ms. Therefore fiber 1 will propagate the impulse (RP 200 ms), but neither fiber 2 nor fiber 3 will propagate the impulse, because each is still refractory. In panel *C*, the S_1S_2 interval is 220 ms. This situation allows for propagation through fiber 2 but not fiber 3. Conduction through fiber 2 is normal, and the impulse arrives at point D in 20 ms (240 ms after the last driven stimulus). Fiber 3 is unable to propagate the impulse even in the retrograde direction, because the RP of fiber 3 is 250 ms and fiber 3 therefore has not recovered the ability to propagate an impulse. In panel *D*, S_1S_2 is again 220 ms (identical to that of panel *C*), but conduction is slowed in fiber 2 such that the impulse arrives at point D 460 ms after the last driven impulse. This is well beyond the RP of fiber 3 (250 ms), and thus fiber 3 conducts retrograde past point C to point A. The impulse arrives at point A 480 − 220 = 260 ms after the last impulse has propagated; thus fiber 2 can again be excited. Thus a reentry circuit is established because two properties coexist: slow conduction (in fiber 2) and "unidirectional block" in a fiber (fiber 3) because of the difference in refractory periods.

AV node, bundle of His) will be referred to as reentry without a bypass tract. Reentry with a bypass tract uses as one of the pathways an abnormal anatomic structure such as an accessory AV connection (Kent bundle), atrio-His fiber (James fiber), or fasciculoventricular connection (Mahaim). In these instances the AV node is usually the antegrade pathway, with a relatively short refractory period and long conduction delay, and the bypass tract is the retrograde pathway, with a relatively long refractory period and rapid conduction.

Abnormal Automaticity. The property of spontaneous self-excitation has been called automaticity.[21] Cells that possess this property are said to be "automatic," and they have the capability of being the pacemaker of the heart. The normal resting membrane potential of such cells is approximately −60 mV; these cells undergo spontaneous diastolic depolarization during phase 4 of the action potential. When the threshold level is reached, a more rapid depolarization begins during phase 0. With normal pacemaker cells, this depolarization during phase 0 is relatively slower than for cells that do not normally spontaneously depolarize (e.g., Purkinje cells) (Fig. 6–13). With normal pacemaker cells the action potential upstroke during phase 0 is caused by a calcium current. This has been called "slow" action potential because the upstroke in these cells is relatively slow. The rate of firing a normal pacemaker cell is determined by three properties of the action potential: the maximum diastolic potential, the threshold potential, and the slope of phase 4. Of these properties, the slope of phase 4 seems to be the most important. Sinus node cells have the most rapid diastolic depolarization and are normally those with the most rapid rate of firing. All other cardiac cells respond to this rapid rate with hyperpolarization. The more rapid the pacemaker rate, the greater is the hyperpolarization of the other cardiac cells. This is the phenomenon of "overdrive suppression." Cells in other areas of the heart (atrium, AV junction, or ventricle) may begin to fire at a rate faster than the sinus node and become the pacemaker. These cells normally have a resting membrane potential of approximately −90 mV and a slower spontaneous diastolic depolarization rate. The depolarization during phase 0 of the action potential is rapid and is largely carried by a sodium current (Fig. 6–13). Because of the rapid upstroke, this type of action has been called "fast" action potential.

These fast action potentials may change either because of cellular injury or through changes in the extracellular fluid composition (e.g., because of body electrolyte changes or drugs). Two types of change may generally be observed in such action potentials: either they can retain their normal maximum diastolic potential of −90 mV and develop spontaneous diastolic depolarization, or they can change the form of the action potential entirely to appear similar to a slow action potential with both reduced maximum diastolic potential and spontaneous diastolic depolarization. Cells that develop only spontaneous diastolic depolarization respond to drugs such as lidocaine that affect fast action potentials. Cells that also develop a change in resting membrane potential respond to verapamil, since it has an effect only on slow action potentials. This response to drugs is the only present method of determining if abnormal automaticity is caused by a cell with a fast or slow action potential.

Triggered Dysrhythmia. When a cell develops diastolic depolarization (automaticity) in response to the introduction of a stimulus (trigger), the result is "triggered dysrhythmia."[22] This type of diastolic depolarization is called a "delayed afterdepolarization" and is caused by an oscillation in membrane potential at the end of phase 3 of the action potential (Fig. 6–14). In cells with delayed afterdepolarization there is an "overshoot" of the resting membrane potential, resulting in a transient hyperpolarization. When membrane potential "rebounds" from this hyperpolarization, the result is a depolarization (the delayed afterdepolarization). This depolarization can be subthreshold or can reach threshold and result in another action potential. The magnitude of the afterdepolariza-

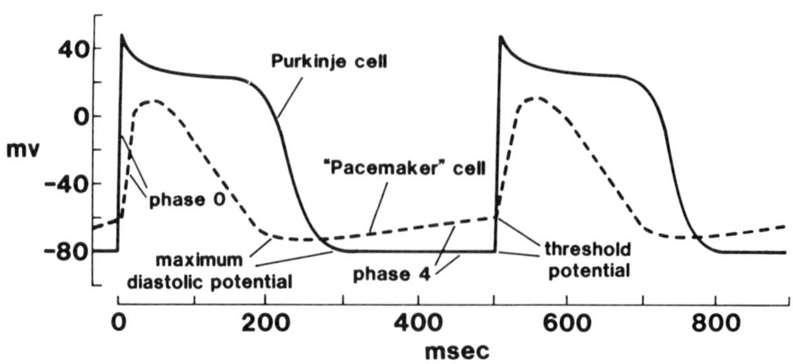

FIGURE 6–13

Diagrammatic action potentials of cardiac cells. The pacemaker cells such as those found in the sinus node (dotted line) have maximum diastolic potential of about —60 mV and undergo spontaneous diastolic depolarization (phase 4 potential moves toward 0). The Purkinje cells (solid line) have a more negative maximum diastolic potential, have a more rapid rise of phase 0 (more vertical), and do not normally undergo significant spontaneous diastolic depolarization.

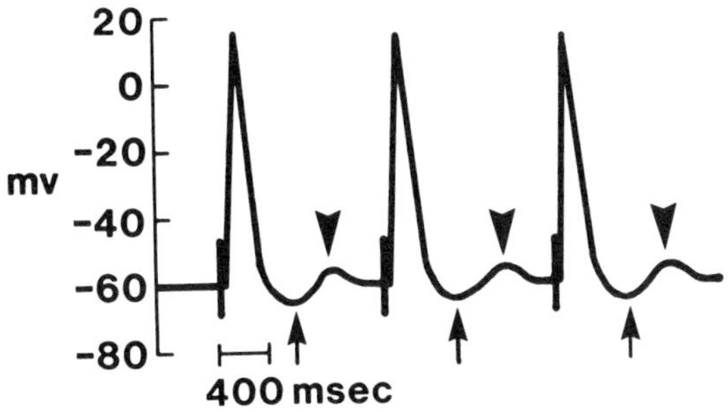

FIGURE 6–14
Diagrammatic action potentials from mitral valve cells being paced at a cycle length of 1250 ms. The arrows show transient hyperpolarization, and the arrowheads show afterdepolarization. (Redrawn from Wit AL, Weiss MB, Berkowitz WD, et al: Patterns of A-V conduction in the human heart. Circ Res 27:345–352, 1970.)

tion depends on the frequency of the stimuli initiating the action potentials: if the drive rate is high, the afterdepolarization is more likely to reach threshold. For this reason a single afterdepolarization that reaches threshold is likely to give rise to a train of afterdepolarizations, because the interval from the last driven action potential to the action potential caused by the afterdepolarization will be shorter than the basic driven interval and an even larger afterdepolarization will result (Fig. 6–15).

Delayed afterdepolarization can occur in normal cardiac muscle fibers isolated from the coronary sinus and mitral valve.[22] Delayed afterdepolarizations are inhibited by acetylcholine and verapamil and enhanced by digitalis and catecholamines; sustained afterdepolarizations are inhibited by overdrive suppression. On the basis of these findings, Wit et al have postulated that delayed afterdepolarizations are at least partially caused by a calcium current and that inhibition of the sodium-potassium pump increases the magnitude of the current.[23]

Clinical Evaluation of Tachydysrhythmias. For the basic scientist studying cardiac cells with microelectrodes, the distinction among mechanisms of SVT is relatively clear-cut compared with the work required of the clinical electrophysiologist, who must infer the mechanisms from studies made during cardiac catheterization. Only rarely can all the basic electrophysiologic criteria be met and the mechanism established with certainty. One such example is the reentry SVT resulting from the classic Wolff-Parkinson-White (WPW) syndrome. The two basic electrophysiologic criteria for reentry are as follows:

1. Unidirectional block can be demonstrated. We have direct evidence of unidirectional block on the surface ECG because this impulse conducts with a normal QRS (without a delta wave) (Fig. 6–16). During SVT, unidirectional block is continually evidenced by a narrow QRS complex.
2. Slow conduction can be shown directly in the reentry circuit, because antegrade conduction through the AV node is demonstrably slowed (evidenced by the abnormally prolonged AH interval). Therefore in this case, reentry can be directly demonstrated.

In most cases, however, the mechanism can be only indirectly demonstrated by observing how the tachycardia is initiated, how the tachycardia responds to electrophysiologic and pharmacologic perturbation, and how the tachycardia is terminated. Table 6–3 contains a series of 10 points that help to differentiate among the types of response observed. We have labeled these clinical responses the same as the basic mechanisms (e.g., reentry, abnormal automaticity, trig-

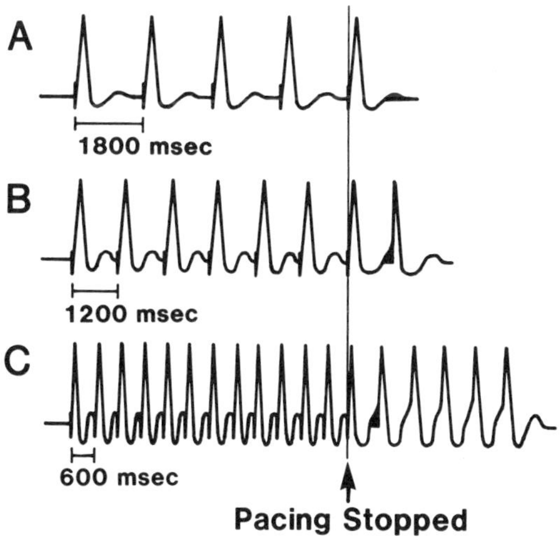

FIGURE 6–15
Diagrammatic representation of change in afterdepolarizations with change in rate of driving stimulus. In panel *A*, the preparation is driven at a cycle length of 1800 ms; when pacing is stopped, a small afterdepolarization results (darkened area). In panel *B*, at a more rapid drive rate, the afterdepolarization (darkened) is sufficient to exceed the threshold, and one action potential is caused by the afterdepolarization. In panel *C*, at the fastest rate, several action potentials occur because of afterdepolarizations that occur when pacing is terminated.

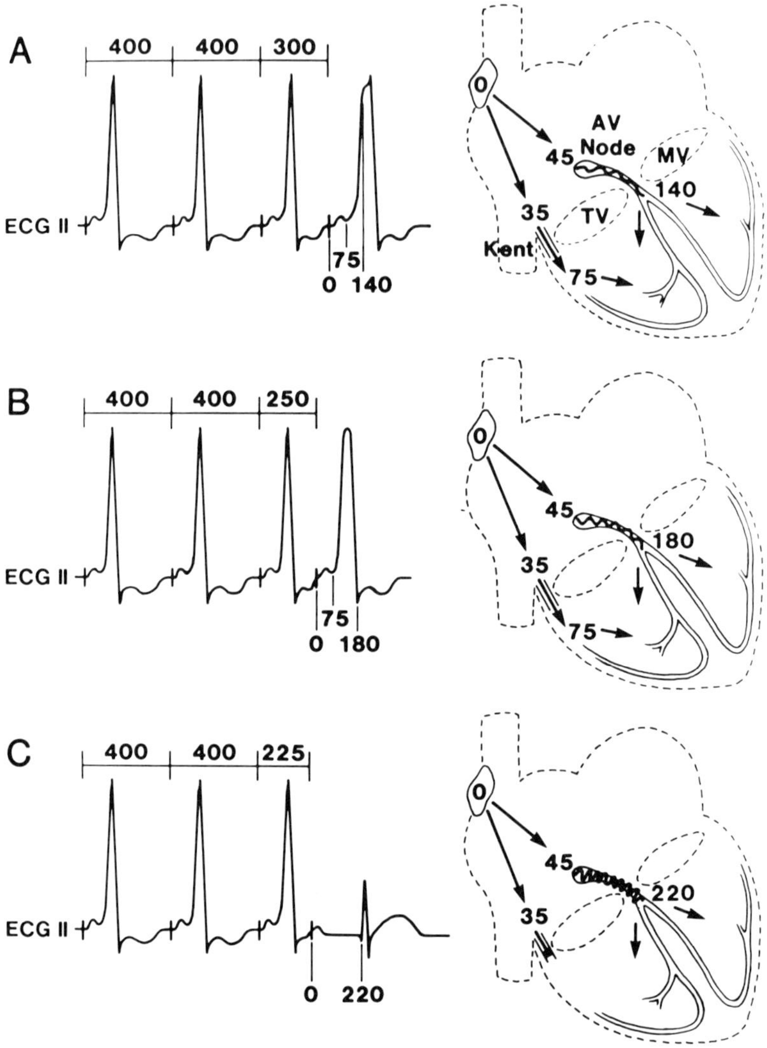

FIGURE 6–16

Determination of Kent bundle effective refractory period. In panel *A*, the atrium is being paced at a cycle length of 400 ms. Note the short PR interval and delta wave. A premature atrial depolarization is introduced 300 ms after the preceding driven atrial stimulus, and the QRS becomes more aberrant. The reason for this is shown in the diagram to the right of the tracing. The activation times for the premature beat are shown. The impulse arrives at the ventricle via the Kent bundle 75 ms after the stimulus, but the ventricle is not activated via the normal His bundle route until 140 ms after the stimulus. This can be seen on the surface ECG, where at 140 ms the QRS becomes a more normal configuration. In panel *B*, with increasing prematurity the conduction time is constant through the Kent bundle but prolonged through the AV node, and the His bundle is not activated until 180 ms after the onset of stimulation. More of the ventricle has been activated via the Kent bundle by this time; thus the QRS appears more aberrant. In panel *C*, there is "unidirectional block," and the effective refractory period of the Kent bundle has been reached. Conduction proceeds slowly entirely through the AV node and His bundle. The resultant QRS complex has a normal configuration.

TABLE 6–3
DIFFERENTIATING POINTS IN CLINICAL ESTIMATION OF TACHYCARDIA MECHANISM

Induction by premature extrastimuli or rapid pacing
Dependency on critical AA, AV, or VA interval for induction
Effect of initiating stimulus cycle length on subsequent rate of SVT
Morphology of initiating P wave compared to subsequent P waves
Cycle length variation of first few beats
Response of SVT to premature stimulation
Response of SVT to overdrive pacing
Response of SVT to dc electrical cardioversion
Effect of the autonomic nervous system on SVT
Response of SVT to drugs

gered dysrhythmia) even though these are not necessarily the same.

DIFFERENTIATING POINTS IN CLINICAL ESTIMATION OF TACHYCARDIA MECHANISM

SVT will be used as the model in the discussion, but the concepts apply to ventricular tachycardia as well. Any discussion of triggered dysrhythmia is speculative; we have never diagnosed a case of triggered dysrhythmia.

Induction by Premature Extrastimuli or Rapid Pacing

Generally, in sinus rhythm at a normal rate the refractory periods of any two areas of the heart are both short enough that conduction occurs through both areas. With the premature extrastimulus technique or with rapid pacing, the conduction system is stressed, and impulses are brought close enough to the preceding depolarization that the second depolarization blocks in one area and conducts through the other area of the heart. Therefore in patients with reentry SVT this mechanism can be started in 90% to 95% of patients by either rapid pacing or the premature extrastimulus technique.[24] If tachycardia is induced by a premature extrastimulus, abnormal automaticity is disproven. Premature stimuli do not induce abnormal automaticity. If SVT is not induced, abnormal automaticity is more likely. Triggered dysrhythmia, on the other hand, is induced by both rapid pacing and premature extrastimuli, presumably from a late afterdepolarization resulting from the short cycle length.

Dependency of Critical AA, AV, or VA Interval for Induction

In reentry there is only a certain prematurity interval (called the "echo zone," because premature stimuli may result in atrial echo beats or SVT) where the refractory periods allow for unidirectional block (Fig. 6–17). This is a relatively constant zone, and stimuli that are too premature or not premature enough (i.e., outside the echo zone) will not induce SVT. Therefore in reentry SVT there is a critical interval for induction. If the reentry circuit is confined to the atrium, the AA interval is critical for induction. If the reentry circuit involves the AV node, the AV interval (or AH interval) is critical for premature stimulation, and the VA interval is critical for premature ventricular stimulation. In abnormal automaticity the interval is unimportant because there is no interval that will induce SVT. In triggered dysrhythmia the interval is critical because the earlier the premature stimulus, the earlier is the first echo beat.

Effect of Initiating Stimulus Cycle Length on Subsequent Rate of SVT

The properties of a reentry circuit are such that once the tachycardia begins, the rate is determined by the conduction times in the circuit and is not dependent on the initiating circumstances. In abnormal automaticity the cycle length is unimportant because it does not initiate SVT. In triggered dysrhythmia, cycle length is inversely proportional to the rate of SVT: the shorter the initiating cycle length, the faster the rate of SVT. This is one of the important differentiating points of reentry and triggered dysrhythmia. For example, if premature stimuli are delivered in one case at 300 ms and in another at 200 ms after the last sinus beat, then both initiate SVT. If the mechanism is reentry, the rates of the two resulting tachycardias should be identical. If the mechanism is triggered dysrhythmia, the rate of the SVT initiated by the 300-ms stimulus will be faster than that initiated by the 200-ms stimulus (Fig. 6–18).

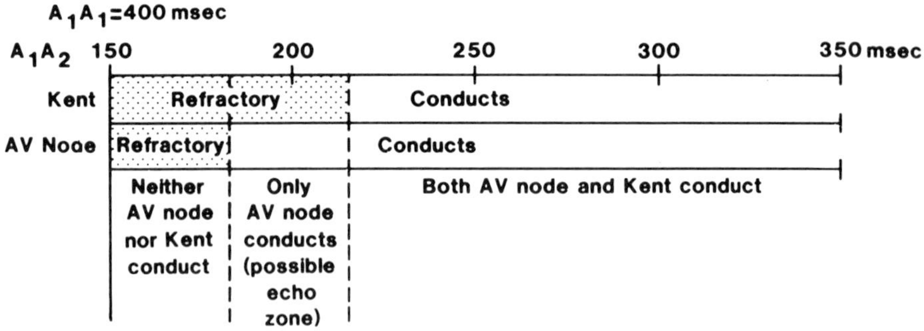

FIGURE 6–17

Example of determination of a possible echo zone in a patient with Wolff-Parkinson-White syndrome. The basic drive rate (S_1S_2 and A_1A_2) is 400 ms, and premature atrial depolarizations are delivered earlier into atrial diastole. These impulses conduct through both the AV node and Kent bundle until the A_1A_2 interval is 210 ms. Between 180 and 210 ms, antegrade impulses block in the Kent bundle and conduct through the AV node His bundle with a narrow QRS configuration (see Fig. 6–20). In this "echo zone," impulses may then travel retrograde through the bundle of Kent and cause an atrial echo beat or SVT. At cycle lengths shorter than 180 ms the impulse blocks in both pathways.

Morphology of Initiating P Wave Compared to Subsequent P Waves

Premature depolarization from any part of the heart may initiate reentry SVT. Therefore the P wave associated with the premature depolarization usually is different from the P waves generated by the reentry circuit. For example, a PAC may originate in the high left atrium (P wave negative in ECG lead I, positive in aVF) and cause reentry in high right atrial muscle (P waves positive in ECG leads I and aVF). One particular type of reentry SVT, that caused by a unidirectional retrograde accessory pathway, may have the same shaped P waves in the initiating and subsequent beats because sinus tachycardia is prone to initiate this type of SVT, and reentry begins with an atrial echo beat that travels to the atria via the AC. In the first beat of SVT, as in subsequent beats, the atria are activated in a retrograde direction from the same place: the point where the AC inserts the atrium (Fig. 6–19). In abnormal automaticity, the initiating P wave must be the same as the subsequent P waves. All beats of the SVT are activated from the same place. If the initiating P wave has a different shape, abnormal automaticity is disproven. In general, the initiating P wave should be different from subsequent P waves in triggered dysrhythmia; however, if the premature impulse originates from a site close to the cell that triggers, the P waves could be identical.

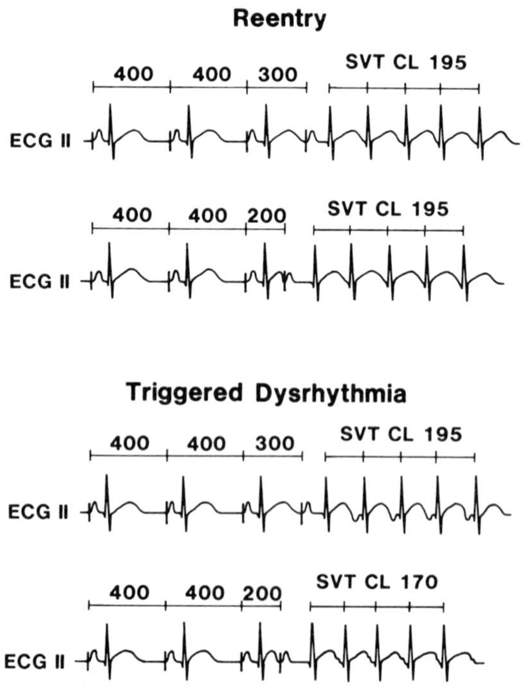

FIGURE 6–18

Effect of initiating cycle length on subsequent cycle length of SVT. In reentry, whether the initiating premature depolarization is 300 ms or 200 ms after the preceding stimulus, the resultant SVT has the same cycle length. With triggered dysrhythmia the cycle length of SVT is shorter if the initiating cycle length is shorter.

Cycle Length Variation of First Few Beats

In reentry the first few cycle lengths of SVT tend to oscillate by 5–10 ms between longer and shorter cycle lengths, because the conduction time of a cardiac structure is

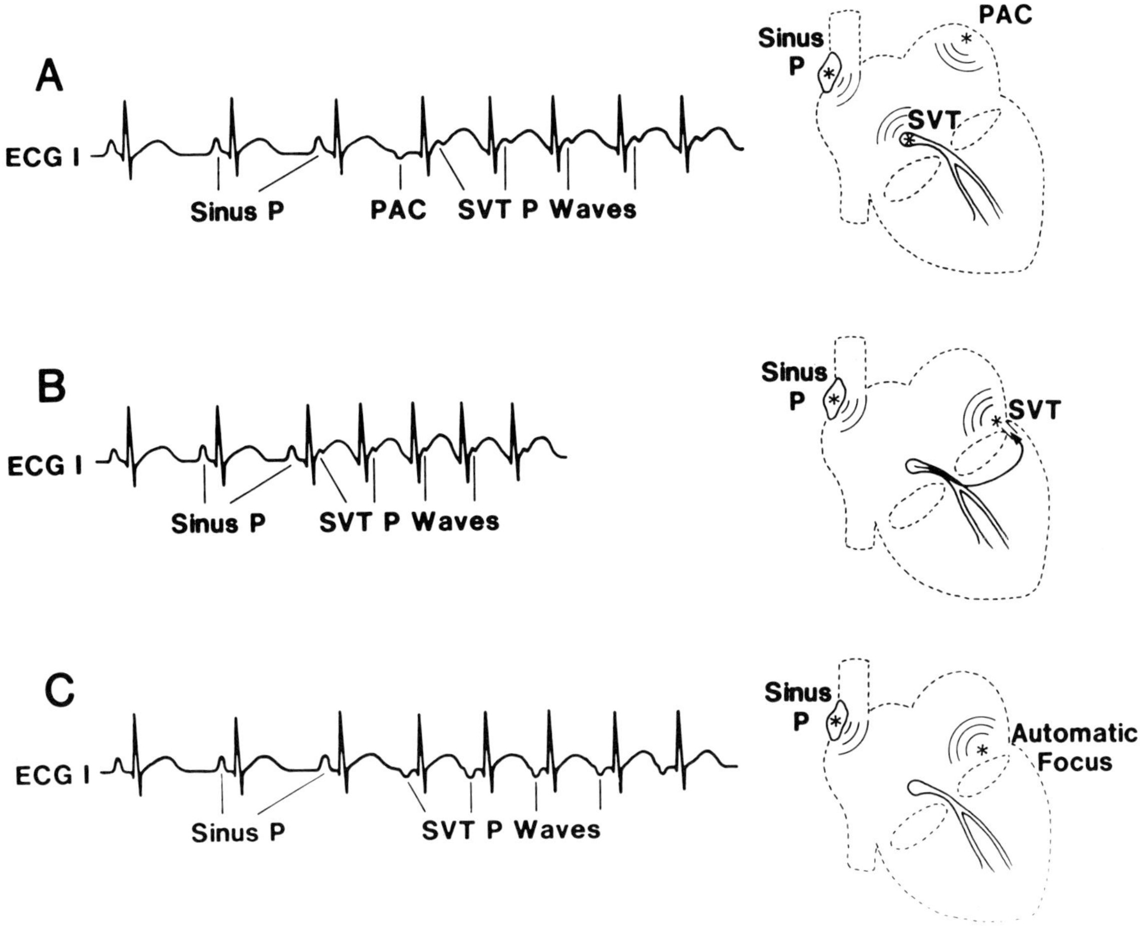

FIGURE 6–19

Panel *A:* A premature atrial contraction originating high in the left atrium can cause the onset of AV node reentry SVT. The shape of the P wave preceding the first QRS of SVT and that of the subsequent P waves are different. Panel *B:* In SVT caused by a left-sided unidirectional retrograde accessory pathway, sinus tachycardia may allow retrograde atrial reentry through the pathway. In this situation the initial and subsequent P waves also are different. Panel *C:* In SVT caused by abnormal automaticity, the initiating and subsequent P waves are identical, because all P waves during SVT originate from the same focus.

dependent on the preceding cycle length.[25] The cycle length between the first two beats of SVT is dependent on the preceding long cycle length (between the premature stimulus and the first beat of SVT), whereas the cycle length between the second and third beats of SVT is dependent on the preceding short cycle length (between the first and second beats of SVT) (Fig. 6–20). In abnormal automaticity the cycle length progressively shortens and the phenomenon of "warm-up" is observed. This is a property of all pacemaker cells, including the sinus node, and is a result of overdrive suppression.[26] Any cell that participates in the propagated action potential will be hyperpolarized by that action potential. If that cell then begins to undergo spontaneous diastolic depolarization, the slope of phase 4 of the action potential will get progressively steeper (and the rate of firing of the cell progressively faster) as the time from the hyperpolarizing stimulus lengthens. Warm-up is also a characteristic of triggered dysrhythmia because the rate of diastolic depolarization is dependent on the preceding cycle length: the shorter the preceding cycle length, the faster the rate of subsequent diastolic depolarization and the sooner the depolarization will reach the threshold potential. Warm-up continues until

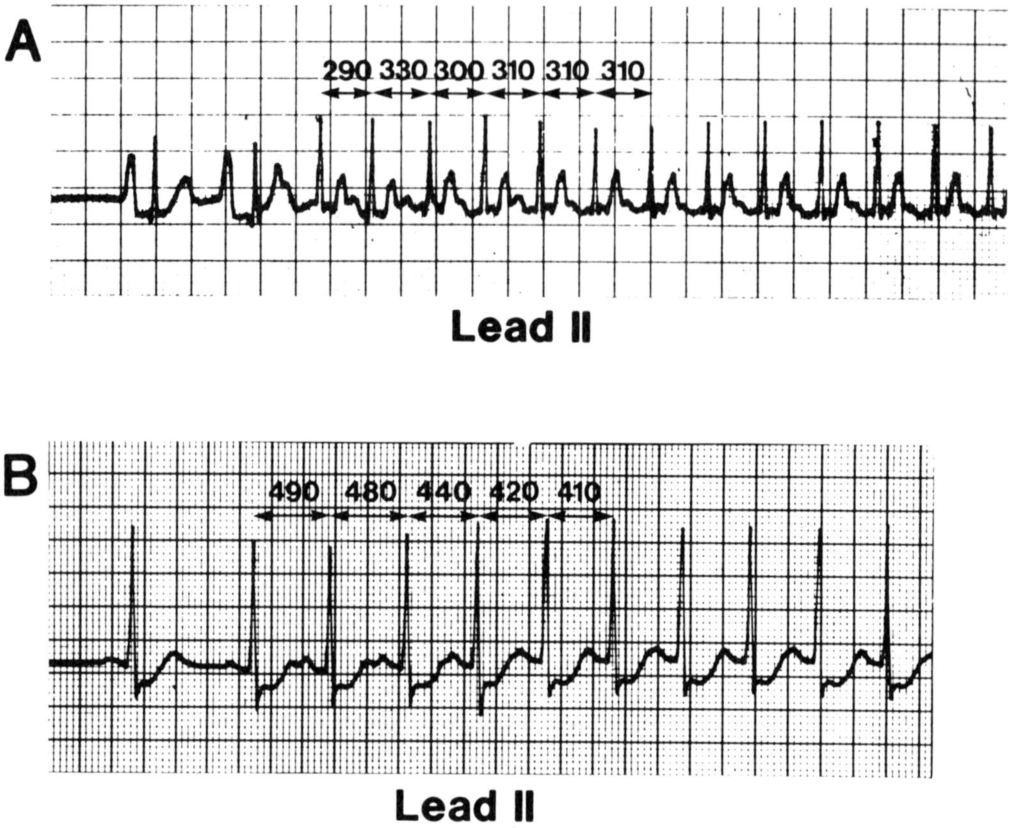

FIGURE 6–20
Panel *A:* Cycle length oscillation at the beginning of SVT. There are alternating short and long cycle lengths until a stable SVT cycle length is reached. The numbers refer to the RR intervals (ms) during SVT. Panel *B:* Cycle length "warmup" at the beginning of SVT caused by abnormal automaticity. The cycle lengths progressively shorten until a stable SVT cycle length is reached.

the maximum rate of firing of that cell is reached, which is dependent on the cycle length of the initiated stimulus.

Response of SVT to Premature Stimulation

SVT can respond to premature stimulation in one of three ways. The premature stimulation can result in a fully compensatory pause in the atrial depolarization, less than a fully compensatory pause, or cessation of the SVT.

The concept of "compensatory pause" is most easily understood by considering sinus rhythm (Fig. 6–21). For example, let us assume the case of sinus rhythm at a rate of 120 bpm (cycle length 500 ms) and an atrial depolarization introduced 450 ms after the last spontaneous impulse. In other words, A_1A_1 is 500 ms and A_1A_2 is 450 ms. The "prematurity index" (A_1A_2/A_1A_1) is 450/500 = 0.90. With a premature stimulus occurring this late in sinus cycle length, the sinus node has already depolarized and the sinus impulse is spreading through the atrium. This collides with the propagated depolarization from the premature stimulus in the atrium, and therefore the premature depolarization does not reach the sinus node. The sinus node is therefore not reset, and it depolarizes at the appropriate time. Thus the interval between the two spontaneous sinus beats on either side of the premature depolarization is exactly equal to twice the basic cycle length—a fully compensatory pause.

On the other hand, a premature impulse delivered 250 ms after the last spontaneous sinus depolarization (A_1A_2/A_1A_1 = 0.5) would be sufficiently early to conduct back into the sinus node and reset the pacemaker (Fig. 6–22). In this instance the sinus node is depolarized early by the impulse propagated from the premature stimulus. The next sinus impulse begins as soon as the sinus node is depolarized, and the interval between the two spontaneous sinus beats on either side of the premature depolarization is less than twice the basic cycle length—less than a fully compensatory pause. In this example the return cycle is 575 ms and the return cycle length index is 1.15. For a less than compensatory pause the prematurity index plus the return cycle length index must be less than 2.0.

If premature atrial stimuli are delivered at decreasing intervals from the preceding sinus impulse and if the prematurity index is graphed on the abscissa with the return length index on the ordinate, a curve can be generated similar to that shown in Figure 6–21. In this figure a line is drawn connecting the points (1.0,1.0) with (0,2.0). Points that fall on this line are those indicating a fully compensatory pause. From the previous example, the premature cycle length is 450 ms ($A_1A_2/A_1A_1 = 0.9$) and the return cycle is 550 ms ($A_2A_3/A_1A_1 = 1.1$); this is point A on the "line of compensatory pause." If the premature cycle is 250 ms ($A_1A_2/A_1A_1 = 0.5$) and the return cycle is 750 ms ($A_2A_3/A_1A_1 = 1.5$), this would be point B' on the "line of compensatory pause." In our example (prematurity index of 0.5), however, the return cycle index was 1.15 (point B), indicating reset and a less than compensatory pause. A series of points such as those shown in Figure 6–21 are typical for the sinus node, with an area of compensatory pause (nonreset) and then, with increasing prematurity, an area of reset with less than a fully compensatory pause. The stimuli can be introduced with increasing prematurity until the atrial effective refractory period is reached at a prematurity index of approximately 0.30.

The same techniques can be used to study SVT, where A_1A_2 is the interval from an atrial depolarization of SVT to the premature stimulus and A_2A_3 the interval to the next atrial depolarization. The responses can help to distinguish among the various mechanisms. In reentry there are two areas of the curve. In the first, the tachycardia continues after the premature stimulus and the pause is compensatory or more than compensatory ($A_1A_2/A_1A_1 + A_2A_3/A_1A_1 > 2.0$). The mechanism for this is shown in Figure 6–22, an example of reentry within the AV node. The pause can be greater than compensatory because conduction time within the AV node lengthens with more premature stimuli. In Figure 6–22, the stimulus is delivered during SVT at a prematurity index of 0.9 from the last atrial depolarization. The impulse propagated from the premature stimulus conducts to the ventricle with a longer AV interval (A_2V_2 = 256 ms) than the impulse before the premature stimulus (A_1V_1 = 224 ms). Delay in the AV node is responsible for the longer return cycle. The premature impulse blocks the returning impulse from the ventricle, but the premature impulse itself is conducted to the ventricles, and the tachycardia continues. Similarly, in Figure 6–22, with a more premature stimulus, there is an even longer delay in the AV node (A_2V_2 = 272 ms), but the tachycardia continues.

The second area of the curve is illustrated by point C in Figure 6–22. With a very early premature stimulus ($A_1A_2/A_1A_1 = 0.5$), the conduction time and the refractory period of the AV node are so prolonged that the premature impulse blocks in the AV node, the reentry circuit is broken, and the tachycardia stops. At point C the return cycle is very long ($A_2A_3/A_1A_1 = 1.95$), and the diagram shows that sinus rhythm has resumed. The first few sinus cycle lengths after cessation of SVT are usually longer (slower heart rate) than the basic sinus rhythm because the rapid rate of SVT typically causes overdrive suppression of the sinus node. This is shown in Figure 6–22, where A_2A_3/A_1A_1 is 1.95 and A_3A_4/A_1A_1 is 1.75. Thus in reentry the points on the curve are on or above the line of compensatory pause until SVT is broken; then there is a discontinuity in the curve, with the long return cycles indicating resumption of sinus rhythm.

In abnormal automaticity the curve shown in Figure 6–23 is identical in shape to that shown for the sinus node in Figure 6–21. This is to be expected because our conception of abnormal automaticity is that it is caused by a single cell that acts just like an "accessory sinus node," except with an abnormally rapid rate.[27] Figure 6–23 shows an ectopic focus in the low lateral right atrium. With greater prematurity indexes ($A_1A_2/A_1A_1 = 0.9$ or 0.8), the impulse from the ectopic focus and that from the premature stimulus collide, and the ectopic focus is not reset, resulting in a fully compensatory pause; however, at point C, with $A_1A_2/A_1A_1 = 0.5$, the stimulus is premature enough to conduct into the ectopic focus, resulting in reset and a less than fully compensatory pause. Just as it is impossible to stop a sinus node with premature

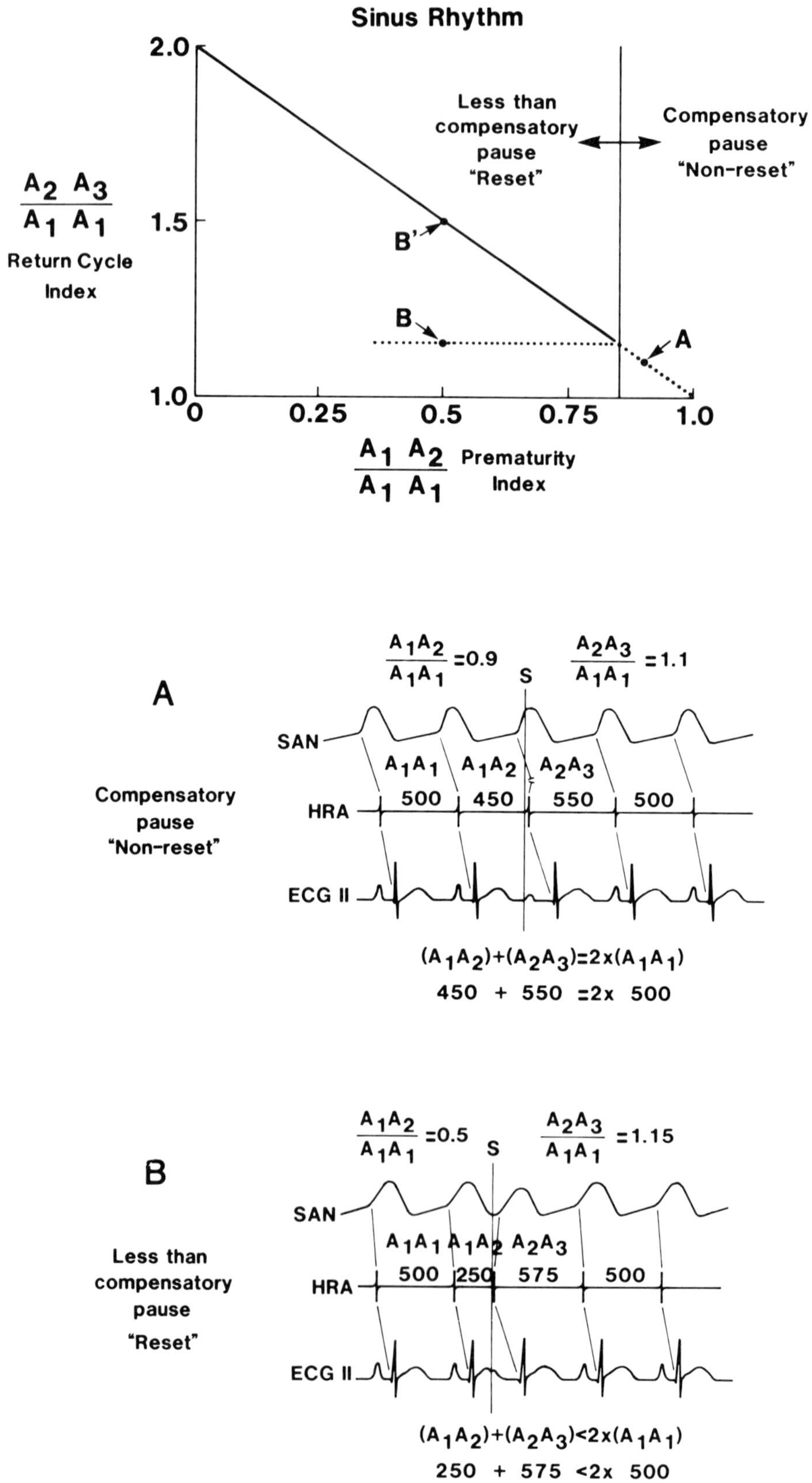

FIGURE 6–21 *See legend on opposite page*

stimulation, it is impossible to stop an ectopic automatic focus with premature stimulation. Therefore although the tachycardia resulting from abnormal automaticity is reset, it does not stop.

Triggered dysrhythmia exhibits behavior that is similar to both reentry and abnormal automaticity. In Figure 6–24 a focus of triggered dysrhythmia is diagrammed as originating in the low lateral right atrium. At longer prematurity indices (A_1A_2/A_1A_1 = 0.9 or 0.8) this responds as an automatic focus, with the impulses from the focus and the stimulus colliding so that reset does not occur, and thus the pause is fully compensatory (Fig. 6–24A and B); however, when an appropriately timed premature impulse does penetrate into the focus of triggered dysrhythmia, instead of resetting it, the premature stimulus depolarizes the area and stops the tachycardia, and sinus rhythm results (Fig. 6–24C). Abnormal automaticity resets because the increased slope of phase 4, which causes abnormal automaticity, is a relatively stable property of the action potential; when the cell is depolarized from an extrinsic stimulus, the next spontaneous action potential will have the same characteristics as previous action potentials. On the other hand, triggered dysrhythmia results from a series of self-regenerating afterdepolarizations. If the delicate balance of the afterdepolarizations is upset by an appropriately timed premature depolarization, the train is interrupted and the dysrhythmia stops. It is a property of cells with triggered dysrhythmia that once the series of afterdepolarizations stops, it is impossible to reinduce tachycardia for a period of several minutes.[23] The basic mechanism for this is poorly understood at present.

From a review of Figures 6–22 through 6–24, it is apparent that all three mechanisms show an area of nonrest (fully compensatory pause) at longer premature lengths; however, the curve for abnormal automaticity differs from the other two at shorter premature cycle lengths, because abnormal automaticity shows reset without cessation of SVT. The other two do not show reset, but the tachycardia will terminate with resumption of sinus rhythm. This would seem to be an excellent way for differentiating abnormal automaticity from the other two; in practice, it is effective in approximately 75% of cases. In the other 25% of cases, the curve generated is similar to that shown in Figure 6–25, in which all the points fall on or slightly above the line of fully compensatory pause. Any of the three mechanisms can respond to premature stimulation in this manner. In the case of reentry the tachycardia is never broken; in both abnormal automaticity and triggered dysrhythmia, "entrance block" exists, and the focus is never reset. In cases such as these, with all the points on or above the line of compensatory pause, the mechanism of SVT cannot be detected by this method.

Response of SVT to Overdrive Pacing

Rapid overdrive pacing both hyperpolarizes and decreases automaticity in cardiac cells. In 95% of reentry circuits, rapid atrial pacing stops the SVT immediately on termination of the stimulation.[24] In the other 5%, a reentry mechanism is demonstrated by other means, and it is thought in these cases that there is a high degree of entrance block into the reentry circuit, so that fewer stimulated impulses arrive in the circuit and the effects of overdrive are diminished. In abnormal automaticity, rapid pacing will capture the atrium and reset the focus, but on termination of stimulation the focus returns, albeit at a slower rate for a few beats (caused by overdrive suppression and a decrease in the slope of phase 4). In triggered dysrhythmia, when the stimulus is stopped, the resultant decrease in the slope of phase 4 slows the rate of the focus; then, usually after several slow beats, the tachycardia terminates.

Response of SVT to dc Electrical Cardioversion

Cardioversion theoretically depolarizes the entire heart. The vast majority of reentry mechanisms are stopped by cardioversion. In

FIGURE 6–21

Response of sinus rhythm to premature atrial stimulation. Panel *A:* Diagrammatic representation of a fully compensatory pause. On the first line sinus node action potentials (SAN) are represented, which in turn conduct to the high right atrium (HRA), depicted as bipolar atrial electrograms. These then conduct to the ventricle, shown as a QRS complex on the surface ECG (lead II). A_1A_1, refers to the interval between basic sinus beats. A_1A_2 refers to the interval between the last sinus beat and the premature stimulus that has been introduced (indicated by the vertical line, marked S). A_2A_3 refers to the "return cycle," or interval from the premature beat to the next sinus beat. All intervals are given in ms. Panel *B:* Diagrammatic representation of a less than compensatory pause. Further explanation is provided in the text.

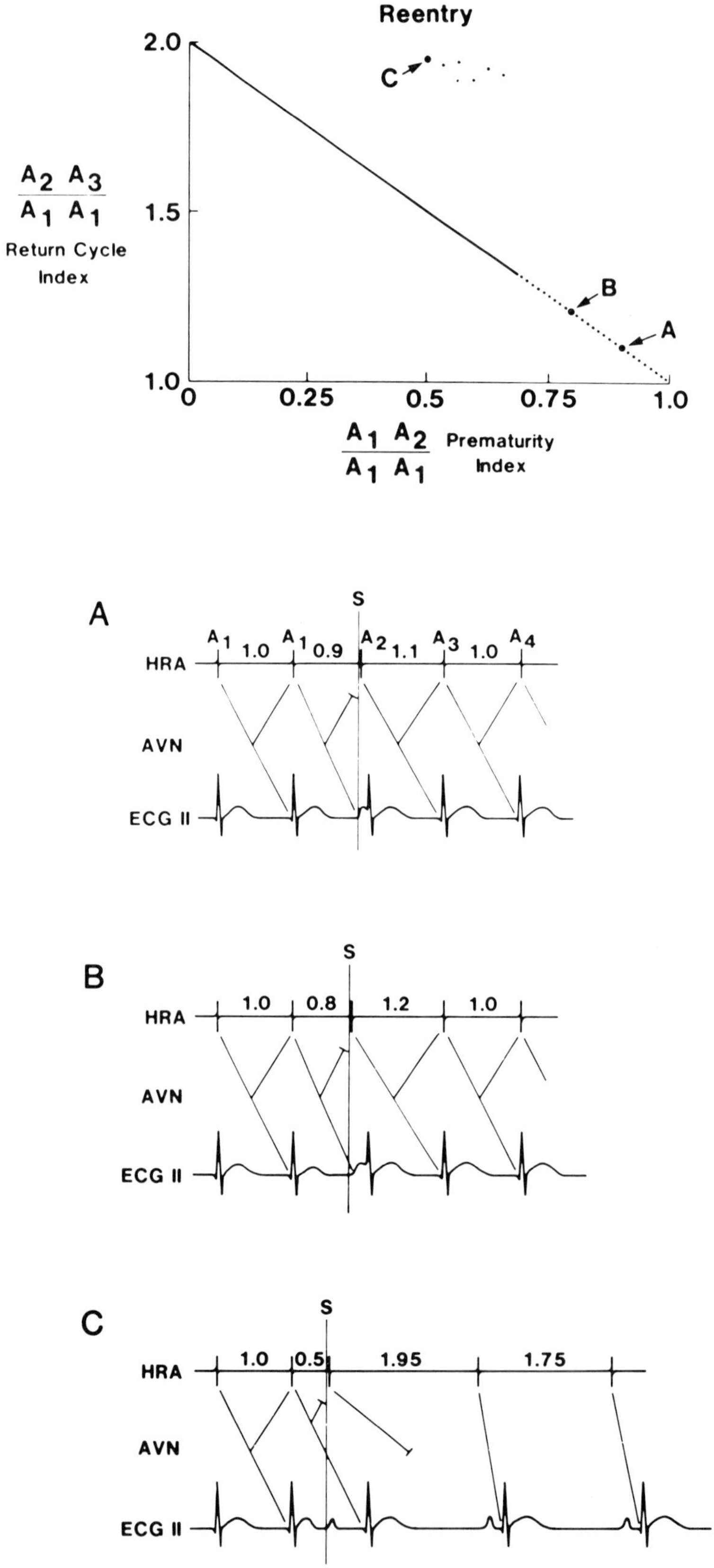

FIGURE 6–22
Response of reentry SVT to premature atrial stimulation. The abbreviations are the same as those in Figure 6–21. See text for explanation.

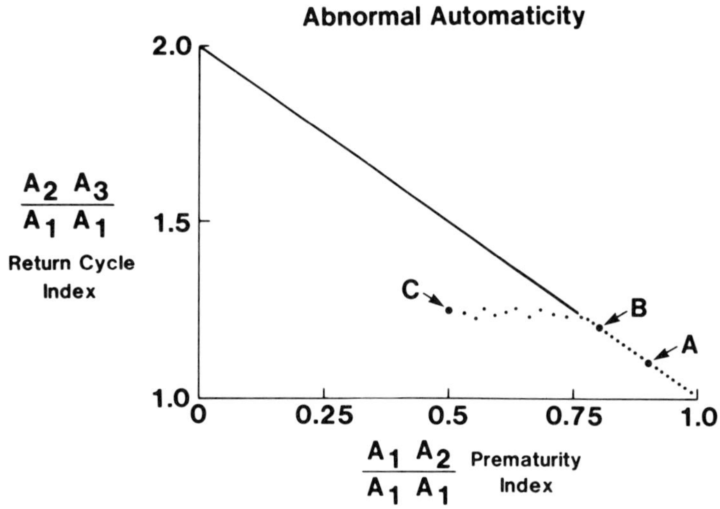

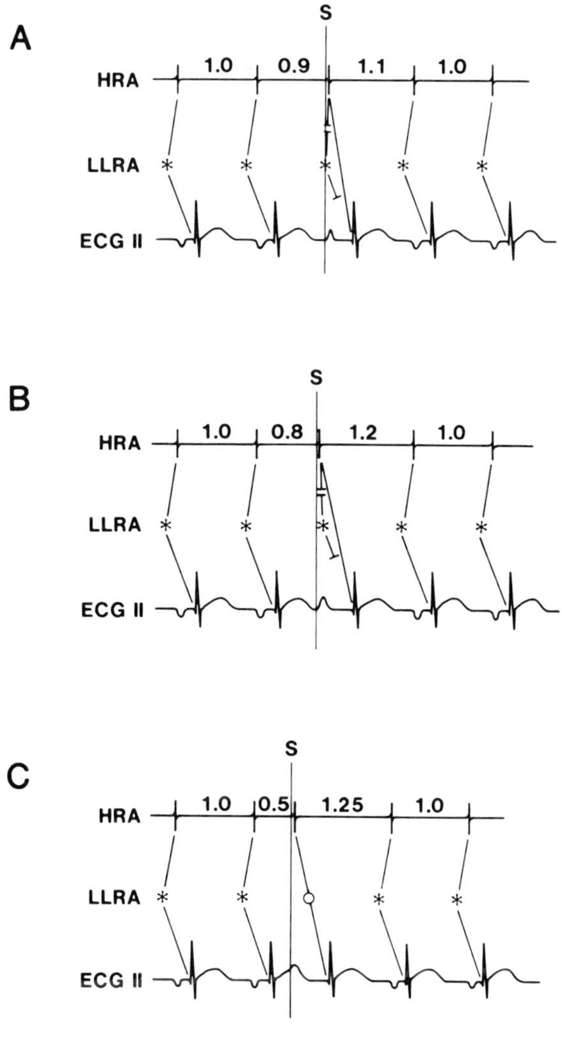

FIGURE 6–23
Response of abnormal automaticity SVT to premature atrial stimulation. The abbreviations are the same as those in Figure 6–21. See text for explanation.

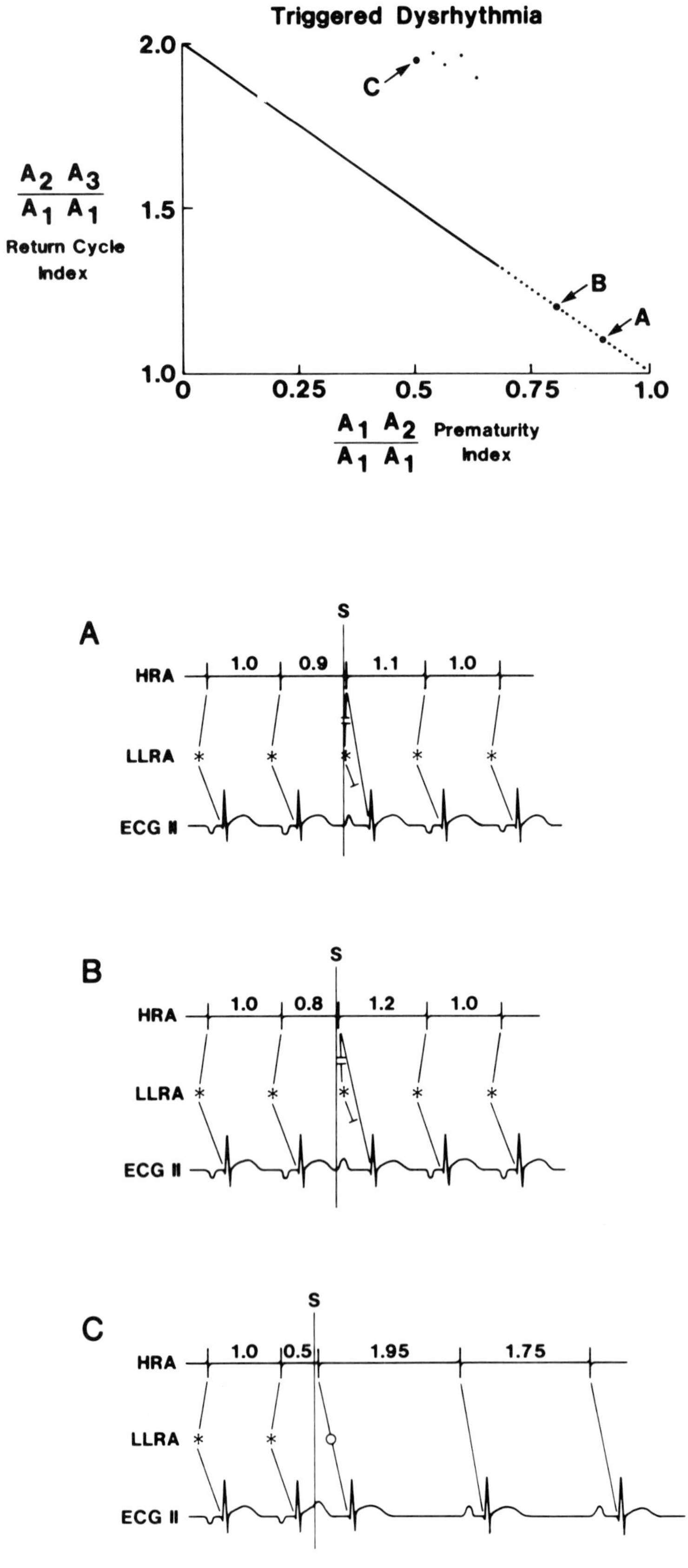

FIGURE 6–24
Response of SVT caused by triggered dysrhythmia to premature atrial stimulation. The abbreviations are the same as those in Figure 6–21. See text for explanation.

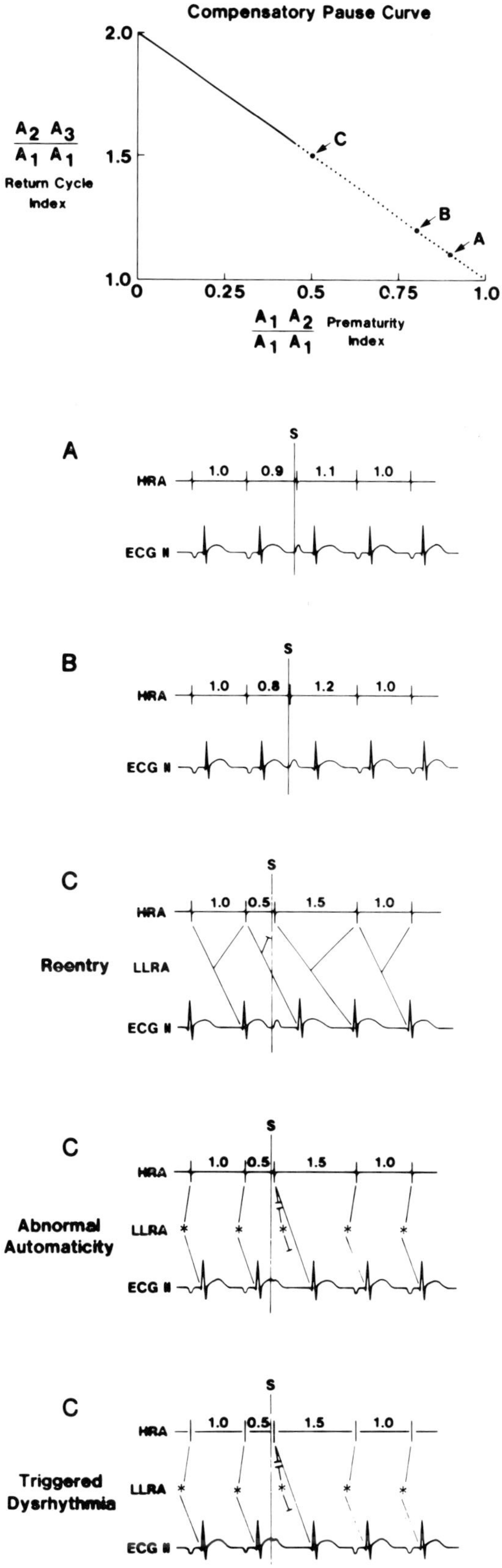

FIGURE 6–25
Response of SVT to premature atrial stimulation, which results in all return cycles falling on or above the line of fully compensatory pause. At points A and B an example of nonreset is shown that would be similar in either reentry, abnormal automaticity, or triggered dysrhythmia. At point C diagrams are shown for the mechanism of nonreset. In reentry the circuit is continued by the stimulus. In abnormal automaticity and triggered dysrhythmia, there is entrance block into the focus.

a very few cases in which cardioversion with adequate current dosage has failed to stop reentry SVT, it has been postulated that the circuit was small and was "insulated" from a cardioversion-induced depolarization.[28] SVT caused by abnormal automaticity responds to cardioversion in the same manner as sinus rhythm.[29] After the heart depolarizes, the abnormal mechanism is unaffected and resumes its rapid rate. Triggered dysrhythmia will stop after cardioversion, because the balance of afterdepolarizations is interrupted.

Effect of the Autonomic Nervous System on SVT

In reentry, the rate of SVT is largely dependent on the refractory periods of the various parts of the reentry circuit. While the refractory periods of atrial muscle and the AV node are influenced to some extent by sympathetic and parasympathetic tone, the rate of reentry SVT is not changed by more than 15% to 20% with exercise or sleep. Increasing vagal tone (e.g., by Valsalva's maneuver) generally slows the rate of reentry SVT, again by only 15% to 20%, and then the SVT usually stops suddenly. The slowing and eventual blocks induced by vagotonia are caused by prolongation of the refractory periods of atrium, AV node, and bundle of His. On the other hand, a marked variation in the rate of SVT (40% or greater) is found in both abnormal automaticity and triggered dysrhythmia in response to autonomic influences. Phase 4 depolarization is responsible for both of these mechanisms, and phase 4 depolarization is affected directly by catecholamines and acetylcholine: norepinephrine increases the rate of phase 4 depolarization, and acetylcholine decreases the rate.[29] Vagal stimulation will markedly slow the rates of SVT stemming from these latter two mechanisms but will not stop the tachycardia.

Response of SVT to Drugs

Digitalis. Digitalis decreases the refractory period of atrial cells and increases the refractory period of the AV node. It therefore changes the balance needed for reentry and prevents many types of reentry SVT in which the AV node is a component of the reentry circuit. Digitalis either has no effect on abnormal automaticity or may theoretically increase the rate of SVT. Triggered dysrhythmia was first discovered in digitalis-intoxicated cells.[22] It is thought that by digitalis inhibition of the sodium-potassium pump, afterdepolarizations are enhanced, thus increasing the likelihood of a sustained rhythm.

Propranolol. Propranolol has marked effects on decreasing automaticity and increasing the refractory periods, primarily of the sinus node and AV node. Propranolol has less effect on atrial muscle. It is effective in stopping reentry SVT because of conduction block in the AV node and atrium and is effective in slowing the rate of (but usually not stopping) abnormal automaticity. Because propranolol inhibits the actions of catecholamines, it may prevent the induction of triggered dysrhythmia by catecholamines. If triggered dysrhythmia is induced, propranolol will slow the rate of SVT because the inducing sinus or junctional rate will be slower.

Isoproterenol. The actions of isoproterenol are directly opposite to those of propranolol: reentry is more likely, and the rate may increase slightly; abnormal automaticity may be slightly more likely, and the rate of SVT is markedly increased; and triggered dysrhythmia is more likely, and the rate of SVT is increased.

Atropine. Atropine increases conduction and shortens the refractory period of the sinus node, atrium, and AV node. Reentry is generally enhanced by atropine. Theoretically, if areas of slow conduction are improved, reentry might be inhibited; in actual practice, atropine makes it easier to introduce reentry SVT. The rate of reentry SVT is increased 15% to 20% with atropine. The rate of abnormal automaticity can increase by 100% in the presence of atropine. Atropine has more of an effect on the sinus node than on automatic ectopic foci; thus it should not allow the appearance of foci caused by abnormal automaticity if the sinus node is normal.[28] In SVT resulting from triggered dysrhythmia, both the likelihood and the rate of SVT are increased by atropine.

Edrophonium. The actions of edrophonium are directly opposite to those of atropine: reentry is less likely, and if it is present, the rate of SVT slows slightly; abnormal automaticity is equally as likely as without the drug, but the rate is slowed; and triggered dysrhythmia is less likely, and if it is present, the rate slows.

Verapamil. Verapamil blocks the inward calcium current and therefore has a profound blocking effect on cells that normally have slow currents (e.g., cells in the sinus node and AV node; cells that, as a resuult of injury, have a lowered maximum diastolic potential and whose action potentials appear similar to slow action potentials; and cells with afterdepolarizations, because calcium is necessary for part of this current). Reentry involving sinus node or AV node is abolished by verapamil. With use of verapamil just before SVT terminates, the rate of SVT slows by 15% to 20%. Theoretically, if abnormal automaticity is caused by an injured cell with primarily a calcium-dependent action potential, verapamil will slow and then stop the SVT. In practice verapamil has been ineffective in treating SVT resulting from abnormal automaticity in most instances. In these cases the mechanism of the abnormal automaticity more than likely involved sodium-dependent action potentials. Verapamil immediately stops SVT caused by triggered dysrhythmia. **Procainamide.** Procainamide blocks the sodium current responsible for phase O of the action potential. By decreasing the rate of rise of phase O (dv/dt) it decreases conduction velocity in tissues of the atrium, ventricle, His-Purkinje system, and AC. Procainamide also prolongs action potential duration and refractory periods of the same tissues. By these actions it may stop tachycardias that involve reentry circuits through the atrium, ventricle, His-Purkinje system, or an AC. Procainamide has no effect on triggered dysrhythmia in isolated tissue. Even though procainamide decreases the slope of phase 4 in abnormal isolated tissues, it has not altered SVT resulting from abnormal automaticity in humans.

VENTRICULAR TACHYCARDIA

We have used SVT as a model for demonstrating the ways to determine the mechanisms of a tachycardia. Many of the same principles are involved in the electrophysiologic diagnosis of ventricular tachycardia. The task is more difficult, however, because there are no specific structures to record from that allow as accurate a localization of the reentry circuit or focus. The specifics of the EPS of ventricular tachycardia are given in Chapter 12.

References

1. Scherlag BJ, Lau SH, Helfant RH, et al: Catheter techniques for recording His bundle activity in man. Circulation 39:13–19, 1969.
2. Gillette PC, Reitman MJ, Gutgesell HP, et al: Intracardiac electrography in children and young adults. Am Heart J 89:36–43, 1975.
3. Brodsky SJ, Mirowski M, Krovetz LJ, et al: Recording of His bundle and other conduction tissue potential in children. J Pediatr 79:61–69, 1971.
4. Roberts NK, Olley PM: His bundle recordings in children with normal hearts and congenital heart disease. Circulation 45:295–301, 1972.
5. Abella JB, Teixeira OHP, Misra KP, et al: Changes of atrioventricular conduction with age in infants and children. Am J Cardiol 30:876–880, 1972.
6. Bekheit S, Morton P, Murtagh JG, et al: Comparison of sinoventricular conduction in children and adults using bundle of His electrograms. Br Heart J 35:507–514, 1973.
7. Roberts NK, Gillette PC: Electrophysiologic study of the conduction system in normal children. Pediatrics 60:858–863, 1977.
8. Gillette PC: Electrophysiologic investigation in children: Indications and techniques. Cardiol Digest 12:9–26, 1977.
9. Wit AL, Weiss MB, Berkowitz WD, et al: Patterns of A-V conduction in the human heart. Circ Res 27:345–352, 1970.
10. Denes P, Wu D, Dhingra R, et al: The effect of cycle length on cardiac refractory periods in man. Circulation 49:32–38, 1974.
11. Gillette PC, Mullins CE, McNamara DG: Functional properties of the atrioventricular node in infants and children. Pediatric Res 9:53, 1975. Abstract.
12. Clapp SK, Driscoll DJ, Gillette PC, et al: The effect of meperidine, promethazine and chlorpromazine on sinus node and atrioventricular node function. Clin Res 26:807A, 1978. Abstract.
13. Hesslein PS, Mullins CE, Kugler JD, et al: Percutaneous sheath brachial vein cardiac catheterization in children. Cath Cardiovasc Diag 6:197–205, 1980.
14. Strauss HC, Saroff AL, Bigger JE, et al: Premature atrial stimulation as a key to the understanding of sinoatrial conduction in man. Circulation 47:86–91, 1973.
15. Hariman RJ, Krongrad E, Boxer RA, et al: Methods for recording electrograms of the sinoatrial node during cardiac surgery in man. Circulation 61:1024–1029, 1980.
16. DuBrow IW, Fisher EQ, Amat-y-Leon F, et al: Comparison of cardiac refractory periods in children and adults. Circulation 51:485–496, 1975.
17. Nasrallah AT, Gillette PC, Mullins CE: Congenital and surgical atrioventricular block within the His bundle. Am J Cardiol 36:914–920, 1975.
18. Driscoll DJ, Gillette PC, Hallman GL, et al: Management of surgical complete atrioventricular block in children. Am J Cardiol 43:1175–1180, 1979.
19. Sung RJ, Tamer DM, Garcia OL, et al: Analysis of surgically induced right bundle branch block pattern using intracardiac recording techniques. Circulation 54:442–449, 1976.
20. Denes P, Wu D, Dhingara RC, et al: Demonstration of dual A-V nodal pathways in patients with paroxysmal supraventricular tachycardia. Circulation 48:549–555, 1973.

21. Cranefield PF, Wit AL, Hoffman RB: Genesis of cardiac arrhythmias. Circulation 47:190–196, 1973.
22. Wit AL, Cranefield PF: Triggered activity in cardiac muscle fibers of the simian mitral valve. Circ Res 38:85–91, 1976.
23. Wit AL, Fenoglio JJ, Hordof AJ, et al: Ultrastructure and transmembrane potentials of cardiac muscle in the human anterior mitral valve leaflet. Circulation 59:1284–1290, 1979.
24. Gillette PC: The mechanisms of supraventricular tachycardia in children. Circulation 54:133–139, 1976.
25. Goldreyer BN, Bigger FT: Site of reentry in paroxysmal supraventricular tachycardia in man. Circulation 43:15–23, 1971.
26. Goldreyer BN, Gallagher JJ, Damato AN: The electrophysiologic demonstration and atrial ectopic tachycardia in man. Am Heart J 85:205–211, 1973.
27. Singer DH, Lazzara R, Hoffman BF: Interrelationships between automaticity and conduction in Purkinje fibers. Circulation 21:537–543, 1967.
28. Moore EN, Jomain SL, Stuckey JH, et al: Studies on ectopic atrial rhythms in dogs. Am J Cardiol 19:676–680, 1967.
29. Gillette PC, Garson A: Electrophysiologic and pharmacologic characteristics of automatic ectopic atrial tachycardia. Circulation 56:571–575, 1977.

SECTION III

ARRHYTHMIAS

CHAPTER 7

SINUS NODE DYSFUNCTION

John D. Kugler

This chapter will encompass all types of sinus node dysfunction. Autonomic nervous imbalance, drug effects, and other disorders that can cause secondary sinus node dysfunction (SND) are discussed in addition to the organic, structural abnormalities of the sinus node. The term "sick sinus syndrome" is avoided, because its implications are imprecise.[1–5] For example, to some clinicians, sick sinus syndrome implies specific arrhythmias (e.g., sinus arrest or bradytachyarrhythmias) or SND but only if associated symptoms (e.g., dizziness, syncope) are documented. To others, the term implies only SND as defined by electrocardiographic criteria[3] or from organic sinus node abnormalities, but autonomic nervous system causes of SND are not considered. Therefore, regardless of cause and to avoid confusion, any disorder of the sinus node in this chapter is described as sinus node dysfunction.

The diagnosis of SND is established by one or more noninvasive or invasive procedures. Documenting the diagnosis as well as determining the clinical significance of the SND occasionally requires several types of testing. The clinical significance of SND is clarified by the documentation of symptoms while recording the electrocardiographic evidence of SND.[4, 5]

NONINVASIVE EVALUATION OF SINUS NODE FUNCTION

Noninvasive testing is commonly used to establish the diagnosis of SND and is virtually always used to assist in determining its severity. Most decisions involving treatment are based on documenting SND during symptoms. Noninvasive testing carries a potentially greater value than invasive testing because it allows a greater chance of documenting symptoms with the associated SND arrhythmia, and the specificity and sensitivity of invasive sinus node evaluation has been disappointing.[6–10] Noninvasive evaluation of SND begins with the surface standard electrocardiogram (ECG) and the ambulatory ECG.

Surface Standard ECG and Ambulatory ECG

Because it is not possible to record sinus node depolarization directly by surface electrocardiograph, sinus node function is assessed by inferring the atrial depolarization (P wave). Impulses are assumed to originate from the sinus node when the resulting P wave axis is approximately +60° (Fig. 7–1). The sinus node is relatively constant in its location at the high right atrial–superior vena caval junction and may extend inferiorly in the lateral right atrial wall to nearly the inferior vena cava.[11] The dominant pacemaker cell normally may be anywhere within the node, and therefore the P wave axis may range from 0° to +90°.[12] Several limb leads (preferably leads I and aVF) are necessary to establish the P wave axis and therefore to infer whether the rhythm is originating within the sinus node or elsewhere in the atria. Ambulatory 24-hour ECG (Holter) monitoring systems used to assess sinus node function ideally should use two perpendicular limb leads to optimize P wave evaluation.[5]

The arrhythmias listed in Table 7–1, alone or in combination, are characteristic of SND. These arrhythmias may be primary (from organic sinus node disease) or secondary (from autonomic imbalance or drug effect).

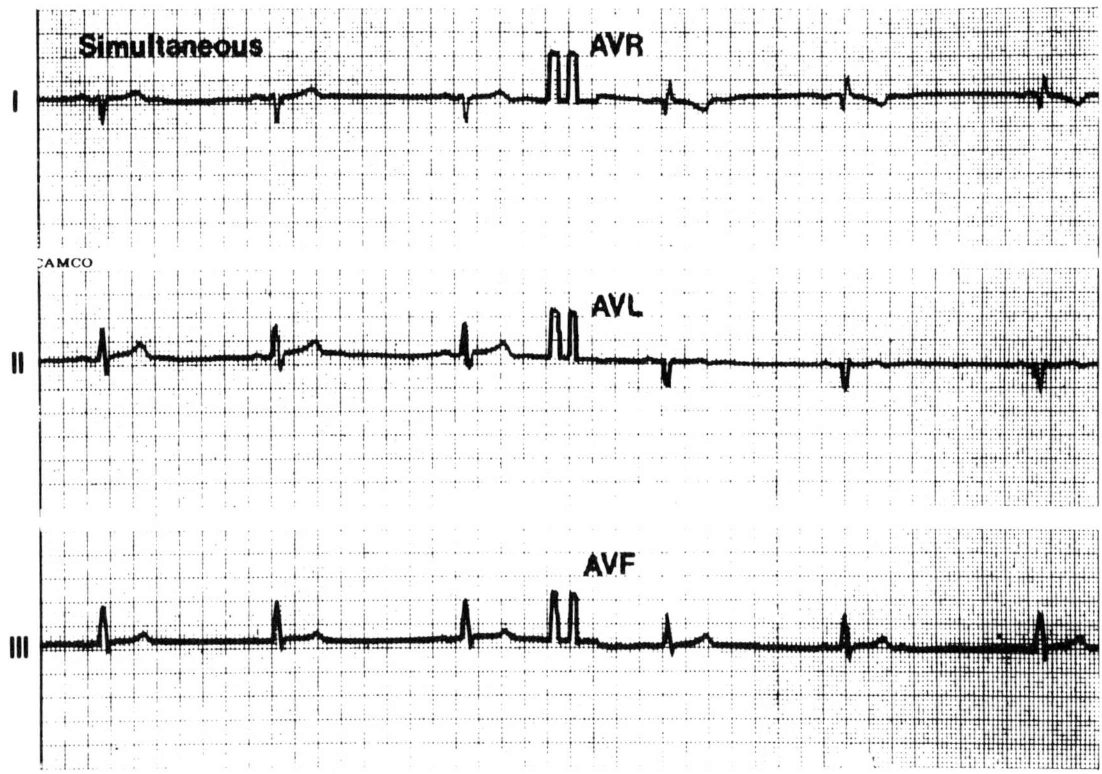

FIGURE 7–1
Sinus bradycardia (rate 40 bpm) was recorded by surface standard ECG in a 15-year-old boy with syncope. Note normal P wave axis (+45°). Paper speed was 25 mm/s; calibration was 1 mV/10 mm.

Sinus bradycardia is present when the sinus rate slows below what is expected for the patient's age. Although more data have become available during the past few years, thoroughly designed studies have not been undertaken to determine the lower limits of normal heart rate for various age groups. Therefore, most clinicians use arbitrary guidelines based partially on the few data available and partially on personal experience.[9, 13, 14] Although some Holter studies have included ranges of heart rate or a mean heart rate without standard deviation,[15–17] Table 7–2 lists four Holter studies in normal children and young adults in which a mean low heart rate was calculated as well as a standard deviation.[18–21] A lower limit of normal heart rate for the ages of subjects in a particular study can be derived by calculating two standard deviations from the mean value of the low heart rate. From these data (see the last column in Table 7–2), it seems reasonable to suggest the following guidelines for the Holter diagnosis of sinus bradycardia relative to age:

1. Neonates: <60 bpm sleeping and <80 bpm awake.
2. Infants: virtually the same, based on the Southall group's[17] study in 110 full-term infants that showed essentially the same mean heart rate at 6 months of age and at all other earlier ages except at 4 months of age, when the mean heart rate was significantly higher (119.3 bpm for males/112.2 bpm for females at birth, 117.3/116.9 at 6 months, and 140.7/131.6 at 4 months, p = 0.002):
3. Children age 2–6 years: <60 bpm.
4. Children ages 7–11 years: <45 bpm.

TABLE 7–1
SURFACE ECG CRITERIA FOR SINUS NODE DYSFUNCTION

1. Sinus bradycardia
2. Severe sinus arrhythmia
3. Sinus pause or arrest
4. Slow escape rhythms
5. Sinoatrial exit block (second degree type I and II)
6. Brady/tachyarrhythmias
7. Sinus node reentry tachycardia
8. Atrial muscle reentry tachycardia* (e.g., atrial flutter-fibrillation)

*May be found in some patients without sinus node dysfunction.

TABLE 7–2
LOW HEART RATE BY 24-HOUR AMBULATORY (HOLTER) ECG IN NORMAL INFANTS, CHILDREN, AND YOUNG ADULTS

INVESTIGATORS	AGE OF SUBJECTS	NUMBER OF SUBJECTS	LOWEST HEART RATE BY HOLTER (bpm)	(−) 2 SD FROM MEAN (bpm)
Montague et al[21]	3.5 d	29	107 ± 15 SD (awake)	77
			92 ± 11 SD (sleep)	70
Southall et al[18]	<1 mon	134	93 ± 12 SD (sleep)	59
Southall et al[19]	7–11 yr	92	56 ± 6 SD	44
Viitasalo et al[20]	23 ± 6.1 SD (endurance athletes)	35	37.7 ± 4.3 SD (sleep)	29
	23 ± 5.8 SD (controls)	35	45.4 ± 6.3 SD (sleep)	39

Abbreviations: bpm = beats per minute; d = days; mo = months; SD = standard deviation from the mean; yr = year.

5. Adolescents and young adults: <40 bpm.
6. Endurance and other highly trained athletes: <30 bpm.

It must be emphasized that these guidelines are derived from Holter studies and that most of the reports did not distinguish between sleeping and waking heart rates. This is relevant to the heart rate found on resting standard ECG. Particularly in infants and young children, substantial anxiety and crying are involved with carrying out a standard ECG. It is therefore practical to assume that these guidelines should be increased somewhat for heart rate determined by standard ECG. On the other hand, the lowest heart rate during sleep may not differ much from the waking heart rate (Fig. 7–2). This was found in the neonate Holter study that evaluated heart rate during both states (Table 7–2)[21] and also in the study in medical students by Brodsky et al.[15] Nevertheless, from available surface ECG data, it appears that sinus bradycardia is present when heart rate is higher at each age when compared to the Holter data listed in Table 7–2. The following guidelines appear reasonable for the diagnosis of sinus bradycardia by surface standard ECG[9]:

1. Infants and children to 3 years of age: <100 bpm.
2. Children age 3–9 years: <60 bpm.
3. Children age 9–16 years: <50 bpm.
4. Children older than 16 years: <40 bpm.

The differential diagnosis of sinus bradycardia should be considered each time the disorder is suspected. First, as with any arrhythmia, artifact should be considered. Fast recordings by Holter tape or by paper speed are confirmed when all intervals appear prolonged and when other recordings from the same patient show normal intervals (Fig. 7–3). Arrhythmias with a regular, slow ventricular rate that show a P wave before each normal QRS make it difficult to distinguish the apparent sinus bradycardia from other causes of regular QRS bradycardia. The key to making the correct diagnosis is to scrutinize the T waves for additional "hidden" P waves. Three arrhythmias with hidden P waves are complete (third degree) AV block, second degree 2:1 AV block, and nonconducted atrial premature beats in a bigeminy pattern (Fig. 7–4). Complete AV block is the easiest to detect; by evaluating longer recordings, it can be seen that usually the P waves occur without any relationship to the QRS. The best technique to distinguish second degree AV block and nonconducted atrial bigeminy is to use multiple ECG leads. In some leads the hidden P waves may not be detectable, but in others it is clear that a P wave is within the T wave. A rare cause of bradycardia is concealed junctional premature extrasystoles in a bigeminy pattern.[22] The diagnosis can be confirmed only by intracardiac electrophysiology study.

Severe sinus arrhythmia may suggest the presence of SND (Fig. 7–5). It is defined by a variation in RR interval of 100% or more.[23] This arrhythmia usually is found in association with sinus bradycardia and is difficult to distinguish from sinoatrial exit block (see below).

Sinus pause or arrest occurs when the sinus node fails to generate an impulse. It is evident by the absence of a sinus-induced P wave for a period that is not equal to a multiple of the sinus PP interval. The latter characteristic distinguishes sinus pause or ar-

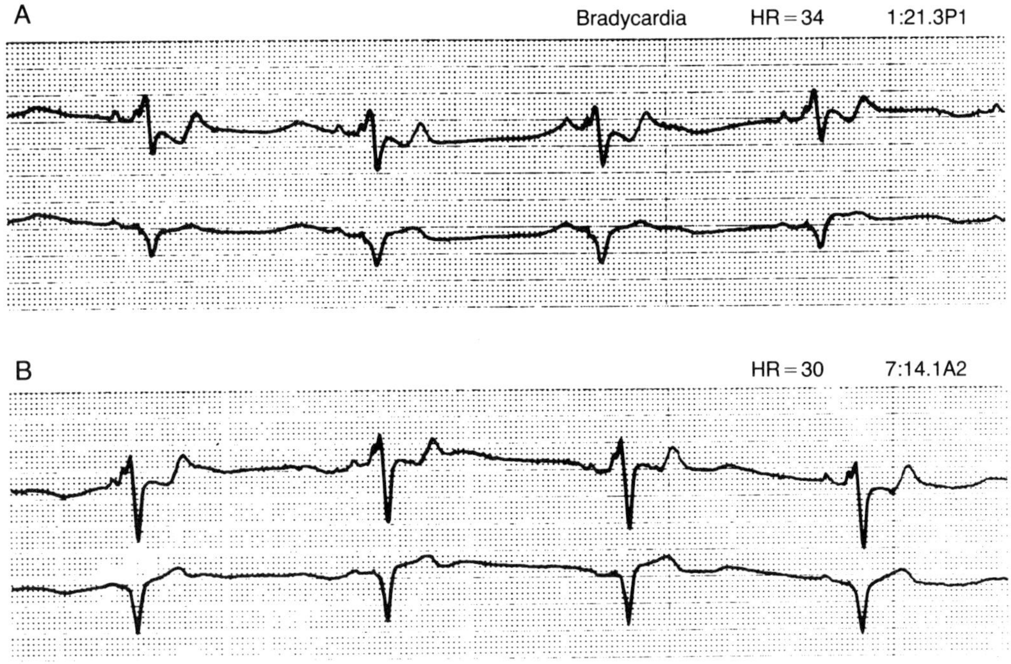

FIGURE 7–2
Sinus bradycardia was recorded by 24-hour ambulatory monitor (Holter) from a 14-year-old boy who previously had undergone plication repair of Ebstein's anomaly and surgical division of accessory atrioventricular connection. Sinus node dysfunction was noted preoperatively but was worse postoperatively, as shown. The degree of sinus bradycardia was approximately the same whether the patient was awake (*A*) or asleep (*B*). Although the patient denied symptoms, parents complained that their son was much less active than his peers. Paper speed was 25 mm/s.

rest from type II second degree sinoatrial exit block (see below). If the sinus arrest is prolonged and sinus rhythm does not resume, an escape focus may act as the pacemaker of the heart for variable periods of time until the sinus node recovers and fires at a rate faster than the subsidiary pacemaker focus.[24–26] Escape beats/rhythm may originate from the right or left atrium, AV junction, or fascicles/ventricles (Fig. 7–6). When more than several consecutive escape beats from a focus other than the sinus node are found, the escape rhythm is referred to as atrial, junctional or ventricular rhythm. The term "by default" may be added, implying that the rhythm exists in default of the sinus node. The interval from the sinus arrest to escape beats depends on the automaticity characteristics and function of the escape pacemaker focus. The presence of long periods without a junctional beat may also imply an abnormality of AV nodal or His bundle (junctional) automaticity. Junctional escape rhythms may be normal at any age and most commonly are found during sinus arrhythmia. The "normal" junctional escape rate is unknown for humans, but Urthaler et al have shown that it approximates 66% of the expected sinus rate in dogs.[27–29] The normal escape interval is unknown, but probably relates to age. Two studies have been carried out: one in healthy children age 7–11 years, and the other in healthy medical students.[15, 18] The mean maximum duration of sinus pause, plus two standard deviations, was 1.82 S for the children and 2.02 S for the young adults.

Escape rhythms at slow rates are signs of SND. Sometimes the onset of sinus arrest is not recorded, and the escape rhythm is the only suggestion of SND (Fig. 7–7). However, it is important to distinguish escape rhythms (i.e., default) from rhythms that result from abnormally increased automaticity (i.e., usurpation). Rhythms of usurpation exist when a rate greater than the sinus rate is present from a focus other than the sinus node. For example, if an adolescent has a resting junctional rhythm at a rate of 95 bpm, it is likely that the junctional pacemaker focus is more rapid than that of the sinus node. That is, the junctional rhythm is by usurpation (so-called "accelerated junctional rhythm") and not by default of the sinus node. Therefore SND is not necessarily present when a junctional rhythm is present. The problem in differentiating between usurpation and de-

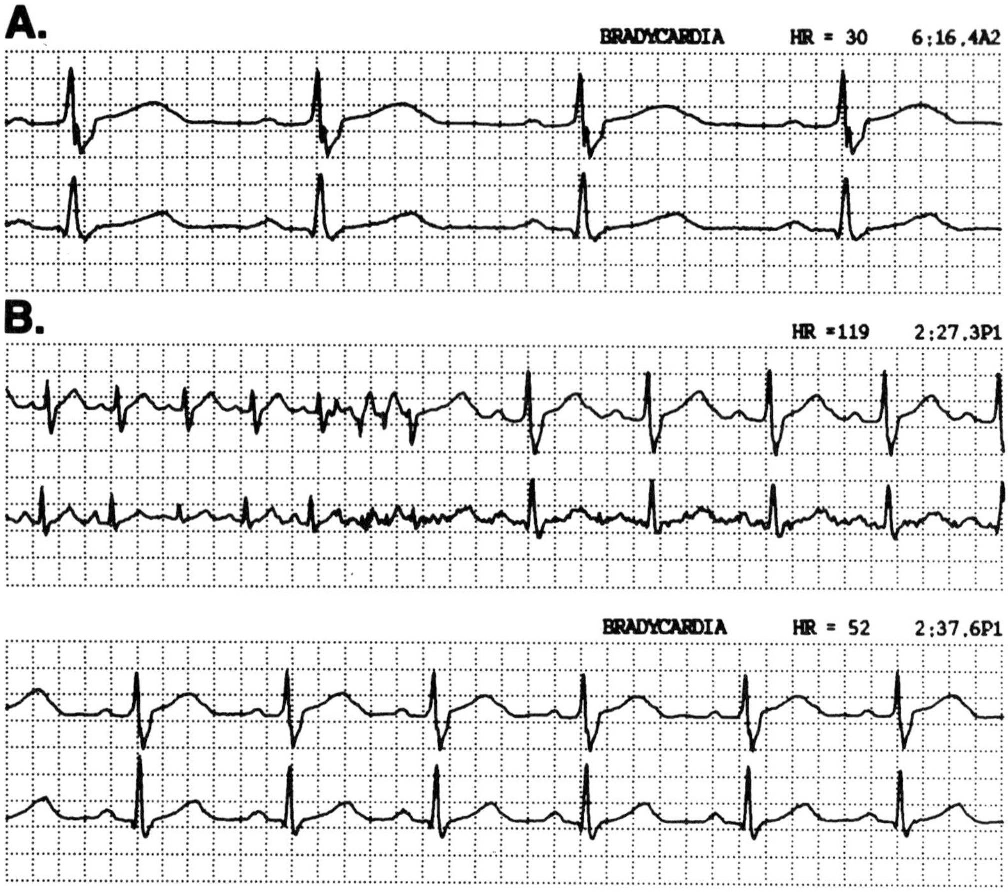

FIGURE 7–3

This apparent sinus bradycardia recorded in a 7-year-old boy actually was artifactual as a result of Holter system malfunction. In *A*, the duration of all ECG intervals was prolonged. The QT especially was notable (1.0 s). In *B*, the recording system malfunction was confirmed by first noting the normal rate of 125 bpm with normal ECG intervals, followed by 3–4 beats of artifactual shortened intervals, then followed again by long intervals. The Holter recorder was found to have a malfunctioning motor (tape drive) that caused variable fast and slow tape recording speeds. Paper speed was 25 mm/s.

fault rhythms is maximized when the rate of the nonsinus focus is only slightly faster or slightly slower than the lower limit of sinus rate for age. In these borderline cases, it is often impossible to determine the site of disease unless the transition from rhythm to rhythm is recorded (Fig. 7–8). Usurpation or default rhythm then can be differentiated: if the sinus node slows, the rhythm is a default rhythm; if the secondary focus increases, the rhythm is an usurpation rhythm.

Arrhythmias that should be considered in the differential diagnosis of sinus pause/arrest include intermittent nonconducted premature atrial beats or concealed junctional premature beats.[22] Another possible cause of an erroneous diagnosis of sinus pause or arrest includes problems associated with recording equipment. The opportunity for artifactual pauses is high when Holter monitoring is carried out in active children. Holter monitor leads can malfunction (e.g., separate from skin), as shown by the recording in Fig. 7–9.

Sinoatrial (SA) exit block, also known as SA block, varies in severity (first, second, or third degree). *First degree SA block* is present when there is prolonged conduction out of the sinus node through the perinodal fibers (SA junction) to the high right atrium. Although the word "block" traditionally is used, first degree SA block means that only prolonged conduction is present, but there is no interruption of the impulse (i.e., normal P wave is generated). Because the sinus nodal impulse is not recordable by surface ECG, first degree SA block is not directly evident. It is possible to diagnose first degree SA block by

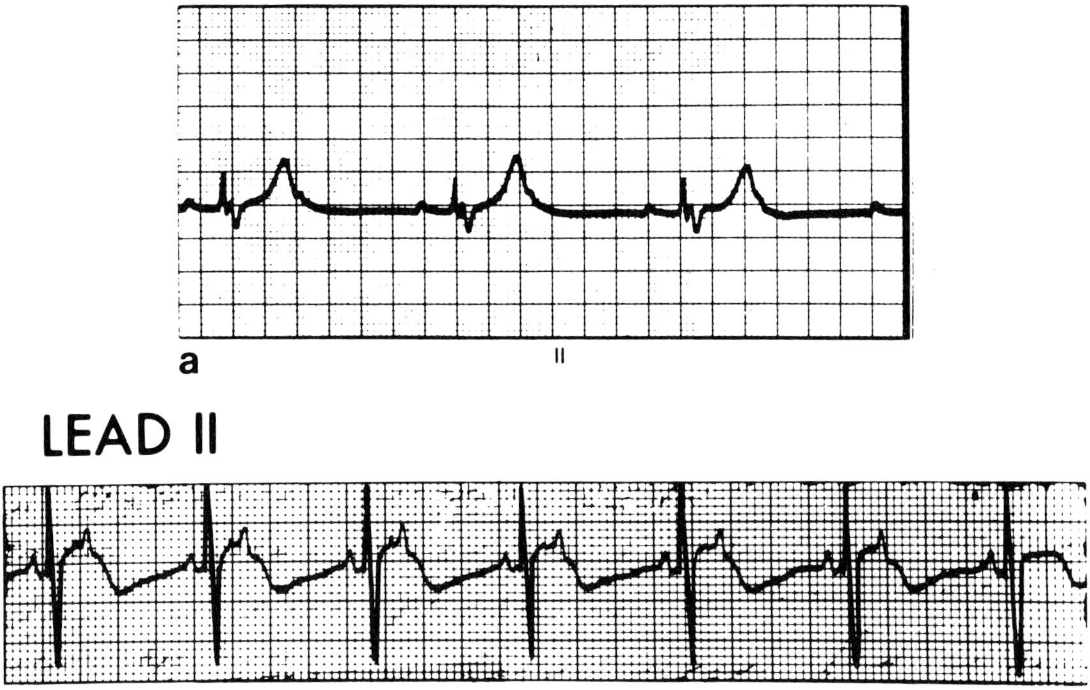

FIGURE 7–4
Two ECG recordings show examples of bradyarrhythmias that can be confused with sinus bradycardia. In *A*, fixed 2:1 second degree AV block accounted for the bradycardia of 42 bpm. The nonconducted P waves were evident within the terminal downslope of the T wave. The rhythm in panel *B* was recorded from a 4-month-old infant who had undergone ventricular septal defect repair 1 day earlier. The bradycardia was a result of nonconducted premature atrial beats in a bigeminy pattern. The infant's condition deteriorated during the bradycardia but markedly improved when the premature atrial beats were controlled. Paper speed was 25 mm/s, and calibration was 1 mV/10 mm.

calculating the sinoatrial conduction time (SACT) indirectly (only when premature atrial beats occur spontaneously); however this is not commonly done. The method is identical to that used to indirectly calculate SACT when premature atrial extra beats are induced into sinus rhythm during electrophysiology study (see section on sinus node function testing).

Second degree SA block may be either type I or type II (Fig. 7–10). Type I SA exit block is synonymously known as SA Wenckebach block and classically is diagnosed when PP intervals shorten by decreasing amounts until SA block occurs (see Fig. 7–10). To understand SA Wenckebach block, it is helpful to begin with the principles of atrioventricular (AV) Wenckebach block: the PP intervals are constant; the PR intervals lengthen progressively until a P wave occurs without a follow-

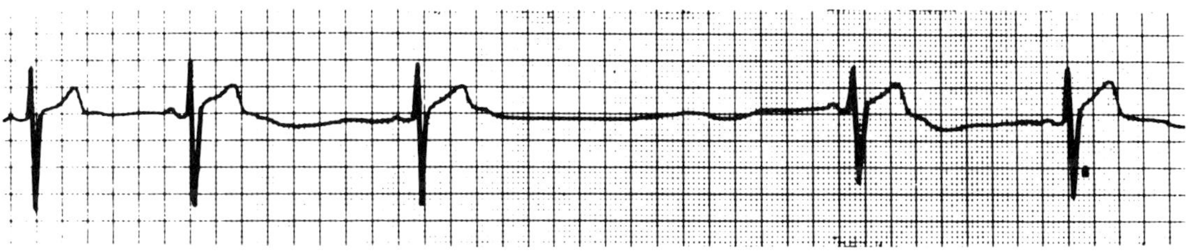

24 Hr Ambulatory ECG - Lead II

FIGURE 7–5
Severe sinus arrhythmia in a 15-year-old boy was detected by a Holter monitor during sleeping and waking (this tracing) hours. The patient also had severe sinus bradycardia with dizziness and syncope. A permanent pacemaker was implanted, and the patient had no further symptoms. Paper speed was 25 mm/s, and calibration was 1 mV/10 mm.

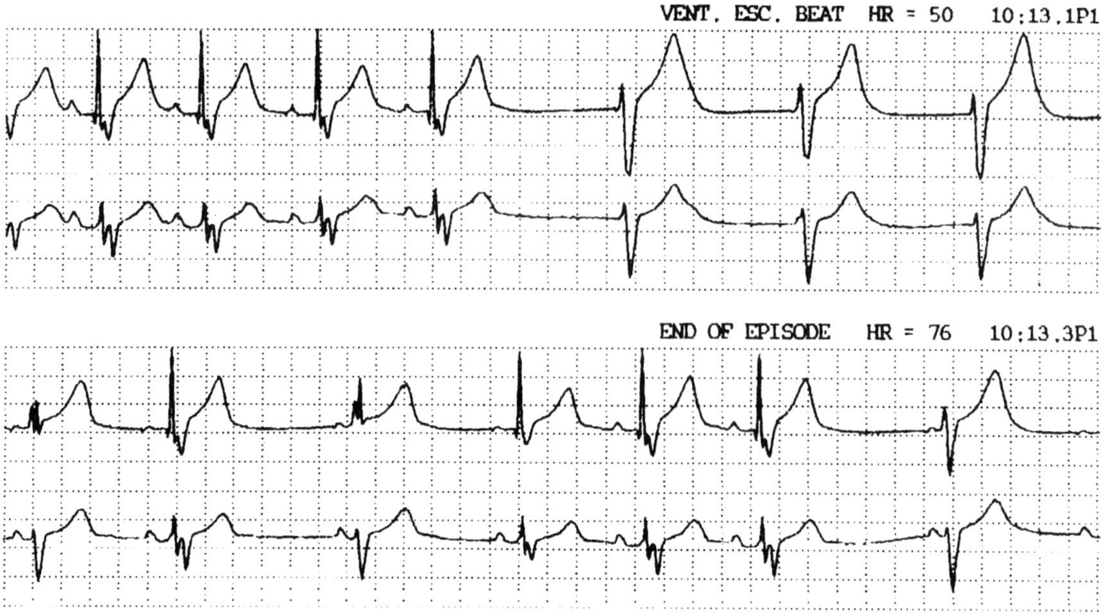

FIGURE 7–6
Holter ECG recording (top, lead II; bottom, lead I) from a 10-year-old boy with preoperative Ebstein's anomaly shows sinus arrest with ventricular escape rhythm. The ventricular escape rate was somewhat faster than expected in this patient. Therefore, junctional disease may not have been present. In the bottom recording, the second and fourth beats were of atrial rather than sinus origin, because the P wave morphology changed, and the first, second, and last beats were atrial and ventricular fusion escape beats. Paper speed was 25 mm/s.

ing QRS complex; the pause in the RR interval containing the nonconducted P wave is less than twice the preceding RR interval; and from the beginning of the sequence, the RR intervals progressively shorten. The reason for the progressive RR shortening is that the increment by which the PR interval lengthens decreases with each successive beat. In SA Wenckebach block (diagrammed in Figure 7–10), (1) the sinus node to sinus node impulse interval is constant; (2) the sinus node impulse to high right atrial intervals lengthens progressively until a sinus node impulse occurs without a following P wave (nonconducted sinus node impulse); (3) the pause in the PP interval containing the nonconducted sinus node impulse is less than twice the preceding PP interval; and (4) from the beginning of the sequence, the PP intervals progressively shorten. Only (3) and (4) can be detected on the surface ECG; (1) and (2) must be inferred. In instances where the sinus PP interval is unknown because of continual SA Wenckebach block, the shortest PP interval occurs immediately before the nonconducted sinus node impulse and in most

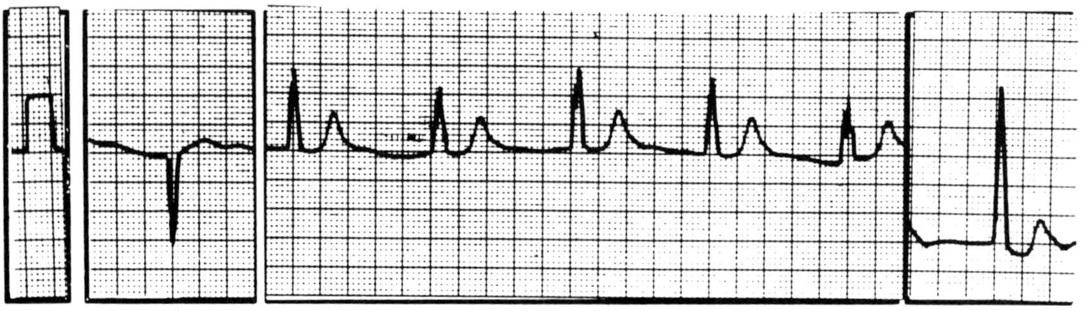

FIGURE 7–7
Leads I, II, and III ECG recording from a 5-year-old boy who had undergone a Mustard operation shows wide QRS junctional or ventricular escape rhythm at 60 bpm. Because of the slow rate for age, it is assumed that this rhythm existed in default of sinus rhythm. Paper speed was 25 mm/s, and calibration was 1 mV/10 mm.

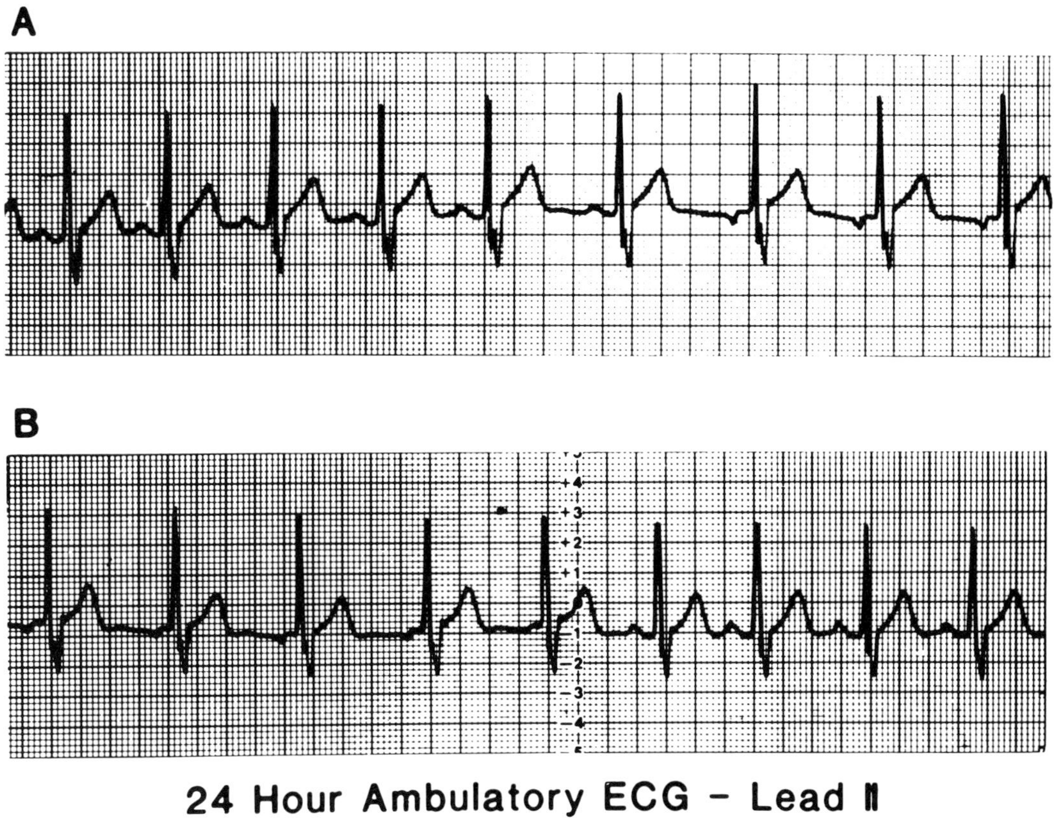

FIGURE 7–8
Transition from sinus to low right atrial rhythm and vice versa was recorded by Holter monitor in a normal 6-year-old child. When the sinus rate decreased only slightly from a rate of 85 bpm (*A*), the atrial pacemaker "escape" rhythm existed (rate of 71 bpm). This patient had normal heart rates (*B*), and there was no evidence of sinus node dysfunction. Paper speed was 25 mm/s, and calibration was 1 mV/10 mm.

cases closely approximates the sinus interval. Schamroth and Dove have explained the calculation of the sinus cycle length from SA Wenckebach sequences.[30]

The differential diagnosis of type I SA block includes sinus arrhythmia and premature atrial beats. Wenckebach SA block in most instances can be distinguished from sinus arrhythmia by carefully noting that in sinus arrhythmia the PP intervals gradually lengthen after a gradual shortening (see Fig. 7–5). Pauses in sinus arrhythmia occur at the end of lengthening PP intervals rather than at the end of shortening PP intervals, as is seen in SA Wenckebach block. When sinus arrhythmia coexists with SA Wenckebach block, the diagnosis of SA Wenckebach is difficult. Schamroth and Dove have noted that it is helpful to plot each PP interval against its succeeding PP interval.[30]

Type II SA exit block is detected by ECG and, perhaps for this reason, is said to be more common than type I SA block. The long PP interval (which includes the nonconducted sinus node impulse) is an exact multiple of the sinus PP interval (see Fig. 7–10). Usually, this is not the case when sinus pause or arrest occurs. Differential diagnosis includes those arrhythmias discussed previously for type I SA block.

Third degree (complete) SA exit block implies normal sinus node impulse generation, but none of the impulses are conducted to the right atrium. This cannot be distinguished on the ECG from sinus arrest caused by automaticity dysfunction. As with complete sinus arrest, an escape rhythm is present on the ECG (either atrial, junctional, or ventricular).

Brady/tachyarrhythmias encompass all arrhythmias that have variable periods of alternating bradycardia and tachycardia (Figs. 7–11 and 7–12).[2, 31] The slow heart rate may be of sinus, atrial, junctional, or even ventricular origin if junctional disease coexists. Most young patients with brady/tachyarrhythmias

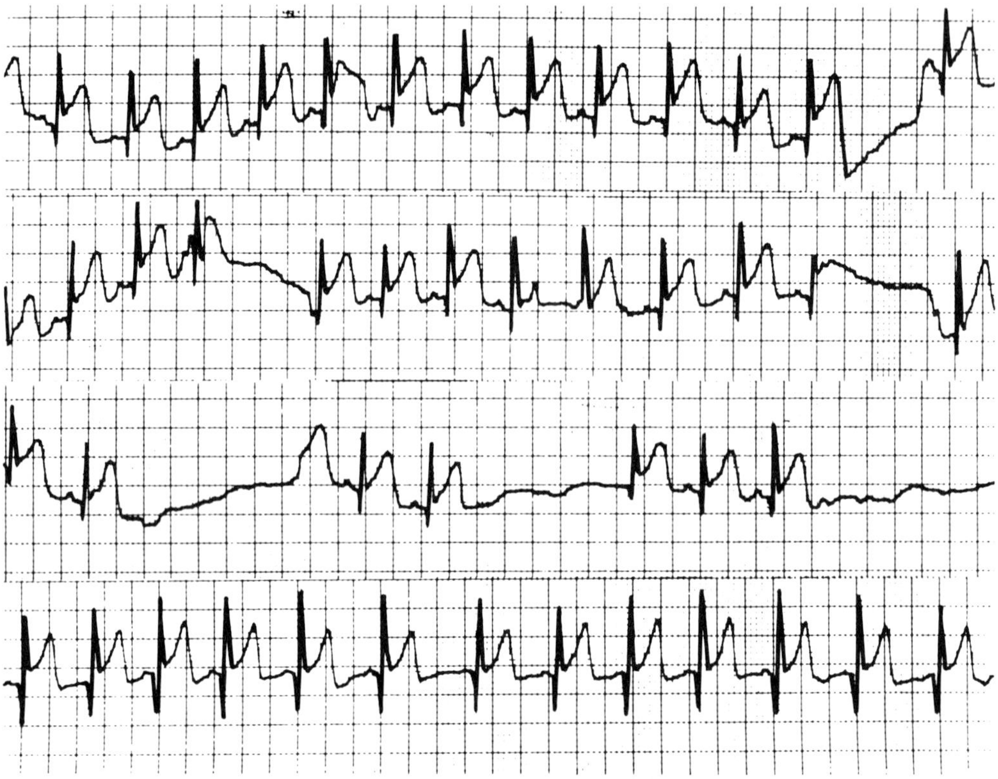

FIGURE 7–9
These ECG recordings by a Holter monitor in an infant demonstrate that sinus arrest can be simulated by intermittent lead malfunction. In this example, the third complex in the third strip shows a T wave without preceding QRS, thus supporting the interpretation that the other pauses were artifactual. The ECG leads were found to be intermittently malfunctioning. Paper speed was 25 mm/s.

at some previous time have undergone an intracardiac operation of one or more of the following types: atrial septal defect repair, atrial repair of transposition of the great arteries, partial or total anomalous pulmonary venous connection, or repair of any defect requiring extensive atrial surgery (e.g., Fontan).[32–45] Operated or nonoperated patients with right atrial (e.g., Ebstein's anomaly) or left atrial (e.g., mitral regurgitation or stenosis) volume/pressure overload also are at risk for these arrhythmias.[46–48]

The mechanism of the tachyarrhythmia typically is atrial muscle reentry.[44, 49, 50] For each patient, the atrial rate is relatively constant, but the ventricular rate ranges from 150 bpm to 350 bpm among patients of different ages. The most common atrial/ventricular rate ratio is 2:1, but with excellent AV conduction and/or slower atrial rates, 1:1 conduction is relatively common. Atrial flutter usually is considered a type of atrial muscle reentry tachycardia.[49] Although the term "atrial flutter" often is used loosely to describe any atrial muscle tachycardia with an atrial rate of 200 bpm to 350 bpm (again, dependent on patient age), classic atrial flutter by ECG shows typical sawtooth "flutter" waves (Fig. 7–12). Atrial fibrillation is uncommon in infants, children, and adolescents.

Sinus nodal reentry tachycardia is thought to involve reentry within the sinus node as part of the microreentry circuit.[50–52] Atrial muscle reentry tachycyardia within the high right atrial muscle would be expected to produce P wave axis and morphology identical to that produced by sinus nodal reentry (Fig. 7–13). Therefore, these two types of tachycardias are virtually indistinguishable by electrophysiology study (see discussion of intracardiac electrophysiologic investigation). Atrial muscle reentry in other parts of the atrium causes P waves with a morphology different from that of the sinus.

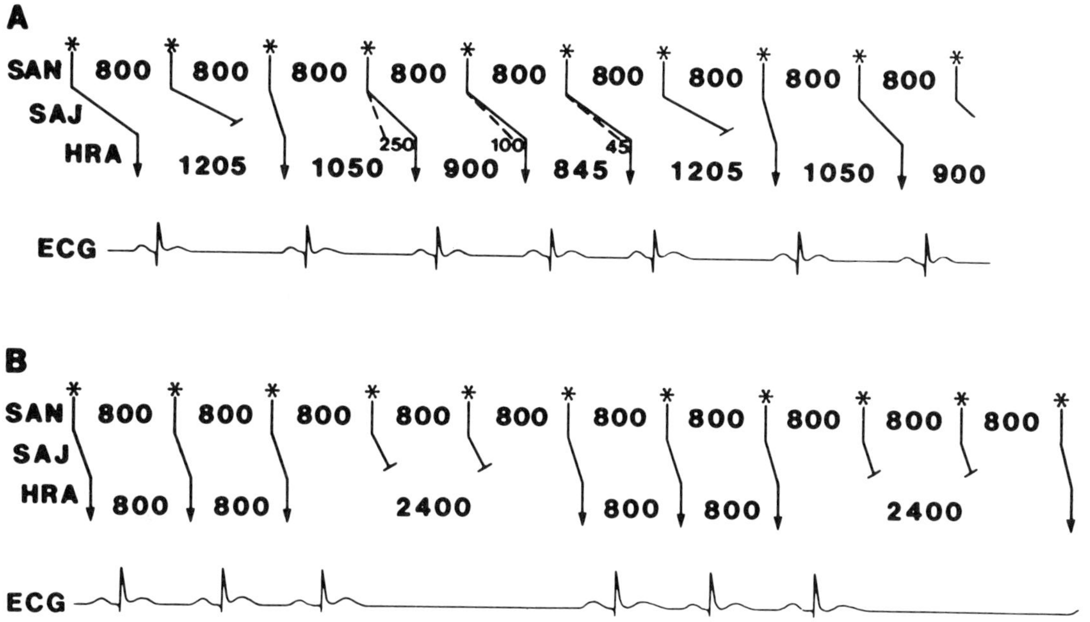

FIGURE 7–10

Second degree sinoatrial (SA) exit block is illustrated by ladder diagram. In *A*, type I (Wenckebach) is characterized by decreasing PP intervals by decreasing amounts (see text). In *B*, type II is more easily diagnosed because the long PP interval is an exact multiple of the sinus PP interval; in the example the SA ratio is 3:2. If the long PP interval was composed of two rather than three sinus PP intervals, the ratio would be 2:1. (SAN, sinoatrial node; SAJ, sinoatrial junction; HRA, high right atrium; all numbers indicate msec.)

Automatic ectopic focus atrial tachycardia from the high right atrium also may be indistinguishable by surface ECG from the various atrial muscle reentry tachycardias and from sinus nodal reentry tachcyardia.[53] This is especially true if the onset and termination are not available for review. The onset and termination of reentry atrial tachycardias (including atrial flutter) are paroxysmal, whereas the automatic ectopic tachycardias typically show a gradual shortening of atrial cycle length during onset and a gradual lengthening during termination.[54]

The mechanism of the bradycardia, regardless of the tachycardia, has been thought by some to be a result of "overdrive suppression" of an abnormal sinus node.[2] Although no data have been reported in children, there are conflicting data in adults. Hattori et al showed that in adults there was no evidence of spontaneous tachycardia-induced overdrive suppression; they found that pauses after tachycardia were not significantly different from spontaneous pauses before tachycardia.[55] These investigators concluded that abnormal sinus node automaticity is independent of the tachycardia episodes. Evaluating sinus node automaticity differently, Gang et al found that spontaneous and postpacing sinus node recovery times correlated closely.[56] These investigators compared sinus node recovery times after spontaneous tachycardia with those after atrial pacing. The postpacing recovery times were more prolonged, suggesting the presence of probable atriosinus entrance block during fast atrial tachycardia. Often the atrial tachycardia is incessant, and the underlying bradycardia is not evident until measures are taken to control the tachycardia. When tachycardia stops, if sinus node automaticity is abnormal, pauses and bradycardia prevail (Figs. 7–11 and 7–12). The type of bradycardia is dependent on the function and automaticity of the sinus node, atria, and AV node/His bundle.

Bradycardia predisposes to the development of ectopy, because longer sinus cycle lengths provide the opportunity for increased automaticity of subsidiary foci (e.g., premature atrial beats). Moreover, these patients often have coexisting atrial muscle disease that provides the substrate for abnormal atrial electrical function. Areas of abnormal atrial conduction and automaticity thus provide the opportunity for spontaneous induction and maintenance of atrial muscle or sinus node reentry tachycardia.[57–59]

Differential diagnosis of brady/tachyar-

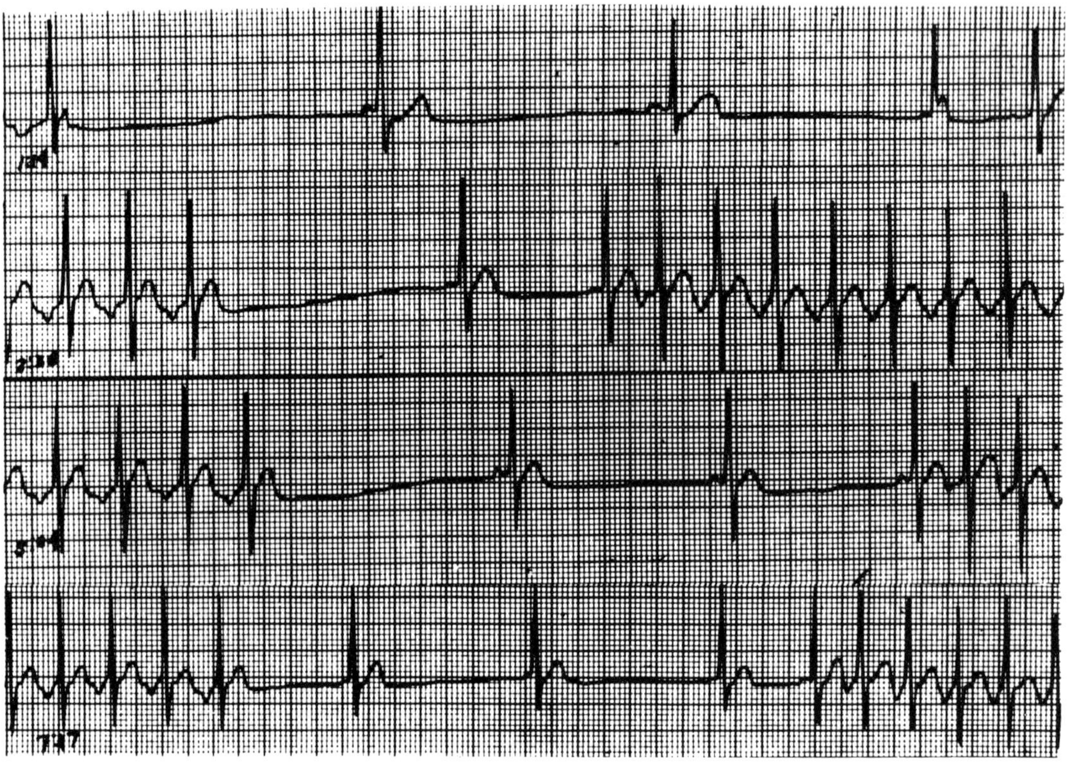

24 Hr Ambulatory ECG - Lead II

FIGURE 7–11
Brady/tachyarrhythmia was recorded by Holter monitor in a patient who had undergone atrial septal defect closure. Sinus/atrial bradycardia is present in the top recording. In each of the other recordings, pauses were interrupted by paroxysmal atrial tachycardia. The atrial tachycardia probably consisted of an atrial rate of 270–300 bpm, and the ventricular rate was 135–150 bpm. Paper speed was 25 mm/s.

rhythmias is primarily made from studying the tachycardias. One of the most overlooked tachyarrhythmias is an atrial muscle tachycardia (discussed previously) with 2:1 AV conduction. Most commonly, the diagnosis of "sinus tachycardia" is made erroneously. A P wave is detected before each QRS, but another P wave is often missed because it is "buried" in the T wave of the preceding QRS (Fig. 7–14). Another helpful clue is to note that the ventricular rate with this tachyarrhythmia varies little with activity or sleep (most commonly, heart rate is approximately 150 bpm). A high index of suspicion is essential to the diagnosis of this subtle tachyarrhythmia. Confirmation in most patients is necessary by either transesophageal (Fig. 7–14) or intracardiac recordings (see section on intracardiac investigation and Fig. 7–28).

Exercise Testing

Exercise testing is a valuable noninvasive technique to evaluate sinus node function in patients older than 4–5 years.[5] The major objective during exercise evaluation of sinus node function is to determine the maximum heart rate response. Therefore, it is imperative that the test is carried out to exhaustion. Also, although both bicycle ergometer and treadmill are accepted methods of exercise testing, the treadmill appears to offer the greatest chance of reaching peak heart rate response. The Bruce protocol as modified by Cumming, Everatt, and Hastman and by Hesslein is an excellent method to use in reaching the goals of exhaustion and maximum heart rate.[60, 61] The major advantages are that it allows continued, progressive speed and load in a relatively short period of time. It is important to record simultaneous limb leads.[5] In this manner, the P wave axis is determined, and sinus rhythm is confirmed before, during, and after exercise.

Exercise testing is most valuable in (1) patients with sinus bradycardia, (2) patients without sinus bradycardia in whom the diagnosis of SND is suspected for other rea-

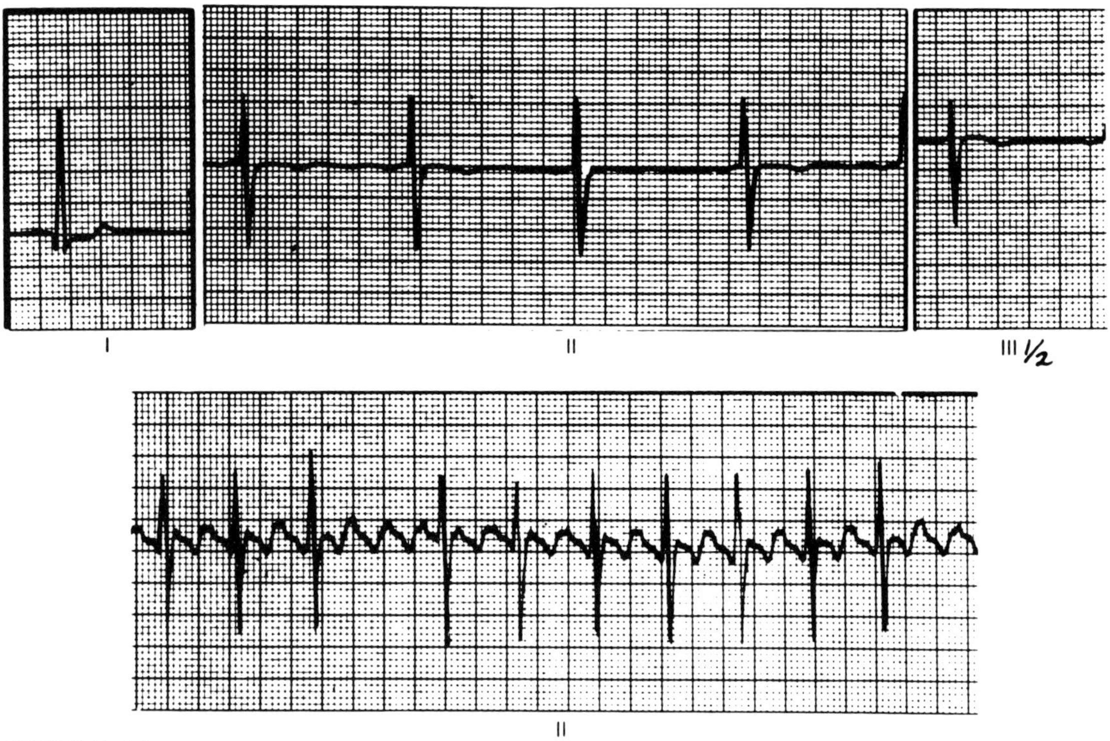

FIGURE 7–12
Rhythm was recorded by ECG at different times and shows brady/tachyarrhythmias in a 5-year-old girl who recently had undergone repair of ostium primum atrial septal defect. In the top recording, low right atrial rhythm at 53 bpm depicts bradycardia, and in the bottom recording, typical atrial flutter with variable AV block depicts the tachyarrhythmia. During electrophysiology study, corrected sinus node recovery time measured more than 4000 ms. Paper speed was 25 mm/s.

sons, and (3) patients in whom SND is known, but severity or clinical significance is unknown.

In patients with sinus bradycardia, the question often arises: Is this a sign of SND or is it merely a clinically insignificant finding? The maximum heart rate response of normal children and adolescents during treadmill testing is frequently greater than 190 bpm and virtually always greater than 180 bpm.[61] Therefore if maximum heart rate is less than 180 bpm during exercise to exhaustion, SND is present. Exercise testing also may be helpful in identifying patients with SND by noting an exaggerated decrease in heart rate after exercise, especially when symptoms correlate.

In patients who have underlying heart disease with a relatively higher incidence of associated SND (e.g., atrial repair of transposition of the great arteries), SND may only become evident during exercise testing. This finding was noted by Hesslein et al when they studied 29 pediatric patients who had previously undergone Mustard repair for transposition of the great arteries.[10] Only two had a resting heart rate less than two standard deviations from normal, but 22 had subnormal heart rate response during maximal treadmill testing. These investigators also found that in these patients, treadmill exercise testing was a more sensitive indicator of SND than electrophysiology testing. This conclusion was based on the finding that of 16 patients having an abnormal exercise heart rate response, only nine were identified by electrophysiology testing as having SND.

Occasionally, further information is needed in patients with known SND. A common problem for clinicians is to assess the significance of "fatigue" in patients who have known mild or moderate SND. Often the information from exercise testing is helpful in determining the severity of dysfunction. For example, if a patient with postoperative atrial septal defect and mild SND (manifested by occasional asymptomatic sinus pauses and mild sinus bradycardia) had a maximum heart rate of 190 bpm with normal exercise tolerance, the complaint of "severe fatigue"

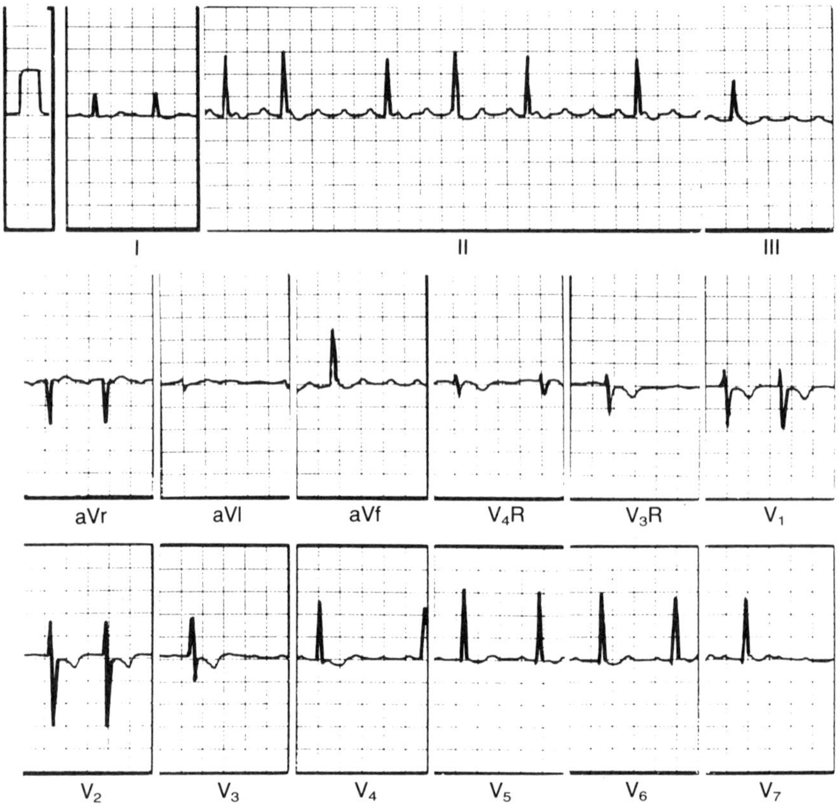

FIGURE 7–13
This 15-lead ECG recorded from an 18-year-old woman who had undergone closure of secundum atrial septal defect 4 years earlier shows sinus node reentry tachycardia or high right atrial muscle tachycardia. The atrial rate was 280 bpm, and the ventricular rate was variable. Paper speed was 25 mm/s.

probably is not related to the SND. Sometimes, however, patients with sinus bradycardia and fatigue have normal responses on treadmill testing, as measured by both endurance and maximum heart rate.

Transtelephonic Electrocardiography

Recording of rhythm by a portable, compact device with memory and then later transmitting data by telephone is an excellent technique to document the presence of infrequent arrhythmia with symptoms.[5, 62, 63] Most often this device helps exclude the presence of arrhythmia. The major limitation is in patients who have infrequent but severe symptoms of syncope, because when symptoms are without warning or are of short duration, the patient or family is unable to physically apply the device in time to record the rhythm.[5] Another practical limitation is that the technique requires close availability of the device at all times.

Transesophageal Atrial Recording and Pacing

Transesophageal atrial recording and pacing is a minimally invasive technique whose utility is greatest with the tachycardia and bradycardia arrhythmias of SND. It is most valuable with the tachyarrhythmias, because often the question arises as to whether atrial tachycardia with 2:1 block is present.[64, 65] With this arrhythmia, the atrial electrogram recorded by transesophageal technique is diagnostic (Fig. 7–14). The technique also is valuable because the atrial tachycardia can be converted by overdrive transesophageal atrial pacing. Although the technique also can be used to determine sinus node recovery time after atrial pacing (see the section on intracardiac electrophysiologic investigation), this

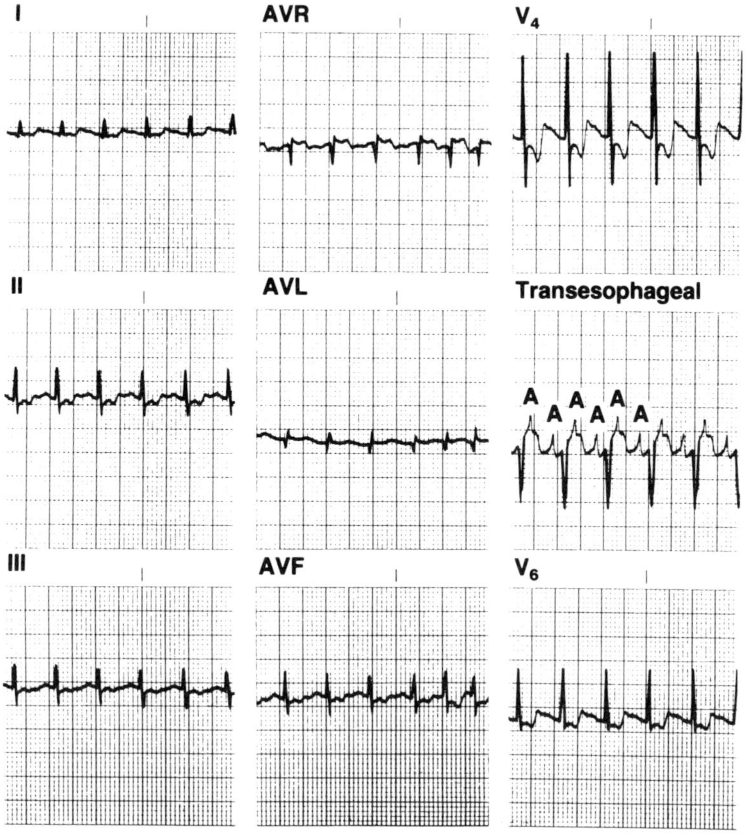

FIGURE 7–14
Simultaneously recorded, three-channel limb leads are shown with chest leads V_4 and V_6 simultaneously recorded with an electrogram from transesophageal electrodes. The surface ECG suggests sinus tachycardia at a rate of slightly faster than 150 bpm in this 2-year-old boy who had undergone Mustard repair for transposition of the great arteries 18 months earlier. However, the rhythm was only correctly identified by recordings from the transesophageal electrodes. High right atrial muscle reentry or sinus node reentry tachycardia at an atrial (A) rate of slightly more than 300 bpm was evident with 2:1 AV block. Paper speed was 25 mm/s.

is not done often. Its major limitation when assessing sinus node function is that the site of atrial pacing is not close to the sinus node, and therefore the results may not be reliable. Also, there are no reported studies using this technique to determine sinus node function in normal children. The specific methodology of transesophageal atrial recording and stimulation has been reviewed by Benson et al.[66]

Atrial Recording and Pacing Using Temporary Epicardial Electrodes

Like transesophageal atrial pacing, atrial recording and pacing using temporary epicardial electrodes is not strictly noninvasive.[5, 67, 68] The epicardial wires are placed during intracardiac operation, but later, when these leads are used for recording and pacing, only a noninvasive technique is utilized.

Similar to transesophageal atrial pacing, this technique is valuable in detecting atrial activity when the surface ECG does not show distinct P waves and when there is a high index of suspicion that "buried" P waves may be present (Fig. 7–15). Sinus node function is assessable with this technique by connecting a pacing stimulator to the temporary leads and then carrying out the same pacing protocol used for intracardiac electrophysiology testing (see section on intracardiac electrophysiology investigation). An example of determining corrected sinus node recovery time is shown in Figure 7–16. The predictive value of later sinus node function is unknown compared to that obtained early postoperatively. Presently, data from the early postoperative assessment of sinus node function are best analyzed as a baseline for later comparison.[69] In a minority of patients, severe SND may be found, possibly requiring longer hospitalization, further evaluation, and/or treatment.

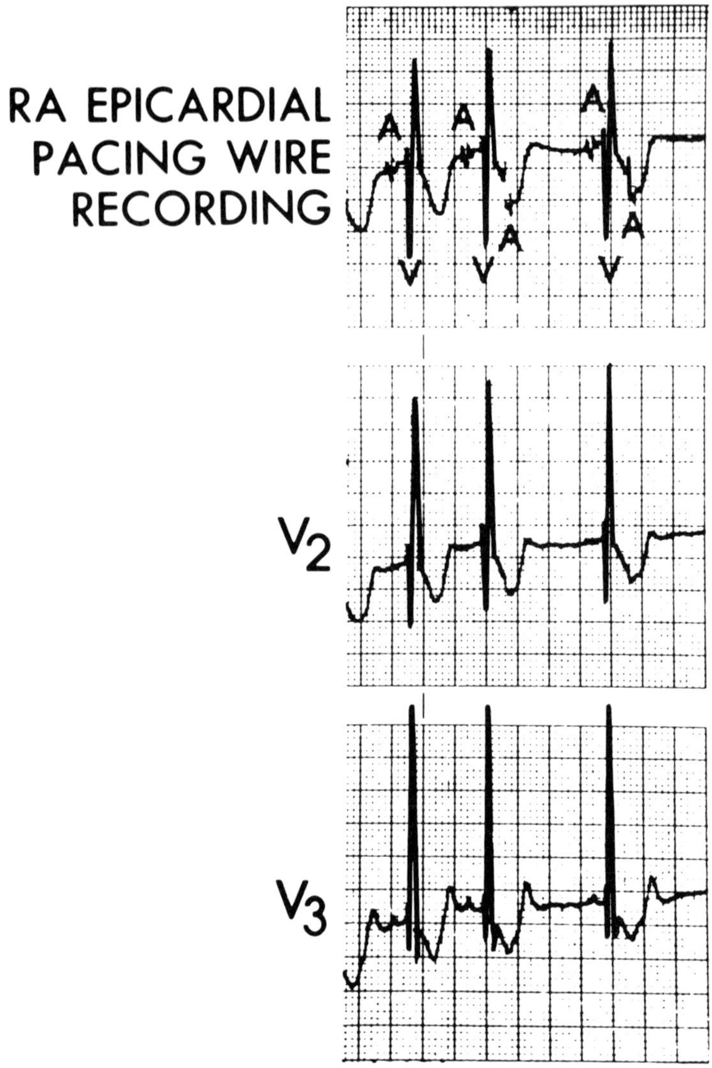

FIGURE 7–15
Electrogram from temporary epicardial right atrial (RA) wires placed at surgery (top) was simultaneously recorded with chest leads V_2 and V_3 from a 2-year-old patient who had just undergone a Mustard operation. Cause of the pauses was not evident until the recordings from the epicardial wires showed nonconducted premature atrial (A) beats (top, after second and third ventricular electrogram). Paper speed was 25 mm/s.

INTRACARDIAC ELECTROPHYSIOLOGIC INVESTIGATION OF SINUS NODE FUNCTION

During intracardiac electrophysiology study (EPS), sinus node activity is assessed directly by recording the sinus node electrogram or indirectly by recording the high right atrial (HRA) electrogram. The sinus node electrogram can be recorded by special techniques (described later) and can be used to directly assess sinus node automaticity and, by measuring the time from the onset of the sinus node electrogram to the onset of the HRA electrogram, to directly measure the sinoatrial conduction time (Fig. 7–17).[70–75] The indirect technique, whether during measurement of sinus node recovery or during calculation of sinoatrial conduction time, always includes the unknown atriosinus conduction time.[76]

The vast majority of electrophysiology laboratories use the indirect methods. The indirect techniques, although associated with many confirmed limitations, have compared favorably to the direct technique in several studies;[74, 77–80] that is, findings from the indirect techniques correspond to those from the direct technique under most circumstances. These results are important, because the direct technique requires more time and effort in the electrophysiology laboratory.

Direct Assessment

Direct recording of the sinus node electrogram is accomplished by using a fluoroscope

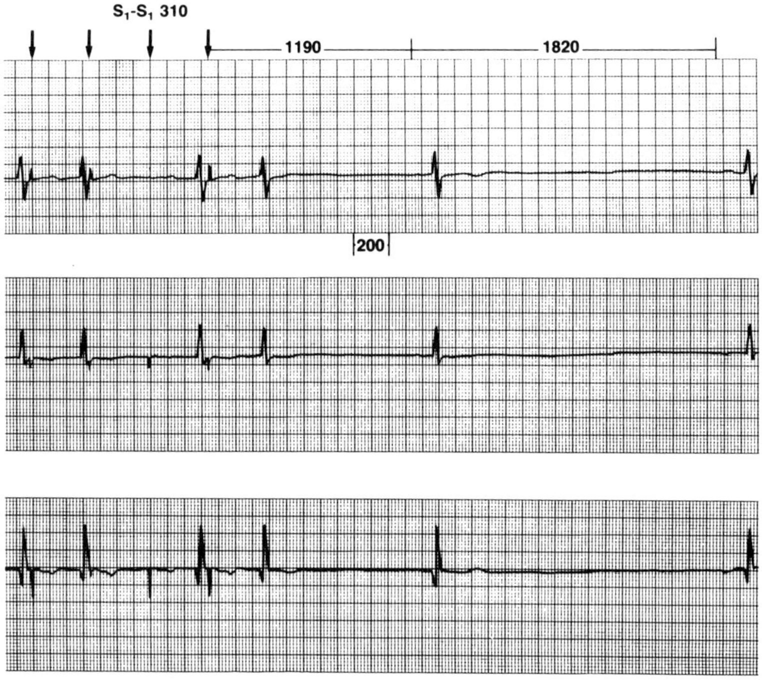

FIGURE 7–16
Simultaneous three-channel ECG (leads I, II, III) was recorded during atrial pacing by temporary epicardial right atrial wires. In this 4-year-old girl who had undergone closure of sinus venosus atrial septal defect 5 days earlier, atrial pacing was carried out to assess sinus node function because of postoperative sinus bradycardia. After 30 seconds of atrial pacing (S_1S_1) at a cycle length of 310 ms, the pacing was terminated, and the sinus node recovery time measured 1190 ms. Because the resting sinus cycle length was 640 ms, the corrected sinus node recovery time was 550 ms (see Fig. 7–18). A secondary pause of 1820 ms interrupted by an atrial escape beat (inverted P wave in II and III) also was found. Paper speed was 50 mm/s.

to achieve a stable catheter position (interelectrode distance, 5–10 mm) in the lateral superior vena caval–HRA junction.[74, 75, 79] Successful stable recordings are enhanced and baseline drift minimized while maintaining the catheter position by looping or by a prefixed catheter contour. High amplitude settings as well as proper filter settings are required. These settings vary among investigators as well as among patients studied by

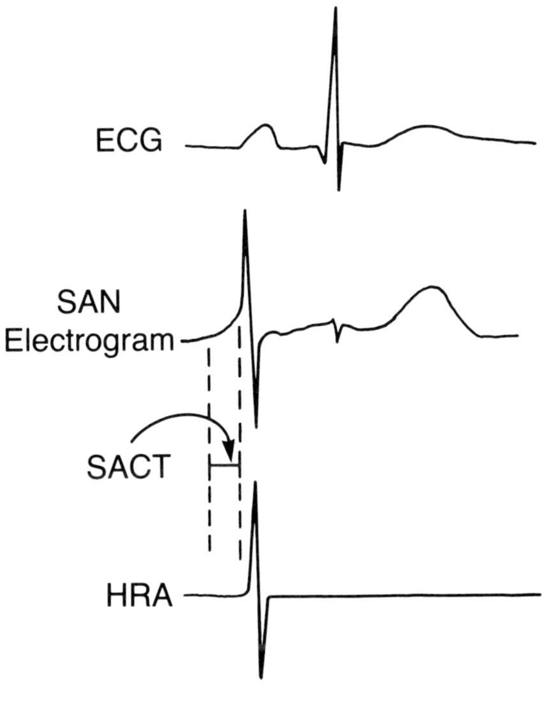

FIGURE 7–17
The measurement of direct sinoatrial conduction time (SACT) is illustrated by depicting diagrammatically simultaneous surface ECG, sinus node (SAN) electrogram, and the high right atrial (HRA) electrogram. The SACT is directly measured from the SAN electrogram onset to the HRA onset. See text for further description of technique.

an individual investigator. The amplification is to approximately 100 μV/cm.

Bethge, Gebhardt-Seehausen, and Mullges preferred unipolar recordings, verifying Irnich's finding that reproducibility potentially is better with the unipolar than with the bipolar technique.[75, 81] Reiffel and Bigger have studied the effect of filter settings and found that low-end settings are more crucial to successful detection of the sinus node electrogram than are high-end settings.[74] They recommend a low- to high-band setting of 0.3–50 Hz or 0.6–50 Hz. However, as pointed out by Bethge et al, lower low-end settings provide for a much higher chance of artifact and other interference such as superimposition of respiratory activity.[75] Thus, interfering "noise" may make it impossible to decipher the sinus node electrogram. Reiffel and Bigger, on the other hand, noted that they could completely eliminate the sinus node electrogram by merely moving the low-end filter setting to 1.0 Hz.[74] These problems, in addition to those involving catheter position, contribute to a major disadvantage of the direct technique: increased time requirement. Moreover, even for the most skilled clinicians, the reported success rate of recording a sinus node electrogram is 80% in adult patients and approximately 50% in pediatric patients.[78, 79, 82] One of the problems inherent in pediatric patients is the relatively faster heart rates, which cause the P wave to merge with the preceding T wave, thus creating difficulty in deciphering onset of the sinus node electrogram.[74] Regardless of age, the onset of the sinus node electrogram is difficult to determine in the same patient, as well as among patients. Specific criteria defining onset have not been decided by investigators.

Indirect Assessment

Indirect assessment of sinus node function means that sinus node activity is assumed to exist by measuring only the resulting HRA electrogram. Thus, the sinus node impulse and the immediate conduction out of the sinus node to the HRA (sinoatrial conduction) can only be indirectly assessed by evaluating the HRA electrogram and its relationship to pacing techniques.[6, 83–88] The specific indirect techniques to calculate sinus node recovery time and sinoatrial conduction are described in detail in later sections.

The catheter technique for all indirect methods is carried out by placing a quadripolar electrode catheter (interelectrode distance, 2–5 mm) in the lateral HRA.[87] Usually the distal pair is used for pacing, and the proximal pair is used for recording. Standard filter settings for intracardiac recordings are used. It is essential to record two perpendicular limb leads simultaneously to verify sinus rhythm by noting high to low right atrial activation. Ideally, atrial activation is evaluated with another electrode catheter across the tricuspid valve by simultaneously recording the His bundle electrogram with its accompanying low right atrial electrogram. Tracings are recorded at 100 mm/s paper speed. In this manner, the demonstration of high to low right atrial sequence of activation supports the presence of sinus rhythm. If this activation sequence is not present, the assessment of sinus node function may not be possible. Instead, the function of the subsidiary atrial pacemaker focus is assessed.

Sinus Node Function Testing

SINUS NODE RECOVERY

Sinus node recovery most often is measured by using the indirect technique.[83–85, 87, 89] Not surprisingly, however, the direct technique has been shown by Gomes, Hariman, and Chowdry to have a major advantage when the testing goal is to eliminate any contribution to the recovery time by atriosinus or sinoatrial conduction.[90]

With either technique, the high right atrium is paced for 30 seconds at a rate slightly faster than the patient's spontaneous rate. The pacing is terminated abruptly, and the interval of time from the last paced captured beat to the first spontaneous sinus beat defines the total sinus node recovery time (SNRT). For the direct technique, the interval is from the last paced beat (to conduct through the atriosinus area to the sinus node) to the first sinus node electrogram. For the indirect technique, the interval is from the last paced beat to the first high right atrial electrogram (Fig. 7–18). These intervals are determined after each pacing rate. The in-

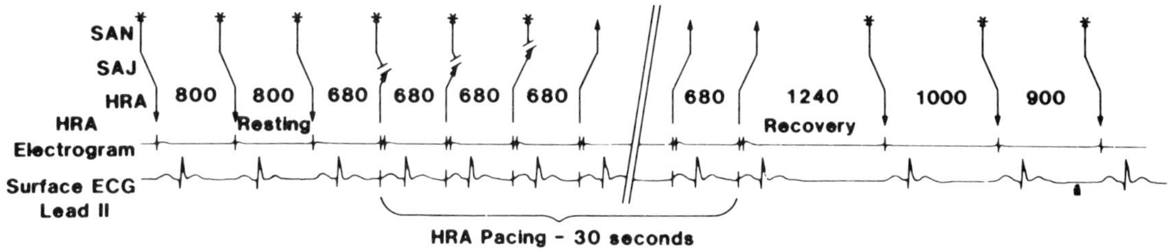

FIGURE 7–18

The explanation of sinus node recovery time is illustrated by ladder diagram. After 30 s of high right atrial pacing has suppressed the sinus node, a 1240-ms interval (sinus node recovery time) is interrupted by a sinus beat. For correction of heart rate, the sinus cycle length (800 ms) is subtracted from the total sinus node recovery time (1240 ms). The corrected sinus node recovery time (CSNRT) is 440 ms. (SNS, sinoatrial node; SAJ, sinoatrial junction; HRA, high right atrium; all numbers indicate ms.)

crement of increase in pacing rate arbitrarily is 10 bpm up to an atrial rate of 200/bpm. It is of utmost importance to monitor the systemic arterial blood pressure, because children have excellent AV conduction. Therefore, at higher atrial pacing rates profound hypotension may occur, and pacing must be discontinued.

The SNRT should be expressed in terms of some relationship to the resting sinus cycle length, so that adequate comparisons of values can be made among subjects with different heart rates.[87, 89] Most investigators subtract the resting sinus cycle length (determined before each pacing increase) from the total SNRT to determine the corrected sinus node recovery time (CSNRT).[83–85, 87] If the sinus node does not recover, and a different focus of atrial, junctional, or ventricular origin recovers first, the interval is termed "pacemaker recovery time" (Fig. 7–19).[85]

Regardless of pacing rate, CSNRT is expressed as the longest or maximum CSNRT that is measured. The upper limit of normal CSNRT for children is 275 ms, and for adults, 525 ms.[83, 87] It is unknown at what age in adolescence adult values should be used.

The atrial pacing rate at which maximum CSNRT occurs is variable among patients. Pop and Fleischman found that in adults the maximum CSNRT occurred most often at atrial pacing rates approximately 15% greater than sinus cycle length.[6] Reiffel et al noted that when maximum CSNRT was found at slow atrial pacing rates, there was a high possibility of atriosinus entrance block during the faster atrial pacing rates.[91] However, shorter CSNRT occurring during faster atrial pacing rates may also involve the reflex autonomic influences secondary to the relative hypotension during the faster pacing rates. This correlation was found in adults by Griebenow et al and confirmed by Nalos et al's autonomic blockade study.[92, 93] These studies showed that the hypotension caused a reflex increase in catecholamines, thus accelerating the sinus node recovery.

Similar studies in children have not been reported, but the related influence of sedation has been studied in the canine model. Clapp et al showed that the sedative combination of meperidine, promethazine, and chlorpromazine shortened the CSNRT by 50% (compared to control) in puppies and in adult dogs.[94] Because chlorpromazine is more likely to have vagolytic/adrenergic action (from hypotension) or antiarrhythmic action, meperidine (2 mg/kg, maximum dose 80 mg) and promethazine (1 mg/kg, maximum dose 40 mg) without chlorpromazine are recommended for sedation before catheterization when assessing sinus node function. When more sedation is required during catheterization, either meperidine (1 mg/kg, maximum dose 50 mg) or promethazine (0.5 mg/kg, maximum dose 25 mg) is recommended. If further sedation is required, diazepam (0.1–0.2 mg/kg, maximum dose 10 mg) is acceptable. Ketamine should be avoided because of its direct sympathomimetic actions.

The effect of atrial pacing on atriosinus and sinoatrial conduction is a major problem when assessing sinus node function by the indirect method of measuring CSNRT, because the atriosinus and sinoatrial conduction cannot be separated from sinus node automaticity assessment with the indirect method. Therefore, sinus node automaticity alone is not assessed. Why, then, is the indirect method of CSNRT used so commonly to assess sinus node automaticity? First, the influence of atriosinus and sinoatrial conduction to the CSNRT has been considered neg-

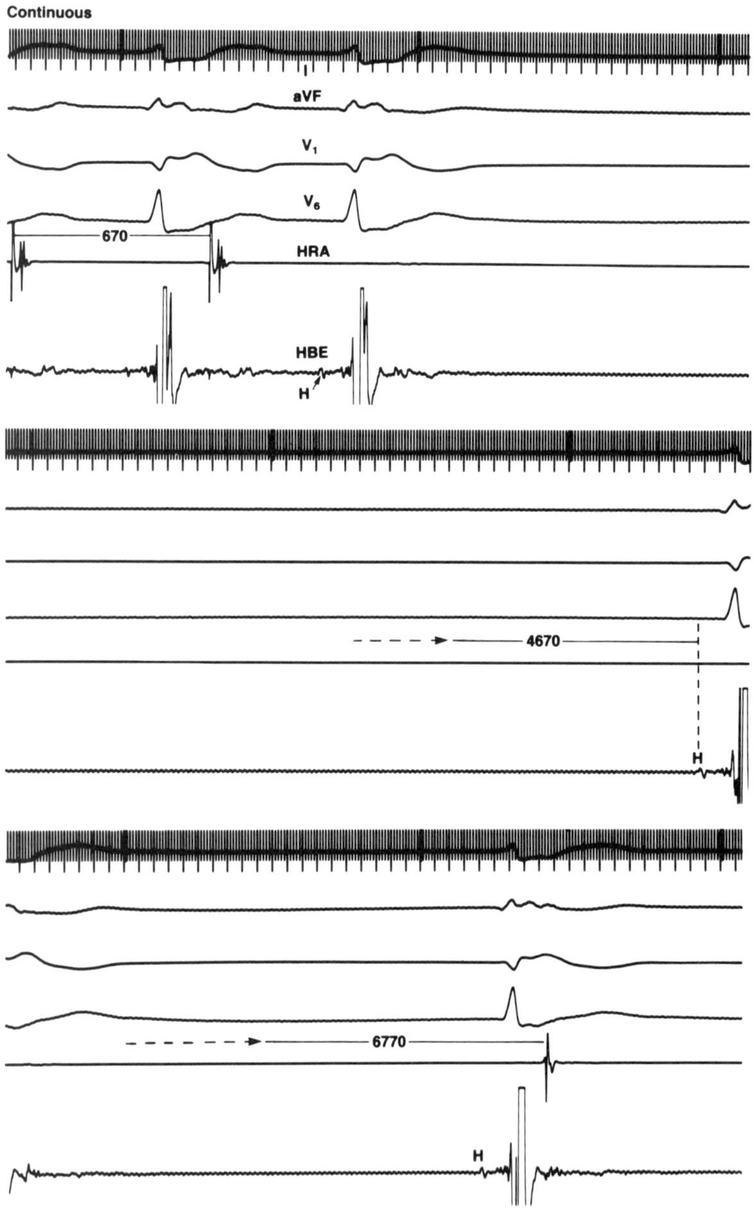

FIGURE 7–19
These continuous intracardiac electrograms simultaneous with surface ECGs show a long pacemaker and sinus node recovery time in a 14-year-old boy with postoperative repair of Ebstein's anomaly and surgical division of accessory atrioventricular connection. Although he had preoperative SND, it was exacerbated postoperatively by flecainide, which was required to suppress an atrial muscle reentry tachycardia. The electrophysiology study was carried out to determine the efficacy and safety of flecainide. In the top recording, high right atrial (HRA) pacing (670-ms cycle length) was terminated after 30 s. Junctional recovery by the AV node or His bundle (H) was noted 4670 ms later (middle recording), and the sinus node recovered 2100 ms later (or 6770 ms after atrial pacing termination). Because the resting cycle length was 950 ms, the corrected "pacemaker" recovery time was 4670 − 950 = 3720 ms. (HBE, His bundle electrogram at high amplication.) Paper speed was 100 mm/s.

ligible relative to the contribution of sinus node automaticity.[74] Second, the technical difficulties involved with the direct technique make it less appealing.

The problems of atriosinus and sinoatrial conduction with the indirect technique must be emphasized, because the limitations are essential in interpretation of the results.[87] During atrial pacing, particularly at faster rates, there is no means of knowing which of the consecutive paced beats are indeed conducting from the catheter electrodes through the atriosinus area to the sinus node pacemaker cell. Therefore when the pacing is terminated, it is unknown whether the last paced beat has actually penetrated into the sinus node. It could be that the previous beat or the second previous beat (or the third, or fourth, etc.) was the last to conduct through the atriosinus area to the sinus node. If the last paced beat to conduct through was not the last paced beat given, the sinus node recovery time (measured from the last paced HRA electrogram) is artifactually shortened because the last time the sinus node was stimulated was many beats before. Atriosinus (often called sinoatrial) entrance block thus causes this artifactual shortened CSNRT.[14, 87, 95]

At more rapid paced rates, only every other or every third stimulus may enter the sinus node, thus causing less suppression. Entrance block should be suspected when the SNRT is less than the sinus cycle length that preceded the onset of atrial pacing.[91]

Atrial pacing also has been found to adversely affect the conduction of the sinus node impulse out to the HRA (sinoatrial conduction). Gomes, Hariman, and Chowdry found that the first beat conducted from the sinus node (after pacing is terminated) often has a longer sinoatrial conduction time.[90] This finding often was associated with normal automaticity in patients with documented clinical SND.[90] Therefore, in many patients a long CSNRT may reflect abnormal sinoatrial conduction rather than sinus node automaticity.[96] It is evident that the direct sinus node recording technique is required when the intent is to evaluate sinus node automaticity independently.

SINOATRIAL CONDUCTION

Sinoatrial conduction is assessable by either of two indirect methods (Strauss and Narula) or by the direct method. Although qualitative evaluation of sinoatrial conduction is often accomplished, calculation of the sinoatrial conduction time (SACT) is the major objective of each method.

Strauss Method. Using single premature atrial depolarization induced into sinus rhythm every 10–20 ms throughout diastole, Strauss et al in 1973 were the first to calculate SACT in adults.[86] An extensive description of the technique also has been reported in children with normal sinus node function as well as in children with documented or suspected SND.[87] The technique is illustrated in Figure 7–20. The SACT is calculated from the A_2A_3 intervals (i.e., the interval from the induced premature impulse to the first sinus return impulse) of the first five well-defined reset responses in each subject. Well-defined reset responses are those that lie on the line parallel to the A_1,A_2/A_1A_1 line (Fig. 7–21). Reset responses that deviate and lie along a down-sloping curve or up-sloping curve (approximately >5% difference in A_2A_3/A_1A_1) should not be used in calculating the SACT. Within each A_2A_3 interval it is assumed that the sinus cycle length (measured A_1A_1) has been unaffected by the premature induced impulse (A_2). With subtraction of A_1A_1 from A_2A_3, the time remaining represents the time it has taken the A_2 to enter the sinus node (conduction from the catheter electrode in HRA to the sinus node) plus the conduction time from the new spontaneous sinus node impulse to the electrode in the HRA. This total time is referred to as the total SACT. Some authors divide this indirectly derived total SACT by two to obtain a SACT that approximates a directly recorded SACT. The five total SACTs calculated from the first five well-defined reset responses are averaged to obtain the value of total SACT in each subject (see Fig. 7–21). It is important to scrutinize the P waves, HRA depolarization, and atrial activation to be certain that the patient has sinus impulses. Because this method is based on the assumption that sinus rhythm is present, the response should not be used for calculation if there is any sign that the atrial depolarization may be from impulses other than those of sinus origin (Fig. 7–22).

To aid in defining reset responses, a plot is made in each subject of normalized A_2A_3 and A_3A_4 (Fig. 7–21). An SACT should not be calculated if no reset responses are identified. The finding of all nonreset responses indicates sinus node entrance block (Fig. 7–23). That is, regardless of the prematurity of A_2 given, the sinus node is not reset (presumably because of very prolonged atriosinus conduction and/or prolonged refractory period of sinus node or perisinus node tissue). In addition, sinus node entrance block may occur intermittently. The SACT can be calculated in most cases of intermittent entrance block because reset responses are present. Most subjects with entrance block have prolonged SACT, if it is measurable.

In addition to the presence of any evidence of entrance block, SND is present in children when the value of total SACT determined by the Strauss method is greater than 200 ms.[87] SACT appears to be unrelated to the sinus cycle length and is slightly longer in normal adults than in children. Most reports have revealed that the upper limit of total SACT in normal adults ranges from 200 ms to 250 ms.[86, 97–99] Methods of calculation, age of study group, sedation, and extent of underlying ischemic heart disease probably account for the wide range of values. In children there is a fair positive correlation of SACT and age (r = 0.62), which would suggest that these two variables are related, but because the relationship is not particularly strong, individual values in children do not need to be corrected for age.[87]

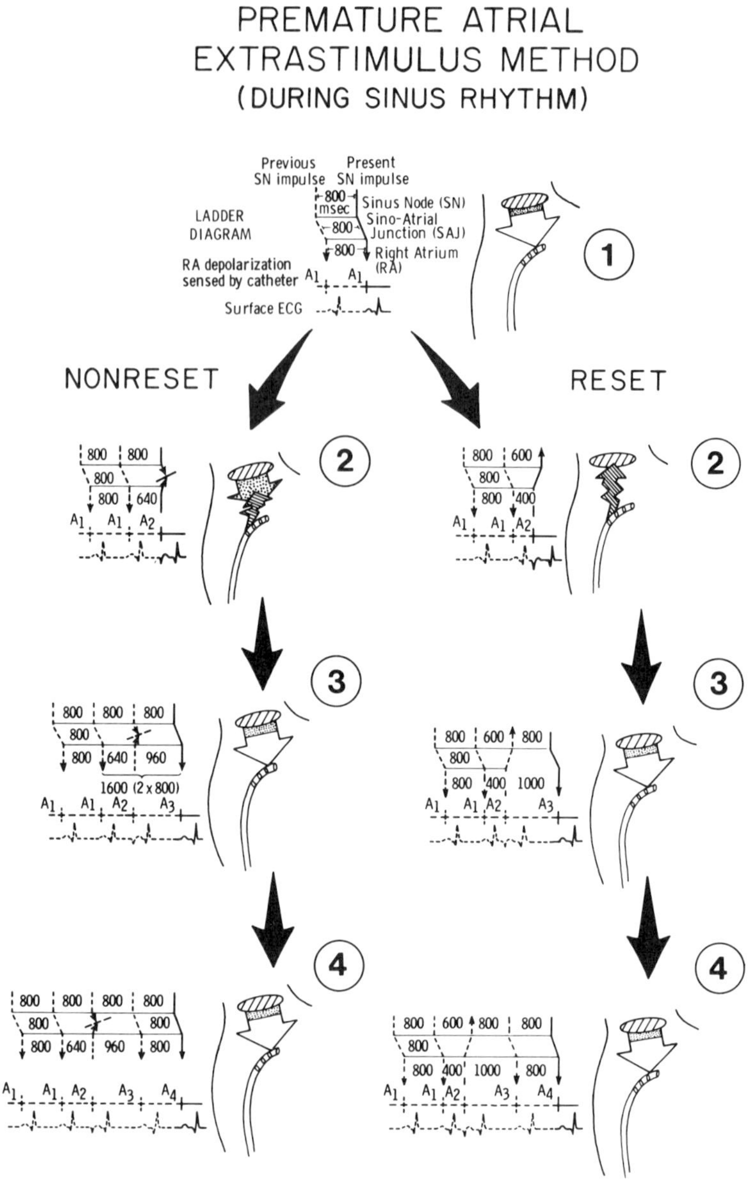

FIGURE 7–20
The atrial extra stimulus technique (Strauss) is illustrated by a ladder diagram with examples of nonreset and reset responses. The structures within the diagrammatic outline of the right atrium (RA) and superior vena cava correspond to those represented in the ladder diagrams. The sinus node (SN), sinoatrial junction (SAJ), RA, RA intracardiac electrogram, and surface ECG lead II are displayed in each step. SN is represented by diagonal lines, SAJ by dots, the sinus depolarization wave by a straight clear arrow, and the electrode induced depolarization (PAC) by a jagged arrow with diagonal lines. The dashed lines indicate previous occurrences in earlier steps; solid lines designate the present event.

Nonreset step 2: A PAC (A_2) is produced 640 ms after a spontaneous sinus cycle length (A_1A_1, 800 ms). Since a second SN impulse has already occurred spontaneously, they collide in the area of SAJ, and SN is not reset. Step 3: Nonreset is not evident, however, until the third SN impulse produces A_3 and the measured A_1A_3 interval is noted to be twice A_1A_1. Step 4: The interval and the A_3 and A_4 P waves are unchanged, suggesting that the SN automaticity has not changed.

Reset step 2: With earlier PAC (A_2A_2, 400 ms), SN has not produced a spontaneous impulse; thus the PAC captures (resets) SN. Step 3: Again reset is not evident until A_3. Now, the A_1A_3 interval is less than twice the A_1A_1 interval, demonstrating reset of SN. When reset has occurred, total SACT may be calculated by subtracting the A_1A_1 interval from the A_2A_1 interval from the A_2A_3 interval (1000 ms − 800 ms = 200 ms). Since it is assumed that the sinus cycle length is unchanged, 200 ms represents the conduction time from PAC into SN plus the conduction time out of SN to the electrodes. Step 4: See nonreset step 4.

(Reprinted by permission of the American Heart Association, Inc., from Kugler JD, Gillette PC, Mullins CE, et al: Sinoatrial conduction in children; An index of sinoatrial node function. Circulation 59:1266, 1979.)

Several limitations of this technique have been extensively reviewed.[14, 87, 100–106] The effect of the induced atrial impulse on sinus node automaticity is the major concern. The method by which the effect on sinus node automaticity is monitored involves measuring the A_3A_4 interval (the interval from the first to the second sinus return beat). If this interval is the same or nearly the same as A_1A_1 (within about ±5%), it is presumed that automaticity is not affected significantly (Fig. 7–21). If sinus arrhythmia is present, A_3A_4 may vary because of variations in spontaneous sinus cycle length and not because a change in automaticity has resulted from the induced atrial impulse. Data in subjects who have sinus arrhythmia during the procedure should be scrutinized carefully. Only reset responses accompanied by normal A_3A_4 intervals should be used for calculating SACT.

Reiffel et al showed that significant depression of sinoatrial conduction may occur from

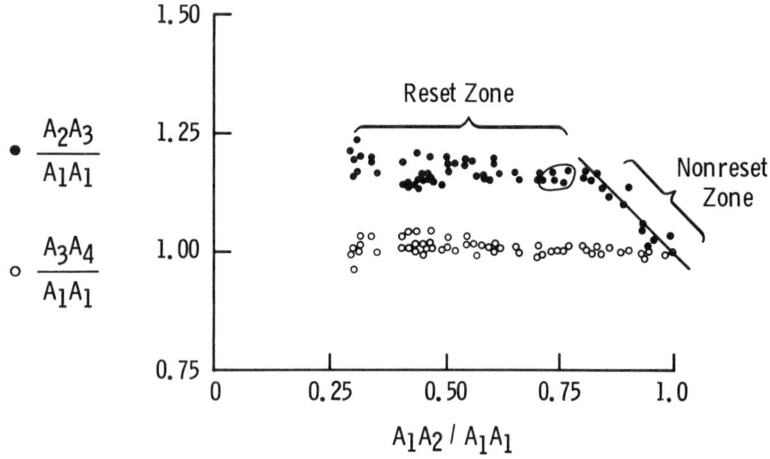

FIGURE 7–21
A graph of A_2A_3/A_1A_1 and A_3A_4/A_1A_1 with corresponding A_1A_1 showing an example of normal responses. The nonreset zone is distinctly separated from the plateau reset zone. The circle around the first five reset points indicates the responses from which the average sinoatrial conduction time was calculated. The closeness to which the A_3A_4/A_1A_1 intervals fall along the 1.00 line suggests that there has been little change in automaticity. (Reprinted by permission of the American Heart Association, Inc., from Kugler JD, Gillette PC, Mullins CE, et al: Sinoatrial conduction in children: An index of sinoatrial node function. Circulation 59:1266, 1979.)

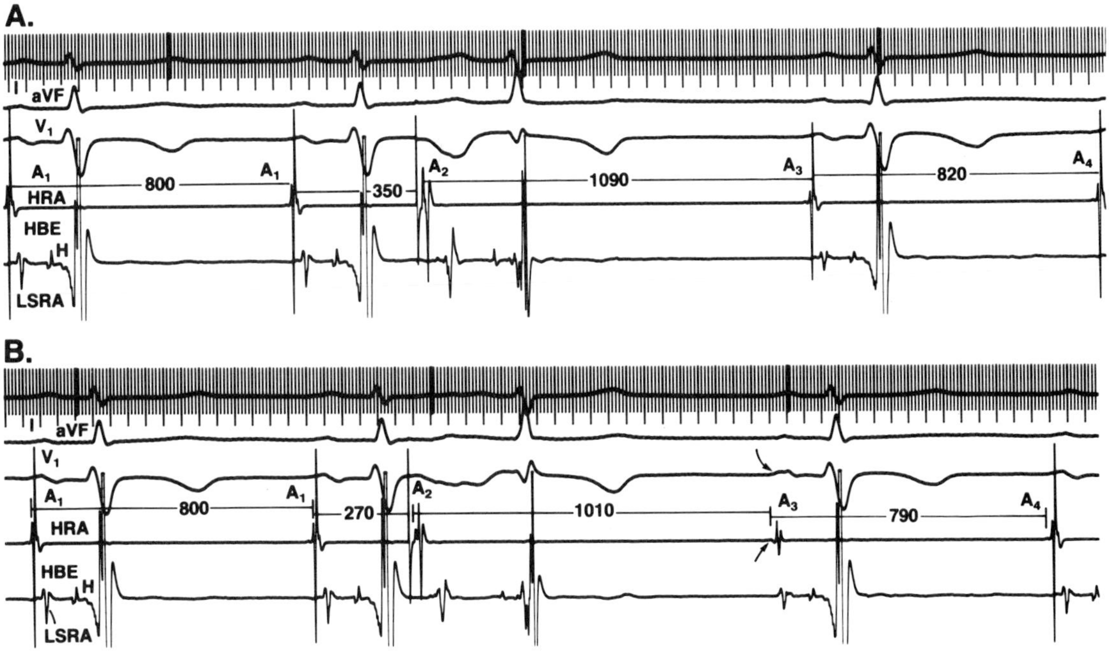

FIGURE 7–22
Two examples of the premature atrial stimulus (Strauss) technique show the importance of evaluating the A_3 electrogram and P wave morphology. In *A*, the premature atrial stimulus (A_2) was induced 350 ms after the last high right atrial depolarization (A_1). The return (A_3) HRA electrogram (assumed to originate from sinus node) and its corresponding P wave were identical in morphology to the resting electrogram and P wave. The A_3A_4 interval was similar to the A_1A_1 interval, and therefore sinus node automaticity appeared essentially unaffected by the A_2. The total SACT was 1090 − 800 = 290 ms.

In *B*, the premature atrial stimulus was given earlier, at 270 ms after A_1. The return A_3 and its corresponding P wave (depicted by arrows) were different in morphology than during previous sinus beats. This strongly suggested that a pacemaker shift occurred, and therefore this response should not be used in calculating sinoatrial conduction time. Paper speed was 100 mm/s. (H, His bundle depolarization; HBE, His bundle electrogram; LSRA, low septal right atrial electrogram.)

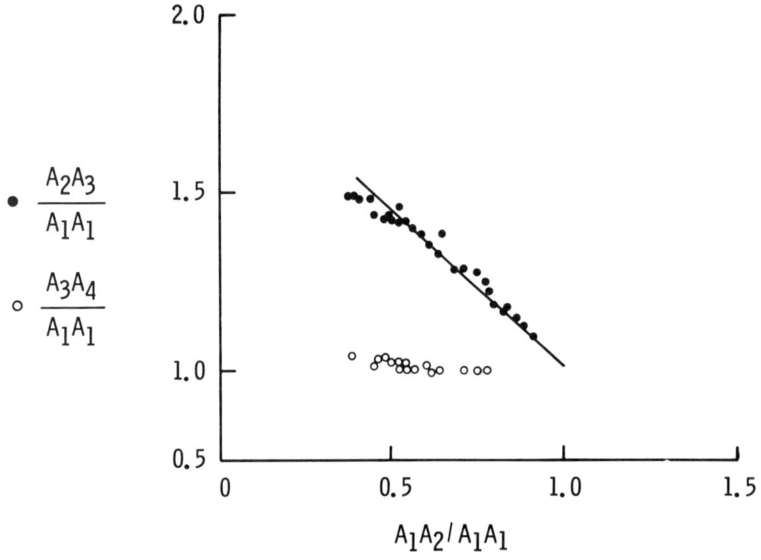

FIGURE 7–23
This graph (same coordinates as in Fig. 7–21) shows an example of sinus node entrance block. In this patient who had undergone a Mustard operation, the decreasing A_1A_2 interval resulted in a continuing nonreset zone with no reset zone. In this patient some A_3A_4 intervals were not recorded, but those that were recorded were similar to the normal response. (Reprinted by permission of the American Heart Association, Inc., from Kugler JD, Gillette PC, Mullins CE, et al: Sinoatrial conduction in children: An index of sinoatrial node function. Circulation 59:1266, 1979.)

the induced atrial impulse.[95] These investigators also found that disturbances of atriosinus conduction (e.g., entrance block) may not predict disturbances in sinoatrial conduction (e.g., exit block). That is, abnormal conduction in either or both directions may occur, and the precise abnormality is not detectable by indirect methods. Despite these well documented limitations, several studies have shown that there are no significant statistical differences between SACT derived by indirect method calculations and those directly measured.[74, 77–80]

Narula Method. Narula et al devised a more simple, rapid, indirect method of calculating SACT (Fig. 7–24).[88] With this technique, HRA pacing is carried out for eight beats at a pacing rate of 5–10 bpm faster than the sinus rate; then the pacing is stopped abruptly. The interval from the last paced beat to the first spontaneous sinus beat (return interval) contains the same three intervals as does the A_2A_3 interval by the Strauss method: conduction from catheter electrodes in HRA to sinus node, and conduction from sinus node back to electrodes. Total SACT equals return interval minus sinus cycle length. The postreturn PP interval is analogous to the Strauss A_3A_4 interval and therefore is used in assessing the effect on sinus node automaticity.

Advantages of the Narula method include shorter time of intracardiac study as well as shorter time for record evaluation, and elimination of apparent, but questionable, reset responses at transition of nonreset-reset zone because no transition exists. Disadvantages are similar to those of the Strauss method

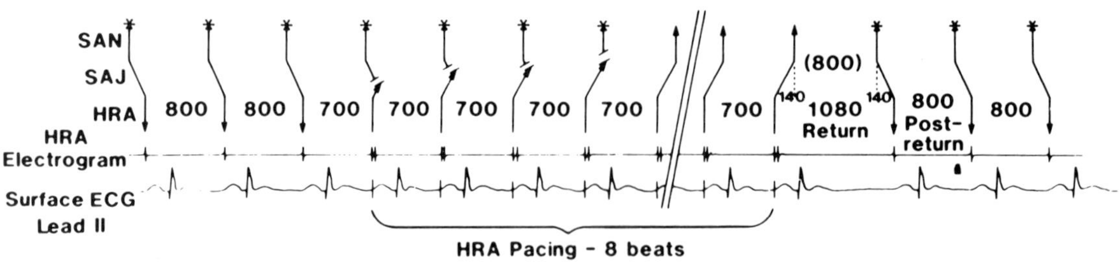

FIGURE 7–24
The slow atrial pacing or Narula method for determining sinoatrial conduction time is illustrated by ladder diagram. HRA pacing is carried out for eight beats at a rate (85 bpm) slightly faster than that of the sinus (75 bpm). Following the last paced beat, the interval ended by the first sinus return beat (return interval) includes conduction from the site of pacing to the SAN, the sinus cycle length (800 ms), and conduction from the SAN back to the catheter (in HRA), which is recording the HRA electrogram. Total SACT (140 + 140 = 280 ms) is derived by subtracting the assumed unchanged sinus cycle length (800 ms) from the measured return cycle (1080 ms). Sinus node automaticity is assumed to be insignificantly affected by the atrial pacing, since the post-return cycle lengths are unchanged. (SAN, sinoatrial node; SAJ, sinoatrial junction; HRA, high right atrium; all numbers indicate ms.)

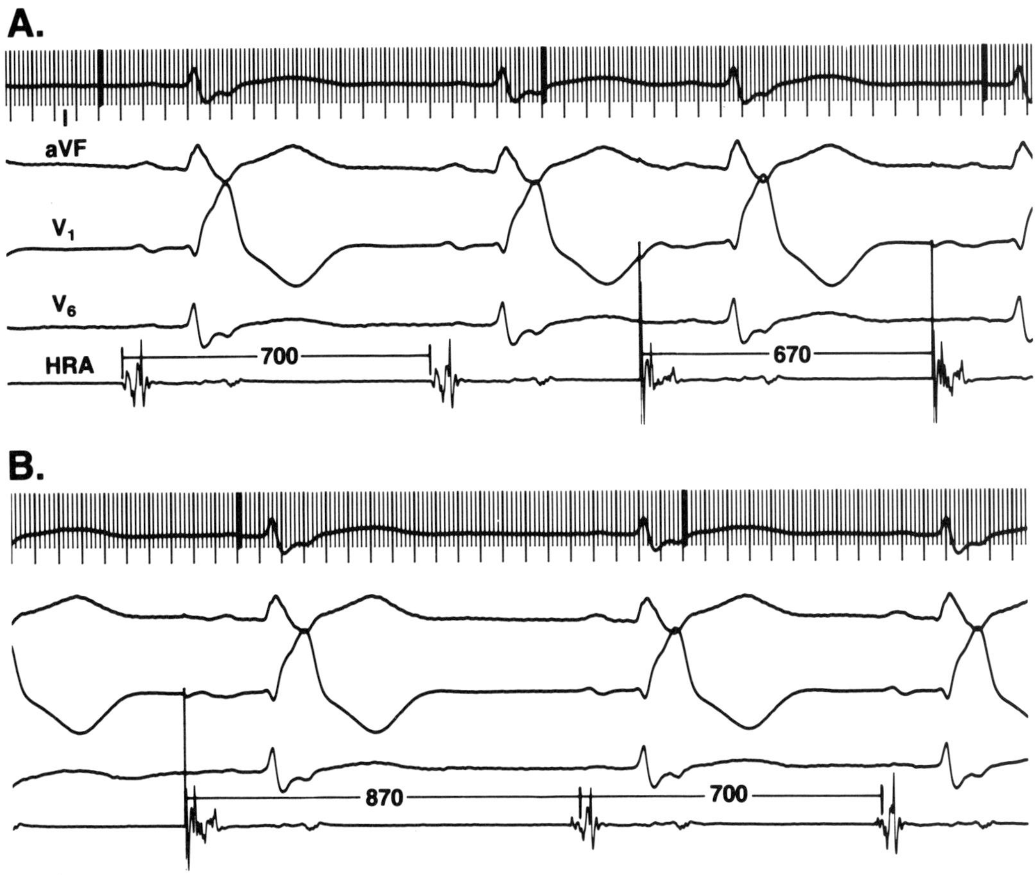

FIGURE 7–25
Two examples of the Narula method of determining sinoatrial conduction time. In *A*, the high right atrial (HRA) pacing (670-ms cycle length) was started in sinus rhythm (700-ms cycle length). In *B*, the pacing was terminated after eight beats. The total sinoatrial conduction time of 170 ms was calculated (870 − 700 ms). The post-return sinus cycle length of 700 ms was unchanged, thus implying that sinus node automaticity was not affected significantly.

(Figs. 7–25 and 7–26). In addition, the effect of eight paced beats on sinus node automaticity often is of greater magnitude than a single induced atrial impulse. When the two methods are compared in the same subject, however, SACT is usually less when calculated by the Narula method.[88, 107] Haberl, Steinbeck, and Luderitz offered an explanation for this difference by noting that sinus node acceleration in rabbits may occur during slow-rate atrial pacing.[108] Normal values by the Narula method have not been established for either adults or children.

Direct Method. The sinoatrial conduction time is obtained directly by measuring from the onset of the sinus node electrogram to the onset of the HRA electrogram (see Fig. 7–17). Development and refinement of the direct sinus node electrogram recording technique has generated much data related to sinoatrial conduction.[70–82, 90, 95, 96] Although a brief early report by Krongrad et al in 14 normal children and adults revealed values ranging from 25 ms to 55 ms (mean 35 ms), no recent data in normal children have been reported.[82] Data from adults without apparent sinus node disease show that the upper limit of normal sinoatrial conduction time as measured by the direct recording technique is approximately 110 ms to 135 ms. Several studies in adults, however, have shown very little difference between sinoatrial conduction times obtained directly compared to those obtained by the indirect methods.[74, 77–80] This is true for patients with normal or abnormal sinus node function. Although no such studies have been reported for children, it may appear reasonable to assume that the same correlation exists in the young. However, the few data available for children do not immediately support this conclusion, but there are problems with the data: only a few subjects were studied by Krongrad et al,[82] and perhaps more importantly, the faster

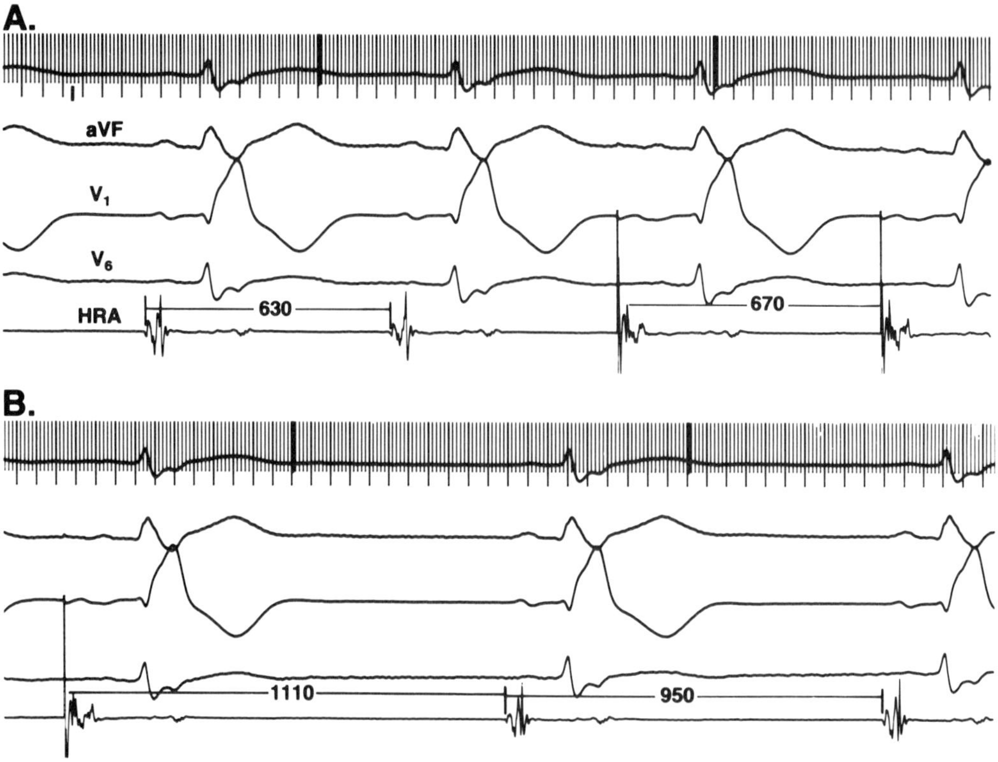

FIGURE 7–26
An example from the same patient shown in Fig. 7–25, illustrating a limitation of the Narula technique. First, the sinus cycle length (630 ms) suddenly shortened more than the pacing cycle length (670 ms). However, high right atrial (HRA) capture was accomplished for the eight beats. After termination of atrial pacing, the return cycle length (1110 ms) was prolonged compared to the response in Fig. 7–25. Also, the post-return interval was 950 ms, much longer than the sinus cycle length, which indicated sinus arrhythmia, suppression of sinus node automaticity, or both. For several reasons, the Narula method was unreliable in this patient.

heart rates in children provide the opportunity to misjudge the onset of the sinus node electrogram.[74] These reasons may explain in part the apparent wider discrepancy between the reported values of directly measured and indirectly calculated sinoatrial conduction time in children.

It is emphasized that the direct sinoatrial conduction time is one-half that obtained by indirect methods, because the latter include atriosinus plus sinoatrial conduction time. Therefore, when comparing times between the methods, it is necessary to halve the indirectly calculated sinoatrial conduction time.

Pharmacologic Autonomic Manipulation

AUTONOMIC BLOCKADE

As mentioned at the outset of this chapter, SND may be secondary to imbalance of the autonomic nervous system (Fig. 7–27); (see also Table 7–5). Moreover, structural SND may be exacerbated by autonomic nervous system imbalance. Pharmacologic autonomic blockade has proven valuable in evaluating autonomic nervous system effects on sinus node function.[109–113]

In 1966 Jose first showed the effects of autonomic blockade in man by administering atropine and propranolol to obtain the intrinsic heart rate (IHR).[114] In 1970, Cumming and Mir[115] applied the technique to children undergoing hemodynamic cardiac catheterization, and in the same year, Jose and Collison[116] studied normal adults and derived the following formula for predicting (p) IHR according to age: IHRp = 118.1 − (0.57 × age).

In 1984, Benson, Dunnigan, and Benditt[117] studied 22 children and adolescents (age 5 days to 18 years) without apparent SND. After intravenous administration of atropine (0.04 mg/kg) and propranolol (0.2 mg/kg),

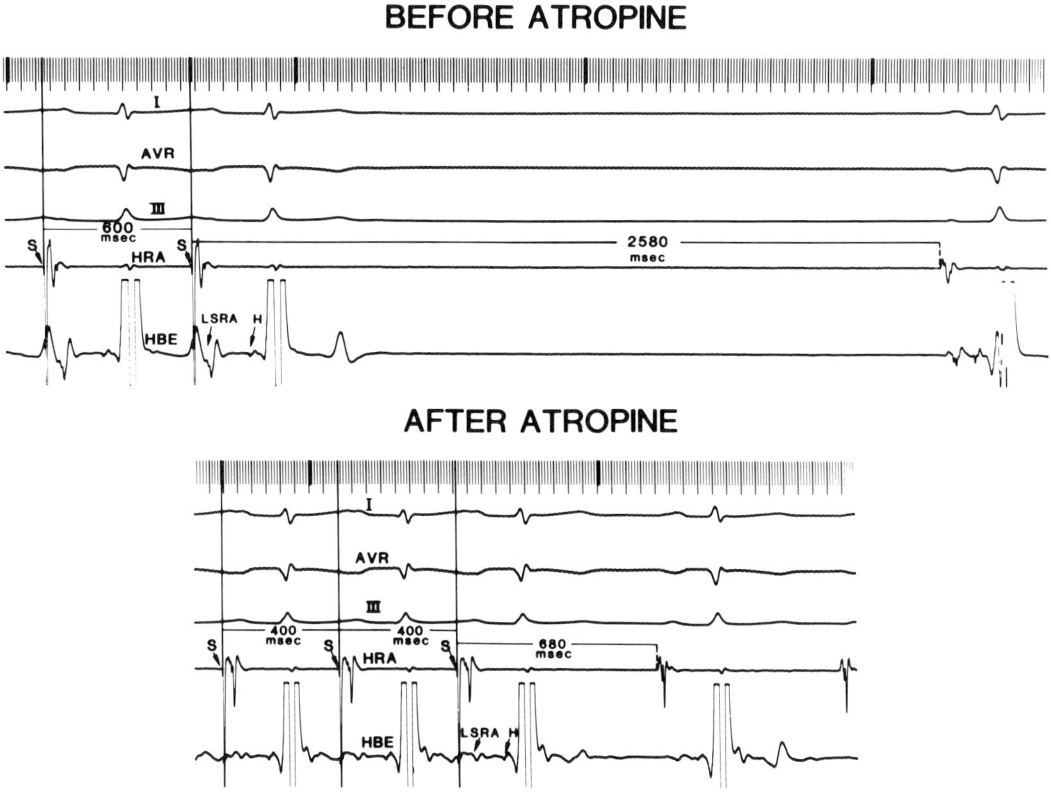

FIGURE 7–27
Intracardiac recordings before and after atropine dosage in an adolescent show that a long sinus node recovery time can be a result of hypervagotonia. The maximum sinus node recovery time was 2580 ms before atropine (corrected to 1310 ms). After 3 mg of intravenous atropine (0.03 mg/kg), the maximum sinus node recovery time shortened to 680 ms (corrected to 100 ms). It is unlikely that sinus node entrance block occurred during HRA pacing. The sinus cycle length decreased to 570 ms (from 1270 ms before atropine), also supporting the diagnosis of hypervagotonia. Paper speed was 100 mm/s. (H, His bundle depolarization; HBE, His bundle electrogram; LSRA, low septal right atrial electrogram.)

they derived a different formula for the pediatric group: IHRp = 139.5 − (2.14 × age in years).

Benson, Dunnigan, and Benditt thus noted that IHR in children, as in adults, decreases linearly as age increases. However, these investigators found that IHR decreases at a faster rate in children than it does in adults. They also evaluated heart rate change after autonomic blockade and discovered that the parasympathetic nervous system influenced heart rate to a similar degree at all ages.

Several autonomic blockade studies have been carried out in patients with SND since the earlier reports of IHR in patients without SND.[109–113] The data show that several combinations of SND are possible. Patients who have normal intrinsic sinus node function but who have hypervagotonia would be expected to have normal IHR and sinus node function after autonomic blockade. Patients with structural SND usually have an abnormal IHR but may have improved sinus node function (indicated by CSNRT or SACT) after autonomic blockade. That is, the SND in these patients may be exacerbated by autonomic nervous imbalance. Patients with structural sinus node disease but in whom sinus node testing after autonomic blockade reveals no further dysfunction, appear to have SND unaffected by the autonomic nervous system. In a few patients with normal IHR, abnormal sinus node function is found by electrophysiology testing after autonomic blockade. Jordan, Yamaguchi, and Mandel offered the explanation that these patients had a catecholamine-dependent type of autonomic disturbance.[109]

These different combinations of sinus node function were similarly found in the two reported studies of children with SND. Marcus et al studied seven patients who had previously undergone Mustard operation, surgery to correct tetralogy of Fallot, or Fontan repair and found that autonomic blockade distinguished patients with autonomic disturbances from those without.[112] In a similar study of 22 children who had undergone repair of congenital heart disease, Ross et al reported that most prolonged sinus node recovery times decreased after autonomic blockade and even improved to normal values, suggesting an additive or exclusive depressant effect of the autonomic nervous system–either increased vagal output/sensitivity or decreased sympathetic output/sensitivity.[113] These preliminary findings from both studies suggest that the technique of autonomic blockade is a valuable adjunct when invasively evaluating sinus node function in children.

AUTONOMIC STIMULATION

In some patients, stimulation of the autonomic nervous system is helpful to demonstrate an autonomic imbalance or hypersensitivity problem. In the older child and adolescent, carotid massage can be carried out to determine if carotid sinus hypersensitivity is present.[118–121] Although this problem is uncommon, it is important to consider the possibility and to carry out carotid sinus massage. If carotid massage is unsuccessful in reproducing symptoms in a patient with suspected hypervagotonia, edrophonium chloride may be administered intravenously. No data exist indicating normal and abnormal responses in children to carotid sinus massage or to edrophonium administration. A tilt table also has been useful for some investigators during autonomic manipulation studies. Whether or not the patient is undergoing EPS, the blood pressure should be continuously monitored during study of the autonomic nervous system. For example, patients with hypervagotonia from carotid sinus hypersensitivity may have a cardioinhibitory (bradycardia) and/or cardiodepressor (hypotension) effect. Moreover, AV nodal dysfunction often accompanies the sinus bradycardia or, in some patients, may occur without evidence of SND.[121] Treatment is based on distinguishing these effects, and therefore detection of the type of vagotonic symptom is imperative.

Electrophysiologic Criteria for SND in Children

Sinus node dysfunction is present in children when any one of the criteria listed in Table 7–3 is present. With the exception of sinus node reentry tachycardia, these indices of sinus node function have been discussed previously.

During EPS, sinus node reentry tachycardia may occur spontaneously, but usually is induced with rapid atrial pacing or with induced premature atrial impulse(s).[50–52] Termination of the tachycardia is accomplished by overdrive rapid atrial pacing. Pauses following termination of tachycardia are similar, whether they occur after atrial pacing or after spontaneous atrial tachycardia.[56] The atrial activation sequence is the key to diagnosis; therefore at least two and preferably four simultaneous atrial electrograms (including coronary sinus or left atrial) are needed to define the site of reentry (Fig. 7–28). Sinus node reentry tachycardia is present when the activation of the atrium during tachycardia is the same as during sinus beats. A P wave axis and morphology during tachycardia that are identical to those of sinus rhythm will confirm the finding. With indirect techniques, high right atrial muscle reentry tachycardia cannot be distinguished from sinus node reentry. When atrial muscle reentry tachycardia originates in areas away from the sinus node, there may or may not be associated SND.[40, 43, 44] The atrial cycle length of sinus node reentry or atrial muscle reentry tachycardia is usually constant within each

TABLE 7–3
ELECTROPHYSIOLOGIC CRITERIA FOR SINUS NODE DYSFUNCTION IN CHILDREN

CSNRT (indirect) > 275 ms[87]
Total SACT (Strauss) > 200 ms[87]
Sinus node entrance block[87]
by Strauss method
by atrial pacing method (e.g., shorter SNRT than resting SCL)[91]
Sinoatrial exit block (direct method)[96]
Sinus node arrest (direct method)[74, 75]
Sinus node reentry tachycardia[44, 52, 58]
Intrinsic heart rate greater than predicted for age[117] [IHRp = 139.5 − (2.14 × age in yr)]

Abbreviations: CSNRT = corrected sinus node recovery time; IHRp = predicted intrinsic heart rate; SACT = sinoatrial conduction time; SNRT = sinus node recovery time (uncorrected); SCL = sinus cycle length.

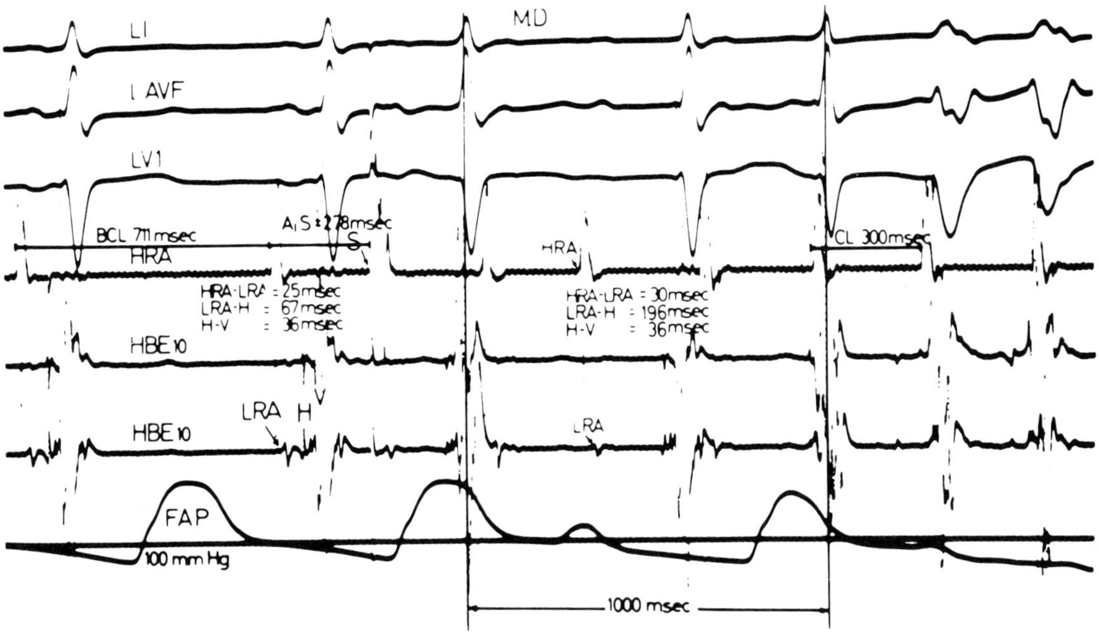

FIGURE 7–28
Intracardiac electrograms demonstrating sinus node reentry tachycardia initiated by an atrial extra stimulus. Surface leads I, AVF and V_1 were recorded with high right atrial (HRA) electrograms, His bundle electrograms (HBE), and femoral artery pressure (FAP). The premature atrial depolarization in the HRA at a coupling interval of 278 ms induced supraventricular tachycardia (cycle length, 300 ms). The atrial activation sequence was from high to low and is seen best in the second beat. The first beat of the tachycardia was blocked, allowing the activation sequence of the second to be easily visualized. The tachycardia P wave configuration was also the same as the sinus P wave. (Reprinted by permission of the American Heart Association, Inc., from Gillette PC: The mechanisms of supraventricular tachycardia in children. Circulation 54:133, 1976.)

patient, but among patients the cycle length is variable. Usually in young children the atrial cycle length of either type of reentry tachycardia often is shorter (174–300 ms) than in older children (200–500 ms). Ventricular response usually is 2:1 at the shorter and 1:1 at the longer atrial cycle lengths. However, characteristics of AV conduction determine the ventricular response (see also the discussion of ECG criteria).

There are other findings not listed in Table 7–3 that may be very suggestive of SND but for which there are no definite normal data available for comparison. For example, no data are reported for Narula SACT in children. Because adult data have shown that Narula SACT is usually shorter than Strauss SACT, it seems reasonable to suspect that SND may exist if the Narula SACT is greater than 200 ms.[88, 107] However, no such studies have been reported to confirm this. The directly measured SACT is another sinus node function index lacking comparative normal data in children.

The sensitivity and specificity of electrophysiologic criteria for SND is an important issue. A few studies in children and several studies in adults have shown many problems with the sensitivity and specificity of intracardiac electrophysiology testing of sinus node function.[6–10, 122] Pop and Fleischman first addressed this problem systematically in four groups of patients with SND (sinoatrial exit block, sinus bradycardia, brady/tachyarrhythmias, and sinus arrest).[6] These investigators, and many others, have found a number of symptomatic patients with clinical evidence of SND but without correlating SND of the same severity during EPS. Conversely, it is not uncommon to find severe SND during EPS in an asymptomatic patient (see Fig. 7–19). Furthermore, SND may be evident by noninvasive testing, but confirmation is not found during EPS, as was demonstrated in children by Hesslein et al.[10] In their study of patients who had undergone Mustard operation, they found treadmill exercise was a more sensitive test than EPS to detect SND. Likewise, Fournier et al carried out EPS in 51 of 104 children with sinus bradycardia and found SND in 39.[9] Moreover, of 27 symptomatic children with sinus bradycardia, four had normal EPS results. These investigators concluded that EPS does not correlate with symptoms and does not add to data from noninvasive studies.

Indications for Intracardiac Electrophysiologic Testing of Sinus Node Function

The lack of high sensitivity and specificity of sinus node function testing during intracardiac EPS has resulted in fewer patients undergoing these invasive studies. Although it was common practice several years ago to study children only for evaluation of sinus node function, it is now uncommon because of the evidence that shows noninvasive testing is often as good as or better than invasive EPS.[9, 10] As will be discussed later, clinical decisions and recommendations are based predominantly on symptoms documented with noninvasive testing. Also, in asymptomatic patients who have an underlying diagnosis associated with a high incidence of SND (e.g., postoperative atrial repair of transposition of the great arteries), clinical decisions and recommendations often can be made without the sometimes unreliable data generated from EPS. Thus indications have changed for sinus node function testing during EPS. Moreover, interpretation of the data from those patients who still undergo EPS sinus node testing has changed. (The interpretation of EPS data is further discussed in the section on treatment.)

There are two situations when sinus node function testing is indicated in all patients during EPS (Table 7–4). One is in patients who undergo EPS to evaluate whether or not an arrhythmia undetected noninvasively is a possible cause of unexplained syncope. The other situation is when patients undergo EPS to evaluate another arrhythmia. Baseline evaluation of sinus node function is important, particularly when antiarrhythmia drug treatment is planned. When an antiarrhythmia drug is used that has a known potential for inducing or exacerbating SND (see Table 7–5), evaluation of sinus node function is indicated. This is not to say that all patients who are treated with these drugs should have invasive sinus node studies, but if the patient is undergoing EPS, and particularly drug EPS, for another reason, then evaluation of sinus node function also should be carried out.[123]

TABLE 7–4
INDICATIONS FOR INTRACARDIAC ELECTROPHYSIOLOGIC TESTING OF SINUS NODE FUNCTION

All patients
for unexplained syncope
to evaluate another arrhythmia (e.g., SVT or VT, especially during drug-EPS)
Selected patients
to assist in determining severity of SND
to determine optimal mode of planned implanted pacemaker
as the sole reason for drug-EPS (i.e., sinus node testing after drug as only reason for EPS)
with CHD that have risk of SND or sudden death who are undergoing hemodynamic/anatomic catheterization

Abbreviations: CHD = congenital heart disease; EPS = electrophysiology study; SND = sinus node dysfunction; SVT = supraventricular tachycardia; VT = ventricular tachycardia.

In other selected patients, assessment of sinus node function may be indicated. (“Selected” means that only some patients may benefit by undergoing invasive evaluation.) In these selected patients, clinically important data are obtained, and thus the pediatric cardiologist can reach a better clinical management decision. The EPS is one additional piece of information that can be used in borderline cases. For many patients, however, the pediatric cardiologist may have sufficient noninvasive and historical data available such that the invasive EPS data, regardless of the potential content, would not alter the clinical decisions for management. Therefore invasive sinus node function testing is not indicated. A good example is the patient who has symptomatic severe SND and mild to moderate AV nodal dysfunction documented by Holter monitoring. Permanent pacemaker implantation is indicated. The patient has marginal ventricular function, and therefore a DDD pacemaker is the optimal choice. In this patient, there are no data obtainable by invasive EPS that would alter management.

Infrequently, severity of SND is not assessable noninvasively, and therefore EPS may be necessary. An example may be the uncommon patient with a complaint of fatigue and/or rare dizziness in whom mild to moderate sinus bradycardia (without symptoms) is the only finding by Holter monitoring. In addition, the exercise tolerance and maximum heart rate by treadmill testing are borderline low. Therefore, more data may be needed before a decision can be made regarding definitive treatment. In one girl with such noninvasive findings, we recorded A 4.7-S CSNRT, thus helping considerably in the decision. In these patients, in addition to EPS of sinus node function, hemodynamic assessment such as cardiac output measurement during various pacing modes is indicated.[124] Similarly, there are some patients in whom the decision to implant a pacemaker has been made (e.g., in a patient with brady/tachyarrhythmias following Mustard operation who has documented syncope but without rhythm documentation), but it is unclear from noninvasive data what type or mode of pacemaker is best. Thus, EPS with hemodynamic evaluation is indicated in these selected patients.

Sinus node function testing also may be carried out in selected patients during cardiac catheterization for hemodynamic/angiographic evaluation. These patients typically have types of congenital heart disease that are associated with an increased risk of SND, and baseline sinus node function may be obtained for possible later comparison. In patients who have undergone Mustard operation, it may be possible to predict who will develop atrial flutter, if it can be induced during EPS. This may provide a rationale for routine postoperative studies. At present, however, routine studies should be considered as research.

CLINICAL SITUATIONS

Symptoms

The emphasis of many studies in children has been on relating the symptomatic patient to the underlying SND arrhythmias.[125–130] In these reports, most patients had symptoms of syncope or near syncope with specific arrhythmias such as sinus arrest with long escape intervals or severe bradycardia. Most reports have not correlated the specific arrhythmia or its severity with severity of symptoms.

Other studies have evaluated groups of patients with specific underlying heart disease or patients with ECG or EPS evidence of SND to determine incidence of SND or symptoms.[9, 32, 34, 41, 42, 131–135] The results have been variable. Most reports of patients with a known risk of SND (Table 7–5, e.g., those patients with postoperative atrial repair of transposition of the great arteries) have provided various incidences of SND but, with the exception of sudden death incidence, few have addressed associated symptoms.[9, 32, 34, 41, 42]

Correlation of symptoms has been evaluated in some studies of children with ECG or EPS evidence of SND. Yebek, Swensson, and Jarmakani and Yabek and Jarmakani in two reports showed that 74% of 30 children were asymptomatic from SND.[133, 134] A recent brief report of sinus or junctional bradycardia by ECG in 104 children revealed only 30 patients (29%) who were symptomatic.[9] In a Holter survey study of 624 healthy children, Roifman et al found 12 children with ECG evidence of SND.[135] The most common arrhythmia (10 patients) was sinus arrest, but no symptoms were present, and no patient had a history of symptoms. These studies, as well as the anecdotal experience of most investigators, suggest that most children with SND are asymptomatic.

Of children with SND who are symptomatic, the most common symptoms appear to be fatigue/exercise intolerance or dizziness/syncope.* The manifestations of fatigue/exercise intolerance are related to the age of the patient. In infants, poor feeding, lethargy, or signs and symptoms of congestive heart failure exist, while in older children, inability to maintain the same level of activity as peers, tiredness in the absence of activity, and frequent naps may be the only signs of fatigue.

Dizziness secondary to SND is probably more common than syncope. Although syncope usually attracts more attention as a potentially life-threatening problem, dizziness or near syncope also should prompt further investigation. Syncope sometimes is difficult to detect in infants and young children. In infants as well as children, seizures may be a secondary problem to unwitnessed syncope. It is imperative to evaluate the patient's rhythm when the presenting symptom is unexplained seizures. This is especially indicated when the patient has an underlying disorder with an associated risk of SND (or risk of any other arrhythmia that causes syncope).[136]

Sudden death is uncommon, but its true incidence relative to SND is very difficult to

*5, 9, 32, 34, 41, 42, 126–135

TABLE 7–5
CAUSES OF SINUS NODE DYSFUNCTION

NONSURGICAL
- Idiopathic/congenital[53, 125–129, 135, 141–146]
- Familial[147–153]
- Congenital Heart Disease
  - Secundum atrial septal defect[154–157]
  - Sinus venosus atrial septal defect[158, 159]
  - Atrioventricular canal[160]
  - Pulmonary stenosis[134]
  - Ventricular septal defect[134–139]
  - Transposition of the great arteries[134]
  - Single ventricle[161]
  - Absent left pulmonary artery[139]
  - Patent ductus arteriosus[134]
  - Coarctation of aorta[162]
  - Wolff-Parkinson-White Syndrome[163, 164]
- Cardiomyopathies
  - Idiopathic (dilated or post-viral)[139]
  - Hypertrophic* (see Fig. 7–31)
  - Infiltrative (amyloidosis, hemosiderosis)[165]
- Inflammatory
  - Immunologic:[140, 166–169] rheumatic fever, collagen vascular disease, muscular dystrophy, Friedreich's ataxia
  - Bacterial: typhoid diphtheria[169, 170]
  - Parasitic: Chagas' disease[171]
  - Viral: those associated with pericarditis, myocarditis[172]
- Ischemic
  - Coronary artery insufficiency:[165, 173–178] Kawasaki disease, right atrial thrombi, traumatic, myocardial infarction, fibromuscular dysplasia of sinus node artery
  - Necrosis:[165] disseminated intravascular coagulopathy, thrombotic thrombocytopenic purpura
- Medications
  - Antiarrhythmia agents:[179–205] digitalis, beta blockers (e.g., propranolol), calcium channel blockers (e.g., verapamil), Type Ia agents (e.g., quinidine, procainamide, disopyramide), Type Ib agents (e.g., lidocaine), Type Ic agents (e.g., flecainide, propafenone), amiodarone, sotalol, adenosine, ethmosine
  - Vagotonic agents: see Hypervagotonia below
  - Others:[206–209] lithium, clonidine, methyldopa
- Endocrine/Metabolic
  - Hypoxia/hypercarbia*
  - Hypothyroidism[169]
  - Hypothermia[140]
  - Hypercalcemia[215, 216]
  - Hyperkalemia[140]
  - Massive weight loss[217]
  - Congenital homocystinuria[165]
  - Pheochromocytoma[165]
  - Hyperthyroidism[218, 219]
- Hypervagotonia
  - Idiopathic[139, 220–222]
  - Nasopharyngeal stimulation/gastroesophageal reflux[223–225]
  - Endurance athletes[226–228]
  - Carotid sinus hypersensitivity[118–120, 229, 230]
  - Coughing (syncope)[231]
  - Swallowing (deglutition syncope)[232–234]
  - Glossopharyngeal neuralgia[235]
  - Vomiting*
  - Sleep[238, 239]
  - Breath-holding[236, 237]
  - Increased intracranial pressure[169, 216]
  - Medications[179, 240, 241]
    - Parasympathomimetic effect
      - Edrophonium
      - Physostigmine
      - Bethanechol
      - Neostigmine
      - Acetylcholine
      - Hyoscyamine
      - Phenylephrine
      - Methoxamine
      - Reserpine
      - Morphine
- Miscellaneous
  - Long QT syndrome[138, 245, 246]
  - Sudden infant death syndrome[247–250]
  - Tumor[251]
  - Coronary angiography[252]
  - Obstructive jaundice[253]
  - Guillain-Barre[254]

SURGICAL
- Atrial operations
  - Mustard[10, 32–48, 84, 87, 131, 255–268, 270, 272, 273]
  - Senning[269, 271, 273]
  - Atrial septal defect[32–34, 46, 132, 156, 158, 274, 275]
  - Fontan[37–39]
  - Endocardial cushion defect[160]
  - Partial or total anomalous pulmonary venous connection[276]
  - Ebstein's anomaly[36, 47]
  - Blalock-Hanlon atrial septectomy[277]
- Cardiac operations[278–280]
  - Requiring superior vena caval cannulation
  - Requiring ischemic arrest

*Personal experience (unpublished data).

document. The primary difficulty in assessing incidence is the possibility of other life-threatening arrhythmias (e.g., tachyarrhythmias) in the same patient.[41, 42, 131, 137, 138] For example, the incidence of sudden death was 2.5% in 372 patients with postoperative Mustard repair for transposition of the great arteries, and the only risk factor identified (weakly) was the presence of tachyarrhythmia, although many of the 372 patients had SND.[41]

The clinical manifestations of SND are directly related to the function of the remaining conduction system and the underlying hemodynamic state. In patients with significant SND (e.g., sinus arrest) at any age, symptoms of dizziness and syncope usually are uncommon when there is adequate AV nodal/His-Purkinje escape rate and no underlying hemodynamic disorder. This is particularly true in infants who usually are recumbent and are therefore not as susceptible to the postural-related effects of relative hypotension, as seen in older children, who are more commonly in upright positions. Regardless of age and status of underlying disease, symptoms of dizziness and syncope are less likely (or if present, less severe) if SND occurs when the patient is supine or sitting. However, children who have undergone surgical repair of congenital heart disease, like the older adult population with ischemic heart disease, have a greater chance of associated conduction system dysfunction and therefore if syncope is severe, may have more severe symptoms, even in recumbent positions.

Any patient with compromised hemodynamic function may have exacerbation during times of SND. Patients who have organ hypoperfusion or a high potential for organ hypoperfusion would be expected to manifest symptoms of dizziness/syncope during times of SND when patients without such underlying problems probably would be asymptomatic. For example, patients with severe congestive heart failure during times of SND may either have worsening general signs of low cardiac output or may have symptoms of cerebral hypoperfusion.

Documentation of symptoms concomitantly with the SND rhythm disturbance is essential. Therefore, 24-hour or more ambulatory ECG (Holter) recording is a valuable test.[5] The Holter monitor is valuable to use in patients without known SND but whose symptoms are compatible with SND. If symptoms do not occur during the time of recording, then documentation is incomplete. Complete documentation is especially important in the patient who has known SND but in whom the symptoms of dizziness or syncope may be from another cause. For further documentation, use of a telephone transmitter may be attempted.

Causes of Sinus Node Dysfunction

Many causes of SND are listed in Table 7–5. There are several types of classification of SND.[1, 3, 14, 139, 140] Because SND from cardiac surgery comprises much of SND in children and adolescents, the causes of SND are best classified as either surgical or nonsurgical.[14, 139] However, it must be emphasized that many of the nonsurgical causes may exacerbate both the surgical types as well as other nonsurgical types of SND. This is particularly important with antiarrhythmia drugs, but is also true of endocrine/metabolic and hypervagotonia causes. The incidence and prevalence of the causes of SND as well as associated severity are unknown, but most children with SND have less than severe SND.

NONSURGICAL CAUSES

"Idiopathic," "primary," and "congenital" are terms that commonly are used to describe SND when no other cause (including hypervagotonia) is found.[53, 125–129, 135, 141–146] Familial occurrences have been reported and are probably uncommon.[147–153] One report revealed an autosomal dominant mode of inheritance associated with mental retardation.[150] Lenegre's disease, a rare, idiopathic, general type of conduction system disease, has been reported in the young.[149] Dysfunction of AV conduction is also part of the pathologic process in Lenegre's disease.

Sinus node dysfunction has been found preoperatively in patients with congenital heart disease.[134, 139, 154–164] Although it is most commonly reported in patients with atrial septal defect, SND has been documented with several types of congenital heart disease. Some patients have presented with SND symptoms (e.g., syncope), and congenital heart disease was detected only secondarily.[130, 154] Concomitant AV nodal dysfunction also has been found in patients with an atrial septal defect.[132, 154–157] This further increases the risk of associated symptoms.

Acquired or familial myocardial disorders such as cardiomyopathies, inflammatory diseases, or ischemic diseases encompass a wide range of potential SND causes.[139, 140, 165–178] The myocardial disease itself often is the direct cause of the SND (e.g., viral myocarditis). However, secondary effects such as coronary artery ischemia (e.g., Kawasaki disease or cardiomyopathy) also may play a role. Furthermore, other secondary problems have been implicated to explain the SND in some of these disorders. An example is vagotonia in rheumatic heart fever.[166]

Medications, particularly antiarrhythmic drugs, are an important cause or exacerbation of SND in children.[179–209] This is more common in children who have undergone surgical repair of congenital heart disease, because these patients more often need antiarrhythmic drug therapy and more often have underlying postoperative SND and/or other conduction system disease. Therefore, any antiarrhythmic drug with potential adverse effects on sinus node function should be administered with caution; in many patients with underlying SND, a permanent pacemaker is needed concomitantly (see section on treatment). Specific documentation of SND from drug studies in children has been reported only for a few drugs.[180, 182, 200] However, sufficient evidence exists from studies of other drugs in adults as well as from case reports in children to provide adequate data indicating the need for proper caution.[179, 199]

Conflicting data as well as other adverse drug effects must not be overlooked. For example, Breithardt, Seipel, and Wiebringhaus found that verapamil has a dual effect on sinus node function: an indirect chronotropic effect often predominates over the direct depressant effect on sinus node function.[210] While quinidine was reported to be safe by Vera, Awan, and Mason in a study of adults with SND,[211] quinidine may actually cause SND. Additionally, quinidine-induced His-Purkinje system dysfunction and *torsades de pointes* are other life-threatening adverse effects, and in many patients may be a potential problem.[212–214]

Other secondary causes of SND include endocrine and metabolic problems.[140, 165, 169, 215–219] Unless a profound and severe insult has occurred, SND from most endocrine and metabolic causes is reversed when the underlying problem is resolved.

Hypervagotonia. Hypervagotonia may occur during a variety of conditions or may be precipitated by a number of events.[139, 220–241] Moreover, it must be emphasized that when hypervagotonia exists from any cause, AV nodal dysfunction may coexist and in some patients may be responsible for the symptoms (e.g., syncope).[222, 226, 228, 231, 232–234, 242]

Nasopharyngeal stimulation is a common cause of hypervagotonia in infants and children who require nasogastric tubes for feeding.[14] In the intensive care unit, endotracheal intubation and nasopharyngeal suctioning often are accompanied by vagotonic bradycardia. There has been much debate as to whether apnea with or without bradycardia is caused by gastroesophogeal reflux.[14] Moreover, there is evidence that gastroesophogeal reflux can cause hypervagotonia with resulting SND.[223–225]

In endurance athletes, it is standard to assume that the ubiquitous finding of marked sinus bradycardia is normal. Although this assumption likely is true for virtually all athletes, evidence suggests that an athlete rarely may also have clinically important SND.[226–228]

Carotid sinus hypersensitivity is more common in older patients.[118–120, 229, 230] When present, however, it is important to distinguish the two types of carotid hypersensitivity effects: cardioinhibitory (bradycardia) and cardiodepressor (hypotensive).[243] Either or both may be present in an individual patient. If only the cardiodepressor effect is present, or if it predominates when both effects are present, treatment likely will fail if efforts are directed only toward the SND (cardioinhibitory bradycardia).

During sleep, it is not surprising to find underlying SND exacerbated by the vagotonia commonly present. However, studies have shown that severe SND may occur in some patients only during sleep.[238, 239] This may manifest as sleep apnea and has been identified in young adults. There are implications, however, for the sudden infant death syndrome. Breath-holding is common in toddlers and rarely may cause syncope by sinus arrest and asystole.[236, 237] In these severe cases, atropine has abolished the sinus arrest, thus proving that hypervagotonia is the mechanism for SND in some children who demonstrate breath-holding.[237] In infants with breath-holding spells who are also taking antiarrhythmic drugs (e.g., for SVT), profound bradycardia may result.

Any cause of increased intracranial pressure may result in SND from hypervagotonia;[169, 216] trauma, tumors, and meningitis are the most common causes in children. Although associated with these central nervous system diseases, vomiting by itself also may cause SND by hypervagotonia.

Parasympathomimetic pharmacologic agents may cause hypervagotonia SND either by direct action (e.g., cholinesterase inhibitors such as edrophonium, or catecholamine depleters such as reserpine) or by indirect reflex action (e.g., α-adrenergic agents such as phenylephrine or methoxamine).[179, 240] Morphine appears to have a direct central nervous system vagotonic effect.[241]

Miscellaneous Causes. Miscellaneous causes of SND are those in which the mechanism is either unknown or is not easily assigned to a category. The long QT syndrome is a perplexing disorder for a number of reasons discussed elsewhere.[244] Regarding SND, recent studies have supported the anecdotal data: SND is found in many patients with long QT syndrome.[138, 245, 246] Vincent found a statistically lower heart rate in children with the long QT syndrome who were less than 3 years old.[245] Investigation of sinus node function in children and adolescents with the long QT syndrome revealed data similar to another recent study in adults: many patients with long QT syndrome have lower-than-expected heart rates during maximal exercise testing.[138, 245] Furthermore, of 10 children and adolescents studied by Kugler, nine had one or more abnormal indices of sinus node function.[138] The mechanism of the SND is unknown in these patients but is likely from autonomic nervous system dysfunction. Therefore, in any patient with bradycardia, the QT interval should be measured carefully.

Other miscellaneous causes of SND include sudden infant death syndrome, tumors, coronary angiography, and obstructive jaundice. The sudden infant death syndrome (SIDS) is listed because SND has been speculated as a cause of this apparent multifactorial disorder.[247–250] In two separate autopsy studies, sinus node arterial diameter was reduced (in five of 40 patients and in three of 30 patients) by intimal thickenings.[248, 249] However, the clinical correlation with SND is unknown. Right atrial wall tumors may interfere with the sinus node artery or by direct invasive action may cause SND.[251] Direct action on the sinus node and/or vagotonia may be involved in SND during angiography.[252] Because the effects are a result of the hyperosmolality, the new contrast agents are expected to be associated with less SND. The mechanism of SND is unknown in obstructive jaundice.[253]

In premature and some full-term infants, bradycardia may occur alone or be accompanied by apnea. These paroxysmal symptoms may persist (resulting in pallor or even seizures) through the first year of life and then usually resolve. Most of these infants respond to stimulation and can be managed with only a home apnea/bradycardia monitor. One recently studied infant had a 20-s sinus pause documented and required a pacemaker.

SURGICAL CAUSES

Sinus node dysfunction (and associated atrial arrhythmias) occurs after several types of surgical procedures for congenital heart disease (Table 7–5).* The incidence is highest in patients who have undergone atrial repair (Mustard or Senning) for transposition of the great arteries.† Several recent studies have shown that sinus rhythm is present in less than 50% of these patients several years after operation. Also, the incidence and prevalence of SND arrhythmias increase with the interval from surgery.[41, 270] Initially, the popularity of the Senning operation was based on the expectation that SND would be less than for the Mustard operation. In a recent prospective study, Deanfield et al found no difference between the two operations in incidence of SND.[273]

In patients who have undergone atrial repair of transposition of the great arteries, the predominant type of arrhythmias are those of sinus arrest and chronic atrial, junctional, or sinus bradycardia. These so-called "passive" arrhythmias of SND are much more common than the "active" arrhythmias of atrial flutter or atrial muscle (or sinus node) reentry tachycardia.[41, 42, 131, 270] The incidence and prevalence of SND arrhythmias vary among reports. Several reasons account for the differences, with surgical technique an important factor. Great attention to avoiding trauma to the sinus node and sinus node artery provides the lowest chance of SND (see discussion on prevention).[262, 263, 265] Also, methods of SND detection and follow-up vary considerably among institutions. While some investigators monitor sinus node function by only the standard ECG, others use periodic Holter recordings, exercise testing, and cardiac catheterization.

Although patients with secundum atrial septal defect may have preexisting SND, postoperative SND may be found.[32–34, 46, 132, 156, 158, 275] In some patients SND resolves after surgical closure, but in others SND may be unchanged or may occur as a result of the repair. Bink-Boelkens et al found that 23% of 204 postoperative atrial septal defect patients had atrial and SND arrhythmias.[34] The chance of SND may be higher with repair of a sinus venosus defect or when repair of

*10, 32–48, 87, 131, 132, 156, 158, 160, 255–280
†10, 40–43, 84, 87, 131, 255–273

partial anomalous pulmonary venous connection to the superior vena cava is also required.

Direct trauma to the sinus node or sinus node artery is the most likely mechanism of SND in patients who have undergone atrial repair of transposition of the great arteries.[40, 280, 281] Pathologic and electrophysiologic correlations have revealed that incisions, sutures, and progressive fibrosis in the area of the sinus node and sinus node artery are definite causes of SND in children who have had the Mustard operation.[281] It is likely that the reason atrial arrhythmias are so common in these patients is that there is a great deal of atrial scarring, and thus subsidiary atrial pacemakers are also likely to be suppressed. However, autonomic effects may also be causative or additive. The same mechanisms are probably responsible in patients who have undergone repair of sinus venosus atrial septal defect or partial anomalous venous connection to the superior vena cava. The mechanism of SND is more speculative in patients who have had closure of secundum or primum atrial septal defect. Some of these patients undoubtedly had preoperative SND.[154–159] Moreover, cannulation of the superior vena caval–high right atrial junction has also been proven to cause SND in any patient who has had cardiopulmonary bypass.[278–280] In patients with atrial septal defect or with complex congenital heart disease, longer cardiopulmonary bypass time, absent or inadequate cardioplegia, and older age at operation also may account for SND arrhythmias.[34] Also, stretching of the right atrium pre-, intra-, or postoperatively may account for SND arrhythmias.[36–39, 46–48] This may explain these arrhythmias in patients who have undergone the Blalock-Hanlon operation, because the site of incision is not near the sinus node or sinus node area.[277]

TREATMENT

Prevention

The surgeon may affect the incidence of SND after operation with attention to three principles during surgery. First, it is imperative that the anatomy of the sinus node and sinus node artery is known. Anderson, Ho, and Anderson have studied 25 infant hearts at necropsy and found that the sinus node location was relatively constant, but the sinus node artery supply was considerably variable (Fig. 7–29).[282] In 22 of the 25 hearts, the location of the sinus node was in the lateral area of the superior vena caval–high right atrial junction. In the other three, it was located at the summit of the crest of the right atrial appendage. The caudal extension of the sinus node was more variable, and in some hearts the border extended inferiorly to the inferior vena caval orifice. These same investigators noted that the connections be-

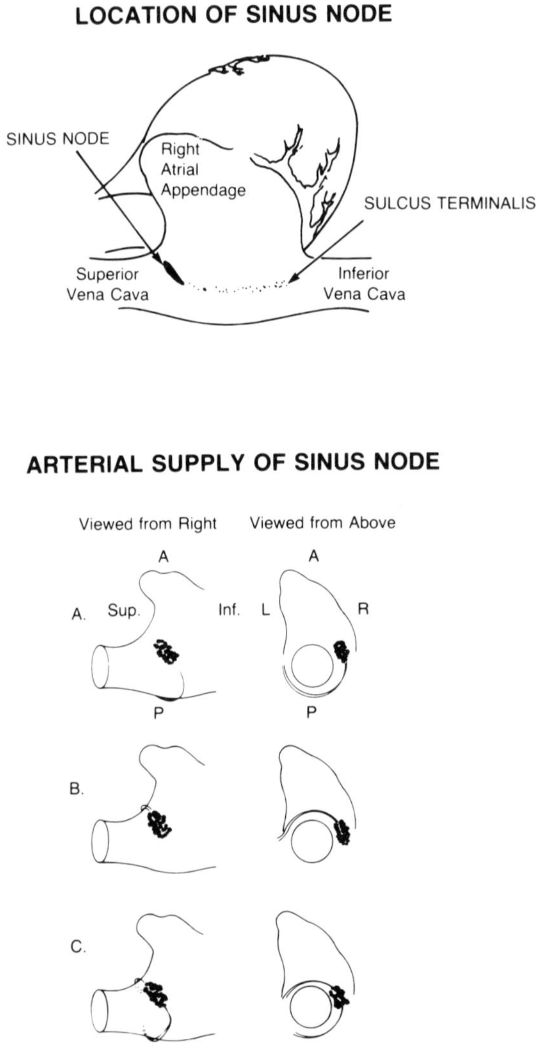

FIGURE 7–29
Diagrammatic illustrations indicate the location of the sinus node and its arterial supply. Anderson, HO, and Anderson[282] found a posterior approaching artery in 11 of 25 hearts (*A*); an anterior approaching artery in 10 (*B*); and an anastomotic ring in 4 (*C*). (A, anterior; Inf, inferior; RAA, right atrial appendage; sup., superior; SVC, superior vena cava.) (Modified from Anderson KR, Ho SY, Anderson RH: Location and vascular supply of sinus node in human heart. Br Heart J 41:28, 1979.)

tween the sinus node and atrial myocardium were diffuse, but no specialized tracts of specialized cells were found in any part of the right atrium. The arterial supply to the sinus node varied considerably (see Fig. 7–29). Anderson, Ho, and Anderson found that the sinus node artery approached the sinus node posteriorly in 40% of the hearts, anteriorly in 40% of the hearts, and by both directions in an anastomotic ring in 16% of the hearts.[282]

Second, the surgeon's attention to superior vena caval cannulation is important, since SND may result from superior vena caval cannulation via the orifice to the high right atrium.[278, 279] This importance was demonstrated by data from Texas Children's Hospital. After cannulation was changed from low to high superior vena cava, the incidence of SND decreased.[262, 270]

Third, myocardial preservation during surgery is an important factor. Bink-Boelkens et al found that lack of cardioplegia and long ischemic time were associated with postoperative SND.[34]

SND arrhythmias can also be prevented by other efforts. Age at operation appears to be an important factor. For example, the optimum age for surgery appears to be between 3 and 12 months for atrial repair for transposition of the great arteries. Also, closure of atrial septal defect in early childhood is associated with a decreased incidence of SND and atrial arrhythmias when compared to closure during adolescence or adulthood.[46] Inducement and exacerbation of SND by antiarrhythmic agents given for atrial or other arrhythmias may be avoided by choosing an alternative agent with less sinus node suppressive effect. In selected patients, electrophysiologic drug studies may be helpful in determining the best choice of antiarrhythmia drug.[123]

Prevention of SND and atrial arrhythmias has been a major impetus to change the type of surgical repair for transposition of the great arteries. Several years ago, the Senning repair gained popularity because the technique appeared to offer less potential damage to the sinus node and atrium. However, a recent prospective study by Deanfield et al has revealed no differences in clinical SND following the Senning procedure when compared to the Mustard operation.[273] The arterial switch repair pioneered by Jatene and recently modified by others has gained strong popularity. Early results seem to indicate that SND is uncommon following this procedure.[283, 284] Late results are needed before it is known whether the total risks and benefits are better for the switch repair than for the atrial repair.

Indications

The decision to recommend treatment is straightforward when symptoms of syncope or near syncope occur during documented arrhythmias of SND. Also it is not difficult to recommend treatment for patients with symptoms of congestive heart failure or severe fatigue that are direct results of SND. However, treatment decisions are complicated when symptoms either are not present or are difficult to document during SND. For these reasons, recommendations for asymptomatic patients and for symptomatic patients with undocumentable SND are somewhat controversial. A major reason for disagreement is that few data exist and therefore recommendations tend to be arbitrary.

One of the most arbitrary recommendations concerns the lower limit of accepted asymptomatic bradycardia.[14, 285] There are no data to show that sleeping sinus or junctional bradycardia is more life-threatening at rates between 20 bpm and 30 bpm than at rates between 30 bpm and 40 bpm. Many variable associated factors and the extent of underlying disease are important. In a multicenter study of 372 patients who had undergone Mustard repair, pacemaker implantation was carried out in all seven patients with rates less than 30 bpm, and each has survived.[41] Because the study did not include an equal number of patients who did not undergo pacemaker implantation and data regarding symptoms (it is implied that they were asymptomatic) in the seven patients is not given, it is not known whether pacemakers are really necessary in similar patients. However, it appears prudent to recommend treatment for such patients, because each of the seven patients survived. It also is important to point out that 11 asymptomatic patients (average age, 6 years) with heart rates between 30 bpm and 40 bpm did not receive a permanent pacemaker, and each has survived (average follow-up, 4.5 years). More data are needed before specific treatment recommendations can be made for asymptomatic patients on the basis of age and heart rate.

Another arbitrary recommendation concerns permanent pacemaker implantation for patients who have tachyarrhythmias, who also are at increased risk of SND (usually because of postoperative atrial repair of transposition of the great arteries), and who require antiarrhythmic drug treatment. Several years ago, an anecdotal association was made between the use of quinidine and sudden death in patients who had previously undergone Mustard repair for transposition of the great arteries.[286] The decision to recommend prophylactic permanent pacemaker implantation in these patients was based on quinidine's known adverse effects on sinus node function and the known high incidence of SND in these patients. Documentation of rhythm at the time of sudden death in this group of patients has never been satisfactorily accomplished. However, the incidence of sudden death probably has decreased (no data are available) in patients who have undergone pacemaker implantation following postoperative atrial repair of transposition of the great arteries when concomitant treatment was required with antiarrhythmic drugs known to produce adverse sinus node effects.

Because of the lack of documentation, there are several problems with this recommendation. Several other alternative explanations exist for sudden death in these patients. Quinidine may have caused life-threatening arrhythmias such as torsades de pointes, or His-Purkinje system dysfunction (complete AV block).[212, 213, 287] By its vagolytic actions, quinidine may accelerate AV conduction during sinoatrial node reentry or atrial muscle reentry tachycardia (e.g., atrial flutter-fibrillation), thus causing a rapid ventricular rate resulting in hypotension, coronary insufficiency, and subsequent ventricular fibrillation.[287] This last possibility is somewhat supported by the multicenter study as well as the studies by Hayes and Gersony and Bink-Boelkens et al.[34, 41, 42] These investigators found a correlation between sudden death and tachyarrhythmia but none between sudden death and bradyarrhythmias.

One patient in Bink-Boelkens et al's study who collapsed suddenly was found to have ventricular fibrillation.[34] The initial arrhythmia, however, may have been a bradyarrhythmia. Beerman et al and Bink-Boelkens et al found that 34% of 87 patients and 22% of 50 patients, respectively, had ventricular ectopy following Mustard repair.[34, 131] Moreover, Scagliotti et al found inducible fast ventricular tachycardia in a patient who presented with syncope following Mustard repair.[137] These data suggest the possibility that ventricular arrhythmias may be a major cause of sudden death in these patients. That quinidine does not have a particularly strong adverse effect on sinus node function (in many patients, the vagolytic effect predominates) also lends support to the possibility that sudden death is unrelated to quinidine's potential adverse effect on sinus node function. Another factor to consider is that AV conduction is normal in most patients who have had atrial repair for transposition of the great arteries. Thus if quinidine's effect is exacerbation of SND, then AV nodal and His-Purkinje system function (assuming nontoxic quinidine serum concentration) would be expected to be normal, and sudden death secondary to bradyarrhythmia would be unlikely because of normal junctional function resulting in tolerable junctional escape rhythm.

Nevertheless, the recommendation for concomitant permanent pacemaker with use of these antiarrhythmic drugs has been made by the Joint Commission on Pacing of the American College of Cardiology and the American Heart Association.[288] Until further data show that these sinus node suppressive drugs are safe without pacemaker implantation in selected patients who have had atrial repair of transposition of the great arteries, the recommendations will remain.

Further caution is emphasized when using quinidine.[212–214] Torsades de pointes occurs only rarely and usually during onset of treatment or during hypokalemia.[212, 213] Hospitalization with ECG telemetry is indicated during the first few days of starting quinidine therapy.[214] Monitoring of serum quinidine and potassium is advised during acute and chronic treatment to decrease the chance of torsades de pointes. Similarly, other type IA drugs and amiodarone are known to cause torsades de pointes, and similar caution and monitoring are advised during therapy with these drugs.

Severe SND without symptoms is also a difficult problem, because there are no indications of SND severity in asymptomatic patients. "Severe" SND implies the presence of symptoms, and the interpretation of severe SND in asymptomatic patients is arbitrary.[41, 285, 286, 289, 290] This is true whether the interpretation is based on ECG criteria or on intracardiac electrophysiologic criteria as listed in Tables 7–1 and 7–3. To one clinician, a sinus pause of 2 s and a CSNRT of 1 s in an asymptomatic 3-year-old child may be severe, while to another clinician these findings may be moderate. Generally, asymptomatic patients with even "severe" SND do not warrant treatment for the SND. The presence of underlying heart disease or requirement of concomitant antiarrhythmic drug therapy, however, may provide a reason to recommend pacemaker implantation in some asymptomatic patients.

The rationale for recommending concomitant pacemaker implantation in patients who have had atrial repair of transposition of the great arteries and who also require antiarrhythmic drug therapy for tachyarrhythmias has been previously discussed. There is less basis for the same recommendation in patients with SND but without similar underlying heart disease. Therefore, a minority of asymptomatic patients with SND who also require treatment with antiarrhythmic drugs known to have adverse sinus node effects benefit from pacemaker implantation. Caution is advised, however, when the antiarrhythmic drug therapy is started. Hospitalization is warranted, with noninvasive monitoring of sinus node function during the initiation of drug treatment. If SND is exacerbated with associated symptoms, then pacemaker implantation is indicated. If SND is exacerbated but no symptoms occur, then the decision for permanent pacemaker is difficult and depends on other factors specific to each patient.

The risk of sudden death does not appear to be great for the asymptomatic patient older than 6 years with sinus or junctional bradycardia at rates greater than 30 bpm.[41] There are no data to show that sudden death is prevented by pacemaker implantation in these patients, including those who have undergone atrial baffle repair for transposition of the great arteries.[41] However, selected asymptomatic patients may develop increasing cardiomegaly resulting from chronic bradycardia. It may be speculated that the cardiomegaly could predispose to life-threatening ventricular arrhythmias, perhaps analogous to patients with long-term bradycardia from congenital complete AV block.[291, 292]

The last category of selected patients is the patient with syncope but in whom only mild SND is found during evaluation. Usually the syncope history is not compatible with an arrhythmogenic cause; frequently the Holter monitor is valuable, because symptoms of dizziness are not associated with an arrhythmia severe enough to cause the reported symptoms.[5] These patients do not require treatment. However, the decision for treatment is complicated in patients with only mild SND who have a syncope history compatible with an arrhythmogenic cause but in whom correlation with SND cannot be documented. It is imperative that complete EPS be carried out to search for other arrhythmia causes of syncope. If none are found, the clinician is faced with a treatment dilemma. Usually the best plan is to make additional efforts to document correlation of symptoms with arrhythmia. However, in some patients circumstances may warrant treatment if further delay is considered dangerous. Chronic medical treatment is an alternative to permanent pacemaker treatment in selected patients.

Medical Treatment

Acute emergency medical treatment is indicated when severe sinus or junctional bradycardia or frequent sinus arrest result in loss of consciousness. Regardless of cause, intravenous atropine (0.04 mg/kg) and/or isoproterenol (0.05–0.5 mg/kg/min) usually are effective. A temporary transvenous pacemaker should be placed if these drugs are unsuccessful in increasing heart rate to a satisfactory level.

Chronic medical treatment has not been acceptable as standard treatment for SND. Several pharmacologic agents are available, but success has been variable and side effects have been prevalent. Atropine and its derivatives (e.g., propantheline bromide) induce parasympathomimetic side effects (dry mouth, urine retention, visual disturbances) that are often intolerable.[179]

Adrenergic stimulatory drugs such as sublingual isoproterenol and oral agents prenalterol, xamoterol, theophylline, and hydralazine have been successful in selected patients.

In the study by Feleke et al, prenalterol, a β-receptor agonist, was given to 10 adult patients with symptomatic SND.[293] Eight patients completed the acute protocol with heart rate significantly increasing after 75 μ/kg of the intravenous drug. However, the heart rate response was not uniform in all patients. Only five patients agreed to chronic therapy (50 mg twice daily), and only three continued the therapy for 3 months. Although prenalterol appears to have mixed results, further data are needed to define its usefulness.

Xamoterol is a β-adrenergic partial agonist.[294] The drug acts as a β-blocker during periods of high sympathetic stimulation and as a β_1-agonist at low levels of sympathetic tone. These actions make xamoterol appealing as an agent for patients with SND. Tseu, Morley, and Mackintosh gave 12 adult patients (11 were symptomatic) 200 mg of oral xamoterol twice daily. The only statistically significant improvement was shortening of the RR interval, but only during sleep (midnight to 8:00 AM). Pauses were eliminated in 3/12 and improved in three others, but four patients had an increase in pauses, with two of them showing worse symptoms. Only six of 12 patients showed ECG improvement. While xamoterol may have theoretical advantages, the indication for its use in patients with SND is not defined.

Hydralazine is another chronotropic agent that has been successful in selected patients with SND (Fig. 7–30).[295–297] The mechanism of hydralazine appears to be both by direct β-adrenergic myocardial stimulation and by reflex cardiac sympathetic stimulation in response to lower blood pressure. Hydralazine has been more successful in SND patients with hypertension than in those without hypertension. Hydralazine increased heart rate by 10% in two of three hypertensive adult patients and in one of two normotensive adult patients. Long-term follow-up has not been reported. It is possible that the short-term beneficial effects of hydralazine are not sustained.

The effect of theophylline has been studied by Benditt et al in 10 patients (age 9–41 years) with recurrent symptomatic bradyarrhythmias believed to be caused by excessive parasympathetic influence on sinus node and/or AV node.[298] Intravenous theophylline significantly shortened sinus cycle length, SACT, and CSNRT. Subsequent chronic oral therapy was tolerated in eight patients, and six had suppression of symptoms. However, the follow-up period was short (5–24 months). In this study, the drawbacks of chronic theophylline therapy were nausea and palpitations. Benditt et al point out another potential important limitation for any of these oral agents in patients with atrial tachyarrhythmias or a potential for atrial tachyarrhythmias: acceleration of AV conduction may occur, and if sinus nodal or atrial muscle reentry tachycardia is present, rapid conduction to the ventricles may result in a life-threatening ventricular arrhythmia.

To summarize medical treatment for patients with SND, the early data show promise for only a few selected patients. The patients who appear to have the greatest chance of benefit are those who have mild to moderate symptoms (e.g., dizziness, fatigue), with hypervagotonia as the major underlying mechanism for SND.[120, 298] Furthermore, hypervagotonia is self-limited in many patients, because symptoms have disappeared in follow-up (see Fig. 7–30).[120] Medical treatment rather than pacemaker implantation offers a valuable alternative to these patients. If many of these patients have an adenosine-mediated disorder, as Watt hypothesizes, theophylline may have the best chance for success.[299] It must be emphasized, however, that these agents are contraindicated in patients with bradyarrhythmias who also have (or are likely to develop) tachyarrhythmias.

Permanent Pacemaker Implantation

When treatment is indicated for infants, children, and adolescents with SND, the accepted mode is permanent pacemaker implantation.[300–304] The pacemaker choices for SND treatment in 1987 include the following types of multiprogrammable generators: ventricular demand (VVI); atrial demand (AAI); dual-chambered demand or triggered (DDD); and activity-detecting, rate-variable ventricular demand (VVI/A).[302–310] The type of pacemaker system recommended is dependent on the underlying arrhythmias, AV conduction function, underlying heart disease (ventricular function), age/body size, and patient preference for location of the pacemaker generator (scar).

When the SND arrhythmia is slow or there is failure of impulse generation or conduction, pacemaker implantation is recommended to maintain a sufficient rate to prevent symptoms. The most simple type of rate support mode is single-chamber pacing (either the VVI or the AAI pacemaker sys-

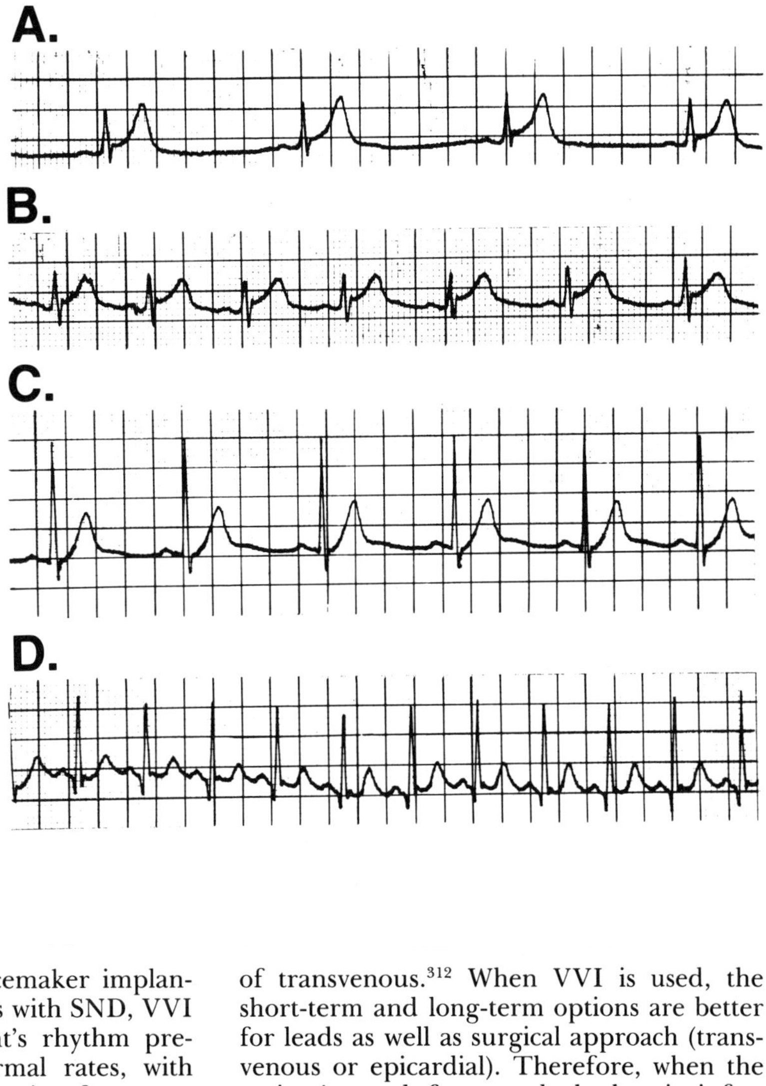

FIGURE 7–30
Four ECG recordings by Holter monitor show the results of SND treatment with hydralazine in a 16-year-old boy who had frequent syncope and documented hypervagotonia. Baseline electrophysiology study (EPS) revealed a long sinus node recovery time (corrected, 795 ms) and Strauss sinoatrial conduction time (310 ms), but each corrected to normal values after atropine dosage. During another EPS, the maximal corrected recovery time was still abnormal (430 ms) after hydralazine dosage (0.5 mg/kg intravenously), but was shorter than baseline. The sinoatrial conduction time was not changed after hydralazine therapy. A trial of oral hydralazine was carried out with Holter monitoring to assess efficacy.

Before hydralazine therapy, the slowest sinus rate during waking hours was 40 bpm (*A*) and the fastest was 80 bpm (*B*). After 2 days of hydralazine dosage the slowest waking heart rate was 65 bpm (*C*) and the fastest was 130 bpm (*D*). Syncope resolved for 1 year but recurred, in part from postural hypotension. Hydralazine therapy was stopped, with two syncopal episodes occurring during the following 3 years, both in the first year after cessation of treatment.

tem). When permanent pacemaker implantation is indicated in patients with SND, VVI is suitable when the patient's rhythm predominantly is sinus at normal rates, with occasional sinus arrest accounting for symptoms. This patient typically also has an AV conduction disorder. Atrioventricular conduction status may be determined during preoperative EPS, during temporary preoperative transvenous pacemaker placement, or at the time of permanent implantation.[301]

In patients with normal AV conduction, AAI is often the ideal choice, because it offers the advantage of the atrial contribution to cardiac output (Fig. 7–31). However, even in the presence of normal AV conduction, the VVI pacemaker offers an excellent choice when the patient's need for pacing is infrequent. The AAI is best suited for transvenous leads, although the subxiphoid approach and the thoracotomy approach are available.[304, 311] Regardless of approach, atrial lead technology is behind that of ventricular leads, and epicardial lead technology is behind that of transvenous.[312] When VVI is used, the short-term and long-term options are better for leads as well as surgical approach (transvenous or epicardial). Therefore, when the patient's need for paced rhythm is infrequent, often the advantages and disadvantages favor the VVI rather than the AAI. Dual-chambered pacemakers are seldom indicated in patients with infrequent bradyarrhythmias, because the infrequent need does not require the vast capabilities of the newer-generation DDD pacemakers.

When the bradyarrhythmia is frequent and the pacemaker need is frequent or continuous, the better pacemaker options are AAI, DDD, or the VVIR.[303–310] The atrial contribution to cardiac output with the AAI and DDD is valuable when underlying ventricular function is decreased or marginal.[124] AAI usually is used with normal AV conduction, and DDD is recommended with abnormal or marginal AV conduction. VVIR appears to be an excellent (and perhaps better) alternative to the DDD or AAI.[308–310] This pace-

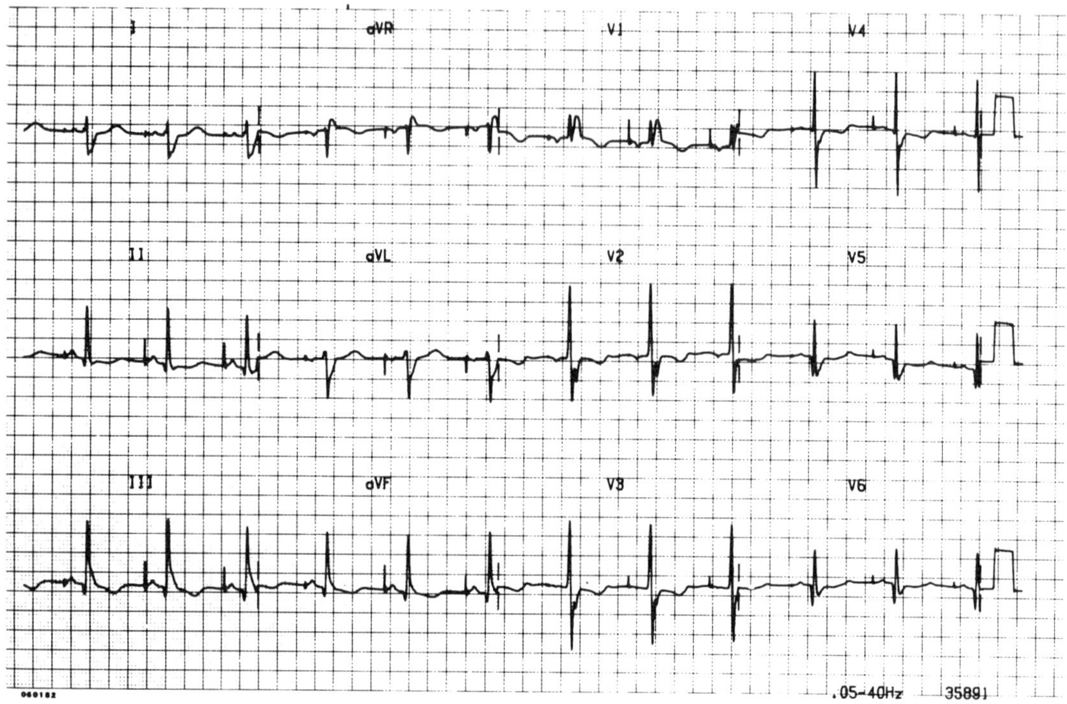

FIGURE 7–31
A surface 12-lead ECG from an 18-year-old woman with SND and hypertrophic obstructive cardiomyopathy shows atrial paced rhythm (70 bpm). Because of excellent AV conduction, an atrial pacemaker was implanted to relieve bradycardia and associated dizziness and fatigue.

maker responds to body activity and in turn increases the ventricular paced rate accordingly. Although more data are needed, it is likely that activity-related rate alone is a more important factor than atrial "kick" alone when increased cardiac output is required in the young patient.[124] A single-chamber pacemaker that is responsive to the activity needs of the patient may be the pacemaker of choice for young patients with SND. If AV conduction is normal, an activity-detecting, rate-responsive atrial demand unit (AAIR) may be implanted. Then both the atrial contribution and the rate contribution to cardiac output optimize hemodynamics. Also, when VA conduction is intact, the AAIR may be indicated instead of the VVIR, because the VVIR pacemaker may induce the pacemaker syndrome with intact VA conduction.[306]

Choosing the type of pacemaker is somewhat more complex when tachyarrhythmias are also a part of the patient's SND bradyarrhythmias. In patients susceptible to tachyarrhythmias, the DVI pacemaker may be contraindicated because atrial activity is not sensed, and therefore an increased risk exists for the induction of sinus node or atrial muscle reentry tachycardias (e.g., atrial flutter-fibrillation). Moreover, with a pacemaker that requires any atrial lead, there is a theoretical increased chance of inducing or exacerbating these atrial tachyarrhythmias, as a result of mechanical stimulation. However, recent data in adult patients have suggested that improved hemodynamics from DDD pacemakers may in fact decrease the incidence of these atrial tachyarrhythmias.[307, 313] Many single and dual-chambered pacemakers can be programmmed for temporary "burst" overdrive pacing of tachyarrhythmias. For atrial arrthymias either an AAT or DDD may be used. In choosing a pacemaker, this capability should be considered. Automatic antitachycardia pacemaker systems are useful in selected patients with SND who have tachyarrhythmias as a major clinical problem.[304, 314–316] In patients with SND, usually the type of tachyarrhythmias (sinus nodal or atrial muscle tachyarrhythmias) are not ideal for antitachycardia pacemakers. The atrial muscle tachyarrhythmias usually are difficult to convert during EPS, and therefore, a high success rate by the antitachycardia device would not be expected.[317] Furthermore, the antitachycardia pacemaker is a mode of treatment that has short-term rather than long-term implications. Thus in children and young adults, this form of treatment usually is used when all other treatment modalities have been exhausted. Before it is considered, a thorough EPS is necessary to be certain the device will be successful.

The type of antiarrhythmic drug being administered is another important factor in patients with bradytachyarrhythmias. For example, flecainide, a new type Ic drug, has the disadvantage of increasing myocardial lead pacing thresholds in some patients.[318]

Underlying structural heart disease is an important consideration when choosing the lead and pacemaker.[300–304, 319, 320] The status of ventricular function has been discussed. Because persistent left superior vena cava is a common associated venous anomaly, it should be identified before transvenous lead placement is carried out, and when detected, the left superior vena cava should not be used.[320] In the child who has undergone surgery to correct congenital heart disease, surgical access is another related problem. Adhesions on and around the heart from previous operations often interfere with placement and the long-term function of epicardial leads. In children who have not had surgery and in whom epicardial leads are used, the subxiphoid approach can be used for atrial as well as ventricular placement.[311] However, with adhesions from previous surgery, the subxiphoid approach may be more difficult.

Transvenous leads also are associated with challenges in patients following surgery for congenital heart disease.[302–304, 321–325] In patients with atrial repair for transposition of the great arteries, the distorted atrial anatomy provides a challenge for successful transvenous lead placement; however, in these patients there appear to be fewer pacing problems with the endocardial approach. Gillette et al have shown that the best technique is to use active fixation leads (screw-in) positioned in the roof of the anatomic left atrium.[322] McGoon et al earlier successfully used a J-tined lead in one patient who had undergone Mustard repair, but in three other patients, they subsequently used active-fixation leads positioned posteriorly in the anatomic left atrium.[319] The active-fixation lead also was used by Vince, Tyers, and Kerr in an 11-year-old patient with univentricular heart who had undergone Fontan repair.[325] Gillette et al also showed that two leads can be passed transvenously.

Patient size is less a problem with transvenous leads currently than it was several years ago. Gillette et al have implanted a pacemaker with transvenous leads in a 3-year-old patient who had undergone Mustard repair for transposition of the great arteries.[304] In a different report, Gillette et al reported transvenous lead placement in children who weighed 15 kg.[302] Holmes, Maloney, and Feldt reported placement of a transvenous pacemaker in an 8.6-kg, 18-month-old infant.[321] Ward, Jones, and Shinebourne reported transvenous pacing in five children, each weighing less than 10 kg.[323] The youngest child was 9 months old.

Patient preference for scar and generator location is an issue that is seldom addressed at the time when the decision for type of pacemaker is discussed with the patient and family. In my experience, this by far is the most important issue with an adolescent. This is best illustrated by a recent case of an 18-year-old young man with bradytachyarrhythmias resulting from Mustard repair. The best choice of pacemaker lead clearly was transvenous, but he insisted on again having the generator placed through the same scar in the lower abdomen where the first pacemaker had been placed 10 years earlier. Even after informing him that another lead placement by thoracotomy was required, he persisted in wanting the generator in the lower abdominal wall rather than the pectoral area. Because this is an important issue with adolescents, it should always be discussed with parents and patients. The advantages and disadvantages of transvenous versus epicardial leads and the ideal type of pacemaker generator for the underlying associated arrhythmias and heart disease are obviously the most important issues involving the physical health of the patient. But psychologically, pacemaker implantation can be a problem, and all issues should be discussed before pacemaker implantation.

Follow-up of Pacemaker Implantation. Follow-up data are readily available because SND is a relatively common indication for pacemaker implantation in children and young adults.[300, 302, 326, 327] Gillette et al found that of 49 symptomatic children, 45 (92%) had relief of symptoms following pacemaker implantation.[302] No early deaths occurred, but two patients died later of causes unrelated to SND. In those with coexisting tachyarrhythmias, symptoms are more difficult to eliminate. Gillette et al found that only 11 of

18 patients (61%) with SND and concomitant tachyarrhythmia were free of symptoms after pacemaker implantation, suggesting that simple bradycardia pacemaker implantation does not prevent tachyarrhythmias in these children. Exercise testing has proven valuable in the follow-up of patients who have a DDD or activity-detecting rate-variable pacemaker.[327] In this manner, the high rate performance can be checked to verify optimum programmed indices.

When atrial pacemakers were initially implanted for SND in patients who had normal AV conduction, investigators were uncertain as to whether late AV conduction dysfunction would appear. Follow-up studies in adults have shown an insignificant incidence of AV conduction disorders.[328, 329] Although similar studies have not been carried out in children, the adult data are supportive of the use of atrial pacemakers in patients with SND without AV conduction dysfunction.

Pacemakers are discussed in further detail in Chapter 17.

ACKNOWLEDGMENTS

I thank Cathy Blodgett, RN, BSN; Cynthia Foreman, RN, BSN; and especially Jeanine Pittman and Lou Larsen for their invaluable time and effort in preparing this chapter.

References

1. Mandel WJ, Laks MM: Overview of the sick sinus syndrome. Chest 66:22, 1974.
2. Kaplan BM, Langendorf R, Lev M, et al: Tachycardia-bradycardia syndrome (so-called "sick sinus syndrome"). Am J Cardiol 31:497, 1973.
3. Ferrer IM: The Sick Sinus Syndrome. Mt Kisco, NY, Futura Publishing Company, 1974, p 37.
4. Dhingra RC: Sinus node dysfunction. PACE 6:1062, 1983.
5. Kugler JD, Yabek SM: Sick sinus syndrome: Clinical features and noninvasive evaluation. In Yabek SM, Gillette PC, Kugler JD (eds): The Sinus Node in Pediatrics. London, Churchill Livingstone, 1984, p 48.
6. Pop T, Fleischman D: Measurement of sinus node recovery time after atrial pacing. In Bonke FIM (ed): The Sinus Node: Structure, Function and Clinical Relevance. The Hague, Martinus Nijhoff, 1978, p 23.
7. Reiffel JA, Bigger JT Jr, Cramer M, et al: Ability of Holter electrocardiographic recording and atrial stimulation to detect sinus nodal dysfunction in symptomatic and asymptomatic patients with sinus bradycardia. Am J Cardiol 40:189, 1977.
8. Thormann J, Schlepper M, Kramer W: Diurnal changes and reproducibility of corrected sinus node recovery time. Cath Cardiovasc Diag 9:439, 1983.
9. Fournier A, Smith RT, Moak JP, et al: Sinus bradycardia in children. Proceedings from the XXII Annual Meeting of the Association of European Paediatric Cardiologists, Dubrovnik, Yugoslavia, May 5–9, 1986. (Abstract).
10. Hesslein PS, Gutgesell HP, Gillette PC, et al: Exercise assessment of sinoatrial node function following the Mustard operation. Am Heart J 103:351, 1982.
11. Anderson RH, Yen HS, Becker AE, et al: The development of the sinoatrial node. In Bonke FIM (ed): The Sinus Node. The Hague, Martinus Nijhoff, 1978, p 166.
12. Gomes JA, Winters SL: The origins of the sinus node pacemaker complex in man: Demonstration of dominant and subsidiary foci. J Am Coll Cardiol 9:45, 1987.
13. Gillette PC: Treatment of sinus node dysfunction. In Yabek SM, Gillette PC, Kugler JD (eds): The Sinus Node in Pediatrics. London, Churchill Livingstone, 1984, p 133.
14. Kugler JD: The sinoatrial node and its dysfunction. In Liebman J, Plonsey R, Rudy Y (eds): New Directions in Pediatric and Fundamental Electrocardiography. The Hague, Martinus Nijhoff, 1987.
15. Brodsky M, Wu D, Denes P, et al: Arrhythmias documented by 24 hour continuous electrocardiographic monitoring in 50 male medical students without apparent heart disease. Am J Cardiol 39:390, 1977.
16. Scott O, Williams GJ, Fiddler GI: Results of 24 hour ambulatory monitoring of electrocardiogram in 131 healthy boys aged 10 to 13 years. Br Heart J 44:304, 1980.
17. Richards JM, Alexander JR, Shinebourne EA, et al: Sequential 22-hour profiles of breathing patterns and heart rate in 110 full-term infants during their first 6 months of life. Pediatrics 74:763, 1984.
18. Southall DP, Richards J, Mitchell P, et al: Study of cardiac rhythm in healthy newborn infants. Br Heart J 43:14, 1980.
19. Southall DP, Johnston F, Shinebourne EA, et al: 24-hour electrocardiographic study of heart rate and rhythm patterns in population of healthy children. Br Heart J 45:281, 1981.
20. Montague TJ, Taylor PG, Stockton R, et al: The spectrum of cardiac rate and rhythm in normal newborns. Pediatr Cardiol 2:33, 1982.
21. Viitasalo MT, Kala R, Eisalo A: Ambulatory electrocardiographic recording in endurance athletes. Br Heart J 47:213, 1982.
22. Nasrallah AT, Gillette PC, Mullins CE, et al: Concealed His bundle extrasystoles in congenital heart disease. Am J Cardiol 35:288, 1975.
23. Garson A Jr, Gillette PC, McNamara DG: A Guide to Cardiac Dysrhythmias in Children. New York, NY, Grune & Stratton, 1980, p 117.
24. Sealy WC, Seaber AV: Surgical isolation of the atrial septum from the atria. J Thorac Cardiovasc Surg 80:742, 1980.
25. Ishikawa S, Sawada K, Tanahashi Y, et al: Experimental studies on sick sinus syndrome: Relationship of extent of right atrial lesions to subsidiary pacemaker shift and its function. Am Heart J 105:593, 1983.
26. Rozanski GJ, Lipsius SL, Randall WC: Functional characteristics of sinoatrial and subsidiary pacemaker activity in the canine right atrium. Circulation 67:1378, 1983.

27. Urthaler F, Katholi CR, Macy J Jr, et al: Mathematical relationship between automaticity of the sinus node and the AV junction. Am Heart J 86:189, 1973.
28. Urthaler F, Katholi CR, Macy J Jr, et al: Electrophysiological and mathematical characteristics of the escape rhythm during complete AV block. Cardiovasc Res 8:173, 1974.
29. Urthaler F, James TN: Hierarchy of supraventricular pacemakers. J Thorac Cardiovasc Surg 80:750, 1980.
30. Schamroth L, Dove E: The Wenckebach phenomenon in sinoatrial block. Br Heart J 28:350, 1966.
31. Bradlow BA: Supraventricular paroxysmal tachycardia interrupted by repeated episodes of total cardiac standstill with syncopal attacks. Chest 58:122, 1970.
32. Reid JM, Stevenson JC: Cardiac arrhythmias following successful surgical closure of atrial septal defect. Br Heart J 29:742, 1967.
33. Esscher E, Michaelsson M: Long-term results following closure of isolated ostium secundum atrial septal defect in children and adults. Eur J Cardiol 6:109, 1976.
34. Bink-Boelkens M, Velvis H, Homan van der Heide JJ, et al: Dysrhythmias after atrial surgery in children. Am Heart J 106:125, 1983.
35. Fox K, Evans T, Rowland E, et al: 'Bradycardia-tachycardia' syndrome 8 yr after correction of Fallot's tetralogy. Eur J Cardiol 10:109, 1979.
36. Oh JK, Holmes DR Jr, Hayes DL, et al: Cardiac arrhythmias in patients with surgical repair of Ebstein's anomaly. J Am Coll Cardiol 6:1351, 1985.
37. Sharratt GP, Johnson AM, Monro JL: Persistence and effects of sinus rhythm after Fontan procedure for tricuspid atresia. Br Heart J 42:74, 1979.
38. Alboliras ET, Porter CJ, Danielson GK, et al: Results of the modified Fontan operation for congenital heart lesions in patients without preoperative sinus rhythm. J Am Coll Cardiol 6:228, 1985.
39. Taliercio CP, Vlietstra RE, McGoon MD, et al: Permanent cardiac pacing after the Fontan procedure. J Thorac Cardiovasc Surg 90:414, 1985.
40. Gillette PC, Kugler JD, Garson A Jr, et al: Mechanisms of cardiac arrhythmias after the Mustard operation for transposition of the great arteries. Am J Cardiol 45:1225, 1980.
41. Flinn CJ, Wolff GS, Dick M II, et al: Cardiac rhythm after the Mustard operation for complete transposition of the great arteries. N Engl J Med 310:1635, 1984.
42. Hayes CJ, Gersony WM: Arrhythmias after the Mustard operation for transposition of the great arteries: A long-term study. J Am Coll Cardiol 7:133, 1986.
43. Vetter VL, Hardy CE: Inducible atrial flutter after the Mustard repair of d-transposition of the great arteries. Am Heart J 112:644, 1986. Abstract.
44. Kugler JD, Pinsky WW, Cheatham JP, et al: Atrial muscle tachydysrhythmia in the young. J Am Coll Cardiol 1:614, 1983. Abstract.
45. Garson A Jr, Bink-Boelkens M, Hesslein PS, et al: Atrial flutter in the young: A collaborative study of 380 cases. J Am Coll Cardiol 6:871, 1985.
46. Brandenburg RO Jr, Holmes DR Jr, Brandenburg RO, et al: Clinical follow-up study of paroxysmal supraventricular tachyarrhythmias after operative repair of secundum type atrial septal defect in adults. Am J Cardiol 51:273, 1983.
47. Ghazi F, Moodie DS, Sterba R, et al: Ebstein's anomaly in adults: Long-term follow-up. Proceedings from Midwest Pediatric Cardiovascular Society Meeting, September, 1986.
48. Flugelman MY, Hasin Y, Katznelson N, et al: Restoration and maintenance of sinus rhythm after mitral valve surgery for mitral stenosis. Am J Cardiol 54:617, 1984.
49. Disertori M, Inama G, Vergara G, et al: Evidence of a reentry circuit in the common type of atrial flutter in man. Circulation 67:434, 1983.
50. Wu D, Amat-Y-Leon F, Denes P, et al: Demonstration of sustained sinus and atrial reentry as a mechanism of paroxysmal supraventricular tachycardia. Circulation 51:234, 1975.
51. Jazayeri MR, Massumi A, Mihalick MJ, et al: Sinus node reentry: Case report and review of electrocardiographic and electrophysiologic features. Texas Heart Inst J 12:249, 1985.
52. Gomes JA, Hariman RJ, Kang PS, et al: Sustained symptomatic sinus node reentrant tachycardia: Incidence, clinical significance, electrophysiologic observations and the effects of antiarrhythmic agents. J Am Coll Cardiol 5:45, 1985.
53. Fox KM, Anderson RH, Hallidie-Smith KA: Hypoplastic and fibrotic sinus node associated with intractable tachycardia in a neonate. Circulation 61:1048, 1980.
54. Gillette PC, Garson A: Electrophysiologic and pharmacologic characteristics of automatic ectopic atrial tachycardia. Circulation 56:571, 1977.
55. Hattori M, Toyama J, Ito A, et al: Comparative evaluation of depressed automaticity in sick sinus syndrome by Holter monitoring and overdrive suppression test. Am Heart J 105:587, 1983.
56. Gang ES, Reiffel JA, Livelli FD Jr, et al: Sinus node recovery times following the spontaneous termination of supraventricular tachycardia and following atrial overdrive pacing: A comparison. Am Heart J 105:210, 1983.
57. Leier CV, Meacham JA, Schaal SF: Prolonged atrial conduction. Circulation 57:213, 1978.
58. Gomes JAC, Kang PS, Matheson M, et al: Coexistence of sick sinus rhythm and atrial flutter-fibrillation. Circulation 63:80, 1981.
59. Cosio FG, Palacios J, Vidal JM, et al: Electrophysiologic studies in atrial fibrillation. Am J Cardiol 51:122, 1982.
60. Cumming GR, Everatt D, Hastman L: Bruce treadmill test in children: Normal values in a clinic population. Am J Cardiol 41:69, 1978.
61. Hesslein PS: Noninvasive diagnosis of dysrhythmias. In Gillette PC, Garson J Jr (eds): Pediatric Cardiac Dysrhythmias. New York, Grune & Stratton, 1981, p 59.
62. Williams RL: Use of transtelephonic electrocardiography in patients with symptoms suggesting cardiac arrhythmias. Pediatrics 61:493, 1978.
63. Dick M II, McFadden D, Crowley D, et al: Diagnosis and management of cardiac rhythm disorders by transtelephonic electrocardiography in infants and children. J Pediatr 94:612, 1979.
64. Dunnigan A, Benson W Jr, Benditt DG: Atrial flutter in infancy: Diagnosis, clinical features and treatment. Pediatrics 75:725, 1985.
65. Butto F, Dunnigan A, Overholt ED, et al: Transesophageal study of recurrent atrial tachycardia after atrial baffle procedures for complete transposition of the great arteries. Am J Cardiol 57:1356, 1986.
66. Benson DW Jr, Dunnigan A, Benditt DG, et al:

Transesophageal cardiac pacing: History, application, technique. Clin Prog Pacing Electrophysiol 2:360, 1984.
67. Yabek SM, Akl BF, Berman W Jr, et al: Use of atrial epicardial electrodes to diagnose and treat postoperative arrhythmias in children. Am J Cardiol 46:285, 1980.
68. Yabek SM, Akl BF, Berman W Jr, et al: Bedside evaluation of postoperative sinus node function in children. J Thorac Cardiovasc Surg 81:691, 1981.
69. Wolff GS, Kaiser G, Casta A, et al: Sinus and atrioventricular nodal function: Preoperative and early postoperative assessment in children. J Thorac Cardiovasc Surg 83:141, 1982.
70. Cramer KM, Hariman RJ, Boxer R, et al: Electrograms from the canine sinoatrial pacemaker recorded in vitro and in situ. Am J Cardiol 42:939, 1978.
71. Mackintosh AF, English MJ, Vincent R, et al: Low voltage electrical activity preceding right atrial depolarization in man. Br Heart J 42:117, 1979.
72. Hariman RJ, Krongrad E, Boxer RA, et al: Methods for recording electrograms of the sinoatrial node during cardiac surgery in man. Circulation 61:1024, 1980.
73. Hariman RJ, Krongrad E, Boxer RA, et al: Method for recording electrical activity of the sinoatrial node and automatic atrial foci during cardiac catheterization in human subjects. Am J Cardiol 45:775, 1980.
74. Reiffel JA, Bigger JT Jr: Current status of direct recordings of the sinus node electrogram in man. PACE 6:1143, 1983.
75. Bethge C, Gebhardt-Seehausen U, Mullges W: The human sinus nodal electrogram: Techniques and clinical results of intra-atrial recordings in patients with and without sick sinus syndrome. Am Heart J 112:1074, 1986.
76. Heddle WF, Jones ME, Tonkin AM: Sinus node sequences after atrial stimulation: Similarities of effects of different methods. Br Heart J 54:568, 1985.
77. Rakovec P, Jakopin J, Rode P, et al: Clinical comparison of indirectly and directly determined sinoatrial conduction time. Am Heart J 102:292, 1981.
78. Reiffel JA, Gang E, Gliklich J, et al: The human sinus node electrogram: A transvenous catheter technique and a comparison of directly measured and indirectly estimated sinoatrial conduction time in adults. Circulation 62:1324, 1980.
79. Gomes JAC, Kang PS, El-Sherif N: The sinus node electrogram in patients with and without sick sinus syndrome: Techniques and correlation between directly measured and indirectly estimated sinoatrial conduction time. Circulation 66:864, 1982.
80. Juillard A, Guillerm F, Chuong HV, et al: Sinus node electrogram recording in 59 patients. Br Heart J 50:75, 1983.
81. Irnich W: Intracardiac electrograms and sensing test signals: Electrophysiological, physical and technical considerations. PACE 8:870, 1985.
82. Krongrad E, Hariman RJ, Boxer RA, et al: A method for recording of sinus node and ectopic atrial pacemaker electrograms during cardiac catheterization in humans. Circulation 58:II–146, 1978. Abstract.
83. Narula OS, Samet P, Javier RP: Significance of the sinus node recovery time. Circulation 45:140, 1972.
84. Gutgesell HP, Gillette PC, McNamara DG: The response of the sinoatrial node to rapid atrial stimulation. Pediatr Res 8:350, 1974. Abstract.
85. El-Said GM, Gillette PC, Mullins CE, et al: Significance of pacemaker recovery time after the Mustard operation for transposition of the great arteries. Am J Cardiol 38:448, 1976.
86. Strauss HC, Saroff AL, Bigger JT, et al: Premature atrial stimulation as a key to the understanding of sinoatrial conduction in man. Circulation 47:86, 1973.
87. Kugler JB, Gillette PC, Mullins CE, et al: Sinoatrial conduction in children: An index of sinoatrial node function. Circulation 59:1266, 1979.
88. Narula OS, Shanth N, Vasquez M, et al: A new method for measurement of sinoatrial conduction time. Circulation 58:706, 1978.
89. Yabek SM, Jarmakani JM, Roberts NK: Sinus node function in children: Factors influencing its evaluation. Circulation 53:28, 1976.
90. Gomes JAC, Hariman RI, Chowdry IA: New application of direct sinus node recordings in man: Assessment of sinus node recovery time. Circulation 70:663, 1984.
91. Reiffel JA, Gang E, Bigger JT Jr, et al: Sinus node recovery time related to paced cycle length in normals and patients with sinoatrial dysfunction. Am Heart J 104:746, 1982.
92. Griebenow R, Saborowski F, Godehardt E, et al: Effect of haemodynamic changes during rapid atrial pacing on determination of sinus node recovery time. Br Heart J 52:87, 1984.
93. Nalos PC, Deng Z, Rosenthal ME, et al: Hemodynamic influences on sinus node recovery time: Effects of autonomic blockade. J Am Coll Cardiol 7:1079, 1986.
94. Clapp SA, Driscoll DJ, Mitrani I, et al: Comparative effects of age and sedation on sinus node automaticity and AV node conduction. Dev Pharmacol Ther 2:180, 1981.
95. Reiffel JA, Gang E, Livelli F Jr, et al: Clinical and electrophysiologic characteristics of sinoatrial entrance block evaluation by direct sinus node electrography: Prevalence, relation to antegrade sinoatrial conduction time, and relevance to sinus node disease. Am Heart J 102:1011, 1981.
96. Asseman P, Berzin B, Desry D, et al: Persistent sinus nodal electrograms during abnormally prolonged postpacing atrial pauses in sick sinus syndrome in humans: Sinoatrial block vs overdrive suppression. Circulation 68:33, 1983.
97. Steinbeck G, Luderitz B: Comparative study of sinoatrial conduction time and sinus node recovery time. Br Heart J 37:956, 1975.
98. Breithardt G, Seipel L, Loogen F: Sinus node recovery time and calculated sinoatrial conduction time in normal subjects and patients with sinus node dysfunction. Circulation 56:43, 1977.
99. Dhingra RC, Wyndham C, Amat-y-Leon F, et al: Sinus nodal responses to atrial extrastimuli in patients without apparent sinus node disease. Am J Cardiol 36:445, 1975.
100. Masini G, Dianda R, Graziina A: Analysis of sinoatrial conduction in man using premature atrial stimulation. Cardiovasc Res 9:498, 1975.
101. Breithardt G, Seipel L: The effect of premature atrial depolarization on sinus node automaticity in man. Circulation 53:920, 1976.
102. Bonke FIM, Bouman LN, van Rijn HE: Change of cardiac rhythm in the rabbit after an atrial premature beat. Circ Res 24:533, 1969.

103. Bonke FIM, Bouman LN, Schopman FJG: Effect of an early atrial premature beat on activity of the sinoatrial node and atrial rhythm in the rabbit. Circ Res 29:704, 1971.
104. Klein HO, Singer DH, Hoffman BF: Effects of atrial premature systoles on sinus rhythm in the rabbit. Circ Res 32:480, 1973.
105. Miller HC, Strauss HC: Measurement of sinoatrial conduction time by premature atrial stimulation in the rabbit. Circ Res 35:935, 1974.
106. Reiffel JA, Gang E, Livelli F, et al: Indirectly estimated sinoatrial conduction time by the atrial premature stimulus technique: Patterns of error and the degree of associated inaccuracy as assessed by direct sinus node electrography. Am Heart J 106:459, 1983.
107. Breithardt G, Seipel L: Comparative study of two methods of estimating sinoatrial conduction time in man. Am J Cardiol 42:965, 1978.
108. Haberl R, Steinbeck G, Luderitz B: Acceleration of sinus rhythm during slow-rate atrial pacing. Circulation 67:1368, 1983.
109. Jordan JL, Yamaguchi I, Mandel WJ: Studies on the mechanism of sinus node dysfunction in the sick sinus syndrome. Circulation 57:217, 1978.
110. Desai JM, Scheinman MM, Strauss H, et al: Electrophysiologic effects of combined autonomic blockade in patients with sinus node disease. Circulation 63:953, 1981.
111. Kang, PS, Gomes JAC, El-Sherif N: Differential effects of functional autonomic blockage on the variables of sinus nodal automaticity in sick sinus syndrome. Am J Cardiol 49:273, 1982.
112. Marcus B, Gillette PC, Smith RT, et al: Electrophysiologic assessment of sinus node dysfunction in postop pediatric patients utilizing combined autonomic blockade. J Am Coll Cardiol 7:50A, 1986. Abstract.
113. Ross BA, Gillette PC, Zinner A, et al: Prospective evaluation of postoperative sinus node function with and without autonomic blockage. PACE 9:289, 1986. Abstract.
114. Jose AD: Effect of combined sympathetic and parasympathetic blockade on heart rate and cardiac function in man. Am J Cardiol 18:476, 1966.
115. Cumming GR, Mir GH: Heart rate and haemodynamics after autonomic blockade in infants and children. Br Heart J 32:766, 1970.
116. Jose AD, Collison D: The normal range and determinants of the intrinsic heart rate in man. Cardiovasc Res 4:160, 1970.
117. Benson DW Jr, Dunnigan A, Benditt DG: Intrinsic heart rate following autonomic blockade in infants and children. Circulation 70(II):321, 1984.
118. Probst P, Muhlberger V, Lederbauer M, et al: Electrophysiologic findings in carotid sinus massage. PACE 6:689, 1983.
119. Gang ES, Oseran DS, Mandel WJ, et al: Sinus node electrogram in patients with the hypersensitive carotid sinus syndrome. J Am Coll Cardiol 5:1484, 1985.
120. Sugrue DD, Gersh BJ, Holmes DR Jr, et al: Symptomatic "isolated" carotid sinus hypersensitivity: Natural history and results of treatment with anticholinergic drugs or pacemaker. J Am Coll Cardiol 7:158, 1986.
121. Stryjer D, Friedensohn A, Schlesinger Z: Ventricular pacing as the preferable mode for long-term pacing in patients with carotid sinus syncope of the cardioinhibitory type. PACE 9:705, 1986.
122. Marneffe MD, Jacobs P, Englert M: Reproducibility of electrophysiologic parameters of extrinsic sinus node function in patients with and without sick sinus syndrome. PACE 9:482, 1986.
123. Kugler JD, Bansal AM, Cheatham JP, et al: Drug-electrophysiology studies in infants, children, and adolescents. Am Heart J 110:144, 1985.
124. Hesslein PS, Williams WG, Rowe RD: Hemodynamic utility of "physiologic" pacing in children. Circulation 66(II):II–170, 1982. Abstract.
125. Radford DJ, Izukawa T: Sick sinus syndrome. Arch Dis Child 50:879, 1975.
126. Ector H, Van der Hauwaert LG: Sick sinus syndrome in childhood. Br Heart J 44:684, 1980.
127. Yabek SM, Dillon T, Berman W Jr, et al: Symptomatic sinus node dysfunction in children without structural heart disease. Pediatrics 69:590, 1982.
128. Rein AJJT, Simcha A, Ludomirsky A, et al: Symptomatic sinus bradycardia in infants with structurally normal heart. J Pediatr 107:724, 1985.
129. Beder SD, Cohen MH, Riemenschneider TA: Occult arrhythmias as the etiology of unexplained syncope in children with structurally normal hearts. Am Heart J 109:309, 1985.
130. Beder SD, Gillette PC, Garson A Jr, et al: Symptomatic sick sinus syndrome in children and adolescents as the only manifestation of cardiac abnormality or associated with unoperated congenital heart disease. Am J Cardiol 51:1133, 1983.
131. Beerman LB, Neches WH, Fricker FJ, et al: Arrhythmias in transposition of the great arteries after the Mustard operation. Am J Cardiol 51:1530, 1983.
132. Bolens M, Friedli B: Sinus node function and conduction system before and after surgery for secundum atrial septal defect: An electrophysiologic study. Am J Cardiol 53:1415, 1984.
133. Yabek SM, Swensson RE, Jarmakani JM: Electrocardiographic recognition of sinus node dysfunction in children and young adults. Circulation 56:235, 1977.
134. Yabke SM, Jarmakani JM: Sinus node dysfunction in children, adolescents, and young adults. Pediatrics 61:593, 1978.
135. Roifman C, Dembo L, Grenadier E, et al: Sinus node dysfunction in a healthy pediatric population. Isr J Med Sci 20:497, 1984.
136. Bricker JT, Garson A Jr, Gillette PC: A family history of seizures associated with sudden cardiac deaths. Am J Dis Child 138:866, 1984.
137. Scagliotti D, Strasberg B, Duffy CE, et al: Inducible polymorphous ventricular tachycardia following Mustard operation for transposition of the great arteries. Pediatr Cardiol 5:39, 1984.
138. Kugler JD: Sinus node dysfunction in young patients with congenital long QT syndrome. Am Heart J 112:650, 1986. Abstract.
139. Beder SD, Gillette PC: Non-surgical etiologies of sick sinus syndrome. In Yabek SM, Gillette PC, Kugler JK (eds): The Sinus Node in Pediatrics. London, Churchill Livingstone, 1984, p 121.
140. Bashour TT: Classification of sinus node dysfunction. Am Heart J 110:1251, 1985.
141. Onat A, Domanic N, Onat T: Sick sinus syndrome in an infant: Severe disturbance of impulse formation and conduction involving the S-A node and the A-V junctional tissue. Eur J Cardiol 2:79, 1974.
142. Trethewie ER: Congenital nodal rhythm. (Letter) Med J Aust 1:281, 1979.
143. Rein AJJT, Ludomirsky A, Sznajderman S, et al:

Suspected sick sinus syndrome in an infant treated by pacemaker implantation. (Letter) Pediatr Cardiol 5:155, 1984.
144. Ho SY, Mortimer G, Anderson RH, et al: Conduction system defects in three perinatal patients with arrhythmia. Br Heart J 53:158, 1985.
145. Bharati S, Nordenberg A, Bauernfiend R, et al: The anatomic substrate for the sick sinus syndrome in adolescence. Am J Cardiol 46:163, 1980.
146. James TN, Froggatt P, Marshall TK: Sudden death in young athletes. Ann Intern Med 67:1013, 1967.
147. Spellberg RD: Familial sinus node disease. Chest 60:246, 1971.
148. Nordenberg A, Varghese PJ, Nugent EW: Spectrum of sinus node dysfunction in two siblings. Am Heart J 91:507, 1976.
149. Dianzumba SB, Singer DH, Meyers S, et al: Lenegre's disease in youth. Am Heart J 94:479, 1977.
150. Lehmann H, Klein UE: Familial sinus node dysfunction with autosomal dominant inheritance. Br Heart J 40:1314, 1978.
151. Schneider MD, Roller DH, Morganroth J, et al: The syndromes of familial atrioventricular block with sinus bradycardia: Prognostic indices, electrophysiologic and histopathologic correlates. Eur J Cardiol 7:337, 1978.
152. Tan ATH, Ee BKH, Mah PK, et al: Diffuse conduction abnormalities in an adolescent with familial sinus node disease. PACE 4:645, 1981.
153. Ward DE, Ho SY, Shinebourne EA: Familial atrial standstill and inexcitability in childhood. Am J Cardiol 53:965, 1984.
154. Clark EB, Kugler JD: Preoperative secundum atrial septal defect with coexisting sinus node and atrioventricular node dysfunction. Circulation 65:976, 1982.
155. Ruschhaupt DG, Khoury L, Thilenius OG, et al: Electrophysiologic abnormalities of children with ostium secundum atrial septal defect. Am J Cardiol 53:1643, 1984.
156. Bagger JP, Thomsen PEB, Bjerregaard P, et al: Intracardiac electrography in patients before and after surgical repair of secundum atrial septal defect. J Electrocardiol 17:347, 1984.
157. Karpawich PP, Antillon JR, Cappola PR, et al: Pre- and postoperative electrophysiologic assessment of children with secundum atrial septal defect. Am J Cardiol 55:519, 1985.
158. Clark EB, Roland JA, Varghese PJ, et al: Should the sinus venosus type ASD be closed? A review of the atrial conduction defects and surgical results in twenty-eight children. Am J Cardiol 35:127, 1975. Abstract.
159. Arensman FW, Boineau JP, Balfour IC, et al: Sinus venosus atrial septal defect and pacemaker requirement in a family. Am J Cardiol 57:368, 1986.
160. Fournier A, Young M-L, Garcia OL, et al: Electrophysiologic cardiac function before and after surgery in children with atrioventricular canal. Am J Cardiol 57:1137, 1986.
161. Radford DJ, Izukawa T: Sick sinus syndrome: Symptomatic cases in children. Arch Dis Child 50:879, 1975.
162. James TN, Jackson DA: De subitaneis morbitus. XXVII. Histological abnormalities in the sinus node, atrioventricular node and His bundle associated with coarctation of the aorta. Circulation 56:1094, 1977.
163. Harper R, Peter T, Vohra J, et al: Sinus node dysfunction and carotid sinus syncope associated with a Wolff-Parkinson-White syndrome. Eur J Cardiol 2:207, 1974.
164. Rakovec P, Rode P, Jakopin J, et al: Latent sinoatrial conduction disturbances in symptomatic patients with Wolff-Parkinson-White syndrome. PACE 6:2, 1983.
165. James TN: The sinus node. Am J Cardiol 40:965, 1977.
166. Keith JD: Overstimulation of the vagus nerve in rheumatic fever. J Med 7:29, 1938.
167. Lenox CC, Zuberbuhler JR, Park SC, et al: Arrhythmias and Stokes-Adams attacks in acute rheumatic fever. Pediatrics 61:599, 1978.
168. Singh S, Shrivastava S: Sinus node suppression in acute rheumatic carditis: A case report. Ind Heart J 31:305, 1979.
169. Swiryn S, McKonough T, Hueter DC: Sinus node function and dysfunction. Med Clin North Am 68:935, 1984.
170. James TN, Reynolds EW Jr: Pathology of the cardiac conduction system in a case of diphtheria associated with atrial arrhythmias and heart block. Circulation 28:262, 1963.
171. Nopre F, Vichi FL, Nogueira JL, et al: The heart rate in chronic Chagas' heart disease. 2. The sinus node rate in Chagas patients with heart failure. Arq Bras Cardiol 31:181, 1978.
172. James TN: Pericarditis and the sinus node. Arch Int Med 110:301, 1962.
173. Fujiwara H, Kawai C, Hamashima Y: Clinicopathologic study of the conduction systems in 10 patients with Kawasaki's disease (mucocutaneous lymph node syndrome). Am Heart J 96:744, 1978.
174. James TN: Thrombi in antrum atrii dextri of human heart as clinically important source for chronic microembolisation to lungs. Br Heart J 49:122, 1983.
175. Loeb JM, Euler DE, Randall WC, et al: Cardiac arrhythmias after chronic embolization of the sinus node artery: Alterations in parasympathetic pacemaker control. Circulation 61:192, 1980.
176. Boenolo DA, Rabow FI, Vijayanaear RR, et al: Traumatic sinus node dysfunction. Ann Emerg Med 11:319, 1982.
177. Parameswaran R, Ohe T, Goldberg H: Sinus node dysfunction in acute myocardial infarction. Br Heart J 38:93, 1976.
178. James TN, Marshall TK: De subitaneis mortibus. XVII. Multifocal stenosis due to fibromuscular dysplasia of the sinus node artery. Circulation 53:736, 1976.
179. Kugler JD: Effects of pharmacologic agents on sinus node function. In Yabek SM, Gillette PC, Kugler JD (eds): The Sinus Node in Pediatrics. London, Churchill Livingstone, 1984, p 84.
180. Kugler JD, Garson A Jr, Gillette PC: Electrophysiologic effect of digitalis on sinoatrial nodal function in children. Am J Cardiol 44:1344, 1979.
181. Strauss HC, Gilbert M, Svenson RH, et al: Electrophysiologic effects of propranolol on sinus node function in patients with sinus node dysfunction. Circulation 54:452, 1976.
182. Yabek SM, Berman W Jr, Dillon T: Electrophysiologic effects of propranolol on sinus node function in children. Am Heart J 104:612, 1982.
183. Williams DO, Tatelbaum R, Most AS: Effective treatment of supraventricular arrhythmias with acebutolol. Am J Cardiol 44:521, 1979.
184. Frishman WH: Atenolol and timolol, two new systemic β-adrenoceptor antagonists. N Engl J Med 306:1456, 1982.

185. Coumel P, Escoubet B, Attuel P: Beta-blocking therapy in atrial and ventricular tachyarrhythmias: Experience with nadolol. Am Heart J 108:1098, 1984.
186. Sung RJ, Tai DY, Svinarich JT: Beta-adrenoceptor blockade: Electrophysiology and antiarrhythmic mechanisms. Am Heart J 108:1115, 1984.
187. Carrasco HA, Fuenmayor PA, Barboza MJS, et al: Effect of verapamil on normal sinoatrial node function and on sick sinus syndrome. Am Heart J 96:760, 1978.
188. Kawai C, Konishi T, Matsuyama E, et al: Comparative effects of three calcium antagonists, diltiazem, verapamil and nifedipine, on the sinoatrial and atrioventricular nodes. Circulation 63:1035, 1981.
189. Valett H, Barnay C, Lopez M, et al: Effects of intravenous diltiazem on sinus node function and atrioventricular conduction in patients. J Cardiovasc Pharmacol 5:62, 1983.
190. Calon AH, Ticzon AR, Akhtar M, et al: Quinidine in sinus node dysfunction. Circulation 54(suppl II):II–231, 1976. Abstract.
191. Shih J-Y, Gillette PC, Kugler JD, et al: The electrophysiologic effects of procainamide in the immature heart. Pediatr Pharmacol 2:65, 1982.
192. Goldberg D, Reiffel JA, Davis JC, et al: Electrophysiologic effects of procainamide on sinus function in patients with and without sinus node disease. Am Heart J 103:75, 1982.
193. LaBarre AN, Strauss HC, Scheinman MM, et al: Electrophysiologic effects of disopyramide phosphate on sinus node function in patients with sinus node dysfunction. Circulation 59:226, 1979.
194. Lippestad CT, Forfang K: Production of sinus arrest by lignocaine. Br Med J 1:537, 1971.
195. Dhingra RC, Deedwania PC, Cummings JM, et al: Electrophysiologic effects of lidocaine on sinus node and atrium in patients with and without sinoatrial dysfunction. Circulation 57:448, 1978.
196. Keidar S, Grenadier E, Palant A: Sinoatrial arrest due to lidocaine injection in sick sinus syndrome during amiodarone administration. Am Heart J 104:1384, 1982.
197. Vik-Mo H, Ohm O-J, Lund-Johansen P: Electrophysiologic effects of flecainide acetate in patients with sinus nodal dysfunction. Am J Cardiol 50:1090, 1982.
198. Connolly SJ, Kates RE, Lebsack CS, et al: Clinical efficacy and electrophysiology of oral propafenone for ventricular tachycardia. Am J Cardiol 52:1208, 1983.
199. Hesslein PS: Amiodarone therapy in children: A cautionary comment. Pediatrics 72:817, 1983.
200. Garson A Jr, Gillette PC, McVey P, et al: Amiodarone treatment of critical arrhythmias in children and young adults. J Am Coll Cardiol 4:749, 1984.
201. Veltri EP, Reid PR: Sinus arrest with intravenous amiodarone. Am J Cardiol 58:1110, 1986.
202. Touboul P, Atallah G, Kirkorian G, et al: Clinical electrophysiology of intravenous sotalol, a beta-blocking drug with class III antiarrhythmic properties. Am Heart J 107:888, 1984.
203. Belhassen B, Pelleg A: Electrophysiologic effects of adenosine triphosphate and adenosine on the mammalian heart. Clinical and experimental aspects. J Am Coll Cardiol 8:1149, 1986.
204. Urthaler F, Rosenshtraukh LV, Hageman GR, et al: Differential modulation of autonomic activity by ethmozine and ethacizin (analog of ethmozine) on the canine sinus node and atrioventricular junction. J Am Coll Cardiol 8:86A, 1986.
205. Shugushev K Kh, Rosenshtraukh LV, Smetnev AS: Electrophysiologic effects of ethmozine on sinus node function in patients with and without sinus node dysfunction. Clin Cardiol 9:443, 1986.
206. Montalescot G, Levy Y, Farge D, et al: Lithium causing a serious sinus-node dysfunction at therapeutic doses. Clin Cardiol 7:617, 1984.
207. Wellens H, Cats VM, Duren D: Symptomatic sinus node abnormalities following lithium carbonate therapy. Am J Med 59:285, 1975.
208. Thormann J, Neuss M, Schlepper M, et al: Effects of clonidine on sinus node function in man. Chest 80:201, 1981.
209. Davis J, Reiffel J, Bigger JT: Sinus node dysfunction caused by methyldopa and digoxin. JAMA 245:1241, 1981.
210. Breithardt G, Seipel L, Wiebringhaus E: Dual effect of verapamil on sinus node function in man. In Bonke FIM (ed): The Sinus Node. The Hague, Martinus Nijhoff, 1978, p 120.
211. Vera Z, Awan NA, Mason DT: Assessment of oral quinidine effects on sinus node function in sick sinus syndrome patients. Am Heart J 103:80, 1982.
212. Barton CW, Dick M, Rosenthal A: Quinidine syncope in children. J Am Coll Cardiol 5:429, 1985. Abstract.
213. Roden DM, Thompson KA, Hoffman BF, et al: Clinical features and basic mechanisms of quinidine-induced arrhythmias. J Am Coll Cardiol 8:73A, 1986.
214. Garson A Jr: Medicolegal problems in the management of cardiac arrhythmias in children. Pediatrics 79:84, 1987.
215. Jimenez O, Johnson CD: Sinus node and atrial dysfunction during hypercalcemia. Bol Assoc Med PR 75:21, 1983.
216. Garson A Jr: The normal electrocardiogram. In Garson A Jr (ed): The Electrocardiogram in Infants and Children: A Systematic Approach. Philadelphia, Lea & Febiger, 1983, p 72.
217. Siegel RJ, Capeen WR Jr, Roberts WC: Prolonged QT interval—ventricular tachycardia syndrome from massive rapid weight loss utilizing the liquid-protein-modified-fast diet: Sudden death with sinus node ganglionitis and neuritis. Am Heart J 102:121, 1981.
218. Wambach G, Schneider M, Saporowski F: Sinus-node syndrome and hyperthyroidism. Deutsch Med Wochenschr 103:1625, 1978.
219. Kramer MR, Shilo S, Hershko C: Atrioventricular and sinoatrial block in thyrotoxic crisis. Br Heart J 54:600, 1985.
220. Green M: Fainting. In Green M, Haggerty R (eds): Ambulatory Pediatrics III. Philadelphia, WB Saunders, 1984, p 154.
221. Sapire DW, Casta A: Vagotonia in infants, children, adolescents and young adults. Int J Cardiol 9:211, 1985.
222. Sapire DW, Casta A, Safley W, et al: Vasovagal syncope in children requiring pacemaker implantation. Am Heart J 106:1406, 1983.
223. Kenigsberg K, Griswold PG, Buckley BJ, et al: Cardiac effects of esophageal stimulation: Possible relationship between gastroesophageal reflux and sudden infant death syndrome. J Pediatr Surg 18:542, 1983.
224. Fontan JP, Heldt GP, Heyman MB, et al: Esophageal spasm associated with apnea and bradycardia in an infant. Pediatrics 73:52, 1984.

225. Guilleminault C, Coons S: Apnea and bradycardia during feeding in infants weighing >2000 gm. J Pediatr 104:932, 1984.
226. Rasmussen V, Haunso S, Skagen K: Cerebral attacks due to excessive vagal tone in heavily trained persons. Acta Med Scand 204:401, 1978.
227. Huston TP, Puffer JC, Rodney WM: The athletic heart syndrome. N Engl J Med 313:24, 1985.
228. Yerg JE II, Seals DR, Hagberg JM, et al: Syncope secondary to ventricular asystole in an endurance athlete. Clin Cardiol 9:220, 1986.
229. Weiss S, Baker JR: The carotid sinus reflex in health and disease: Its role in the causation of fainting and convulsions. Medicine 12:297, 1933.
230. Walter PF, Crawley SI, Dorney ER: Carotid sinus hypersensitivity and syncope. Am J Cardiol 42:396, 1978.
231. Wenger TL, Dohrmann ML, Strauss HC, et al: Hypersensitive carotid sinus syndrome manifested as cough syncope. PACE 3:332, 1980.
232. Woody RC, Kiel EA: Swallowing syncope in a child. Pediatrics 78:507, 1986.
233. Kunis RL, Garfein OB, Pepe AJ, et al: Deglutition syncope and atrioventricular block selectively induced by hot food and liquid. Am J Cardiol 55:613, 1985.
234. Engelhardt W, Kotlarek F, von Bernuth G: Deglutition syncope in childhood with complete atrioventricular block. Am J Cardiol 58:1113, 1986.
235. Khero BA, Milins CB: Cardiac syncope due to glossopharyngeal neuralgia. Arch Intern Med 128:806, 1971.
236. Lombroso CT, Lerman P: Breathholding spells (cyanotic and pallid infantile syncope). Pediatrics 39:563, 1967.
237. Stephenson JBP: Reflex anoxic seizures ("white breathholding"): Nonepileptic vagal attacks. Arch Dis Child 53:193, 1978.
238. Guilleminault C, Pool P, Motta J, et al: Sinus arrest during REM sleep in young adults. N Engl J Med 311:1006, 1984.
239. Thorpy MJ, Spielman AJ, Abbott ML: Sleep apnea and sinus node dysfunction. JAMA 251:2514, 1984.
240. Taylor P: Cholinergic agonists and anticholinesterase agents. In Gilman AG, Goodman LS (eds): The Pharmacological Basis of Therapeutics. New York, Macmillan, 1985, pp 100, 110.
241. Hariman RJ, Hoffman BF: Ouabain effects on sinus node function in conscious dogs. Circulation 58(suppl II):II–106, 1978. Abstract.
242. Sapire DW, Shah JJ, Black IFS: Prolonged atrioventricular conduction in young children and adolescents: The role of increased vagal tone. S Afr Med J 55:669, 1979.
243. Almquist A, Gornick C, Benson W Jr, et al: Carotid sinus hypersensitivity: Evaluation of the vasodepressor component. Circulation 71:927, 1985.
244. Schwartz PJ: Idiopathic long QT syndrome: Progress and questions. Am Heart J 109:399, 1985.
245. Vincent GM: The heart rate of Romano-Ward syndrome. Am Heart J 112:61, 1986.
246. Vincent GM, Skach L: The exercise heart rate of long QT syndrome subjects is lower than normals. Circulation 74(suppl II):II–31, 1986. Abstract.
247. Cole S, Lindenberg LB, Galioto FM Jr, et al: Ultrastructural abnormalities of the carotid body in sudden infant death syndrome. Pediatrics 63:13, 1979.
248. Anderson KR, Hill RW: Occlusive lesions of cardiac conduction tissue arteries in sudden infant death syndrome. Pediatrics 69:50, 1982.
249. Kozakewich HPW, McManus B, Vawter GF: The sinus node in sudden infant death syndrome. Circulation 65:1242, 1982.
250. Colan SD, Liberthson RR, Cahen L, et al: Incidence and significance of primary abnormalities of cardiac rhythm in infants at high risk for sudden infant death syndrome. Pediatr Cardiol 5:267, 1984.
251. Bini RM, Westaby S, Bargeron LM Jr, et al: Investigation and management of primary cardiac tumors in infants and children. J Am Coll Cardiol 2:351, 1983.
252. Higgins CG: Effects of contrast media on the conducting system of the heart. Radiology 124:599, 1977.
253. Bashour TT, Antonini C Sr, Fisher J: Severe sinus node dysfunction in obstructive jaundice. Ann Intern Med 103:384, 1985.
254. Narayan D, Huang MTC, Mathew PK: Bradycardia and asystole requiring permanent pacemaker in Guillain-Barre syndrome. Am Heart J 108:426, 1984.
255. Aberdeen E, Waterston DJ, Carr I, et al: Successful "correction" of transposed great arteries by Mustard's operation. Lancet 1:1233, 1965.
256. Khoury GH, Shaher RM, Fowler RS, et al: Preoperative and postoperative electrocardiogram in complete transposition of the great vessels. Am Heart J 72:199, 1966.
257. Zuberbuhler JR, Bauersfeld SR: Unusual arrhythmias after corrective surgery for transposition of the great vessels. Am Heart J 73:752, 1967.
258. Waldhausen JA, Pierce WS, Rashkind WJ, et al: Total correction of transposition of the great arteries following balloon atrial septostomy. Circulation 41:123, 1970.
259. El-Said G, Rosenberg HS, Mullins CE, et al: Dysrhythmias after Mustard's operation for transposition of the great arteries. Am J Cardiol 30:526, 1972.
260. Gillette PC, El-Said GM, Sivarajan N, et al: Electrophysiological abnormalities after Mustard's operation for transposition of the great arteries. Br Heart J 36:186, 1974.
261. Clarkson PM, Barratt-Boyes BG, Neutze JM: Late dysrhythmias and disturbances of conduction following Mustard operation for complete transposition of the great arteries. Circulation 53:519, 1976.
262. El-Said GM, Gillette PC, Cooley DA, et al: Protection of the sinus node in Mustard's operation. Circulation 53:788, 1976.
263. Lewis AB, Lindesmith GG, Takahashi M, et al: Cardiac rhythm following the Mustard procedure for transposition of the great vessels. J Thorac Cardiovasc Surg 73:919, 1977.
264. Saalouke MG, Rios J, Perry LW, et al: Electrophysiologic studies after Mustard's operation for d-transposition of the great vessels. Am J Cardiol 41:1104, 1978.
265. Ullal RR, Anderson RH, Lincoln C: Mustard's operation modified to avoid dysrhythmias and pulmonary and systemic venous obstruction. J Thorac Cardiovasc Surg 78:431, 1979.
266. Southall DP, Keeton BR, Leanage R, et al: Cardiac rhythm and conduction before and after Mustard's operation for complete transposition of the great arteries. Br Heart J 43:21, 1980.
267. Hayes CJ, Boxer RA, Krongrad E, et al: Cardiac

rhythm after the Mustard operation for transposition of the great arteries. Am J Cardiol 45:430, 1980. Abstract.
268. Vetter VL, Horowitz LN: Electrophysiologic consequences of Mustard repair of transposition of the great arteries. Am J Cardiol 45:430, 1980. Abstract.
269. Martin TC, Smith L, Hernandez A, et al: Dysrhythmias following the Senning operation for dextrotransposition of the great arteries. J Thorac Cardiovasc Surg 85:928, 1983.
270. Duster MC, Bink-Boelkens MThE, Wampler D, et al: Long-term follow-up of dysrhythmias following the Mustard procedure. Am Heart J 109:1323, 1985.
271. Byrum CJ, Bove EL, Sondheimer HM, et al: Hemodynamic and electrophysiologic results of the Senning procedure for transposition of the great arteries. Am J Cardiol 58:138, 1986.
272. Stark SI, Rosenfeld LE, Kleinman CS, et al: Atrial dissociation: An electrophysiologic finding in a patient with transposition of the great arteries. J Am Coll Cardiol 8:236, 1986.
273. Deanfield JE, Macartney FJ, Bull C, et al: Arrhythmia and late mortality after Mustard and Senning operations for transposition: A 7-year prospective study. Circulation 74(suppl II):II–50, 1986. Abstract.
274. Portman MA, Beder SD, Ankeney JL, et al: A 20-year review of ostium primum defect repair in children. Am Heart J 110:1054, 1985.
275. Bricker JT, Gillette PC, Cooley DA, et al: Dysrhythmias after repair of atrial septal defect. Texas Heart Inst J 13:203, 1986.
276. Byrum CJ, Dick M, Behrendt DM, et al: Repair of total anomalous pulmonary venous connection in patients younger than 6 months old. Circulation 66(suppl I):I–208, 1982. Abstract.
277. Hamilton SD, Bartley TD, Miller RH, et al: Disturbances in atrial rhythm and conduction following the surgical creation of an atrial septal defect by the Blalock-Hanlon technique. Circulation 38:73, 1968.
278. Smith PK, Buhrman WC, Levett JM, et al: Supraventricular conduction abnormalities following cardiac operations. J Thorac Cardiovasc Surg 85:105, 1983.
279. Marin-Neto JA, Carneiro JJ, Maciel BC, et al: Impairment of baroreflex control of the sinoatrial node after cardiac operations with extracorporeal circulation in man. J Thorac Cardiovasc Surg 86:718, 1983.
280. Kugler JD: Effect of cardiac surgery for congenital heart disease on sinus node function. In Yabek SM, Gillette PC, Kugler JD (eds): The Sinus Node in Pediatrics. London, Churchill Livingstone, 1984, p 104.
281. Edwards WD, Edwards JE: Pathology of the sinus node in d-transposition following the Mustard operation. J Thorac Cardiovasc Surg 75:213, 1978.
282. Anderson KR, Ho SY, Anderson RH: Location and vascular supply of sinus node in human heart. Br Heart J 41:28, 1979.
283. Arensman FW, Bostock J, Radley-Smith R, et al: Cardiac rhythm and conduction before and aftter anatomic correction of transposition of the great arteries. Am J Cardiol 52:836, 1983.
284. Scott WA, Dick M, Bove EL: Decreased incidence of early sinus node dysfunction following the arterial switch procedure. Circulation 74(suppl II):II–178, 1986. Abstract.
285. Gillette PC: Treatment of sinus node dysfunction. In Yabek SM, Gillette PC, Kugler JD (eds): The Sinus Node in Pediatrics. London, Churchill Livingstone, 1984, p 135.
286. Kugler JD: Sinoatrial node dysfunction. In Gillette PC, Garson A Jr (eds): Pediatric Cardiac Dysrhythmias. New York, Grune & Stratton, 1981, p 265.
287. Hoffman BF, Rosen MR, Wit AL: Electrophysiology and pharmacology of cardiac arrhythmias. VII. Cardiac effects of quinidine and procainamide, part B. Am Heart J 90:117, 1975.
288. Frye RL, Collins JJ, DeSanctis RW: Guidelines for permanent cardiac pacemaker implantation. Circulation 70:331A, 1984.
289. Hilgard J, Ezri MD, Denes P: Significance of ventricular pauses of three seconds or more detected on twenty-four-hour Holter recordings. Am J Cardiol 55:1005, 1985.
290. Dreifus LS, Michelson EL, Kaplinsky E: Bradyarrhythmias: Clinical significance and management. J Am Coll Cardiol 1:327, 1983.
291. Molthan ME, Miller RA, Hastreiter AR, et al: Congenital heart block with fatal Adams-Stokes attacks in childhood. Pediatrics 30:32, 1962.
292. Winkler RB, Freed MD, Nadas AS: Exercise-induced ventricular ectopy in children and young adults with complete heart block. Am Heart J 99:87, 1980.
293. Feleke E, Ryden L, Smedgard P, et al: Prenalterol in symptomatic sinus node dysfunction. Am Heart J 109:185, 1985.
294. Tseu FL, Morley CA, Mackintosh AF: Oral xamoterol in patients with sinoatrial disease. Br Heart J 56:469, 1986.
295. Engel TR, Leddy C, Gonzalez AD, et al: Electrophysiologic effects of hydralazine on sinoatrial function in patients with sick sinus node syndrome. Am J Cardiol 41:763, 1978.
296. Weiss AT, Rod JL, Gotsman MS, et al: Hydralazine in the management of symptomatic sinus bradycardia. Eur J Cardiol 12:261, 1981.
297. Lewis BS, Rozenman Y, Merdler A, et al: Chronotropic effect of hydralazine and its mechanism in symptomatic sinus bradycardia. Am J Cardiol 59:93, 1987.
298. Benditt DG, Benson W Jr, Kreitt J, et al: Electrophysiologic effects of theophylline in young patients with recurrent symptomatic bradyarrhythmias. Am J Cardiol 52:1223, 1983.
299. Watt AA: Sick sinus syndrome: An adenosine-mediated disease. Lancet 1(8432):786, 1985.
300. Fleming WH, Sarafian LB, Kugler JD, et al: Changing indications for pacemakers in children. Ann Thorac Surg 31:329, 1981.
301. Gillette PC: Recent advances in mechanisms, evaluation, and pacemaker treatment of chronic bradydysrhythmias in children. Am Heart J 102:920, 1981.
302. Gillette PC, Shannon C, Garson A Jr, et al: Pacemaker treatment of sick sinus syndrome in children. J Am Coll Cardiol 1:1325, 1983.
303. Albin G, Hayes DL, Holmes DR Jr: Sinus node dysfunction in pediatric and young adult patients: Treatment by implantation of a permanent pacemaker in 39 cases. Mayo Clin Proc 60:667, 1985.
304. Gillette PC, Wampler DG, Shannon C, et al: Use of cardiac pacing after the Mustard operation for transposition of the great arteries. J Am Coll Cardiol 7:138, 1986.
305. Stone JM, Bhakta RD, Lutgen J: Dual chamber

sequential pacing management of sinus node dysfunction: Advantages over single-chamber pacing. Am Heart J 104:1319, 1982.
306. Van Mechelen R, Hagemeijer F, de Boer H, et al: Atrioventricular and ventriculo-atrial conduction in patients with symptomatic sinus node dysfunction. PACE 6:13, 1983.
307. Rosenqvist M, Brandt J, Schuller H: Atrial versus ventricular pacing in sinus node disease: A treatment comparison study. Am Heart J 111:292, 1986.
308. Benditt DG, Mianulli M, Fetter J, et al: Normalization of exercise heart rate responses in sinoatrial node dysfunction by an activity-detecting rate-variable pacing system. Circulation 74(suppl II):II–387, 1986. Abstract.
309. Bren GB, Wasserman AG, El-Bayoumi J, et al: Comparison of DDD and rate responsive VVI pacing during exercise. Circulation 74(suppl II):II–388, 1986. Abstract.
310. Benditt DG, Mianulli M, Fetter J, et al: Single-chamber cardiac pacing with activity-initiated chronotropic response: Evaluation by cardiopulmonary exercise testing. Circulation 75:184, 1987.
311. Ott DA, Gillette PC, Cooley DA: Atrial pacing via the subxiphoid approach. Texas Heart Inst J 9:149, 1982.
312. Hanglein D, Gillette PC, Shannon C, et al: Long-term follow-up of pulse width threshold of transvenous and myo-epicardial leads. PACE 7:203, 1984.
313. Stone JM, Bhakta RD, Lutgen J: Dual chamber sequential pacing management of sinus node dysfunction. Advantages over single chamber pacing. Am Heart J 104:1319, 1982.
314. den Dulk K, Kersschot IE, Brugada P, et al: Is there a universal antitachycardia pacing mode? Am J Cardiol 57:950, 1986.
315. Saksena S, Pantopoulos D, Parsonnet V, et al: Usefulness of an implantable antitachycardia pacemaker system for supraventricular or ventricular tachycardia. Am J Cardiol 58:70, 1986.
316. Luceri RM, Castellano A, Thurer RJ, et al: Non-invasive conversion of atrial flutter using a multi-programmable DDD pulse generator. PACE 9(1):137, 1986.
317. Campbell RM, Dick M II, Jenkins JM, et al: Atrial overdrive pacing for conversion of atrial flutter in children. Pediatrics 75:730, 1985.
318. Hellestrand KJ, Burnett PJ, Milne JR, et al: Effect of the antiarrhythmic agent flecainide acetate on acute and chronic pacing thresholds. PACE 6:892, 1983.
319. McGoon MD, Maloney JD, McGoon DC, et al: Long-term endocardial atrial pacing in children with postoperative bradycardia-tachycardia syndrome and limited ventricular access. Am J Cardiol 49:1750, 1982.
320. Westerman GR, Dungan WT, van Devanter SH: Permanent pacing in children: Should the persistent left superior vena cava be used for permanent pacing? Clin Prog Electrophysiol Pacing 4:100, 1986.
321. Holmes DR Jr, Maloney JD, Feldt RH: The use of the percutaneous subclavian technique for permanent cardiac pacing in childhood. Mayo Clin Proc 55:579, 1980.
322. Gillette PC, Shannon C, Blair H, et al: Transvenous pacing in pediatric patients. Am Heart J 105:843, 1983.
323. Ward DE, Jones S, Shinebourne EA: Long-term transvenous pacing in children weighing less than 10 kg. Circulation 72(suppl III):III–340, 1985. Abstract.
324. Epstein ML, Knauf DG, Alexander JA: Long-term follow-up of transvenous cardiac pacing in children. Am J Cardiol 57:889, 1986.
325. Vince DJ, Tyers GFO, Kerr CR: Transvenous atrial pacing in the management of sick sinus syndrome following surgical treatment of the univentricular heart: Case Report and Review. PACE 9:441, 1986.
326. Kay R, Estioko M, Wienier I: Primary sick sinus syndrome as an indication for chronic pacemaker therapy in young adults: Incidence, clinical features, and long-term evaluation. Am Heart J 103:338, 1982.
327. Bricker JT, Garson A Jr, Traweek MS, et al: The use of exercise testing in children to evaluate abnormalities of pacemaker function not apparent at rest. PACE 8:656, 1985.
328. Hayes DL, Furman S: Stability of AV conduction in sick sinus node syndrome patients with implanted atrial pacemakers. Am Heart J 107:644, 1984.
329. Rosenqvist M, Vallin H, Edhag O: Clinical and electrophysiologic course of sinus node disease: Five-year follow-up study. Am Heart J 109:513, 1985.

CHAPTER 8

FIRST AND SECOND DEGREE ATRIOVENTRICULAR BLOCK

Bertrand A. Ross

This chapter will deal with the definition and features, both clinical and experimental, of first degree atrioventricular (AV) block and second degree AV block (Mobitz type I and II), which, although they share a common feature (conduction changes from sinus node activation to ventricular activation), may be much different in cause and clinical significance.

FIRST DEGREE AV BLOCK

First degree AV block is defined as a PR interval greater than established norms. This interval is more age dependent than rate dependent, so normal intervals have been determined based on the age of the patient. A number of causes or associations between first degree AV block and disease states have been reported (Table 8–1). It has generally been proposed that those structural heart lesions that produce first degree AV block do so by stretching the atria in the area of the AV node. It has also been reported to occur in up to 6% of neonates.[1] Narula et al found that the delay occurs at more than one site in adults, but the AV node was the dominant site, occurring in 83% of patients.[2] There is no clinical significance of first degree AV block when it is found.

TABLE 8–1
DISEASE STATES ASSOCIATED WITH FIRST DEGREE AV BLOCK

Rheumatic fever
Diphtheria
Trichinosis
Chagas' disease
Rubella
Mumps
Hypothermia
Increased parasympathetic tone
Electrolyte abnormalities: hypo/hyperkalemia, hypo/hypercalcemia, hypoglycemia, hypomagnesemia
Congenital heart disease: PDA, ASD (primum and secundum), Ebstein's anomaly, TAPVC
Duchenne muscular dystrophy
Myotonic dystrophy

SECOND DEGREE AV BLOCK

Second degree AV block was described by Wenckebach first in 1899 and again in 1906 when he timed jugular venous pulsations and associated atrial beats with blocked ventricular beats.[3, 4] Hay also reported the same findings in 1906.[5] Wenckebach described one type of periodicity in which the AC interval gradually prolonged, with the eventual dropping out of the C wave (thought to be a result of impaired atrioventricular conduction) and a second type consisting of dropped beats not associated with AC lengthening, but instead resulting from decreased ventricular excitability. After the introduction of electrocardiography, Mobitz described these two types of conduction abnormalities as type I (progressive prolongation of the PR interval until a dropped ventricular beat occurs) and type II (a constant PR interval with dropped ventricular beats).[6] By 1927, Wenckebach and Winterburg were suggesting that there were frequent variations from the typical periodicity.[7] Mobitz then called attention to the association of Adams-Stokes disease with Type II block.[8]

Mobitz Type I (Wenckebach) Block

Wenckebach described type I block as (1) progressive PR lengthening, (2) the greatest increase in the PR occurring between the first and second conducted beats, (3) progressive shortening of the RR intervals, and (4) a pause equal to less than twice the preceding PP interval (Fig. 8–1).[7] The incidence of type I second degree AV block appears to be low for both adults and children, although there is much more information available about adults. However, the incidence rate is affected by how the data were obtained (by Holter monitoring or electrocardiogram) and by whether the myocardium is normal or damaged. Johnson, Averill, and Lamb reported electrocardiogram findings of 67,375 healthy soldiers and found only one case of Wenckebach periodicity.[9] Brodsky et al reported Holter results in 50 healthy medical students and found a 6% incidence of Wenckebach periodicity during sleep.[10] The greatest incidence of Wenckebach periodicity occurs after an inferior myocardial infarction, but is transient (lasting 3 to 5 days), and generally requires no treatment. Experimental studies for the most part have localized the point of block to the AV node itself. In children, Wenckebach block periodicity is found during sleep or in situations that produce relative parasympathetic dominance, such as increased intracranial pressure.

The periodicity that meets the four criteria originally described by Wenckebach has been labeled *typical Wenckebach.* However, there are numerous cases of *atypical Wenckebach* in which one or more of these criteria are not met, but the general pattern of a lengthening PR interval followed by a nonconducted P wave occurs.[11–16] Denes et al determined the frequency of typical and atypical Wenckebach (both spontaneous and pacing-induced) in a group of adults. In naturally occurring Wenckebach, 86% was atypical and 14% typical.[17] In addition, the incidence of atypical Wenckebach was 100% when the Wenckebach ratio increased to greater than 4:3. (The

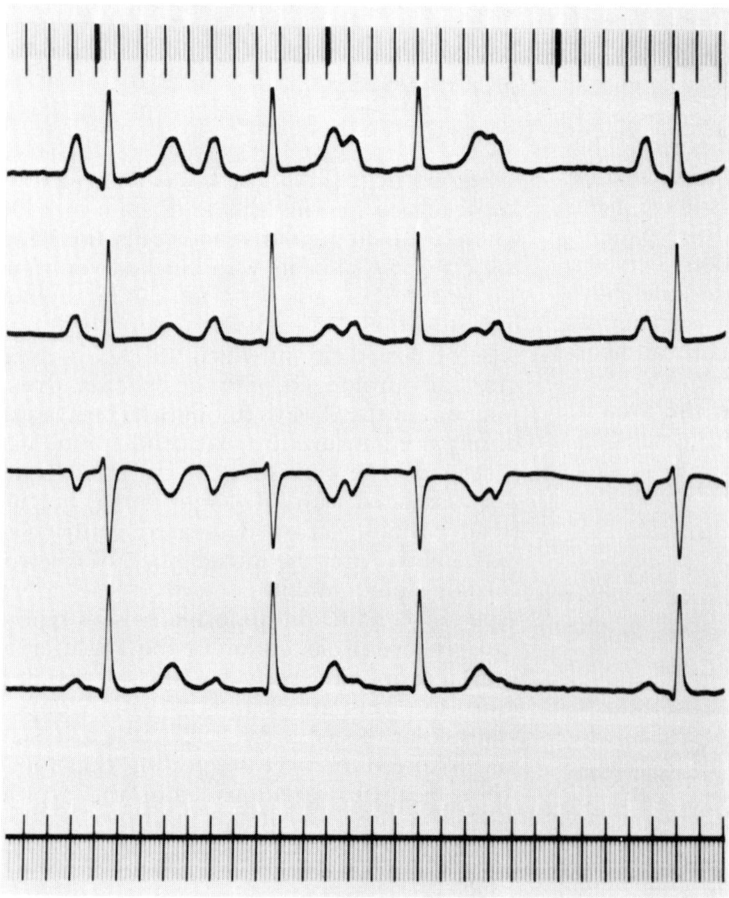

FIGURE 8–1
This ECG shows 4:3 Wenckebach periodicity. Note that there is a gradual increase in the PR interval leading to the eventual dropped beat. Leads I, AVF, V_1, and V_6 are shown from top to bottom, respectively.

TABLE 8–2
TYPES OF ATYPICAL WENCKEBACH

1. Last increment increased from the previous increment.
2. Last increment was the largest increment.
3. PR interval repeated at least once during the period.
4. PR interval decreasing at least once during the cycle.
5. Incremental increase in the PR interval not the greatest between the first and second conducted P waves.

4:3 ratio was the most common ratio spontaneously.) It should be noted that the spontaneous Wenckebach periods were secondary to myocardial infarction or digitalis excess. However, even in those patients who had Wenckebach block periods produced by atrial pacing during routine EPS testing, the atypical type was more common (66% vs 34%). Once again, the atypical form was more common with the higher ratios. Five types of atypical Wenckebach have been described and are listed in Table 8–2. Kinoshita and Konishi in the early 1980s showed other variants as well.[18] Wenckebach periodicity has been reported to occur at an increased rate in highly trained athletes, and in this group the atypical form also appears to predominate.[18, 19] El-Sheriff et al described a type of atypical Wenckebach that appeared to mimic Mobitz type II block.[20] However, this has less relevance in pediatric patients as this entity was associated with an acute inferior myocardial infarction.

The exact pathophysiologic mechanism of type I second degree AV block is unknown, but there are numerous theories (Table 8–3). All of the presented theories are affected by hemodynamics and variation in autonomic nervous system tone as well as by the very complex anatomic and electrophysiologic characteristics of the AV node. Clearly the association of Wenckebach periodicity with individuals with a predominance of vagal tone implicates the autonomic nervous system at least at some point in the production of Wenckebach periodicity. However, the exact interaction between autonomic tone and cellular mechanisms is unknown and may not be the same for all Wenckebach periodicity.

TABLE 8–3
THEORIES OF WENCKEBACH

Increased vagal tone (absolute or relative)
Increase in conduction time
Longitudinal dissociation
Concealed dissociation
Concealed reentry
Fatigue
Accumulation of extracellular potassium ions
Encroachment of succeeding impulses
Electrotonus

Mobitz Type II AV Block

Second degree Mobitz type II AV block is defined as the intermittent loss of atrioventricular conduction without a preceding lengthening of the PR interval. In addition, the first PR interval after the dropped beat should be no shorter than the PR interval of the last conducted P wave. It has been stated that a shortening of greater than twenty ms in the first PR interval after the dropped beat is more likely to be indicative of Wenckebach block.[21] However, as Zipes points out, this approach may be too simplistic.[22]

The inability of alternating atrial impulses to conduct to the ventricles is termed *2:1 AV block*. This can be caused by block either in the AV node or the proximal His-Purkinje system. However, 2:1 block cannot be classified as type I or type II, because the surface electrocardiogram cannot determine whether there is any degree of PR lengthening before the dropped beat. Therefore, a variation must be found in the conduction pattern from 2:1 to be certain of the true nature of the block. Type II AV block is uncommon and, if present, usually implies an abnormal conduction system. In children it may be found in normally structured hearts or in patients with a damaged conduction system from surgery for structural congenital heart disease. In both cases there is usually progression to complete heart block. In adults it most commonly occurs after an anterior myocardial infarction. The concern regarding type II AV block is its association with Adams-Stokes attacks and sudden death.[23–25]

Advanced Mobitz type II block is the loss of atrioventricular conduction for several consecutive P waves. When one atrial impulse is conducted to the ventricle, followed by two nonconducted impulses, it is termed 3:1 conduction; conduction of one out of four atrial impulses is 4:1 conduction. This type of block generally goes on to complete heart block.

CLINICAL SIGNIFICANCE

The concern regarding any type of heart block centers around the symptoms it produces and the likelihood of sudden death. Clearly, first degree AV block does not have any such concerns. Second degree AV block, however, is a classic example in which the clinical diagnosis of type I vs type II has significant repercussions regarding potential for serious problems and the need for treatment, potentially prophylactic in nature. Mobitz type II is associated with Adams-Stokes attacks, sudden death, and/or progression to complete heart block, whereas type I is for the most part an incidental finding of little long-term significance.

The clinical significance of type I or II block may also be dependent on whether it is associated with a wide QRS. Second degree AV block in the presence of intraventricular conduction delay is usually associated with Mobitz type II and may have a more ominous prognosis.[26] Therefore, differentiating type I from type II is clinically important, but the difficulty lies in the fact that the surface electrocardiogram is just an approximation of what occurs endocardially. Type I has for the most part been localized to the AV node, whereas type II occurs more distally in the His bundle. However, this point has been open to much debate.

The association of symptoms of syncope with type II AV block is primarily based on studies of adult patients following myocardial infarction. However, Kelly, Brodsky, and Krovetz documented two pediatric cases of Mobitz type II block that progressed to complete heart block.[27] One patient had undergone surgery to repair tetralogy of Fallot, while the other patient was without structural defect. Both patients also had associated right bundle-branch block. In these two patients, type II block preceded the development of complete heart block. One patient had symptoms while suffering from Mobitz II block, and one had no symptoms until the development of complete heart block. Because type II block is uncommon in children, its natural history is unclear; however, available information indicates that type II block produced by surgery or that develops as an idiopathic abnormality of the conduction system mirrors the experience in adults, progressing to high grade block and complete atrioventricular block.

TREATMENT

Treatment consists of an implantable pacemaker and is generally only necessary for those patients with type II AV block. However, the timing of the intervention depends on the clinical situation and must be individualized for each patient. We recommend treatment for the postoperative patient with type II block if it continues for more than 10 days, especially if the ventricular escape rate is low. The patient with type II block of only a few dropped beats should be watched closely, and should not need treatment if there appears to be evidence of an acceptable underlying junctional or ventricular escape rate. However, this type of patient is rare. In a child with a structurally normal heart, development of type II AV block probably indicates advancing conduction system disease. This patient should be followed very closely until such time that the ventricular response rate is so affected as to produce symptoms. Permanent pacing should then be instituted.

References

1. Ferrer PL: Arrhythmias in the neonate, infant, and child. In Roberts NK, Gelband H (eds): Arrhythmias in the Neonate. New York, Appleton-Century-Crofts, 1977, pp 265–316.
2. Narula OS, Scherlag BJ, Samet P, et al: Atrioventricular block: Localization and classification by His bundle recordings. Am J Med 50:146, 1971.
3. Wenckebach KF: Zur Analyse des unregel massigen Pulses. Z Klin Med 37:475–488, 1899.
4. Wenckebach KF: Beitrage zur Kenntnis der menschlichen Herztatigkeit. Arch Anat Physiol (Physiol Abth) 1–2:1–10, 1907.
5. Hay J: Bradycardia and cardiac arrhythmia produced by depression of certain functions of the heart. Lancet 1:139, 1906.
6. Mobitz W: Uber die unvollstandige storung der erregungsuberleitung zwischen Vorhof und Kammer des menschlichen Herzens. Z Ges Exp Med 41:180, 1924.
7. Wenckebach KF, Winterberg H: Die unregelmassige Herztatigkeit. Leipzig, W Engelmann, 1927, pp 313–320.
8. Mobitz W: Uber den partiellen Herzblock. Z Klin Med 107:449, 1928.
9. Johnson RL, Averill KH, Lamb LE: Electrocardiographic findings in 67,375 asymptomatic subjects. VII. Atrioventricular block. Am J Cardiol 6:153–177, 1960.
10. Brodsky M, Wu D, Denes P, et al: Arrhythmias documented by 24 hour continuous electrocardiographic monitoring in 50 male medical students without apparent heart disease. Am J Card 39:390–395, 1977.
11. Katz LN, Pick A: Clinical electrocardiography, part I. In The Arrhythmias. Philadelphia, Lea & Febiger, 1956.
12. Dressler W, Swiller SL: Atypical Wenckebach peri-

ods with dropped atrial beats. Am J Cardiol 2:575, 1958.

13. Watanabe Y, Dreifus LS: Second degree atrioventricular block. Cardiovasc Res 1:150–158, 1967.
14. Castillo C, Maytin O, Castellanos A Jr: His bundle recordings in atypical A-V nodal Wenckebach block during cardiac pacing. Am J Cardiol 27:570–574, 1971.
15. Gambetta M, Denes P, Childers RW: Vagally induced second degree A-V block, Mobitz type I, and the hyperactive S-A node. Chest 62:152–154, 1972.
16. Friedman HS, Gomes JAC, Haft JI: An analysis of Wenckebach periodicity. J Electrocardiol 8:307–314, 1975.
17. Denes P, Levy L, Pick A, et al: The incidence of typical and atypical A-V Wenckebach periodicity. Am Heart J 89(1):26–31, 1975.
18. Kinoshita S, Konishi G: Atrioventricular Wenckebach periodicity in athletes: Influence of increased vagal tone on the occurrence of atypical periods. J Electrocardiol 20(3):272–279, 1987.
19. Meytes I, Kaplinsky E, Yahini JH, et al: Wenckebach A-V block: A frequent feature following heavy physical training. Am Heart J 90(4):426–430, 1975.
20. El-Sherif N, Aranda J, Befeler B, et al: Atypical Wenckebach periodicity simulating Mobitz II AV block. Br Heart J 40:1376–1383, 1978.
21. Langendorf R, Cohen H, Gozo EG Jr: Observations on second degree atrioventricular block, including new criteria for the differential diagnosis between type I and type II block. Am J Cardiol 29:111–118, 1972.
22. Zipes DP: Second-degree atrioventricular block. Circulation 60:465–472, 1979.
23. Johansson B: Adams-Stokes syndrome, a review and follow-up of forty-two cases. Am J Cardiol 8:76–93, 1961.
24. Donoso E, Adler L, Friedberg C: Unusual forms of second degree atrioventricular block, including Mobitz type II block, associated with the Morgagni-Adams-Stokes syndrome. Am Heart J 67:150–157, 1967.
25. Kaufman J, Wachtel F, Rothfield E, et al: The association of complete heart block and Adams-Stokes syndrome in two cases of Mobitz type of block. Circulation 23:253–256, 1961.
26. Watanabe Y, Dreifus L: Atrioventricular block: Basic concepts. In Mandel W (ed): Cardiac Arrhythmias: Their Mechanisms, Diagnosis, and Management. Philadelphia, JB Lippincott, 1987, pp 297–320.
27. Kelly DT, Brodsky SJ, Krovetz LJ: Mobitz type II atrioventricular block in children. J Pediatr 79(6):972–976, 1971.

CHAPTER 9

COMPLETE ATRIOVENTRICULAR BLOCK

Bertrand A. Ross, William W. Pinsky & David J. Driscoll

Complete atrioventricular (AV) block is defined as the inability of an atrial impulse to be propagated to the ventricles. The diagnosis is therefore dependent on electrocardiographic proof that no atrial impulse that should conduct to the ventricles actually does conduct. Care must be taken to ensure that the AV dissociation seen on an EKG is caused by complete AV block and not by a junctional or ventricular rate faster than the atria, as may be seen in accelerated junctional rhythm or severe sinus bradycardia with an appropriate junctional rate. Generally, a long rhythm strip will be helpful in making this distinction (Fig. 9–1).

Concern about congenital AV block in children appears to have begun at the turn of the century. In 1901 Morquio reported a familial incidence of children with low heart rates and fainting. He is generally credited with the first description of congenital complete heart block.[1] Graphic proof of AV block in children had to wait until 1908 when Van den Heuvel reported the EKG findings.[2] Yater in 1929 reported a case of congenital third degree AV block diagnosed in utero and established criteria for making the diagnosis of congenital complete heart block.[3] Fetal electrocardiography was attempted for many years but was too unreliable to prove useful unless electrodes were placed in the fetal scalp, which restricted its use to during labor. However, the recent addition of fetal ultrasonography has allowed for the prenatal diagnosis and observation of congenital complete AV block.[4–7]

CONGENITAL COMPLETE ATRIOVENTRICULAR BLOCK

Incidence

The incidence of congenital complete AV block has generally been reported to be between 1/15,000 and 1/25,000 live births, with most estimates at 1/22,000 live births.[8–12] In addition, congenital complete AV block may present as familial clusters. The cooperative study of Michaelson and Engle showed 14 families in which two siblings were affected and in which examples of congenital complete AV block in more than one generation were evident.[9] Congenital complete AV block spanning three generations has also been reported by Winkler, Nora, and Nora.[13] Approximately 25% to 33% of the cases of congenital complete AV block will have associated structural heart disease. By far the most commonly associated lesion is L-transposition of the great arteries with ventricular inversion. However, congenital complete AV block is also frequently seen in abnormalities of atrial and ventricular septum formation as well as in isolated cases with other cardiac abnormalities.

Etiology

The etiology of congenital complete AV block is not fully understood at this time but

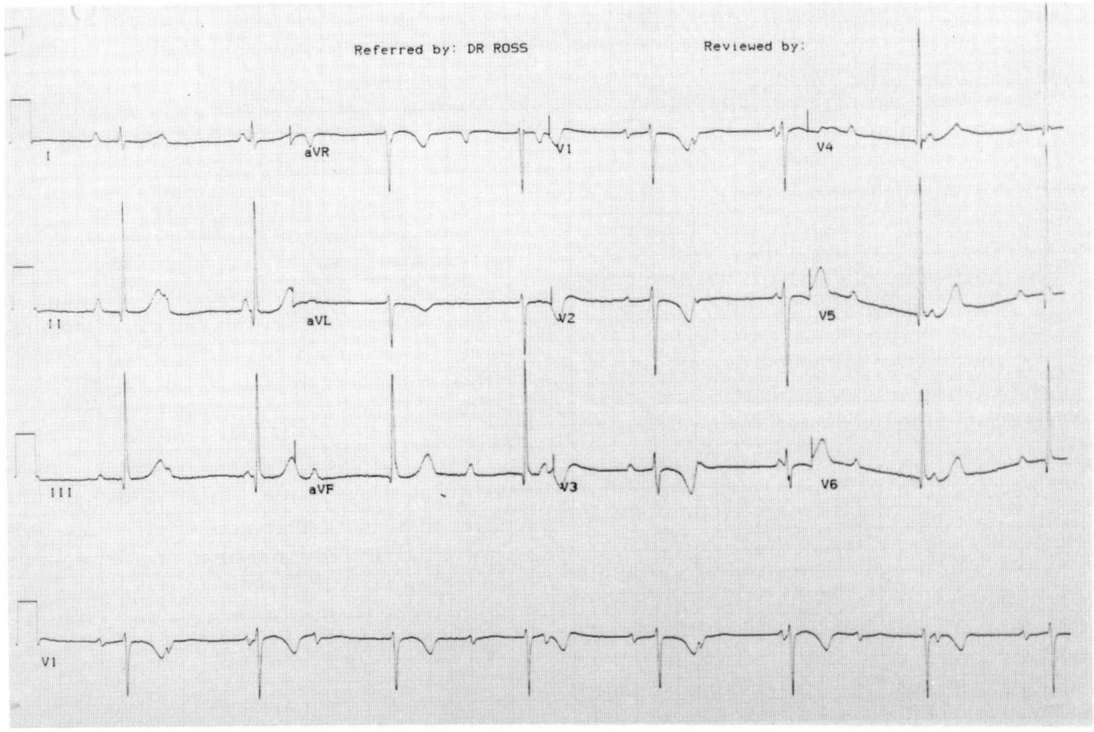

FIGURE 9–1
An example of complete AV block. Note the lack of conduction to the ventricle of P waves occurring after the T wave.

appears to center around two concepts. The first is the association of collagen vascular abnormalities (either overt or subclinical) in the mothers of children with congenital complete AV block. The majority of these patients have structurally normal hearts. This association was first commented on by Hull, Binns, and Joyce in 1966, but no causality was investigated.[14] McCue et al and Chameides et al in separate reports in 1976 appear to be the first to have reported a demonstrable association between congenital complete AV block in infants and clinical or laboratory evidence of connective tissue disease in the mothers.[15, 16] However, not all of the cases listed in the McCue et al study were complete heart block. Nonetheless, this area has recently seen a large amount of study lending further credence to this association.

There now appears to be a clear association between SS-A/Ro or SS-B/La autoantibodies in the mother and the development of congenital complete AV block in the child.[17–20] The antibodies are of the IgG class and can therefore cross the placental barrier and enter the fetal circulation. The timing of the antibody transfer is unknown, although the onset has been reported as early as the sixteenth week and twenty-third week.[21, 22] The antibodies continue to be present in the neonatal circulation up to 3 months after birth. Scott found that 75% of asymptomatic mothers who had infants with congenital complete AV block had anti-Ro (SS-A) antibodies—more than 600 times the expected incidence. However, not all anti-Ro positive mothers had children with congenital complete AV block.[23] Litsey et al demonstrated IgG deposits only in the conduction system of a fetus with congenital complete AV block.[24] Singsen et al, and more recently Taylor et al, could not demonstrate any antibody specific for the conduction system.[25] Taylor et al demonstrated via immunofluorescence staining deposition of immunoglobulin and complement components in all cardiac tissues of fetal specimens. Reactivity of maternal antibody to fetal cardiac tissue was positive in 51% of mothers of infants with congenital complete AV block versus only 10% for controls.[26]

Although these studies show a correlation between immunologic abnormalities and congenital complete AV block, and although the description of the pathology of the AV node in these patients is similar to the changes seen in the AV node of adults with connective tissue disease, the causality has yet to be shown; that is, the proof of the cytotoxic nature of the antibodies on the AV node has not been demonstrated. Not all mothers with immunologic abnormalities have children with congenital complete AV block. Some other factor such as HLA type, in utero environment, or timing of antibody transfer to the fetus may be necessary.

On these same lines, there has been work done which indicates that there may be an association between certain HLA types (HLA-DR3, B8, DRw52, DQw2) in the mother or the fetus that increases the likelihood of neonatal lupus, whose sole manifestation may be congenital complete AV block.[27, 28] More work needs to be done in this area before any definitive statements can be made.

The second possible cause of congenital complete AV block is abnormal embryonic development of the AV node from atrioventricular canal musculature. Lev postulated that the various types of pathology seen in congenital complete AV block may be a result of abnormal development of the central fibrous body, lack of union between the AV node and AV bundle (assuming separate development), or formation of conduction system from anterior endocardial tissue (L-transposition of the great arteries with ventricular inversion).[29]

Pathology

Much of the work on the pathology of congenital complete AV block has been by Lev and associates. His work has generally described three pathologic patterns (Figs. 9–2 through 9–4):

1. Lack of communication between the atria and the AV node. The AV node may be totally absent. This pathology is seen in normal hearts as well as fibroelastosis and transposition of the great arteries with single ventricle.
2. Interruption of the AV bundle. The penetrating part of the bundle is interrupted, yet the distal bundle branches are intact. This pathologic type can be seen in normal hearts and in ventricular septal defect and ostium primum atrial septal defect, among others.
3. Aberrant conduction system. The AV node and distal conduction system may be formed from anterior endocardial tissue, producing an anterior AV node in the right AV groove. This is most commonly seen in L-transposition of the great arteries with ventricular inversion.

Anderson et al postulated that the AV node origins may be multiple (i.e., there may be a deep region of AV canal origin with a superficial atrial component derived from musculature from venous valves).[30] They postulated that sulcus tissue may separate atria from ventricle during fetal development, with abnormal development leading to congenital complete AV block.

Those individuals with congenital complete AV block and neonatal lupus who have died have shown replacement of the AV node with granulation tissue or dense collagen networks encroaching on the AV node.[31] It may be that Lev's necropsy specimens without an AV node represent similar cases.

Clinical Features

The symptoms of patients with a structurally normal heart and congenital AV block range from a total lack of symptoms to syncope, exercise intolerance, or congestive heart failure. This great diversity in symptoms is directly related to the baseline junctional or ventricular escape rate of each patient. Those with a faster underlying rate will generally demonstrate less fatigue or exercise intolerance. However, the baseline heart rate is only one factor. A second is the ability of the underlying pacemaker to increase its rate in response to various physiologic demands (i.e., exercise). Normally the increase in cardiac output with exercise is produced by an increase in both stroke volume and heart rate; however, heart rate is the main component of the cardiac output increase. As can be seen from Figure 9–5 there are significant differences among various patients with congenital AV block in their ability to increase their heart rate with exercise. This ability does not seem to be related to resting heart rate, atrial rate, or heart size. Clearly those individuals who can increase their ventricular rates are better able to handle the oxygen delivery demands that are produced by an increase in activity than those who cannot. Patients with complete AV block compensate for reduced resting heart rates by an increase

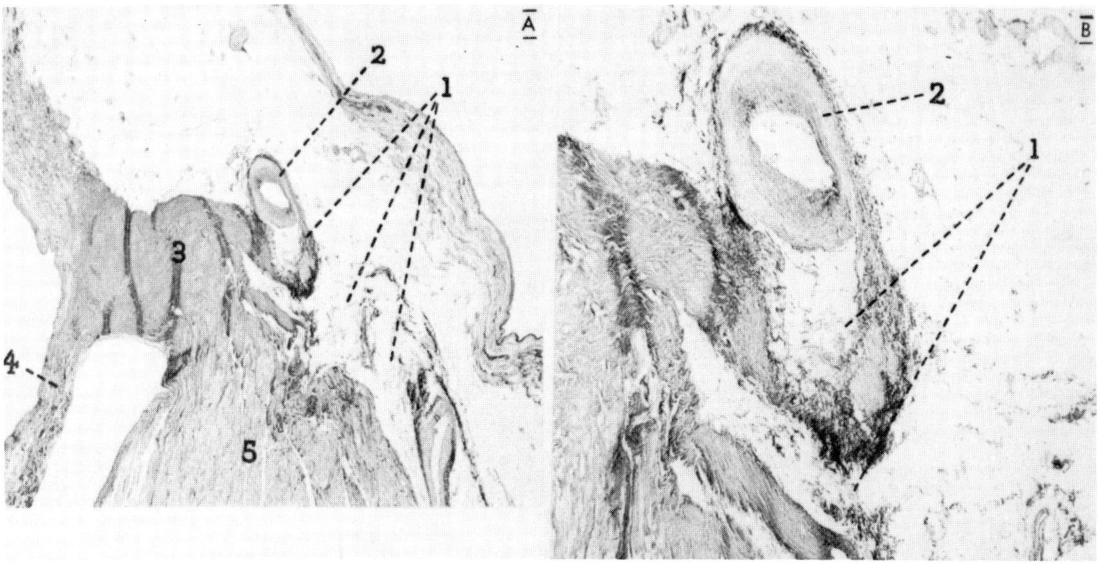

FIGURE 9–2
Lack of communication between the atria and the more peripheral conduction system. Weigert-van Gieson stain. (*A*)×15; (*B*) ×48; 1, region of AV node; 2, branch of ramus septi fibrosi; 3, central fibrous body; 4, mitral valve; 5, ventricular musculature. (Reprinted from Lev M: Pathogenesis of congenital atrioventricular block. Prog Cardiovasc Dis 15:146, 1972.)

in stroke volume and left ventricular end diastolic volume.[32] Even though heart rate increases vary among these patients, there is evidence that the cardiac output response to exercise is blunted in all of them.[32] One of the difficulties in determining symptomatology in a child is that he or she has never experienced any other situation for comparison and may have no complaints. Once pacemaker therapy has been implemented, the child usually feels much better, presumably because of improved cardiac output or decreased atrial pressures.

In addition to ventricular rate, the incidence of premature ventricular contractions (PVCs) in patients with complete AV block has been a clinical feature of some concern. However, the clinical implications of this finding are still unclear. Winkler, Freed, and Nadas and Chawla et al have presented different opinions regarding the incidence of ventricular ectopy. Chawla et al found an association between lower resting heart rates and ventricular ectopy during exercise, whereas Winkler, Freed, and Nadas found an association between increasing age of the patient and premature ventricular beats.[33, 34]

The infant with isolated congenital complete heart block may be asymptomatic or may present with varying degrees of decreased cardiac output or even congestive heart failure. The age of presentation is important when considering the clinical features in this group of patients. The newborn infant with congestive heart failure requires intense medical support and treatment. These neonates may have significant anasarca, hepatomegaly, and lactic acidosis. Clearly more severe symptoms indicate a more critical need for emergent pacing. However, the neonate with a structurally normal heart and a borderline reduction in peripheral perfusion may stabilize over a 24-hour period following the birth process and, with an appropriate ventricular escape rate, have normal perfusion. Neonates who are clinically asymptomatic do not require treatment, but instead can be followed clinically in an intensive care unit as long as the baseline heart rate is above the rate considered to be at risk for sudden death (55 bpm).

The child with a structurally normal heart or a physiologically insignificant structural defect will have symptoms based on the ventricular or junctional escape rate. Symptoms will usually present as fatigue or exercise intolerance. Syncope may also occur. However, the child with congenital complete AV block (CCAVB) may be asymptomatic, and the block may only be discovered on a routine well child evaluation.

The infant or child with structural heart disease and congenital complete AV block is in a much different situation than the patients previously described. This group of

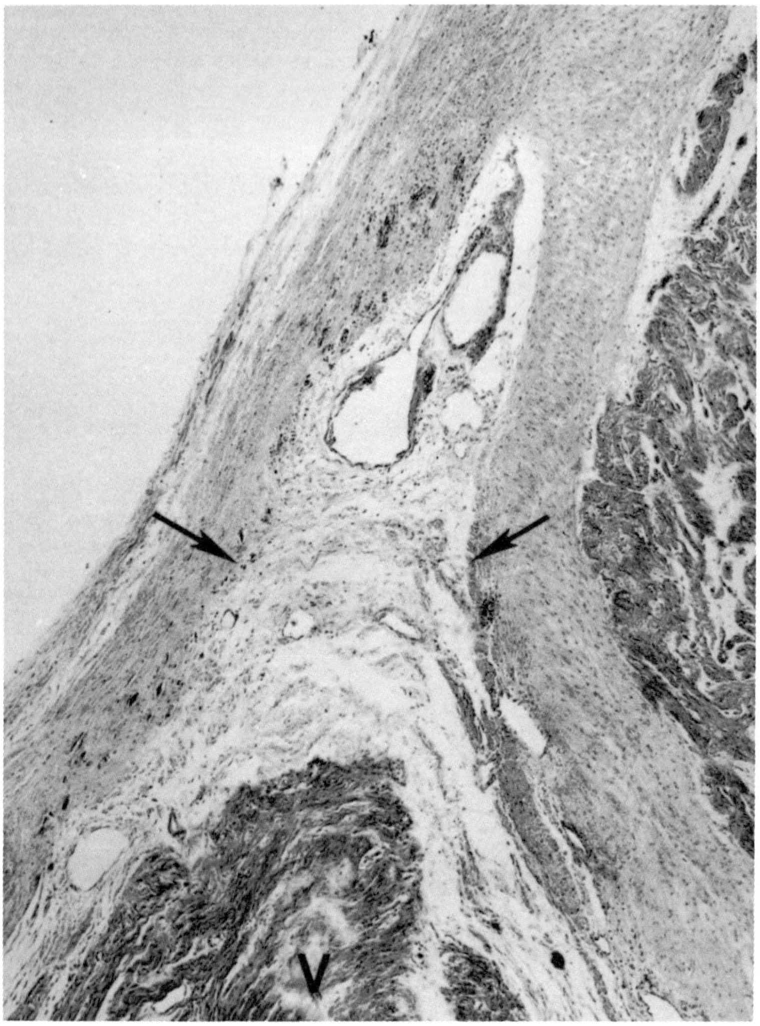

FIGURE 9–3
Interruption of the penetrating portion of the bundle of His, which is replaced by space and loose connective tissue. Hematoxyline-eosin stain, × 50. Arrows point to region of penetrating portion of AV bundle. V, ventricular muscle. (Reprinted from Lev M: Pathogenesis of congenital atrioventricular block. Prog Cardiovasc Dis 15:147, 1972.)

patients requires the highest and most responsive cardiac output, yet has the least ability to respond appropriately. For this reason, this group presents the earliest in life (three times more likely to present in the first week of life compared to those with isolated complete AV block) and is in the most need of care and treatment.[9] Even with appropriate therapy, a number of these patients die in infancy. An exception is the patient with CCAVB and a structural abnormality that is not hemodynamically significant who can respond in a manner similar to the infant with CCAVB and a structurally normal heart (i.e., those with L-TGA or mild Ebstein's anomaly).

In summary, the clinical features of patients with congenital complete heart block primarily involve the effect of the heart rate on cardiac output and the risk of sudden death. Treatment is based on the ability of pacing to improve symptoms or prevent sudden death.

Diagnostic Techniques

PRENATAL

Until the 1970s, fetal monitoring for arrhythmias had consisted mostly of auscultation of the fetal heart rate. This obviously left much unknown, not the least of which was the type of rhythm. Fetal electrocardiography, which consisted of trying to obtain a fetal EKG through the maternal abdomen, was cumbersome and inaccurate until shortly before birth, when electrodes could be placed on the fetal scalp. Even with this method, however, the type of rhythm was still uncertain.[35] However, with the advent of fetal

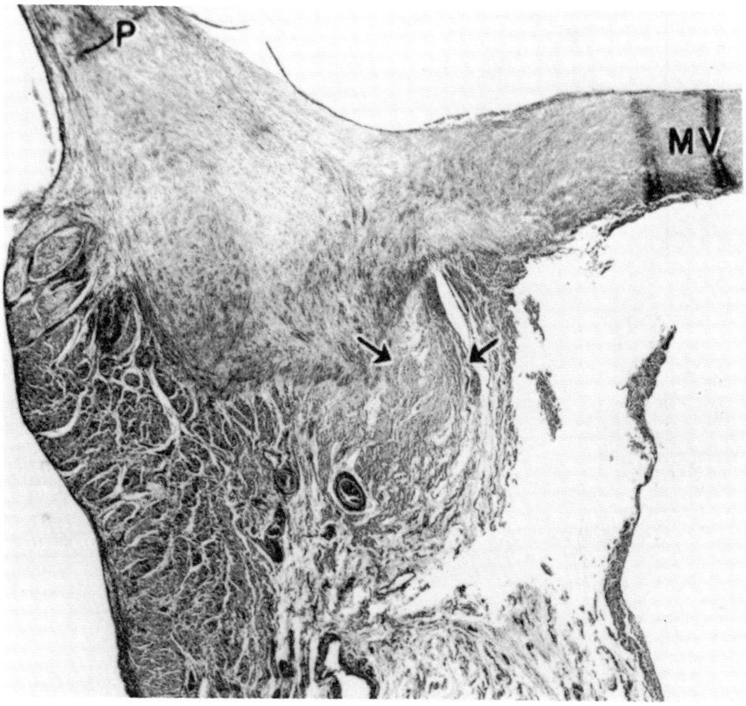

FIGURE 9–4
Abnormal conduction system in a case of mixed levocardia with ventricular inversion (corrected transposition) with fetal coarctation and ventricular septal defect. Normally situated AV node. Weigert-van Gieson stain, ×27. P, pars membranacea; MV, annulus of mitral valve. Arrows point to node. (Reprinted from Lev M: Pathogenesis of congenital atrioventricular block. Prog Cardiovasc Dis 15:148, 1972.)

echocardiography, a method was available to determine the heart rate and the relationship of atrial and ventricular contractions by timing mitral valve opening and ventricular contraction.

POSTNATAL

EKG and Holter Monitor

A surface EKG is all that is needed to make the diagnosis of congenital complete AV block. However, because the EKG represents an isolated event in time, it does not give enough information to determine the junctional or ventricular escape rate. A 24-hour Holter monitor is ideal for this, as the heart rate can be monitored over a spectrum of times and conditions, and the incidence and severity of ectopy can be evaluated. Because there may be an association between increasing age and ventricular ectopy in patients with congenital complete AV block, the ability to monitor the rhythm for 24 hours, encompassing a variety of situations and activities, is invaluable.[33]

Intracardiac Electrophysiology

Evaluation by invasive electrophysiologic testing has been used in the past to determine the site of block. It was thought that the site of block could help predict stability of the cellular pacemaker. This, however, has not proven to be the case.[36] Benson et al have presented evidence that evaluating the automaticity of the pacemaker by using pacemaker recovery times may be helpful.[37] A junctional or ventricular recovery time of greater than 3 seconds in children may be correlated with clinical symptoms or sudden death.

Exercise Testing

Exercise testing is an important adjunct in the evaluation of the seemingly asymptomatic child with congenital complete AV block. In this way some objective criteria can be employed to help document symptomatology and to determine if any ectopy is present. Although the significance of exercise-induced ventricular ectopy has not been proven, it has been suggested that ventricular ectopy may increase the risk of sudden death in some patients with congenital complete AV block.[33]

Treatment

Treatment of patients with congenital complete AV block falls into two main categories:

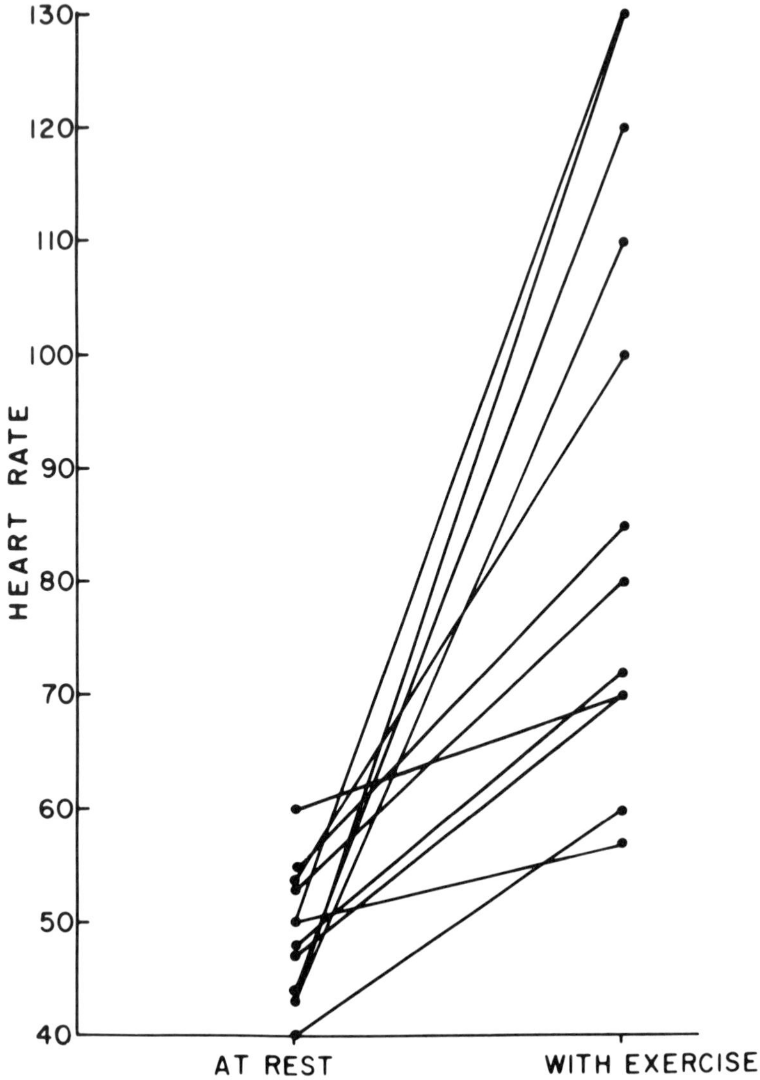

FIGURE 9–5
Change of ventricular rate with maximal exercise in 12 children. In 10 of 12, the rate increased more than 20 bpm and in 5 of 12 the rate increased more than 40 bpm. (Pinsky WW: Diagnosis and management of congenital complete atrioventricular block. Gillette PC, Garson A Jr [eds]: Pediatric Cardiac Dysrhythmias. New York: Grune & Stratton, 1981, p 393.

treatment of the patient with low cardiac output and treatment of those patients thought to be at risk of sudden death. Treatment for the most part centers around temporary and permanent pacing, as chronotropic drugs appear to have only modest success at best.[38] However, if the patient is in extremis, chronotropic agents such as isoproterenol or atropine may be used while arrangements are being made for pacing. The use of external transthoracic pacing has been little studied in children, but in emergency situations, it may be appropriate to attempt this modality.

The fetus with severe congestive heart failure and congenital complete AV block should be delivered as soon as is considered safe from an obstetric viewpoint. Transuterine pacing of a fetus in extremis but too young to deliver has been tried; however, after a short period of capture, pacing capability was lost, and the fetus died.[39] Infants with complete congenital AV block seem to tolerate vaginal delivery fairly well unless they are in distress or in congestive heart failure; in these cases an emergency cesarean section is indicated. Arrangements should be made prior to delivery for treatment of the congestive heart failure soon after birth with inotropic agents and diuretics as well as with temporary or permanent pacing. Placement of some type of pacing modality should have the highest priority.

Occasionally, an infant with very mild signs of low cardiac output can be stabilized with a temporary pacing catheter in place and may not need permanent pacing if the heart rate and output improve following birth.

The fetus or newborn with asymptomatic congenital complete AV block should be placed in an intensive care setting with the heart rate monitored very closely. The decision to pace this group of patients depends on the baseline ventricular rate and the likelihood of sudden death. Michaelson and Engle showed only one death in patients who had a ventricular rate greater than 55 bpm and an atrial rate less than 140 bpm.[9] It should also be noted that there were no deaths in those with a ventricular rate greater than 60 bpm and an atrial rate less than 140 bpm, but there were also fewer patients who met these criteria. Karpawich et al found similar data in an older age group, with no infant or child with a heart rate greater than 50 bpm having syncope.[36] In the past the need for a permanent pacemaker in an infant was reason for grave concern and implantation of a pacing system occasionally resulted in the patient's demise. However, current thought is that any patient considered to be at risk of sudden death from congenital complete AV block should have a pacemaker implanted. In the asymptomatic infant, this would include an infant with a persistent ventricular rate less than 55 bpm. As confidence in pacemakers rises, the cut-off rate may be raised to 60 bpm, as only one child in the collaborative study died with a ventricular rate greater than 60 bpm, regardless of the atrial rate.

The newborn with congenital heart disease and complete heart block, regardless of symptoms, should probably be paced, as the incidence of death in infancy in this group is exceedingly high (29%, compared to 8% in those without congenital heart disease in the Michaelson and Engle series, and only an 80% first-year survival rate in patients in the Pinsky et al series).[40]

The child with congenital complete AV block presents a slightly different set of circumstances. The decision if and when to pace these patients is much less clear. Generally, the older child is followed with exercise testing and Holter monitoring to look for increasing exercise intolerance, arrhythmias, and/or very low baseline heart rate. Individual patients whose activity level is impaired because of decreased exercise tolerance should be paced. Exercise testing is helpful in determining tolerance as well as in eliciting ventricular arrhythmias. This is important, as syncope and sudden death in children with congenital complete AV block may be caused by ventricular arrhythmias as well as by severe bradycardia. Molthen et al reported patients with congenital complete AV block having Adams-Stokes attacks and ventricular tachycardia.[41] Studies of patients with congenital complete AV block undergoing exercise testing have shown an increased rate of ectopy.[34, 36, 42] There is disagreement as to the cause, whether increased age of the patient or an inadequate chronotropic response. However, it is unclear whether ventricular ectopy increases the risk of sudden death in these patients or if permanent pacing is protective. It may be that the increase in heart size in these patients (a compensatory mechanism for low heart rate) may through the years predispose them to the development of ventricular arrhythmias, just as atrial dilatation predisposes to atrial flutter. If so, pacing at a younger age may be somewhat protective, but more work will need to be done in this area. Holter and EKG monitoring in children with congenital complete AV block has been used not only to determine the low heart rate, but also to help guide therapy. The consensus is that average awake heart rates in children of less than 50 bpm are an indication for pacing. A random rate of less than 45 bpm is also considered an indication for a pacemaker. Although the sleeping heart rate can dip to quite low levels, there are as yet no criteria for determining if and when to pace based on this parameter.

SURGICAL COMPLETE ATRIOVENTRICULAR BLOCK

One of the complications of surgical correction of congenital heart defects is postsurgical complete heart block. This may be transient or permanent, or may be transient in the immediate postoperative period, only to reappear in a permanent form at a later time. Transient postsurgical AV block may last as long as 10 days to 2 weeks. As in congenital complete AV block, diagnosis requires proof that atrial impulses that should conduct to the ventricle do not. This may be somewhat complicated in postoperative patients, as many have a markedly accelerated junctional rhythm. If atrial wires are present, intact conduction can be proven by pacing the atria at a rate sufficiently fast to overdrive the existing junctional rate.

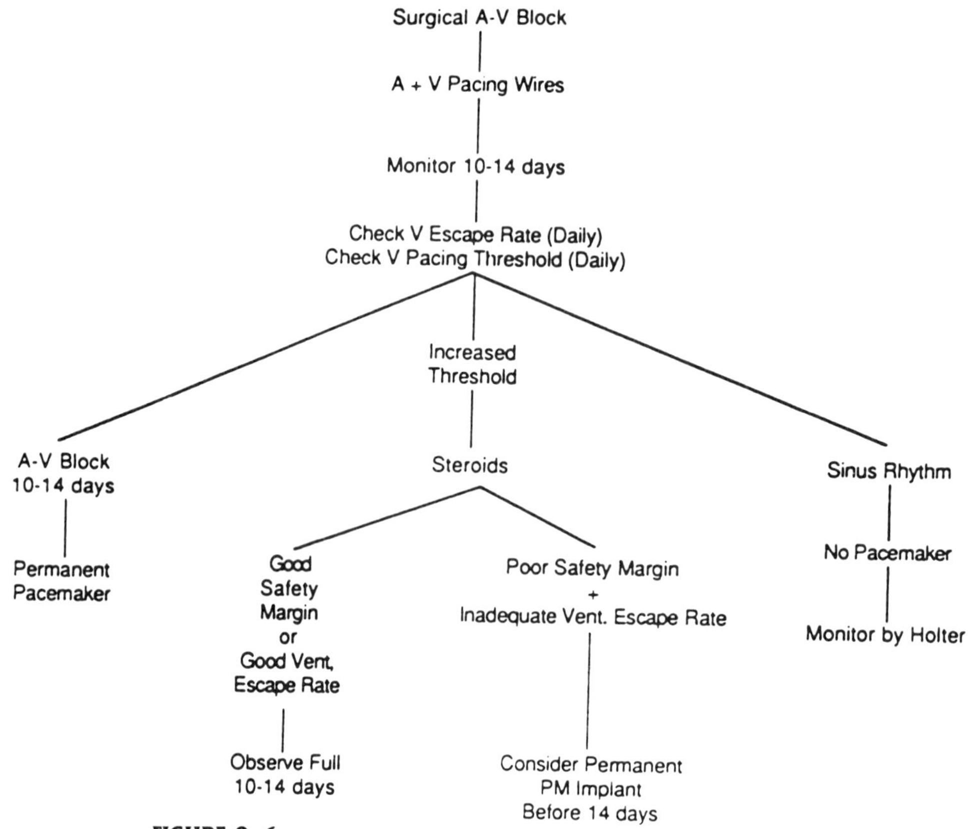

FIGURE 9–6
Flow chart outlining a management protocol for post-surgical AV block.

Because of an increased awareness of the location of the AV node and the His bundle, the incidence of postsurgical AV block is much lower than that of even 10 years ago. However, any surgery involving the AV node area (e.g., surgical repair of ventricular septal defect, AV canal, or L-transposition of the great arteries with or without a ventricular septal defect, or a Fontan procedure requiring oversewing of the tricuspid valve) is still a risk for producing complete AV block.

Treatment

Once it has been ascertained that AV block has occurred, it is advisable to have both atrial and ventricular wires placed. This will aid in distinguishing complete AV block from an accelerated junctional rhythm and will allow for AV synchrony in the immediate recovery period. In addition, any patient suspected of having postsurgical block should be watched closely, with backup pacing readily available in the event the junctional ectopic focus suddenly slows without a sufficient ventricular escape rhythm. We have had at least one patient arrest in a similar situation. The patient should be watched closely for any sign of intact AV conduction, and the threshold of the temporary pacing wires should be checked each day. This is especially important if the patient is pacemaker dependent with an inadequate ventricular escape rate. The ventricular output should be kept at twice the capture threshold. Unless forced to place a permanent pacemaker because of markedly elevated ventricular thresholds in a postoperative pacemaker-dependent patient, any decision regarding a permanent pacemaker should be delayed for 10 days to 2 weeks, since sinus rhythm may return (Fig. 9–6).

Although disagreement still exists regarding the need for permanent pacing in the postsurgical AV block patient, the consensus is to pace all these patients. Lillehei et al reported a 60% mortality rate in postsurgical AV block patients during the first postoperative year alone.[43] However, Hurwitz reported a much lower incidence of death in postoperative AV block patients.[44] In that series, only one of every three patients who had a pacemaker implant died. As with other types of AV block, the indications for pacemaker implants will, to a large extent, depend on the confidence the physician has in permanent pacing and the concern regarding battery changes and lead problems. In the past 5 to 10 years, the capability to pace children effectively has improved markedly, as evidenced by the reports of Waelkens, Beder et al, and Gillette et al.[45–47] We generally install a permanent pacemaker in any postsurgical AV block patient who has complete block lasting 10 to 14 days without performing electrophysiologic testing to determine the site of block.

References

1. Morquio L: Sur une maladie infantile et familiale caracteristique et la mort subite. Arch Med Enfantes 4:467–475, 1901.
2. Van den Heuvel GCJ: Die ziekle van Stokes-Adams en een genal van aangeboren hart block (profschrift aan de ryks universitat). Gronigen, 1908.
3. Yater WM: Congenital heart block. Review of the literature: Report of a case with incomplete heterotaxy; the electrocardiogram in dextrocardia. Am J Dis Child 38:112–136, 1929.
4. Kleinman CS, Donnerstein RL, Jaffe CC, et al: Fetal echocardiography—A tool for evaluation of in utero cardiac arrhythmias and monitoring of in utero therapy: Analysis of 71 patients. Am J Cardiol 51:237–243, 1983.
5. Sokol RJ, Hutchison P, Krouskop RW, et al: Congenital complete heart block diagnosed during intrauterine fetal monitoring. Am J Obstet Gynecol 120:1115–1119, 1974.
6. Steinfeld L, Rappaport HL, Rossbach HC, et al: Diagnosis of fetal arrhythmias using echocardiographic and Doppler techniques. JACC 8:1425–1433, 1986.
7. Allan LD, Anderson RH, Sullivan ID, et al: Evaluation of fetal arrhythmias by echocardiography. Br Heart J 50:240–245, 1983.
8. Gochberg SH: Congenital heart block. Am J Obstet Gynecol 88:238–241, 1964.
9. Michaelson M, Engle MA: Congenital complete heart block: An international study of the natural history. In Brest AN, Engle MA (eds): Cardiovascular Clinics. Philadelphia, FA Davis, 1972, pp 85–101.
10. Landtmann B, Linder E, Hjelt L, et al: Congenital complete heart block. I. A clinical study of 37 cases. Ann Paediatr Fenn 10:99–104, 1964.
11. Linton D, Human D: Peri-operative management and administration of anesthesia in children with congenital complete heart block. A case report and review. S Afr Med J 66:875–876, 1984.
12. Camm AJ, Bexten RS: Congenital heart block. Eur Heart J Suppl A:115–117, 1984.
13. Winkler RB, Nora AH, Nora JJ: Familial congenital complete heart block and maternal systemic lupus erythematosus. Circulation 56(6):1103–1106, 1977.
14. Hull D, Binns BAO, Joyce D: Congenital heart block and widespread fibrosis due to maternal lupus erythematosus. Arch Dis Child 41:688–690, 1966.
15. Chameides L, Truex RC, Vetter V, et al: Association of maternal systemic lupus erythematosus with congenital complete heart block. N Engl J Med 297:1204–1207, 1977.
16. McCue CM, Mantakas ME, Tinglestad JB, et al: Congenital heart block in newborns of mothers with connective tissue disease. Circulation 56(1):82–90, 1977.
17. Reed BR, Lee LA, Harmon C, et al: Autoantibodies to SS-A/Ro in infants with congenital heart block. J Pediatr 103(6):889–891, 1983.
18. Parke A, Rothfield NF: Congenital heart block, systemic lupus erythematosus and anti-Ro antibodies. (Letter) Arth Rheum 28(9):1077–1078, 1985.
19. Harley JB, Kaine JL, Fox OF, et al: Ro (SS-A) antibody and antigen in a patient with congenital complete heart block. Arth Rheum 28(12):1321–1325, 1985.
20. Franco HL, Weston WL, Peebles C, et al: Autoantibodies directed against Sicca syndrome antigens in the neonatal lupus syndrome. Am Acad Dermatol 4:67–72, 1981.
21. Lee LA, Weston WL: New findings in neonatal lupus syndrome. Am J Dis Child 138(3):233–236, 1984.
22. Herreman G, Betous F, Batisse P, et al: Intra-uterine detection of atrioventricular block in two children whose mother had Sjogren's syndrome. Nouv Presse Med 11(9):657–660, 1982.
23. Scott JS, Maddison PJ, Taylor PV, et al: Connective tissue disease, antibodies to ribonucleoprotein, and congenital heart block. N Engl J Med 309:209–212, 1983.
24. Litsey SE, Noonan JA, O'Connor WN, et al: Maternal connective tissue disease and congenital heart block. Demonstration of immunoglobulin in cardiac tissue. N Engl J Med 312(2):98–100, 1985.
25. Singsen BH, Akhter JE, Weinstein MM, et al: Congenital complete heart block and SSA antibodies: Obstetric implications. Am J Obstet Gynecol 152:655–658, 1985.
26. Taylor PV, Scott JS, Gerlis LM, et al: Maternal antibodies against fetal cardiac antigens in congenital complete heart block. N Engl J Med 315:667–672, 1986.
27. Lee LA, Bias WB, Arnett FC, et al: Immunogenetics of the neonatal lupus syndrome. Ann Intern Med 99(5):592–596, 1983.
28. Watson RM, Lane AT, Barnett NK, et al: Neonatal lupus erythematosus. A clinical serological and immunogenetic study with review of the literature. Medicine 63(6):362–378, 1984.
29. Lev M: Pathogenesis of congenital atrioventricular block. Prog Cardiovasc Dis 25(2):145–162, 1972.
30. Anderson RH, Wenick AC, Losekoot TG, et al: Congenitally complete heart block: Developmental aspects. Circulation 56(1):90–101, 1977.
31. Bharati S, de la Fuente DJ, Kallen RJ, et al: Conduction system in systemic lupus erythematosus with atrioventricular block. Am J Cardiol 35:299–304, 1975.
32. Manno BV, Hakki AH, Eshaghpour E, et al: Left ventricular function at rest and during exercise in

congenital complete heart block: A radionuclide angiographic evaluation. Am J Cardiol 52(1):92–94, 1983.
33. Winkler RB, Freed MD, Nadas AS: Exercise-induced ventricular ectopy in children and young adults with complete heart block. Am Heart J 99:87–92, 1980.
34. Chawla K, Serratto M, Cruz J, et al: Response to maximal and submaximal exercise testing in patients with congenital complete heart block. Circulation 56(suppl III):171, 1977.
35. Shenker L: Fetal cardiac arrhythmias. Obstet Gynecol Surv 34(8):561–572, 1979.
36. Karpawich PP, Gillette PC, Garson A, et al: Congenital complete atrioventricular block: Clinical and electrophysiologic predictors of need for pacemaker insertion. Am J Cardiol 48:1098–1102, 1981.
37. Benson DW, Edwards SB, Serwer GA, et al: Heart block in children: Evaluating pacemaker recording times. Circulation 60:11–114, 1979. Abstract.
38. Nakamura F, Nadas A: Complete heart block in infants and children. N Engl J Med 270(24):1261–1268, 1964.
39. Strasburger J, Carpenter R, Smith RT, et al: Fetal transthoracic pacing for advanced hydrops fetalis secondary to complete atrioventricular block. PACE 9:295, 1986.
40. Pinsky WW, Gillette PC, Garson AT, et al: Diagnosis, management and long-term results of patients with complete atrioventricular block. Pediatrics 69(6): 728–733, 1982.
41. Molthen ME, Miller RA, Hastreiter AR, et al: Congenital heart block with fetal Adams-Stokes attacks in childhood. Pediatrics 30:32–41, 1962.
42. Ikkos D, Hanson JS: Response to exercise in congenital complete atrioventricular block. Circulation 22:583–590, 1960.
43. Lillihei C, Sellers RD, Bonnabeau RC, et al: Chronic post-surgical complete heart block. J Cardiovasc Surg 46:436–456, 1973.
44. Hurwitz RA, Riemenschneider TA, Moss AJ et al: Chronic postoperative heart block in children. Am J Cardiol 21:185–189, 1968.
45. Waelkens JJJ: Cardiac pacemakers in infants and children. Pediatr Cardiol 3:337–340, 1982.
46. Beder SD, Hanisch DG, Cohen MH, et al: Cardiac pacing on children: A 15 year experience. Am Heart J 109(1):152–156, 1985.
47. Gillette PC, Shannon C, Blair H, et al: Transvenous pacing in pediatric patients. Am Heart J 105(5):843–847, 1983.

CHAPTER 10

BUNDLE-BRANCH AND FASCICULAR BLOCKS

Lesley Ewing

The QRS complex represents depolarization of the right and left ventricles but the QRS pattern that is visible on the surface ECG represents only a portion of the total electrical forces. Because of their vectors, up to 95% of the electrical forces generated by ventricular depolarization cancel each other. Normal ventricular depolarization requires conduction through the intact bundle of His and its three major fascicles. Disruption of this pathway causes the electrocardiographic pattern of bundle-branch block (BBB). Block in the normal interventricular conduction pathway results in depolarization of one ventricle after the other; therefore there is asynchronous ventricular activation. This is manifest on the electrocardiogram as prolonged ventricular depolarization (QRS duration) and repolarization (QT interval). The normal QRS duration is age related, being shorter in younger children.

ANATOMY OF THE HIS-PURKINJE SYSTEM

The ventricular conduction system is composed of the distal bundle of His and the right and left bundle branches and their radiations. The proximal His bundle connects the atria to the ventricular conduction system as the direct continuation of the atrioventricular (AV) node.[1] Purkinje fibers are longitudinally aligned within the bundle, supported by a collagen network, and are joined by transverse crossover connections.[2] The proximal His bundle traverses the fibrous AV ring through the central fibrous body, and then travels in the posterior inferior margin of the membranous interventricular septum adjacent to the noncoronary cusp of the aortic valve. Just inferior to the membranous portion of the septum, the His bundle bifurcates into the right and the left bundle branches. The right bundle branch (RBB) is the direct continuation of the His bundle.[1]

The RBB lies just beneath the endocardium of the interventricular septum.[3] It continues as a discrete bundle, passing beneath the septal band and through the moderator band.[1] At the origin of the anterior papillary muscle, the RBB splits into numerous distal branches.[4]

The left bundle branch (LBB) sends fanlike radiations at right angles to the common bundle. The course of the LBB varies greatly among individual hearts.[3] The pathology literature does not support the clear delineation of discrete fascicles of the LBB,[5] but a recognition of anterior and posterior fascicles (conduction pathways) is clinically useful.[6]

The shorter posterior fascicle of the LBB arises proximal to the anterior fascicle; it leaves the sub–aortic valve region and approaches the posterior papillary muscle. The posterior fascicle then branches diffusely into the Purkinje network. The longer anterior fascicle of the LBB arises distally from the LBB and courses across the left ventricular outflow tract toward the anterior papillary muscle.[1] A third (septal) fascicle initiating septal depolarization has also been described.[1, 3, 6]

BLOOD SUPPLY TO THE HIS-PURKINJE SYSTEM

A branch of the right coronary artery (RCA) supplies the AV node in most people.[1]

The His bundle receives its blood from the RCA and from the septal branches of the left anterior descending artery (LAD). Rarely, the LAD is the only blood supply to the His bundle. The proximal RBB is supplied by branches of the RCA and the remainder of the RBB by septal perforating branches of the LAD. Branches from both the LAD and the posterior descending coronary arteries supply the posterior fascicle of the LBB; the anterior fascicle receives its blood from septal perforating branches of the LAD.[1]

NORMAL VENTRICULAR DEPOLARIZATION

Extensive electrical mapping of in situ and excised, perfused hearts have described the sequence of interventricular conduction in some detail.[4, 7–9] The initial endocardial depolarization does not occur along the His bundle or its fascicles; it begins distally at the junction of the Purkinje fibers and the ventricular myocardium.[4] Muscle depolarization begins in the interventricular septum on the left side and at the anterior paraseptal wall of the left ventricle.[4] It then spreads from left to right through the septum in an anterior and apical direction. Right ventricular endocardial depolarization begins near the origin of the anterior papillary muscle 10 ms or less after initiation of left ventricular depolarization.[10] Right ventricle depolarization begins slightly later, because the RBB is longer than the LBB. Depolarization traverses the ventricular walls from the endocardial surface to the epicardium. Both ventricular free walls are depolarized at the same time, but in opposite directions. The last regions to be depolarized are the basal left and right epicardial surfaces of the ventricles.[4]

COMPLETE RIGHT BUNDLE-BRANCH BLOCK

ECG

In complete right bundle-branch block, the QRS duration is prolonged (total duration more than 90 ms in children younger than 3 years, and more than 100 ms in those older than 3 years). There is an RSR′ pattern in the right chest leads (V_{3r}, V_{4r}, V_1) with initial (40 ms) rapid deflection and slow terminal deflection. There is a deep, wide, terminal S wave in standard leads I and aVL, and in the left lateral precordial leads, V_5 and V_6. Impulses are transmitted to the interventricular septum through the LBB, so septal activation is normal, as indicated by a normal initial R wave in V_1 and a normal Q wave in V_6. There are no Q waves in leads I or aVL unless there are additional conduction disturbances. The major QRS deflection in leads II, III, and aVF is positive. The T waves are inverted in the anterior precordial leads (Fig. 10–1).

Etiology

Right bundle-branch block in children is most commonly an acquired condition following surgical repair of congenital heart defects, most frequently ventricular septal defect (VSD), tetralogy of Fallot (TOF), and complete atrioventricular canal.[11–14] RBBB is rarely an isolated, primary anomaly.[15–19] It can be seen in association with many heritable and acquired diseases (Table 10–1).

Most children with RBBB have had open heart surgery. Following VSD repair, some centers report an incidence of RBBB as low as 32% and others as high as 100%.[13] The reported incidence is less (ranging from 32% to 44%) at centers that repair the VSD through the tricuspid valve.[12, 25] RBBB occurs in most patients undergoing repair of a complete atrioventricular septal defect,[12] and it is uncommon not to have RBBB after TOF repair.[12, 13] Repair of a double-chambered right ventricle also usually results in RBBB.

The vulnerability of the His-Purkinje system to injury during surgery for VSD or TOF results from the anatomic proximity to the area involved in the repair.[13] Pathologic studies of hearts following VSD repair show hemorrhage, necrosis, and inflammatory changes in the base of the membranous septum and the superior edge of the muscular septum.[26] Investigators have also shown that the RBBB pattern can be caused by a ventriculotomy[27] rather than by surgical trauma at the margins of the VSD (i.e., distal rather than proximal damage to the RBB). Gelband et al recorded ECGs and ventricular mapping by direct electrograms in patients

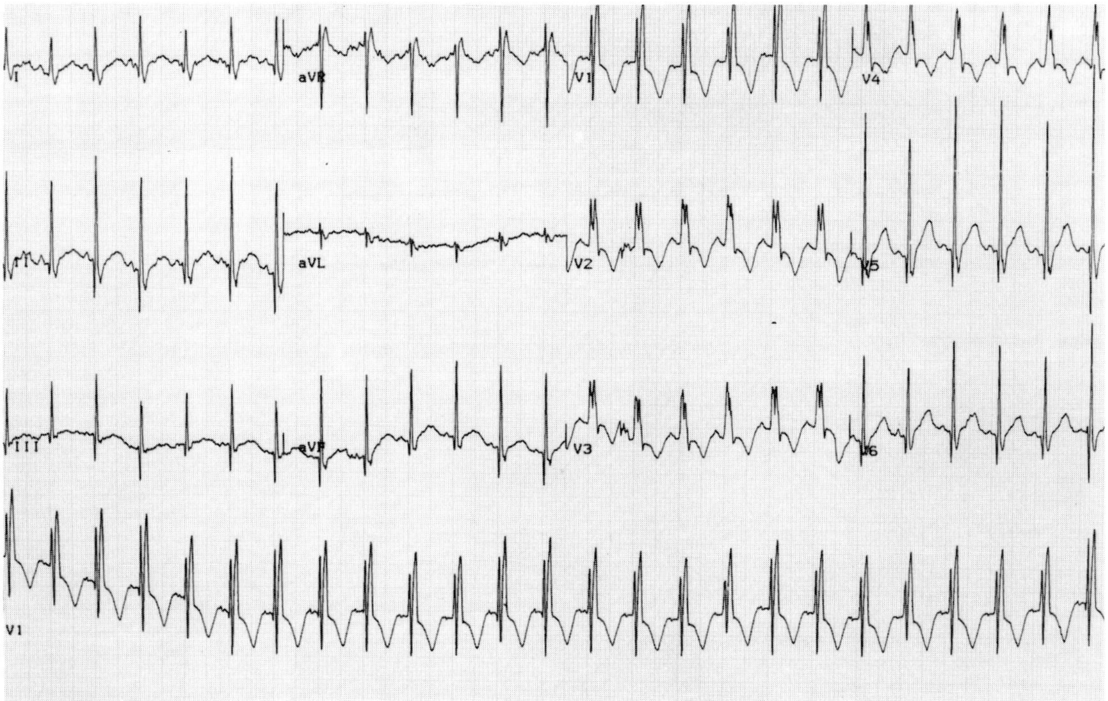

FIGURE 10–1
Right bundle branch block after repair of tetralogy of Fallot. Paper speed was 25 mm/s; calibration was 1 mV/10 mm.

at the time of repair of VSD, TOF, or pulmonic stenosis (PS).[27] The surgery was performed in stages to determine when RBBB occurred. RBBB was recorded after the ventriculotomy was performed in each patient who developed RBBB. Whether distal or proximal damage causes RBBB on the ECG and the mechanism of damage caused by a distal lesion are not completely understood.[13, 29–31]

Differentiating between distal and proximal RBBB is possible during electrophysiologic study.[13, 32] The interval between ventricular activation seen on surface ECG and the intracardiac electrode at the RV apex is normal (less than 30 ms)[33] in distal lesions of the RBBB but prolonged in proximal lesions (Figs. 10–2 and 10–3).[13, 32, 34] Intracardiac mapping of the ventricular conduction system[13, 35] or comparison between right and left ventricular activation times can also distinguish proximal from distal lesions.[36]

TABLE 10–1
NONSURGICAL CONDITIONS ASSOCIATED WITH RBBB

Heritable
Isolated RBBB[15–19]
RBBB, with left anterior fascicular block[20]
Myotonic dystrophy[21]
Kearns-Sayre syndrome[1]
Duchenne's muscular dystrophy[22]
Infection
Myocarditis[11]
Trauma
Blunt chest trauma[23]
Idiopathic
Cardiomyopathy
Miscellaneous
Congestive heart failure, dilatation of cardiac chambers[11]
Polymyositis[24]
Structural heart disease
Ebstein's anomaly of the tricuspid valve[11]
Atrial septal defect

Prognosis and Natural History of RBBB

The true significance of RBBB, especially postsurgical RBBB, is unknown. A clinically significant hemodynamic effect has not been associated with RBBB in the normal heart. Investigations in which hypertrophied and normal canine right ventricles were compared following section of the RBB demonstrated a decline in cardiac output in the hypertrophied ventricles.[37]

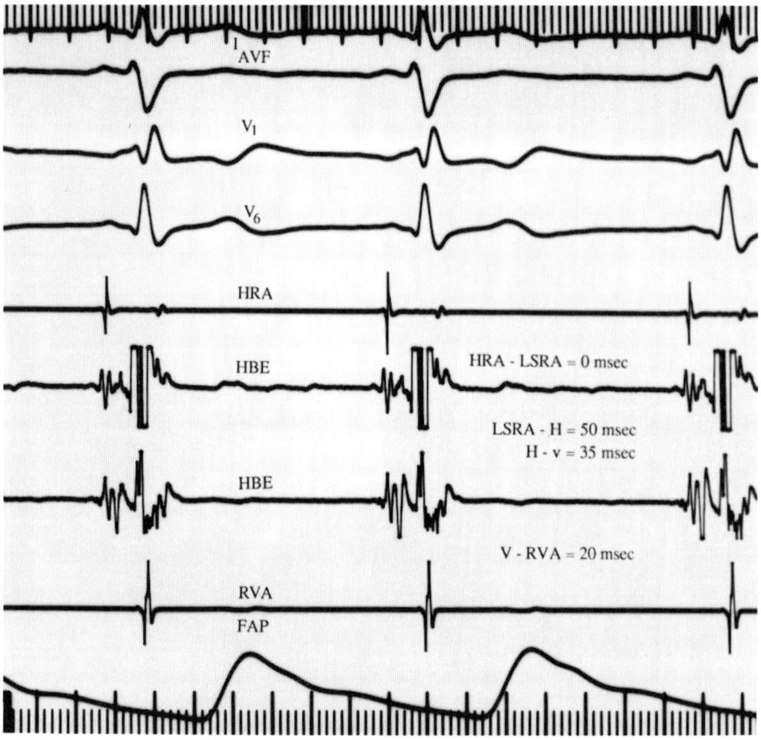

FIGURE 10–2
Surface electrocardiogram recorded simultaneously with high right atrial (HRA), low septal right atrial (LSRA), His bundle (H), and right ventricular apex (RVA) electrograms and femoral artery pressure (FAP), demonstrating distal right bundle branch block. Intracardiac right ventricular electrogram is not delayed (i.e., the V-RVA interval is 20 ms).

The prognostic importance of RBBB derives from its potential to progress to complete AV block and the possibility of sudden death. There are no long-term studies on prognosis after surgery to assess the incidence of progressive conduction system disease. Moss, Klyman, and Emmanoulides reported late-onset (permanent) complete AV block in 20 patients after repair of structural heart disease.[38] Eleven of the 20 had RBBB with left anterior hemiblock, four had only right bundle-branch block, and two had no bundle-branch block. A period of transient complete AV block during the immediate postoperative period was seen in 14 of the 20 patients. Permanent complete AV block was diagnosed from 1 month to 14 years after the operation. Friedli, Bolens, and Taktak reported electrophysiologic studies on 57 patients after repair of TOF.[39] Seven patients had a prolonged HV interval, and two of these developed permanent complete AV block several years after the repair. Both of the latter patients had transient AV block

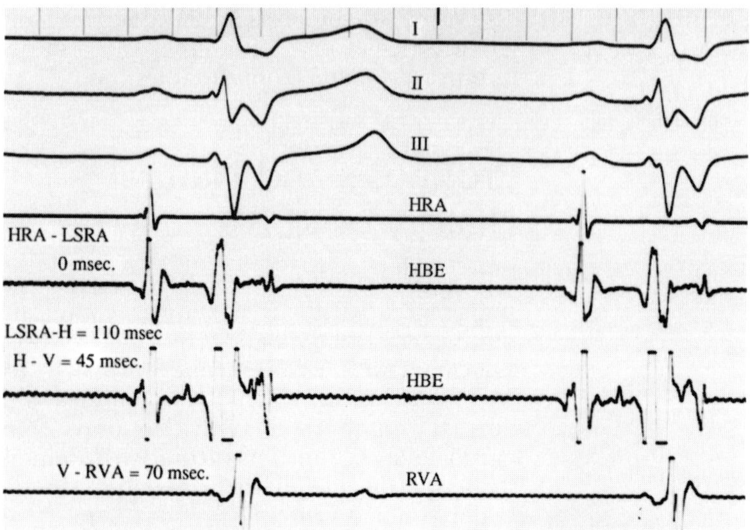

FIGURE 10–3
Surface electrocardiogram demonstrating proximal right bundle branch block. Intracardiac right ventricular electrogram is delayed. The V-RVA interval is 50 ms.

after surgery; four other patients also had had transient heart block. Mehran-Pour et al described nine patients who had resolution of postsurgical RBBB, one patient after 3 years, and one after 12 years.[40]

Familial isolated RBBB appears to be nonprogressive,[16, 17] but congenital RBBB associated with other rhythm disturbance can progress to complete AV block and sudden death.

Variation in the position of injury to the conduction system makes predictions for an individual patient difficult. The prognostic significance of the proximal versus distal damage in RBBB remains to be evaluated. Theoretically, if isolated distal RBBB exists, the patient is at less risk for future development of complete atrioventricular block.

Treatment

Isolated right bundle-branch block never requires any specific treatment. Right bundle branch block with first degree AV block is equally benign and also requires no treatment.

INCOMPLETE RIGHT BUNDLE-BRANCH BLOCK

The term "incomplete RBBB" has been used to describe any electrocardiogram with an RSR′ pattern in the anterior precordial leads and normal or only slightly prolonged QRS duration (Fig. 10–4). This term is confusing in light of the controversy surrounding proximal and distal RBBB and recognizing that there may be varying degrees of RBBB.[32] In the QRS pattern usually described by incomplete RBBB, the duration of the R′ is approximately equal to the duration of the RS wave (i.e., there is no terminal conduction delay).[11] Approximately 7% of normal children older than 6 months have this ECG pattern.[11]

The RSR′ pattern is also usually seen in patients with terminal right ventricular conduction delay. It is seen most often in patients with right ventricular volume overload such as in ostium secundum atrial septal defect (ASD) or pulmonary or tricuspid regurgitation.[41] This QRS pattern is seen in more than 85% of patients with ASD.[41] In children with ASD, the proximal right bundle-branch conduction time is normal,[42] and the conduction delay appears to be distal.[11] The lesion may result from hypertrophy of the right ventricular outflow tract, stretching of the peripheral conduction fibers, or both.[11, 43]

LEFT BUNDLE-BRANCH BLOCK

ECG

Complete left bundle-branch block (LBBB) results from impaired conduction either in the main LBB or in both the anterior and posterior fascicles. The entire QRS complex is abnormal. Its duration is longer than 90 ms in children younger than 4 years, and longer than 100 ms in children aged 4 to 16 years. The QRS complex is usually notched; leads I and aVL show an rR′ or rSR′ pattern. V_1 has a deep QS, and R waves in V_6 are tall. Because septal depolarization is aberrant, Q waves are absent in the left precordial leads (Fig. 10–5).[11]

Etiology

Complete LBBB is infrequent in childhood. Most commonly, LBBB follows surgery of the aortic valve or subvalvular area.[11] Nonsurgical causes include myocarditis, endocarditis, hypertrophic cardiomyopathy, hemochromatosis, and myocardial infarction.[11, 32, 44, 45] Fuhrman reported three siblings who had syncope associated with LBBB, which progressed to complete AV block.[46] Echocardiograms of the involved family members showed subtle findings of cardiomyopathy.

Treatment

Left bundle-branch block itself does not require treatment, but it does lead to complete AV block in a percentage of patients. This is particularly true in those with muscular dystrophy or cardiomyopathy. Thus a full cardiovascular evaluation is indicated in pediatric patients with LBBB, and a pace-

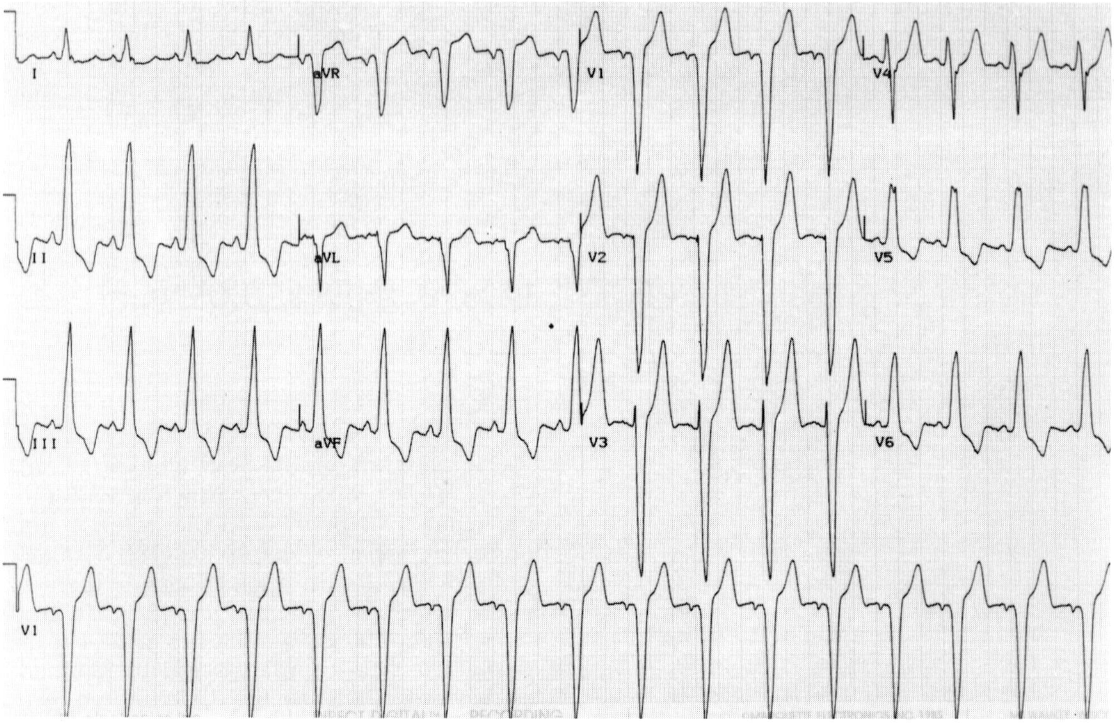

FIGURE 10–4
Left bundle branch block in a 7-year-old boy after resection of subaortic stenosis. Paper speed was 25 mm/s; calibration was 1 mV/10 mm.

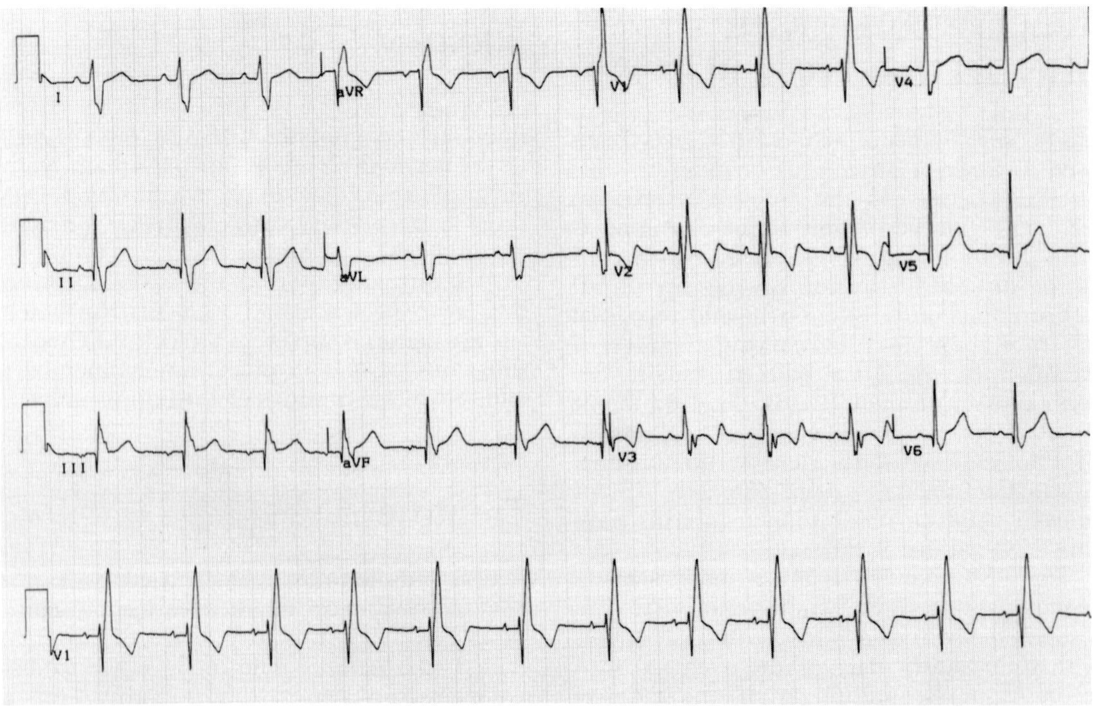

FIGURE 10–5
Right bundle branch block with left anterior hemiblock in a patient after repair of tetralogy of Fallot.

maker should be inserted in those patients experiencing syncope or near syncope.

RATE-DEPENDENT BUNDLE-BRANCH BLOCK

Bundle-branch block may be caused by either tachycardia or bradycardia. This type of BBB rarely occurs in childhood. Tachycardia-dependent BBB could result from abnormal prolongation of the action potential in diseased conduction tissue. The shortened cycle length of tachycardia would not be associated with a concomitant decrease in the refractory period, so depolarization would occur during the relative refractory period (phase 3). The net effect is the appearance of BBB when a critical heart rate is reached.[47, 48]

Bradycardia-dependent BBB, also referred to as phase 4 block, results from enhanced automaticity of the bundle branch because of ischemia or metabolic disorder. The enhanced automaticity causes a decrease in membrane potential, so depolarization occurs when the membrane potential of the bundle is high, resulting in a lower dv/dt and impaired conduction.[1]

EXERCISE-RELATED BUNDLE-BRANCH BLOCK

The incidence of exercise-related BBB in the adult population is approximately 0.4% to 0.9%.[49] Exercise-related BBB is uncommon in children; the incidence in a group of 2761 children, including 264 normal children, was 0.2%.[50] None of the children with exercise-related BBB had a normal heart, with the most common anomaly being aortic stenosis. In 1- to 8-year follow-up of the children with exercise-related BBB, there were no deaths.

OTHER CONDITIONS SIMULATING BUNDLE-BRANCH BLOCK PATTERN

Two conditions simulate BBB pattern on ECG but are not related to interrupted conduction in the bundle-branch system. The abnormal QRS complex seen in the Wolff-Parkinson-White syndrome represents a fusion between impulses conducted normally and early activation from an anomalous pathway. The resultant wide QRS may be confused with BBB, but it is actually formed by early initial activation rather than by delay. Ventricular pacemakers produce asynchronous ventricular activation with BBB pattern on surface ECG.

FASCICULAR BLOCK

Lesions of either the anterior or posterior fascicles of the LBB cause fascicular block. In fascicular block, ventricular activation (and therefore QRS duration) is nearly normal. Asymmetric depolarization of the left ventricle shifts the QRS frontal plane vector.

Left Posterior Hemiblock

Lesions of the left posterior fascicle are difficult to diagnose in children. The QRS is normal or minimally prolonged, with an axis of greater than 100° and Q waves in leads II, III, and aVF. These ECG findings also occur in normal children. Left posterior hemiblock can be diagnosed if the frontal plane QRS axis is between 120° and 180° in a child older than 1 year and occurs in the absence of anatomic causes of right axis deviation (e.g., hypertrophy). The rare instances in which it has been reported in childhood were associated with surgery, myocarditis, or endocarditis.[11]

Left Anterior Hemiblock

Left anterior hemiblock (LAH) results in asynchronous left ventricular activation in which the posterior inferior wall is activated before the anterior superior wall. The QRS duration is prolonged by less than 20 ms. The QRS axis is shifted leftward between −30° and −90°.[11] Q waves are usually present in leads I and aVL. The major QRS forces are negative in lead aVF. Delay in conduction supplied by the left anterior fascicle is seen by a late R wave (>45 ms) in aVR or a slurred terminal R wave in aVL.[51] There are also slurred S waves in the left precordium.[51]

ETIOLOGY

Left axis deviation alone cannot be used to diagnose left anterior hemiblock, as left axis deviation may be a normal variant in children. Although healthy adults may have LAH,[52] it is suggestive of organic heart disease in children. LAH in childhood has both acquired and congenital causes.[11] LAH is found among members of families with the autosomal dominant form of familial bundle-branch disease[16, 20, 46] and is associated with lentiginosis.[53] Isolated injury to the left anterior fascicle has been postulated as the cause of the left axis deviation in congenital rubella syndrome.[11] LAH may indicate anomalous origin of the left coronary artery from the pulmonary artery. The ischemia resulting from this anomaly resembles that seen in adults in whom myocardial infarction is a leading cause of LAH. In children with anomalous origin of the left coronary artery, the associated left axis deviation may also result from hypertrophy of noninfarcted myocardium.[11]

In congenital heart disease, left axis deviation is seen most often in patients with complete endocardial cushion defect and Down's syndrome.[41] It is also seen in tricuspid atresia, single ventricle, double outlet right ventricle, and transposition with VSD.[11, 41, 52] In tricuspid atresia, selective hypertrophy of the basal anterolateral left ventricle delays conduction sufficiently to cause the ECG appearance of LAH.[52]

Septal myectomy, subvalvular aortic resection, or surgical correction of VSD or TOF can be followed by LAH. This conduction defect may be seen with any injury to the interventricular septum.[51]

TREATMENT

No treatment is indicated for isolated or postoperative LAH. Even that related to surgery on the ventricular septum is unlikely to progress.

Bifascicular Block

Bifascicular block is caused by lesions affecting the RBB and the anterior fascicle, the RBB and the posterior fascicle, or both the anterior and posterior fascicles. By this criterion, complete LBBB can be viewed as bifascicular block. Bifascicular block caused by combined lesions of the RBB and the posterior fascicle is rarely diagnosed in children; most often bifascicular block in children is RBBB with left anterior hemiblock. The QRS pattern is that of RBBB with left axis deviation greater than $-30°$ (Fig. 10–6).

The most common cause of combined RBBB and LAH in children is surgery for tetralogy of Fallot, in which there is an 8% to 23% incidence.[12, 13, 36] This type of bifascicular block may follow injury to the distal portion of the bundle of His.[13] Nonsurgical causes include myocarditis, cardiomyopathy, and endocarditis.[54] Familial bifascicular block occurs and may progress to complete AV block.[20]

Combined RBBB and LAH represents the most common ECG pattern seen before complete AV block in adults.[32] The possibility that the presence of bifascicular block increases the risk of complete AV block in children has not yet been supported.[13] The RBBB-LAH type of bifascicular block may possibly be predictive of future complete AV block in those cases in which complete block occurred in the perioperative period[12] or in those patients with central damage to the right bundle branch, but even this has not been proven conclusively.

TREATMENT

No specific treatment is needed for bifascicular block, even postoperative bifascicular block. Even patients with transient surgical AV block or prolonged HV intervals have not been shown to develop complete AV block or have a significant risk of sudden death. The only exception is the Kearn-Sayre syndrome, in which bifascicular block commonly precedes complete AV block. In this situation, pacemaker implantation is clearly indicated.

Trifascicular Block

Trifascicular block, or delay in all three fascicles, can only be diagnosed by a prolonged HV interval on intracardiac electrogram measurement. It cannot be diagnosed

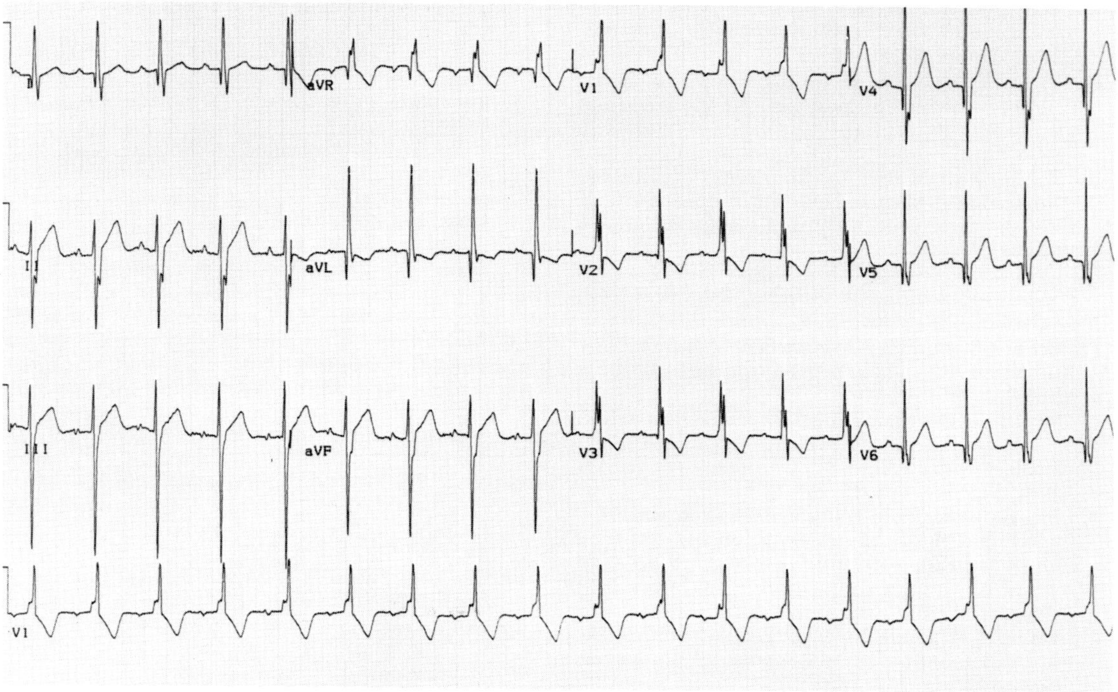

FIGURE 10–6
Right bundle branch block and left anterior fascicular block in an 11-year-old girl after repair of tetralogy of Fallot. Paper speed was 25 mm/s; calibration was 1 mV/10 mm.

from the surface ECG.[36] The ECG pattern of PR prolongation with RBBB and left axis deviation has been called trifascicular block, but intracardiac studies have shown that this pattern may be seen in patients with no delay in right ventricular depolarization and with conduction delay in the AV node rather than the His-Purkinje system.[36] Some studies in adults have reported the need for prophylactic pacing in these patients,[55] but other studies have reported no difference in symptoms or incidence of sudden death with prophylactic pacing.[32]

SUMMARY

Bundle-branch and fascicular blocks are rare in children. They are most often seen in children after open heart correction of congenital heart disease, although there are reports of congenital BBB in children with normal hearts. The real clinical significance of these conduction blocks is not known.

References

1. Scheinman MM, Goldschalager NF, Peters RW: Bundle branch block. Cardiovasc Clin 11:57–80, 1980.
2. James TN, Sherf L: Fine structure of the His bundle. Circulation 44:9–18, 1971.
3. Massing GK, James TN: Anatomical configuration of the His bundle and bundle branches in the human heart. Circulation 53:609–612, 1976.
4. Scher AM, Spach MS: Cardiac depolarization repolarization and the electrocardiogram. In Handbook of Physiology, The Cardiovascular System I. Washington, DC, American Physiological Society, pp 357–391.
5. Rossi L: Histopathology of conducting system in left anterior hemiblock. Br Heart J 38:1304–1311, 1976.
6. Flowers NC: Left bundle branch block: A continuously evolving concept. Seminar on the changing role of electrocardiography in clinical practice, IV. J Am Coll Cardiol 9:3:684–697, 1987.
7. Wyndham CR, Meeran MK, Smith T, et al: Epicardial activation of the intact human heart without conduction defect. Circulation 59:161–168, 1979.
8. Kastor JA, Godreyer BN, Moore N, et al: Interventricular conduction in man studied with an endocardial electrode catheter mapping technique. Circulation 51:786–796, 1975.
9. Nagao K, Toyama J, Kodama I, et al: Role of the conduction system in the endocardial excitation spread in the right ventricle. Am J Cardiol 48:863–870, 1981.
10. Garson A: Derivation of the electrocardiogram. In The Electrocardiogram in Infants and Children. Philadelphia, Lea & Febiger, 1983, pp 39–48.
11. Garson A: Interventricular conduction disturbances. In The Electrocardiogram in Infants and Children. Philadelphia, Lea & Febiger, 1983, pp 119–142.
12. Krongrad E: Postoperative arrhythmias in patients with congenital heart disease. Chest 85:107–113, 1984.

13. Vetter VL, Horowitz LN: Electrophysiologic residua and sequelae of surgery for congenital heart defects. Am J Cardiol 50:588–604, 1982.
14. Krongrad E: Prognosis for patients with congenital heart disease and postoperative intraventricular conduction defects. Circulation 57:867–870, 1978.
15. Simonsen EE, Madsen EG: Four cases of right-sided bundle branch block and one case of atrioventricular block in three generations of a family. Br Heart J 32:501–504, 1970.
16. Husson GS, Blackman MS, Rogers MC, et al: Familial congenital bundle branch system disease. Am J Cardiol 32:365–369, 1973.
17. Esscher E, Hardell L, Michaelson M: Familial isolated complete right bundle branch block. Br Heart J 37:745–747, 1975.
18. Stephan E: Hereditary bundle branch system defect. Am Heart J 95:89–95, 1978.
19. Stephan E: Hereditary bundle branch defect. Am Heart J 97:708–718, 1979.
20. Schaal SF, Seidensticker J, Goodman R, et al: Familial right bundle branch block, left axis deviation, complete heart block and early death. A heritable disorder of cardiac conduction. Ann Intern Med 79:63–66, 1973.
21. Komajda M, Frank R, Vedel J, et al: Intracardiac conduction defects in dystrophia myotonica. Br Heart J 43:315–320, 1980.
22. Sanyal S, Johnson W: Cardiac conduction abnormalities in children with Duchenne's progressive muscular dystrophy. Circulation 66:853–863, 1982.
23. Harris LK: Transient right bundle branch block following blunt chest trauma. Am J Cardiol 23:884, 1969.
24. Kehoe RF, Bauernfeind R, Tommaso C, et al: Cardiac conduction defects in polymyositis: Electrophysiologic studies in four patients. Ann Intern Med 94:41–43, 1981.
25. Schneider JF, Thomas HE, Kreger BE, et al: Newly acquired right bundle branch block. Ann Intern Med 92:37–42, 1979.
26. Krongrad E, Bharati S, Steinfeld L, et al: Histologic observations of the cardiac conduction system in a patient with postoperative bilateral bundle branch block. Am J Cardiol 40:635–640, 1977.
27. Gelband H, Waldo AL, Kaiser GA, et al: Etiology of right bundle branch block in patients undergoing total correction of tetralogy of Fallot. Circulation 44:1022–1033, 1971.
28. Krongrad E, Hefler SE, Bowman FO, et al: Further observations on the etiology of the right bundle branch block pattern following right ventriculotomy. Circulation 50:1105–1113, 1974.
29. Goor DA, Lavee J, Smolinshky A, et al: Correction of tetralogy of Fallot with reduced incidence of right bundle branch block. Am J Cardiol 48:892–896, 1981.
30. VanLier TAR, Harinck E, Hitchcock JF, et al: Complete right bundle branch block after surgical closure of perimembranous ventricular septal defect. Eur Heart J 6:959–962, 1985.
31. Hazan E, Bizal O, Bax JP, et al: Is right bundle branch block avoidable in surgical correction of tetralogy of Fallot? Circulation 62:852–854, 1980.
32. Josephson ME: Intraventricular conduction disturbances. In Clinical Cardiac Electrophysiology. Philadelphia, Lea & Febiger, 1979, pp 103–118.
33. Mehta AV, Wolff GS, Tamer DF, et al: Right ventricular activation time in children. Pediatr Cardiol 2:47–49, 1982.
34. Snug RJ, Tamer DM, Garcia OL, et al: Analysis of surgically induced right bundle branch block pattern using intracardiac recording techniques. Circulation 54:442, 1976.
35. Horowitz LN, Alexander JA, Edmunds LH: Postoperative right bundle branch block. Identification of three levels of block. Circulation 62:319–328, 1980.
36. Friedli B, Bolens M: Intraventricular conduction disturbance after correction of tetralogy of Fallot: Can bifascicular and trifascicular block be diagnosed from the surface ECG? Pediatr Cardiol 6:133–136, 1985.
37. Yasui H, Yoshitoshi M, Komoni M, et al: Cardiodynamic effects of experimental right bundle branch block in canine hearts with normal and hypertrophied right ventricles. Am Heart J 109:69–77, 1985.
38. Moss AJ, Klyman G, Emmanoulides GC: Late onset complete heart block: Newly recognized sequela of cardiac surgery. Am J Cardiol 30:884–887, 1972.
39. Friedli B, Bolens M, Taktak M: Conduction disturbances after correction of tetralogy of Fallot: Are electrophysiologic studies of prognostic value? J Am Coll Cardiol 11:1:162–165, 1988.
40. Mehran-Pour M, Borkat G, Liebman J, et al: Resolution of surgically induced right bundle-branch block. Ann Thorac Surg 23:139–144, 1977.
41. Liebman J, Plonsey R, Gillette PC: Interpretation of Conduction Abnormalities in Pediatric Electrocardiography. Baltimore, Williams and Wilkins, 1985, pp 172–191.
42. Snug RJ, Tamer DM, Agha A, et al: Etiology of the electrocardiographic pattern of "incomplete right bundle branch block" in atrial septal defect: An electrophysiologic study. J Pediatr 87(6;2):1182–1186, 1975.
43. Moore EN, Boineau JP, Patterson DF: Incomplete right bundle branch block: An electrocardiographic enigma and possible misnomer. Circulation 44:678–687, 1971.
44. Barson WJ, Craenem J, Hosier DM, et al: Survival following myocarditis and myocardial calcification associated with infection by coxsackie virus B-4. Pediatrics 68:79–82, 1981.
45. Cohen HC, Singer DH: Bundle branch block and other forms of aberrant intraventricular conduction: Clinical aspects. In Cardiac Arrhythmias. Philadelphia, JB Lippincott, 1987, pp 413–451.
46. Fuhrman BP, Bass JL, Laurence C, et al: Progressive cardiac conduction defect and cardiomyopathy in siblings with syncope. Pediatr Cardiol 2:57–62, 1982.
47. Kinoshita S: Mechanism of tachycardia-dependent bundle branch block. Am J Cardiol 53:1456–1457, 1984.
48. Jalife J, Antzelevitch C, Lamanna V, et al: Rate-dependent changes in excitability of depressed cardiac Purkinje fibers as a mechanism of intermittent bundle branch block. Circulation 67:912–922, 1983.
49. Wayne VS, Bishop RL, Cook L, et al: Exercise induced bundle branch block. Am J Cardiol 52:283–286, 1983.
50. Bricker JT, Traweek MS, Danford DA, et al: Exercise related bundle branch block in children. Am J Cardiol 56:796–797, 1985.
51. Milliken JA: Isolated and complicated left anterior fascicular block: A review of electrocardiographic criteria. J Electrocardiol 16:199–212, 1983.

52. Perloff JD, Roberts NK, Cabeen WR: Left axis deviation: A reassessment. Circulation 60:12–15, 1979.
53. Sharratt GP, Virmani S: Left axis deviation in otherwise healthy children. Pediatr Cardiol 6:7–10, 1985.
54. Kulbertus HE, deLaval-Rutten F, Dubois M: Prognostic significance of left anterior hemiblock and right bundle branch block in mass screening. Am J Cardiol 41:305, 1978.
55. Pine MB, Oxen M, Ciafone R, et al: Excess mortality and morbidity associated with right bundle branch and left anterior fascicular block. J Am Coll Cardiol 1:1207–1212, 1983.

CHAPTER 11

PREMATURE ATRIAL CONTRACTIONS AND ATRIAL TACHYARRHYTHMIAS

Co-burn J. Porter

PREMATURE ATRIAL CONTRACTIONS

Criteria

A premature atrial contraction (PAC) is defined as a recognizable premature P wave on the surface electrocardiogram, generally with morphology and mean vector that are different from those of a sinus P wave. If a regular sinus rhythm is present, any P wave occurring more than 0.08 s before the expected sinus P wave is considered premature. When sinus arrhythmia is present, a premature atrial beat is more difficult to diagnose. An abrupt decrease in the PP interval must be differentiated from a gradually increasing and decreasing PP interval, as is found in sinus arrhythmia. Generally, if the underlying rhythm is irregular, the diagnosis of a PAC is most easily made on the basis of a different morphology rather than simply by the timing.

Frequently, a PAC enters the sinus node, depolarizes the pacemaker cells in the node, and resets the timing interval. If this happens, the interval from the PAC to the next sinus P wave should be the same as the interval between the normal sinus P waves. However, two factors prevent this from occurring.[1] First, there is a certain finite time for the conduction from the focus of the PAC through the atrium and perinodal cells to the pacemaker cells in the sinus node to discharge them, after which spontaneous phase 4 depolarization occurs, again allowing the impulse to travel through the perinodal cells to re-emerge in the atrium. This finite period will lengthen the basic interval from the PAC to the next sinus P wave by 10–100 ms. Second, premature discharge of a pacemaker such as the sinus node by a PAC may depress the sinus node's automaticity and delay its return. When this occurs, there can even be a change in the morphology of the sinus P wave because of a shift in the pacemaker locus within the sinus node to an ectopic locus or to alteration in the intra-atrial conduction.

A PAC is conducted to the ventricle normally, aberrantly, or is blocked. In general, the refractory period of the atrioventricular node exceeds that of the atria; therefore, a very premature P wave may find the atrioventricular node refractory to conducting an impulse to the ventricles ("nonconducted" or "blocked" PAC). However, a slightly later PAC may find the atrioventricular node ready to conduct the impulse through the His-Purkinje system to the ventricles. If the impulse is conducted rapidly through the atrioventricular node, it may find one of the bundle branches refractory to conduction, resulting in aberrancy of the QRS complex (Fig. 11–1). The duration of the refractory period of the bundle branches is directly related to the preceding RR interval; a long RR interval results in a long refractory period of the bundle branches. However, if the PAC occurs relatively late, there may have been enough time for the bundle branches to repolarize completely, and the impulse will be conducted with a normal narrow QRS complex. Frequently, the PAC will be buried in the T wave, and careful inspection, including

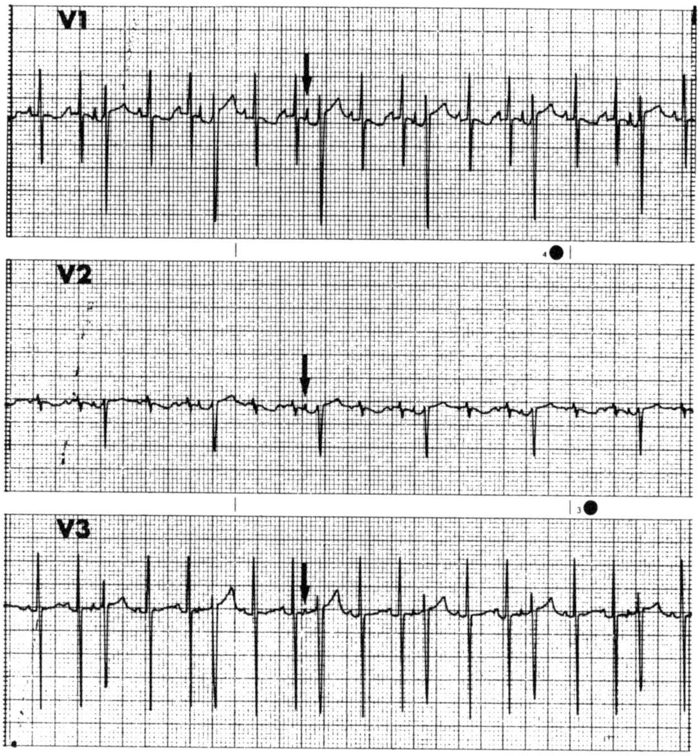

FIGURE 11–1
Electrocardiogram of leads V_1, V_2, and V_3 recorded simultaneously. Frequent premature atrial beats are seen in a trigeminal pattern. Arrows indicate the third premature P wave. All premature P waves are followed by a wide QRS complex with a morphology different from that of the normal narrow QRS complexes. These are examples of aberrant conduction.

the use of multiple leads, is necessary to find it. Buried PACs may be the basis for unexplained "sinus bradycardia" (blocked atrial bigeminy) or "single premature ventricular contractions" (aberrant conduction) (Fig. 11–2). It is rare for PACs and premature ventricular contractions to occur together, and if a tracing is encountered that appears to have both arrhythmias, the T waves should be especially scanned for buried P waves; most often, the wide QRS beats are PACs with aberrancy if there are other PACs with normal QRS. This is extremely common in newborns.

Clinical Manifestations

In most patients, the cause of PACs is unknown. Usually, they are of such a benign nature that no systematic invasive studies need be performed. Using 24-hour ambulatory monitoring, Southall, Richards, Mitchell, Johnston, Shinebourne, et al[2, 3] and Scott, Williams, and Fiddler[4] studied healthy children. PACs occurred in 14% of infants (all having fewer than 12 PACs per hour) and in 13% to 21% of older children. Salice, Segantini, Locati, et al[5] prospectively followed up 6900 infants who had 24-hour ambulatory monitoring at 4 days of age and at 2, 4, and 6 months of age. At 4 days of age, 47 of the 6900 (0.68%) had PACs; of these, 33 were available for regular follow-up. PACs were still present in five of the 33 at 2 months, in two at 6 months, and in one at 1 year. All patients remained asymptomatic. Of 5618 infants who had no PACs at 4 days old and who were available for long-term follow-up, 17 (0.3%) developed PACs by 2 months. Eight of the 17 were followed for up to 1 year, after which time only one still had PACs.

Causes of PACs can be divided into acute and chronic factors.[6] Acute causes include mechanical factors (e.g., central venous catheters), hypokalemia, hypercalcemia, hypoxia, hypoglycemia, and drugs (digitalis, sympathomimetic agents, and imipramine). The chronic causes include atrial enlargement and the state of the atrium after atrial surgery. Most often, the heart is otherwise normal.

Management

Once PACs are found on a standard electrocardiogram, a search should be made for

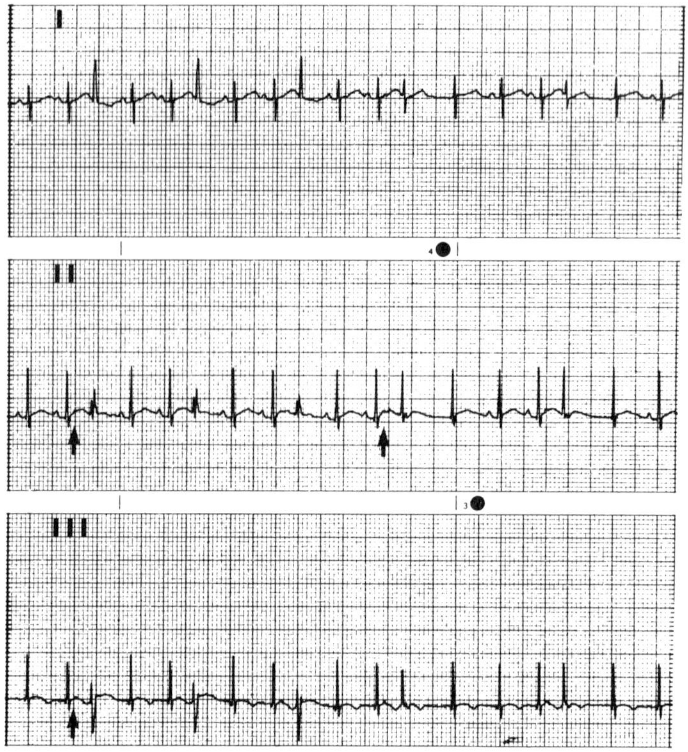

FIGURE 11–2
Electrocardiogram of leads I, II, and III recorded simultaneously. In lead I, premature P waves are not seen, and the premature wide QRS complexes appear to be premature ventricular beats. However, close inspection of leads II and III reveals P waves (*arrows*) preceding the premature QRS complexes, indicating premature atrial beats with aberrant conduction.

mechanical, metabolic, medicinal, or hemodynamic causes. If these factors are ruled out, 24-hour ambulatory monitoring may be performed, looking for episodes of supraventricular tachycardia. If older children who can give a symptom history are asymptomatic, and only have PACs, 24-hour ambulatory monitoring is probably not necessary. As long as PACs are single and do not predispose to supraventricular tachycardia, they do not require treatment. If, however, they are the trigger event for supraventricular tachycardia or atrial flutter or fibrillation, they should be prevented. Generally, treatment with digoxin may be enough, but rarely a combination of digoxin and a type I or II agent may be necessary (see section on treatment of atrial flutter).

CHAOTIC ATRIAL RHYTHM

Criteria

In 1969, Phillips, Spano, and Burch[7] reported 31 patients who had a rhythm the authors called "chaotic atrial mechanism." The arrhythmia was characterized by (1) clearly recognizable P waves of at least three waveforms in one lead of the electrocardiogram; (2) absence of a single, persistent, dominant atrial pacemaker (distinct from normal sinus rhythm with multiple and multiform premature atrial beats); and (3) variable PP intervals, RR intervals, and PR intervals (Fig. 11–3). The atrial impulses could be blocked or conducted (either normally or with aberrancy). Before this time, Shine, Kaston and Yurchak[8] had reported studies in patients with an arrhythmia that they called "multifocal atrial tachycardia." As a part of the criteria for diagnosis, they included an atrial rate greater than 100 bpm; otherwise the criteria were essentially the same as those of Phillips, Spano, and Burch. Since several of their patients had atrial rates of less than 100 bpm, Phillips, Spano, and Burch preferred the term "chaotic atrial mechanism." In 1972, Berlinerblau and Feder[9] combined all of the criteria and called the arrhythmia "chaotic atrial rhythm," or CAR.

Clinical Manifestations

The early reports of CAR were on adult patients. The 31 patients reported by Phillips, Spano, and Burch were found in a review of

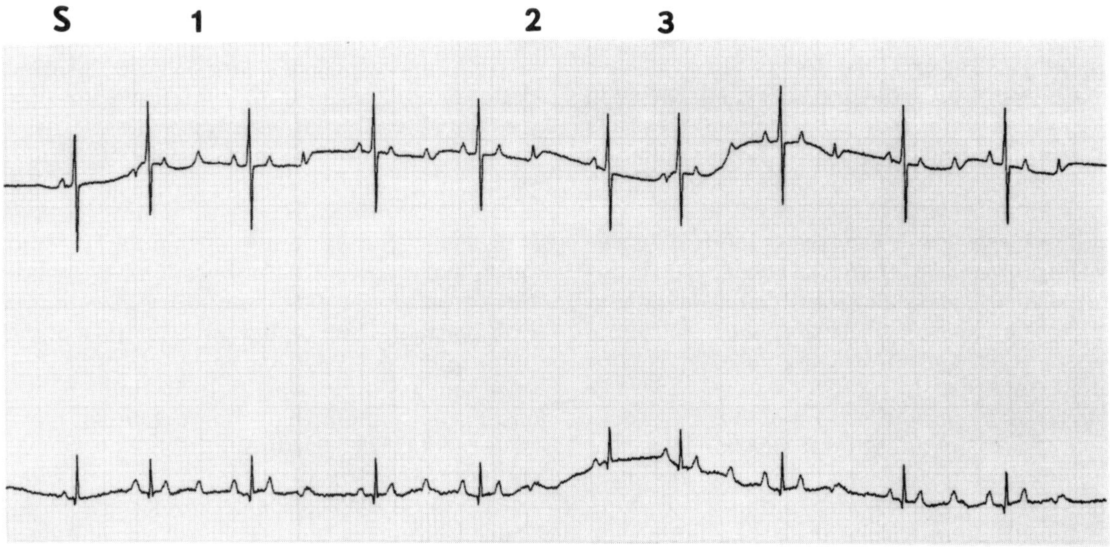

FIGURE 11–3
Electrocardiogram of two surface leads recorded simultaneously, demonstrating chaotic atrial rhythm. A normal sinus P wave (*S*) is seen first, then there are three different P-wave morphologies (1,2,3), with variable PP, PR, and RR intervals.

approximately 24,000 electrocardiograms during a 2-year period.[7] The patients ranged in age from 53 to 80 years, with an average age of 68.5 years. The ventricular rate was between 56 bpm and 200 bpm, with 61% of the patients having a rate of 101–150 bpm. The arrhythmia lasted from a few seconds to months or even years. Many patients complained of dyspnea associated with the arrhythmia, and many had pulmonary disease and diabetes mellitus. Other atrial arrhythmias were common, including atrial flutter, atrial fibrillation, and paroxysmal atrial tachycardia with atrioventricular block. Fifty-eight percent of patients were receiving digitalis when CAR occurred, and in 29%, digitalis toxicity was suspected. In two patients, digitalization resulted in cessation of the arrhythmia, with no recurrence. Quinidine, procainamide, and phenytoin were not helpful in the few instances in which they were tried. Sixteen of the 31 patients (51.6%) died during hospitalization; however, this was not unexpected, considering the age and associated cardiac and pulmonary problems. Five of the 16 patients who died (31%) had clinical evidence of digitalis toxicity. Twelve of the patients who died had CAR at the time of death.

In a review of 60,000 electrocardiograms taken during a 6-year period, Lipson and Naimi[10] found 31 adult patients with CAR. The longest episode lasted 1 week, but recurrences were common. In addition, they found that 58% of patients eventually developed atrial fibrillation or flutter. Again, a high percentage of patients (39%) had significant acute or chronic pulmonary disease. Only two patients were suspected of having digitalis toxicity, and most patients showed little response to digitalis therapy. There was some improvement in 11 of 24 patients. Berlinerblau and Feder,[9] using the same criteria for CAR, found 31 patients with CAR among 8000 patients (0.4%) seen during a 1-year period. The average age of the group was 74 years, and there was a high incidence of bronchopulmonary disease. Seventeen patients were receiving digitalis when CAR occurred, and in three, discontinuation of digitalis resulted in conversion to sinus rhythm. In 13 patients, continuation or initiation of digitalis had no effect on the arrhythmia, while in seven patients, digoxin seemed to convert the arrhythmia to sinus rhythm. CAR did not appear to be a precursor to atrial fibrillation in their study, nor did it appear to be a cause of death.

More recently, there have been several reports of CAR occurring in pediatric patients.[11–16] The earliest report was by Farooki and Green, who described two infants with "multifocal atrial tachycardia."[11] Both infants were younger than 5 days old, and both had irregular heart rates without evidence of heart failure. The atrial rates were between

115 bpm and 500 bpm, with a ventricular rate of 115 to 250 bpm. The PP, RR, and PR intervals were variable, and multiple P wave shapes were present (five in one and three in the other). Both patients were treated orally with digoxin, and by 1 week after initiation of therapy, both were in sinus rhythm. Both patients survived.

Using the same criteria of at least three different P-wave shapes, variable PP intervals, isoelectric baseline between P waves, and a mean atrial rate of greater than 150 bpm, Bisset et al[12] found 10 patients with "chaotic atrial tachycardia"; there was a wide age range at presentation (1 day to 18 years). Five patients had normal hearts, four had congenital heart disease (three had had previous intracardiac repair), and one had rheumatic carditis. Eight of the 10 patients were asymptomatic, and two complained of palpitations; no patient had signs or symptoms of congestive heart failure. In addition, half of the patients had premature atrial contractions or paroxysmal atrial tachycardia. All patients received digoxin for treatment, but only one (the patient with rheumatic carditis) may have benefited from it. However, that patient had also received quinidine simultaneously. No patient demonstrated a slowing of the atrial rate or decrease in conduction of atrial impulses after digoxin therapy, and one patient may have died because of digoxin toxicity. All patients except the one who died had reversion to a normal sinus rhythm.

More recent reports have noted only young patients. Liberthson and Colan[13] found nine patients who were between 1 day and 5 months of age; Toussaint, Hofstetter, and von Bernuth[14] found four patients, all younger than 4 months of age; and Ming-yi, Zhi-fang, and Xiu-yu[15] found 22 infants, all younger than 2 years (17 were between the ages of 1 month and 6 months). In Liberthson and Colan's group, two infants were born with paroxysmal atrial tachycardia and heart failure requiring digoxin therapy.[13] In these two patients and an additional one, CAR developed while the patients were taking digoxin. A total of four infants had intermittent sustained atrial tachycardia with rates from 140 bpm to 270 bpm, and these four were treated with digoxin; two of the four also received quinidine, and three of the four also received propranolol. In no patient did medical therapy seem to convert CAR to sinus rhythm. In eight patients, CAR reverted spontaneously 1 day to 20 months after onset; in one patient, CAR persisted at the age of 7 months and alternated with periods of paroxysmal atrial tachycardia. Also, all nine patients had periodic sinus arrest with slow junctional escape rates as low as 40 bpm during ambulatory monitoring. However, no patient died during follow-up.

Of the 22 infants reported by Ming-yi, Zhi-fang, and Xiu-yu and colleagues, 19 had pulmonary disease manifested as bronchopneumonia or upper respiratory infection.[15] Five patients had congenital heart disease manifested as a ventricular septal defect, but only one of these was in heart failure. An additional patient had heart failure from endocardial fibroelastosis. Of the 22 patients, six had short runs of atrial flutter, with rates from 375 bpm to 430 bpm, and six had sinus arrest lasting 1.0–1.2 s. Because many antiarrhythmic medications, including digoxin, propranolol, practolol, phenytoin, and verapamil, were ineffective in the first 10 patients, eight of the 12 later patients were not treated with any medication. The remaining four patients received amiodarone or propranolol (or both) for a brief time, without effect. CAR reverted to sinus rhythm in 20 patients and remained unchanged in two patients, both of whom had ventricular septal defects. Overall, 19 patients survived; two patients with ventricular septal defect died of unknown cause at home, and one died of respiratory failure in the hospital.

Recently, Yeager, Hougen, and Levy reported the sudden deaths of three infants with CAR.[16] One infant had multiple congenital anomalies, including hydrocephalus, micrognathia, hypospadias, undescended testes, and tetralogy of Fallot. When the patient was 3 weeks of age, digoxin therapy was started for CAR. At 3 months of age, the patient developed sudden respiratory distress during a feeding. A roentgenogram of the chest showed bilateral infiltrates, and death occurred before an electrocardiogram could be performed. The second infant was discovered to have an irregular rhythm at 6 weeks of age. An electrocardiogram showed CAR, and oral digoxin therapy was started. Four weeks later, an electrocardiogram showed normal sinus rhythm, and the digoxin therapy was stopped. Two weeks later, a repeat electrocardiogram showed normal sinus rhythm, and at 7 months of age, the child was found dead in his crib. Findings at autopsy were unremarkable. The third infant had intrauterine supraventricular tachycardia; the tachycardia was still present at birth. Digoxin and propranolol were required to control the rhythm. Despite frequent episodes of "ectopic atrial tachycardia," the propranolol therapy was discontinued at 2 months, and the digoxin therapy was stopped at 3 months. At 5 months, the child experienced symptoms of an upper respiratory infection, and while waiting to be examined in an emergency room, she became pale and unresponsive. An electrocardiogram showed periods of "ectopic atrial tachycardia" at a rate of 200 bpm, alternating with periods of sinus bradycardia as slow as 50 bpm. The heart rate became progressively slower despite treatment, and she died. At autopsy, the heart showed mild-to-moderate enlargement, mild diffuse endocardial thickening of both the left atrium and the left ventricle, and hypertrophy and dilatation of the left atrial appendage. Microscopic evaluation revealed interstitial inflammation and patchy fibrosis.

Treatment

In pediatrics, CAR seems to be a disease primarily of infants. Overall, there is a better prognosis for the infant than for the adult. Frequently, infants with CAR also manifest other atrial arrhythmias, such as premature atrial contractions, paroxysmal atrial tachycardia, and atrial flutter.[11–15] The exact mechanism is unknown. Many infants with CAR are asymptomatic; even those with rapid atrial rates may not show signs or symptoms of heart failure. Perhaps symptoms are lacking because the rapid atrial rates are not sustained. Those infants who do experience heart failure have sustained episodes of atrial tachycardia or atrial flutter. Many authors recommend not treating patients who have CAR.[12, 15, 16] Digoxin alone is usually not an effective agent to convert or prevent CAR, although it may allow for a reduced ventricular rate in infants with CAR and a rapid ventricular rate. For infants with episodes of rapid sustained atrial tachycardia or those with atrial flutter, treatment is indicated. To prevent these arrhythmias, a type Ia or Ic antiarrhythmic agent should be used (see section on atrial flutter treatment). Recently, Garson and colleagues have used encainide (type Ic) for treatment of infants with CAR and atrial flutter.* Because atrial flutter can result in rapid conduction through the atrioventricular node, especially after treatment with a type Ia agent, digoxin should be used to slow atrioventricular conduction. Because some patients with CAR may have sinus node dysfunction, 24-hour ambulatory monitoring is necessary, especially if antiarrhythmic agents, which further depress sinus node function, are used. Rarely, amiodarone has been used to control CAR in pediatric patients with signs of congestive heart failure.[17]

ATRIAL FLUTTER

Classically, atrial flutter has been defined as the presence of a characteristic electrocardiographic pattern consisting of a "sawtooth" appearance of the atrial depolarization ("flutter" waves), seen best in leads II, III, aVF, and V_1 (Fig. 11–4). In addition, in adults, the atrial rate is approximately 300 bpm. However, some variations are often seen and are still consistent with a diagnosis of atrial flutter. Frequently, the P waves are more undulating (Fig. 11–5) than "sawtooth," and occasionally, atrial rates of 350 bpm to 600 bpm in infants and 250 bpm to 350 bpm in older children are seen. While it is rare to have 1:1 atrioventricular conduction in adults, rapid atrioventricular conduction can be seen in children.

Mechanism

Atrial flutter is classified generally as a primary atrial tachyarrhythmia, a tachyarrhythmia confined solely to atrial tissue. There is no participation of the atrioventricular node structure, His-Purkinje tissue, or ventricular myocardium in the primary mechanism. During the past 60 years, several different mechanisms have been proposed to explain atrial flutter. However, no one mechanism explains all of the unique characteristics of spontaneous atrial flutter, and most likely it is the result of a complex multifactorial process. Although "atrial flutter" is the term applied to a group of atrial tachyarrhythmias with atrial rates from 240 bpm to 300 bpm in adults and with undulating P

*Personal communication.

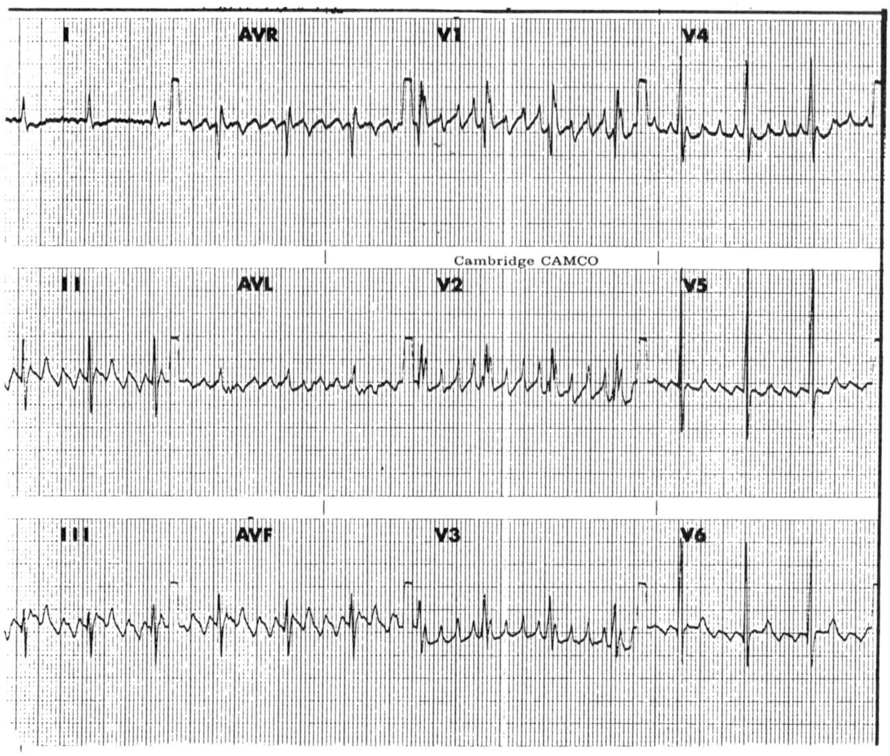

FIGURE 11–4
Standard 12-lead electrocardiogram showing atrial flutter with classic "sawtooth" flutter waves in leads II, III, aVF, V_1, V_2, and V_3. There is 4:1 atrioventricular conduction.

waves, this designation tells nothing about the mechanism and does not add specificity to the electrocardiographic findings. In spite of much research into the mechanisms of atrial flutter, a gap exists between the mechanisms and the findings on the electrocardiogram.

At present, there are three proposed electrophysiologic mechanisms for tachyarrhythmia: (1) automaticity, (2) reentry, and (3) triggered activity. To date, research into the mechanism of atrial flutter has focused on reentry. It is now generally accepted that atrial flutter is not an automatic rhythm, and there is no supporting evidence for triggered activity.

Both animal and human studies in atrial flutter have shown that there are two types of reentry or circus motion: a microreentrant loop (also known as "focal" or intramyocardial reentry), and a macroreentrant loop (also known as "obstacle atrial flutter").[18] In order for reentry to occur in the atrium, certain causal factors should be present: (1) an anatomic, or geometric, substrate abnormality in the atrial myocardium (that is, an obstacle or fibrosis creating a discontinuity in conduction); (2) a functional substrate resulting in inhomogeneous repolarization of the myocardium within or near a potential reentry circuit; (3) an abnormal unifocal eccentric impulse origin as opposed to a normal multicentric impulse origin (a single site of origin produces slow, uneven initial depolarization with islands of conduction delay); (4) an initiating or trigger event, represented by an atrial premature depolarization; and (5) interactions among components 1 through 4.[18, 18a]

In the mid 1970s, Allessie, Bonke, and Schopman published a series of papers showing that sustained circus movement tachycardia could be produced in an isolated segment of left atrium of the rabbit after addition of carbamoyl.[19, 20] The reentrant circuit was small and moved about a central area of converging wavelets, which served as an "obstacle" for the impulse to move around. These researchers referred to this mechanism of repolarization inhomogeneity and vortical reentry as the "leading circle" concept: the "head" of excitability chases the "tail" of refractoriness, such that there is no excitable gap. Boineau found similar results in his animal experiments but believed that the circuit was too small and that the rate

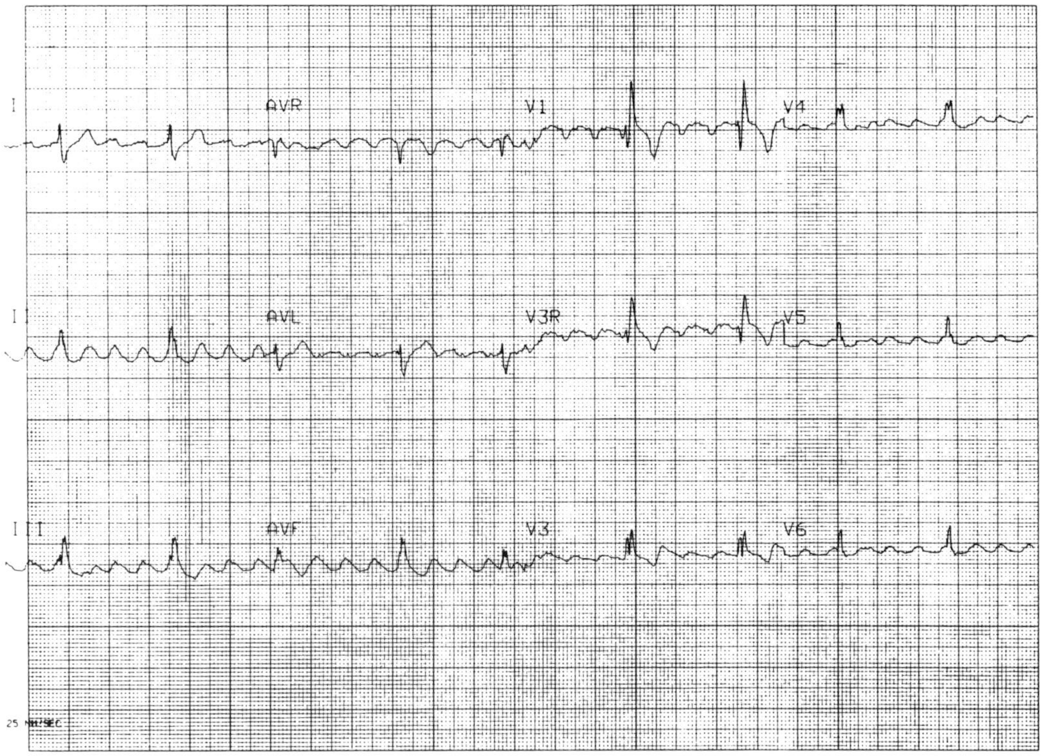

FIGURE 11–5
Standard 12-lead electrocardiogram showing atrial flutter with undulating P waves in all leads.

was faster than the rate found in spontaneous atrial flutter.[18] Because of short cycle lengths, the reentrant circuits terminated spontaneously or degenerated into atrial fibrillation. However, recent work in clinical electrophysiology laboratories by Watson and Josephson,[21] Gomes et al,[22] Friedman et al,[23] and Cosio et al[24] has provided support for a focal reentry circuit in humans. Gomes et al[22] reported a patient whose surface electrocardiogram showed atrial flutter at 240 bpm while the intracardiac electrograms showed simultaneous (1) sinus-like rhythm around the sinus node, (2) flutter or fibrillation (or both) of the remaining right atrium, (3) fibrillation of the left atrium, and (4) transient degeneration of flutter into fibrillation and back to flutter in other areas of the right atrium. Friedman et al[23] studied two patients who had spontaneous atrial flutter and demonstrated interatrial dissociation or conduction delay, suggesting that a significant portion of the right atrium is not essential for maintaining the arrhythmia. In addition, rapid atrial pacing from different sites in the atrium did not terminate or alter the flutter cycle.

Macroreentrant circuits have been postulated for years as a mechanism of atrial flutter. Rytand[25] noted the classic studies of Mayer, Mines, Garrey, Lewis et al, Rosenbleuth and Garcia-Ramos, Kimura et al, and Hayden, which showed the importance of circulating depolarization waves propagating around artificial obstacles and natural orifices in cardiac muscle. For circus motion to occur, the tissue ahead of the wave had to have repolarized. This required a sufficiently large obstacle or orifice, a small orifice with slow conduction of the wave in the circuit, or a short wavelength caused by a uniformly short repolarization time. In 1980, Boineau et al[26] reported a dog that had spontaneous stable atrial flutter. Two forms of atrial flutter were present, and both forms had a consistent reproducible rate and electrocardiographic pattern. Extensive investigation revealed that both forms of atrial flutter were caused by a macroreentrant circuit and that the basic substrate for both forms of reentry was a region of myocardial band discontinuity (with decremental conduction) in the right atrium, which combined with the contiguous vena cava to form a large anatomic obstacle, creating a sufficiently long pathway for stable atrial flutter. If viewed anteriorly, one wave front had a counterclockwise motion around the combined region of discontinuity in the superior and inferior vena cava, traveling cephalad in the atrial septal wall and caudally in the atrial free wall. The atrial rate was 343 bpm, and the surface electrocardiogram showed flutter waves identical to the pattern seen in man and referred to as type I or typical atrial flutter. In the other form, the wave front traveled in a clockwise fashion over the same tissues with an atrial rate of 397 bpm. The surface electrocardiogram showed type II or atypical atrial flutter waves. Work by Inoue et al[27] and Disertori et al[28] has provided evidence for a macroreentrant circuit in humans by showing that properly timed extrastimuli from multiple sites in the atria could enter the circus pathway earlier than expected and shorten the flutter cycle. Both studies have proven the existence of an "excitable gap," which is necessary for a macroreentrant circuit.

Waldo, Plumb, and Henthorn have provided further support for a mechanism of reentry and an excitable gap by demonstrating transient entrainment and interruption of atrial flutter.[29] Transient entrainment of a tachycardia by overdrive pacing is defined as an increase in a tachycardia rate to equal the pacing rate (which is faster than the original tachycardia rate), with resumption of the original rate when pacing is stopped abruptly or slowed below the original intrinsic tachycardia rate. Transient entrainment indicates there is an excitable gap that can be entered. If the pacing rate is increased to a point at which the morphology of the flutter wave changes, then the pacing wave has resulted in orthodromic and antedromic waves that collide. When pacing is stopped, the original tachycardia has ceased. These characteristics support a reentry mechanism. Waldo's group defined two types of atrial flutter independent of flutter wave morphology or polarity: type I (classic 240 bpm to 340 bpm), which can always be influenced by rapid atrial pacing from sites high in the right atrium; and type II (very rapid, 340 bpm to 433 bpm), which cannot be influenced by pacing but does convert spontaneously to type I. Type I is more consistent with circus movement, having an excitable gap, and type II is more consistent with the "leading circle" concept, having no excitable gap. Recently, Beckman et al have shown that classic transient entrainment can be demonstrated in typical and atypical atrial flutter in a human, lending support to a reentry mechanism for either type.[30] In addition, their findings were in agreement with Boineau's[18]—that is, the circus movement is counterclockwise in typical atrial flutter and clockwise in atypical flutter.

Frame, Page, and Hoffman have developed an interesting canine model of atrial flutter that could be consistent with the postoperative state in humans.[31] In one group of dogs, they made an incision that extended from the superior to the inferior vena cava and sutured the incision back together; in a second group of dogs, they made, in addition to the first incision, a second incision contiguous with the first, running parallel to the atrioventricular groove to the base of the right atrial appendage. In the first group, only a transient atrial flutter could be induced with rapid atrial pacing; however, in the second group, rapid pacing induced a stable flutter with cycle lengths of 140 ms to 188 ms. Interestingly, the atrial activation sequence showed that part of the reentrant impulse traveled around the tricuspid valve in the atrial tissue above the tricuspid ring. The tachycardia could be terminated by tightening a ligature looped around atrial tissue just above the tricuspid valve; this caused the authors to conclude that the reentrant pathway was localized primarily, if not totally, to the atrial tissue around the tricuspid ring. In addition to the anatomic barrier necessary for the perpetuation of flutter, these authors found incomplete recovery of excitability at the end of the excitable gap, implying that factors affecting refractoriness influence the cycle length of a tachycardia. Finally, in their model the left atrium had no part in the reentry circuit.

Human studies have emphasized the importance of intra-atrial conduction delay as a predisposing factor to atrial flutter.[32, 33] Buxton et al found pronounced intra-atrial conduction delay in response to premature stimuli in adults with spontaneous and inducible atrial flutter, as compared to adults without these arrhythmias.[32] However, there was no difference in atrial effective or relative refractory periods between the two groups. Dobmeyer et al had similar findings in a group of patients with induced atrial flutter.[33] However, in their patients with mitral valve prolapse and induced atrial flutter, the intra-atrial conduction times were normal, but atrial effective refractory periods were longer, suggesting various degrees of autonomic influence on right atrial tissue.

Boyden developed a canine model of stable

atrial flutter by causing right atrial enlargement after producing tricuspid insufficiency and pulmonary stenosis.[34] With this model, she attempted to answer the question of whether atrial flutter was caused by delayed afterdepolarization-dependent triggered activity or by reentrant excitation. During sustained atrial flutter, she administered various medications. Initially, she tested agents affecting the parasympathetic nervous system. Atropine (a parasympatholytic agent) increased the ventricular rate but did not change the atrial rate, nor did it terminate flutter. Phenylephrine (a parasympathomimetic agent) shortened the atrial cycle length slightly but not significantly. In all trials, methacholine (another parasympathomimetic agent) produced a significant decrease in atrial cycle length, and in two trials it terminated the rhythm. In one trial, atrial fibrillation occurred before termination.

Next, agents that affect the sympathetic nervous system were tested. Propranolol (a β-adrenergic blocking agent) caused a significant decrease in ventricular rate and atrial rate, but it did not terminate the flutter. In all trials, infusion with isoproterenol (a β-adrenergic stimulating agent) produced a pronounced shortening of the atrial cycle length, but it did not terminate the rhythm.

Third, a calcium channel blocking agent, verapamil, was given intravenously at a 0.2 mg/kg dose to five dogs. A variable response was found: termination of flutter occurred in two dogs; there was a slight increase in atrial and ventricular rates in one dog, and a significant decrease in ventricular rate and no change in atrial rate in another dog; the fifth dog showed a decrease, then an increase, in atrial rate before conversion to normal sinus rhythm.

Fourth, agents that increase the refractory period of atrial tissue were given. In four of five trials, *N*-acetylprocainamide increased the atrial cycle length, terminated atrial flutter, and restored sinus rhythm with the first dose. Both bretylium and clofilium increased the atrial cycle length before causing conversion to normal sinus rhythm.

Finally, a standard type I agent, procainamide, which decreases atrial conduction velocity, prolongs the atrial refractory period, and abolishes delayed afterdepolarizations, was used. Procainamide produced a significant increase in cycle length of atrial flutter and in three of five trials converted flutter to normal sinus rhythm.

The results with the parasympathomimetic agents phenylephrine and methacholine, which decrease the flutter cycle length, are opposite to what would be expected if the sustained flutter were a result of a delayed afterdepolarization mechanism. In cellular electrophysiology studies, parasympathomimetic agents slow or terminate arrhythmias caused by delayed afterdepolarization-dependent activity. In addition, the results of verapamil are not consistent enough to support this mechanism. In the results presented, the atrial flutter was more sensitive to agents that alter atrial refractoriness, all lending support to a reentrant mechanism.

Recently, Pagé et al developed a canine model of atrial flutter by inducing sterile pericarditis, resulting in a situation very similar to human atrial flutter after open heart surgery, regardless of the type of surgery or underlying heart disease.[35] There were no intracardiac manipulations, only a pericardiotomy, after which sterile talcum powder and gauze were placed on the right and left atrial free walls, followed by closure of the pericardiotomy. Within 4 days, sustained atrial flutter could be induced. There was no relationship between atrial effective refractory periods or intra-atrial conduction times and inducibility. Fractionated electrograms and double potentials were recorded at some sites and were postulated to reflect local reentry, collision of wave fronts in the center of the reentry circuit, or localized fibrillation in that part of the atrium, with flutter in the remainder of the atrium.

Atrial Flutter in the Fetus, Newborn, and Infant

There have been numerous reports of atrial flutter occurring in the fetus and the newborn infant. Documentation of the specific type of intrauterine arrhythmia often was not possible, and it was only after the child was delivered that flutter was documented. In 1931, Carr and McClure reported what probably was the first case of intrauterine atrial flutter.[36] Using fetal electrocardiography, Blumenthal et al documented intrauterine flutter in 1968.[37] However, this technique is difficult to perform, and usually the type of arrhythmia has to be inferred from the fetal heart rate, lack of rate variability, or abrupt change in rate. Generally, the ventricular rate is between 150 bpm and 200 bpm, and rarely can be as much as 220 bpm. More recently, echocardiography and Doppler have been used to determine the presence of fetal flutter by comparing atrial and ventricular contraction patterns.[38]

Early reports emphasized the features of atrial flutter in the fetus and newborn.[39–41] The intrauterine ventricular rate was rapid and irregular. Shortly after birth, the infant's electrocardiogram showed typical flutter waves. Digoxin was not effective in converting the rhythm to normal sinus rhythm. The prognosis was poor if the infant had a cardiac malformation or if atrial fibrillation alternated with atrial flutter. Moller, Davachi, and Anderson were the first to note increased birth weight and suggested that this is caused by edema resulting from intrauterine cardiac failure secondary to the arrhythmia.[41] However, van der Horst[42] was the first to report a case of hydrops fetalis secondary to intrauterine atrial flutter; the child improved rapidly after postnatal digitalization, and conversion to normal sinus rhythm occurred 8 hours after the last digitalizing dose.

The report by Moller, Davachi, and Anderson reviewed the outcomes in 36 infants with atrial flutter; nine infants died, six of whom had failed to respond to digitalis therapy.[41] They suggested that electrical cardioversion should be performed for atrial flutter that is not responsive to digitalis. Hassenrück, Chojnacki, and Barker[43] reported the first successful direct current cardioversion of a newborn with atrial flutter. The next successful outcome was not reported until 1972, when Barclay and Barr[44] used direct current cardioversion to achieve sinus rhythm in a 10-day-old infant who had not responded to digoxin. They later used practolol. After cardioversion, the child immediately went into sinus rhythm and remained in this rhythm while oral practolol was resumed.

In reviewing their cases of supraventricular tachycardia occurring within the first 12 months of life, Lubbers et al[45] found eight cases of atrial flutter, two of which also exhibited type A Wolff-Parkinson-White syndrome. In the two patients with Wolff-Parkinson-White syndrome, atrioventricular conduction during flutter occurred by way of the atrioventricular node–His-Purkinje system and, alternately, the accessory pathway. One of the two patients had many recurrences in spite of digoxin and propranolol treatment. Personal experience has corroborated the difficulty of treating these patients medically.

Newborn atrial flutter and congenital cardiac malformations seem to occur together infrequently. Most newborns with atrial flutter have structurally normal hearts. Pearl[46] described a patient with atrial flutter and tetralogy of Fallot and reviewed the literature, finding only seven other patients with combined flutter and congenital heart defect (three with atrial septal defect, one with multiple fenestrations of the interatrial septum, one with subendocardial fibroelastosis, one with ventricular septal defect, and one with pulmonary atresia and intact ventricular septum). Known birth weights exceeded the mean birth weight of normal full-term infants, suggesting that hydrops fetalis might have occurred in these patients.

The fetus with atrial flutter can provide a challenge to the attending obstetrician and pediatrician. Frequently, the arrhythmia is detected before term, and a course of medical management is necessary before delivery. Anderson, Simmons, and Hallide-Smith described a patient who had reduced fetal movement and sustained tachycardia with reduced variability in the baseline heart rate, but not in the beat-to-beat pattern, suggestive of fetal hypoxia.[47] However, oxytocin challenge failed to show evidence of fetal hypoxia, and atrial flutter was considered the probable diagnosis. Because the condition of the fetus seemed to be stable, medication was not started, and the pregnancy progressed another 4 weeks, when an elective cesarean section was performed. For most patients, however, echocardiography is currently used to diagnose atrial flutter and check for hydrops, and treatment with digoxin is started immediately in the mother.[48] The infant often has to be delivered early because of inadequate response to treatment or extenuating circumstances, such as ruptured membranes. Fetal atrial flutter was noted in one of a set of twins, starting 5 days after tocolytic therapy was begun to prevent premature delivery.[49] At birth one twin was normal, and the other was hydropic with severe heart failure.

Early reports attempted to separate atrial flutter in newborns and infants into a "congenital" form (presenting during the first week of life and responding well to digitalis therapy) and a "paroxysmal" form (presenting later in infancy and responding poorly to digitalis therapy).[41] However, more recent papers have questioned this distinction and the prognosis. Rowland et al[50] described eight infants younger than 2 years with atrial flutter, all of whom survived and seven of whom were in normal sinus rhythm without medication 1 to 7 years after onset of flutter. The other infant was in normal sinus rhythm but had multiple episodes of supraventricular tachycardia in addition to atrial flutter, which required several medications for control. Two of the infants did not respond to digoxin alone, and quinidine therapy was started. Both of these infants required direct current cardioversion: one for ventricular fibrillation and cardiac arrest and the other for 1:1 atrioventricular conduction. Cardioversion in these two patients resulted in normal sinus rhythm. Ten patients with atrial flutter were reported by Martin and Hernandez;[51] seven had flutter at or near birth, and three had flutter after 6 weeks of age. In all 10 patients, conversion to normal sinus rhythm was achieved, and only one patient (who presented at 9 weeks of age) died (death from endocardial fibroelastosis occurred at 6 months of age). In six of the patients, normal sinus rhythm was achieved by direct current cardioversion. Recently, Dunnigan, Benson, and Benditt described eight infants younger than 2 months of age who presented with atrial flutter.[52] Interestingly, in six of the eight patients, atrial flutter was not suspected from the surface electrocardiogram because of the absence of classic flutter waves. Transesophageal studies were performed, which documented atrial flutter and allowed atrial overdrive pacing in five patients to convert the rhythm to a normal sinus mechanism. All eight patients survived, and in six patients, medication was not used to prevent recurrences after cardioversion. These reports suggest that atrial flutter presenting in the newborn has a favorable prognosis.

Currently, little is known about why the human fetus or newborn develops atrial flutter and what trigger events or susceptibility factors are present. In attempting to evaluate this, Pickoff et al studied atrial vulnerability in the immature canine.[53] They showed that the effective and functional refractory periods of the atrium of the neonatal dog are much shorter than those of puppies or adult dogs. In addition, the neonatal canine atrium was more likely to respond to a single extrastimulus by demonstrating paroxysms of nonsustained atrial flutter-fibrillation than was that of the puppy or the adult dog.

Treatment of atrial flutter in the newborn may vary with the clinical situation. However, virtually all infants will respond to direct current synchronized cardioversion, and this should be attempted if transesophageal pacing is not available or is unsuccessful. Once flutter is converted to sinus rhythm, one may elect to wait and watch to see if it recurs.[52] If atrial flutter recurs, digoxin should be started and maintained for 6 months, then discontinued. Again, a wait and watch posture should be adopted.

Atrial Flutter in the Older Child and Adolescent

CLINICAL PROFILE

In 1985, Garson et al reported the findings in a collaborative study of 380 patients who had the onset of atrial flutter when they were between 12 months and 25 years of age.[54] Atrial flutter was defined as the presence of flutter waves on the surface electrocardiogram; an atrial rate was not specified, because it can vary from 200 bpm to 500 bpm, depending on the patient's age and clinical situation. This study produced a definite clinical profile of the older patient with atrial flutter. Among the 380 patients, seven diagnoses accounted for more than 75% of the patients. In descending order of prevalence they were (1) dextrotransposition of the great arteries (20.5%); (2) complex congenital heart disease (e.g., single ventricle with or without pulmonary stenosis) (17.8%); (3) atrial septal defect (80% ostium secundum) (12.1%); (4) pulmonary stenosis (with or without ventricular septal defect), pulmonary atresia (with or without ventricular septal defect), and tetralogy of Fallot as a single category (92% with tricuspid insufficiency) (7.9%); (5) normal heart (6.3%); (6) congestive cardiomyopathy (5.8%); and (7) complete atrioventricular canal defect (5.0%). When the diagnoses were considered by categories, 60.4% of the patients had repaired congenital heart disease, 13.3% had palliated congenital heart disease, 7.6% had unoperated congenital heart disease, 7.6% had a normal heart, 6.2% had congestive cardiomyopathy, and 4.9% had other lesions. Seventy-five percent of the 380 patients had had at least one cardiac operation before the onset of flutter.

The five most commonly performed operations were Mustard or Senning (27.6%), Blalock-Hanlon (16.1%), repair of atrial septal defect (11.1%), repair of pulmonary atresia/tetralogy of Fallot (7.9%), and aorticopulmonary anastomosis (6.6%).

CONGENITAL HEART DEFECTS

Patients with dextrotransposition of the great arteries begin having trouble with atrial flutter after they undergo intracardiac repair, by either a Mustard or a Senning procedure. Early reports concentrated more on bradyarrhythmias after complete repair of transposition of the great arteries and less on the tachyarrhythmias.[55–58] However, sudden deaths of patients with both arrhythmias were reported. To determine the mechanisms of cardiac arrhythmias seen after the Mustard operation for transposition, Gillette et al performed intracardiac electrophysiologic studies in 52 children aged 1 to 8 years after surgery.[59] In three patients, there was delayed conduction from the high right atrium to the low lateral right atrium, and one of the three patients had an atrial muscle reentry supraventricular tachycardia. In three other patients, typical atrial flutter was induced, and an additional four patients had sinus node reentry tachycardia, which may be a variant of atrial flutter. Bink-Boelkens et al obtained follow-up data on 50 patients who had had Mustard repair between 1969 and 1980.[60] Twenty-five percent of patients developed atrial flutter; 50% of these also had junctional escape rhythm, and 25% had sinus node dysfunction. There was a high late mortality: eight of the 50 (16%) died suddenly, and two of these had a normal functioning pacemaker. There was a significant relationship between the type of arrhythmia and the occurrence of sudden death. For all 50 patients, the late mortality for those with sinus node dysfunction was 19%; for those with junctional escape rhythm, 40%; and for those with atrial flutter, 62%. Flinn et al reported a similar finding in a collaborative study of 372 patients after Mustard repair.[61] Of 29 patients with a dominant (primary arrhythmia) supraventricular tachyarrhythmia, 64% had atrial flutter, and there was a significant association between a dominant tachyarrhythmia and sudden death. More recent reports have noted the sudden deaths of patients manifesting supraventricular tachycardias after the Mustard operation.[62] Because of the increased risk of atrial flutter and the poor outcome after the Mustard repair, Duster et al[63] recommended lifelong digoxin therapy. Patients with transposition of the great arteries who undergo a Senning repair (atrial switch) have similar problems. However, those who have anatomic correction (arterial switch) are apparently at low risk of supraventricular tachyarrhythmias, specifically atrial flutter.[64–66]

There is a common association between atrial septal defect and atrial flutter. Of the 380 patients with atrial flutter reported by Garson et al, 47 (12.4%) had an atrial septal defect and 87% of these had undergone repair.[54] Bink-Boelkens et al.[60] reported the results in a series of 204 patients who underwent closure of a secundum atrial septal defect between 1967 and 1980. During the postoperative period, 18% of these patients developed atrial flutter, and the only late (and sudden) death was that of a patient with atrial flutter. The data of Esscher and Michaëlsson[67] suggest that atrial flutter is related to patient age at repair of atrial septal defect. The postoperative incidence of atrial flutter was 4.5% (four of 88 patients) if repair was performed in patients who were younger than 20 years, but 25.6% (20 of 78 patients) if repair was performed in patients older than 20 years.

Patients with congenital heart defects characterized by an enlarged right atrium seem to be more susceptible to the development of atrial flutter. Tricuspid atresia and Ebstein's abnormality of the tricuspid valve are two such lesions. In the former, flow from the right atrium is obstructed, and in the latter, there is regurgitant flow into the right atrium and (less frequently) associated obstructed flow through the tricuspid valve. In either situation, an increased right atrial volume or pressure (or both) predispose to atrial flutter, requiring medical and frequently surgical therapy.[68, 69] Those patients with tricuspid atresia who have undergone a Fontan procedure are at increased risk of atrial flutter, both in the immediate postoperative period and long term.[69a] Approximately one-fourth of these patients will develop a significant supraventricular tachyarrhythmia, predominantly atrial flutter, by 5 years after surgery.

AGE AT ONSET

In the report by Garson et al, the mean age at onset of atrial flutter was 10.3 years, with an age range of 1.1 years to 25 years.[54] In patients whose flutter developed after operation, the mean postoperative interval was 3.6 years, and in 23% of these patients, the flutter developed within the first 2 weeks after surgery. Patients who were youngest at onset of flutter were those with transposition of the great arteries (mean age, 5.5 years), followed by those with an atrial septal defect (mean age, 10.3 years) and normal heart (mean age, 12.8 years).

SYMPTOMS WITH FIRST EPISODE

Garson et al[54] determined the presence or absence of symptoms in 364 of 380 patients: 30% were asymptomatic, 28% had dyspnea or other symptoms of congestive heart failure, 24% had palpitations, 9% had syncope, and 8% had presyncope with dizziness. In three patients (1%) without previous episodes of atrial flutter, the flutter was found during attempted resuscitation from sudden death. Syncope was significantly more common in patients with a normal heart and in those with Wolff-Parkinson-White syndrome. Overall symptoms were more common when flutter had its onset after 5 years of age.

ANATOMY AND HEMODYNAMICS

Garson et al[54] had M-mode echocardiographic data on 134 of 380 patients with atrial flutter. Sixty-four percent of patients had a left atrial dimension exceeding the upper limit of normal for age, but no information was obtained for right atrial dimension. In a group of 18 adult male patients (mean age, 59 years) who had undergone electrical cardioversion for pure atrial flutter, Pozen et al found that the left atrial size and left ventricular ejection fraction, as measured by M-mode echocardiography, were the most reliable predictors of a recurrence of flutter.[70] Patients with a large left atrial size and lower ejection fraction ($<45\%$) were at greater risk of recurrence of atrial flutter by 6 months after cardioversion. Thus atrial size and ventricular function may be co-predictors of the likelihood of atrial flutter. The cardiac catheterization data obtained by Garson et al did not show an elevated left or right atrial pressure in a large number of patients with atrial flutter.

TACHYCARDIA-BRADYCARDIA SYNDROME

The tachycardia-bradycardia syndrome is not a pure clinical or electrocardiographic entity but rather is a conglomerate of various combinations of cardiac arrhythmias and their clinical manifestations. The tachycardia component of the syndrome in patients with sick sinus syndrome is usually manifested as supraventricular tachycardia, atrial flutter, or atrial fibrillation. This syndrome can be found after repair of a congenital heart defect (e.g., after the Mustard procedure for dextrotransposition of the great arteries) or after repair of an atrial septal defect. Tachycardia can be initiated by bradycardia. Coumel et al[71] described a group of adult males who had bradycardia-induced recurrent paroxysmal atrial tachycardia. Vagal activity results in slowing of the sinus rate and shortening of the atrial refractory period. However, the vagally induced changes in the action potentials and refractory periods in the atrium are not homogeneous, and this imbalance of refractory periods in the atrium provides a substrate for intra-atrial reentry. A second mechanism for inducing atrial flutter could operate during a junctional escape rhythm, which would conduct retrogradely to the atrium when the atrium was partially depolarized as a result of a preceding sinus beat. With this combination, the retrogradely conducted atrial impulse could initiate a reentry circus movement. Conversely, the bradycardia can be initiated by tachycardia. Probably the most common mechanism for this is overdrive suppression, an episode of supraventricular tachycardia or atrial flutter that terminates spontaneously and results in a long pause before the next spontaneous beat or in a persistent bradycardia. Electrophysiologic studies in isolated superfused fibers with pacemaker activity have shown that depression of pacemaker activity after overdrive is the result of hyperpolarization and depression of phase 4 diastolic depolarization.[72]

ATRIAL FLUTTER INDUCED BY DIGITALIS

Digitalis toxicity causes both tachyarrhythmias and bradyarrhythmias. Of the digitalis-induced tachycardias, sinus tachycardia and atrial flutter are exceedingly rare, but there is a possible cause-and-effect relationship.[73] Digitalis should be suspected as the causative agent when atrial flutter occurs only during administration of large doses of the drug or during rapid digitalization, and then disappears after discontinuation of the use of the drug.

ATRIAL FLUTTER SECONDARY TO HYPOKALEMIA

Varriale, Kwa, and Parikh[74] described a 76-year-old woman who at presentation had atrial flutter with 2:1 atrioventricular conduction and hypokalemia (potassium, 2.4 mEq/L) secondary to diuretic treatment for mild hypertension. A roentgenogram of the chest revealed a normal cardiac silhouette, and M-mode echocardiography showed normal left atrial and ventricular dimensions. Endocardial atrial overdrive pacing converted the rhythm to normal sinus with multiple atrial premature beats; rapid atrial pacing could reinduce atrial flutter. After 48 hours of treatment, the serum potassium level was 4.0 mEq/L. Repeat electrophysiologic testing revealed the following: the atrial effective refractory period was 85 ms longer than in the first study, and multiple stimulation techniques failed to induce atrial flutter. The researchers concluded that significant hypokalemia could cause (1) an inhomogeneous refractory period distribution in the atrium and (2) the generation of frequent premature atrial beats, which could interact to initiate and sustain atrial flutter.

ATRIAL FLUTTER AND RAPID ATRIOVENTRICULAR CONDUCTION

Generally during atrial flutter, 2:1 atrioventricular conduction is present, but if atrioventricular conduction is impaired, there can be 3:1 or 4:1 atrioventricular conduction (see Fig. 11–4). However, in children and occasionally in adults, atrioventricular conduction can be accelerated, resulting in sustained 1:1 atrioventricular conduction at rates of 250 bpm to more than 300 bpm. Obviously, these ventricular rates could have deleterious consequences, leading to syncope or sudden death. This may, in fact, be a common mechanism for sudden death in patients after the Mustard or Senning operation.

Occasionally, children undergoing electrophysiologic testing will manifest 1:1 atrioventricular conduction during atrial pacing at rates as high as 250 bpm. But one would have to postulate some other mechanism to account for 1:1 atrioventricular conduction at rates as high as 300 bpm. One such factor is emotional stress: a 15-year-old boy who had a Mustard procedure for dextrotransposition of the great arteries in early childhood presented for a routine outpatient visit in atrial flutter with 2:1 atrioventricular conduction. When told that he was going to be hospitalized for electrical cardioversion, he began conducting 1:1 at 300 bpm (Fig. 11–6) and rapidly deteriorated, requiring direct-current cardioversion without the benefit of an intravenous line in place. Type Ia antiarrhythmic medications, such as quinidine and procainamide, will increase atrioventricular conduction and result in 1:1 ventricular conduction during atrial flutter. Therefore, it is mandatory to administer digitalis therapy before a type I medication is given for control of atrial flutter. Occasionally in adults an anatomic abnormality such as an atrio-His bundle fascicle is present and would account for rapid atrioventricular conduction.[75]

Another group of patients susceptible to rapid atrioventricular conduction during atrial flutter are those with preexcitation syndromes demonstrating the Wolff-Parkinson-White patterns on the surface electrocardiogram. Benditt, Pritchett, and Gallagher[76] reported 163 patients with accessory atrioventricular pathways who underwent clinical electrophysiologic testing. During the study, 26 patients had a regular tachycardia with a QRS pattern of apparent ventricular preexcitation and 1:1 atrioventricular conduction. In 15 of the 26 (58%), atrial flutter with 1:1 atrioventricular conduction over the accessory pathway was present. Heart rates were documented at 188 bpm to 340 bpm. It is known that atrial flutter occurs in approximately 5% of patients with Wolff-Parkinson-White syndrome, a figure higher than that in the general population.[77]

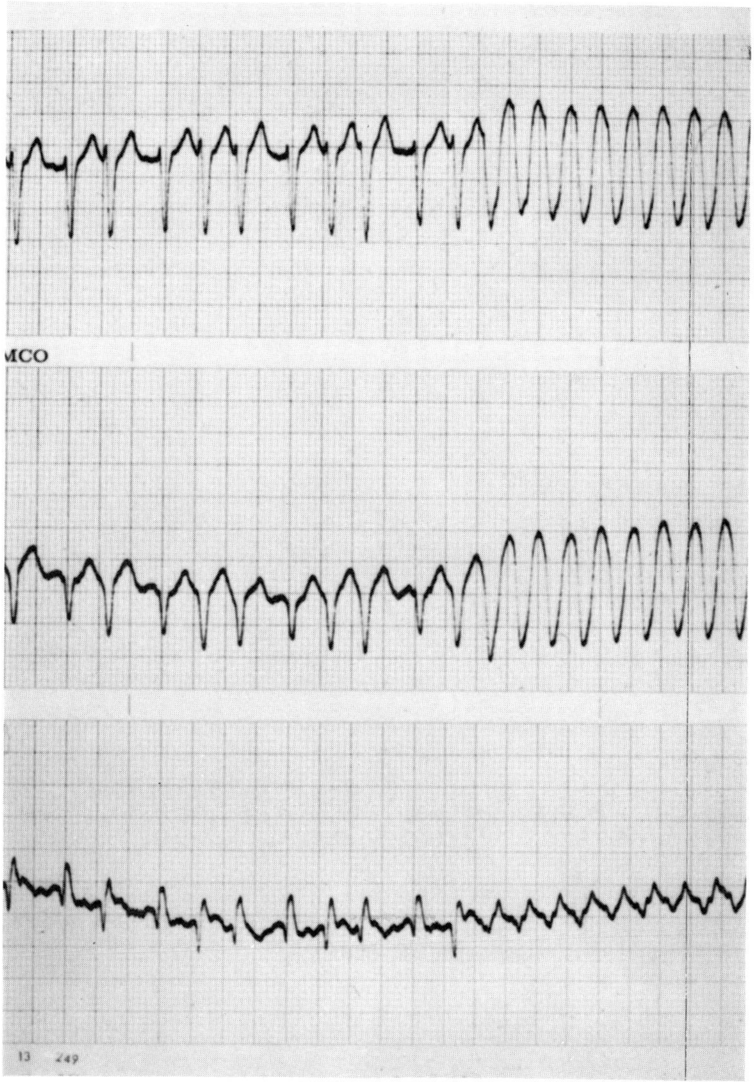

FIGURE 11–6
Surface electrocardiogram of leads I, II, and III. Left side of the tracing shows atrial flutter with variable atrioventricular conduction. Right side shows abrupt change to 1:1 atrioventricular conduction of 300 bpm with aberrant ventricular conduction.

INAPPARENT ATRIAL FLUTTER

Recently there have been reports of atrial flutter seen on the atrial electrogram in which the surface electrocardiogram showed only a supraventricular tachycardia believed to be junctional or atrioventricular nodal reentrant in origin, or a normal sinus tachycardia (Figs. 11–7 and 11–8). Humes et al[78] reported their findings in a study of 20 pediatric patients who had undergone intracardiac repair of a congenital heart defect and had temporary atrial epicardial wires left in place for diagnosis and therapy. Surface electrocardiograms from these patients were reviewed by five pediatric cardiologists, and a diagnosis of the rhythm was made. These rhythms were compared with those diagnosed by use of atrial electrograms. Five of the rhythms were atrial flutter, but only one (that in a patient with atrial flutter and 1:1 atrioventricular conduction) was correctly identified from the surface tracing (Fig. 11–9). The other four patients had 2:1 atrioventricular conduction with inapparent flutter waves (Fig. 11–10). Atrial flutter with inapparent flutter waves is seen rarely in pediatric patients with structurally normal hearts and no surgery, but may occur more commonly in those after the Mustard, Senning, or Fontan repair, perhaps since the sinus P waves are also of low voltage.[79]

Inapparent flutter waves are seen in older patients who have sick sinus syndrome. Rakovec et al[80] studied two older patients who had suspected sick sinus syndrome and induced nonsustained atrial flutter, which was seen on the atrial electrogram while the sur-

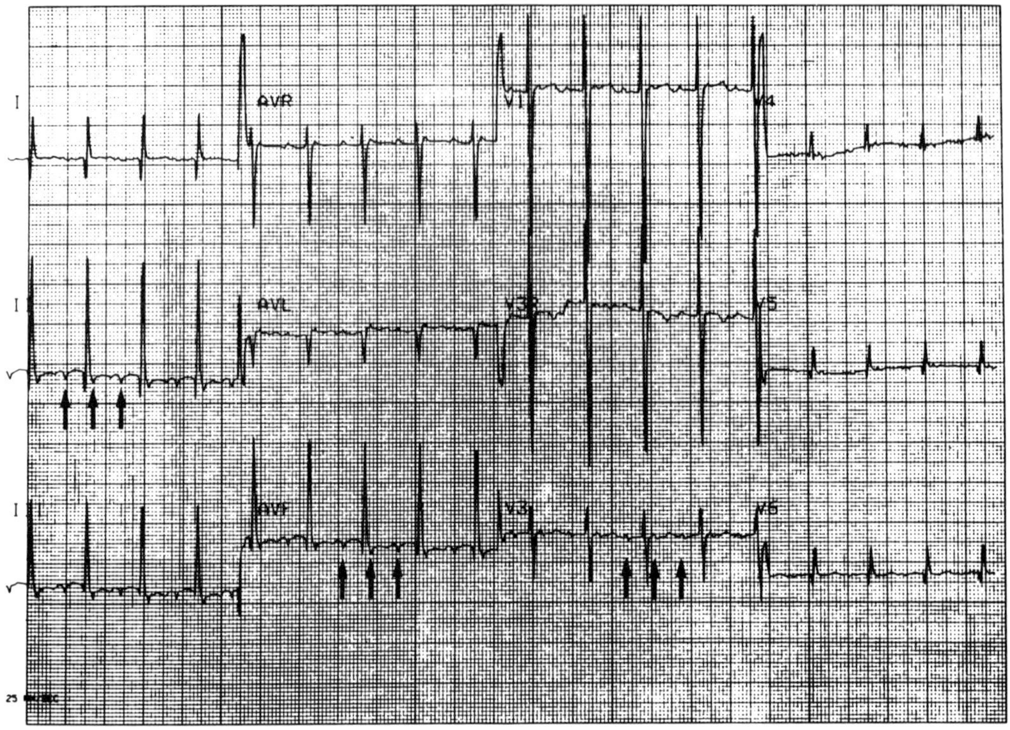

FIGURE 11–7
Standard 12-lead electrocardiogram of patient believed to have a low atrial rhythm at 100 bpm. Careful inspection of leads II, III, aVF, and V_3 reveals a second P wave immediately after the QRS complexes (arrows point to P waves), indicating atrial flutter with 2:1 atrioventricular conduction.

face electrocardiogram showed only normal sinus rhythm. They referred to this as a "concealed dissimilar atrial rhythm."

TRANSESOPHAGEAL STUDY

Because of the difficulty in diagnosing some forms of supraventricular tachycardia, especially atrial flutter, there has been greater use of atrial electrograms recorded by placement of transesophageal electrodes. This approach is relatively noninvasive, allows analysis of atrial rate and atrioventricular relationship for accurate diagnosis of the rhythm, and provides a means for atrial overdrive pacing for conversion. Early reports in adults by Kerr et al[81] showed the importance of the transesophageal approach for initiation as well as termination of atrial flutter in the patient with Wolff-Parkinson-White syndrome. Recently, Butto et al[82] demonstrated the utility of the transesophageal approach for diagnosing and treating recurrent atrial tachycardias, including atrial flutter, in pediatric patients who had undergone an atrial baffle procedure for dextrotransposition of the great arteries.

Electrophysiology Testing

INVASIVE TESTING

The percutaneous technique allows multiple electrode catheters to be manipulated into the right atrium for stimulation and recording. Generally, the distal pair of electrodes are placed high in the right atrium, near the sinus node, for stimulation. The more proximal electrodes are used for recording the atrial electrograms. This catheter can be manipulated to other sites for pacing and recording or can be left in one position while additional catheters are positioned for use. Atrial extrastimuli are delivered by a programmable stimulator.

The two most frequent techniques for induction of atrial flutter are (1) single or double premature atrial extrastimuli delivered into a sensed rhythm or an atrially paced rhythm (cycle length: 600, 500, and 400 ms)

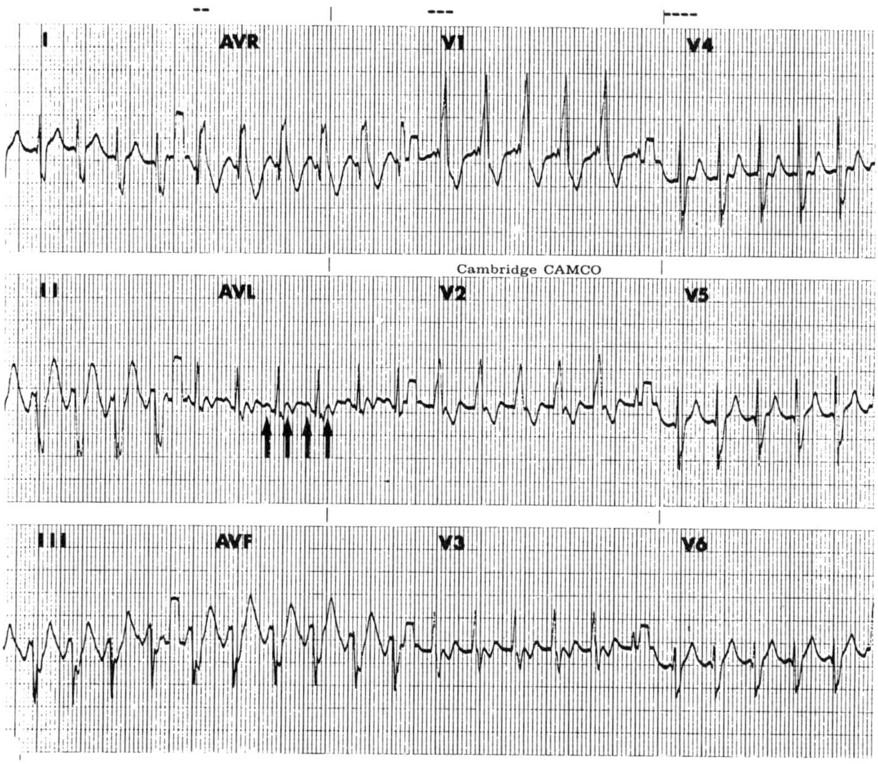

FIGURE 11–8
Standard 12-lead electrocardiogram from patient after repair of ventricular septal defect. Leads II, III, and aVF do not show easily visible P waves. Close inspection of lead aVL reveals two P waves for every QRS complex (arrows point to P waves).

and (2) rapid atrial pacing (cycle length: 600 ms, decreasing to 200 ms). Watson and Josephson[21] studied 525 consecutive adults in the clinical electrophysiology laboratory. Forty-one adults had sustained atrial flutter; of these, 31 had previously documented spontaneous atrial flutter or fibrillation (or both), and 10 had paroxysmal palpitations without documented cause. Atrial flutter was induced by one or two atrial extrastimuli in 31 patients and by rapid atrial pacing in 29 of 35 patients in whom it was attempted. Casta et al[83] induced nonsustained (0.45 to 60 s) atrial flutter in six (4%) of 137 children with preoperative congenital heart defects who underwent electrophysiologic testing as a part of cardiac catheterization. No patient had electrocardiographic or clinical documentation of an arrhythmia. Thus, in the pediatric patient who has congenital heart disease but who has not had intracardiac repair, induction of atrial flutter seems to be rare and usually not sustained. Limited data are available for postoperative patients. However, in 65 patients who had undergone Mustard repair for dextrotransposition of the great arteries, Vetter, Burton, and Hardy[84] found that 31 (48%) had inducible sustained atrial flutter during electrophysiology testing, and the majority of these either had had clinical atrial flutter or developed atrial flutter within 1 year of the electrophysiology study. Spontaneous atrial flutter occurs more often in patients with congenital heart defects following surgery.[54]

NONINVASIVE TESTING

As mentioned, Kerr et al[81] used transesophageal pacing in an attempt to induce atrial flutter in adult patients with Wolff-Parkinson-White syndrome in order to examine properties of anterograde conduction across accessory connections. Atrial flutter or fibrillation was successfully induced in 23 of 23 patients. There has been no systematic study reported attempting to induce atrial flutter by this technique in pediatric patients.

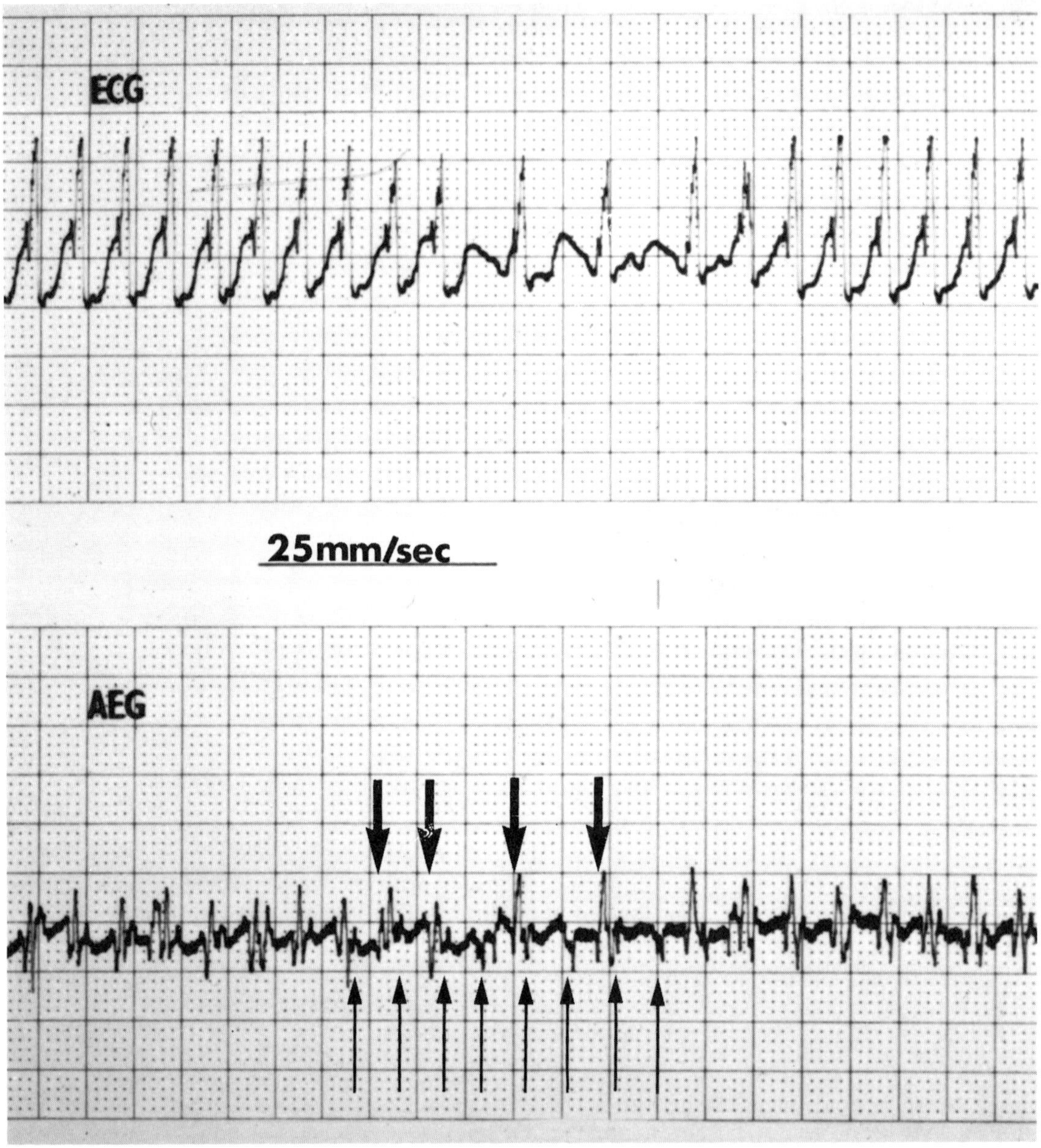

FIGURE 11–9
Atrial flutter with 1:1 atrioventricular conduction. *Top panel:* Surface electrocardiogram (ECG). *Bottom panel:* Atrial electrogram (AEG). Small arrows show the atrial activity at approximately 300 bpm; the atrial polarity changes midway through the tracing, initially the atrial deflections are positive, and later they are negative. Large arrows point to ventricular activation.

Follow-up

In the collaborative study reported by Garson et al, follow-up data were collected on 357 of the original 380 patients entered in the study.[54] Of the 357 patients, 297 (83%) were alive at an average follow-up time of 6.5 years. Sixty patients (17%) had died an average of 2.4 years after the first episode of flutter, and 88% of the deaths occurred within 5 years of the onset. In 33% of the patients, atrial flutter occurred only once, and in an additional 21%, the duration of flutter was only 1 year or less. But in the remaining 56%, episodes of flutter continued for more than 1 year, and about half of these patients were still having episodes of flutter at the time of follow-up study.

The final status of 360 of the 380 patients

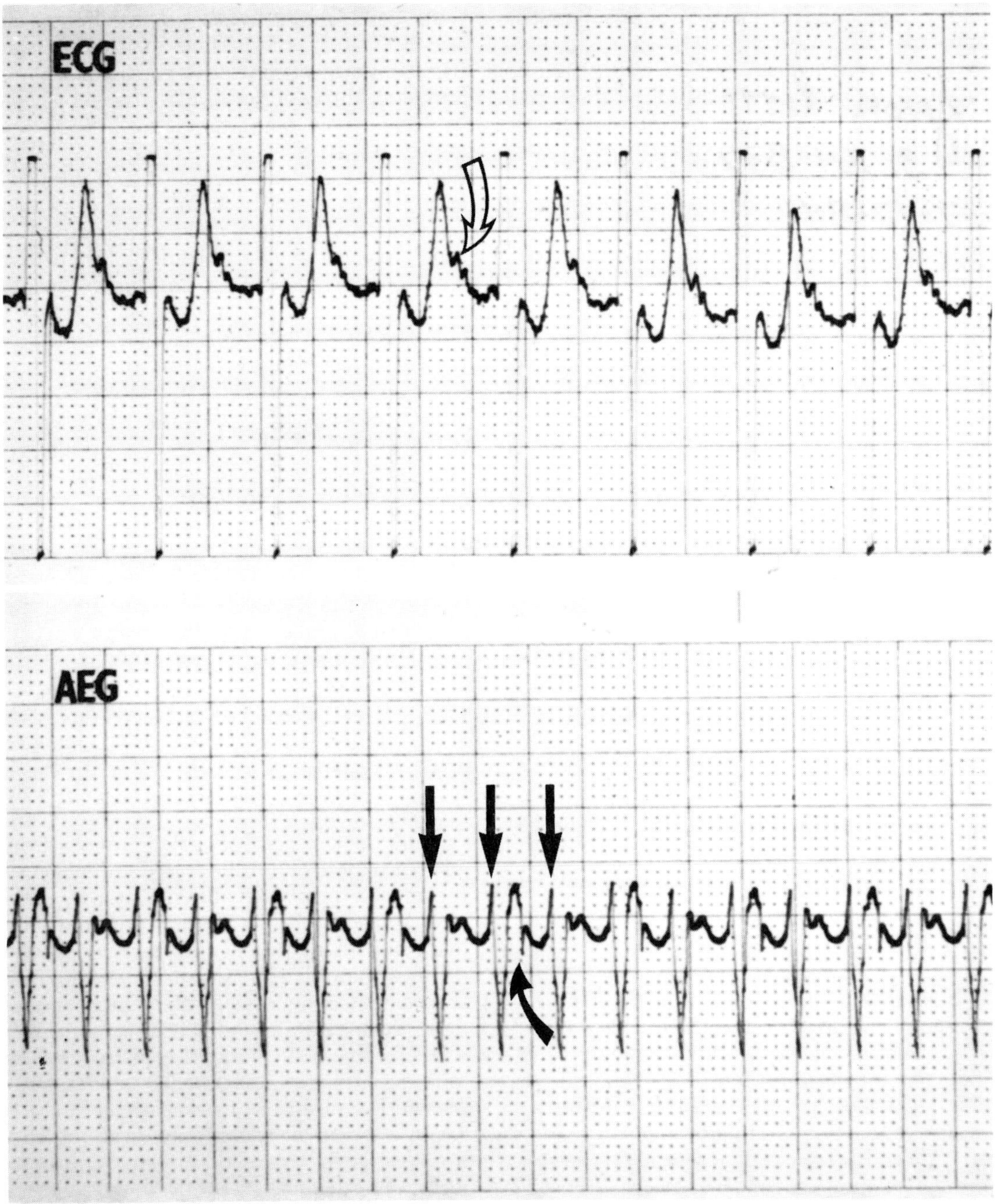

FIGURE 11–10
Inapparent atrial flutter. *Top panel:* Surface electrocardiogram (ECG) shows apparent sinus tachycardia with first degree atrioventricular block (open arrow shows apparent sinus P wave). *Bottom panel:* Atrial electrogram (AEG) shows atrial flutter waves (*black straight arrows*) at 260 bpm with 2:1 atrioventricular block (black curved arrow points to ventricular activation). Paper speed, 25 mm/s.

was determined; 83.4% of the patients were alive at an average age of 14.5 years. Most (48.6%) were not having episodes of atrial flutter, but 34.8% had flutter, even with treatment. At follow-up, 16.6% had died at an average age of 15.5 years, and most of the deaths were sudden.

Four variables seemed to have a role in the likelihood of death: (1) cardiac diagnosis, (2) echocardiographic left atrial size, (3) pacemaker implantation, and (4) unsuccessful drug treatment. Patients with cardiomyopathy and complex heart disease had a significantly higher overall death rate than did other groups, and the rate of sudden death was significantly greater in those with complex congenital heart defects. With increasing left atrial dimension, the incidence of sudden and nonsudden death increased; this was especially true for patients with left atrial dimension greater than 150% of the upper limits of normal. Seventeen percent of patients had pacemaker implantation, and sudden death occurred in 7% of patients without and 10% with a pacemaker. The difference was not significant. Thus, a pacemaker does not seem to be protection from sudden death in a patient with atrial flutter. Finally, sudden death occurred more often in patients in whom drug treatment of atrial flutter was unsuccessful (18 of 91, or 20%), compared to those with successful complete elimination of flutter (8 of 169, or 5%). The same was true for episodes of nonsudden cardiac death: 12% in those without effective control, compared to 5% in whom flutter was eliminated. Thus, unlike in adults, episodes of atrial flutter in children should not be allowed to continue. It is not acceptable to simply "control the ventricular rate."

Treatment

DRUG THERAPY

Digitalis has long been the main drug for treatment of atrial flutter. It exerts a direct effect on the cardiac cell membrane by inhibiting the magnesium-dependent, the adenosine triphosphate–dependent, and the sodium- and potassium-activated transport enzyme complex and by influencing the slow inward calcium current.[85] However, most of its antiarrhythmic properties are a result of its indirect actions mediated through the autonomic nervous system. At low concentrations, digitalis causes increased parasympathetic tone and withdrawal of sympathetic tone. In the atrium at low concentrations, digitalis causes increased parasympathetic tone and, possibly, sympathetic withdrawal, which shorten the atrial refractory periods and conduction; but at higher concentrations, the direct effects and increased sympathetic tone favor spontaneous depolarizations and arrhythmias. The direct and indirect effects of digitalis on the atrioventricular node prolong the refractory period and slow the conduction. Hearts denervated by cardiac transplantation show little prolongation of atrioventricular nodal refractory period or conduction time after digitalization. In the ventricle, the increased parasympathetic tone and the decreased sympathetic tone from low concentrations are antiarrhythmic, while higher concentrations are arrhythmogenic.

Digitalis may be used in an attempt to convert atrial flutter or to prevent recurrences. Its efficacy as an agent to convert atrial flutter is unpredictable, because conversion depends on the ability of digitalis to lengthen or shorten the atrial refractory period, and this effect depends on interaction of digitalis with the autonomic nervous system. In animal models, if the vagus nerve is intact, shortening of the atrial refractory period occurs and the atrial rate increases and degenerates into atrial fibrillation.[86] If the vagi are blocked, the atrial refractory period is prolonged and the flutter rate is slowed, favoring conversion to sinus rhythm. In general, digitalis is not an effective drug for the acute conversion of atrial flutter. In the collaborative study reported by Garson et al, digoxin used alone was successful in preventing recurrences of atrial flutter in only 44% of patients.[54] Of the conventional agents, the most effective treatment for preventing recurrences (53%) was the combination of digoxin with a type I agent, such as quinidine or procainamide. Thus, although digitalis has several advantages—low cost, once or twice daily dosing, and relatively few noncardiac side effects—it has limited effectiveness as a lone antiarrhythmic agent for conversion or prevention of atrial flutter.

Type I antiarrhythmic medications function primarily by decreasing membrane sodium conductance; recently they have been subdivided into three groups: type Ia agents (quinidine, procainamide, and disopyramide), which prolong refractoriness and decrease conduction velocity; type Ib agents (lidocaine, tocainide, mexiletine, and phenytoin), which increase membrane potassium conductance and shorten refractoriness without slowing conduction; and type Ic agents (flecainide and encainide), which slow conduction, with minimal effects on refractoriness and action potential duration. Of these medications, only the type Ia and Ic antiarrhythmic agents are useful for the treatment of atrial flutter, because of their effect on the atrial tissue. Because of their vagolytic properties, type Ia medications need to be given in combination with digitalis preparations to prevent 1:1 atrioventricular conduction if atrial flutter should occur. Garson et al found that, of the conventional agents, a combination of digoxin and a type I antiarrhythmic agent was the second most effective treatment to prevent recurrences of atrial flutter in pediatric patients; yet the combination was only effective in 53% of patients.[54] Unfortunately, quinidine has a high frequency of gastrointestinal side effects, such as nausea, vomiting, and diarrhea (thereby making absorption erratic), and when used with digoxin, it displaces digoxin from muscle-binding sites and reduces renal clearance, thus increasing the risk of digitalis toxicity. Procainamide seems to be a much more effective medication, because it does not cause gastrointestinal side effects or interact with digoxin, and it can be administered easily intravenously. However, even in the long-acting form, it usually needs to be given four times per day. The newer type Ic agents, flecainide, and encanide, may be promising agents for prevention of atrial flutter.

Type II drugs interfere with the sympathetic nervous system and are known as β-adrenergic blocking agents, the prototype being propranolol. These antiarrhythmic agents do not seem to be very effective for the acute treatment or prevention of atrial flutter. In the collaborative study by Garson et al, propranolol, whether used alone or in combination with digoxin, was the least effective of the conventional agents for preventing recurrences of atrial flutter.[54] It was effective in 33% of patients when used alone and in 43% of patients when used in combination with digoxin.

Type III agents exert their action primarily by prolonging action potential duration and refractoriness without affecting conduction significantly. The agents in this category are amiodarone and sotalol. Garson et al had an opportunity to use amiodarone in a group of 39 patients with congenital heart disease, critical tachyarrhythmias, and arrhythmias not responsive to conventional agents.[87] Of these, 16 had recurrent atrial flutter, and of the 16, 15 experienced complete elimination of the flutter following amiodarone therapy. In Garson et al's collaborative study, amiodarone was the most effective agent in preventing atrial flutter recurrence.[54] The authors cautioned about the side effects in pediatric patients who take amiodarone: keratopathy, skin rash, hyperthyroidism or hypothyroidism, hepatic and pulmonary toxicity, and bradyarrhythmias significant enough to warrant pacemaker insertion. Interestingly, amiodarone given intravenously in adults has not been effective for acute conversion of atrial flutter.[88]

Type IV drugs (for example, verapamil) cause blocking of the slow, inward calcium channels, resulting in slowed conduction, prolonged refractoriness, and reduced automaticity in slow-response fibers such as the sinus or atrioventricular nodes. Verapamil has been used almost exclusively as an acute intervention given intravenously to the patient with atrial flutter. Conversion of atrial flutter to normal sinus rhythm occurs rarely after the intravenous use of verapamil; however, what does occur is a lowering of the ventricular rate secondary to (1) delayed conduction through the atrioventricular node or (2) conversion from atrial flutter to atrial fibrillation with a reduction in conducted impulses.[89–91] Verapamil may be an effective agent for a patient with atrial flutter and 1:1 atrioventricular conduction whose condition is deteriorating rapidly (as long as the patient does not have Wolff-Parkinson-White syndrome, in which case verapamil is contraindicated for atrial flutter). In general, verapamil should be administered very cautiously in young children. Abinader, Borochowitz, and Berger described a neonate who was born with atrial flutter.[92] Six hours before the birth, the mother was given propranolol (5 mg intravenously) and 14 hours after birth, the infant was given verapamil (1.5 mg intravenously), which resulted in sinus rhythm at 125 bpm. Immediately thereafter the infant experienced low output and required cardiopulmonary resuscitation for 2 hours before recovery. A recent report has suggested giving calcium chloride before the intravenous administration of verapamil in order to prevent hemodynamic complications, although because of the study design, the conclusions require confirmation on a larger group of patients.[93]

Pacemaker Indications. It has been recommended that in any child with a potential for sinus bradycardia (e.g., following Mustard repair), if any antiarrhythmic drug is used for treatment of atrial flutter, other than digitalis, that could suppress the sinus node (especially quinidine, propranolol, and amiodarone), a pacemaker should be implanted.[106] While this is clearly the safest route, many physicians, patients, and parents have difficulty with such prophylactic treatment. If a pacemaker is not implanted, the child should be observed extremely carefully for progressive bradycardia.

DIRECT-CURRENT SYNCHRONIZED CARDIOVERSION

Direct-current cardioversion was first reported in 1962 by Lown, Amarasingham, and Neuman[94] and was met with enthusiasm as an emergent form of therapy for various life-threatening arrhythmias. In 1968, Bjerkelund and Orning[95] reported their results in a series of 437 patients (including pediatric patients) undergoing cardioversion for atrial arrhythmias only. In 80% of their patients, reversion to sinus rhythm was achieved with 100–400 watt-seconds. In addition, they found that of 46 patients with atrial flutter, 41 (89%) achieved reversion to sinus rhythm with direct current cardioversion. Significant complications occurred in 13 patients (all 437 patients had received digitoxin before conversion): eight patients had ventricular fibrillation requiring resuscitation (transient with spontaneous conversion in four patients, and lasting 1 to 20 minutes in four patients), and five had transient bradycardia (three with complete atrioventricular block lasting as long as 2 hours, and two with pronounced sinus bradycardia). All 13 patients with complications survived, and there were no deaths during direct current shock. Frithz and Åberg[96] reviewed their results for 29 adults with atrial flutter who underwent direct current cardioversion between 1963 and 1968. All 29 patients had successful conversion to sinus rhythm, and 23 patients required only 80–100 watt-seconds for conversion. One patient experienced asystole and required brief resuscitation before sinus bradycardia resumed; six patients had junctional rhythm, and three of these had return to sinus rhythm without additional measures.

Direct current synchronized cardioversion is an effective means of converting atrial flutter to sinus rhythm (Fig. 11–11). In the past, concern was expressed about possible complications, including induction of ventricular fibrillation, especially if the patient had been taking digitalis. In the author's experience, this complication occurs rarely and generally is a result of inappropriate sensing or machine malfunction, with delivery of the shock after the QRS complex. If the child has received digitalis, some physicians may prefer to administer lidocaine (1 mg/kg) intravenously immediately before cardioversion. In a patient with potential sick sinus syndrome (e.g., following Mustard repair), cardioversion for atrial flutter should be done with the knowledge that asystole may develop immediately after the shock, and methods should be available to increase the ventricular rate (e.g., with isoproterenol or esophageal pacing) should this occur. For this reason, overdrive pacing is preferred in children with atrial flutter if there is potential for sick sinus syndrome; this is especially true the first time flutter is converted, since the response is unknown.

For atrial arrhythmias, an even lower energy level than that used for ventricular defibrillation frequently will convert the rhythm to sinus rhythm and avoid complications.[97] Current recommendation is 0.5–1.0 watt-second/kg for the initial trial. Recently, Atkins et al[98] showed that transthoracic impedance is relatively high with "pediatric" paddles and could contribute to cardioversion failure. They recommended using "adult" paddles whenever a child's thorax is large enough to accommodate them.

OVERDRIVE PACING

In the late 1960s and early 1970s, rapid atrial stimulation was found to be useful in converting supraventricular tachycardia, including atrial flutter.[99] In 1983, Waldo[100] summarized a number of factors that were important determinants for the efficacy of overdrive suppression of type I atrial flutter:

1. Critical atrial pacing rate that was 115% to 125% of the spontaneous flutter rate.
2. Transient entrainment (see mechanism of atrial flutter) that progressed to complete interruption of the reentry circuit.
3. A change in polarity and morphology of the atrial complexes on the surface electrocardiogram, occurring during progression from transient entrainment to complete interruption of the circuit.
4. Critical duration of pacing, usually from 2 s to 22 s, with a mean of 10 s.
5. Critical pacing threshold between 10

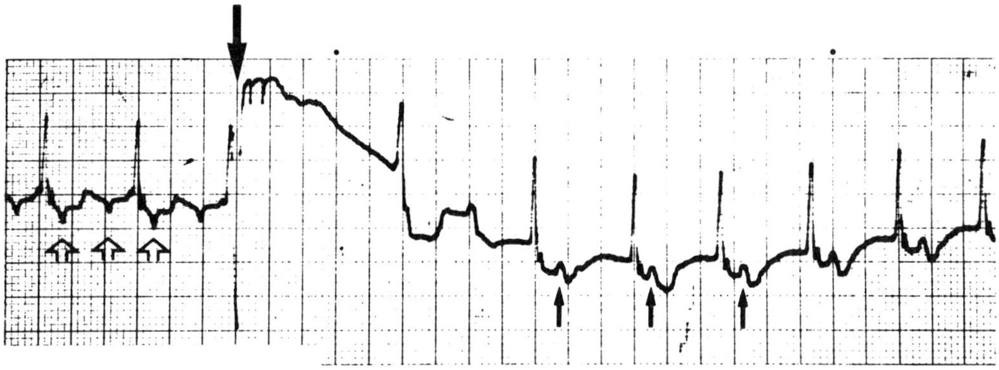

FIGURE 11–11
Electrocardiogram showing direct current synchronized cardioversion. Atrial flutter waves (*open arrows*) are seen at left. Synchronized direct current energy was applied during the QRS complex (*large dark arrow*), and within 1 s, conversion was achieved to a junctional rhythm with retrograde P waves (*small dark arrows*).

and 20 mA using atrial epicardial wire electrodes.

Recently, several reports have demonstrated the effectiveness, safety, and convenience of atrial overdrive pacing for conversion of atrial flutter in adults and children by endocardial, epicardial, and transesophageal approaches (Fig. 11–12).[82, 101–104] This technique can be performed at the bedside, with or without the use of sedation or anesthesia, and provides a means of atrial pacing if the patient should manifest a bradyarrhythmia after conversion. Using either intracardiac or transesophageal techniques in pediatric patients, Campbell et al[103] successfully converted atrial flutter to sinus rhythm in 63% and 73% of patients, respectively. There were no complications by either technique. Butto et al[82] recommended a protocol for use with transesophageal pacing:

1. Determine the atrial cycle length.

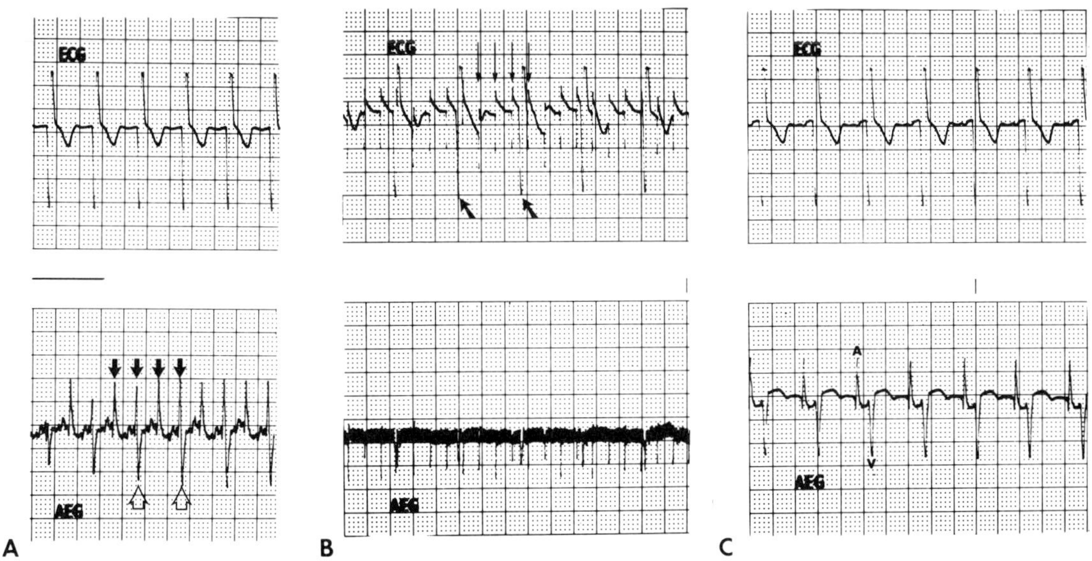

FIGURE 11–12
Demonstration of atrial overdrive pacing to convert atrial flutter to normal sinus rhythm. (*A*, top panel) Surface electrocardiogram (ECG) shows inapparent atrial flutter with ventricular rate at 155 bpm. (*A*, bottom panel) Atrial electrocardiogram (AEG) shows atrial flutter waves (*small black arrows*) with 2:1 atrioventricular block (large open arrows point to ventricular activation). (*B*, top panel) ECG shows atrial pacing spikes (*small arrows*) at 430 bpm and QRS complexes (*larger arrows*) at 111 bpm. (*B*, bottom panel) Temporary atrial wires are being used for pacing. (*C*, top panel) ECG shows small P waves preceding QRS complexes; ventricular rate is 125 bpm. (*C*, bottom panel) AEG shows one atrial activation (A) for every ventricular activation (V), indicating the presence of sinus rhythm.

2. Use stimuli of 9.9 ms in duration.
3. Begin at 50 ms less than the atrial cycle length, with four stimuli at 20 mA.
4. Shorten the pacing cycle length by 10 ms, until conversion or minimum of 100 ms.
5. Then increase the number of stimuli by two and start again; if necessary, go to a maximum of 10 stimuli.
6. Increase to 24 or 28 mA and start the pattern over again.

The object is to use the minimal number of stimuli and the lowest current for conversion. Using this technique, they were successful in 51 of 51 episodes of tachycardia.

ANTITACHYCARDIA PACEMAKER THERAPY

Recent technologic advances have resulted in newer implantable pacemakers that have been used to achieve pacing out of supraventricular tachycardia and, specifically, atrial flutter. Depending on the pacemaker, the techniques for conversion vary greatly from underdrive to overdrive pacing, and from programmed extrastimuli to scanning methods.[105] Some pacemakers are manually activated, whereas others sense tachycardia and are automatically activated. Antitachycardia pacing is generally chosen if an arrhythmia is refractory to medication, the patient is intolerant of medication, or the attacks are frequent and of long duration. An additional advantage is that many patients have the tachycardia-bradycardia syndrome, and after pacing out of atrial flutter is achieved, the pacemaker is on standby to begin pacing if the patient's spontaneous rate is not adequate. Nathan et al[107] reported their experience with the Intermedics Intertach 262-12 model, which seems to be a promising antitachycardia pacemaker. Luceri et al[108] and Fröhlig et al[109] reported the use of a DDD pacemaker (Medtronic Symbios 7005) in the AOO mode to achieve pacing out of atrial flutter. The patients reported by these two groups and two additional patients reported by Greenspon, Greenberg, and Frankl[110] demonstrate an interesting problem encountered in patients with recurrent atrial flutter and the sick sinus syndrome who have implantation of a DDD pacemaker. When these patients had reversion to atrial flutter, a pacemaker-mediated tachycardia developed. There was atrial sensing of every other flutter wave with ventricular tracking, resulting in a ventricular rate of half the atrial flutter rate. All patients became symptomatic, with palpitations, from the faster ventricular rate.

SURGERY FOR ATRIAL FLUTTER

Atrial flutter may be eliminated or easier to treat if a patient's hemodynamics improve. In the collaborative study reported by Garson et al, 66 patients underwent some type of intracardiac repair after the onset of atrial flutter.[54] The most frequently performed procedures were mitral valve surgery (14 patients), reoperation for ventricular septal defect closure (11 patients), tricuspid valve surgery (8 patients), reoperation for Mustard repair (5 patients), ventricular septal defect closure (first operation) (5 patients), and atrial septal defect closure (first operation) (4 patients). In 34 of the 66 patients (52%), the atrial flutter either ceased completely without further medication after operation or the flutter responded to antiarrhythmic agents that had been ineffective before. Only 6% of patients had an increase of flutter episodes after surgery. The best results were obtained in patients undergoing ablation of an accessory pathway, closure of an atrial septal defect, and reclosure of a ventricular septal defect. Among the five patients with reoperation for Mustard repair, only two had improvement. The least successful results occurred in the patients who had mitral or tricuspid valve surgery. It would seem that, for selected patients, intracardiac repair may improve hemodynamics and eliminate or lessen episodes of atrial flutter.

In 1986, Klein et al[111] reported an operative procedure to eliminate the common type of atrial flutter (negative flutter waves in leads II, III, and aVF). Two patients presented with long-standing atrial flutter that was resistant to conventional and investigational drugs. A macroreentrant circuit was mapped in the right atrium, with the orifice of the coronary sinus as the site of earliest activation, resulting in a spreading of activation to the region of the His bundle, high lateral aspect of the right atrium, and low lateral aspect of the right atrium. While the patients were on normothermic cardiopulmonary bypass and after the atrioventricular fat pad was dissected from the right inferior atrial wall, a cryoprobe was applied to the tissue in the posteroseptal atrium between the atrioventricular ring and the orifice of the coronary sinus and inferior edge of the inferior vena cava. After surgery, one patient was free of atrial flutter while not taking medication, and the other was free of arrhythmia while taking a combination of quinidine and verapamil.

ATRIAL FIBRILLATION

Atrial fibrillation is an infrequent occurrence in the pediatric age group. It is characterized by irregular, disordered, and desynchronized activation of the atrial fibers, with rates from 400 bpm to 700 bpm. The electrical wave fronts travel in a chaotic and random fashion, thereby preventing effective atrial contractions. The surface electrocardiogram shows high-frequency "f waves" without a true isoelectric baseline.

Mechanisms

Like atrial flutter, atrial fibrillation has many causes. Several wave fronts circulate through the atrium concurrently, and perpetuation of these wave fronts is dependent on three factors: a critical mass of atrial tissue, the duration of the atrial refractory period, and the rapidity of atrial conduction velocity.[112] Generally, fibrillation will be sustained if the atrium is enlarged, the refractory period is short, and the conduction velocity is slow. In addition, the greater the heterogeneity of the refractory periods, the more likely it is that fibrillation will be spontaneously initiated and sustained.

Cellular electrophysiology studies of right atrial fibers removed at open heart surgery in patients with moderately to greatly dilated atria and arrhythmias revealed that the action potentials showed less negative resting membrane potentials (-50.3 ± 5.7 mV), decreased upstroke velocity, and depressed maximal amplitude.[113] These factors predispose to fibrillation, because they tend to slow or fractionate the activation wave front and lead to reentry.

The role of the autonomic nervous system in the initiation and perpetuation of atrial fibrillation is slowly being uncovered. In the canine atrium, vagal stimulation results in dispersion of the refractory periods, which predisposes to fibrillation.[114] Coumel[115] described patients with chronic intermittent atrial fibrillation that occurred at night, at rest, or postprandially and that was preceded by progressive sinus bradycardia, often immediately preceded by a further lengthening of the sinus cycle length, all presumably caused by relative increased vagal tone. Vagal maneuvers or injection of vagotonic drugs confirmed the mechanism. A less common form of atrial fibrillation occurs in patients who have attacks of palpitations during daytime, after exercise, or during emotional stress, and the fibrillation is preceded by a progressively increasing sinus rate until fibrillation supervenes.

Waldo, Henthorn, and Plumb described four distinct types of atrial fibrillation in adults based on bipolar atrial electrogram morphology and nature of the baseline between atrial electrograms.[116] Type I atrial fibrillation electrograms show discrete complexes of variable morphology separated by an isoelectric baseline without electrical activity; mean atrial rate is 335 bpm, with a range of 291 bpm to 405 bpm. In type II atrial fibrillation, there are discrete complexes of variable morphology, but the baseline is not isoelectric, having high-frequency waves of various degrees; the mean atrial rate of the larger complexes is 383 bpm, with a range of 263 bpm to 436 bpm. Type III electrograms are not characterized by any discrete complexes or isoelectric intervals; they show only chaotic electrical activity. Type IV atrial fibrillation is a combination of type III alternating with type I or type II (or both types). The significance of these four types remains to be determined, but it may have application in treatment, response to medication, or ability to control with the use of pacemakers/defibrillators.

Clinical Manifestations

In 1977, Radford and Izukawa reported a 22-year experience in children with atrial fibrillation at the Hospital for Sick Children in Toronto.[117] Only 35 patients with pure atrial fibrillation were found, 23 of whom (66%) were males. Fibrillation was sustained in 14, paroxysmal in 14, and transient in 7. The ages at onset ranged from 1 day to 19 years, with an average of 8 years. At follow-up, 18 patients were alive and 13 were known to have died; 3 of the survivors had had cerebral embolism with residual neurologic deficits. Of the 35 patients, 17 had congenital heart disease, and of these, 13 (77%) had had intracardiac repair. Five children had cardiomyopathy, and three had rheumatic heart disease with severe mitral regurgitation. There were four patients with atrial tachycardia and atrial fibrillation in infancy: one neonate had atrial flutter and fibrillation in utero and immediately after birth, one infant developed supraventricular tachycardia and atrial fibrillation at age 3 months, and two other infants developed atrial flutter and fibrillation at 3 months. Only one patient was classified as having idiopathic paroxysmal atrial fibrillation; she had a normal heart. In their series, the authors advocated the use of digoxin (all 35 patients) as the mainstay of treatment, with only a few patients requiring propranolol (five patients) or quinidine (four patients). In addition, they recommended the aggressive use of cardioversion and surgery when appropriate to eliminate or control the atrial fibrillation.

Atrial fibrillation in infancy is rare, and recurrences in early childhood are extremely rare. Zaldivar et al[118] reported on an infant with a normal heart who presented with atrial fibrillation at 8 months of age and had recurrences at 15 and 18 months of age. The first two episodes were associated with the administration of a decongestant for an upper respiratory illness, whereas an association with the third episode could not be determined. Each time, the patient was given digoxin, and sinus rhythm was achieved.

Although atrial fibrillation has been reported with some frequency in adults who have hyperthyroidism, there have been few pediatric patients reported. Perry and Hung[119] described a 14-year-old boy who presented with atrial fibrillation and congestive heart failure and who subsequently was found to have an enlarged thyroid gland and laboratory evidence of hyperthyroidism.

Rheumatic fever with or without significant cardiac involvement has been a vanishing disease in the United States, and therefore there are few cases of severe mitral regurgitation causing atrial fibrillation. However, in countries in which rheumatic heart disease is a problem, atrial fibrillation can present in early adolescence as a result of significant mitral valve disease.[120]

Atrial fibrillation is associated with both dilated and hypertrophic cardiomyopathy. The combination of atrial fibrillation and hypertrophic cardiomyopathy can be lethal. Stafford et al[121] reported a 15-year-old boy who collapsed while jogging in a school gymnasium; when the emergency personnel arrived, he was in ventricular fibrillation. After resuscitation and hospitalization, he was found to have diffuse left ventricular hypertrophy with mild systolic anterior motion of the mitral valve on echocardiogram—findings consistent with a hypertrophic cardiomyopathy. He underwent invasive electrophysiology study with incremental pacing and programmed stimulation using single, double, and triple extrastimuli at two cycle lengths from the right ventricular apex and the outflow tract. Ventricular arrhythmias were not induced. Rapid atrial pacing was performed at progressively shorter cycle lengths until atrial fibrillation was induced and the ventricular rate was 180 bpm to 192 bpm. At this time, ST-segment changes had occurred, and the systolic blood pressure had decreased to 70 mm Hg. The patient complained of substernal chest discomfort, and after 100 seconds of this arrhythmia, he suffered a sudden degeneration of the rhythm to ventricular fibrillation, requiring immediate cardioversion. After treatment with a β-adrenergic blocking agent and verapamil, he was re-studied. Although atrial fibrillation could be reinduced, a rapid ventricular response or ST changes did not develop.

Another group of patients at high risk of developing ventricular fibrillation after an episode of atrial fibrillation are patients with accessory atrioventricular pathways (Wolff-Parkinson-White pattern) that have short effective refractory periods, allowing rapid atrioventricular conduction during atrial fibrillation. Atrial fibrillation becomes more common as children with Wolff-Parkinson-White approach adolescence. There have been several reports of patients with Wolff-Parkinson-White patterns who develop ventricular fibrillation after the onset of atrial fibrillation.[122–125] Occasionally, out-of-hospital cardiac arrest is the presenting complaint. There is a definite risk of ventricular fibrillation after onset of atrial fibrillation in those patients with Wolff-Parkinson-White pattern who are given digoxin to prevent or control atrial fibrillation.

Sellers, Bashore, and Gallagher described nine patients with accessory atrioventricular pathway who developed ventricular fibrillation after receiving digoxin for control or prevention of atrial fibrillation.[126] Four patients were given digoxin intravenously while having an attack of atrial fibrillation, and the other five patients were taking digoxin orally long-term to prevent arrhythmia. By analyzing the electrocardiograms done during the conversion from atrial fibrillation to ventricular fibrillation, they found a tendency toward a shorter cycle length of the shortest preexcited RR interval after digoxin was given. This indicated more rapid conduction to the ventricle over the accessory pathway. Significantly, in each case, the shortest RR interval before digoxin was given was less than 220 ms. Also, using invasive electrophysiologic testing, they evaluated 11 additional patients who had preexcitation, some of whom had atrial fibrillation but no ventricular fibrillation. Nine patients received digoxin intravenously during the electrophysiology study, and subsequently atrial fibrillation was induced; three had a decrease in the shortest RR interval, one had no change, and five had an increase in the shortest RR interval. The two other patients received digoxin orally until a steady state was achieved before the electrophysiology study; one had an increase and one had a decrease in the shortest RR interval during atrial fibrillation after digoxin was given. Five of the 11 patients received digoxin both intravenously and orally, and the results of oral administration could not be predicted for either the shortest or the average RR intervals from the results of acute intravenous administration of digoxin. They concluded that digoxin has the potential to cause ventricular fibrillation if atrial fibrillation occurs and the shortest RR interval in the control state is 220 ms or less. In patients with preexcitation, the effect of digoxin on the accessory pathway cannot be predicted a priori because some patients have an increase in the ventricular rate, others have a decrease, and still others have no change. Their final recommendation was to avoid the use of digitalis in patients whose shortest RR interval in atrial fibrillation is less than 300 ms. In patients with clinical atrial fibrillation and Wolff-Parkinson-White syndrome, it is probably best to avoid treatment with digoxin.

Treatment

In general, many of the principles in the treatment of atrial flutter may be applied to the treatment of atrial fibrillation. However, the most effective rapid conversion is by direct current synchronized cardioversion. There is no place for atrial overdrive pacing in the conversion of atrial fibrillation. There are reports of the intravenous administration of procainamide to effect conversion to sinus rhythm. In adults, Fenster et al[127] reported successful conversion by the intravenous administration of procainamide in 15 of 26 patients (58%), and two patients developed nonsustained ventricular tachycardia. If the patient has a rapid ventricular response and does not have Wolff-Parkinson-White syndrome, verapamil may be given intravenously to decrease the ventricular response; however, it should not be given intravenously to infants, those in heart failure, or those taking β-blocking agents. The long-term prevention of atrial fibrillation should include the concomitant administration of digoxin and a type Ia antiarrhythmic agent, the administration of a type Ic agent alone, or possibly the administration of amiodarone alone. If the recurrence of atrial fibrillation cannot be prevented, then digoxin and either verapamil or propranolol can be used to control the ventricular rate. It is probably best to avoid digoxin or verapamil in treatment of children with atrial fibrillation and Wolff-Parkinson-White syndrome. Frequently, the sick sinus syndrome or other bradyarrhythmias coexist with atrial fibrillation, and in order for treatment with potent antiarrhythmic agents to be given, a demand pacemaker may need to be implanted.

References

1. Zipes DP, Fisch C: Premature atrial contraction. Arch Intern Med 128:453–455, 1971.
2. Southall DP, Richards J, Mitchell P, et al: Study of cardiac rhythm in healthy newborn infants. Br Heart J 43:14–20, 1980.
3. Southall DP, Johnston F, Shinebourne EA, et al: 24-hour electrocardiographic study of heart rate and rhythm patterns in population of healthy children. Br Heart J 45:281–291, 1981.
4. Scott O, Williams GJ, Fiddler GI: Results of 24 hour ambulatory monitoring of electrocardiogram in 131 healthy boys aged 10 to 13 years. Br Heart J 44:304–308, 1980.
5. Salice P, Segantini A, Locati E, et al: The prognosis of premature atrial beats in infancy: A prospective study of 6900 infants. Circulation 68 (suppl 3): 395, 1983. Abstract.
6. Garson A Jr: The Electrocardiogram in Infants and Children: A Systematic Approach. Philadelphia, Lea & Febiger, 1983, pp 210–211.

7. Phillips J, Spano J, Burch G: Chaotic atrial mechanism. Am Heart J 78:171–179, 1969.
8. Shine KI, Kastor JA, Yurchak PM: Multifocal atrial tachycardia: Clinical and electrocardiographic features in 32 patients. N Engl J Med 279:344–349, 1968.
9. Berlinerblau R, Feder W: Chaotic atrial rhythm. J Electrocardiol 5:135–144, 1972.
10. Lipson MJ, Naimi S: Multifocal atrial tachycardia (chaotic atrial tachycardia): Clinical associations and significance. Circulation 42:397–407, 1970.
11. Farooki ZQ, Green EW: Multifocal atrial tachycardia in two neonates. Br Heart J 39:872–874, 1977.
12. Bisset GS III, Seigel SF, Gaum WE, et al: Chaotic atrial tachycardia in childhood. Am Heart J 101:268–272, 1981.
13. Liberthson RR, Colan SD: Multifocal or chaotic atrial rhythm: Report of nine infants, delineation of clinical course and management, and review of the literature. Pediatr Cardiol 2:179–184, 1982.
14. Toussaint R, Hofstetter R, von Bernuth G: Multifokale atriale Tachykardie im Säuglingsalter. Klin Padiatr 196:118–120, 1984.
15. Ming-yi W, Zhi-fang W, Xiu-yu C: Chaotic atrial tachycardia in 22 infants. Chin Med J (Engl) 97:500–503, 1984.
16. Yeager SB, Hougen TJ, Levy AM: Sudden death in infants with chaotic atrial rhythm. Am J Dis Child 138:689–692, 1984.
17. Zeevi B, Berant M, Sclarovsky S, et al: Treatment of multifocal atrial tachycardia with amiodarone in a child with congenital heart disease. Am J Cardiol 57:344–345, 1986.
18. Boineau JP: Atrial flutter: A synthesis of concepts. Circulation 72:249–257, 1985.
18a. Boineau JP, Wylds AC, Autry LJ, et al: Mechanisms of atrial flutter as determined from spontaneous and experimental models. In Josephson ME, Wellends JHH (eds): Tachycardia: Mechanisms, Diagnosis, Treatment. Philadelphia, Lea & Febiger, 1984, pp 91–111.
19. Allessie MA, Bonke FIM, Schopman FJG: Circus movement in rabbit atrial muscle as a mechanism of tachycardia. Circ Res 33:54–62, 1973.
20. Allessie MA, Bonke FIM, Schopman FJG: Circus movement in rabbit atrial muscle as a mechanism of tachycardia. III. The "leading circle" concept: A new model of circus movement in cardiac tissue without the involvement of an anatomical obstacle. Circ Res 41:9–18, 1977.
21. Watson RM, Josephson ME: Atrial flutter. I. Electrophysiologic substrates and modes of initiation and termination. Am J Cardiol 45:732–741, 1980.
22. Gomes JAC, Kang PS, Matheson M, et al: Coexistence of sick sinus rhythm and atrial flutter-fibrillation. Circulation 63:80–86, 1981.
23. Friedman PL, Brugada P, Kuck K-H, et al: Inter- and intraatrial dissociation during spontaneous atrial flutter: Evidence for a focal origin of the arrhythmia. Am J Cardiol 50:756–761, 1982.
24. Cosio FG, Arribas F, Palacios J, et al: Fragmented electrograms and continuous electrical activity in atrial flutter. Am J Cardiol 57:1309–1314, 1986.
25. Rytand DA: The circus movement (entrapped circuit wave) hypothesis and atrial flutter. Ann Intern Med 65:125–159, 1966.
26. Boineau JP, Schuessler RB, Mooney CR, et al: Natural and evoked atrial flutter due to circus movement in dogs: Role of abnormal atrial pathways, slow conduction, nonuniform refractory period distribution and premature beats. Am J Cardiol 45:1167–1181, 1980.
27. Inoue H, Matsuo H, Takayanagi K, et al: Clinical and experimental studies of the effects of atrial extrastimulation and rapid pacing on atrial flutter cycle: Evidence of macro-reentry with an excitable gap. Am J Cardiol 48:623–631, 1981.
28. Disertori M, Inama G, Vergara G, et al: Evidence of a reentry circuit in the common type of atrial flutter in man. Circulation 67:434–440, 1983.
29. Waldo AL, Plumb VJ, Henthorn RW: Observations on the mechanism of atrial flutter. In Surawicz B, Reddy CP, Prystowsky EN (eds): Tachycardias. Boston, Martinus Nijhoff Publishing Company, 1984, pp 213–229.
30. Beckman K, Ta-Lin H, Krafchek J, et al: Classic and concealed entrainment of typical and atypical atrial flutter. PACE 9:826–835, 1986.
31. Frame LH, Page RL, Hoffman BF: Atrial reentry around an anatomic barrier with a partially refractory excitable gap: A canine model of atrial flutter. Circ Res 58:495–511, 1986.
32. Buxton AE, Waxman HL, Marchlinski FE, et al: Atrial conduction: Effects of extrastimuli with and without atrial dysrhythmias. Am J Cardiol 54:755–761, 1984.
33. Dobmeyer DJ, Stine RA, Leier CV, et al: Electrophysiologic mechanisms of provoked atrial flutter in mitral valve prolapse syndrome. Am J Cardiol 56:602–604, 1985.
34. Boyden PA: Effects of pharmacologic agents on induced atrial flutter in dogs with right atrial enlargement. J Cardiovasc Pharmacol 8:170–177, 1986.
35. Pagé PL, Plumb VJ, Okumura K, et al: A new animal model of atrial flutter. J Am Coll Cardiol 8:872–879, 1986.
36. Carr JG, McClure WB: Auricular flutter in a newly born infant: Report of a case. Am Heart J 6:824–829, 1931.
37. Blumenthal S, Jacobs JC, Steer CM, et al: Congenital atrial flutter: Report of a case documented by intra-uterine electrocardiogram. Pediatrics 41:659–661, 1968.
38. Losure TA, Roberts NS: In utero diagnosis of atrial flutter by means of real-time-directed M-mode echocardiography. Am J Obstet Gynecol 149:903–905, 1984.
39. McDonagh BJ: Congenital atrial flutter. Arch Dis Child 43:731–733, 1968.
40. Rodriguez-Coronel A, Sueblingvong V, Hastreiter AR: Clinical forms of atrial flutter in infancy. J Pediatr 73:69–76, 1968.
41. Moller JH, Davachi F, Anderson RC: Atrial flutter in infancy. J Pediatr 75:643–651, 1969.
42. van der Horst RL: Congenital atrial flutter and cardiac failure presenting as hydrops foetalis at birth. S Afr Med J 44:1037–1039, 1970.
43. Hassenrück A, Chojnacki B, Barker HJ: Cardioversion of auricular flutter in a newborn infant. Am J Cardiol 15:726–731, 1965.
44. Barclay RPC, Barr DGD: Direct current cardioversion in a case of congenital atrial flutter. Arch Dis Child 47:833–834, 1972.
45. Lubbers WJ, Losekoot TG, Anderson RH, et al: Paroxysmal supraventricular tachycardia in infancy and childhood. Eur J Cardiol 2:91–99, 1974.
46. Pearl W: Cardiac malformations presenting as congenital atrial flutter. South Med J 70:622–624, 1977.

47. Anderson KJ, Simmons SC, Hallidie-Smith KA: Fetal cardiac arrhythmia: Antepartum diagnosis of a case of congenital atrial flutter. Arch Dis Child 56:472–474, 1981.
48. Hirata K, Kato H, Yoshioka F, et al: Successful treatment of fetal atrial flutter and congestive heart failure. Arch Dis Child 50:158–160, 1985.
49. Beitzke A, Winter R, Zach M, et al: Kongenitales Vorhofflattern mit Hydrops fetalis durch mütterliche Tokolytikamedikation. Klin Padiatr 191:410–417, 1979.
50. Rowland TW, Mathew R, Chameides L, et al: Idiopathic atrial flutter in infancy: A review of eight cases. Pediatrics 61:52–56, 1978.
51. Martin TC, Hernandez A: Atrial flutter in infancy. J Pediatr 100:239–242, 1982.
52. Dunnigan A, Benson DW Jr, Benditt DG: Atrial flutter in infancy: Diagnosis, clinical features, and treatment. Pediatrics 75:725–729, 1985.
53. Pickoff AS, Singh S, Flinn CJ, et al: Atrial vulnerability in the immature canine heart. Am J Cardiol 55:1402–1406, 1985.
54. Garson A Jr, Bink-Boelkens M, Hesslein PS, et al: Atrial flutter in the young: A collaborative study of 380 cases. J Am Coll Cardiol 6:871–878, 1985.
55. El-Said G, Rosenberg HS, Mullins CE, et al: Dysrhythmias after Mustard's operation for transposition of the great arteries. Am J Cardiol 30:526–532, 1972.
56. El-Said GM, Gillette PC, Cooley DA, et al: Protection of the sinus node in Mustard's operation. Circulation 53:788–791, 1976.
57. Champsaur GL, Sokol DM, Trusler GA, et al: Repair of transposition of the great arteries in 123 pediatric patients: Early and long-term results. Circulation 47:1032–1041, 1973.
58. Hagler DJ, Ritter DG, Mair DD, et al: Clinical, angiographic, and hemodynamic assessment of late results after Mustard operation. Circulation 57:1214–1220, 1978.
59. Gillette PC, Kugler JD, Garson A Jr, et al: Mechanisms of cardiac arrhythmias after the Mustard operation for transposition of the great arteries. Am J Cardiol 45:1225–1230, 1980.
60. Bink-Boelkens MTE, Velvis H, van der Heide JJH, et al: Dysrhythmias after atrial surgery in children. Am Heart J 106:125–130, 1983.
61. Flinn CJ, Wolff GS, Dick M II, et al: Cardiac rhythm after the Mustard operation for complete transposition of the great arteries. N Engl J Med 310:1635–1638, 1984.
62. Hayes CJ, Gersony WM: Arrhythmias after the Mustard operation for transposition of the great arteries: A long-term study. J Am Coll Cardiol 7:133–137, 1986.
63. Duster MC, Bink-Boelkens MTE, Wampler D, et al: Long-term follow-up of dysrhythmias following the Mustard procedure. Am Heart J 109:1323–1326, 1985.
64. Matherne GP, Razook JD, Thompson WM Jr, et al: Senning repair for transposition of the great arteries in the first week of life. Circulation 72:840–845, 1985.
65. Arensman FW, Bostock J, Radley-Smith R, et al: Cardiac rhythm and conduction before and after anatomic correction of transposition of the great arteries. Am J Cardiol 52:836–839, 1983.
66. Lange PE, Sievers HH, Onnasch DGW, et al: Up to 7 years of follow-up after two-stage anatomic correction of simple transposition of the great arteries. Circulation 74(suppl 1):47–52, 1986.
67. Esscher E, Michaëlsson M: Long-term results following closure of isolated ostium secundum atrial septal defect in children and adults. Eur J Cardiol 6:109–116, 1977.
68. Alboliras ET, Porter CJ, Danielson GK, et al: Results of the modified Fontan operation for congenital heart lesions in patients without preoperative sinus rhythm. J Am Coll Cardiol 6:228–233, 1985.
69. Oh JK, Holmes DR Jr, Hayes DL, et al: Cardiac arrhythmias in patients with surgical repair of Ebstein's anomaly. J Am Coll Cardiol 6:1351–1357, 1985.
69a. Porter CJ, Battiste CE, Humes RA, et al: Risk factors for supraventricular tachyarrhythmias after Fontan procedure for tricuspid atresia. Am Heart J 112:645, 1986. Abstract.
70. Pozen RG, Pastoriza J, Rozanski JJ, et al: Determinants of recurrent atrial flutter after cardioversion. Br Heart J 50:92–96, 1983.
71. Coumel P, Attuel P, Lavallée J, et al: Syndrome d'arythmie auriculaire d'origine vagale. Arch Mal Coeur 71:645–656, 1978.
72. Lu H-H, Lange G, Brooks C McC: Factors controlling pacemaker action in cells of the sinoatrial node. Circ Res 17:460–471, 1965.
73. Fisch C: Digitalis-induced tachycardias. In Surawicz B, Reddy CP, Prystowsky EN (eds): Tachycardias. Boston, Martinus Nijhoff Publishing Company, 1984, pp 401–402.
74. Varriale P, Kwa RP, Parikh N: Atrial flutter secondary to hypokalemia. PACE 6:8–12, 1983.
75. Blanc JJ, Fontaliran F, Gerbaux A, et al: Atrial flutter with 1-1 atrioventricular conduction: Electrophysiologic and histologic correlations. Am Heart J 107:1044–1049, 1984.
76. Benditt DG, Pritchett ELC, Gallagher JJ: Spectrum of regular tachycardias with wide QRS complexes in patients with accessory atrioventricular pathways. Am J Cardiol 42:828–838, 1978.
77. Newman BJ, Donoso E, Friedberg CK: Arrhythmias in the Wolff-Parkinson-White syndrome. Prog Cardiovasc Dis 9:147–165, 1966.
78. Humes RA, Porter CJ, Danielson GK, et al: The utility of temporary atrial epicardial electrodes in postoperative pediatric cardiac patients. J Am Coll Cardiol 5:427, 1985. Abstract.
79. Luca C, Petrescu LP: Atrial flutter with inapparent flutter waves on the surface electrocardiogram. Acta Cardiol (Brux) 40:477–483, 1985.
80. Rakovec P, Horvat M, Jakopin J, et al: Induced concealed dissimilar atrial rhythms. PACE 5:523–528, 1982.
81. Kerr CR, Gallagher JJ, Smith WM, et al: The induction of atrial flutter and fibrillation and the termination of atrial flutter by esophageal pacing. PACE 6:60–72, 1983.
82. Butto F, Dunnigan A, Overhold ED, et al: Transesophageal study of recurrent atrial tachycardia after atrial baffle procedures for complete transposition of the great arteries. Am J Cardiol 57:1356–1362, 1986.
83. Casta A, Wolff GS, Mehta AV, et al: Induction of nonsustained atrial flutter by programmed atrial stimulation in children: Incidence, mechanisms, and clinical implications. Am Heart J 107:444–448, 1984.
84. Vetter VL, Burton DA, Hardy CE: Inducible atrial flutter after the Mustard repair of d-transposition of the great arteries. Am Heart J 112:644, 1986. Abstract.

85. Simpson RJ Jr, Foster JR, Woelfel AK, et al: Management of atrial fibrillation and flutter: A reappraisal of digitalis therapy. Postgrad Med 79:241–253, June 1986.
86. Prystowsky EN, Naccarelli GV, Jackman WM, et al: Enhanced parasympathetic tone shortens atrial refractoriness in man. Am J Cardiol 51:96–100, 1983.
87. Garson A Jr, Gillette PC, McVey P, et al: Amiodarone treatment of critical arrhythmias in children and young adults. J Am Coll Cardiol 4:749–755, 1984.
88. Storelli A, Andriulo C, Chisena A, et al: L'amiodarone endovena nella terapia delle tachiaritmie parossistiche sopraventricolari. G Ital Cardiol 15:290–297, 1985.
89. Aronow WS, Ferlinz J: Verapamil versus placebo in atrial fibrillation and atrial flutter. Clin Invest Med 3:35–39, 1980.
90. Plumb VJ, Karp RB, Kouchoukos NT, et al: Verapamil therapy of atrial fibrillation and atrial flutter following cardiac operation. J Thorac Cardiovasc Surg 83:590–596, 1982.
91. Tommaso C, McDonough T, Parker M, et al: Atrial fibrillation and flutter: Immediate control and conversion with intravenously administered verapamil. Arch Intern Med 143:877–881, 1983.
92. Abinader E, Borochowitz Z, Berger A: A hemodynamic complication of Verapamil therapy in a neonate. Helv Paediatr Acta 36:451–455, 1981.
93. Haft JI, Habbab MA: Treatment of atrial arrhythmias: Effectiveness of verapamil when preceded by calcium infusion. Arch Intern Med 146:1085–1089, 1986.
94. Lown B, Amarasingham R, Neuman J: New method for terminating cardiac arrhythmias: Use of synchronized capacitor discharge. JAMA 182:548–555, 1962.
95. Bjerkelund C, Orning OM: An evaluation of DC shock treatment of atrial arrhythmias: Immediate results and complications in 437 patients, with long-term results in the first 290 of these. Acta Med Scand 184:481–491, 1968.
96. Frithz G, Åberg H: Direct current conversion of atrial flutter. Acta Med Scand 187:271–274, 1970.
97. Gutgesell HP, Tacker WA, Geddes LA, et al: Energy dose for ventricular defibrillation of children. Pediatrics 58:898–901, 1976.
98. Atkins DL, Sirna S, Charbonnier F, et al: Transthoracic impedance in pediatric defibrillation: Importance of paddle electrode size. Circulation 74(suppl 2):177, 1986. Abstract.
99. Haft JI, Kosowsky BD, Lau SH, et al: Termination of atrial flutter by rapid electrical pacing of the atrium. Am J Cardiol 20:239–244, 1967.
100. Waldo AL: Some observations concerning atrial flutter in man. PACE 6:1181–1189, 1983.
101. Henthorn R, Roberts WS, Kelly K, et al: Conversion of atrial flutter: Rapid atrial pacing as a bedside technique. PACE 3:202–206, 1980.
102. Sen S, Rettig G, Fröhlig G, et al: Sustained atrial flutter after cardiac surgery: Successful termination by rapid atrial pacing. Thorac Cardiovasc Surg 32:41–44, 1984.
103. Campbell RM, Dick M II, Jenkins JM, et al: Atrial overdrive pacing for conversion of atrial flutter in children. Pediatrics 75:730–736, 1985.
104. Greenberg ML, Kelly TA, Lerman BB, et al: Atrial pacing for conversion of atrial flutter. Am J Cardiol 58:95–99, 1986.
105. Fisher JD, Johnston DR, Kim SG, et al: Implantable pacers for tachycardia termination: Stimulation techniques and long-term efficacy. PACE 9:1325–1333, 1986.
106. Joint American College of Cardiology/American Heart Association Task Force on Assessment of Cardiovascular Procedures (Subcommittee on Pacemaker Implantation): Guidelines for permanent cardiac pacemaker implantation, May 1984. J Am Coll Cardiol 4:434–442, 1984.
107. Nathan AW, Creamer JE, Davies DW, et al: Clinical experience with a software based tachycardia reversion pacemaker. PACE 9:1312–1315, 1986.
108. Luceri RM, Castellanos A, Thurer RJ, et al: Noninvasive conversion of atrial flutter using a multiprogrammable DDD pulse generator. PACE 9:137–140, 1986.
109. Fröhlig G, Sen S, Rettig G, et al: Termination of atrial flutter during DDD pacing by rapid overdrive stimulation using the implanted pacemaker lead system. Am J Cardiol 57:483–485, 1986.
110. Greenspon AJ, Greenberg RM, Frankl WS: Tracking of atrial flutter during DDD pacing: Another form of pacemaker-mediated tachycardia. PACE 7:955–960, 1984.
111. Klein GJ, Guiraudon GM, Sharma AD, et al: Demonstration of macroreentry and feasibility of operative therapy in the common type of atrial flutter. Am J Cardiol 57:587–591, 1986.
112. Simpson RJ Jr, Foster JR, Mulrow JP, et al: The electrophysiological substrate of atrial fibrillation. PACE 6:1166–1170, 1983.
113. Hordof AJ, Edie R, Malm JR, et al: Electrophysiologic properties and response to pharmacologic agents of fibers from diseased human atria. Circulation 54:774–779, 1976.
114. Alessi R, Nusynowitz M, Abildskov JA, et al: Nonuniform distribution of vagal effects on the atrial refractory period. Am J Physiol 194:406–410, 1958.
115. Coumel P: Atrial fibrillation. In Surawicz B, Reddy CP, Prystowsky EN (eds): Tachycardias. Boston, Martinus Nijhoff Publishing Company, 1984, pp 231–244.
116. Waldo AL, Henthorn RW, Plumb VJ: Relevance of electrograms and transient entrainment for antitachycardia devices. PACE 7:588–600, 1984.
117. Radford DJ, Izukawa T: Atrial fibrillation in children. Pediatrics 59:250–256, 1977.
118. Zaldivar N, Gelband H, Tamer D, et al: Atrial fibrillation in infancy. J Pediatr 83:821–822, 1973.
119. Perry LW, Hung W: Atrial fibrillation and hyperthyroidism in a 14-year-old boy. J Pediatr 79:668–671, 1971.
120. Ternova TI, Nagaibekova AS: Auricular fibrillation in rheumatic heart defects in children. Pediatriia no. 11:30–33, 1974.
121. Stafford WJ, Trohman RG, Bilsker M, et al: Cardiac arrest in an adolescent with atrial fibrillation and hypertrophic cardiomyopathy. J Am Coll Cardiol 7:701–704, 1986.
122. Touche M, Jouvet M, Touche S: Fibrillation ventriculaire au cours d'un syndrome de Wolff-Parkinson-White: Réduction par choc électrique externe. Arch Mal Coeur 59:1122–1133, 1966.
123. Kaplan MA, Cohen KL: Ventricular fibrillation in the Wolff-Parkinson-White syndrome. Am J Cardiol 24:259–264, 1969.
124. Dreifus LS, Haiat R, Watanabe Y, et al: Ventricular fibrillation: A possible mechanism of sudden death

in patients with Wolff-Parkinson-White syndrome. Circulation 43:520–527, 1971.
125. Dreifus LS, Wellens HJ, Watanabe Y, et al: Sinus bradycardia and atrial fibrillation associated with the Wolff-Parkinson-White syndrome. Am J Cardiol 38:149–156, 1976.
126. Sellers TD Jr, Bashore TM, Gallagher JJ: Digitalis in the pre-excitation syndrome: Analysis during atrial fibrillation. Circulation 56:260–267, 1977.
127. Fenster PE, Comess KA, Marsh R, et al: Conversion of atrial fibrillation to sinus rhythm by acute intravenous procainamide infusion. Am Heart J 106:501–504, 1983.

CHAPTER 12

PREEXCITATION SYNDROMES

Paul C. Gillette, Henry L. Blair, & Fred A. Crawford

Preexcitation has been defined as a condition in which the ventricular myocardium is activated earlier than would be expected had the impulse reached the ventricle by way of the normal atrioventricular (AV) conduction system.[1] We will add to this definition conditions in which the atrial muscle is preexcited—for example, during supraventricular tachycardia (SVT) or ventricular paced rhythm—earlier than would be expected had the impulse reached the atrium retrograde by way of the normal AV conduction system. Thus we will include not only classic Wolff-Parkinson-White (WPW) and Lown-Ganong-Levine (LGL) syndromes but also the more recently recognized concealed WPW syndrome resulting from a unidirectional retrograde accessory pathway (URAP).[2–5]

Preexcitation in adults was brought to clinical recognition by Wolff, Parkinson, and White in 1930.[6] The clinical features of WPW syndrome in children have also been described extensively.[7–14] The importance of the WPW syndrome has increased following recent observations that preexcitation is responsible for SVT in about half of the children with this dysrhythmia.

ANATOMIC BASIS

The anatomic basis for WPW is now firmly established as being a direct muscular connection between the atrium and ventricle.[15] Direct muscular AV connections were described first by Paladino[16] in 1876 and by Kent[17] in 1893 and were considered to be responsible for normal AV conduction. Holzmann and Scherf consolidated the concepts of Wolff, Parkinson, and White and of Paladino and Kent when they suggested in 1932 that direct AV muscular connections could be responsible for the WPW syndrome.[18] Wood, Wolferth, and Geckeler were the first to demonstrate accessory muscular connections in a patient with WPW syndrome.[19]

Many adults and children with the WPW syndrome have since been shown to have an anatomic muscular connection.[20] Accessory AV muscle bundles have been found on the right and left free walls as well as in the septum. The pathways are small, usually 10 mm in length and 1 mm in diameter. They are usually made up of normal working atrial or ventricular myocardium, but they may also be made of specialized cells resembling the normal AV node. The pathways may be multiple, with two or more occurring on the same free wall or with one pathway on one free wall and another on the opposite free wall.

Histopathologic studies have not yet been published of patients with the concealed WPW syndrome (i.e., having accessory connections that conduct only in the ventriculoatrial direction).

The LGL syndrome, characterized by a short PR interval and normal QRS, has been less well studied histopathologically.[21] Brechenmacher published one case of a patient with definite LGL and SVT who had an accessory connection that bypassed the AV node and inserted in the bundle of His.[22]

NOMENCLATURE

The European Society of Cardiology proposed a new nomenclature for the anatomic substrates of preexcitation.[23] The terminology has varied in the past, partly because eponyms have been used for structures that differ from those originally described by the authors. We will use the following nomenclature in this chapter:

Accessory atrioventricular muscle bundles (also called *Kent bundles*) are bundles that originate in the atrial myocardium and terminate in the ventricular myocardium. This term will apply irrespective of the direction of the conduction. The abbreviated term for these fibers is *accessory connection* (AC).

Atriofascicular fibers (also called *atrio-Hissian fibers* or *James fibers*) originate in the atrial myocardium and insert into the bundle of His or one of the bundle branches.

Intranodal pathways (also called *James fibers*) are faster conducting pathways through the AV junctional area without decremental conduction.

Accessory nodoventricular muscle bundles (also called *Mahaim fibers*) are defined as muscle bundles that originate in the AV node and insert directly into the ventricular myocardium.

Fasciculoventricular connections (also called *Mahaim fibers*) originate in the ventricular specialized conduction system (i.e., the bundle of His or bundle branches) and insert directly into the ventricular myocardium.

SURFACE ECG AND RECOGNITION

Wolff-Parkinson-White Syndrome

The WPW syndrome is defined electrocardiographically as an abnormally short PR interval with an abnormally prolonged QRS duration. The QRS complex is a fusion between electrical activation of the ventricles by the bundle of His and the AC. The initial slurred part of the QRS (delta wave) is caused by activation of the ventricles by the AC, while the normal terminal part of the QRS is caused by activation of the remainder of the ventricles via the bundle of His. For adults, WPW is defined as a PR interval less than 0.12 s and a QRS duration greater than 0.12 s. For pediatric patients, our criteria are a PR interval ≤0.08 s in infants younger than 2 years, <0.10 s in children 2 to 10 years of age, and <0.12 s in older children; and a QRS duration >0.08 s in infants younger than 2 years, ≥0.10 s in children 2 to 10 years of age, and ≥0.12 s in children older than 10 years (Fig. 12–1). Some patients may have the anatomic substrate of WPW without the usual ECG criteria. On the surface ECG, WPW with a normal PR interval may be found in patients with intra-atrial conduction delay or in those taking drugs that prolong AV conduction of the AC.

The degree of preexcitation of the ventricles in WPW varies from moment to moment and from day to day in many patients. At times a patient with proven WPW syndrome may have a normal ECG. Some cases of WPW are subtle on the surface ECG during sinus rhythm, especially in patients with left lateral ACs, in whom the delta wave may become apparent only on careful search of the PR segment in multiple ECG leads (Fig. 12–2). This may be proved by pacing the right or left atrium and causing marked preexcitation. Alternatively, vagotonic or sympathomimetic effects may unmask a delta wave.[24]

Patients thought to have concealed WPW may manifest if vagal stimulation maneuvers are applied. In our series (Gillette, unpublished observations) of 105 children with WPW syndrome, 72 had evidence of WPW on each ECG, whereas 33 had at least one ECG with no evidence of WPW.

WPW has been subclassified into types A, B, and C based on the shape of the QRS in the precordial leads. Type A mimics right bundle-branch block, with positive delta waves and QRS forces in lead V_1 (Fig. 12–3). Type B mimics left bundle-branch block, with a positive delta wave in lead V_6 (Fig. 12–1). Type C has a mainly positive delta wave and QRS forces in V_1 through V_6. We have not found this to be a useful classification, because the location of the AC is not always as predicted by the ECG. However, for historical purposes we will provide these data. Of our 105 patients, 29 had type A, 62 had type B, and 11 had type C.

The vectorcardiographic (VCG) manifestation of WPW syndrome consists of slowing of the initial QRS forces, corresponding to the delta wave (Fig. 12–4).

Lown-Ganong-Levine Syndrome

The LGL syndrome is characterized by a short PR interval (as defined in WPW syndrome) and a normal QRS complex.

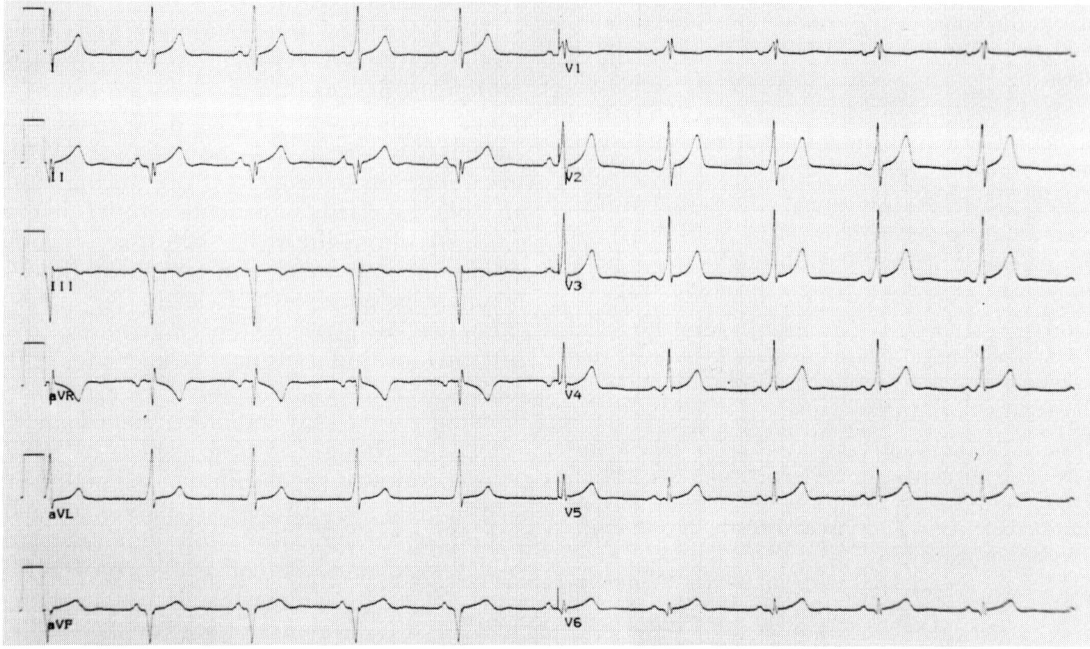

FIGURE 12–1
Demonstration of Wolff-Parkinson-White syndrome, showing 12 simultaneously recorded surface ECG leads at standard calibration. The delta wave is most apparent in lead I, aVL, and the mid-precordial leads.

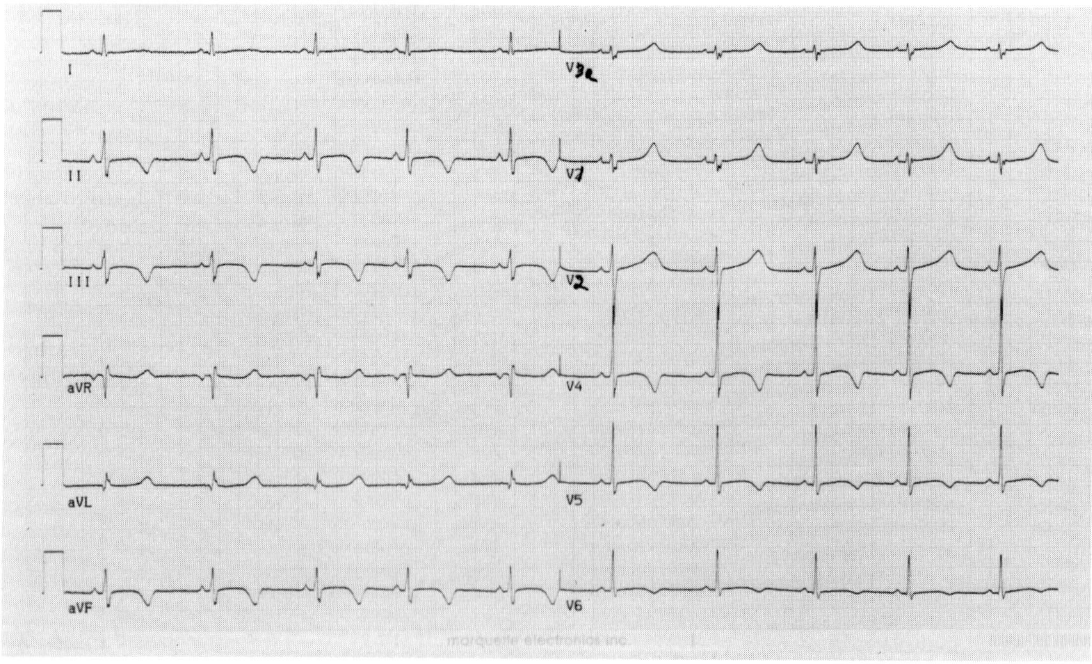

FIGURE 12–2
A demonstration of a more subtle form of WPW syndrome with the same recording technique. The delta wave is only apparent in V_4 and V_5, but the absence of a Q wave in V_6 is also suggestive of abnormal depolarization.

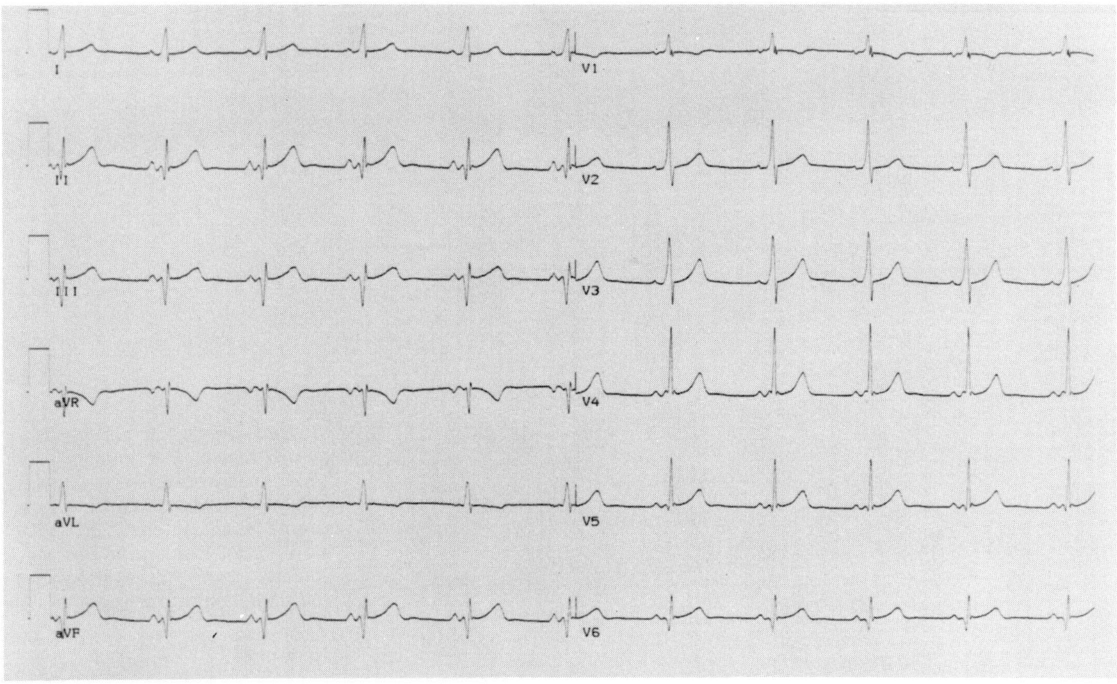

FIGURE 12–3
Wolff-Parkinson-White syndrome, type A, with the most positive delta wave being at surface lead V_1. Abnormal depolarization can also be seen well on leads II and aVF.

CLINICAL IMPLICATIONS AND NATURAL HISTORY OF WPW IN CHILDREN

Scherf and Neufeld reviewed the prevalence of the WPW syndrome in children and adults, combining four reports taken from random surface ECG tracings in children without known heart disease who were between birth and 16 years of age.[14] The prevalence of WPW was found to be 0.15%. In two series of children from heart clinics, the prevalence was 0.5%. In two random groups of ECGs from patients aged 16 to 50 years, it was 0.16%. Thus approximately 1.5 patients in 1000 will show classic WPW syndrome on surface ECG. The threefold increased incidence in the pediatric heart clinic series probably indicates that WPW is associated with various types of congenital heart disease.

WPW syndrome appears to be more common in males than females. Scherf and Neufeld reviewed 23 series from the literature and found that 65% of the cases of WPW occurred in males.[14] In our series of 105 patients (Gillette, unpublished observations), 57% of the patients were male.

The WPW syndrome may be inherited. An adequate family history was available in 56 of our 105 patients. Of these 56 patients, 13 had a history of dysrhythmia or WPW in the immediate family; nine had WPW syndrome, and the other four had SVT. The anatomic substrate can be inherited with no surface ECG evidence of WPW. We have reported a case of a boy with severe, repetitive SVT that was eventually proven by electrophysiologic studies (EPS) and surgical division to be caused by a concealed AC.[25] The father and a cousin of the boy had classic WPW on surface ECG; two of his aunts had SVT. We have recently investigated another family in which a daughter had a concealed AC, and the mother had WPW with SVT. Each had an AC proved by EPS and epicardial mapping at the time of surgery. Both pathways were on the left posterolateral surface of the heart.

Of our 105 patients with WPW, 36 had congenital heart disease (CHD). Virtually every type of defect was represented in this group; the most common were ventricular septal defect (six), Ebstein's anomaly of the tricuspid valve (four), and endocardial cushion defect (three). Other types of heart disease were found in only one or two patients each. The finding of four patients with Eb-

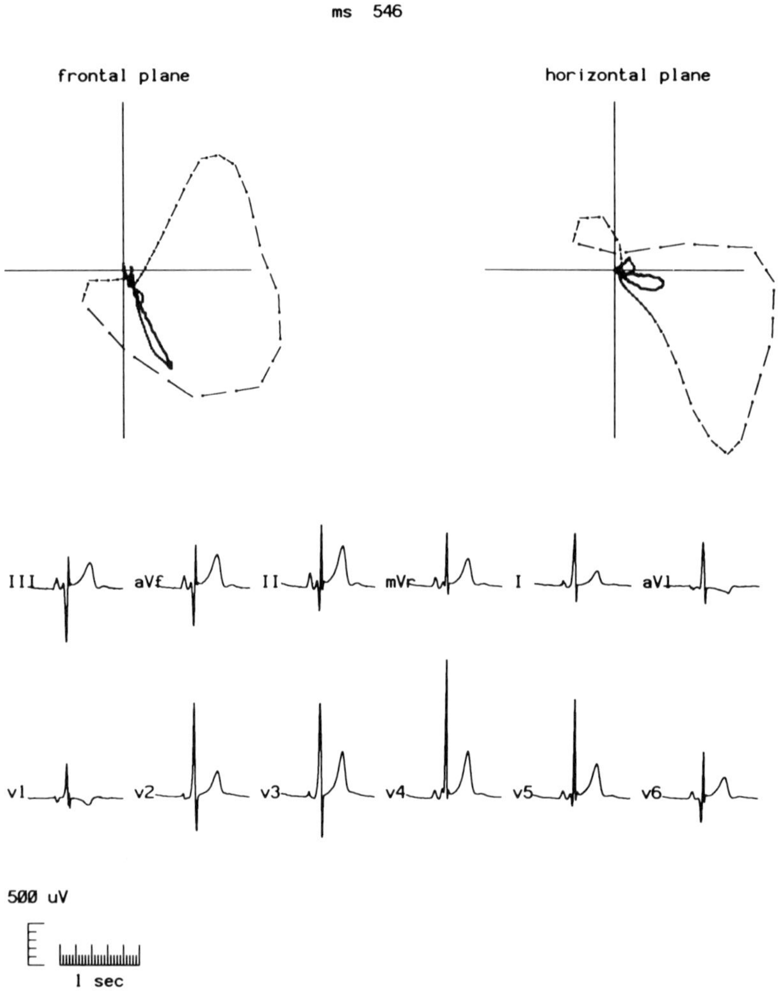

FIGURE 12–4
Vectorcardiographic and electrocardiographic presentation of Wolff-Parkinson-White syndrome. The Wolff-Parkinson-White syndrome is characterized by initial slow depolarization. In the vectorcardiogram, this is shown by the dots being close together.

stein's anomaly and WPW out of a total of 72 cases of Ebstein's anomaly seen in our institution indicates a statistical ($p < 0.05$) association of these two defects. The finding of six cases of WPW and ventricular septal defect out of 1675 ventricular septal defects does not represent a statistical association.

WPW on the surface ECG may either mimic or mask CHD. Type A WPW may be mistaken for right ventricular hypertrophy. A 9-year-old girl was referred to us for evaluation of Ebstein's anomaly and WPW diagnosed clinically at the age of 3 years. The physical examination was not typical of Ebstein's anomaly. Echocardiography showed no evidence of a tricuspid valve anomaly but did indicate that the patient had pulmonary hypertension. After catheterization she was found to have a large ventricular septal defect with pulmonary hypertension and irreversible pulmonary vascular disease. The right ventricular hypertrophy that should have manifested on her surface ECG had been masked by the WPW syndrome, although it was seen on the ECG when SVT was induced in the catheterization laboratory. When WPW is present on the surface ECG, its mimicking/masking properties effectively remove one of our most useful clinical tools. Since one-third of patients with WPW have CHD, care must be taken to search for associated heart defects.

The natural history of the WPW syndrome has been of interest to pediatric cardiologists for many years and is now assuming increasing importance because of the possibility of surgical treatment of the associated dysrhythmias. In 1973 Moene and Roos[12] reported an infant in whom WPW was first recognized at 1 month of age following an episode of SVT. After the second month of life he no longer showed either WPW or SVT, despite frequent ECGs over a 10-month period. Wolff, Parkinson, and White[6] suggested that this resolution occurs because of anatomic maturation of the conduction system, the development of adrenergic innervation, and a decrease in cholinergic dominance.

We have followed several infants with catheterization-proven WPW syndrome who lost the WPW pattern on ECG and ceased having SVT within the first year of life. Of our 98 patients with WPW syndrome (excluding the seven patients who had had surgical treatment of the WPW syndrome), 28 (29%) had no WPW on multiple follow-up ECGs. The age of the patient when WPW disappeared from the ECG ranged from 2 weeks to 18 years (median, 15 months). Of these 28 patients, six continued to have intermittent SVT after disappearance of the WPW syndrome; 14 patients had no further SVT, but seven of these were still receiving medical treatment; and eight never had SVT. Of the 79 patients with WPW who had SVT, seven had surgical treatment; in the remaining 72, SVT resolved in 35; 22 patients still had WPW pattern on ECG, but 13 no longer had it.

Patients who no longer have WPW syndrome but who continue having SVT may have converted from a bidirectional AC to a unidirectional AC conducting only from ventricle to atrium. In patients who no longer have SVT but who continue having WPW syndrome, a pathway that formerly conducted in both antegrade and retrograde directions may now conduct only in the antegrade direction. As will be documented later in this chapter, most ACs that are part of a reentry circuit for SVT conduct at least in the retrograde direction. This study shows that 29% of the patients with WPW syndrome lost the ECG manifestation; 70% of these stopped having SVT. Of patients in whom WPW did not disappear, 40% stopped having SVT. Therefore the disappearance of WPW was significantly ($p < 0.05$) related to the cessation of SVT.

ELECTROPHYSIOLOGY OF ACCESSORY CONNECTIONS

The electrophysiologic substrate of the WPW syndrome was predicted correctly many years ago to be an AC, or preexcitation of the ventricle by way of a Kent bundle. This hypothesis has been substantiated in recent years with the use of new electrophysiologic recording and stimulating techniques (Fig. 12–5). Surgical interruption of ACs with resulting elimination of SVT has been the final proof.[26–34]

As the term "preexcitation" implies, at least part of the ventricle is activated before the His bundle is depolarized. This is documented by recording electrical activity from one or both ventricles before depolarization of the His bundle (Fig. 12–6). Therefore in sinus rhythm the low septal right atrial to His (LSRA-H) interval is usually normal and His to ventricle (HV) interval is short. The electrophysiologic explanation for the observations during atrial pacing relies on the fact that AV node conduction is slowed at rapid paced rates, while the AC usually does not have this property of decremental conduction (Fig. 12–7). With incrementally more rapid atrial pacing, the conduction velocity remains the same. Since the AC continues conducting at the same velocity and the AV node conducts at a slower velocity during

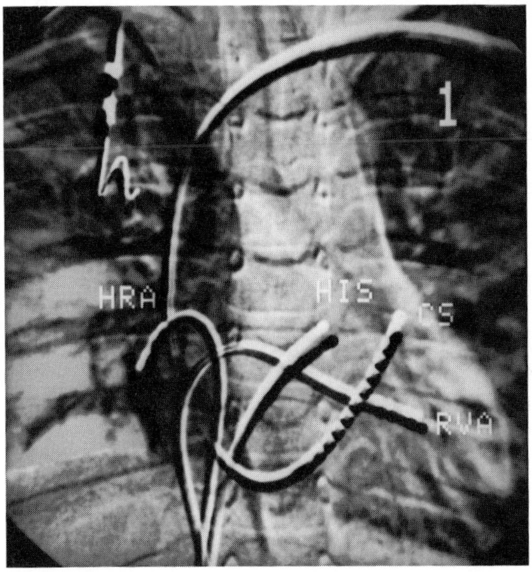

FIGURE 12–5
Digital subtraction image of catheter positions during a study of Wolff-Parkinson-White syndrome. Surface ECG lead VI is seen overlying the fourth rib. The high right atrial (HRA) quadripolar catheter is positioned near the sinus node. The His bundle catheter (HIS) is positioned just across the septal leaflet of the tricuspid valve. The right ventricular apex (RVA) catheter is positioned across the tricuspid valve against the right ventricular septum. The coronary sinus (CS) catheter is positioned from the left brachial vein into the coronary sinus to the left heart border.

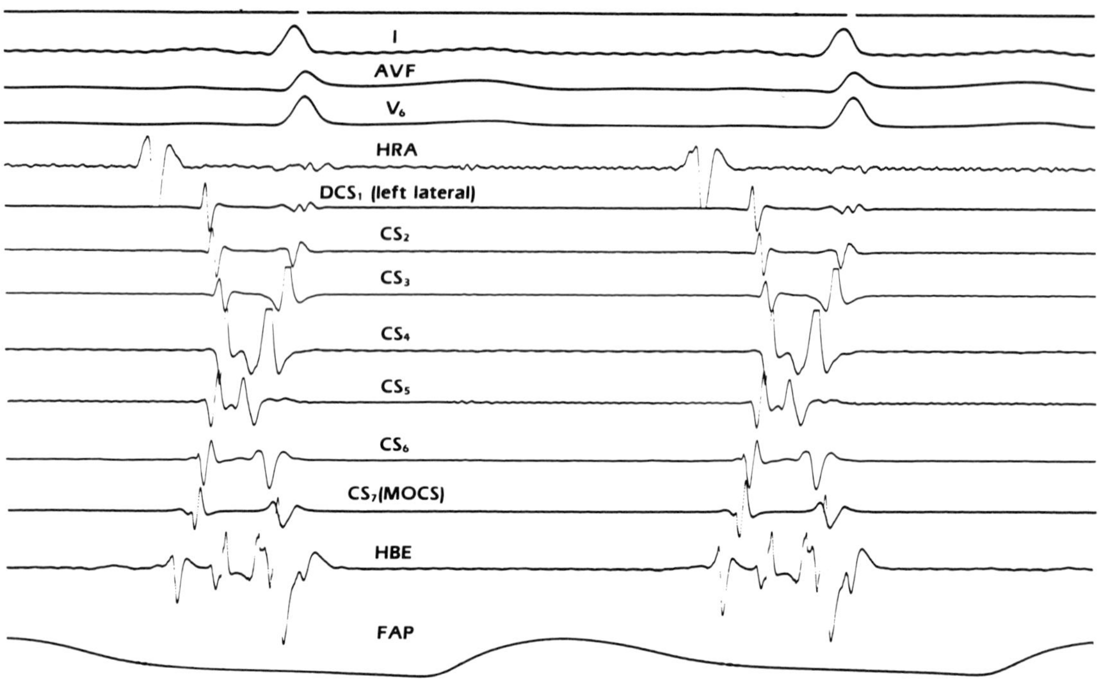

FIGURE 12–6
Surface ECG leads I, aVF, and V_6 recorded simultaneously with the high right atrial (HRA) electrogram, seven coronary sinus electrograms, His bundle electrogram (HBE), and femoral artery pressure (FAP). These recordings were done in a patient with very subtle Wolff-Parkinson-White syndrome. On intracardiac electrograms, it can be seen on coronary sinus pair 5 (CS_5) that atrial ventricular conduction is very rapid in that area, and the ventricular depolarization occurs before ventricular depolarization on the surface ECG and before termination of His bundle depolarization on the His bundle electrograms. This localizes the area of accessory connection to the mid-coronary sinus.

rapid atrial pacing, more and more of the ventricle is activated by the AC. The fact that the QRS on the surface ECG is a fusion complex may be also shown during programmed premature stimulation when the His to delta interval becomes progressively shorter and then negative (Fig. 12–8). In some cases the His bundle depolarization even occurs after the termination of the QRS complex at rapid atrial pacing rates. Again, the ventricle is depolarized through the AC, whereas the His bundle depolarization occurs at increasingly longer intervals because of increasing antegrade delay in the AV node.

The property of nondecremental conduction through an AC can be demonstrated in the retrograde direction as well when, with more and more rapid ventricular pacing or earlier and earlier premature ventricular stimulation, the ventriculoatrial (VA) conduction time remains constant (Fig. 12–9). This is in contrast to patients without an AC and retrograde conduction entirely through the AV node: The VA conduction time increases with more premature (earlier) ventricular stimulation. A few cases have recently been reported in which VA conduction occurred over a structure other than the normal AV node, but decremental VA conduction was present.[35] The physiology of the AC was assumed to be similar to that of the AV node in these patients.

In a study of 28 pediatric patients with WPW syndrome,[27] we compared the conduction properties and refractory periods of the AC in antegrade and retrograde directions; we also compared the properties of the AC with those of the normal AV conduction system. In two of the 28 patients, although there was antegrade conduction over the AC, no retrograde conduction was present. In the other 14 patients in whom retrograde conduction was evaluated, the retrograde effective and functional refractory periods of the AC were shorter than the antegrade effective and functional refractory periods in each case. The mean retrograde effective refractory period (ERP) of the AC was 231 ms; the mean antegrade ERP of the AC was 310 ms. The antegrade ERP of the AV node was shorter than the antegrade ERP of the AC in 18 of the 20 patients in whom both could

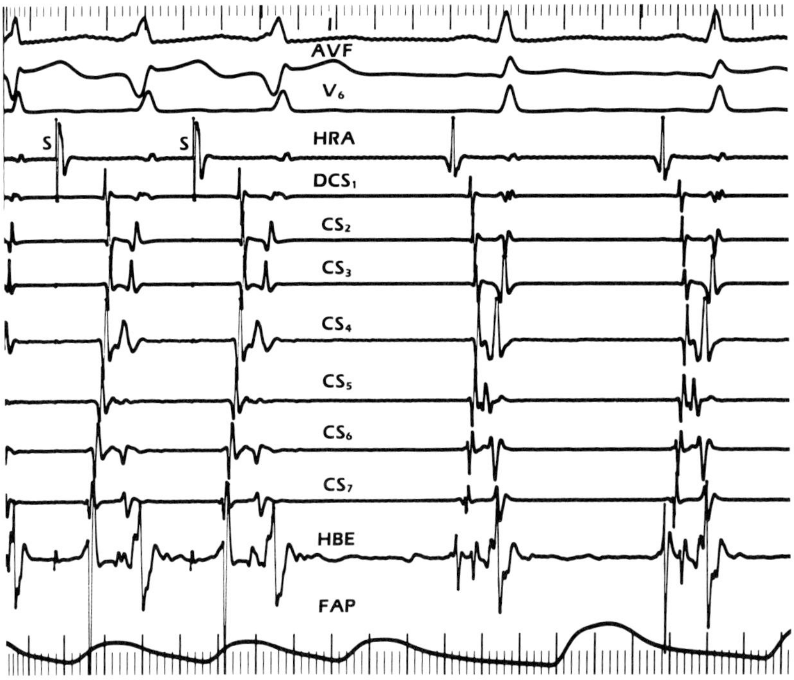

FIGURE 12–7

Surface ECG leads I, aVF, and V_6 recorded simultaneously with a high right atrial electrogram (HRA), seven coronary sinus electrograms, and a His bundle depolarization during high right atrial pacing and sinus rhythm. The first two beats on the left are paced from the high right atrium. Earliest ventricular activation can be seen on CS_5. During right atrial pacing a large delta wave appears that is positive in lead I and negative in lead aVF. The His bundle depolarization occurs further after ventricular depolarization. During sinus rhythm the delta wave is inapparent, but early activation of the ventricle can still be seen in the left ventricular leads.

FIGURE 12–8

Single premature atrial stimulation enhances the delta wave and further shortens the HV interval. Shown are surface leads I, aVF, V_1, and V_6 recorded simultaneously with a high right atrial (HRA) electrogram, six coronary sinus electrograms, two His bundle electrograms, a right ventricular apex (RVA) electrogram and femoral artery pressure (FAP). During sinus rhythm, His bundle depolarization occurs simultaneously with ventricular depolarization on the coronary sinus lead and the surface electrocardiogram lead, after a single premature stimulus, which conducts to a greater extent over the accessory connection. The His bundle depolarization occurs midway into ventricular depolarization on the surface electrocardiogram.

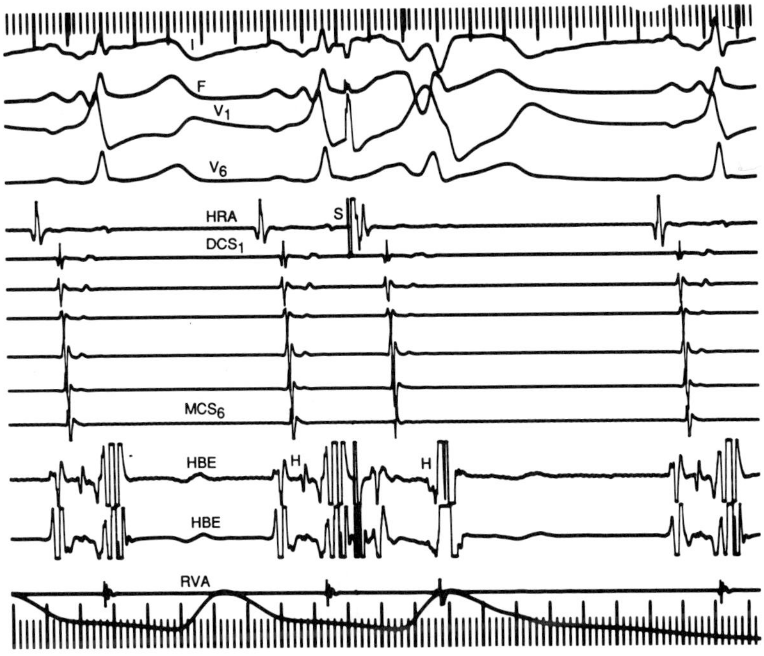

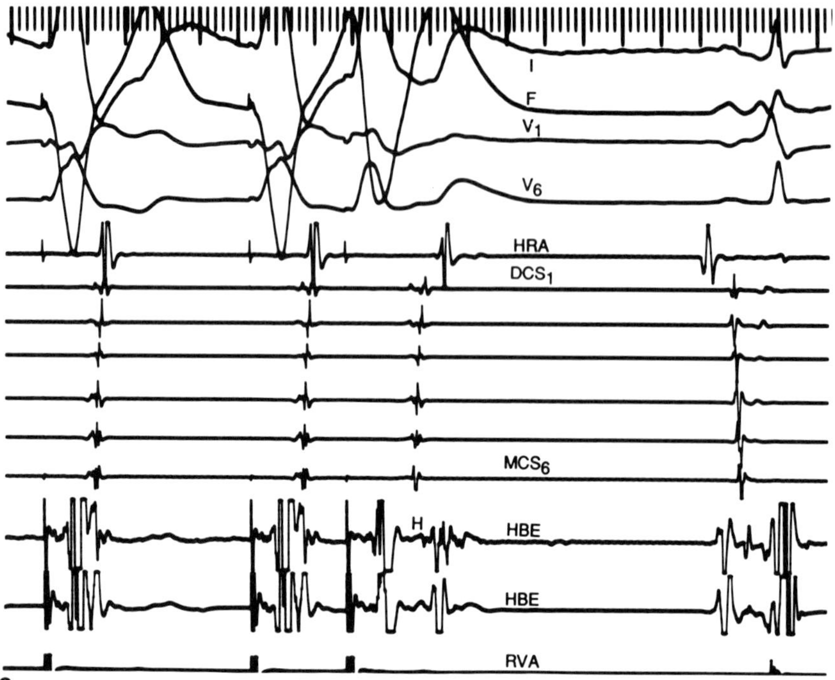

FIGURE 12–9

A demonstration of fusion conduction in a retrograde manner. Shown are simultaneously recorded leads I, aVF, V_1, and V_6 together with a high right atrial (HRA) electrocardiogram, six coronary sinus electrograms, two His bundle electrograms (HBE), and a right ventricular apex (RVA) electrogram. During ventricular pacing (i.e., the first two beats), the activation of the atrium is purely through the coronary sinus electrodes. After the premature stimulus, there is slowed ventricular conduction to the left ventricle as evidenced by the further widening of the QRS and the fact that the left ventricular depolarization is very late. This results in part of the atrium being activated by the accessory connection (i.e., the left atrium), and part of the atrium being activated by way of His bundle and the AV node (i.e., the low septal right atrium). It can be seen that the coronary sinus depolarization occurs before His bundle depolarization. The His bundle depolarization still occurs and appears to activate the low septal right atrium.

be measured. Thus although the conduction times of the AC were always faster than those of the AV node, the antegrade ERPs of the AC were usually longer than those of the AV node, with the difference ranging from 20 ms to 510 ms. We have found a statistical association between the presence of a left-sided AC and a short LSRA-H interval with lower than normal decremental conduction.

Our findings in children were qualitatively similar to those in adults. Adults usually had a longer refractory period of the AC than of the AV node and a shorter retrograde ERP of the AC than of the antegrade ERP. DuBrow et al showed that the refractory period of the AV node is shorter in children than it is in adults.[36] In our study we also found short refractory periods of the AV node in children; however, the mean antegrade ERP of the AC was longer than that reported in adults. We did not find as high a frequency of short antegrade ERPs as Tonkin et al found in adults.[28] We do not know if there is a change in refractory periods between the pediatric age group and adulthood, because patient groups were selected based on their refractory periods. Our patients were chosen for study in the catheterization laboratory predominantly because of the presence of SVT. Patients with a relatively long antegrade ERP of the AC and a relatively short AV node ERP are predisposed to SVT, because they have a large window in which a premature atrial beat can start the SVT (Fig. 12–10). On the other hand, although many of the adults studied by Gallagher's group[26] were studied because of SVT, a greater percentage was selected for study because of atrial fibrillation. It may be that patients with a large window for SVT induction present earlier (thus they are studied by pediatric cardiologists), and patients with shorter refractory periods have less frequent episodes of SVT but are more prone to rapid response to atrial fibrillation. Whether the atrial fibrillation is caused by the WPW syndrome or is secondary to ischemic or hypertensive heart disease is not known.

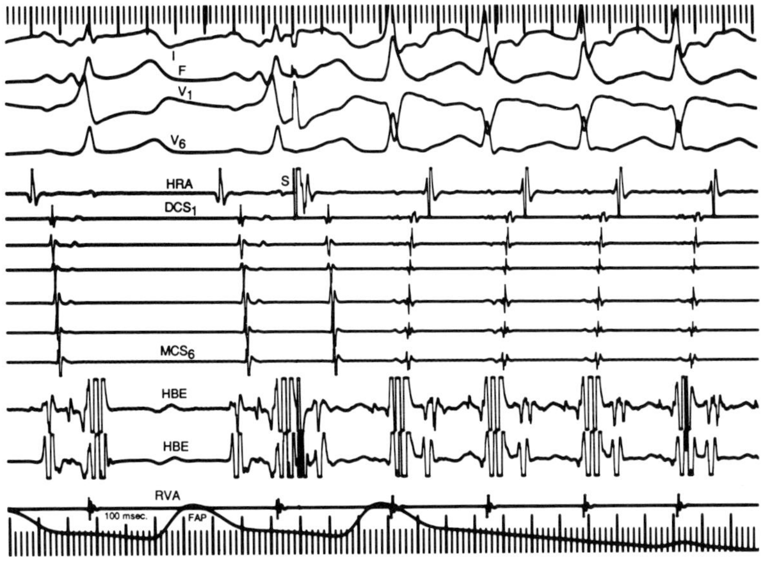

FIGURE 12–10
Induction of supraventricular tachycardia by single premature right atrial depolarization. The premature depolarization results in refractoriness in the accessory connection and slow conduction over the AV node. It can be seen that there is now a long period of time between left atrial depolarization and left ventricular depolarization. There is a narrow normal QRS on the surface electrocardiogram as compared to a large delta wave in the sinus beats. The HV interval is now normal. As soon as the left ventricle is activated, the left atrium is reactivated, and a reentrant supraventricular tachycardia with an antegrade conduction over the AV node His axis and retrograde conduction over the accessory connection is started and perpetuated.

MECHANISMS OF SVT

The mechanisms of supraventricular tachydysrhythmias in patients with WPW vary, but the AC is usually involved. The tachydysrhythmia seen most often in this syndrome is reciprocating SVT with a normal QRS complex. In our clinical series of 105 patients, 79 had documented SVT (Fig. 12–11). The ECG recorded during their first episode of SVT was available in 41 of these 79. In 38 of the 41, the QRS complex was normal during SVT. Three patients had a wide QRS during tachycardia that appeared to be the same as the WPW QRS complex during sinus rhythm.

In our series of 28 patients studied by catheter electrophysiologic techniques,[27] reciprocating tachycardia (defined as a reentrant SVT in which both the atrium and the ventricle form part of the reentry circuit) was induced in 26. In 22 of these 26 the QRS complex was normal during tachycardia, and the reentry circuit was as follows: antegrade through the AV node, bundle of His, and bundle-branch system to the ventricular myocardium, then retrograde through the AC to the atrium and back to the AV node (Fig. 12–12)—so-called orthodromic tachycardia. In each of these 22 subjects, the method of induction was a premature atrial depolarization that did not conduct antegrade through the AC but did conduct antegrade through the AV node. Since the AC had not been used in the antegrade direction, it was available for retrograde conduction and completed the reentry circuit. In each case the antegrade ERP of the AC was longer than that of the AV node. In 11 of these 22 patients, the QRS morphology showed a bundle-branch block pattern at the onset of tachycardia, but none had a consistent, continuous bundle-branch block pattern during SVT.

Three subjects had a QRS morphology during tachycardia similar to the WPW QRS seen during sinus rhythm—so-called antidromic tachycardia (Fig. 12–13).[37] Each had reciprocating SVT with the following reentry circuit: antegrade through the AC to the ventricular myocardium and retrograde through the bundle of His and AV node or through a second AC to the atrium and back to the AC. The mechanism of induction of SVT in two of these three patients was by a premature atrial depolarization that blocked antegrade in the AV node but conducted through the AC, leaving the AV node available for retrograde conduction to complete the reentry circuit.

On the surface ECG this type of SVT can mimic ventricular tachycardia, and two of these three patients had been diagnosed ini-

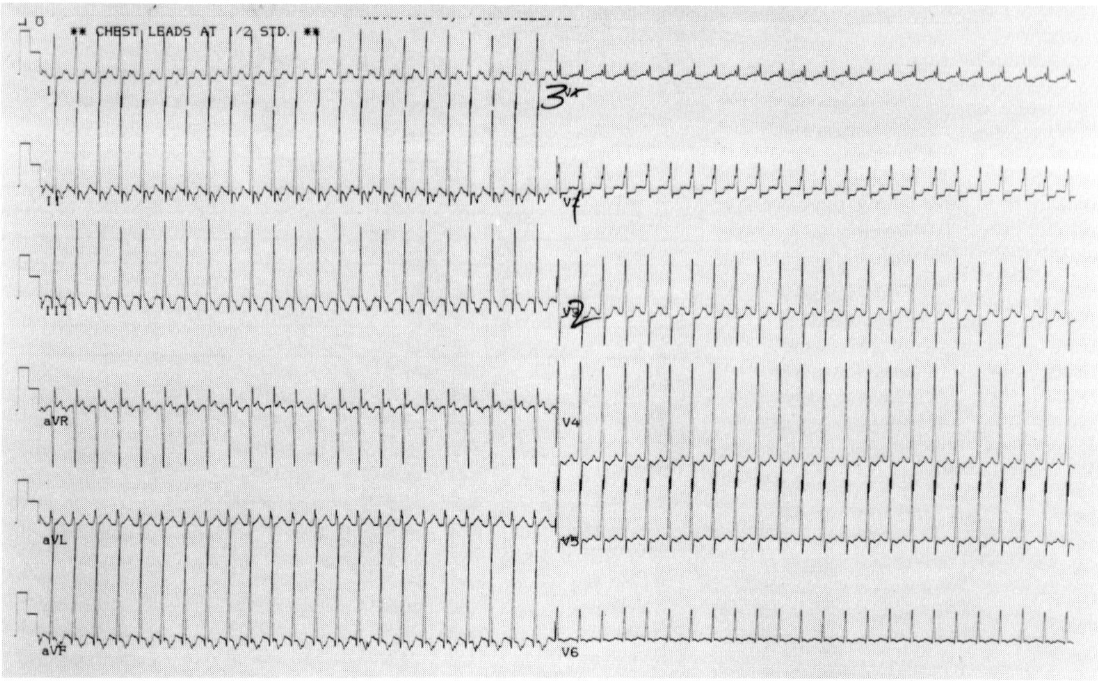

FIGURE 12–11
12-lead surface electrocardiogram with full calibration of the limb leads and half calibration of the chest leads taken from a infant with a posterior septal accessory connection. A rapid normal narrow QRS tachycardia can be seen, with clear retrograde activation of the atrium. Retrograde activation is most clearly defined in surface lead II.

tially as having ventricular tachycardia. In one of these three patients, SVT could be induced only by ventricular premature stimulation (Fig. 12–14). If antidromic tachycardia is found, multiple pathways should be suspected.

It is important to remember that not all supraventricular tachydysrhythmias in patients with WPW syndrome are the result of an AC. One patient in our series of 28 had only AV nodal reentry tachycardia. This was demonstrated by a normal atrial activation sequence during tachycardia and 2:1 block below the His bundle during SVT.[27] We have since seen another patient with WPW syndrome who had two types of SVT; one type of tachycardia involved antegrade conduction through the AV node-His bundle pathway and retrograde conduction through an AC, and the other involved both antegrade and retrograde conduction through the AV node (AV node reentry).

Patients with the permanent form of junctional reciprocating tachycardia (incessant tachycardia with normal QRS and a low atrial P wave) have a specific type of accessory connection with decremental properties. These ACs preexcite the atrium during SVT.

There are other dysrhythmias in which the AC is important in the patient's response, even though it may not play a primary role in the genesis of the dysrhythmia. Two examples are atrial fibrillation and atrial flutter (Figs. 12–15 and 12–16).[38, 39] The AC, if it has a short refractory period, allows rapid transmission of the supraventricular impulses to the ventricles.[40, 41] In our clinical series of 105 patients, two patients had atrial fibrillation, two had atrial flutter, and one had both. The patient with both atrial flutter and fibrillation also frequently developed ventricular fibrillation when the rapid impulses penetrated the ventricles.

Two of our 28 patients who had EPS had atrial fibrillation as the predominant clinical dysrhythmia. Both exhibited an extremely rapid, irregular, wide QRS tachycardia clinically and had severe symptoms. The antegrade ERP of the AC was less than 200 ms in each. The antegrade ERP and FRP of the AC correlate with the rapidity of the ventricular responses to atrial fibrillation. In Gal-

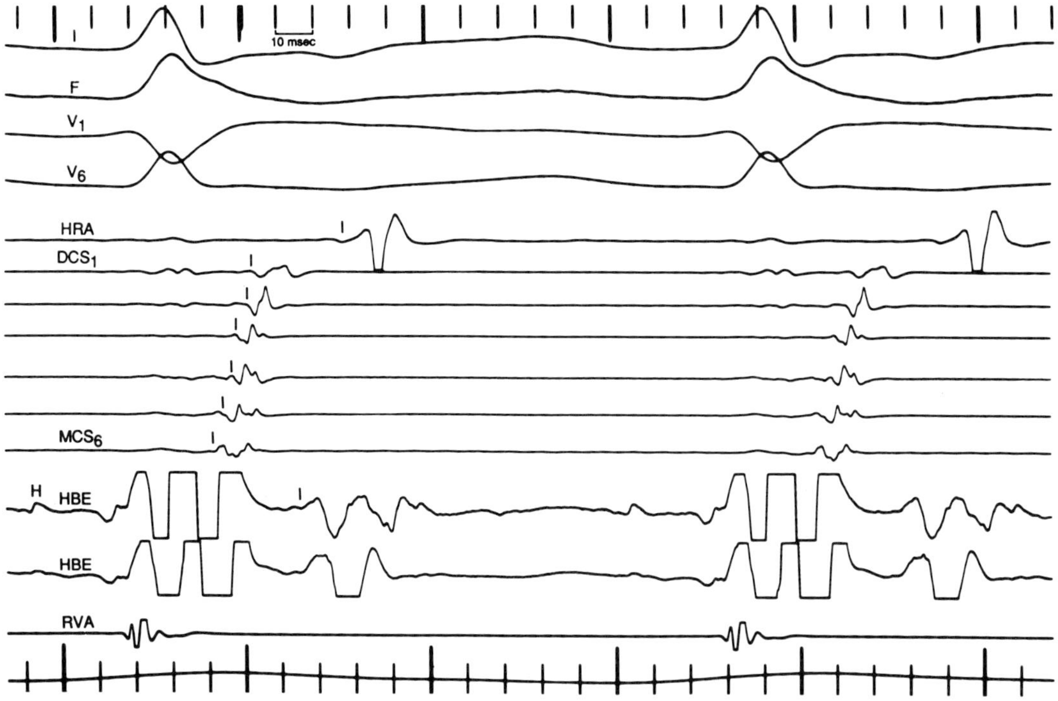

FIGURE 12–12

Rapid paper speed in a patient with a left posterior accessory connection during supraventricular tachycardia. Shown are simultaneously recorded surface ECG leads I, F, V_1, and V_6 together with a high right atrium (HRA) electrogram, six coronary sinus electrograms, two His bundle electrograms, right ventricular apex (RVA) electrogram, and femoral artery blood pressure. Tick marks have been placed on the beginning of atrial activation. It can be seen that the earliest atrial activation occurs on coronary sinus pair 6, which is positioned in the mid coronary sinus. This activation is clearly earlier then the low septal right atrium and the high right atrium.

lagher's series[26] a correlation coefficient of 0.74 was obtained between the antegrade ERP of the AC and the shortest cycle length of the ventricular response during atrial fibrillation.

The anatomic location of the AC may be determined by EPS. The most accurate method to localize an AC is to observe the atrial activation sequence at a time when the AC is depolarizing the atria retrograde. This is best determined during reciprocating SVT with retrograde conduction over the pathway (Figs. 12–17 and 12–18). Four catheters are used: one with six pairs of electrodes in the coronary sinus to record distal to proximal coronary sinus electrograms, one in the high right atrium for high right atrial recording, one in the His bundle area for recording low septal right atrial activity, and one in the right ventricle apex for recording and pacing. The catheter that we insert initially in the apex of the right ventricle may be moved to various sites in the right atrium during SVT so that the entire endocardial surface may be mapped. The earliest site of the atrium activated during SVT or ventricular pacing with retrograde conduction over the accessory pathway is the atrial insertion of the AC. We have found that if SVT cannot be induced, the atrial end of the pathway is best delineated by introduction of premature ventricular stimuli. In this manner the atrial electrograms can be separated from the ventricular electrograms. In our series, as well as in those of Gallagher, Gilbert, and Svenson[42] and others, catheter localization of the pathway has correlated well with the site found during surgical mapping and division.

Pacing the atrium from different sites also may help localize the pathway.[43, 44] The closer the pacing electrodes are placed to the atrial end of the AC, the larger is the component of the ventricle that is activated by way of the AC and the larger is the delta wave. Thus if left atrial pacing enhances the delta wave more than does right atrial pacing at a similar cycle length, we can presume a left-sided pathway. Pacing from the right and left atria has had nearly equal effects in cases of septal ACs.

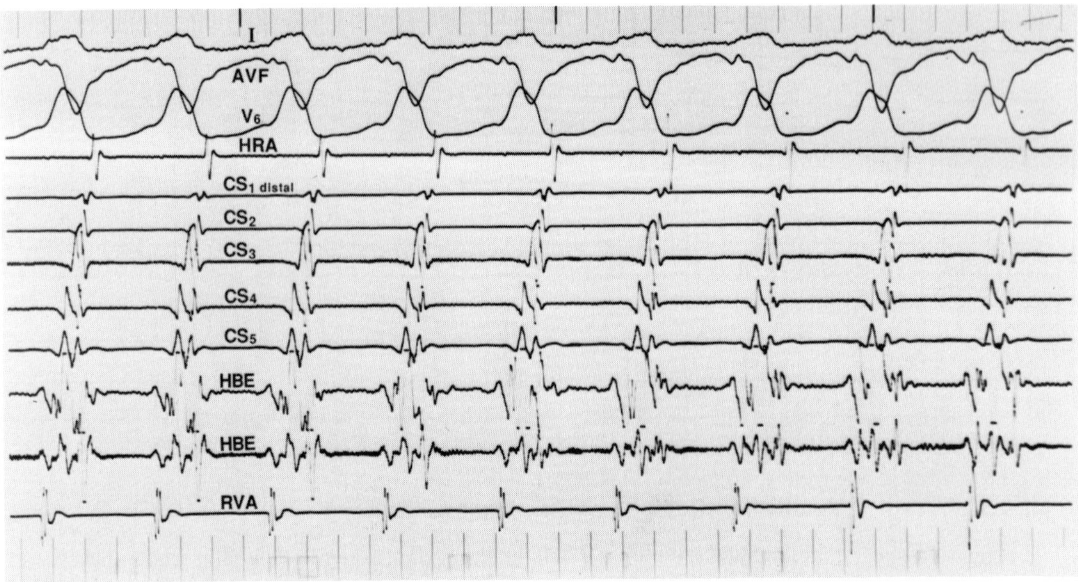

FIGURE 12–13
Antidromic reciprocating tachycardia recorded in a patient with two accessory connections. Antegrade conduction is proceeding down the right atrial accessory connection, and retrograde conduction is proceeding up a left atrial accessory connection. Shown are simultaneously recorded surface ECG leads I, aV, F, and V_6 together with a high right atrial (HRA) electrogram, 5 coronary sinus electrograms, two His bundle electrograms (HBE), and right ventricular apex (RVA) electrogram. A left bundle branch block pattern is occurring, indicating anterograde conduction through a right-sided accessory connection. No His bundle depolarization is seen. Retrograde conduction is earliest in coronary sinus pair 3, with nearly simultaneous activation of the atrium and ventricle, indicating retrograde conduction over a left-sided accessory connection.

One of the best methods for localizing the pathway (right, left, or septal) is available if a bundle-branch block occurs.[45] If a right-sided AC is responsible for the retrograde limb of the SVT and right bundle-branch block occurs, the VA conduction time and the cycle length of the tachycardia will increase, because the right bundle branch is an integral part of the reentry circuit. If the right bundle branch is blocked, the reentry circuit is lengthened, because the impulse has to travel down the left bundle branch and

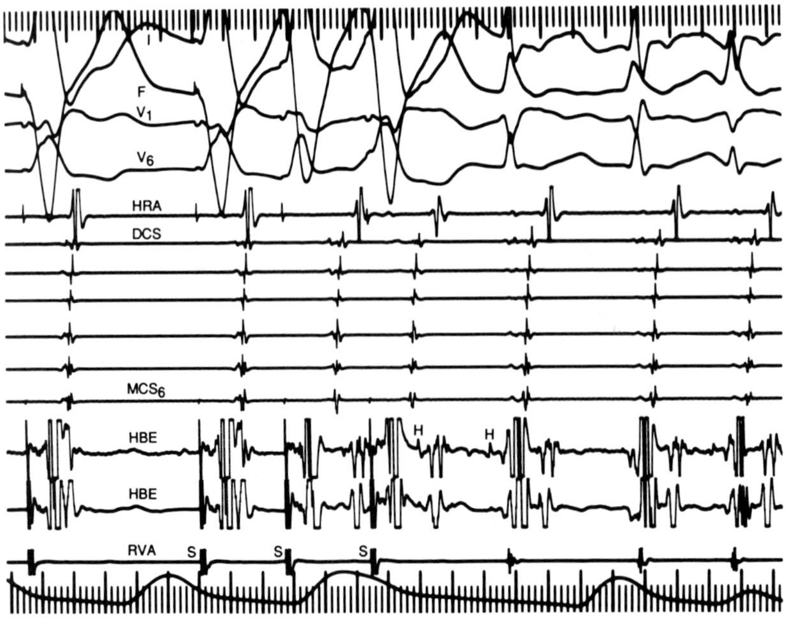

FIGURE 12–14
Induction of supraventricular tachycardia by paired ventricular premature stimuli. Each of the two premature ventricular stimuli results in retrograde conduction. The second one creates enough delay in the AV node that reentry may occur over the left-sided accessory connection.

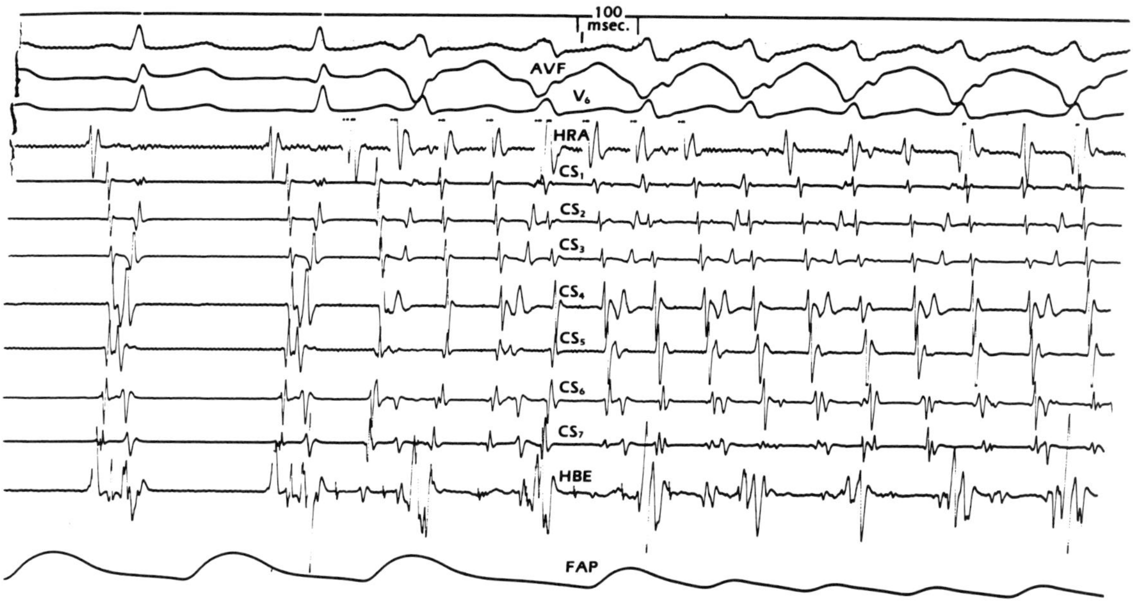

FIGURE 12–15

Induction of atrial flutter/fibrillation in a patient with Wolff-Parkinson-White syndrome, resulting in anterograde conduction over the accessory connection. Shown are surface leads I, aVF, and V_6 recorded simultaneously with a high right atrial (HRA) electrogram, seven coronary sinus electrograms, and a His bundle electrogram (HBE). A burst of rapid atrial pacing results in a disorganized high right atrial activity, indicating atrial fibrillation. The left atrium as manifested by the coronary sinus is more organized and may be in atrial flutter. Antegrade conduction is occurring over the accessory connection, as indicated by the wide QRS complexes.

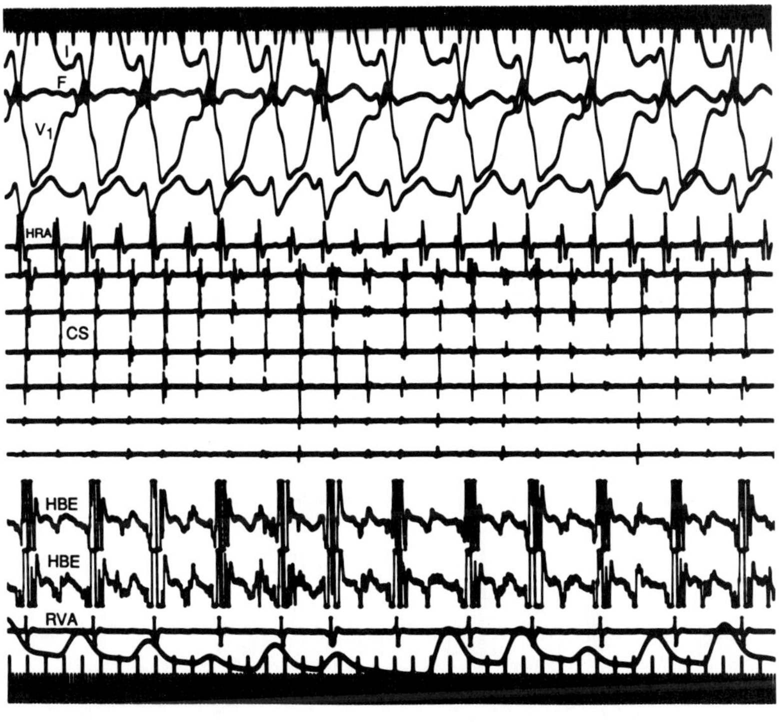

FIGURE 12–16

Atrial flutter in a patient with Wolff-Parkinson-White syndrome. Shown are simultaneously recorded leads I, F, V_1, and V_6 together with a high right atrial (HRA) electrogram, six coronary sinus (CS) electrograms, two His bundle electrograms (HBE), and one right ventricular apex (RVA) electrogram. Rapid regular activity is seen in each of the atrial leads, and rapid wide QRS complex is seen in the surface ECG, indicating atrial flutter with 2:1 conduction through the accessory connection.

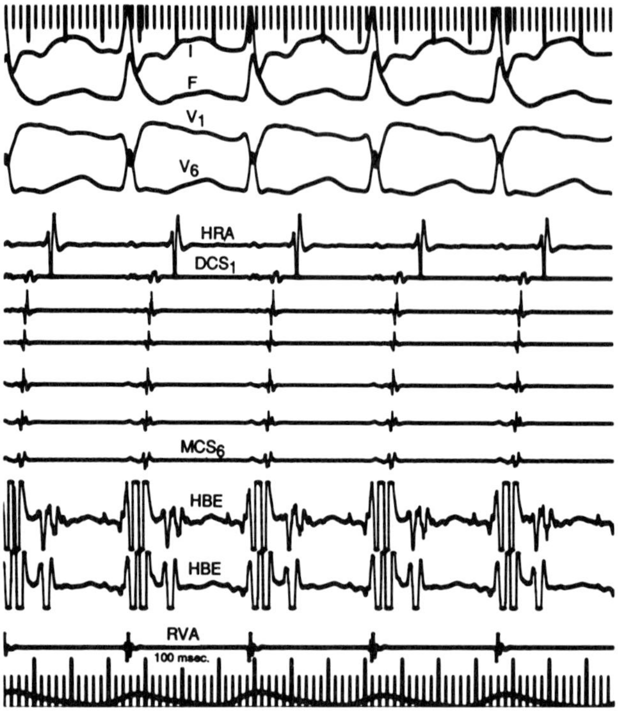

FIGURE 12–17
Mapping of retrograde activation in a patient with a left sided accessory connection during supraventricular tachycardia. Shown are simultaneously recorded surface ECG leads I, aVF, V_1, and V_6 together with a high right atrium, six coronary sinus electrograms, two His bundle electrograms (HBE), and a right ventricular apex (RVA) electrogram. The earliest activation is occurring in the mid coronary sinus, that is coronary sinus pair 6. From these electrograms it cannot be determined whether there is an earlier point in the coronary sinus farther toward the septum.

through the septal myocardium before activating the right ventricular-Purkinje network and then the right ventricular AC. Left bundle-branch block does not affect the VA conduction time or the tachycardia cycle length in patients with right-sided pathways, but it does cause slowing of VA conduction and cycle length in patients with a left-sided AC. A patient with a septal AC has no change in VA conduction or cycle length with either right or left bundle-branch block. Slowing of VA conduction time and cycle length second-

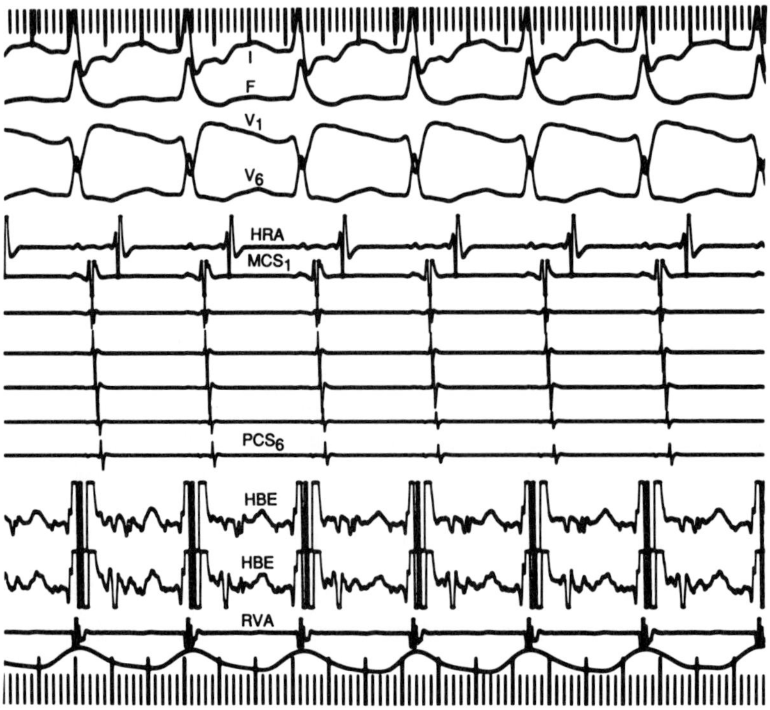

FIGURE 12–18
Mapping of the site of an accessory connection in a patient with a mid left atrial accessory connection. Shown are simultaneously recorded surface ECG leads I, F, V_1, and V_6 together with the high right atrial (HRA) electrogram, six coronary sinus electrograms, two His bundle electrograms (HBE), and a right ventricular apex (RVA) electrogram. The catheter has been pulled back from its position in Figure 12–17 so that the distal pair of electrodes now lie where the proximal pair of electrodes formerly were. This is now the side of earliest activation. All other more proximal coronary sinus positions are activated later, indicating that the pair of electrodes MCS_1 is on the site of the accessory connection.

ary to ipsilateral bundle-branch block also proves that the AC is part of the reentry circuit.

Premature stimulation of the ventricle at a time when the His bundle is refractory is another good method for proving the presence of an AC and determining its participation in the reentry circuit. If the atrium can be preexcited—that is, if the atrial cycle length can be shortened by a premature ventricular extrastimulus when the His bundle is refractory—then an AC is present. If the atrial activation sequence stays the same as that during SVT, the AC is part of the reentry circuit. If the atrium cannot be preexcited by right ventricular premature stimulation in a patient with a presumed left-sided AC, then the AC cannot be ruled out, because the time required for conduction through the septum and across the ventricle to the AC may be such that the ventricular end of the pathway has already been activated by the natural reentry. In this case left ventricular stimulation may be used to prove that an AC is present (Fig. 12–19).

EFFECTS OF DRUGS ON THE AC IN WPW SYNDROME

Studies in the catheterization laboratory have given us a better understanding of the effects of antidysrhythmic drugs on the AC. Digitalis glycosides, frequently used to treat SVT in patients with WPW syndrome, were found to shorten the antegrade effective refractory period of the AC and increase the rate of the ventricular response to atrial fibrillation in six of 21 adult patients studied in the catheterization laboratory.[46] In seven of 21 patients the reverse was true, while in five no difference was elicited. The effect could not be determined in three patients. We administered ouabain intravenously in the catheterization laboratory to eight children; in three of them the antegrade ERP of the AC lengthened, and in five it shortened, but only in two of these patients was the ERP shortened to 220 ms or less.[27] In these two we felt it wisest not to use digitalis in the clinical treatment of their SVT. Further investigation is needed of the effects of digitalis preparations on the refractory period and the ventricular response during atrial fibrillation. Digitalis, to some degree in all patients, slows conduction and increases refractoriness of the AV node.

Propranolol has been found to have little or no effect on the refractory period of the AC.[47] It lengthens the refractory period and slows conduction in the AV node and thus is of some use in the treatment of SVT in the WPW syndrome. The effects of procainamide, quinidine, flecainide, encainide, and amiodarone on the conduction properties of the AC have been studied extensively in adults but not in children.[48, 49] These drugs tend to prolong the antegrade and retrograde refractory periods and conduction times of the AC. The degree of prolongation varies markedly among patients; in general, the patients with the shortest refractory periods tend to have the least response to procainamide and quinidine. Thus in patients with atrial flutter and/or fibrillation and a rapid ventricular response through a Kent bundle, digitalis is contraindicated, and flecainide or procainamide is the drug of choice. It is important to test the patient's response with regard to slowing the ventricular response to atrial flutter or fibrillation in the hospital, since this is a life-threatening dysrhythmia and the response is not uniform.

Several new drugs are available for treating the tachycardias related to the WPW syndrome. Disopyramide[50] and aprindine[51] are quinidine congeners that seem to have effects similar to those of quinidine on the refractory period. Amiodarone lengthens the refractory period of the AC; it has been used extensively in Europe to treat these tachycardias, with excellent results, but its diversity of side effects may not permit its use in this country.[52, 53]

TREATMENT OF DYSRHYTHMIAS ASSOCIATED WITH WPW SYNDROME

In the past, treating SVT associated with the WPW syndrome in children was simply a matter of using digitalis glycosides. In the majority of patients digitalis was either successful in preventing the reciprocating tachycardia or caused no harm if the tachycardia continued. It may be that digitalis amelio-

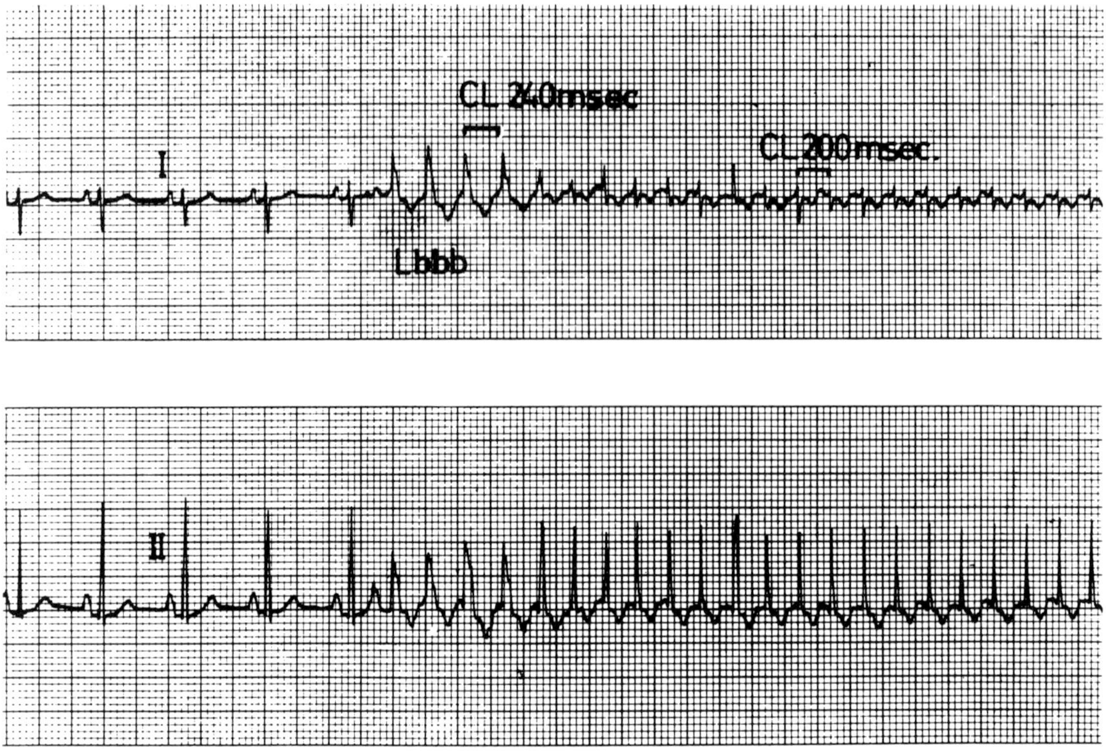

FIGURE 12–19
Surface electrocardiogram demonstrating the presence of a left accessory connection. Shown are surface leads I and II recorded simultaneously on a patient with spontaneous onset of supraventricular tachycardia. In lead I, a premature atrial contraction can be seen on the ST segment preceeding the onset of tachycardia. There are four wide QRS left bundle branch block beats with a cycle length of 240 ms, but when the QRS normalizes, the cycle length shortens to 200 ms. This indicates that there is an accessory connection, despite the fact that no Wolff-Parkinson-White syndrome was indicated on the surface ECG and that it does participate in the reentry circuit. (Reprinted from Gillette PC: The preexcitation syndromes. In Gillette PC, Garson A Jr (eds): Pediatric Cardiac Dysrhythmias. New York, Grune and Stratton, 1981, p 171.)

rated the symptoms of tachycardia, even when the tachycardia did not stop, by slowing the tachycardia and by increasing the heart's ability to withstand the fast rates. Physicians treating adult patients with WPW syndrome have been less than satisfied with the use of digitalis for many years, even before it was known that in some patients digitalis shortened the antegrade ERP of the AC. It was known that adults with WPW syndrome who developed atrial fibrillation were more likely to have an extremely fast ventricular response, and perhaps ventricular fibrillation, when they were taking digitalis. This clinical response has not been clearly defined in pediatric patients; however, there have been reports of sudden unexpected death in adults with the WPW syndrome, some of whom were taking digitalis.[7, 8, 10, 54–57] Because WPW syndrome is rare in the pediatric age group and only a small percentage of the patients seem to develop life-threatening dysrhythmias, it is possible that deaths from rapid ventricular response to supraventricular rhythms do occur but have not been brought to the attention of pediatric cardiologists. In the large pediatric cardiology clinic at Texas Children's Hospital we have seen only slightly more than 100 patients with WPW syndrome in 25 years; two of these patients experienced ventricular fibrillation, and both were receiving digitalis. One had a univentricular heart, and the other had a normal heart. These and other patients have been reported in a combined series from Texas Children's and Boston Children's Hospitals.

These findings, together with the findings in adults and the EPS of Sellers, Bashore, and Gallagher[46] demonstrating possible shortening of the Kent bundle refractory period by digitalis, call into question the current practice of most pediatric cardiologists to treat all children with SVT and WPW with digitalis. Ideally, a patient with WPW and

SVT who requires treatment should have an EPS to determine the antegrade ERP of the AC at rest and after intravenous administration of ouabain or digoxin. It is currently our policy to investigate each such patient older than 1 year in this manner. Digitalis is not used clinically to treat SVT in patients with an antegrade ERP of the AC that is less than 220 ms (either at rest or after digoxin administration) unless an overriding need exists, such as a severe cardiomyopathy. In patients with a short ERP of the AC, propranolol may be used as an alternate treatment, although it must be given four times per day. In infants younger than 1 year, we used propranolol because of the difficulties of performing detailed EPS in infants.

In a patient of any age who does not respond to single drug treatment of SVT associated with WPW syndrome, we recommend EPS to determine the mechanism of the SVT and the anatomic and physiologic characteristics of the pathway. The combination of quinidine and propranolol has been extremely effective in several infants in our series who had severe, repetitive SVT. The most frequently successful medication for our overall group of patients was digitalis. The second most effective drug was propranolol alone. Verapamil successfully controlled SVT in one patient in our series after digoxin, propranolol, quinidine, and combinations of the three had failed. Recently, flecainide has been used with great success.

There are two other methods used to treat SVT in patients with WPW syndrome. One is a pacemaker, particularly a radiofrequency rapid atrial pacemaker, that can be used by the patient or parent to override the SVT after it occurs.[58, 59] We have used this on one patient with good success, and another such patient has been reported by Dreifus et al.[60] Pacemakers have been developed that will be able to sense the rapid rate of the SVT and automatically induce one or several premature atrial extrastimuli to terminate the tachycardia. Patients with WPW syndrome are not the best candidates for this treatment, however, since they are prone to rapid 1:1 conduction of the atrial overdrive impulses to the ventricle.

A more direct surgical treatment has been popularized by Sealy, Gallagher, and their colleagues at Duke University in which the AC—or, more rarely, the normal AV conduction system—is divided surgically, thereby interrupting the reentry circuit.[61–64] The AC, rather than the normal system, must be divided in patients in whom the primary dysrhythmia is atrial flutter or fibrillation. In all such patients who may undergo surgery, it must first be proven that the AC is part of the reentry circuit, and the AC must be localized by endocardial mapping in the catheterization laboratory. The AC is pinpointed by epicardial mapping in the operating room and is divided surgically while the patient is on cardiopulmonary bypass. We have used this technique in 67 pediatric patients, with complete cure of the SVT in 62 (93%) of them. The surgical technique as it is used in our institution is described in detail in chapter 16.

We recommend direct surgical division of the AC when a single low-risk drug does not control the SVT, or in patients predisposed to sudden death. We believe the open heart surgical procedure is preferable to long-term treatment with multiple drug regimens. We recommend medical therapy be carried out more aggressively in infants in hope that the AC will cease to function and the WPW syndrome and SVT will disappear. In resistant cases, however, successful surgical interruption of ACs has been carried out in infants as young as 1 month. A surgeon who routinely performs surgery on neonates and infants with congenital cardiac defects has a decided advantage in performing surgery on infants with WPW syndrome.

References

1. Durrer D, Schuilenburg RM, Wellens HJJ: Preexcitation revisited. Am J Cardiol 25:690–697, 1970.
2. Coumel P, Attuel P: Reciprocating tachycardia in overt and latent preexcitation. Influence of functional bundle branch block on the rate of the tachycardia. Eur J Cardiol 1:423–436, 1974.
3. Wellens HJJ, Durrer D: The role of an accessory atrioventricular pathway in reciprocal tachycardia. Observations in patients with and without the Wolff-Parkinson-White syndrome. Circulation 52:58–72, 1975.
4. Orzan F, Gillette PC: Reciprocating tachycardia due to a right-sided unidirectional retrograde anomalous pathway. PACE 1:306–312, 1978.
5. Gillette PC: Concealed anomalous cardiac conduction pathways: A frequent cause of supraventricular tachycardia. Am J Cardiol 40:848–852, 1977.
6. Wolff L, Parkinson J, White PD: Bundle branch block with short PR interval in healthy young people prone to paroxysmal tachycardia. Am Heart J 5:686–692, 1930.
7. Engle MA: Wolff-Parkinson-White syndrome in in-

fants and children. Am J Dis Child 84:692–698, 1952.
8. Shiebler GL, Adams P, Anderson RC: Wolff-Parkinson-White syndrome in infants and children. Pediatrics 24:585–591, 1959.
9. Swiderski J, Lees MH, Nadas AS: Wolff-Parkinson-White syndrome in infancy and childhood. Br Heart J 24:561–569, 1962.
10. Giardina ACV, Ehlers KH, Engle MA: Wolff-Parkinson-White syndrome in infants and children. Br Heart J 34:839–m846, 1972.
11. Wolff GS, Han J, Curran J: Wolff-Parkinson-White syndrome in the neonate. Am J Cardiol 41:559–563, 1978.
12. Moene RJ, Roos JP: Transient Wolff-Parkinson-White syndrome and neonatal reciprocating tachycardia. Circulation 48:443–447, 1973.
13. Wellens HJJ, Lubbers WJ, Losekoot TG: Preexcitation. In Roberts NK, Gelband H (eds): Cardiac Arrhythmias in the Neonate, Infant and Child. New York, Appleton-Century-Crofts, 1977, pp 231–263.
14. Scherf L, Neufeld HN: Prognosis. In The Pre-Excitation Syndrome: Facts and Theories. New York, Yorke Medical Books, 1978, pp 162–178.
15. Becker AE, Anderson RH, Durrer D, et al: The anatomical substrates of the WPW syndrome. Circulation 57:870–879, 1978.
16. Paladino G: Contribuzione all'anatomia, istologia e fisiologia del cuore. Mov Med-Chir (Napoli) 8:428–434, 1876.
17. Kent AFS: Researches on the structure and function of the mammalian heart. J Physiol 14:233–246, 1893.
18. Holzmann M, Scherf D: Ueber elektrocardiogramme mit verkurzter vorhof-kammer-distanz und positiven P-zacken. Z Klin Med 121:404–422, 1932.
19. Wood FC, Wolferth CC, Geckeler GD: Histologic demonstration of accessory muscular connections between auricle and ventricle in a case of short P-R interval and prolonged QRS complex. Am Heart J 24:454–459, 1943.
20. Rosenberg HS, Klima R, McNamara DG, et al: Atrioventricular communication in the WPW syndrome. Am J Clin Pathol 56:79–86, 1971.
21. Lown B, Ganong WF, Levine SA: The syndrome of a short P-R interval, narrow QRS complex and paroxysmal rapid heart action. Circulation 5:663–670, 1952.
22. Brechenmacher C: Atrio-His bundle tracts. Br Heart J 37:853–855, 1975.
23. Anderson RH, Becker AE, Brechenmacher C, et al: Ventricular preexcitation. A proposed nomenclature for its substrates. Eur J Cardiol 3:27–36, 1975.
24. Hariman RJ, Krongrad E, Boxer RA, et al: Methods for recording electrograms of the sinoatrial node during cardiac surgery in man. Circulation 61:1024–1029, 1980.
25. Gillette PC, Gallagher JJ, Sealy W: Concealed anomalous cardiac conduction pathway: An operable cause of supraventricular tachycardia. J Pediatr 90:427–430, 1977.
26. Gallagher JJ, Gilbert M, Svenson RH, et al: WPW syndrome. The problem, evaluation and surgical correction. Circulation 51:767–774, 1975.
27. Gillette PC, Garson A, Kugler JD: WPW syndrome in children: Electrophysiologic and pharmacologic characteristics. Circulation 60:1487–1495, 1979.
28. Tonkin AM, Miller HC, Svenson RH, et al: Refractory periods of the accessory pathway in the WPW syndrome. Circulation 52:563–569, 1975.
29. Castillo CA, Castellanos A: His bundle recordings in patients with reciprocating tachycardias and WPW syndrome. Circulation 42:271–285, 1970.
30. Gallagher JJ, Kasell J, Sealy WC, et al: Epicardial mapping in the WPW syndrome. Circulation 57:854–866, 1978.
31. Gallagher JJ, Pritchett ELC, Sealy WC, et al: The preexcitation syndromes. Prog Cardiovasc Dis 20:285–327, 1978.
32. Wellens HJJ: Value and limitations of programmed electrical stimulation of the heart in the study and treatment of tachycardias. Circulation 57:845–852, 1978.
33. Waldo AL, MacLean WAH, Karp RB, et al: Sequence of retrograde atrial activation of the human heart: Correlation with P wave polarity. Br Heart J 39:634–640, 1977.
34. Amat-y-Leon F, Dhingra RC, Wu D, et al: Catheter mapping of retrograde atrial activation. Observations during ventricular pacing and AV nodal reentrant paroxysmal tachycardia. Br Heart J 38:355–362, 1976.
35. Narula OS: Retrograde pre-excitation. Comparison of antegrade and retrograde conduction intervals in man. Circulation 50:1129–1143, 1974.
36. DuBrow IW, Fisher EA, Amat-y-Leon F, et al: Comparison of cardiac refractory periods in children and adults. Circulation 51:485–496, 1975.
37. Benditt DG, Pritchett ELC, Gallagher JJ: Spectrum of regular tachycardias with wide QRS complexes in patients with accessory atrioventricular pathways. Am J Cardiol 42:828–838, 1978.
38. Campbell RWF, Smith RA, Gallagher JJ, et al: Atrial fibrillation in the preexcitation syndrome. Am J Cardiol 40:514–520, 1977.
39. Dreifus LS, Wellens HJ, Watanabe Y, et al: Sinus bradycardia and atrial fibrillation associated with the Wolff-Parkinson-White syndrome. Am J Cardiol 38:149–156, 1976.
40. Dreifus LS, Haiat R, Watanabe Y, et al: Ventricular fibrillation: A possible mechanism of sudden death in patients with WPW syndrome. Circulation 43:520–527, 1971.
41. Klein GJ, Bashore IM, Sellers TD, et al: Ventricular fibrillation in the WPW syndrome. N Engl J Med 301:1080–1085, 1979.
42. Gallagher JJ, Gilbert M, Svenson RH: WPW syndrome. The problem, evaluation, and surgical correction. Circulation 51:767–785, 1975.
43. Castellanos A, Aranda J, Gutierrez R, et al: Effects of pacing site on QRS morphology in WPW syndrome. Br Heart J 38:363–368, 1976.
44. Morris A, Cohn K, Scheinman MM: Right atrial versus left atrial echo zones: A proposed new criterion for determining the atrial site of retrograde preexcitation. J Electrocardiol 9:357–363, 1976.
45. Pritchett ELC, Tonkin AM, Dugan FA, et al: Ventriculo-atrial conduction time during reciprocating tachycardia with intermittent bundle-branch block in WPW syndrome. Br Heart J 38:1058–1064, 1976.
46. Sellers TD, Bashore TM, Gallagher JJ: Digitalis in the pre-excitation syndrome. Analysis during atrial fibrillation. Circulation 56:260–267, 1977.
47. Rosen KM, Barwolf C, Ehsani A, et al: Effects of lidocaine and propranolol on the normal and anomalous pathways in patients with preexcitation. Am J Cardiol 30:801–809, 1972.
48. Sellers TD, Campbell RWF, Bashore TM, et al: The effects of procainamide and quinidine sulfate in the WPW syndrome. Circulation 55:15–22, 1977.

49. Wellens HJJ, Durrer D: Effect of procainamide, quinidine, and ajmaline in the WPW syndrome. Circulation 50:114–120, 1974.
50. Spurrell RAJ, Thorburn CW, Camm J, et al: Effects of disopyramide on electrophysiological properties of specialized conduction system in man and on accessory atrioventricular pathway in WPW syndrome. Br Heart J 37:861–867, 1975.
51. Zipes DP, Gaum WE, Foster PR, et al: Aprindine for treatment of supraventricular tachycardias with particular application to WPW syndrome. Am J Cardiol 40:586–596, 1977.
52. Wellens HJJ, Lie KI, Bar FW, et al: Effect of amiodarone in the WPW syndrome. Am J Cardiol 38:189–194, 1976.
53. Rosenbaum B, Chiale PA, Ryba D, et al: Control of tachyarrhythmias associated with WPW syndrome by amiodarone hydrochloride. Am J Cardiol 34:215–223, 1974.
54. Wellens HJJ, Lubbers WJ, Losekoot TG: Preexcitation. In Roberts NK, Gelband H (eds): Cardiac Arrhythmias in the Neonate, Infant and Child. New York, Appleton-Century-Crofts, 1977, pp 231–263.
55. Becker AE, Anderson RH, Durrer D, et al: The anatomical substrates of WPW syndrome. A clinicopathologic correlation in seven patients. Circulation 57:870–879, 1978.
56. Duvernoy WFC: Sudden death in WPW syndrome. Am J Cardiol 39:472–478, 1977.
57. Scherf L, Neufeld HN: Prognosis. In The Pre-Excitation Syndrome: Facts and Theories. New York, Yorke Medical Books, 1978, pp 162–178.
58. Kahn A, Morris JJ, Citron P: Patient-initiated rapid atrial pacing to manage supraventricular tachycardia. Am J Cardiol 38:200–204, 1976.
59. Ryan GF, Easley RM, Zaroff LI, et al: Paradoxical use of a demand pacemaker in treatment of supraventricular tachycardia due to the WPW syndrome. Circulation 38:1037–1083, 1968.
60. Dreifus LS, Arriaga J, Watanabe Y, et al: Recurrent WPW tachycardia in an infant. Successful treatment by radio-frequency pacemaker. Am J Cardiol 28:586–591, 1971.
61. Wallace AG, Sealy WC, Gallagher JJ, et al: Surgical correction of anomalous left ventricular preexcitation: WPW (type A). Circulation 49:206–213, 1974.
62. Sealy WC, Anderson RW, Gallagher JJ: Surgical treatment of supraventricular tachyarrhythmias. J Thorac Cardiovasc Surg 73:511–522, 1977.
63. Harrison L, Gallagher JJ, Kasell J, et al: Cryosurgical ablation of the A-V node His bundle. A new method of producing A-V block. Circulation 55:463–470, 1977.
64. Gallagher JJ, Sealy WC, Anderson RW, et al: Cryosurgical ablation of accessory atrioventricular connections. A method for correction of the preexcitation syndrome. Circulation 55:471–479, 1977.

CHAPTER 13

SUPRAVENTRICULAR TACHYCARDIA

Achi Ludomirsky & Arthur Garson, Jr.

Supraventricular tachycardia (SVT) is the most common symptomatic arrhythmia in children. An estimated incidence of one in 25,000 was made in 1967,[1] but in the intervening 20 years, methods of detection have improved and awareness of the condition has increased. For example, the prevalence of Wolff-Parkinson-White syndrome in children is approximately two in 1000.[2] In addition, the number of children who have had cardiac surgical procedures has increased in the past decade, and SVT has become recognized as one of the late sequelae of these procedures. For these reasons we believe that SVT is much more common than originally estimated, and its incidence probably ranges from one in 250 to one in 1000 children.

For the purposes of this discussion, SVT is defined as tachycardia resulting from an abnormal mechanism that requires structures in the heart proximal to the bifurcation of the bundle of His for its perpetuation and that does not have the morphology of atrial flutter on the surface electrocardiogram (ECG). Several clarifications need to be made:

1. The definition of tachycardia depends on the age of the patient and the specific site of origin of the rapid heartbeat. We consider a rhythm that originates in the atrium to be abnormally rapid if, for example, the rate is more than 200 beats per minute (bpm) in a newborn infant or more than 110 bpm in a 10-year-old child. Similarly, a rhythm that originates in the atrioventricular (AV) junction is abnormally rapid if the rate exceeds 100 bpm in a newborn or 80 bpm in a 10-year-old child.
2. SVT is generally defined by the atrial rate and not necessarily by the ventricular rate, because in certain kinds of SVT confined to the atrium AV block may occur, and the ventricular rate will be less than the atrial rate. Two difficulties are encountered with this definition: First, P waves are not always visible on the surface ECG during SVT. In these cases, if the QRS complex is normal and the ventricular rate is abnormally rapid, we infer that the diagnosis is SVT. Second, the ventricular rate may exceed the atrial rate in SVT that has its origin in the AV junction. This situation will exist if there is partial or complete retrograde block in the AV node of impulses that originate in the AV junction. The ventricles will be depolarized once for each impulse, but the atria may be completely dissociated and producing P waves that originate from the sinus node. Again, in this case if the QRS complex is narrow and the ventricular rate is abnormally rapid, we infer that the diagnosis is SVT.
3. This definition of SVT as "tachycardia resulting from an abnormal mechanism" specifically excludes sinus tachycardia.
4. The distinction between SVT and atrial flutter depends on the morphology of atrial depolarization on the surface ECG. Intracardiac recordings may not be helpful. We have therefore included in the definition of SVT absence of flutter waves on the surface ECG (Fig. 13–1).

In this chapter we will consider first the clinical features, surface electrocardiographic findings, and response to treatment of patients with SVT. These features have changed little since the comprehensive review by Nadas et al[3] in 1952. What has evolved in the past quarter century is our concept of the mechanisms of SVT. Knowledge of the mechanisms in a patient with SVT can be important, because different mechanisms re-

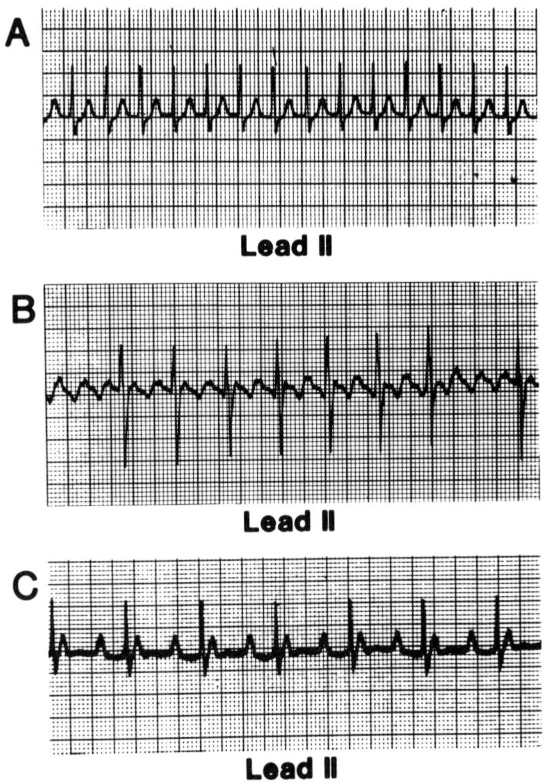

FIGURE 13–1
(*A*) SVT, at a rate of 210/min. P waves are not visible. (*B*) Atrial flutter with varying 2:1 and 3:1 AV block; atrial rate is 260/min. Note angular, "sawtooth" baseline of flutter waves. (*C*) SVT with 2:1 AV block; atrial rate is 195/min. The baseline is isoelectric between P waves. Note: All surface ECG tracings in this chapter were taken at the usual paper speed (25 mm/s) with usual standardization (1 mV/10 mm).

spond differently to treatment. After providing some basic electrophysiologic concepts that are essential to the understanding of the mechanisms of SVT, we will discuss the possible methods of determining the mechanism in the clinical electrophysiology catheterization laboratory. The four clinically separate mechanisms (re-entry with a bypass tract, re-entry without a bypass tract, automatic ectopic focus, and triggered arrhythmia) will then be differentiated with respect to clinical features, surface ECG, intracardiac studies, and response to treatment.

CLINICAL FEATURES OF SVT

In 1952 Nadas et al[3] provided the first comprehensive analysis of SVT in 29 infants and children. We have recently reviewed our data on 346 children under 18 years of age with SVT (Table 13–1) and have found that the data gathered in 1952 are quite similar to the more recent information.

Of 346 patients in the Texas Children's Hospital (TCH) series, 207 of them (60%) lived fewer than 100 miles (160 km) from the Medical Center (the "Houston" patients), and 78 (40%) lived at a distance of 100 miles or greater (the "referred" patients). These 346 patients represent 1% of the 35,000 seen by the TCH Cardiology Section between 1954 and 1989. Despite the two groups having a similar age at onset of SVT, more of the referred patients had their onset of SVT after surgery for congenital heart disease than did the Houston patients.

The referred patients also had a higher percentage of SVT that did not respond to acute treatment within 48 hours, a high recurrence rate, and a higher incidence of SVT that was still present on follow-up (mean 9.7 years). The two groups did not differ with respect to the incidence of congestive heart failure, preexcitation, surface ECG features of SVT, or type of SVT as determined by intracardiac electrophysiologic study.

We have included all 346 patients in the remainder of the analysis. The bias of this study is that 139 patients had difficult-to-control SVT and were referred from other parts of the state and country; however, "simple" cases of SVT have not been omitted. Most pediatricians in Houston refer children with the first episode of SVT to our clinic. Our group of 346 patients therefore is similar to groups seen in other major referral centers but not necessarily to those encountered by hospitals that treat patients only from a small geographic area.

Age at Onset

Our 346 patients ranged in age from 1 day to 17.5 years (median, 22 months) when SVT began. SVT appeared at 1 month of age or less in 18%, by the age of 3 months in 26%, and by the age of 1 year in 36% (Fig. 13–2). The remaining 20% were greater than 1 year of age at onset. The study reported by Nadas et al from the Children's Hospital Medical Center in Boston (CHMC) found that 60% of their patients with SVT were 4 months of age or younger, while the other 40% were between 5 months and 13 years of age.

TABLE 13–1
SUMMARY OF TEXAS CHILDREN'S HOSPITAL STUDY OF CHILDREN WITH SVT (N = 346)

History	
Age at onset	mean: 3.25 yr (range: in utero to 17.8 yr)
Sex	182 male, 164 female
Normal heart (no predisposing factors)	191/346 (55%)
Preoperative CHD	53/346 (18%)
Postoperative CHD	45/346 (13%)
Family history of SVT	41/181 (22%)
Congestive heart failure	73/331 (22%)
ECG in SVT	
QRS rate	mean: 235/bpm (range: 118 to 330)
Prolonged QRS duration	17/172 (10%)
Visible P wave	90/172 (53%)
Normal P wave axis	32/172 (18%)
ECG in sinus rhythm	
WPW	88/346 (25%)
Treatment	
Acute treatment stopped SVT within 48 hrs	142/241 (60%)
Chronic treatment given after first episode	269/331 (81%)
Follow-up	
Recurrence more than 7 days after initial episode	170/228 (75%)
SVT present on long-term follow-up	202/330 (62%)
Died	4/346 (1%)
Duration of follow-up	mean: 9.5 yr (range: 3 mo to 26 yr)
Recurrence of SVT	mean: 2.2 yr (range: 20 mo to 25 yr)

Abbreviations: CHD = congenital heart disease; ECG = electrocardiogram; WPW = Wolff-Parkinson-White.

As with the CHMC study, we found 4 months to be the best dividing line (Table 13–2). Infants whose SVT began at 4 months of age or less had fewer predisposing factors (e.g., myocarditis, drugs, congenital heart disease, thyrotoxicosis, sepsis) and thus a more normal heart, a higher incidence of Wolff-Parkinson-White (WPW) syndrome, more rapid heart rates during SVT, and a greater degree of congestive heart failure. These data are qualitatively similar to those of the CHMC study. Acute treatment was equally

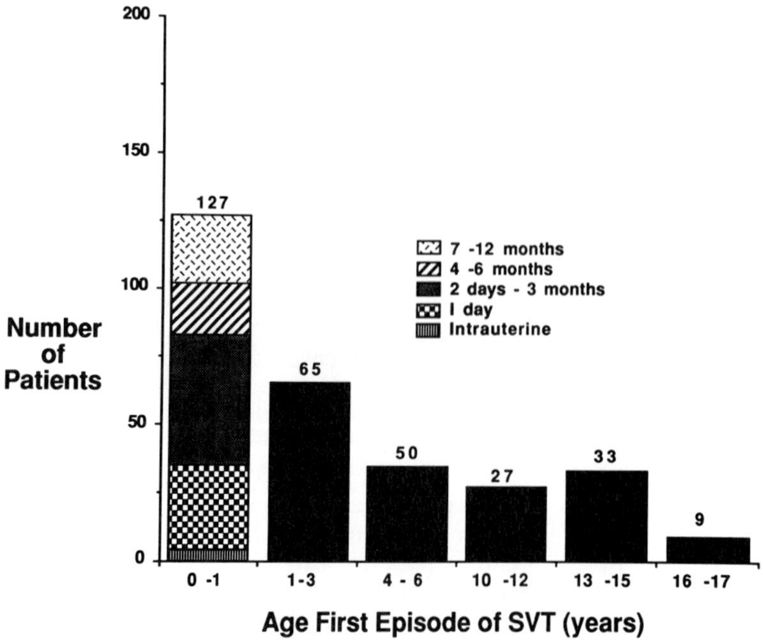

FIGURE 13–2
Age of patients at first episode of SVT.

TABLE 13–2
SUMMARY OF THE EFFECTS OF AGE AT ONSET OF SVT

	AGE AT ONSET		
	≤ 4 mo	*>9 mo*	*p*
Predisposing factors	14/94 (15%)	108/252 (93%)	p <0.01
CHF	33/94 (35%)	40/252 (16%)	p <0.01
Heart rate*	271 ± 9	211 ± 5	p <0.0001
WPW	30/90 (34%)	58/245 (23%)	p <0.02
Acute treatment success	75/91 (82%)	182/231 (79%)	NSD
Recurrent SVT	71/89 (80%)	191/225 (85%)	NSD
SVT at follow-up	37/92 (40%)	159/234 (64%)	p <0.005

*Beats per minute ± standard error of mean.
Abbreviations: CHF = congestive heart failure; NSD = no significant difference; *p* = probability.

successful (i.e., first episode terminated within 48 hours) in the two groups.

We found that at least one recurrence of SVT after the first episode was likely in almost all patients. Age at onset did not affect the recurrence rate; however, age at onset did affect the presence or absence of SVT on long-term follow-up. We found that if SVT began before the age of 4 months, it was less likely to be present on long-term follow-up. This supports the CHMC finding that recurrences are more likely within the first year after the initial episode. The two studies were also in agreement that if a child was older than 4 months when the initial episode occurred, SVT was more likely to continue for longer than 1 year. Nonetheless, 40% of infants in whom SVT began at less than 4 months of age continued to have SVT at follow-up.

Sex Distribution

The striking male:female ratio of 3:1 reported in the CHMC study was not confirmed in our study with a larger number of patients. Our group consisted of 182 males and 164 females (1.12:1). The CHMC study also included a group of patients who had a low risk of late recurrence; this group consisted of males whose SVT began at less than 5 months of age. We have found that age is the most important factor, and we found no significant difference between males and females with respect to history, ECG, response to treatment, or follow-up.

Predisposing Factors

The majority of children with SVT have an otherwise normal heart. In our series 55% of patients had a normal heart, and 45% had a factor present that might predispose to tachyarrhythmias. We have not included WPW syndrome as a predisposing factor, which could partially account for our slightly lower incidence of predisposing factors compared with the 46% reported by the CHMC study, which did include WPW as a factor. The factors from our patient group are listed in Table 13–3. In our study patients without predisposing factors were younger when SVT began, had a greater degree of congestive heart failure, and had faster heart rates. A similar percentage of those with and without predisposing factors still had SVT on follow-up.

Congenital heart disease occurred in 28% of the patients. All types of congenital heart defects occurred, generally following the expected incidence of the various defects found in children without SVT. Two defects that were overrepresented in the SVT group were Ebstein's anomaly (10% of our patients with congenital heart disease) and L-transposition of the great arteries (8% of our patients with congenital heart disease). WPW on surface ECG was present in three of the 10 patients with Ebstein's anomaly and in two of the eight with L-transposition of the great arteries.

The 53 patients with congenital heart disease who had SVT before any surgery had congestive heart failure more frequently than did those patients without congenital heart disease (Table 13–4). Fewer patients in the group with congenital heart disease had SVT on follow-up than did those without congenital heart disease. In 11 of the patients with congenital heart disease, SVT was present before cardiac surgery but was absent afterward. In four of these 11, a Kent bundle was divided at the time of the operation for congenital heart disease. In the seven others

TABLE 13–3
PREDISPOSING FACTORS FOR SVT (N = 155)

APPEARANCE OF SVT			
Preoperative (N=53)	*Postoperative (N=45)*	*Drugs (N=16)*	*Other Factors (N=30)*
VSD=10	Mustard =12	Epinephrine=5	Cardiomyopathy=11
LTGA=8	ASD=6	Methylphenidate=3	Fever=6
AVC=2	AVC=5	Ephedrine=2	Back sepsis=8
ASD=4	ASD=5	Other=2	Myocarditis=6
AS=5	PAB=3	Caffeine=4	Hyperthyroidism=3
PDA=4	BAS=4		Encephalitis=3
EA=6	Other=10		Chest trauma=1
MVP=5			Hypoglycemia=1
Tumors=3			RDS=3
Other=6			Muscular dystrophy=1
			Acidosis=2

Abbreviations: AS = aortic stenosis; ASD = atrial septal defect; AVC = AV canal; EA = Ebstein's anomaly; LTGA = L-transposition of the great arteries; MVP = mitral valve prolapse; PAB = pulmonary artery banding; PDA = patent ductus arteriosus; RDS = respiratory distress syndrome; VSD = ventricular septal defect.

it is possible that correction of congenital heart disease played a part in cessation of SVT.

Among the 42 patients whose first episode of SVT occurred more than 2 weeks after surgery for congenital heart defect, the most common operations were the Mustard operation for d-transposition of the great arteries and repair of atrial septal defects. The mean age at operation for the group whose SVT began after surgery was 61 months (range: 3 days to 15.4 years), and SVT began a mean of 23 months after operation (range: 25 days to 10 years). When we compared the postoperative group to patients without congenital heart disease, we found that patients in the operated group were older when SVT began.

The postoperative patients also had more additional arrhythmias than nonoperated patients. The tachycardia-bradycardia ("sick sinus") syndrome caused 42% of the total arrhythmias in postoperative patients.

Family History

SVT, rapid regular palpitations, or sudden, unexpected death was found in a relative (sibling, father, mother, aunt, uncle, cousin, grandparent) in 41 of 181 families (22%) of patients with SVT in which a family history was available. Twenty-one (12%) of these included a first-degree (immediate) relative. Paternal and maternal sides were equally affected. One family in our group had three girls, each with SVT; in each girl the SVT began within the first month of life. On the surface ECG two of the three had AV dissociation (probable junctional ectopic tachycardia), and the third had visible P waves with a normal PR interval (probable atrial ectopic tachycardia). This was the only family with more than one member in the study. In three other families, siblings were reported to have had SVT, but the arrhythmias had disappeared by the time of our study. SVT has been reported to occur in families.[4] Our data indicated that a positive family history suggestive of SVT is significantly more common than a positive family history of congenital heart disease. If only documented cases of SVT found in first-degree relatives of our patients are counted, the incidence of a positive family history is 7%, only slightly higher than that for congenital heart disease. This information should be made available to prospective parents.

Congestive Heart Failure

Congestive heart failure (CHF), marked by restlessness, tachypnea, pallor, diaphoresis, and cough, occurred in 73 of 331 patients (22%) (see Table 13–4). We found that those with CHF were younger, had more rapid heart rates, and had a higher incidence of congenital heart disease (both pre- and postoperatively) than those without CHF.

The major determinant of CHF, however, appeared to be age rather than heart rate. The younger the patient, the more frequently CHF was present, regardless of

TABLE 13–4
EFFECT OF CONGESTIVE HEART FAILURE

	CONGESTIVE HEART FAILURE *(N=73)*	NO CONGESTIVE HEART FAILURE *(N=258)*	*p*
Age of onset (yr)	1.9 ± 0.4*	4.1 ± 0.2*	<0.005
Heart rate (bpm)	254.2 ± >1*	234 ± 4.2*	<0.005
Congenital heart disease (pre- and postop)	30/73 (41%)	46/258 (16%)	<0.0001
SVT at follow-up	35/70 (50%)	110/245 (45%)	NSD

*± Standard error of mean.
Abbreviations: NSD = no significant difference; *p* = probability.

whether the heart rate was markedly elevated or the patient had congenital heart disease. For patients less than 1 year of age, CHF was present in 32% of those with a heart rate greater than 280 bpm or less.

Another factor that appeared to be important from the CHMC study was duration of tachycardia. In their study, none of those patients whose first attack lasted 24 hours or less developed CHF. One-fifth of those whose episode lasted at least 36 hours and half of those whose SVT lasted at least 48 hours showed evidence of CHF. From our study the presence of CHF at the onset of SVT was not related to prognosis. The same percentage of those with and without CHF still had SVT on follow-up (see Table 13–4).

HEART RATE

The mean heart rate during SVT was 235 bpm (range, 128 bpm to 325 bpm). This was identical to that found in the CHMC study. More rapid heart rates were found in younger infants and in those with CHF (Table 13–4).

QRS COMPLEX

The QRS complex during SVT had a normal duration and configuration in 155 of 172 patients (90%) in whom the ECG during the first episode of SVT was available. In eight patients the QRS duration was frankly prolonged, with a complete right bundle-branch block (CRBBB) morphology in all eight (Table 13–5). In four of the eight, CRBBB resulted from surgery and was present in sinus rhythm; the other four had WPW in sinus rhythm. Overall, in five of the 172 patients (2.9%), the QRS complex during SVT had a different morphology from sinus rhythm, indicating a rate-dependent change in conduction (Fig. 13–3). This phenomenon is rare in children, and therefore if rate-dependent bundle-branch block is seen with tachycardia in a child, ventricular tachycardia should be suspected.

P WAVES

P waves were visible on the surface ECG in 90 of 172 patients (53%) during SVT. We found P waves much more frequently than did the CHMC study, which reported that 10% of patients with SVT had visible P waves. We attribute this difference largely to the development of improved recording instruments for ECGs. We inferred a presence of a P wave if the T wave was quite pointed or if a notch was visible on the T wave (Fig. 13–4). The surface ECG was interpreted without knowledge of the intracardiac electrophysiology; however, in 91 cases, comparison between the surface ECG and intracardiac electrophysiology was made after interpretation of the surface ECG. The surface ECG interpretation of both the existence and location of P waves was confirmed in 82 of the 91 cases. The P wave axis could be estimated in 80 of 84 patients (Table 13–6). The most common P wave axis was 270° to 359° (i.e., inverted in leads II, III, and aVF and positive in leads I and aVL).

P-QRS RELATIONSHIP

The PR interval was calculated in 71 patients with visible P waves and 1:1 AV conduction. Different heart rates could be compared by dividing the PR interval by the RR interval (Fig. 13–5). Therefore PR/RR indicates how close the P wave is to the next QRS complex. The majority of the PR/RR intervals were long, indicating that most P waves were

TABLE 13–5
ABNORMAL QRS MORPHOLOGY DURING SVT

QRS COMPLEX				
SVT	*NSR*	*Heart Rate (bpm)*	*Age at Onset*	*Congenital Heart Disease*
IRBBB	IRBBB	220	6 yr	PO-TOF
IRBBB	IRBBB	225	3 yr	ASD
IRBBB	IRBBB	215	4 yr	None
IRBBB	IRBBB	210	11 yr	PO-ASD
IRBBB	CLBBB (WPW)	295	2 wk	VSD
IRBBB	IRBBB	315	1 wk	None
IRBBB	IRBBB	310	1 yr	None
ILBBB	ILBBB	210	7 mo	ASD
ILBBB	ILBBB	230	15 mo	None
CRBBB	CRBBB	310	4 yr	PO-TOF
CRBBB	CRBBB	290	7 yr	None
CRBBB	CRBBB	295	3 yr	None
CRBBB	CLBBB (WPW)	310	1 mo	AVC
CRBBB	CRBBB	265	2 yr	VSD
CRBBB	CRBBB(WPW)	255	9 yr	None
CRBBB	CLBBB (WPW)	210	7 yr	ASD
CRBBB	CLBBB (WPW)	230	5 yr	None

Abbreviations: ASD = atrial septal defect; AVC = AV canal; CLBBB = Complete left bundle-branch block; CRBBB = Complete right bundle-branch block; ILBBB = Incomplete left bundle-branch block; IRBBB = Incomplete right bundle-branch block; NSR = normal sinus rhythm; PO = postoperative; TOF = tetralogy of Fallot; VSD = ventricular septal defect; WPW = Wolff-Parkinson White syndrome.

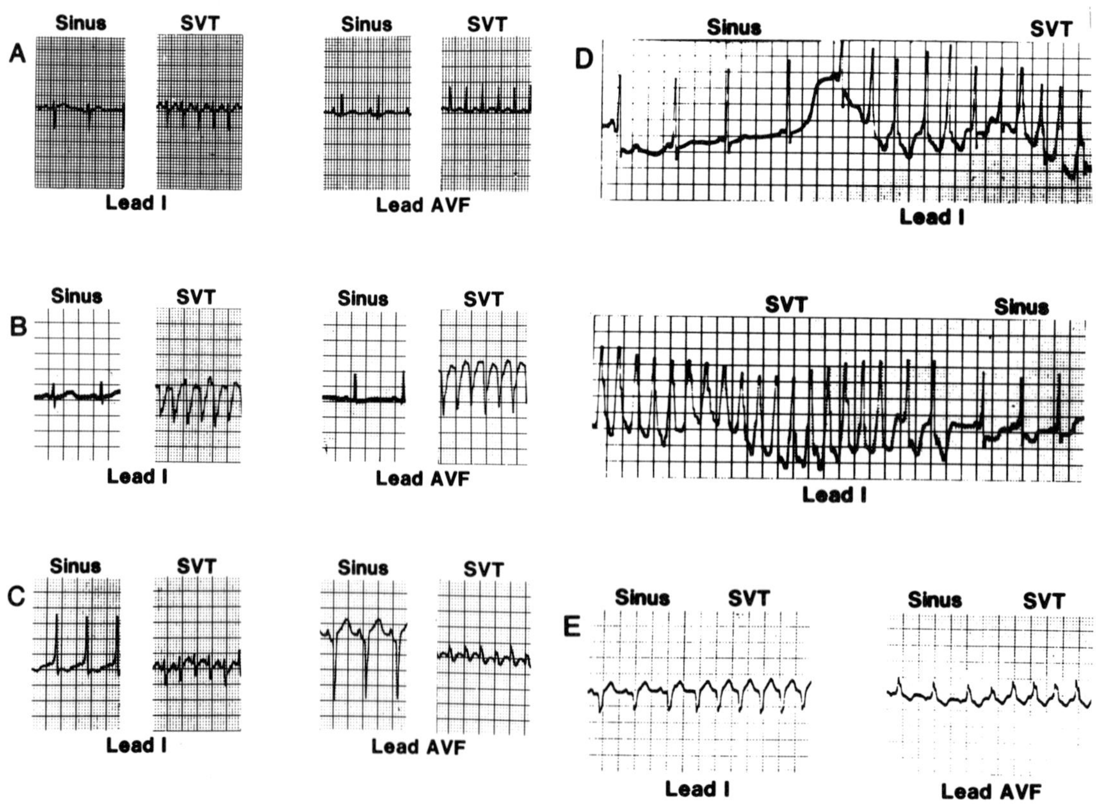

FIGURE 13–3
(*A*) Similar QRS configurations from same patient: sinus rhythm, normal QRS; SVT, normal QRS. (*B*) Different QRS configurations from same patient: sinus rhythm, normal QRS; SVT, complete right bundle-branch block. (*C*) Different QRS configurations from same patient: sinus rhythm, WPW; SVT, normal QRS configuration. (*D*) Same QRS configuration from a patient with WPW showing onset and termination of SVT with the same aberrant QRS as that found in sinus rhythm. (*E*) Same QRS configuration (right bundle-branch block) in sinus rhythm from a patient who developed SVT.

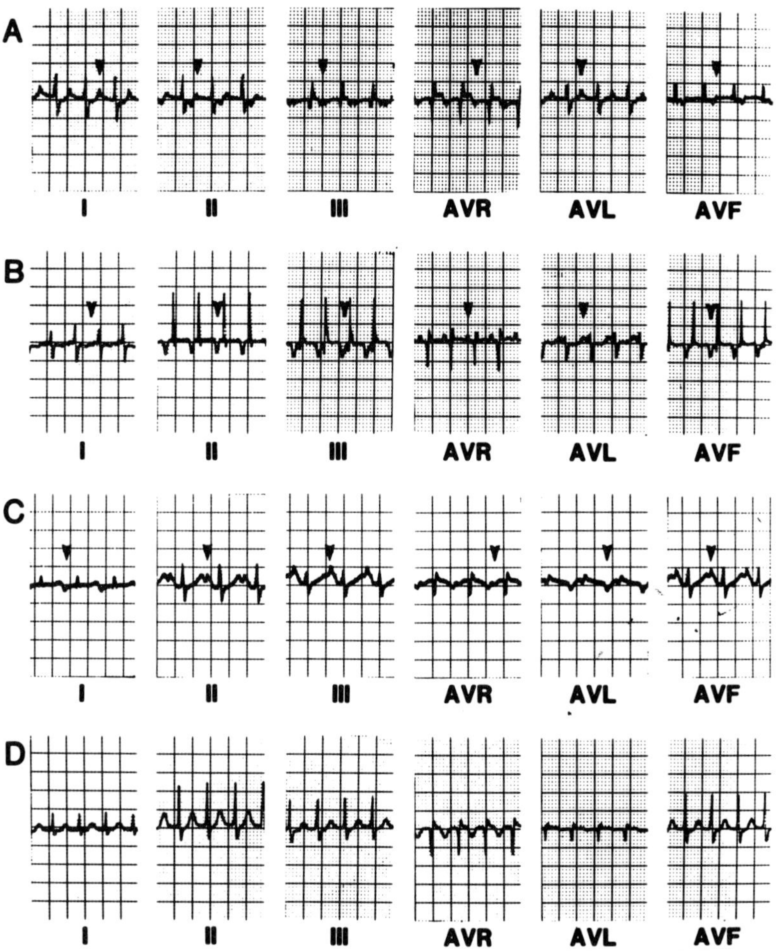

FIGURE 13–4
(*A*) SVT with P wave axis approximately +45° (high right atrial). Arrows mark P waves. (*B*) SVT with P wave axis approximately −90° (low right atrial). (*C*) SVT with P wave axis approximately −60° (high left atrial). (*D*) SVT without visible P waves.

closest to the preceding QRS complex (Fig. 13–6).

Second degree AV block was found before treatment of SVT in 12 of 172 patients (7%). In seven of these the block was type I, and in five it consisted of 2:1 conduction. The block was unrelated to age or heart rate.

TABLE 13–6
P WAVE DURING SVT

	NUMBER	PERCENTAGE
P wave not visible	82	47
P wave visible axis undetermined	14	8
P wave axis 0° to 90° (high RA)	34	20
P wave axis 90° to 270° (LA)	12	8
P wave 270° to 360° (low RA)	30	17
Total	172	100

Abbreviations: LA = left atrium; RA = right atrium.

Complete AV dissociation (no relationship of P waves to QRS complexes, with QRS rate more rapid than P wave rate) occurred in 7 of 172 patients (Fig. 13–7).

PREEXCITATION

A WPW pattern was found on the surface ECG in 88 of 346 patients (25%) who had SVT. When those patients who had WPW on the surface ECG were compared to those without preexcitation, we found no difference. Although there was a tendency for patients with WPW to have the first episode at a younger age, there was no significant difference with respect to age at onset, recurrence rate, or final status (Table 13–7).

A Lown-Ganong-Levine (LGL) pattern was found in 10 patients (3%) with SVT. Although the small number did not permit quantitative comparison, there were no qual-

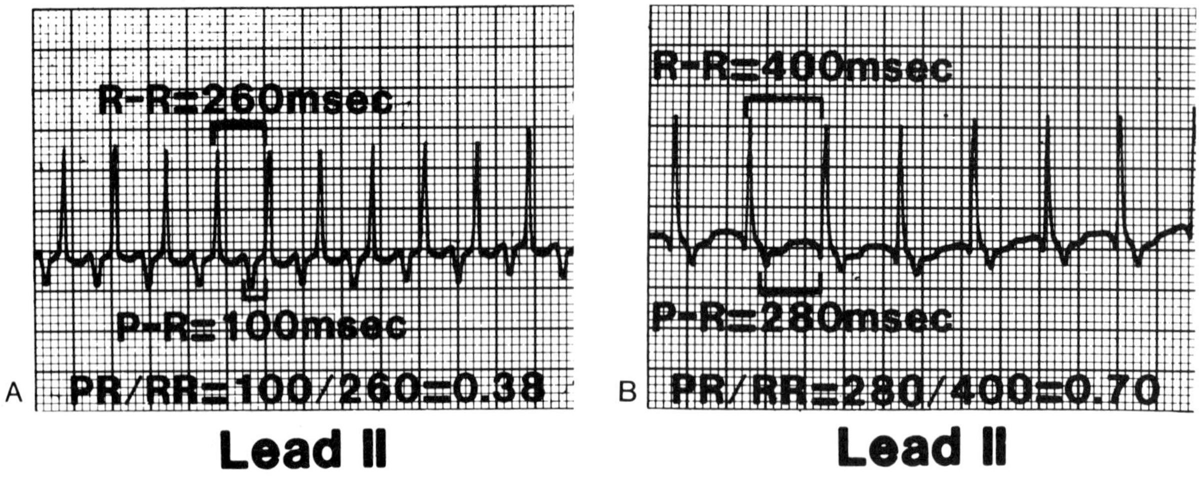

FIGURE 13–5
Calculation of the PR/RR ratio. The onset of the P wave and the onset of the QRS complex are used. In tracing *A*, the RR interval is 260 ms, and the PR interval is 100 ms. Therefore PR/RR = 0.38. The shorter the PR interval, the lower will be the value for PR/RR.

itative differences between those with LGL and those without preexcitation.

OTHER ARRHYTHMIAS

Arrhythmias other than SVT were present in 93 of 346 patients (27%). The most common arrhythmias were premature ventricular contractions (PVCs). Atrial flutter and atrial fibrillation occurred rarely in patients with SVT. Tachycardia-bradycardia syndrome was most common in postoperative patients.

Treatment Results

ACUTE TREATMENT

Data on acute treatment of the first episode were available for 321 of 346 patients. In 80 of the 321 (21%), the SVT stopped spontaneously before any treatment was instituted. The other 291 patients were treated (Fig. 13–8). Acute treatment was successful in terminating any SVT within 48 hours in 142 of 241 patients (60%).

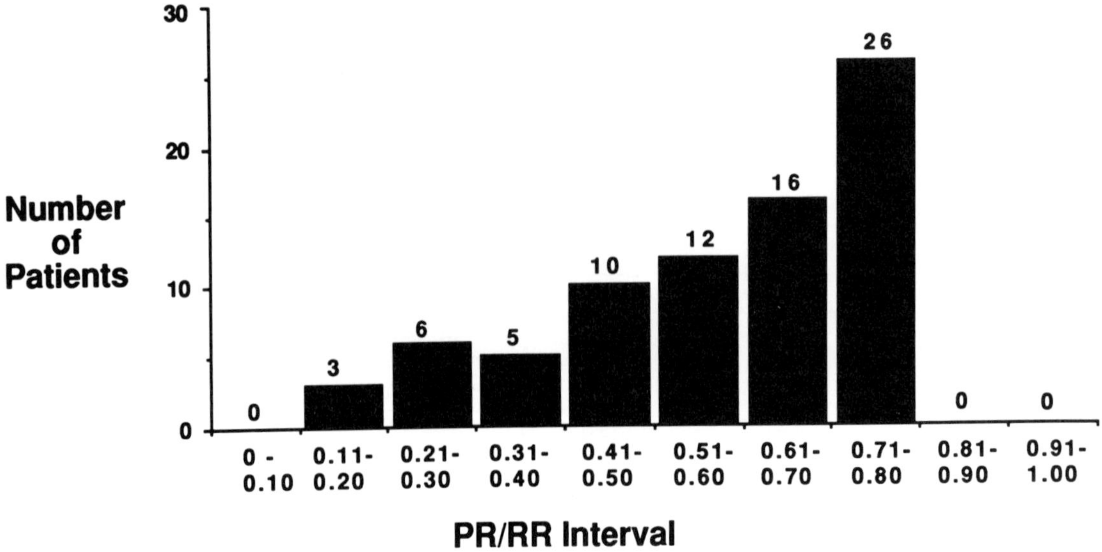

FIGURE 13–6
Distribution of PR/RR intervals.

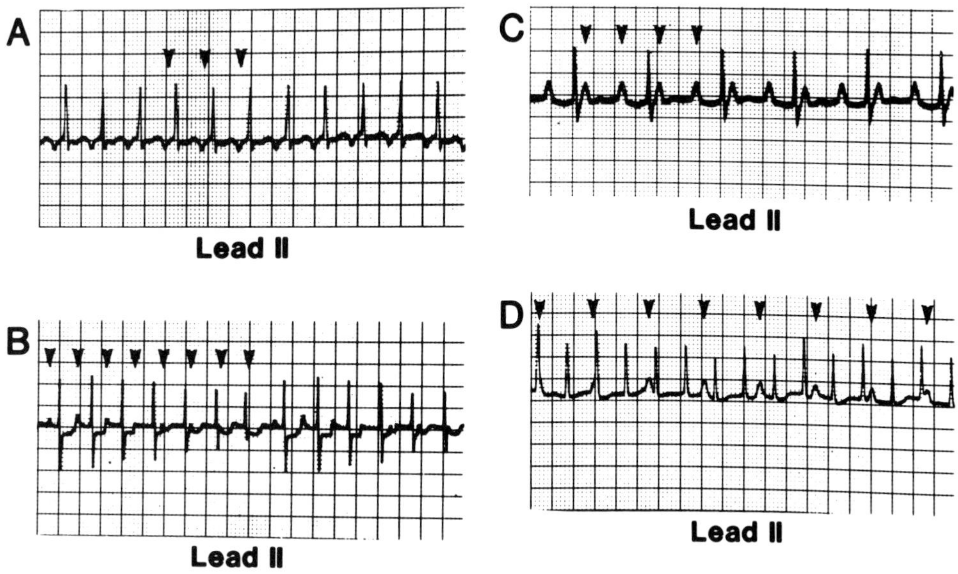

FIGURE 13–7
(*A*) SVT with 1:1 AV conduction. P waves are marked by arrows. (*B*) SVT with type I 2 AV block (8:7 Wenckebach). P waves are marked by arrows. The PR interval begins at 0.10 s and prolongs to 0.23 s before a P wave is not followed by a QRS complex. (*C*) SVT with 2:1 AV block. P waves are marked by arrows. (*D*) SVT with AV dissociation. P waves are marked by arrows.

Intravenous digoxin was most frequently used for treatment and was successful in 70% of patients. The median time from digoxin administration to cessation of SVT was 6 hours. Digoxin success was unrelated to age or to presence of CHF, heart rate, or other ECG features. Acute therapy with digoxin was significantly (p <0.01) more effective in patients with WPW (90%) than in those without WPW (66%).

Synchronized direct current (DC) electrocardioversion was successful in interrupting SVT in only 16 of 29 patients (55%) in whom it was used. The energy dose that was applied was unavailable in three of 13 patients in whom cardioversion failed. Therefore it is possible that in these three patients the dose was inadequate. In the other 13 the dose was appropriate but was still ineffective. The effectiveness of cardioversion was unrelated to age, CHF, or heart rate. The presence of P waves during SVT was related to success of cardioversion: cardioversion was successful in nine of 12 (75%) of those without visible P waves and in only 25% of those with a P wave axis of 0° to 90°. One of these patients had AV dissociation; it is likely that many of the others had ectopic SVT.

Vagal maneuvers (e.g., carotid sinus massage, Valsalva) were reported to be successful in 26 of 42 patients (62%). The only significant factor related to vagal success was age; vagal maneuvers were ineffective in infants and young children. The mean age of those in whom vagal maneuvers were successful was 4.2 years (youngest: 3 months), compared with a mean age of 1.1 years (range: 9 days to 27 years) for those in whom vagal maneuvers were unsuccessful.

Similar results were found for phenylephrine treatment, which was successful in four of 11 patients (36%). Age was the differen-

TABLE 13–7
EFFECT OF PREEXCITATION

	WPW (N=88)	NO PREEXCITATION (N=250)	DIFFERENCE
Age at onset (yr)*	3.2 ± 0.3*	3.7 ± 0.4	NSD
Recurrence	71/86 (81%)	203/238 (85%)	NSD
SVT present on follow-up	37/88 (42%)	93/239 (39%)	NSD

*± Standard error of mean.

tiating factor; the youngest infant in whom phenylephrine was successful was 1.5 years old. The mean age of those in whom the drug was successful was 3.7 years, compared to 1.2 years (range: 4 days to 4.5 years) for those in whom phenylephrine failed.

Overdrive atrial pacing was the most successful treatment used. It was effective in eight of 10 patients (80%). Overdrive pacing was also the most invasive method and was used infrequently as the initial acute treatment. The only failure of overdrive pacing was in a patient with AV dissociation during SVT.

Intravenous verapamil was used in three patients and was successful in two of them. All three patients were older than 1 year. Propranolol was administered to four patients and was successful in stopping SVT in two. Quinidine failed in two patients, and procainamide was successful in terminating SVT in one of two patients.

In summary, acute treatment was unsuccessful in terminating SVT within 48 hours in 49 of 241 patients (40%). Younger patients responded poorly to vagal maneuvers and phenylephrine. Visible P waves, especially in the presence of AV dissociation, are indicators of a poor prognosis for successful acute treatment.

CHRONIC TREATMENT

After acute treatment, 252 of 336 patients (75%) were begun on chronic treatment. Those who were not treated were older, had a lower percentage of CHF, and had slower heart rates than those who were treated. Among those who were treated, digoxin was the most common drug initially employed, either by itself or in combination with another drug.

Twenty-one patients with incessant SVT were treated with encainide or ethmozine.

RECURRENCE

SVT recurred at least once more than 7 days after the initial episode in 194 of 240 patients (81%) (Table 13–8). Therefore in only 46 patients (19%), SVT did not recur. The recurrence appeared within 1 month in 88 of 160 patients (55%) and within 3 months in 123 of 160 (76%). In 18 of 160 (11%), more than 1 year elapsed before the second episode of SVT (Fig. 13–9). The other 34 patients had recurrence between 3 months and 1 year of age.

Those patients who received no initial chronic treatment had a higher recurrence rate than those who received treatment. Among those who were treated, none of the drug regimens used proved significantly superior than others in delaying or preventing recurrence (see Table 13–8).

Ten patients had demand pacemakers implanted to aid in treatment of SVT; six received an atrial pacemaker, and four received a ventricular pacemaker. One patient had a radiofrequency-controlled, rapid overdrive atrial pacemaker inserted. All of these patients were also treated with drugs. Seven of the 11 patients with pacemakers had no SVT on follow-up. One patient with a demand pacemaker continued to have SVT despite therapeutic digoxin, propranolol, and quinidine. This 6-year-old boy and nine other children aged 6 months to 15 years had undergone surgical division of a bundle of Kent for SVT that was unresponsive to medical therapy; SVT was abolished in none of the 10.

FINAL STATUS

Follow-up data were available for 330 of 346 patients (95%). The follow-up period ranged from 2 days (in one of the patients who died) to 27.2 years, with an average follow-up of 4.8 years. The age at end of follow-up ranged from 2 months to 27.6 years (mean: 9.1 years).

SVT was present on long-term follow-up in 62% of the patients (Table 13–9). Those 30 patients (9%) who continued to have SVT but who were not on drug therapy had fewer than two episodes per year. Only 12% of the patients (36 of 330) were free from SVT without treatment on follow-up.

Four patients died. Two of the four were infants aged 1 week and 3 weeks. Each had SVT with AV dissociation. The 1-week-old child had coarctation of the aorta and ventricular septal defect and died from low cardiac output associated with SVT. The 3-week-old infant died suddenly and unexpectedly at home; he was being treated with digoxin and propranolol. Another death was in a 24-month-old child who had had surgery for multiple ventricular septal defects and division of a bundle of Kent. Death occurred

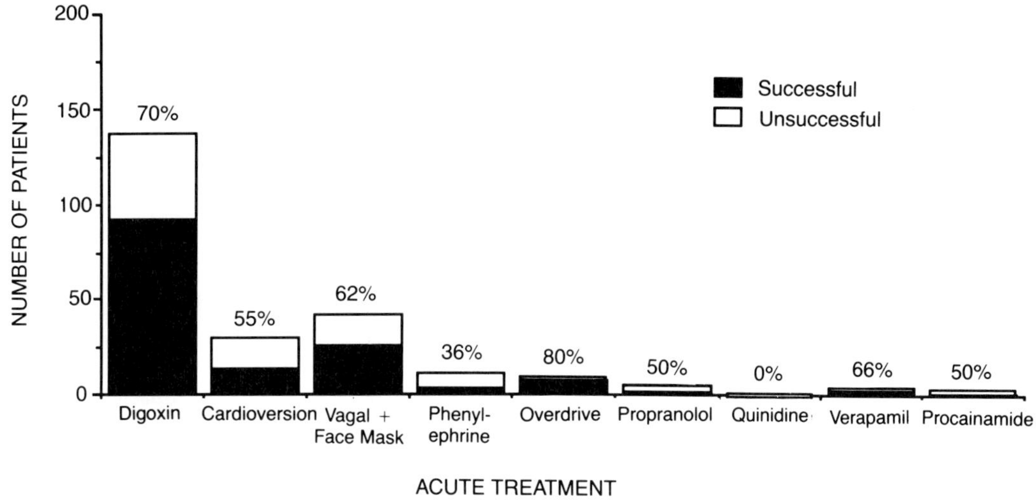

FIGURE 13–8
Results of acute treatment.

TABLE 13–8
RECURRENCE WITH CHRONIC TREATMENT

TREATMENT	RECURRENCE *Number*	RECURRENCE *Percent*	MEDIAN TIME TO RECURRENCE (days)
Digoxin only	119/155	76	12
Digoxin and propranolol	28/36	77	16
Digoxin and quinidine	7/8	88	11
Propranolol	10/12	83	18
Quinidine	3/7	76	9
Verapamil	2/3	66	15
Digoxin and verapamil	1/2	50	10
All treated	170/228	75	12
No treatment	61/68	89	34

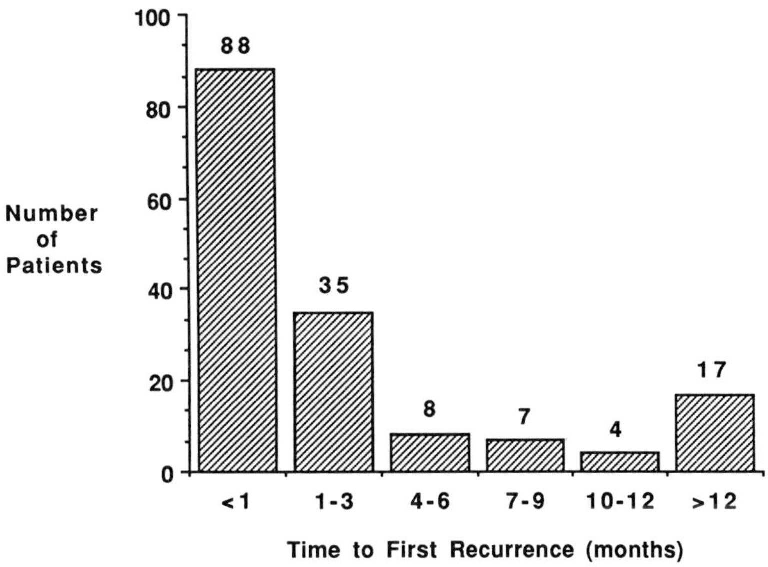

FIGURE 13–9
Time to first recurrence of SVT.

TABLE 13–9
RESULTS OF FOLLOW-UP (MEAN = 4.8 YR)

	NUMBER OF PATIENTS	PERCENTAGE
SVT present		
With drug therapy	168	51
Without drug therapy	30	9
SVT absent		
With drug therapy	89	27
Without drug therapy	39	12
Died	4	1
Total	330	100

3 days after surgery and resulted from a cerebrovascular accident. An embolus was thought to have originated from the large dacron patch used to close the ventricular septum. There had been no SVT in the 3 days after surgery. The final patient died after surgery for congenital heart disease.

It is difficult to predict the final status of a patient with SVT. Data from the history, ECG, and initial response to treatment are not helpful, with four exceptions:

1. Patients whose SVT began earliest in life (4 months of age or younger) had a lower incidence of SVT on follow-up than those whose SVT began later (see Table 13–3).
2. Patients with congenital heart defects whose SVT began before any operation had a lower incidence of SVT at follow-up (see Table 13–6).
3. SVT with AV dissociation has a poor prognosis. Acute therapy failed to stop SVT in all four cases. Two of these four patients died. These were the only two deaths that were directly related to SVT, except for one patient who died as a direct result of surgery to correct a Kent bundle.
4. Initial recurrence is not a poor prognostic sign. SVT recurred at least once in 70 of 228 patients without SVT at follow-up.

DIFFERENTIAL DIAGNOSIS OF SVT ON THE SURFACE ECG

In the majority of cases, sinus tachycardia is a narrow QRS tachycardia (Fig. 13–10). SVT in our series was a narrow QRS tachycardia in 90% of the cases. The QRS rate may be helpful in distinguishing between the two. In sinus tachycardia the rate is virtually always less than 230 bpm in infants who are younger than 2 months and less than 210 bpm in older infants and children. We have encountered three infants, each younger than 6 months, who had sinus tachycardia at rates up to 265 bpm. Each was extremely ill with sepsis.[5] On the other hand, more than 60% of children with SVT have QRS rates of 230 bpm or more.

The presence and axis of the P waves may also help (see Fig. 13–10); for this reason a 15-lead ECG is indispensable for diagnosis. In the vast majority of patients with sinus tachycardia, P waves are visible with a normal (0° to 90°) axis. P waves with a normal axis were found in only 20% of our cases of SVT. Therefore the presence of P waves with a normal axis is a strong indication of sinus tachycardia; the absence of visible P waves favors a diagnosis of SVT.

If the patient's history is available, certain clinical clues may be helpful. The four most common clinical situations in which marked sinus tachycardia are found are hypovolemia, sepsis, fever of any cause, and iatrogenic overdose with isoproterenol or epinephrine. While any of these conditions can predispose to SVT, sinus tachycardia is much more common in such situations. It is rare to observe the initiation of tachycardia, but observance of the cessation of tachycardia can be planned. If, in response to an intervention such as phenylephrine or vagal maneuvers, the heart rate changes abruptly, the problem is most likely SVT. If the heart rate slows gradually in response to an intervention, the diagnosis is more than likely sinus tachycardia. If the heart rate is unaffected, it could be either sinus tachycardia or SVT. The lack of change of the heart rate in response to maneuvers that increase vagal tone is the rule rather than the exception in younger children. If a hypovolemia patient's intravascular volume was increased or a febrile patient's fever decreased and the heart rate gradually decreased, then the retrospective diagnosis is sinus tachycardia. If the heart rate continued to be elevated at the same rate with amelioration of the clinical condition, the diagnosis most likely is SVT.

The final method of establishing the diagnosis is by the response to specific treatment for SVT. We are not suggesting that antiarrhythmic treatment be employed simply to make the diagnosis; however, if the heart rate is over 200 bpm and peripheral perfusion is poor or the patient is in distress, a

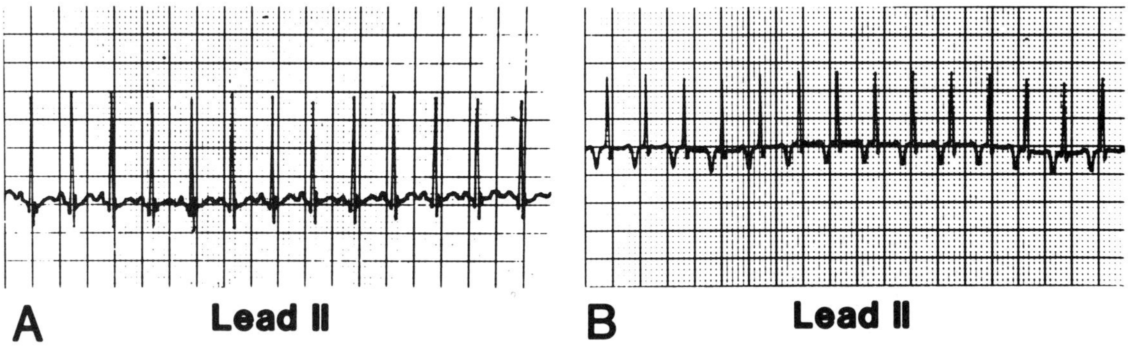

FIGURE 13–10
(*A*) Sinus tachycardia, rate 200–230/min. P waves are clearly visible, with a normal P wave axis. (*B*) SVT, rate 230/min. P waves are clearly visible with an abnormal P wave axis.

trial of phenylephrine or synchronized DC electrical cardioversion is indicated. If the rhythm abruptly converts to a slower sinus rhythm after cardioversion, the diagnosis is SVT. If the rhythm continues unchanged, the diagnosis may be SVT but is most likely sinus tachycardia, and the search for the cause of sinus tachycardia should be continued.

Atrial Flutter

The usual rate for atrial flutter with 1:1 AV conduction in infants and children is 300 bpm or more. This rate was also the most common rate for SVT in our series. The distinction between atrial flutter and SVT can be made by observation of flutter waves on the surface ECG. A 15-lead ECG is mandatory for making this distinction, since flutter waves may not be present in all leads (Fig. 13–11). If flutter waves are absent in all leads, the diagnosis is SVT.

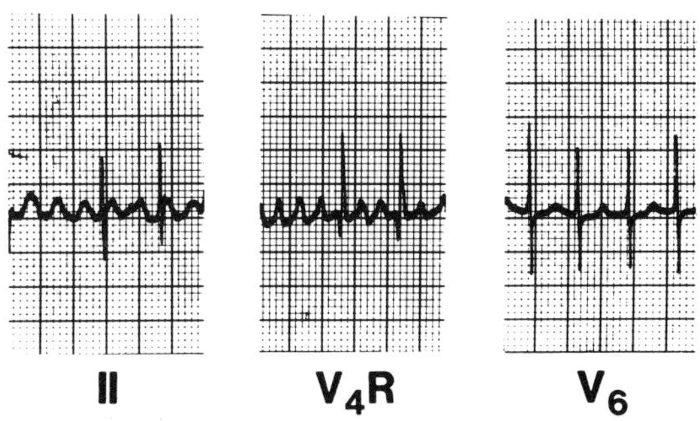

FIGURE 13–11
Atrial flutter with varying second degree AV block. Flutter waves are clearly visible in leads II and V_4R but are not apparent in lead V_6.

Ventricular Tachycardia

In ventricular tachycardia, the QRS complex is virtually always from the sinus QRS. Most of the time, the QRS is also prolonged for age; however, in infants younger than 2 years with ventricular tachycardia, the mean QRS duration was normal for age.

Rarely, SVT is associated with a wide QRS in children; therefore in any wide QRS tachycardia a ventricular origin should be suspected. In any patient with a wide QRS tachycardia, it is helpful to locate an ECG from that patient that was taken prior to the onset of the tachycardia. In 14 of 17 cases of SVT with a wide QRS, the QRS was wide before the SVT started. If the QRS was narrow before tachycardia began and was wide during tachycardia, there was only a 5 of 170 (2.9%) chance that this was SVT (from our data). Fusion complexes (Fig. 13–12) establish the diagnosis of ventricular tachycardia, but the absence of fusion complexes is not helpful. The morphology of the wide QRS (complete right bundle-branch block or complete left bundle-branch block) is not helpful in children, with one exception: if

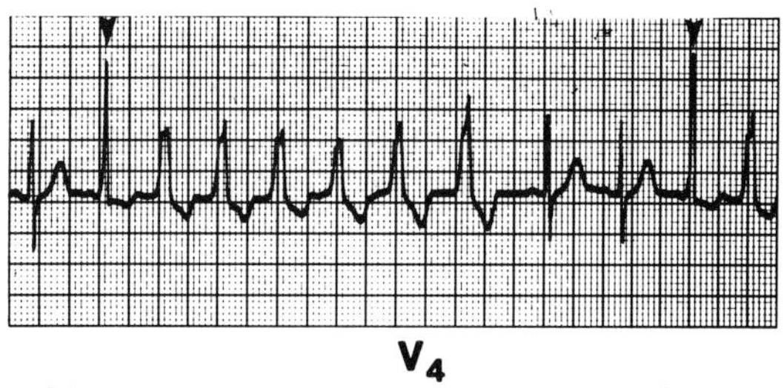

FIGURE 13–12
Ventricular tachycardia alternating with sinus rhythm. Arrows mark fusion complexes.

the wide QRS is mainly positive and has a similar morphology in all chest leads, this most likely represents conduction of a supraventricular rhythm antegrade through a bundle of Kent, rather than ventricular tachycardia (Fig. 13–13). The rate of a tachycardia is rarely helpful, except that most ventricular tachycardia is slower than 300 bpm (except in infants, where it may be more than 400 bpm). AV dissociation, if present, is a useful differentiating point. AV dissociation is much more common in ventricular tachycardia than in SVT. Only 7 of 172 patients (4%) with SVT had AV dissociation, with sinus P waves continuing without interruption through the rapid QRS complexes, and all of these patients with SVT had narrow QRS complexes.

The clinical condition of the patient may be helpful in establishing the diagnosis. Cardiovascular collapse is more frequently associated with ventricular than with supraventricular tachycardia, although patients with either disorder may be entirely asymptomatic. If a patient is symptomatic from a wide QRS tachycardia, the response to DC electrical cardioversion will not establish the specific diagnosis but will aid in the alleviation of symptoms.

MANAGEMENT OF SVT BASED ON NONINVASIVE ASSESSMENT

The initial steps in management are directed at both diagnosis and treatment. At the same time acute treatment is being instituted, a search for a predisposing factor should begin. It is helpful to obtain information about what the child was doing when SVT began. Most frequently SVT is not precipitated by exercise or fright. Parents should be questioned about drug ingestion (including caffeine) or antecedent history suggestive of infection, hyperthyroidism, or prior evidence of congenital heart disease. A history should be taken to find other family members with SVT or rapid palpitations or a family history of sudden, unexpected death. Physical examination should be directed at assessment of distress in degree of CHF and signs of congenital heart disease, infection, or hyperthyroidism. Laboratory data should include a 15-lead ECG, chest radiograph, and echocardiogram.

Renal function must be assessed to determine if antiarrhythmic drug dosages need to be adjusted. After the initial episode has been converted, a 15-lead ECG should be repeated to determine whether WPW or evidence of congenital heart disease is apparent on the tracing. Frequently, children with otherwise normal hearts may demonstrate right atrial enlargement on the ECG immediately after an episode of SVT. This regresses over several hours to several days. If an echocardiogram and a repeat chest radiograph are normal, congenital heart disease is unlikely. The treadmill exercise test is not performed routinely on these children, because so few episodes of SVT are exercise induced. After chronic treatment has been instituted, the best method of follow-up is by the parents' and patient's observation. The chances that SVT will occur in any 24-hour period are so small that Holter monitoring may be unrewarding.

Acute Treatment

The first episode of SVT should be treated in all patients. The type of acute treatment depends on the condition of the patient. If a patient of any age is acutely ill with congestive symptoms and/or symptoms of low cardiac output, treatment may consist of facial im-

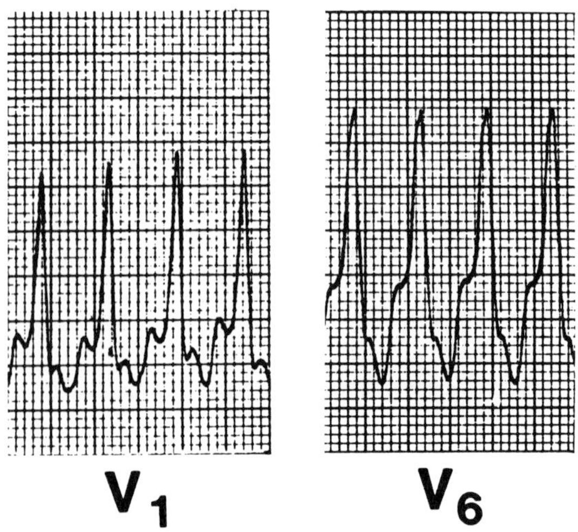

FIGURE 13–13
SVT with aberrant conduction resulting from antegrade conduction through a posterior Kent bundle. The QRS complexes are mainly positive throughout the precordium.

mersion, vagal maneuvers, esophageal pacing, cardioversion, drug therapy (verapamil, phenylephrine, edrophonium, or propanolol), overdrive atrial pacing, or cooling the patient (Table 13–10).

FACIAL IMMERSION

Facial immersion in cold water (5° to 15°C) for 10 to 30 s has been effective in stopping SVT. This maneuver elicits the diving reflex, which results in a strong vagal stimulation. It has been effective in small infants, but care must be taken to pinch the nose and mouth to prevent aspiration. A variation of this technique that is also effective in younger infants and children is to (without warning) place either a cold wet washcloth or an ice bag on the face of the patient.

Bisset, Gaum, and Kaplan described the ice bag technique for interruption of SVT.[6] The study involved 10 patients converted to sinus rhythm within 15 s after initiation of this technique. Because of the remote risk of ventricular arrhythmias or severe bradycardia, we recommend that this procedure be performed with resuscitation and monitoring equipment close at hand.

VAGAL MANEUVERS

Carotid sinus massage may be undertaken for 5 to 10 s, and only on one side at a time. The carotid sinus is located in the internal carotid artery just superior to the bifurcation of the common carotid artery in the anterior triangle of the neck. It can be located by palpating for arterial pulsations lateral to the superior border of the thyroid cartilage. Valsalva's maneuver can be used in infants; older children may be asked to strain. Gagging the patient with a tongue depressor is another frequently employed maneuver. Administration of syrup of ipecac to induce vomiting may also be tried. We strongly recommend against ocular pressure because damage to the eye may occur. Each recommended vagal maneuver may be tried in succession but will most likely not be successful in children younger than 4 years.

TABLE 13–10
ACUTE TREATMENT OF SVT

Patient seriously ill
Washcloth/facial immersion (water temperature, 5°–18° C)
Vagal maneuvers
Esophageal pacing
Cardioversion (0.25–1.0 J/kg)
Phenylephrine 0.01–0.1 mg/kg IV
Edrophonium 0.2 mg/kg IV
Patient cooling
Propranolol 0.01–0.1 mg/kg IV
Intracardiac overdrive atrial pacing
Patient not acutely distressed
Washcloth immersion
Vagal maneuvers
If young, esophageal pacing
IV verapamil (no CHF, >1 year old, no β-blockers)

ESOPHAGEAL PACING

Benson et al[7] reported their experience in terminating SVT by esophageal pacing in a series of 38 pediatric patients. The procedure is safe and effective for interruption of reentrant SVT, but in our experience, it is less successful for converting atrial flutter and automatic SVT. The tip of the catheter should pass through the esophagus to a point adjacent to the left atrium. Then the atrial electrogram should be recorded by connecting the two catheter leads to the left arm and the right arm jacks of the ECG, recording simultaneous leads I, II, and III. The atrial bipolar electrogram will be recorded on lead I. Overdrive pacing is accomplished with a pulse duration of 10 ms. The atrium is paced for 10 to 30 s; if capture does not occur, the pulse duration and/or output amplitude may be increased (maximum 18 ms, 20 A). If capture still does not occur, the electrodes should be adjusted.

CARDIOVERSION

Synchronized DC electrical cardioversion should be successful in converting the arrhythmia in the majority of patients with SVT. In our series, it was only successful in 55% of patients; however, it is possible that cardioversion was used more commonly in patients with difficult-to-treat SVT. For example, cardioversion is uniformly unsuccessful in those with SVT and AV dissociation (junctional ectopic tachycardia) or those with atrial ectopic focus SVT. The initial energy dose used is 0.25 J (watt-seconds)/kg, and this may be increased to 1.0 J/kg (Fig. 13–14).[6] If synchronized cardioversion is performed on a patient who has a therapeutic serum con-

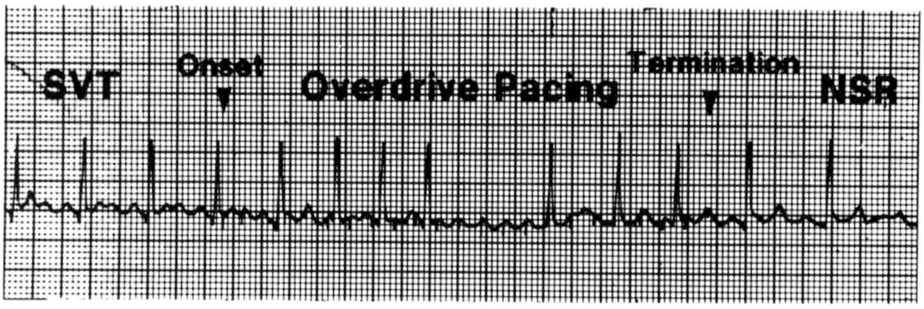

FIGURE 13–14
Overdrive pacing. SVT at a rate of 280/min is interrupted by overdrive atrial pacing (arrows) at a rate of 375/min, with resultant sinus rhythm when pacing is terminated. Note advanced second degree AV block with rapid atrial pacing.

centration of digitalis, ventricular tachycardia or ventricular fibrillation may rarely result. Therefore, in such patients lidocaine should be administered (1.0 mg/kg) immediately before cardioversion as prophylaxis against ventricular arrhythmias. All but the smallest infants (i.e., less than 1 month of age) should be sedated for cardioversion. Ketamine (1 mg/kg intravenously) or diazepam (0.3 mg/kg intravenously, maximum dose 10 mg) may be used. We have also found that anesthesia with a short-acting barbiturate (e.g., sodium pentobarbital) administered by an anesthesiologist is an excellent method.

DRUG THERAPY

Verapamil. The antiarrhythmic effect of verapamil appears to be caused by blockade of the slow channel. Verapamil slows AV conduction and prolongs the effective refractory period within the AV node in a rate-related manner. Acute cardiovascular adverse reactions have been reported with intravenous verapamil and include symptomatic hypotension, bradycardia, AV block, asystole, rapid ventricular rates caused by antegrade conduction in atrial flutter-fibrillation with WPW, and apnea. Severe hemodynamic side effects have occurred in neonates and infants following the intravenous administration of verapamil. For this reason, we do not recommend the use of IV verapamil in infants younger than 1 year. In older patients, verapamil should be given as a slow intravenous injection over at least a 2-minute period. Intravenous verapamil should not be given to patients with congestive heart failure who are on calcium channel or β-blocking agents. The initial dose for children age 1 year to 15 years is 0.1–0.3 mg/kg (not to exceed a total of 5 mg). This dose may be repeated twice within 30 minutes after the initial dose. It has been suggested that pretreatment with calcium chloride improves hemodynamics while maintaining the electrophysiologic effect of verapamil.[8] This form of treatment has not been used in a sufficient number of infants under 1 year of age to recommend its use at present.

Phenylephrine. Phenylephrine is less commonly used now than previously. The initial IV bolus of phenylephrine should be 0.01 mg/kg. If in 5 minutes the systolic blood pressure is less than twice the initial systolic blood pressure, give an additional 0.02 mg/kg. The dose may be doubled every 5 minutes (e.g., 0.04 mg/kg, 0.08 mg/kg, etc.) until the systolic blood pressure is twice the initial blood pressure. Alternatively, an intravenous drip at an initial rate of 0.01 mg/kg/min (10 μg/kg/min) can be instituted and the rate of the drip increased until the blood pressure responds. If SVT remains after blood pressure response has been achieved, vagal maneuvers may be tried. When SVT does terminate, frequently because of overdrive suppression of the sinus node and the increase in vagal tone, a pause lasting several seconds may occur before cardiac rhythm is reestablished. Slow junctional rhythm may occur for several beats or last for up to a few minutes. In the vast majority of cases, normal sinus rhythm is established in from <30 s to 1 min. If the slow cardiac rate (less than 90 bpm in an infant under 1 year of age or 55 bpm in a child) persists for longer than 1 minute, a single IV dose of atropine (0.01 mg/kg) should abolish residual vagotonia and restore normal cardiac rate. For this reason, when vagotonic maneuvers are employed, atropine should be close at hand and the proper dose already calculated.

Treatment with phenylephrine may also be ineffective in younger infants. In our series the youngest patient in whom this drug was effective was 18 months old. A possible hazard associated with the use of phenylephrine is an acute elevation of blood pressure. If a patient has a borderline cardiac output, elevation of systemic vascular resistance may, by increasing afterload, worsen the congestive heart failure. This applies especially in the period immediately following cardiac surgery. In this period, when bleeding is a potential problem, elevation of the blood pressure may in certain instances also increase bleeding. Therefore phenylephrine should be used with caution in such patients, and the potential risks must be weighed against the benefit to be achieved with cessation of SVT.

Edrophonium. Edrophonium is used only extremely rarely. This cholinesterase inhibitor is directly vagotonic and has the advantage that it does not rely on reflex stimulation from hypertension for its mechanism of action. The dose is 0.2 mg/kg intravenously. One-fifth of this should be given as a test dose; if the SVT does not stop, the remaining 0.16 mg/kg should be given in four divided IV doses every 30 to 45 s. If this dose is ineffective, vagal maneuvers may be tried. When SVT stops after administration of edrophonium, sinus bradycardia may be extreme and prolonged. For this reason a syringe containing 0.01 mg/kg of atropine should be at the bedside before administration of edrophonium. Edrophonium may also be ineffective in younger infants and children. Either phenylephrine or edrophonium can be used in an individual patient, but not both in rapid succession. The vagotonic effect provided by the two may be additive; if the SVT does stop, severe sinus bradycardia and AV block may result.

Propranolol. If all other measures have failed, IV propranolol may be given. The total IV dose of propranolol is 0.1 mg/kg. We recommend dividing the total dose by four, giving one-quarter dose every 5 minutes with close observation of the blood pressure and heart rate. We administer IV propranolol only if a pacing catheter is present in the right atrium, since propranolol can cause severe sinus bradycardia. If the SVT converts and sinus bradycardia results, atrial pacing can then be instituted immediately. Intravenous propranolol can also severely depress myocardial contractility. If blood pressure falls, an IV drip of isoproterenol (0.05–0.5 μg/kg/min) may be necessary.

OVERDRIVE ATRIAL PACING

In overdrive pacing, an electrode catheter is placed in the right atrium and pacing at a rate faster than the SVT is carried out. The most common use of overdrive pacing is to stop the SVT. The pacing rate should be at least 10 to 15 bpm more than the rate of SVT and should be carried out for 5 to 15 s (see Fig. 13–14). The current used should be at least twice that which results in atrial capture; 5 to 10 mA is generally sufficient. Several pacing rates may be tried. If overdrive pacing is still unsuccessful in stopping SVT, then the catheter can be moved to a different location in the atrium and several rates tried again. If this is still unsuccessful and all other acute measures to stop SVT have been tried, the atrium may be paced chronically (for hours or days) at a rapid rate that is both faster than the SVT and rapid enough that 2:1 AV block occurs. This rate is usually from 300 bpm to 350 bpm in infants and from 250 bpm to 300 bpm in older children. The ventricular rate will be lowered sufficiently that symptoms can be relieved and chronic antiarrhythmic treatment begun. Ater several hours a trial of cessation of pacing may be instituted. If the tachycardia persists, pacing is reinstituted and chronic treatment continued.

We have used a method of paired pacing developed by Waldo et al[9] for the acute management of refractory SVT with AV dissociation. This type of SVT is seen most commonly in the immediate postoperative period after surgery for congenital heart disease; however, this method is applicable to all types of SVT with a rapid, regular ventricular response. (While such pacing can be performed, cardiac output may not increase; other methods such as cooling the patient have largely replaced paired pacing.) The catheter is placed in the right ventricle, and paired stimuli are delivered. Initially, the S_1S_2 interval is set equal to the S_2S_1 interval (S_1S_2 is half of S_1S_1, and the S_1S_2 interval is slightly shorter than the tachycardia cycle length). For example, for SVT with a heart rate of 300 bpm (cycle length, 200 ms), S_1S_2 is 190 ms, S_1S_1 is 380 ms, and therefore S_2S_1 is 190 ms. Pacing in this mode will result in a regular ventricular rate that is slightly faster than that of SVT. Next the S_1S_2 interval is progressively shortened until S_2 captures the ventricle electrically (QRS complex visible) but there is no mechanical contraction (i.e., no blood pressure response). At this point ventricular contraction occurs after every S_1, or every 380 ms. With the effective ventricular rate almost halved, chronic treatment can proceed.

COOLING THE PATIENT

In "automatic" tachycardias such as postoperative junctional tachycardia, cooling the patient to 31°–34°C has been effective in reducing the rate.

SUMMARY

We suggest that acute treatment of SVT be initiated with facial immersion in cold water for 5 to 10 s, followed by simple vagal maneuvers. If SVT does not terminate, proceed with esophageal pacing and cardioversion in the order listed in Table 13–12. Intracardiac atrial overdrive pacing should be the last option of acute treatment.

If the patient is less severely ill, the same order of acute treatment may be employed. We prefer to terminate the SVT with one of the treatments listed; however, it is certainly acceptable to use digoxin to convert SVT if the child is not in acute distress. The total IV digitalizing dose is 0.04–0.05 mg/kg (maximum, 0.8 mg). One-half should be given immediately; one-quarter may be given in 6 hours, and the last quarter may be given in another 6 hours. Then, 6 hours following the last dose, a dosage of 0.004 mg/kg IV every 12 hours can be instituted. The oral doses should be calculated at 1.25 times the IV dose. In our patients with SVT who had digoxin therapy as primary acute treatment, SVT stopped in a median of 6 hours after the first dose of digoxin. We recommend that if the SVT has not converted 18 hours after the initiation of digoxin, the other acute treatments should be tried in the order previously listed. If cardioversion is employed in such patients, pretreatment should be given with lidocaine (see above).

Chronic Treatment

After the initial episode of SVT has been converted, chronic therapy should be begun in all cases and continued for at least 12 months (Table 13–11).

Our data indicate that SVT recurs in most children regardless of whether the initial episode was provoked by a predisposing factor (e.g., by an episode of fever, sepsis, or thyrotoxicosis), but it recurs significantly less frequently in treated patients.

TABLE 13–11
CHRONIC DRUG TREATMENT OF SVT

	DOSE (mg/kg)	DOSAGE SCHEDULE
Digoxin	0.005–0.0075	bid
Propranolol	0.5–1.5	q6h
Quinidine sulfate	7.5–10.0	q6h
Encainide	0.3–2.0	q8h
Flecainide	1.5–3	bid
Ethmozine	1.5–5.0	q4h
Verapamil	1–3	q8h
Phenytoin	2.5–3.0	bid
Procainamide	10–20	q4h

CHRONIC DRUG THERAPY

Digoxin. In patients without WPW on the surface ECG, digoxin should be the initial drug administered. The total oral digitalizing dose is 0.05–0.06 mg/kg (maximum, 1.0 mg) given first as 0.025–0.030 mg/kg, then 0.0125–0.015 mg/kg 8 hours later, and the final 0.0125–0.015 mg/kg in another 8 hours. Maintenance therapy with 0.005–0.0075 mg/kg orally twice a day (usual maximum, 0.125 mg orally twice a day) is begun 12 hours later. In 75% of our patients, this was the only drug used for chronic treatment.

The use of digoxin in infants and children with WPW is controversial. In the study by Deal et al[10] of 85 infants with WPW and SVT treated with digoxin, there were four sudden deaths. In two of the four, the patient had congenital heart disease and could have died suddenly for other reasons. The other two patients each had a normal heart and died suddenly, perhaps implicating digoxin as a contributor to the deaths. Digoxin may decrease the antegrade functional and effective refractory periods of the bundle of Kent, either (1) allowing for an early PAC to conduct to the ventricles, perhaps occurring during the "ventricular vulnerable period" and causing ventricular tachycardia and/or ventricular fibrillation; or (2) allowing for a more rapid ventricular response during atrial fibrillation, perhaps precipitating ventricular tachycardia or ventricular fibrillation. If digoxin decreased the retrograde function or effective refractory period of the bundle of Kent, this could allow for a more rapid rate of SVT; rapid SVT could then induce atrial fibrillation with rapid ventricular response. Finally, since digoxin may lower the ventricular fibrillation threshold, this consequence may be more common.

For all of these reasons, there is a theoretic

basis for concern in giving digoxin. However, balanced against this are the numerous pediatricians and pediatric cardiologists who have used digoxin to treat infants who have WPW without problems. It may be that the risk of sudden death is low enough that most pediatric cardiologists have simply been "lucky." It would be helpful to predict the possible dangers of digoxin in an individual patient. Electrophysiology studies have been performed both before and after a digitalis preparation and the measurement of refractory period (marked shortening or absolute value <220 ms following digitalis administration) used as the criterion to avoid digitalis. However, the number of patients managed this way has been small, and the follow-up has been too short to determine if this is an effective test. Similarly, assessment before and after digoxin administration by esophageal pacing techniques or treadmill exercise tests (delta wave disappeared prior to digoxin therapy but did not disappear following digoxin, suggesting a shortening of the refractory period) may be predictive, but long-term follow-up is not yet available.

At the present time, avoid the use of digoxin in children with WPW. This is especially true in children older than 8 years, when atrial fibrillation becomes more likely. As the newer antiarrhythmic drugs such as the class Ic agents become available, their relative efficacy and toxicity will need to be compared to digoxin. Only further study will help to settle some of these unknowns. Other physicians may reasonably choose to continue to treat with digoxin.

In some patients with or without WPW, digoxin is ineffective in preventing repeated episodes of SVT. In these patients, if the rate of SVT has not been demonstrated, we recommend continuing digoxin and adding another drug. The reason for this is that chronic SVT is generally associated with cardiomegaly and mild-to-moderate CHF. While digoxin may be ineffective in treating the SVT, it should be continued to treat CHF. The other antiarrhythmic drugs are all negatively inotropic, and digoxin may be useful in increasing contractility in the presence of these drugs.

Propranolol. The combination of digoxin and propranolol was the second most common regimen employed in our patients with SVT. The dose of propranolol required to produce an effective serum concentration of 40 to 200 ng/mL varies widely among patients. Generally, 0.5–1.5 mg/kg every 6 hours orally is effective (2.0–6.0 mg/kg/d). All patients should be observed for signs of decreased myocardial contractility: systemic hypotension, symptoms of CHF, or decreased echocardiographic left ventricular shortening fraction. If none of these develop and severe sinus bradycardia does not occur, the dosage may be increased further, with continued monitoring of contractility and heart rate. On occasion we have given as much as 4.5 mg/kg every 6 hours without observable side effects. The goal of treatment is permanent cessation of SVT; however, in some patients with AV dissociation and other chronic types of SVT, the best result obtainable has been continuing SVT with a markedly reduced rate. With a reduced rate the patients were asymptomatic, and cardiomegaly improved.

Quinidine. Quinidine, especially in combination with digitalis or propranolol, may be effective in patients with Kent bundles (digitalis should only be used with "concealed" Kent bundles). Quinidine is not effective in SVT with AV dissociation. The dosage of quinidine sulfate is 7.5–10 mg/kg every 6 hours orally (30–40 mg/kg/d). The same total daily dosage can be given as quinidine gluconate, which may be given in two or three divided doses. With quinidine, it is important to keep the patient's serum concentration within the known effective serum concentrations for the particular laboratory. In our TCH laboratory, this is 2.5–6.0 μg/mL. At levels below 2.5 μg/mL, quinidine is ineffective; at levels above 6.0 μg/mL, abnormalities of ventricular conduction and depolarization become more likely, with increased susceptibility to ventricular tachycardia and ventricular fibrillation. The QT interval prolongs in most patients following quinidine administration, but if the QRS duration prolongs by more than 25% (e.g., from 0.10 s to 0.125 s) or if ventricular arrhythmia occurs, quinidine should be discontinued, even if the serum concentration is within the effective range. Patients should be hospitalized for initiation of quinidine therapy, because there is an increased risk of torsades de pointes during the early phases of quinidine treatment. Late development of quinidine toxicity has been associated with hypokalemia.[11]

Verapamil. Porter, Garson, and Gillette[12] studied seven children ranging in age from 2.8 years to 15.3 years (median, 10.8 years). All had SVT controlled by long-term oral verapamil treatment at doses of 0.5–2.9 mg/kg (mean dose, 1.36 mg/kg). These doses achieved a blood level of 248 ± 117 ng/mL. We treated five patients with verapamil alone or in combination with digoxin. The drug controlled SVT in two of the five. Because of the very rapid removal of orally administered verapamil by the liver (80% first-pass elimination), the oral dose is much larger than the intravenous dose. While intravenous verapamil may be dangerous in young infants, it appears that oral verapamil may be better tolerated. The patient should be closely assessed for development of CHF.

Other Drugs. We have used digoxin, propranolol, and quinidine singly or in combination as chronic drug treatment in more than 84% of the patients who received drug therapy for SVT. In patients with refractory SVT who were unresponsive to various combinations of digoxin, propranolol, and quinidine, digoxin was usually continued. The new antiarrhythmic drugs encainide, flecainide, and ethmozine were mainly used to treat incessant SVT.

Encainide. Encainide hydrochloride is a benzanoid derivative similar in action to other class I antiarrhythmic agents. It is from four to 14 times more effective than quinidine and procainamide in abolishing various atrial and ventricular arrhythmias.

Oral administration of encainide prolongs the PR, QRS, and QT intervals. However, in clinical trials less than 10% of the patients have required discontinuation of the drug because of prolongation of any interval. The pediatric dose is initiated at 60 mg/m²/d (three or four times daily). The dose may be increased by 30 mg/m²/d every 72 to 96 hours to a maximum dosage of either 120 mg/m²/d or 200 mg/d. In Strasburger et al's study, encainide prolonged the PR interval by 35%, the QRS interval by 44%, and the corrected QT interval by 10%.[13] Because encainide was required four times daily in the majority of children, flecainide has become more commonly used.

Flecainide. Flecainide acetate is a relatively new benzamide that has been classified as a class Ic antiarrhythmic agent. Flecainide's primary effect is to slow the rate of rise of "fast" action potentials and delay recovery from inactivation of the fast sodium channel, resulting in significant slowing of conduction throughout the heart (including accessory pathways) and prolongation of the PA, AH, and HV intervals. The drug appears to be more effective in suppressing ventricular ectopy than are quinidine, disopyramide, mexiletine, tocainide, and proprafenone.[14] Flecainide suppresses ventricular tachycardia in approximately 80% of adult patients and has proven effective in re-entrant supraventricular tachycardias complicating Wolff-Parkinson-White syndrome.[15] The dose for children begins at 100 mg/m²/d and may be increased to 200 mg/m²/d. Therapeutic plasma levels are in the 0.2–1.0 mg/L range. Flecainide has been very successful in all types of childhood SVT.

Ethmozine. Ethmozine is a phenothiazine derivative, and is most similar in action to class Ib antiarrhythmic agents. Ethmozine was developed as an antiarrhythmic drug in the USSR, with preliminary results demonstrating efficacy in ventricular rhythm disturbances.[16] There are significant changes in atrial and right ventricular refractory periods, AV conduction, and uncorrected QT interval.[17] In addition, ethmozine reduces abnormal automaticity. The average effective dosage was 5–15 mg/kg/d, divided into three daily doses.

Ethmozine occasionally prolongs the PR and/or QRS intervals and corrected QT interval. Side effects associated with ethmozine are lightheadedness, dizziness, numbness or tingling, headache, and dry mouth. Ethmozine has been used successfully in children with atrial ectopic SVT.

DIAGNOSIS OF SVT BY INTRACARDIAC ELECTROPHYSIOLOGIC STUDY

Indications

The indications for the use of intracardiac electrophysiologic study in patients with SVT include the following:

1. To determine the mechanism of SVT in patients with drug-resistant SVT for the purposes of surgical treatment;
2. For mapping prior to surgery (WPW, unidirectional retrograde accessory pathway [URAP], sinoatrial node [SAN] re-entry, atrial ectopic tachycardia [AET], junctional ectopic tachycardia [JET], atrioventricular node [AVN] re-entry);

3. For ablation (SAN re-entry, AET, JET, AVN re-entry);
4. For drug testing (SAN re-entry, James or Mahaim fibers, AVN re-entry, digitalis in WPW);
5. To evaluate antitachycardia pacemaker (SAN re-entry, AVN re-entry, or James or Mahaim fibers);
6. To establish diagnosis in a patient with documented tachycardia but uncertain specific diagnosis;
7. To evaluate a patient with recurrent symptomatic episodes of SVT;
8. For research (new antiarrhythmic drugs, partial AV node ablation, AV node physiology in a child, autonomic blockade, autonomic stimulation); and
9. For pacemaker implantation.

Technique

The overall plan for diagnosis of SVT is shown in Table 13–12. Basic measurements are made with the patient in sinus rhythm, and then maneuvers are performed to induce SVT. After tachycardia is induced and a supraventricular origin is confirmed, the SVT is characterized by basic measurements and response to certain perturbations. Finally, the response to measures used to terminate SVT is recorded.

TABLE 13–12
INTRACARDIAC ELECTROPHYSIOLOGIC STUDY OF SVT

Basic measurements in NSR
Intracardiac conduction intervals
CSNRT
Pace HRA, LLRA, LSRA, PCS, DCS to uncover a delta wave
Induce SVT
From HRA single premature atrial stimuli into NSR: scan diastole
Double premature atrial stimuli into NSR
Rapid atrial pacing
Single and double premature atrial stimuli into atrial paced rhythm:scan diastole
Move catheter and repeat above previous steps from LLRA and CS
Single premature ventricular stimuli into NSR (also determine atrial activation sequence)
Single premature ventricular stimuli into ventricular paced rhythm
Isoproterenol
Atropine
Characterize SVT
Is it SVT?
QRS duration and morphology
Flutter waves on surface ECG
HV interval
Atrial activation sequence
Atrial cycle length in first few beats
Change in atrial cycle length with spontaneous BBB
Change in atrial cycle length with PVC
Terminate SVT
Overdrive atrial pacing
Premature atrial stimuli into SVT
Synchronized DC electrical cardioversion
Reinduce SVT
Induce atrial fibrillation (if WPW)
Note response to drugs

BASIC MEASUREMENTS

In children older than 18 months, four catheters are used, one each in the high right atrium (HRA), low septal right atrium, right ventricular apex, and coronary sinus (Fig. 13–15). In infants younger than 18 months, three catheters are generally used. Intracardiac conduction intervals in sinus rhythm are measured, and with the high atrial catheter, a corrected sinus node recovery time (CSNRT) is calculated. This information is used in planning therapy. If the CSNRT is prolonged, drugs that lead to sinus bradycardia should probably be avoided, although data on their use in patients with a prolonged CSNRT are not available. Then, at a heart rate 10 to 20 bpm faster than the patient's sinus rhythm, several supraventricular areas are paced and a delta wave is sought on the surface ECG. Pacing near the atrial region of a Kent bundle will bring out a delta wave. It is possible during pacing to observe a delta wave that had never been observed on routine ECGs taken previously in the patient's life.

SVT INDUCTION

Several methods are available to induce SVT. Usually the most reliable method is to use the extrastimulus technique to induce premature stimuli at increasingly earlier intervals into the HRA during normal sinus rhythm (NSR). Even if SVT is not induced by this method, the stimuli should be continued until the atrial refractory period is reached. If WPW is present, the QRS complex will be narrow at shorter cycle lengths. The point of transition between a narrow QRS and a wide QRS with a delta wave is the effective refractory period of the bundle of Kent. From the data on AV conduction, dual AV node pathways or a bypass tract that

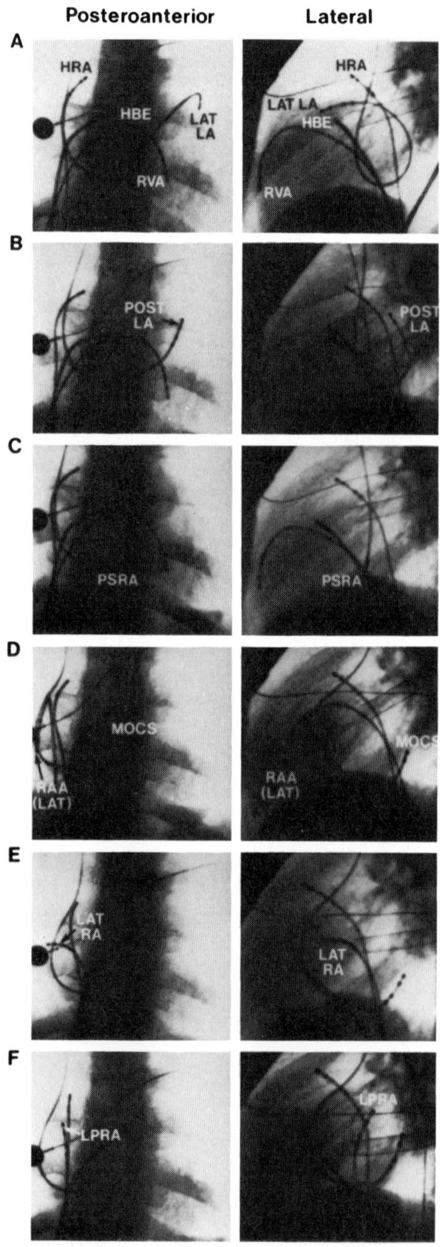

FIGURE 13–15
Catheter positions for recording intracardiac electrograms. The high right atrial (HRA) catheter and the catheter that records the low septal right atrium (LSRA) and His bundle electrogram (HBE) remain stationary, while the other two catheters are moved. (*A*) Anterolateral left atrium (LAT LA), RV apex (RVA), high right atrium (HRA), low septal right atrium (LSRA), and His bundle (HBE) electrograms. (*B*) Posterior left atrium (POST LA), RVA, HRA, LSRA/HBE. (*C*) Posterior septal right atrium (PSRA), RVA, HRA, LSRA/HBE. (*D*) Mouth of coronary sinus (MOCS), lateral right atrial appendage (RAA LAT), HRA, LSRA/HBE. (*E*) Midlateral right atrium (LAT RA), MOCS, HRA, LSRA/HBE. (*F*) Low posterior right atrium (LPRA), MOCS, HRA, LSRA/HBE.

conducts in an antegrade direction may be revealed.

If single premature atrial stimuli do not induce SVT, paired premature atrial stimuli may do so. The S_1S_2 interval is set 40 ms longer than the atrial effective refractory period, and the S_2S_3 interval is set at 50 ms longer than S_1S_2; then S_2S_3 is progressively shortened.

Rapid atrial pacing at rates of 150 to 400 bpm may induce SVT. The systemic blood pressure should be monitored carefully during this procedure, because some children with excellent AV conduction may conduct all atrial stimuli to the ventricle and become hypotensive because of the rapid ventricular rate.

Introduction of premature atrial stimuli (single or paired) into an atrial paced rhythm that is 40 to 50 bpm faster than normal sinus rhythm is tried next. With the faster paced rhythm, the atrial and AV node refractory periods will change and possibly induce SVT.

If none of these maneuvers has been successful with high right atrial stimulation, the site should be changed to the low right atrium or the left atrium, and the maneuvers repeated. Wellens and Durrer[18] have shown that the closer a stimulus is to the site of tachycardia, the more likely it is to be successful in initiating the tachycardia.

Premature ventricular stimuli may sometimes initiate SVT when atrial stimuli will not. Stimuli may be introduced into the ventricle (into normal sinus rhythm or ventricular paced rhythm) at progressively earlier intervals in ventricular diastole until the ventricular effective refractory period is reached. The retrograde atrial activation sequence (see later discussion) can be determined from the ventricular beats that conduct to the atrium. From data on ventriculoatrial conduction intervals, a bypass tract that conducts in a retrograde direction may be revealed.

If none of these maneuvers has initiated SVT, an intravenous infusion of isoproterenol (0.05–0.5 μg/kg/min) or an intravenous atropine bolus (0.01–0.03 mg/kg) may alter conduction and refractoriness sufficiently to allow initiation of SVT.

CHARACTERIZATION OF SVT

When tachycardia is initiated, the supraventricular origin must be confirmed. If the QRS duration is normal and the morphology is identical to that observed in normal sinus rhythm (NSR), the diagnosis is most likely SVT. If flutter waves are visible on the surface ECG, the diagnosis is atrial flutter, not SVT. If the HV interval is the same as or longer than that recorded during NSR, regardless of the QRS duration, the diagnosis is SVT. There is one exception to this rule, and that is in patients who have an AV node bypass tract (Kent, Mahaim, or James) and who have the rare antidromic type of SVT in which the impulse travels antegrade over the bypass tract and retrograde through the AV node. In these patients the QRS complex will be identical to that observed during NSR, and the diagnosis of SVT is made on this basis.

The relationship of the atrial depolarization to the ventricular depolarization should be determined. SVT that has the AV node as part of the re-entry circuit almost never continues in the presence of AV block, since the re-entry circuit is broken. This is virtually always true for SVT caused by a Kent bundle. Very rarely, block below the bundle of His may exist while either AV node re-entry or SVT resulting from James fiber continues. If AV dissociation occurs with a narrow QRS tachycardia, the most likely diagnosis is junctional tachycardia caused by an ectopic focus in the bundle of His. However, it is possible to have His bundle re-entry SVT. This diagnosis would be made on the basis of SVT with AV dissociation that oscillated at the onset.

Atrial Activation Sequence

After SVT is diagnosed, it is important to determine the atrial activation sequence. To accomplish this, endocardial recordings are made from several areas within the right and left atrium. Recordings are taken from several sites within the coronary sinus to estimate posterior or left atrial activation. These recordings can be done with one catheter that is moved to all the different sites, but the preferred method is to use four catheters simultaneously. The catheter that records the low right atrial depolarization and the bundle of His potential remains stationary, as does the catheter that records the high right atrium (HRA) potential. These are held constant so that other activation times can be compared to two fixed points (Fig. 13–16). The catheter in the coronary sinus is advanced as distally as possible, so that it is pointing anteriorly and records from the anterolateral left atrium. This catheter is then withdrawn, and recordings are made from the posterior left atrium (proximal and distal coronary sinus) and then from the mouth of the coronary sinus (MOCS). Next the right ventricular catheter is withdrawn and moved throughout the right atrium. The first position is in the right atrial appendage; the catheter is then moved from the right atrial appendage to the midlateral right atrium and then to the low posterior right atrium as well as to other sites such as the anterior septum or the atrial septum between the His bundle catheter and the MOCS.

As an introduction to the methodology, consider sinus rhythm (see Fig. 13–16). The normal antegrade atrial activation sequence in sinus rhythm begins with the HRA (1 in the figure). There may be preferential spread of excitation inferiorly along the terminal crest so that the anterior low lateral right atrium (LLRA) and posterior LLRA are depolarized almost simultaneously (2). At approximately the same time or shortly thereafter, the lateral right atrial appendage, medial right atrial appendage, and low septal right atrium depolarize (3). Very shortly thereafter, the posterior septal right atrium and MOCS depolarize (4), followed by the midcoronary sinus and the distal coronary sinus (5). Several of these electrograms may occur almost simultaneously, but the general order is maintained (e.g., LLRA should not occur before HRA).

On the other hand, if the apex of the right ventricle is stimulated with an electrode catheter and retrograde activation of the atria proceeds normally through the bundle of His and AV node, we observe the normal retrograde atrial activation sequence. The first part of the atria to be activated normally is the low septal right atrium (LSRA) (shown on the atrial electrogram recorded with the catheter that also records the bundle of His depolarization). If the LSRA is not the first to be activated, the retrograde activation sequence is abnormal. From the LSRA (1, Fig. 13–17), the impulse spreads radially from the AV node; 2 is the MOCS; 3 is the LLRA, posterior septal right atrium, and coronary sinus; and 4 is the HRA and the right atrial appendage.

A normal retrograde activation sequence during SVT implies that the tachycardia enters the atrium near the AV node. Numerous

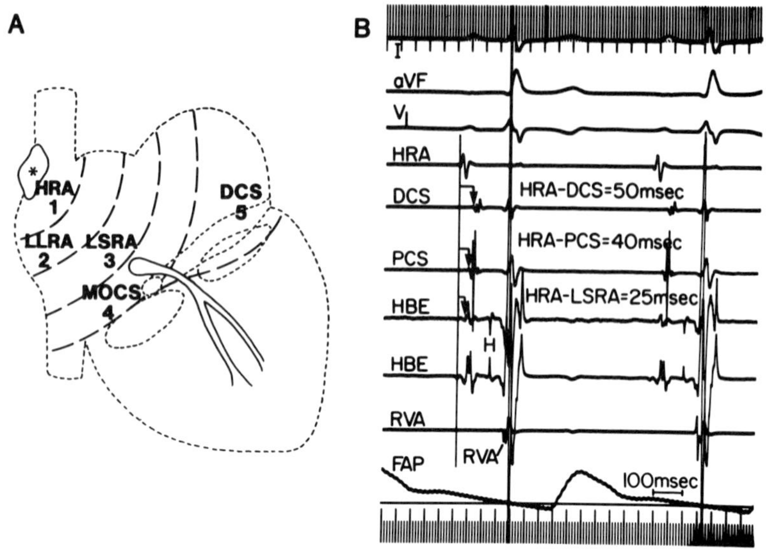

FIGURE 13–16
(*A*) Diagram showing atrial activation sequence during normal sinus rhythm beginning with HRA and spreading to DCS; the area indicated by 1 is first to be activated, and the area indicated by 5 is last to be activated. (*B*) Recording made during intracardiac electrophysiologic study with three surface ECG leads (I, aVF, and V_1) and six bipolar intracardiac electrograms. Arterial pressure is shown at the bottom of the tracing. The difference in activation times shows that the HRA was activated first, followed by the LSRA, PCS, and DCS. DCS = distal coronary sinus; H and HBE = His bundle electrogram; HRA = high right atrium; LLRA = low lateral right atrium; LSRA = low septal right atrium; MOCS = mouth of coronary sinus; PCS = proximal coronary sinus; RVA = right ventricular apex.

types of SVT have a normal retrograde sequence; these are listed in Table 13–13.

If the atrial activation sequence does not begin with the LSRA, either an atrial ectopic focus or atrial muscle re-entry may be occurring at the site with the earliest atrial activation (Fig. 13–18). The other possibility is that the atria are being activated eccentrically by an accessory connection that forms the retrograde limb for re-entry SVT. Only further testing can distinguish among these possibilities.

If the atrial activation sequence is different on the first beat from subsequent beats, ectopic SVT is extremely unlikely. If the atrial activation sequence is the same on the initi-

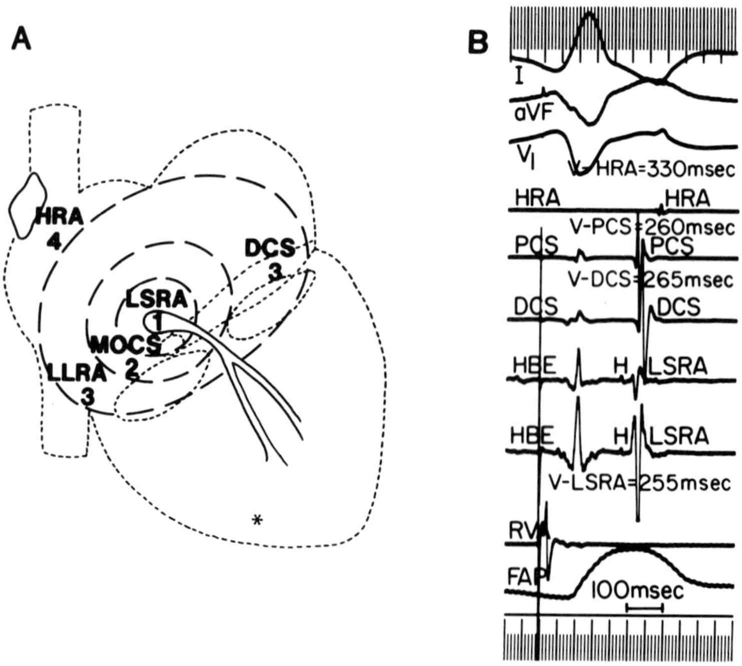

FIGURE 13–17
(*A*) Diagram showing normal retrograde atrial activation sequence from right ventricular pacing. Activation spreads radially from the AV node, beginning at the low septal right atrium and finally spreading to the HRA and DCS. (*B*) Recordings made during intracardiac electrophysiologic study during premature stimulation of the right ventricular apex showing a normal retrograde activation sequence. The difference in activation times shows that the LSRA is activated first, followed by the PCS, DCS, and HRA.

TABLE 13—13
ATRIAL ACTIVATION SEQUENCE IN SVT

SITE OF FIRST ATRIAL ACTIVATION	TYPE OF SVT
Low septal right atrium (LSRA)	AVN re-entry Antegrade Kent—retrograde AVN Reentry via atrio-His fiber JET His bundle re-entry AET (LSRA) Atrial muscle re-entry (LSRA) Antegrade AVN—retrograde Kent (septal) Mahaim
Mouth of coronary sinus (MOCS)	Antegrade AVN—retrograde Kent (posterior septal) AET—septal Atrial muscle re-entry (MOCS) PJRT
Right paraseptal	Antegrade AVN—retrograde Kent (right paraseptal) AET (right paraseptal) Atrial muscle re-entry (right paraseptal)
Midcoronary sinus	Antegrade AVN—retrograde Kent (left posterior) AET (left posterior) Atrial muscle re-entry (left posterior)
Distal coronary sinus	Antegrade AVN—retrograde Kent (left lateral) AET (left lateral) Atrial muscle re-entry (left lateral)
Low lateral right atrium	Antegrade AVN—retrograde Kent (right lateral) AET (right lateral) Atrial muscle re-entry (right lateral)
Low posterior right atrium	Antegrade AVN—retrograde Kent (right posterior) AET (right posterior) Atrial muscle re-entry (right posterior)
Right atrial appendage	Antegrade AVN—retrograde Kent (right anterior) AET (right anterior) Atrial muscle re-entry (right anterior)
High right atrium (identical to sinus rhythm)	SAN re-entry AET
High right atrium (sinus rhythm with AV dissociation)	JET His bundle re-entry

ating and subsequent beats, any type of SVT is possible.

Atrial Cycle Length

When SVT is initiated, it is important to observe also the changes that occur in atrial cycle length during the first few beats: in re-entry the cycle lengths oscillate, whereas in ectopic focus and triggered arrhythmia the cycle lengths shorten progressively.

Effect of Bundle-Branch Block

If a Kent bundle is located in the free wall of either ventricle, the usual pathway of the impulse is to go from the atrium through the AV node, specialized conduction system, ventricular muscle, and bundle of Kent back to the atrium. If bundle-branch occurs on the same side as the Kent bundle, the atrial cycle length will be prolonged. For example, if a patient with a right anterior Kent bundle developed right bundle-branch block that reverted to normal conduction with a narrow QRS, the atrial cycle length would be longer when right bundle-branch block was present than when there was normal conduction. The reason for this is that the right bundle branch is in the tachycardia circuit; if delay or block occurs in the right bundle branch, the rate of the tachycardia will decrease. If, on the other hand, this patient with a right anterior Kent bundle developed left bundle-branch block, the cycle length of the tachycardia would not change, because the left bundle branch would not be part of the re-entry circuit (Fig. 13–19). In patients whose Kent bundles are located in the septum, bundle-branch block does not affect the cycle length.

Introduction of PVCs

The best way of proving that a bypass tract is participating as the retrograde limb of an

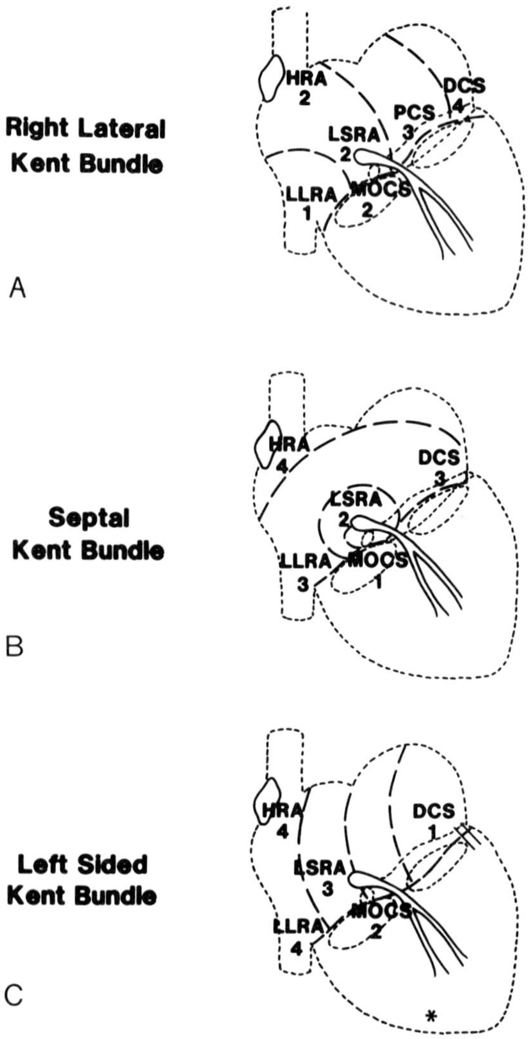

FIGURE 13–18

(*A*) Diagram showing atrial activation sequence in a right lateral Kent bundle. The LLRA is activated first. (*B*) Diagram showing atrial activation sequence in a septal Kent bundle. The MOCS is usually activated before the LLRA. (*C*) Diagram showing atrial activation sequence in a left lateral Kent bundle. The DCS is activated first.

SVT is by introduction of PVCs into the tachycardia. If PVCs are introduced at decreasing intervals into ventricular diastole, eventually one will fall at the time that the bundle of His deflection is recorded (Fig. 13–20). At that instant the SVT had just traversed the AV node and the bundle of His in an antegrade direction just before stimulating the ventricles. Therefore at the time that the His deflection is recorded, the bundle of His must be refractory and will not conduct a stimulated impulse either antegrade or retrograde. In a patient without a bypass tract, stimulating the ventricles simultaneously with the His deflection will not result in capture of the atrium because the only way for the impulse to get from the ventricle to the atrium is through the His bundle, and this is refractory; however, if there is a bypass tract, this tract may not be refractory at the time of the His potential and will conduct an impulse from ventricle to atrium.

The manifestation of the stimulated ventricular impulse capturing the atrium is a shortening of the atrial cycle length of SVT for that beat. The atrium in essence has been prematurely stimulated. Because conduction time of the stimulated impulse through the ventricles can be significant (and therefore, although the impulse started at the time of the His deflection, it might not arrive at the Kent bundle prematurely), the atrial cycle length is shortened maximally if the stimulus arises close to the ventricular end of the bypass tract. Therefore if a right-sided bypass tract is suspected from atrial activation sequence, the PVCs should be delivered in the right ventricle. If a left-sided bypass tract is suspected, the PVCs should be delivered in the left ventricle.

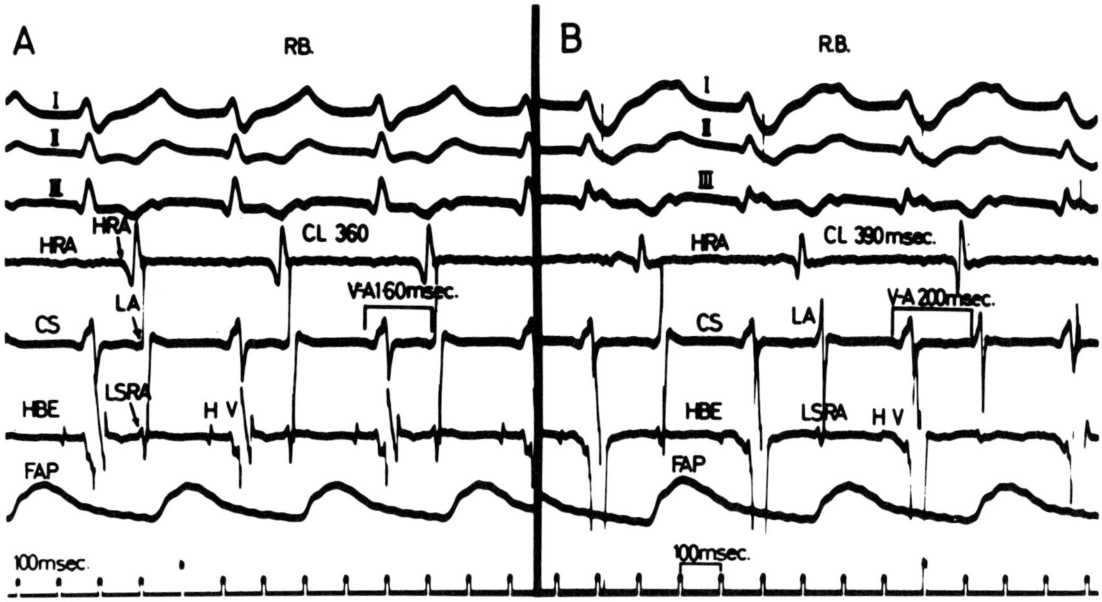

FIGURE 13–19
Effect of bundle-branch block during SVT caused by a right-sided Kent bundle. (*A*) With normal conduction, the cycle length is 360 ms, and the ventriculoatrial (VA) conduction time is 160 ms. (*B*) During complete right bundle-branch block, the cycle length prolongs to 390 ms and the VA time to 200 ms. The fact that right bundle-branch block prolonged the VA time showed that the Kent bundle was on the right side of the heart (see text).

Since permanent junctional reciprocating tachycardia (PJRT) appears to be caused by a bypass tract, it also may be possible to preexcite the atrium with PVCs in PJRT.

SVT TERMINATION

The response to overdrive atrial pacing at a rate 10 to 20 bpm faster than the SVT helps to classify SVT: re-entry stops immediately, triggered arrhythmia stops several beats later, and ectopic focus may slow for a few beats but does not stop. If there is no effect on SVT, then different pacing sites, different current amplitudes, or different pacing rates should be tried.

An appropriately timed premature atrial stimulus will generally stop re-entry or triggered arrhythmia SVT, but will not stop an ectopic focus SVT. Premature atrial stimuli should be introduced at decreasing cycle lengths beginning at a cycle length slightly shorter than that of the SVT. By plotting the response of SVT to this maneuver (reset or nonreset), the mechanism may be established. Only ectopic SVT will reset.

Synchronized DC electrical cardioversion (0.25–1.0 J/kg) may be used both diagnostically and therapeutically. If the patient becomes symptomatic from SVT, cardioversion may be necessary. Seen as a diagnostic tool, cardioversion will not stop ectopic focus SVT, but in the majority of cases it will terminate SVT resulting from re-entry or triggered arrhythmia.

SVT REINDUCTION

The major reason for reinducing SVT is to find the range of stimuli that will cause SVT (e.g., to find the cycle lengths of PACs that will induce tachycardia). These cycle lengths can then be compared before and after a drug is given to see if a different range of cycle lengths will cause SVT. If SVT is more difficult to induce after drug administration, then the drug's effect is beneficial; if SVT is easier to induce, then the drug's effect is detrimental.

ATRIAL FIBRILLATION INDUCTION

In patients with WPW it is important to determine the functional refractory period of the bundle of Kent by inducing atrial fibrillation. The shortest R-R interval defines the functional refractory period.

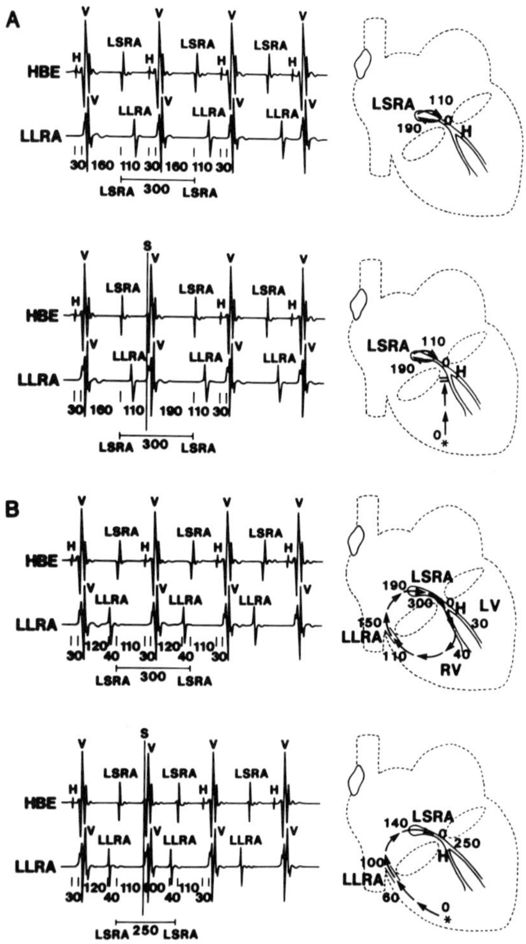

FIGURE 13–20
Effect of ventricular stimulation during His bundle depolarization. (*A*) Top tracing shows diagrammatic representation of intracardiac recordings on a patient with AV node re-entry SVT. Recordings are shown from catheters with electrograms in the His bundle area and the low right atrium. During SVT the cycle length (LSRA = LSRA) is 300 ms. From the activation sequence, the LSRA is activated before the LLRA, which is consistent with AV node re-entry SVT. The diagram to the right indicates that the time for the impulse to pass from the LSRA to the His bundle is 110 ms. Since the cycle length is 300 ms, it takes approximately 190 ms for the impulse to return to the LSRA. The re-entry circuit is entirely within the AV node and does not involve the His bundle. In the bottom pair of tracings, a stimulus (S) is introduced into the ventricle at the time that the His bundle is depolarized. The His bundle is refractory and will not propagate the impulse from the ventricular stimulation. Therefore the impulse does not propagate back to the atria and the SVT is unaffected. (*B*) Top tracing shows diagrammatic representation of SVT caused by re-entry through a right-sided Kent bundle. The numbers on the diagram at the right refer to activation times of various cardiac structures after the His bundle is activated. In the bottom pair of tracings, a stimulus is introduced into the right ventricle at the time that the His bundle is depolarized. As in Figure 13–21(A), the impulse cannot pass retrograde through the His bundle; however, if another means is available for ventriculoatrial conduction, the atria can be stimulated. In this instance the Kent bundle is not refractory when the His bundle is refractory. The prematurely stimulated impulse arrives at the atrium before the next atrial impulse is due from SVT, and the atrial cycle length is shortened to 250 ms.

Response to Drug Therapy

The administration of drugs during the study can be of both diagnostic and therapeutic use. Patients with WPW may receive digoxin (one-half the "digitalizing" dose) to assess its effect on the antegrade refractory periods of the bundle of Kent. The acute effects of intravenous propranolol, procainamide (which may be given intravenously and which has effects similar to those of quinidine), or verapamil provide acute information that may be useful in planning chronic therapy. Generally, the response of re-entry SVT to a drug is either to stop or to remain unchanged. The response of an ectopic SVT is to slow or to remain unchanged. It is rare for an ectopic SVT to stop in response to acute drug administration.

Types of SVT

In the cardiac catheterization laboratory at least three major mechanistic categories of SVT can be identified: re-entry without a bypass tract, re-entry with a bypass tract, and ectopic focus. These major types can be further classified primarily on the basis of the site of SVT.

We have performed intracardiac electrophysiologic study (EPS) in 178 children with SVT, aged 2 days to 17.5 years at the time of cardiac catheterization. The types of SVT found are shown in Table 13–14. The first three categories of SVT listed are all represented; we have not yet identified a patient with triggered arrhythmia. The 178 children who underwent electrophysiologic study differed in several important ways from the other 168 patients with SVT that we have seen in Houston (Table 13–15). Although the EPS patients had the same age at onset of SVT, they had more congenital heart disease and more congestive heart failure, were more often treated with a "complex regimen" (i.e., a regimen other than digoxin alone), and had more recurrences and more SVT present on follow-up.

TABLE 13—14
FREQUENCY OF OCCURRENCE OF TYPES OF SVT (N = 178)

TYPE OF SVT	NUMBER	PERCENTAGE
Re-entry without bypass tract		
Sinus node re-entry	12	7
Atrial muscle re-entry	2	1
AV node re-entry	29	16
Re-entry with bypass tract		
Wolff-Parkinson-White	40	23
Unidirectional accessory pathway	22	12
Lown-Ganong-Levine	7	4
Permanent junctional reciprocating pathway	23	13
Ectopic focus		
Atrial	32	18
Junctional	7	4
Type undetermined	4	2

In summary, the patients who underwent EPS were more severely ill and more difficult to treat than patients who did not undergo EPS. Therefore in this group the response to acute and chronic treatment and the recurrence and presence of SVT on follow-up are biased in favor of nonresponders.

The specific types of SVT will now be described, based on our patients who underwent electrophysiologic study. For each type the clinical features (Table 13–16), surface ECG characteristics (Table 13–17), intracardiac electrophysiologic criteria for diagnosis (Table 13–18), results of acute therapy and initial chronic drug therapy, rate of recurrence, and final status at follow-up will be described.

RE-ENTRY WITHOUT BYPASS TRACT

In this broad category criteria must be met for re-entry, with no evidence that a bypass tract participates in the SVT. Of our patients with SVT who underwent electrophysiologic study, 35% met these criteria. Re-entry can occur in any supraventricular site, and this category of SVT has been subclassified according to where the SVT occurs.

Reentry that occurs within the sinus node or in the perisinus tissue (SAN re-entry) and re-entry that occurs elsewhere in the atrial muscle (atrial muscle re-entry) are basically indistinguishable electrophysiologically with the exception of the site of origin. If a re-entry tachycardia without a bypass tract has an identical activation sequence to that seen during sinus rhythm, then this is SAN re-entry SVT. If the atrial activation sequence originates from any other atrial site except the LSRA, or if atrial activation begins in the LSRA and AV block is present during SVT with block above the His bundle, then this is atrial muscle re-entry SVT. If a critical A_1A_2 is necessary for initiation of SVT, generally re-entry is within the atrium or SAN. On the other hand, if a critical A_2H_2 is necessary for induction, generally re-entry is within the AV node. If the atrial activation sequence begins in the LSRA and the graphs of A_1A_2 versus H_1H_2 (or V_1V_2 versus A_1A_2) are discontinuous, suggesting dual AV node pathways, we may infer the area of re-entry as the AV node.

Sinus Node Re-entry SVT

Clinical Features. Sinus node re-entry SVT was found in 12 of 178 patients (7%). No patient was younger than 2 years at the time of onset, and the mean age of onset (6.7 years) was the oldest among all the types. This was one of the two types found most commonly in patients after surgery for a congenital cardiac defect. The incidence of CHF was the lowest among all the types, possibly because of the older age at onset or because atrial contraction preceded each ven-

TABLE 13—15
SUMMARY OF FINDINGS IN PATIENTS WITH SVT

	EPS (N = 178)	NO EPS (N = 168)	*p*
Age at onset (years)	3.9 ± 0.4	4.1 ± 0.4	NS
Preop CHD	28/178 (15%)	14/168 (8%)	0.01
Postop CHD	24/178 (13%)	10/108 (7%)	NS
CHF	69/178 (39%)	35/165 (20%)	0.01
Complex treatment	54/164 (33%)	18/155 (12%)	0.005
Recurrence	151/168 (89%)	95/152 (63%)	0.005
SVT on follow-up	121/164 (74%)	86/154 (50%)	0.01

Abbreviation: EPS = electrophysiology study.

TABLE 13–16
CLINICAL FEATURES OF PATIENTS WHO UNDERWENT EPS (N = 178)

	TYPE OF SVT								
	SAN	*AM*	*AVN*	*PJRT*	*WPW*	*URAP*	*LGL*	*AET*	*JET*
Age SVT began (yrs)	7.1 ± 1.4	8.1	4.7 ± 0.3	3.9 ± 0.4	3.4 ± 0.7	3.9 ± 1.1	4.5 ± 1.2	7.7 ± 2.1	2.3 ± 1
Predisposing factors									
None	5/12	1/2	16/29	10/23	19/40	15/22	7/7	6/32	0/7
Pre-op CHD	1/12	0/2	1/29	1/23	10/40	4/22	0/7	5/32	6/7
Post-op CHD	4/12	0/2	11/29	0/73	6/40	1/22	0/7	2/32	1/7
Cardiomyopathy	0/12	1/2	1/29	12/23	2/40	2/22	0/7	14/32	0/7
CHF	2/12	1/2	4/29	13/20	11/40	7/19	1/7	25/32	5/7
Positive family history	2/10	0/2	6/27	4/23	7/40	4/19	3/7	12/32	3/7

Abbreviations: AET = atrial ectopic tachycardia; AM = atrial muscle re-entry; AVN = atrioventricular node re-entry; JET = junctional ectopic tachycardia; LGL = Lown-Ganong-Levine; PJRT = permanent junctional reciprocating tachycardia; SAN = sinus node re-entry; URAP = unidirectional retrograde accessory pathway; WPW = Wolff-Parkinson-White.

tricular contraction in all cases, allowing for an appropriate atrial contribution to cardiac output.

Surface ECG During SVT. Only four ECGs during SVT were available for review. The QRS rate ranged from 170 to 270 bpm; P waves were visible in each, with a long PR interval.

Five of the 12 patients had tachycardia-bradycardia syndrome. The other major type of SVT found in patients with tachycardia-bradycardia syndrome was AV node re-entry.

Intracardiac Electrophysiology. Sinus node re-entry SVT can be induced or terminated by rapid atrial pacing or premature atrial stimulation. Induction depends on a critical A_1A_2 interval and is not related to the AH, AV, or VA intervals.[19] SVT can be induced from ventricular premature extrastimuli when a critical retrograde A_1A_2 is reached. Because the AV node does not form a necessary part of the re-entry circuit, SVT can be induced by a PAC that blocks above the bundle of His. The atrial activation sequence and the P wave shape in the surface ECG must be identical to that found in sinus rhythm in order for the condition to be classified as SAN re-entry SVT (Fig. 13–21).

Treatment. In seven of our 12 patients, the first episode of SVT converted spontaneously. Therefore the response to acute therapy involves a small number of patients. Success was found with digoxin in one of 5, with overdrive pacing in one of one, and with cardioversion in one of one. Quinidine failed in the one patient to whom it was given. Chronic drug therapy was given initially to only five of the 12 patients; two more patients eventually required therapy.

We recommend initial treatment with digoxin. If the patient is relatively asymptomatic, it may be best to avoid adding other drugs that could depress sinus node function. If treatment is required and if both normal sinus node automaticity and sinoatrial conduction are demonstrated at cardiac catheterization, a trial of propranolol, quinidine, encainide, or amiodarone is indicated, with

TABLE 13–17
SUMMARY OF ECG DATA IN PATIENTS WITH SVT

	TYPE OF SVT*								
	SAN	*AM*	*AVN*	*PJRT*	*WPW*	*URAP*	*LGL*	*AET*	*JET*
QRS rate (±SEM)	231 ± 32	255	221 ± 14	167 ± 31	261 ± 13	238 ± 14	255†	143 ± 25	181 ± 33
PR/RR	−0.74	0.43	261 ± 0.01	—	0.41 ± 0.08	0.68 ± 0.04	0.70†	0.45 ± 0.06	—
P waves									
Not visible	0/4	0/1	4/15	0/23	4/19	5/13	1/2	0/23	0/5
Axis 0°–90°	3/4	0/1	0/15	0/23	0/19	21/13	0/2	6/23	4/5
Axis 90°–270°	3/4	0/1	0/15	14/23	2/19	1/13	0/2	2/23	0/5
Axis 270°–360°	0/4	1/1	14/15	9/23	7/19	1/13	1/2	13/23	0/5
Visible, ? axis	1/4	0/1	0/15	0/23	6/19	2/13	0/2	0/23	0/5
P-QRS									
Second degree AV block	1/4	0/1	0/15	0/23	0/19	0/13	0/2	4/13	0/5
AV dissociation	0/4	0/1	0/15	0/23	0/19	0/13	0/2	0/13	4/5

*See Table 13–16 for abbreviations of types of SVT.

TABLE 13–18
INTRACARDIAC ELECTROPHYSIOLOGIC CRITERIA FOR DIAGNOSIS*

	TYPE OF SVT†										
	SAN	*AM*	*AVN*	*HIS REE*	*PJRT*	*WPW*	*URAP*	*LGL*	*MAHAIM*	*AET*	*JET*
Delta wave with atrial pacing	–	–	–	–	–	+	–	–	+	–	–
Fixed AV interval with AE	–	–	–	–	–	+	–	+	–	–	–
Discontinuous AH	–	–	±	±	–	–	–	–	±	–	–
Fixed VA interval during VE	–	–	–	–	–	+	+	+	±	–	–
SVT inducible with atrial pacing or AE	+	+	+	+	+	+	+	+	+	–	–
Reset response during AE	–	–	–	–	–	–	–	–	–	±	±
Earliest atrial activation	Same as NSR	Different from NSR	LSRA	LSRA (If VA conduction)	MOCS	Most not LSRA	Most not LSRA	LSRA	LSRA (if VA conduction)	Any	LSRA (if VA conduction)
Atrial activation of first and subsequent beats same	–	–	–	–	±	–	–	–	–	+	+
CL of first few beats oscillate	±	±	±	±	±	±	±	±	±	–	–
Longer atrial CL with ipsilateral BBB	–	–	–	–	–	+	+	–	–	–	–
Shorter atrial CL with PVC on HBE	–	–	–	–	+	+	+	–	–	–	–
SVT possible with AV block	+	+	±	–	–	–	–	±	–	±	±
AV dissociation	–	–	–	±	–	–	–	–	±	–	+
SVT usually terminates with overdrive atrial pacing AE or CV	+	+	+	+	+	+	+	+	+	–	–
SVT response to drugs	Stops or no effect	Stops or no effect	Stops or no effect	Stops or no effect	Stops or no effect	Stops or no effect	Stops or no effect	Stops or no effect	Stops or no effect	Stops or no effect	Stops or no effect

*+ = helpful in including diagnosis; – = helpful in ruling out diagnosis; ± = sometimes helpful.
†See Table 13–16 for abbreviations of types of SVT.
Abbreviations: AE = atrial extrastimulation; AV = atrioventricular; BBB = bundle branch block; CL = cycle length; CV = cardioversion; HBE = His bundle electrogram; LSRA = low septal right atrium; MOCS = mouth of coronary sinus; NSR = normal sinus rhythm; PVC = premature ventricular contraction; VA = ventriculoatrial.

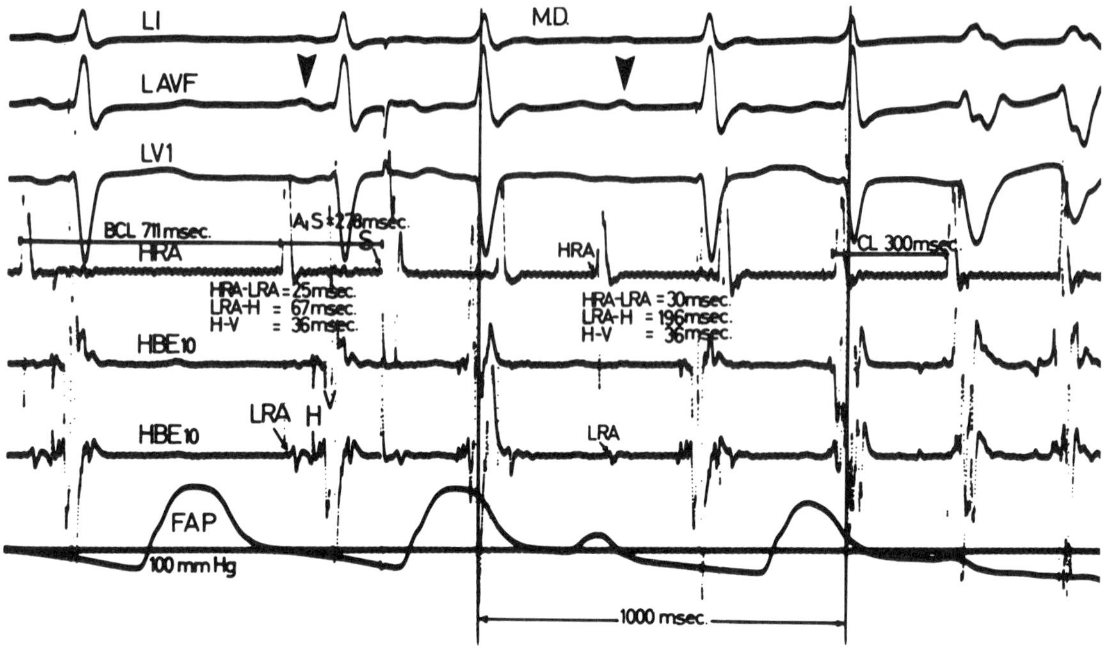

FIGURE 13–21
Recordings made during intracardiac electrophysiologic study in a patient with sinus node re-entry SVT. The first two beats are spontaneous sinus beats. The basic cycle length (BCL) of sinus rhythm is 711 ms. The atrial activation sequence has been measured on the second complex, and the HRA to LRA time is 25 ms. A premature atrial depolarization is introduced into the HRA 278 ms after the preceding HRA depolarization. In the lead labeled HRA, note that SVT occurs immediately after the pacemaker stimulus. The atrial activation sequence of SVT and the P waves during SVT are similar to those found in sinus rhythm (arrowheads). The sinus node re-entry tachycardia continues despite AV block and left bundle-branch block.

close attention to resting heart rate. If SAN function is abnormal and further treatment is required, an atrial pacemaker should be implanted to guard against bradycardia.

Patient Follow-up. SVT recurred at least once in 11 of 12 patients (92%) and was still present at follow-up (approximately 5 years) in eight of 11 (73%). These are approximately the same percentages as for other types of SVT.

Atrial Muscle Re-entry

Clinical Features. Only two of our 178 patients had atrial muscle re-entry SVT. Therefore it is difficult to generalize about this entity in children. Both of these patients were older than 3 years at the onset of SVT. One of the two had cardiomyopathy with CHF following viral illness. This illness was presumed to be myocarditis.

Surface ECG During SVT. Only one ECG during SVT was available. The P waves were visible with an axis toward the left shoulder, and the PR interval was shorter than that found in SAN re-entry SVT.

Intracardiac Electrophysiology. The intracardiac findings are identical to those of SAN re-entry SVT except that the atrial activation sequence and P waves during SVT are different from those found in sinus rhythm (Fig. 13–22).

Treatment. The SVT stopped spontaneously in one patient, and the other responded to digoxin. Both eventually received combination therapy with digoxin and quinidine. We recommend beginning treatment with digoxin. If this is unsuccessful, quinidine, flecainide, or amiodarone may be added if sinus node function is normal. If sinus node function is abnormal, encainide may be preferable.

Patient Follow-up. One of the two patients continues to have SVT.

AV Node Re-entry

AV node re-entry is the second most common type of SVT in children and was found

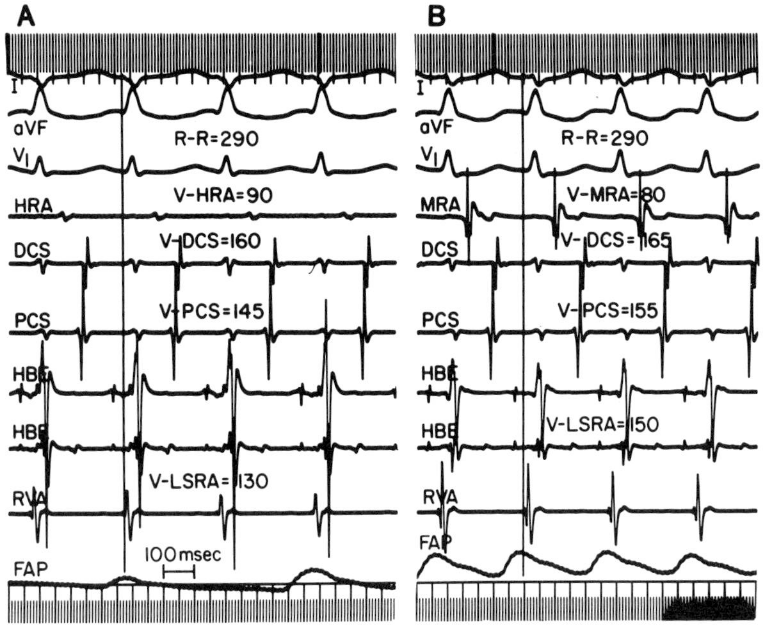

FIGURE 13–22
Recordings made during intracardiac electrophysiologic study in a patient with atrial muscle re-entry SVT. (*A*) Using the onset of the preceding QRS complex as the reference point, we find the earliest atrial activation to be in the region of the sinus node (HRA). (*B*) However, when the catheter is moved to the mid right atrium (MRA), with the same cycle length, V-MRA is shorter than V-HRA, indicating that the earliest point of atrial activation is the mid right atrium. The activation sequence therefore is MRA, HRA, LSRA, PCS, DCS.

in 29 of our 178 patients (16%). It can occur at any age but was the most common type of SVT with onset occurring after the age of 4.1 years. It was relatively uncommon to find a predisposing factor in AV node re-entry SVT (only 16 of 29 patients had predisposing factors); however, in 15 of 29 patients (51%) with AV node re-entry SVT, the first episode began a mean of 10.7 months after an operation for a congenital cardiac defect. This was the most common type of SVT to be found in children following surgery to correct congenital heart defects.

Surface ECG During SVT. AV node re-entry SVT can have any heart rate, but the heart rates tended to be lower than those in WPW and URAP. Contrary to reports showing that most adults with AV node re-entry SVT have the P wave occuring during QRS complex,[19] we found that in children P waves were visible in 11 of 16 ECGs (69%) during SVT (see Fig. 13–22). This is similar to the findings reported by Wolff et al.[20] The PR interval varied widely among different patients, and all visible P waves had an axis of 270° to 359°. We can explain the difference between children and adults only in terms of the different properties of the AV node in children and adults. It is probable that the antegrade pathway in children is relatively faster than that in adults and therefore the retrograde pathway is relatively more refractory, thus slowing conduction in the retrograde direction.

Intracardiac Electrophysiology. AV node re-entry SVT can usually be induced or terminated by rapid atrial pacing or premature extrastimuli. In both of these situations induction of SVT is dependent on a critical AV nodal delay in the impulse (AH delay with atrial extrastimuli and VA delay with ventricular extrastimuli).[19]

Helpful in the diagnosis (but not essential) is the demonstration of a discontinuous A_1A_2/H_1H_2 curve suggesting dual AV node pathways. This can also be demonstrated using ventricular extrastimuli and finding a discontinuous V_1V_2/A_1A_2 curve. Demonstration of dual AV node pathways is not sufficient evidence to diagnose AV node re-entry SVT, since 41% of children without SVT have dual AV node pathways. Participation of the dual pathways in the SVT is suggested by induction of SVT at the same cycle length at which block occurs in the fast pathway. All of these findings, however, are also compatible with a septal URAP. Therefore in addition to positive evidence of AV node re-entry SVT, evidence proving that a URAP does not exist must also be found. In AV node re-entry SVT, the earliest site or retrograde activation is the LSRA (Fig. 13–23); however, in SVT resulting from a septal URAP, it is possible that atrial activation begins so close to the LSRA that the distinction is impossible. The only additional evidence that makes a URAP unlikely is the finding of progressive VA delay in response to ventricular extrastimuli or ventricular pacing. This finding suggests

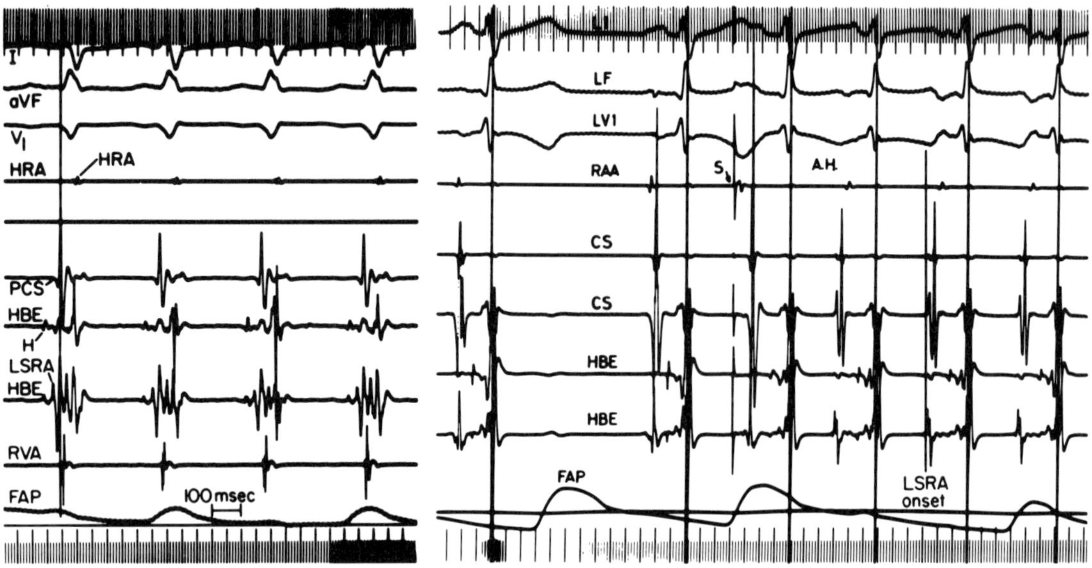

FIGURE 13–23

(*A*) Recordings made during intracardiac electrophysiologic study in a patient with AV node re-entry SVT. This is the type of AV node re-entry SVT in which atrial and ventricular depolarization occur simultaneously. Vertical line represents ventricular activation. LSRA is activated first. (*B*) Recordings made during intracardiac electrophysiologic study in another patient with AV node re-entry SVT. The patient is in sinus rhythm; then a premature stimulus delivered into the right atrial appendage causes the onset of SVT. P waves are visible in the surface ECG (lead aVF). Atrial activation occurs after the QRS complex, with initial activation in the LSRA. The vertical line marked LSRA onset shows that all other atrial electrograms follow the LSRA.

that retrograde conduction is occurring through the AV node, although in rare instances bypass tracts may exhibit progressive conduction delay.[21]

Treatment. AV node re-entry SVT converted spontaneously in 14 of 29 patients (48%). Only 11 patients received acute treatment, with digoxin being effective in only six of the 11 patients to whom it was given. Vagal maneuvers were successful in all four patients who received this type of acute therapy; each was older than 5 years. If digoxin is not effective, oral verapamil, encainide, flecainide, or amiodarone may be tried.

Patient Follow-up. AV node SVT is extremely resistant to treatment. It recurred in 25 of 28 patients (89%) and 95% of these still have SVT on follow-up. Drug therapy has been discontinued in only two of 22 patients with AV node re-entry SVT.

His Bundle Re-entry

Two patients were studied with His bundle re-entry.

Surface ECG During SVT. Re-entrant SVT oscillates with AV dissociation. It is also possible to have 1:1 retrograde conduction that looks like AV node re-entry.

Intracardiac Electrophysiology. The mechanism for His bundle re-entry is similar to the AV node re-entry mechanism.

Treatment. If digoxin is not effective, drugs such as quinidine, encainide, flecainide, or amiodarone should be tried.

RE-ENTRY WITH BYPASS TRACT

In this broad category criteria must be met for re-entry with evidence that a bypass tract both exists and participates in the SVT. This was the largest category and included 48% of our patients.

The existence of a bypass tract is suggested by the finding of a fixed AV interval during atrial extrastimulus testing or a fixed VA interval during ventricular extrastimulus testing. This behavior is different from that of a normal AV node that, with increasing prematurity of stimuli, responds with progressive prolongation of conduction. Rarely, conduction through a bypass tract may prolong with increasing prematurity.[21] The participation of a bypass tract as the retrograde limb of re-entry SVT is suggested by the findings during SVT of an eccentric retrograde activation sequence and of atrial capture with a PVC delivered when the bundle of His is refractory.

Of the numerous types of bypass tracts in children, there are three major types that cause SVT: SVT can be caused by a Kent bundle that conducts both antegrade and retrograde (WPW type of SVT), and by a Kent bundle that conducts only retrograde (URAP type of SVT), or that conducts antegrade only on certain clinical occasions or only in the catheterization laboratory ("intermittent" or "shy" WPW type of SVT). URAP type of SVT has also been called "concealed" WPW. In concealed WPW, the Kent bundle *never* conducts antegradely, even during cardiac catheterization. It is important to make the distinction between concealed and intermittent WPW, because digoxin therapy should be safe in those patients with concealed WPW. Third, it has been hypothesized that SVT in a short PR interval during sinus rhythm may result from a "James" fiber that conducts both antegrade and retrograde (LGL type of SVT). The presence of these James fibers is controversial.

In the WPW type of SVT, the re-entry circuit is usually antegrade through the AV node and retrograde through the bundle of Kent, and the QRS complex during SVT is narrow; however, in 5% to 10% of patients, the QRS complex during SVT is wide and similar to that seen in sinus rhythm. The re-entry circuit in this type begins antegrade through the bundle of Kent and retrograde through the AV node. With electrophysiologic study during normal sinus rhythm a delta wave is demonstrated, and the AV and HV intervals are short. The AH interval is normal. During narrow QRS SVT, the atrial activation sequence is abnormal; during wide QRS SVT, the retrograde atrial activation sequence is normal and begins in the LSRA.

In the URAP type of SVT, the Kent bundle conducts only in a retrograde direction. Therefore preexcitation does not occur in normal sinus rhythm, and a delta wave is not observed during either NSR or SVT. Only one type of re-entry circuit is possible: antegrade through the AV node and retrograde through the Kent bundle (Fig. 13–24).

In the LGL type of SVT, the re-entry circuit is usually antegrade through the AV node and retrograde through the James fiber. Electrophysiologic study during NSR demonstrates an AV node bypass with ventricular preexcitation. The AV interval is short, with a short AH and normal HV. During both NSR and SVT, the ventricles are activated normally through the bundle of His, so that a delta wave does not occur.

In another type of SVT with a bypass tract, known as permanent junctional reciprocating tachycardia (PJRT), the circuit passes antegrade through the AV node and retrograde through a slowly conducting septal bypass tract.

WPW Syndrome

Clinical Features. A Kent bundle that could conduct both antegrade and retrograde formed part of the re-entry circuit in 40 of 178 patients (23%). This was the most common type of SVT found in children. Although SVT resulting from WPW can begin at any age, the most common time for SVT to occur is in the first month of life. Of those with WPW and SVT, 66% had unoperated congenital cardiac defect. Patients with WPW had the highest incidence of CHF among those with re-entry SVT. A major factor in the high incidence of CHF is the young age of most patients at presentation. Of 25 patients younger than 1 year who presented with SVT, 16 had CHF. By contrast, of 15 patients who presented at an age older than 1 year, only three had CHF.

Surface ECG During SVT. In 26 of 31 patients (84%) in whom an ECG was available, the QRS complex during SVT was different from that observed during NSR. In 24 of 28 patients, the morphology and duration of QRS complex normalized during SVT. In two of 17, functional bundle-branch block developed during SVT. In all 28 of these patients the SVT was found to use the AV node as the antegrade limb and the Kent bundle as the retrograde limb. The heart rates during SVT in these patients were the most rapid found in any type of SVT, probably because of the large number of infants with this type of SVT. The heart rates of older children with WPW SVT were not different from those found in patients with other types of SVT. P waves were visible during SVT in 17 of 25 patients. The most common P wave axis was 270° to 359°. The PR interval varied widely among different patients and was similar to that found in other types of SVT.

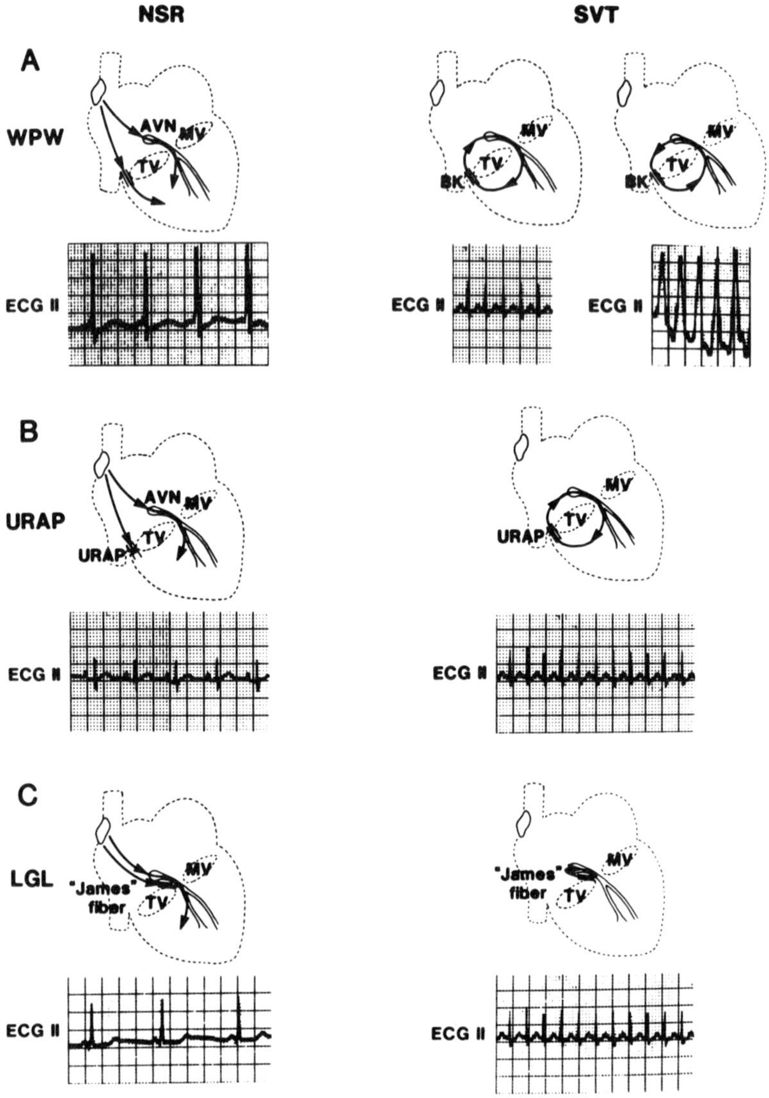

FIGURE 13–24
Re-entry circuits and ECG during sinus rhythm and SVT caused by bypass tracts. (*A*) In WPW, during sinus rhythm the QRS is a fusion resulting from activation of the ventricles through both the bundle of Kent (BK) and AV node (AVN). In SVT, in the majority of patients (left diagram), the QRS complex is narrow because the re-entry circuit is antegrade through the AV node. In approximately 5% to 10% of patients (right diagram), the QRS complex is prolonged, simulating ventricular tachycardia, because the re-entry circuit is antegrade through the Kent bundle. (*B*) With a unidirectional retrograde accessory pathway (URAP), no delta wave is visible during sinus rhythm because the impulse does not conduct antegrade through the URAP. The PR interval is normal. During SVT the only possible re-entry circuit is antegrade through the AV node. (*C*) With a James fiber in the Lown-Ganong-Levine (LGL) syndrome, during sinus rhythm the AV node is bypassed and a short PR interval is found, but the ventricles are activated normally. During SVT the re-entry circuit is usually antegrade through the AV node, and the QRS complex is normal.

In the two patients with wide QRS SVT with a morphology similar to that seen in NSR (one complete left bundle-branch block and one complete right bundle-branch block), heart rates were 210 bpm and 230 bpm, respectively. P waves were not visible in either of these patients during SVT.

Intracardiac Electrophysiology. To make the diagnosis of WPW type of SVT, a delta wave must be visible on the surface ECG either during NSR or with atrial pacing. Pacing near the atrial end of the Kent bundle will cause more preexcitation and bring out a delta wave. As in any other re-entry SVT, preexcitation can be induced and terminated with rapid atrial pacing or premature extrastimuli. Induction is related to a critical AV conduction time; if the prematurity interval is shortened, preexcitation will increase as the conduction time through the AV node is lengthened, but the conduction time through the Kent bundle remains constant. For this reason more of the ventricle will be excited by the bypass tract before the impulse reaches the ventricle through the AV node. Therefore the QRS becomes wider with a short PR interval, with increasingly premature impulses—up to a point. At a critical premature interval, the Kent bundle will become refractory, and all conduction will proceed through the AV node. At this point the PR interval will be long and the QRS complex will be narrow. Re-entry SVT usually begins at this critical interval. (This is the case for the 90% of patients with a narrow QRS during SVT. In the 10% of patients with a wide QRS, the effective refractory period of the bundle of Kent is unusually short, shorter than that of the AV node. In these patients the QRS complex continues to widen until SVT continues with a similar QRS.)

In patients with a narrow QRS during SVT, evidence of bypass tract conduction must be demonstrated both in the antegrade and retrograde directions, because the bypass tract is used antegrade in sinus rhythm and retrograde during SVT. In atrial extrastimulus testing, the AV interval is usually fixed, and in ventricular extrastimulus testing, the VA interval is usually fixed. In patients with wide QRS SVT, the bypass tract is used only in the antegrade direction. The bypass tract may also conduct in a retrograde direction, but proof of this is unnecessary, because the re-entry circuit does not require retrograde bypass conduction.

Proof that the bypass tract participates in SVT can be found in two ways. If, during SVT, a PVD is introduced when the bundle of His is refractory, and the resulting premature impulse conducts back to the atrium (resetting and therefore shortening the atrial cycle length), then retrograde conduction must have occurred through a pathway other than the His bundle–AV node, (i.e., through a bypass tract). This proves that a bypass tract is present and available for VA conduction. If the atrial activation sequence caused by conduction of the premature stimulus is identical to that found during SVT, then the bypass tract may also be involved in the tachycardia circuit.

The second way of proving the participation of a bypass tract in SVT is by observing an eccentric atrial activation sequence (beginning at a point other than the LSRA) during SVT. The earliest atrial activation marks the point of atrial insertion of the Kent bundle in patients with narrow QRS SVT. In those with wide QRS SVT, the retrograde atrial activation sequence is normal because the retrograde limb of the SVT is the His bundle and AV node. In these patients the location of the bypass tract can be found by pacing the atrium at different points and determining that point with the shortest AV interval (most preexcitation). This marks the atrial end of the bypass tract. In our patients with WPW SVT, we located the Kent bundle at the right atrial free wall in 31%, at the left ventricular free wall in 38%, and at the septum in 31%. The locations of Kent bundles for patients with WPW and URAP in our series were not significantly different. SVT occurs at a significantly younger age in patients with a left-sided Kent bundle than in those with Kent bundles found in the other two locations. Congenital cardiac defects occurred in 15% of those with left-sided pathways, in 27% of those with right-sided pathways, and in 54% of those with septal pathways. During SVT the heart rates of patients with left-sided and septal pathways were more rapid than those of patients with right-sided pathways. The rapid heart rates of those with left-sided pathways can be explained on the basis of younger age, but those with septal pathways were significantly older than those with left-sided pathways, and yet the heart rates were equally rapid. This can be explained on the electrophysiologic basis that the re-entry circuit with a septal pathway is shorter, because the impulse is not required to go through ventricular muscle to complete the circuit. P waves were not particularly helpful in distinguishing the location of the bypass tract. Most commonly in right-sided Kent bundles, the P waves were not visible. In left-sided Kent bundles, an axis of 270° to 359° was most common in children, compared to the 91°–269° axis reported in adults.[22] Septal Kent bundles produced all types of P waves.

The last characteristic of WPW SVT found during intracardiac electrophysiology studies was the response of the atrial cycle length to ipsilateral bundle-branch block. In a free wall pathway, the re-entry circuit includes the His bundle and bundle-branch system on the side of the pathway (see Fig. 13–20). Therefore if conduction delay or block occurs in that bundle-branch system, the SVT cycle length will be slower than when bundle-branch block does not occur. This change is approximately 10 ms to 20 ms in children. Therefore, while it is helpful in the cardiac catheterization laboratory, it usually cannot be observed on the routine surface ECG recorded at 25 mm/s.

Treatment. WPW SVT responds well to acute therapy (83% success rate). Success was most often attained with digoxin therapy, vagal maneuvers, or cardioversion. Digoxin alone was used most commonly as the initial chronic therapy, followed by propranolol alone and then by a combination of digoxin and propranolol. Our recommendations for chronic management of SVT caused by WPW are given in the section on management.

Patient Follow-up. SVT recurred in 80% of the patients with SVT resulting from WPW. Although this percentage is not significantly different from that found in other types of SVT, it is the lowest recurrence rate. This may be because more patients with WPW (84%) received initial chronic treatment than did patients with either SAN re-entry SVT (41%), AV node re-entry (43%), or URAP (70%). The CHMC study stated that SVT recurs more frequently in patients with WPW, and the influence of this study may have caused us to treat more patients with WPW initially and therefore actually reduce the number of recurrences.

On long-term follow-up, SVT was still present in 67% of patients. This was not different from the recurrence rates found in patients with other types of SVT. WPW remained on the surface ECG in 36 of 40 patients. Therefore, although regression of the WPW pattern has been reported in children,[22] this was an uncommon occurrence in our patients with SVT.

URAP SVT

Clinical Features. Of our 178 patients with SVT, 22 (12%) had URAP, making this the third most common type of SVT in children. The clinical features were similar to those of patients with the WPW type of SVT. In patients with unoperated CHD, URAP was slightly more common than WPW; 22% of those with URAP had unoperated CHD, compared with 18% of those with WPW.

Surface ECG During SVT. The surface ECG during SVT in patients with URAP was similar to that seen in patients with WPW. None of the patients had a wide QRS during SVT, since with a URAP, by definition, conduction does not occur in an antegrade direction through the Kent bundle. The only significant difference was in the PR/RR interval, which was significantly longer ($p > 0.01$) in URAP than in WPW. This difference is most likely a result of the location of the pathways rather than an intrinsic difference in conduction between WPW and URAP. The longest PR/RR intervals were seen in URAP and were the result of right anterior pathways, while the shortest PR/RR intervals were found in WPW and were the result of left lateral pathways. This can be explained by relatively longer intraventricular conduction in left lateral pathways than in right anterior pathways.

Treatment. Treatment results were similar to those found in the WPW type of SVT. Our recommendations for patients with URAP type of SVT are similar to those for patients with WPW, except that in URAP, digoxin should be the first drug used in all patients. These Kent bundles do not conduct in an antegrade direction and there is therefore no danger that digoxin will enhance antegrade conduction.

Patient Follow-up. SVT recurred in 17 patients with URAP type of SVT and was still present at follow-up in 70% of them. The characteristics, response to therapy, and prognosis were therefore similar in all patients with SVT caused by Kent bundles, whether the bypass tracts conducted in an antegrade direction and caused WPW on the surface ECG or conducted only in the retrograde direction, producing URAP.

LGL SVT

Clinical Features. It is uncertain if SVT truly involves an AH bypass tract. Only seven patients (4%) had SVT that might have used a "James" AV node bypass tract as part of the re-entry circuit.[23] There was no particular age at which onset was more likely to occur. All patients had otherwise normal hearts, and only one of the seven (a 3-week-old child with a heart rate of 300 bpm) had CHF. A family history of SVT was present in three of the seven patients, making this one of the types of SVT that most often had a positive family history.

Surface ECG During SVT. The surface ECG during tachycardia was available in only two patients. In one the P wave was not visible, and in the other the P wave axis was 270° to 359°. A P wave axis other than 270° to 359° is incompatible with a diagnosis of SVT caused by LGL.

Intracardiac Electrophysiology. Ventricular preexcitation is evident with a short AV interval in sinus rhythm. The AH interval is short, but HV is normal, indicating bypass of the normal AV nodal delay with normal conduction through the His bundle to the ventricular muscle. Because the ventricles are activated normally, a delta wave is not observed. This is a re-entry SVT and can be both induced and terminated by rapid atrial pacing or premature extrastimuli. As in WPW SVT, conduction of this form of SVT is related to a critical AV or VA delay. During atrial extrastimuli, the AH interval remains short and fixed until the James fiber becomes refractory. Then the AH interval suddenly prolongs, as all AV conduction occurs through the AV node. This cycle length is the effective refractory period of the James fiber and is generally the point at which SVT is induced. Ventricular extrastimuli also reveal a short, fixed VA interval in these patients.

The retrograde activation sequence is normal in patients with the LGL type of SVT. Therefore the major problems in differential diagnosis are a septal URAP and AV node re-entry SVT. The electrophysiologic findings in septal URAP may be identical to those in LGL SVT except for the following:

1. The AH interval during NSR is short in LGL and may be either normal or short in URAP. Some patients with URAP may have rapid antegrade AV node conduction.
2. AV block may occur during SVT caused by LGL, with block occurring below the His bundle. SVT will continue because the distal bundle of His is not part of the re-entry circuit; however, in septal URAP, block below the His will terminate the SVT.
3. A PVC delivered during SVT when the His bundle is refractory will not change the atrial cycle length in LGL but may affect SVT caused by a URAP. In AV node re-entry SVT, the AH interval is not short and prolongs during atrial extrastimulus testing.

Treatment. Digoxin alone was not an effective treatment of SVT caused by LGL. Digoxin was tried only once as acute therapy and failed. None of our patients received digoxin alone for chronic therapy; all who were treated have required the addition of quinidine or propranolol.

We recommend acute treatment with cardioversion, vagal maneuvers, or phenylephrine. Digoxin may be given initially, but propranolol or quinidine should be added if a short trial of digoxin proves ineffective. Verapamil was used successfully in termination of acute episode.

Patient Follow-up. SVT recurred in all seven patients. In one patient SVT had stopped and drugs had been withdrawn; in the other six patients, SVT continued despite drug therapy. SVT resulting from LGL was therefore the least responsive type of SVT to drugs.

PJRT SVT

Permanent junctional reciprocating tachycardia (PJRT) is the most common form of incessant SVT in children. This type of tachycardia has also been called the atypical form of AV node re-entrant tachycardia. The current consensus is that the mechanism involves an AV re-entrant circuit in which the retrograde limb is an extranodal structure with decremental retrograde properties. PJRT was first described by Critelli et al in 1978.[24]

Clinical Features. Twenty-three patients seen at TCH met the ECG criteria of PJRT. The age at diagnosis ranged from in utero to 10 years, with a mean of 3.8 years. Symptoms and signs were varied. Ten of 23 patients had presyncopal episodes, and 3 of 23 described palpitations. CHF was present in 13 of 23. Cardiomegaly was present on the initial radiograph in 13 of 23 patients, and in 20 patients with available M-mode echocardiography, 10 had a decreased shortening fraction of 28%.

Surface ECG During SVT. The electrocardiographic pattern of PJRT consists of: (1) an RP interval longer than the PR interval, with the PR interval being normal or short; (2) negative P waves in leads II, III, and aVF; and (3) the absence of "warm-up" at SVT onset.

The SVT rate determined on the initial ECG ranged from 125 bpm to 230 bpm, with a mean of 167 bpm. The frequency of SVT (defined as the percentage of the day in which SVT was present) ranged from 10% to 75% in five patients and was greater than 75% in 18 patients.

Intracardiac Electrophysiology. Certain electrophysiologic characteristics support the concept of AV re-entry through an anatomically distinct AV pathway and the concept that this pathway is the retrograde limb of the tachycardia loop. These characteristics include (1) a point of earliest retrograde atrial activation during SVT at a location other than the LSRA (usually just inside the MOCS), (2) interruption of SVT by premature atrial and ventricular stimuli, and (3) evidence of decremental retrograde accessory pathway conduction. The PJRT is more specifically defined when the earliest point of activation retrograde endocardial-atrial activation is close to or within the mouth of the coronary sinus. This activation sequence, when associated with low decremental retrograde pathway conduction properties, is typical for PJRT (Fig. 13–25).

Treatment. All patients initially received medical treatment. A wide range of medications was given; all patients received digoxin

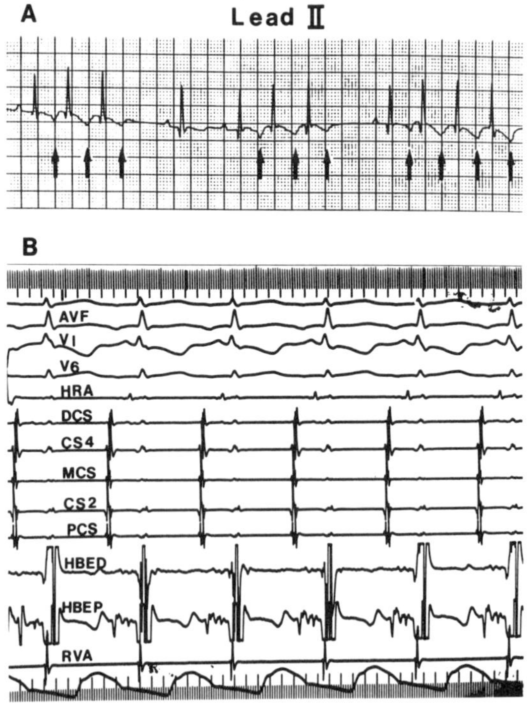

FIGURE 13–25
(*A*) Typical ECG example of PJRT. Lead II rhythm strip demonstrates periods of sinus rhythm and PJRT, and arrows indicate the typical P waves of PJRT. (*B*) Electrophysiologic demonstration of PJRT, evident in the normal PR interval and the long RP interval. Earliest site of retrograde activation during supraventricular tachycardia is the proximal coronary sinus (PCS).

initially, with improvement of congestive heart failure but no suppression of SVT. A β-blocker was added to the digoxin, with no resulting response. Verapamil was also added in 13 patients, with complete suppression of SVT reported in only one. Six of the 17 patients were improved but continued to have recurrent episodes of SVT. Procainamide, quinidine, phenytoin, and disopyramide were administered in thirteen patients, with no improvement of SVT frequency. Encainide was given to nine patients; PJRT was completely controlled in five, partially controlled in two, and had no effect in two.

Surgical procedures were performed in eight patients; two had dissection of the posterior septum and developed complete atrioventricular block. Most recently, six patients had cryoablation of the posterior septum, now have normal AV conduction, and are cured of PJRT.

We recommend surgical treatment of PJRT in all patients except the smallest infants who could develop AV block with cryoablation; for these we recommend encainide or flecainide therapy.

Mahaim SVT

Mahaim SVT was found in three of the 178 patients, making it the least common type of SVT in children.

Surface ECG During SVT. In sinus rhythm, patients with Mahaim fibers have a normal PR interval with a delta wave, almost always with a type B (left bundle-branch block) pattern. During SVT, a prolonged QRS is usually present, giving a "wide QRS" SVT. Frequently there is AV dissociation.

Treatment. Drug therapy for patients with Mahaim SVT is conceptually similar to that for patients with URAP type of SVT.

ECTOPIC FOCUS SVT

Twenty-two percent of our patients (39 of 178) had SVT resulting from an ectopic focus. Abnormal automaticity can develop in a cell in any part of the heart. If this automatic ectopic focus is in the atria, the resultant SVT is called atrial ectopic focus SVT; if the automatic focus is in the area of the AV node–His bundle, it is called junctional ectopic focus SVT. Certain electrophysiologic criteria must be met for a diagnosis of automatic ectopic focus. Atrial ectopic foci can be distinguished from junctional ectopic foci by the atrial activation sequence and the AH interval. In atrial ectopic tachycardia (AET), atrial activation may begin at any point, but in junctional ectopic tachycardia (JET) with 1:1 retrograde activation of the atria, atrial activation is through the AV node and begins with the LSRA. JET and His bundle re-entry are the only two types of SVT in children in which AV dissociation has been found. In patients with AV dissociation, the atria are activated at the normal sinus rate and the atrial activation is from the sinus node. In AET, the AH interval is normal or long; in JET or His bundle re-entry with 1:1 retrograde atrial activation, either the AH interval is short or the atrial depolarization begins just following the His bundle electrogram.

Atrial Ectopic Focus

Clinical Features. Atrial ectopic focus SVT occurred in 32 of 178 (18%) of patients. The age at onset was the second youngest among all the types, with no patient experiencing onset after 6 years of age. A family history of SVT was found in 12 of 32 patients in whom a family history was available, making this and JET the most common forms of SVT to have a positive family history. A major clinical difference between ectopic SVT and re-entry SVT is the number of hours or days a patient spends actually having tachycardia. In re-entry SVT, a patient with frequent episodes may have three or four episodes per week, each lasting 30 to 60 minutes. In a patient with an ectopic focus, the SVT is generally always present. In most patients with ectopic focus tachycardia, conventional drugs, at best, can only slow the rate. Therefore it is not surprising that 25 of 32 patients (82%) with AET had CHF; 16 of the 32 had a cardiomyopathy evidenced by chronic cardiomegaly and an abnormal echocardiographic left ventricular shortening fraction. It is not clear whether the cardiomyopathy is caused by the SVT. After elimination of SVT by surgery, all patients have had normalization of their ventricular function.

Surface ECG During SVT. AET is recognized on ECG by P waves at an abnormally rapid rate (with any axis, although not usually originating from the low right atrium), with progressive shortening in the PP interval at the onset of SVT ("warm-up"); it may occur with AV block. Atrial rate is between 90 bpm and 220 bpm (mean, 143 bpm). The P axis originates from the HRA in 77%, the LA in 20%, and the LRA in 3% of patients. Seventy-five percent of patients had a long PR interval, and 28% had blocked P waves (Fig. 13–26).

Intracardiac Electrophysiology. An important criterion for an automatic ectopic focus is that it cannot be induced or terminated by rapid atrial pacing or premature extrastimuli. If atrial extrastimuli are introduced into the SVT, the most common type of response to be found is the "reset" phenomenon, where at relatively short prematurity intervals a less-than-compensatory pause occurs in the return cycle. Entrance block into the focus may occur, in which case a fully compensatory pause will be observed at all cycle lengths. Rapid atrial pacing at a rate faster than SVT will capture the atrium, but on termination of pacing the tachycardia immediately resumes without an intervening sinus beat (Fig. 13–27).

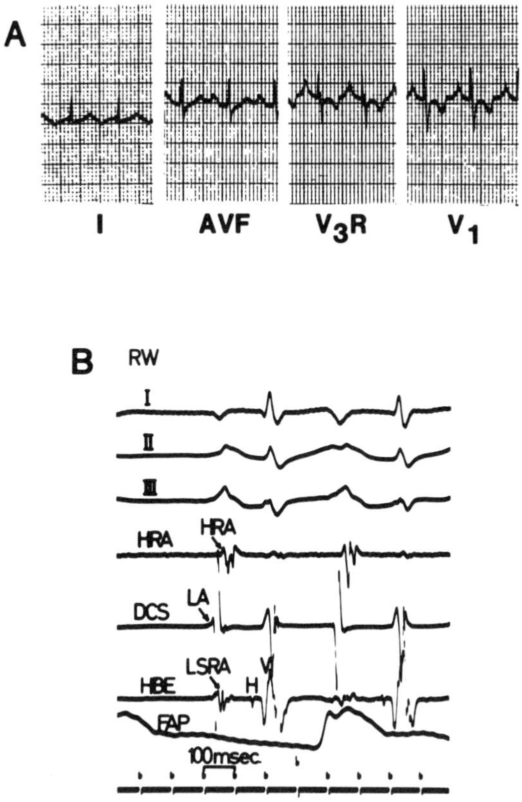

FIGURE 13–26
(*A*) Surface ECG of left atrial ectopic focus tachycardia with a typical "dome and dart" P wave in V_{3R} and V_1. Note negative P wave in lead I. (*B*) Intracardiac recordings from the same patient with a left atrial ectopic focus SVT. Note that the left atrium is activated first.

The atrial activation sequence may begin from any point in either atrium. If the atrial activation sequence and P wave shape are identical to those found in sinus rhythm, then it may be difficult to distinguish an automatic ectopic focus from sinus tachycardia. It is also possible that sinus rhythm may not even be observed during an electrophysiologic study; this makes the distinction even more difficult. If there is no explanation for sinus tachycardia (e.g., fever, sepsis, dehydration), if the atrial rate is 230 bpm or greater, or if SVT is observed to start and stop suddenly without provocation, then the diagnosis is probably not sinus tachycardia.

If the onset of SVT is observed, the atrial activation sequence and P wave of the first beat are identical to the subsequent beats of SVT in AET. This may be true of other types of re-entry SVT; however, if the first and subsequent beats are different, the diagnosis is not AET. If the cycle lengths of the first four or five beats progressively shorten (by

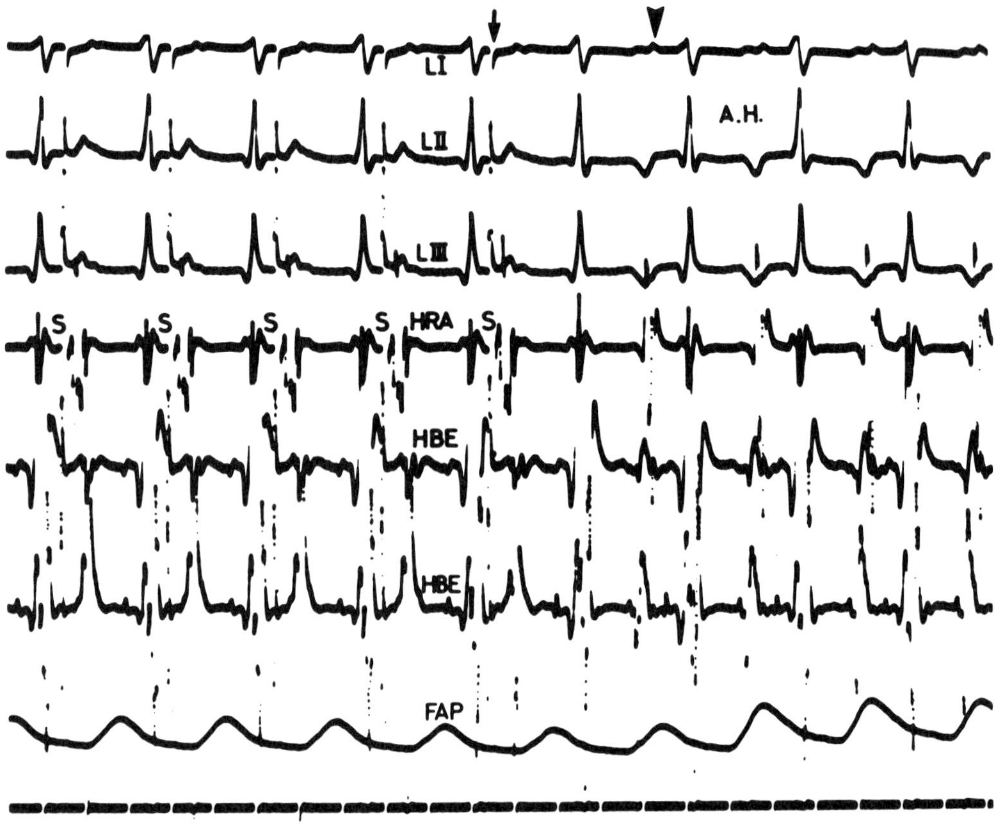

FIGURE 13–27
Attempt at overdrive pacing in a patient with a low right atrial ectopic focus SVT. The tracing begins with overdrive pacing of the high right atrium (P waves positive in leads II and III). When pacing is terminated (small arrow), the tachycardia resumes immediately with low atrial ectopic focus evidenced by negative P waves in leads II and III (arrowhead).

10 ms to 20 ms each beat), a diagnosis of an ectopic focus is likely. This warm-up behavior is distinct from the "oscillatory" behavior of most types of re-entry SVT.

As in the other types of SVT in which the AV node is not involved in sustaining SVT, AV block can occur in the presence of SVT.

The response of AET to drugs administered during the electrophysiologic studies is different from that of re-entry SVT. If a drug is given to a patient with AET, the rate of the tachycardia sometimes will slow, perhaps by as much as 40% to 50%, with continuing SVT. AET rarely terminates with acute drug administration. Re-entry SVT is generally not sustained at a wide range of rates. In re-entry SVT the circuit is critically balanced; if a drug has any effect on the re-entry circuit, the SVT will generally stop rather than slow.

Treatment. AET is difficult to treat, both acutely and chronically, because of its resistance to conventional drug therapy. Digoxin, verapamil, quinidine, procainamide, and amiodarone were used with only minimal success. Propranolol suppressed AET in three patients. Ethmozine has been quite successful in seven of eight patients with AET, and flecainide has been successful in three of six patients. Surgical ablation was performed in 25 patients. Sixteen were found to have a single focus, and surgery stopped the tachycardia in all of them. In nine patients, after surgical removal of the first focus, multiple foci became apparent, and surgery was effective in only four of the nine. Patients with a single focus had slower atrial rates than did those with multiple foci; 100% had rates of 70/min at night, compared with only 11% of those with multiple foci ($p < 0.05$).

Junctional Ectopic Focus

Clinical Features. SVT resulting from an ectopic focus in the AV node–His bundle region is one of the rarest types of SVT in children (7 of 178 patients). The average age at which JET began was the youngest among all of the groups. Five of the seven patients had CHF, probably because of their young age, and three of the seven patients in whom a family history was available had a sibling with SVT.

Surface ECG During SVT. The most distinctive characteristic of JET is AV dissociation, with normal sinus P waves continuing through the tracing unrelated to the more rapid QRS complexes (Fig. 13–28).[25] AV dissociation was present in all patients with catheterization-proven JET. In one patient with JET, P waves (axis 300°) immediately followed each QRS complex, indicating 1:1 retrograde capture of the atria. The QRS rates varied from 128 bpm to 270 bpm. His bundle re-entry can also have AV dissociation on the surface ECG; however, JET warms up at initiation and His bundle re-entry oscillates.

Intracardiac Electrophysiology. Findings in JET are similar to those in AET. Criteria for an ectopic focus must be met. During SVT in six of seven cases, the atrial depolarizations were slower than (and unrelated to) the ventricular depolarization (AV dissociation). In these cases the atrial depolarization had an activation sequence that began in the high right atrium and represented sinus impulses. Each ventricular depolarization was preceded by a His bundle electrogram with a normal HV interval (Fig. 13–29). In the seventh case, atrial activation beginning in the LSRA immediately followed each ventricular depolarization (PR/RR = 0.78). In this case, the diagnosis had to be distinguished from AET originating in the LSRA. AET was less likely, because the atrial depolarization in AET should precede the His electrogram and ventricular depolarization with a PR/RR interval less than 0.60.

Rapid pacing of the atrium or ventricles in each of these cases captured the ventricles, but as soon as the pacing was stopped or the rate was decreased to below that of the SVT, the SVT resumed.

Treatment. Conventional acute drug therapy was unsuccessful in all cases. We successfully treated one patient with acute paired pacing, and hemodynamics were stabilized. In terms of chronic therapy, one patient had a QRS rate of 128 and received no therapy, two patients received digoxin and propranolol, and one patient received digoxin and chlorpromazine. Two patients received ethmozine without success. We recommend that chronic therapy be instituted as early as possible with combination digoxin and propranolol. If this combination is unsuccessful, then therapy with procainamide, flecainide, or amiodarone may be tried; these have been successful in selected patients. In severely symptomatic patients, surgical ablation of the bundle of His may be undertaken.

Patient Follow-up. JET did not stop acutely, either spontaneously or with treatment, in any patient. One patient died from low cardiac output associated with continuing junctional tachycardia and a large ventricular septal defect with coarctation of the aorta. Three are taking amiodarone; JET continues, but the QRS rates are 130 bpm to 150 bpm.

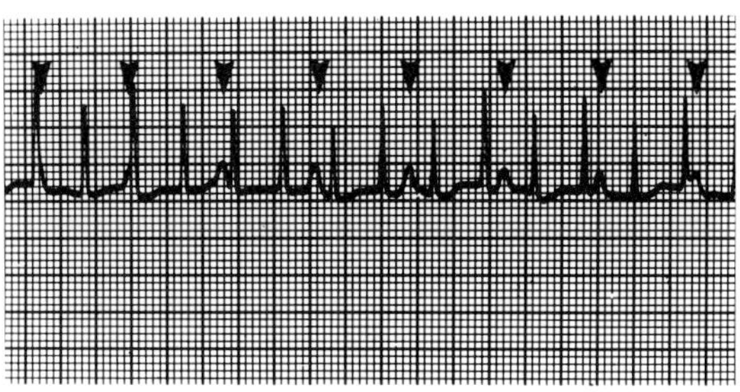

Lead II

FIGURE 13–28
Surface ECG of junctional ectopic focus SVT. AV dissociation is evident, with P waves marked by arrows. The QRS complexes are normal.

Noninvasive Estimation of SVT Type

Knowledge of the type of SVT that is present in an individual patient is helpful in planning therapy and assigning prognosis; however, intracardiac electrophysiologic techniques are not available or absolutely necessary in all patients. We have developed a method for predicting the type of SVT based on noninvasive assessment using the ECG (P waves, PR/RR ratio, QRS rate, presence of AV block), the age at which SVT began, and the presence and type of predisposing factors (Table 13–19).

The most common types of SVT are WPW and AV node re-entry, followed by URAP, AET, and PJRT. Therefore if nothing is known about the patient, a guess of WPW,

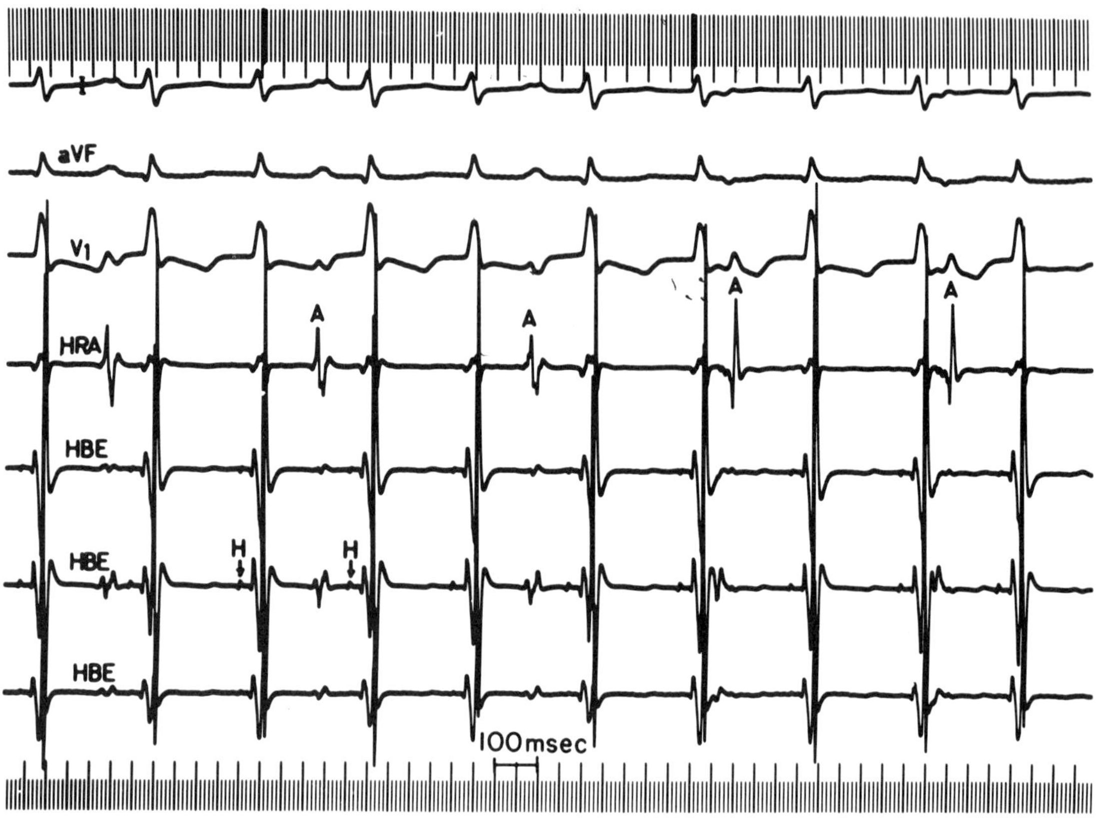

FIGURE 13–29
Intracardiac recordings taken from a patient with junctional ectopic focus SVT. The atrial depolarization in the HRA lead (A) are unrelated to the QRS complexes. The HV interval (H, in HBE lead) is normal at 35 ms.

AET, AV node re-entry, or URAP would be correct half of the time. However, with information about the patient, the estimation accuracy is improved. The analysis begins with the ECG.

P Wave Not Visible. The most commonly found type of SVT without a P wave visible during tachycardia is AV node re-entry, although WPW and URAP may not have a clearly visible P wave. The clinical distinction among these types is difficult, and the age at presentation is noncontributory. In this group the most rapid QRS rates are found in WPW and the slowest in AV node re-entry, with URAP in between. If the patient has an otherwise normal heart, all are equally likely. If the patient has unoperated congenital heart disease, URAP and WPW are likely, but AV node re-entry is unlikely. If SVT begins after an operation, the most likely diagnosis is AV node re-entry.

P Wave Visible with Normal Axis (0° to 90°) and 1:1 AV Conduction. The most commonly found SVT with this morphology is AET, followed by SAN re-entry and URAP. If the QRS rate is 270 bpm or greater, the most likely diagnosis is WPW or URAP. If PR/RR is less than 0.50, URAP and SAN re-entry are unlikely, and the best possibility is AET or WPW. If PR/RR is 0.75 or more, then AET, SAN re-entry, and WPW are unlikely, and URAP is the most probable diagnosis. If AV block is present during SVT, either AET or SAN re-entry is the best choice. If the age at onset is less than 3 months, SAN re-entry is unlikely, and if the age is greater than 6 years, AET is unlikely. If the patient has a normal heart or unoperated CHD, then the most likely diagnosis is URAP or WPW; if SVT began after surgery for congenital heart disease, WPW or SAN re-entry is most likely. If a cardiomyopathy is present, the most likely diagnosis is AET.

P Wave Visible with Normal Axis and AV Dissociation. The only type of SVT with this morphology that we have found in children is JET.

P Wave Visible with Low Right Atrial Axis (270° to 359°). The most common type of

TABLE 13–19
NONINVASIVE ESTIMATION OF SVT TYPE*,†

	P WAVES					PR/RR			QRS RATE (bpm)			AGE AT ONSET			FACTORS					
	Not Vis	*NL Axis 1:1*	*NL Axis AV Dis*	*INV*	LA	*<0.50*	*0.51–0.79*	*>0.80*	*<170*	*170–299*	*>300*	*<3M*	*3 Mo–6 Yrs*	*>6 Yrs*	*NL Heart*	*Preop CHD*	*Postop CHD*	*CM*	*FH*	*AV Block*
SAN re-entry	–	+	–	–	–	–		–	–	+	–	–						–		+
AM re-entry	–		–	–			–	–	–		–	–				–	–			+
AVN re-entry	+	–	–	–	–			+	+				+	+	+	–	+	–	–	–
WPW	±	+	–	+	+		+	–	–		+	+		+	+	+			+	–
URAP	±	+	–	+	+	–	+	+	–	+		+		+	+	+	–	–	+	–
LGL		–	–	+	–	–		–			–					–	–	–		–
AET	–	+	–	–	+		+	–			–			–				+		+
JET	–	–	–	–	–	–	–				–			–	–	+	–	–	+	–
PJRT	–	–	–	+		+			+				+		–			+	–	–

*See Table 13–16 for abbreviations of types of SVT.
†+ = helpful in including diagnosis; – = helpful in ruling out diagnosis; ± = variable help.
Abbreviations: AV Dis = atrioventricular dissociation; CHD = congenital heart disease; CM = cardiomegaly; FH = family history; INV = inverted in II, III, aVF; LA = left atrium; NL = normal; Vis = visible.

SVT with this morphology is PJRT, followed by WPW and (only occasionally) AET. If the QRS rate is less than 170 bpm, WPW is unlikely; if the rate is 300 bpm or more, AET is unlikely. If PR/RR is 0.50 or less, the most likely diagnosis is PJRT; if PR/RR is 0.51–0.75, it is most likely AET; if PR/RR is 0.75 or greater, it is most likely WPW. If SVT continues during AV block, the diagnosis is AET. If the age at onset is more than 6 years or if the patient has an otherwise normal heart, AET is unlikely. If the patient has unoperated congenital heart disease, WPW is most likely. If a cardiomyopathy and CHF are present, AET or PJRT are more common.

P Wave Visible with Left Atrial Axis (91° to 269°). The most common SVT with this morphology is AET, followed by WPW and URAP. If the QRS rate is less than 170 bpm, WPW and URAP are unlikely. If the QRS rate is 300 bpm or more, AET is unlikely. If PR/RR is 0.50 or less, URAP is unlikely and AET is likely; if PR/RR is 0.75 or more, the SVT is unlikely to be WPW or AET. If AV block occurs during SVT, the diagnosis is not WPW or URAP. If the age at onset is more than 6 years, AET is unlikely. If the heart is otherwise normal, AET is unlikely, but if the patient has a cardiomyopathy, AET is most likely. If the patient has had an operation for CHD, WPW is the most likely. If the P wave is positive in leads II, III, and aVF (and negative in lead I), left AET is most likely.

References

1. Keith JD, Rowe RD, Vlad P: Heart Disease in Infancy and Childhood. New York, Macmillan, 1967, p 1056.
2. Garson A Jr, Gillette PC, McNamara DG: Supraventricular tachycardia in children: Clinical features, response to treatment, and long-term follow-up in 217 patients. J Pediatr 98(6):875–882, 1981.
3. Nadas AS, Daeschner CW, Roth A, et al: Paroxysmal tachycardia in infants and children. Pediatrics 9:167–181, 1952.
4. Gillette PC, Freed D, McNamara DG: A proposed autosomal dominant method of inheritance in the Wolff-Parkinson-White syndrome and supraventricular tachycardia. J Pediatr 93:257–258, 1978.
5. Fisher DJ, Gross DM, Garson, A Jr: Rapid sinus tachycardia: Differentiation from supraventricular tachycardia. Am J Dis Child 137:164–169, 1983.
6. Bisset GS, Gaum WE, Kaplan S: The ice bag: A new technique for interruption of supraventricular tachycardia. J Pediatr 97:593–595, 1980.
7. Benson DW Jr, Dunnigan A, Benditt DG, et al: Transesophageal study of infant supraventricular tachycardia: Electrophysiologic characteristics. Am J Cardiol 52(8):1002–1006, 1983.
8. Abinader E, Borochowitz Z, Berger A: A hemodynamic complication of verapamil therapy in a neonate. Helv Paediatr Acta 36(5):451–455, 1981.
9. Waldo AL, Krongrad E, Kupersmith J, et al: Ventricular paired pacing to control rapid ventricular heart rate following open heart surgery. Circulation 53:176–180, 1976.
10. Deal BJ, Keane JF, Gillette PC, et al: WPW syndrome with supraventricular tachycardia during infancy: Management and follow-up. J Am Coll Cardiol 5:130–135, 1985.
11. Ludomirsky A, Klein HO, Teitelman U, et al: Prolongation of the QT interval and polymorphous ventricular tachycardia associated with organophosphorus poisoning. Am J Cardiol 49:1654–1658, 1982.
12. Porter CJ, Garson A Jr, Gillette PC: Verapamil: An effective calcium blocking agent for pediatric patients. Pediatrics 71:748–754, 1983.
13. Strasburger JF, Moak JP, Smith RT, et al: Encainide for refractory supraventricular tachycardia in children. Am J Cardiol 58:49C–54C, 1986.
14. Perry JC, McQuinn R, Smith RT, et al: Flecainide acetate for resistant arrhythmias in the young: Efficacy and pharmacokinetics. J Am Coll Cardiol (in press).
15. Ward DE, Jones S, Shinebourne EA: Use of flecainide acetate for refractory tachycardias in children with the Wolff-Parkinson-White syndrome. Am J Cardiol 57:787–790, 1986.
16. Ruggio JM, Somberg JC: New therapy focus: Ethmozine. Cardiovasc Rev Rep 5:738–741, 1984.
17. Evans VL, Garson A Jr: Ethmozine: A promising drug for "automatic" atrial ectopic tachycardia. Am J Cardiol 60:83–86, 1987.
18. Wellens HJJ, Durrer D: The role of an accessory atrioventricular pathway in reciprocal tachycardia: observation in patients with and without the Wolff-Parkinson-White syndrome. Circulation 52:58–72, 1975.
19. Wu D, Denes P, Amat-y-Leon F, et al: Clinical, electrocardiographic and electrophysiologic observations in patients with paroxysmal supraventricular tachycardia. Am J Cardiol 41:1045–1051, 1978.
20. Wolff GS, Sung RJ, Pickoff A, et al: The fast-slow form of atrioventricular nodal reentrant tachycardia in children. Am J Cardiol 43:1181–1188, 1979.
21. Epstein ML, Stone FM, Benditt DG: Incessant atrial tachycardia in childhood: Association with rate-dependent conduction in an accessory atrioventricular pathway. Am J Cardiol 44:498–504, 1979.
22. Benditt DG, Pritchett ELC, Smith WM, et al: Ventriculo-atrial intervals: Diagnostic tools in patients with reciprocating tachycardia. Circulation 57/58:II–10, 1978. Abstract.
23. Wolff GS, Han J, Curran J: Wolff-Parkinson-White syndrome in the neonate. Am J Cardiol 45:559–563, 1978.
24. Critelli G, Gallagher JJ, Monda V, et al: Anatomic and electrophysiologic substrate of the permanent form of junctional reciprocating tachycardia. J Am Coll Cardiol 4(3):601–610, 1984.
25. Garson A Jr, Gillette PC: Junctional ectopic tachycardia in children: Electrocardiography, electrophysiology and pharmacologic response. Am J Cardiol 44:298–302, 1979.

CHAPTER 14

VENTRICULAR ARRHYTHMIAS

Arthur Garson, Jr.

Most of the information concerning ventricular arrhythmias in the young has been learned in the past 10 years, and much of it in the past 5 years. Ventricular arrhythmias, defined as those rhythm disturbances that originate distal to the bifurcation of the bundle of His, can be either completely benign or lethal, depending on the type of arrhythmia and the clinical situation. Included in this chapter are premature ventricular contractions (PVCs), ventricular tachycardia, and ventricular fibrillation. Despite the fact that Schamroth has written that "the term 'premature ventricular contraction' is nonspecific, vague, inadequate and undesirable,"[1] this is the term with the most familiarity and will be used here. Since the clinical situations and treatment are similar for both PVCs and ventricular tachycardia, these two entities will be discussed together, followed by a discussion of ventricular fibrillation. We have specifically excluded ventricular escape rhythms that arise normally in association with atrioventricular block. Accelerated ventricular rhythm will be included in the discussion of ventricular tachycardia.

PREMATURE VENTRICULAR CONTRACTIONS

ECG Characteristics

A premature ventricular contraction may be recognized electrocardiographically by the following five criteria:

1. The QRS complex is premature. It is difficult to define "premature," since this term refers to the underlying rhythm; this is discussed in detail elsewhere.[2] For this discussion, premature is defined as occurring before the next expected QRS in a regular rhythm (Fig. 14–1).
2. The morphology of the QRS complex is virtually always different from that of the regular QRS. It is important to obtain simultaneous three-channel ECG recordings from patients in whom PVCs are suspected. It is possible for a PVC to have a morphology similar to the regular QRS in one lead, but have an entirely different morphology in other simultaneous leads. PVCs in children are not always "wide," but have a different QRS morphology (Fig. 14–2).
3. The QRS complex usually, but not always, has a prolonged duration (>0.08 s in an infant or >0.09 s in a child older than 3 years) (Fig. 14–3).
4. There are usually ST segment and T wave abnormalities after the QRS complex, with the direction of the T wave usually opposite to that of the QRS complex.
5. There is no premature atrial depolarization (P wave or flutter wave) preceding the premature QRS complex.

PVCs may show fusion, thus confirming their ventricular origin. A fusion complex is one in which the QRS morphology is intermediate between two distinct QRS morphologies. Therefore, in any case of fusion, it is important to identify the two "pure" QRS morphologies and indicate that there is a fusion between these two complexes (Fig. 14–4). In order for fusion to occur between two different types of QRS complex, the ventricles must be activated simultaneously from two directions. In sinus rhythm, a fusion occurs between the normal QRS and a prolonged duration QRS; the complexes with the prolonged duration must have come from the ventricle in order to collide with the normal QRS (which is being activated by the bundle of His) and produce an intermediate fusion QRS. It is also possible to see how fusion can occur between two types of

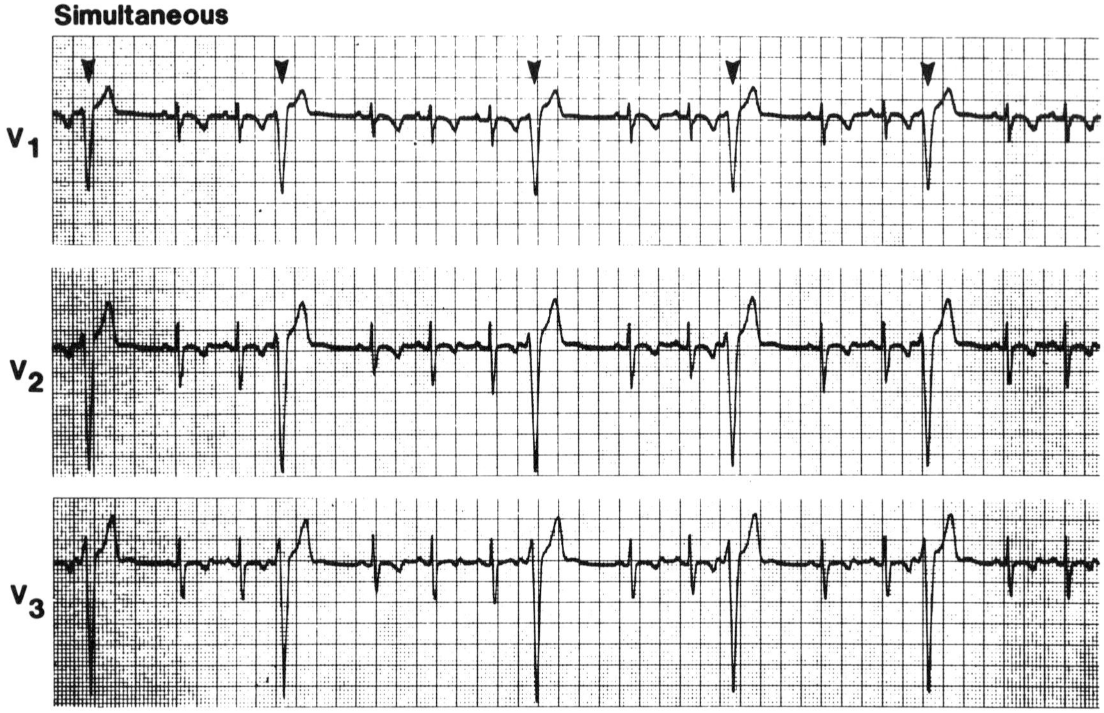

FIGURE 14–1
Premature ventricular contractions (*arrows*). Each ventricular beat occurs 0.22 s before the next expected QRS in sinus rhythm. Simultaneous leads V_1, V_2, V_3; paper speed 25 mm/s; calibration, 1 mV/10 mm. *Note:* all surface electrocardiograms in this chapter are the same paper speed and calibration. Leads are indicated on each figure.

PVC, or between sinus rhythm with normal conduction and sinus rhythm with conduction through a bundle of Kent in the Wolff-Parkinson-White syndrome.

There are three common arrhythmias in the differential diagnosis of PVCs: premature atrial contractions with aberrant ventricular conduction, premature junctional contractions with aberration, and intermittent antegrade conduction through a Kent bundle.

Premature Atrial Contractions (PACs) With Aberrant Ventricular Conduction. In children, about half of PACs are conducted with aberration. Therefore, it is difficult to rely on the QRS duration or morphology to distinguish PACs from PVCs. All PACs are preceded by a premature P wave. The axis or morphology of the P wave may be different from those of the sinus P wave (Fig. 14–5). The T wave preceding the beat in question must be scanned for possible differences from other T waves that might indicate the presence of a superimposed P wave (Fig. 14–6). If there is no preceding premature P wave and the QRS morphology of the premature beat is different from the regular QRS, the diagnosis is premature ventricular contraction.

The morphology of the QRS complex has been helpful in identifying aberrant conduction in adults. However, in children, the refractory periods of the right and left bundle branches are so similar that a PAC with aberration may have any morphology. PVCs in children may also have any morphology, so differentiation on this basis is impossible.[3]

The effect on sinus rhythm has been used to distinguish PAC with aberrancy from PVC. PVCs were generally thought to produce "a fully compensatory pause" (e.g., the sum of the RR interval before the beat, plus the RR interval after the beat, is equal to the sum of two basic RR intervals). PACs were generally thought to produce less than a fully compensatory pause. However, we know that a PAC may cause a fully compensatory pause, and PVCs may cause less than a fully compensatory pause (Fig. 14–7). The situation is analogous to that seen with premature atrial stimulation delivered into sinus rhythm or supraventricular tachycardia (see chapter 13). If a PVC conducts retrogradely to the atrium, depolarizing and resetting the sinus

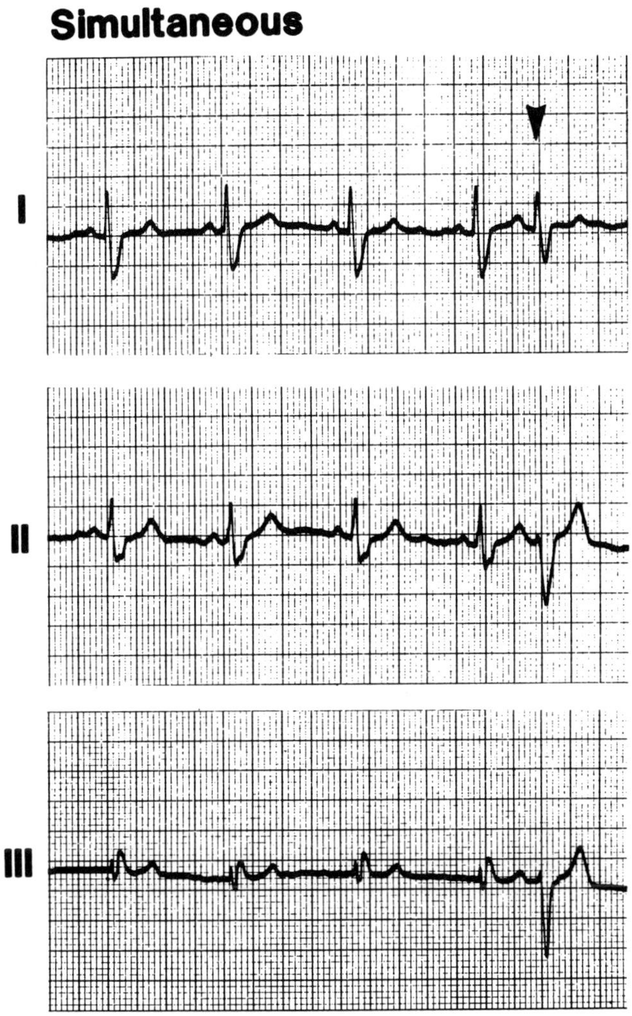

FIGURE 14–2
QRS morphology of premature beat (*arrow*) in lead I is almost identical to the sinus beats. In leads II and III, the marked difference is apparent.

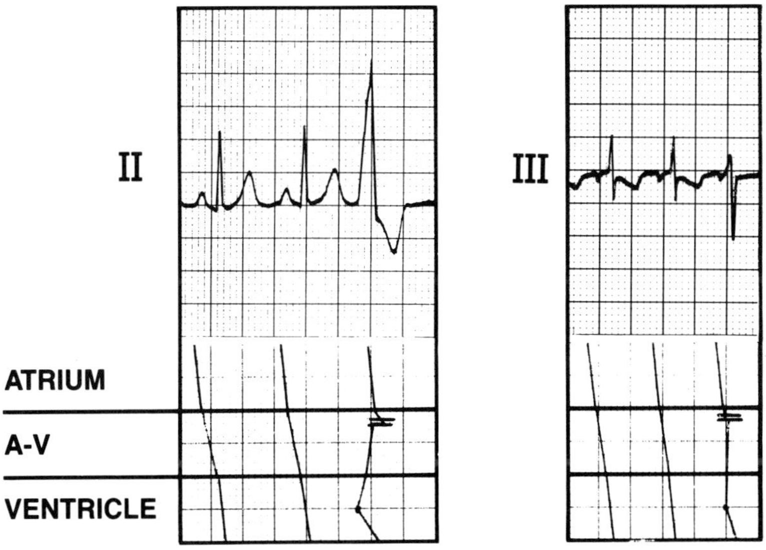

FIGURE 14–3
On the left, the third beat is a premature ventricular contraction. The QRS duration is 0.11 s, which is abnormal for a 2-year-old. In the tracing on the right, the third beat is a premature ventricular contraction. The QRS duration of the premature ventricular contraction is 0.50 s, not abnormally prolonged for this newborn infant. However, note the difference in morphology from the other two sinus beats.

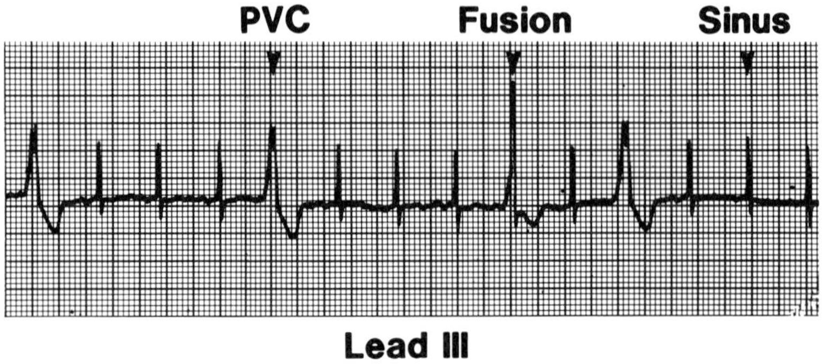

FIGURE 14–4
Fusion complex is marked. The morphology is intermediate between the sinus QRS and the QRS of the PVC.

node, there will be less than a fully compensatory pause. If a PAC occurs late enough in atrial diastole that the sinus node is already depolarized, then the PAC will not reset the sinus node and a fully compensatory pause will result.

Both PACs with aberrancy and PVCs may be interpolated. This means that the basic rhythm is not disturbed, and the premature impulse falls between two regular QRS complexes. In this situation, the sinus node does not reset, and conduction of the next sinus impulse is not blocked (Fig. 14–8).

A special situation exists when a supraventricular rhythm is not sinus, but instead is atrial flutter or atrial fibrillation. In this case, it is possible either to have aberrant conduction of the supraventricular rhythm or to have PVCs, and a correct diagnosis is important. Schamroth[1] has listed four differentiating points applicable to children. Favoring aberrant conduction are:

1. A relatively fast mean ventricular rate. PVCs tend to occur more often with slower ventricular rates.
2. QRS variability. The rapid atrial impulses occur during all stages of the cardiac cycle and therefore encounter different phases of recovery in the conduction system. This results in varying degrees of aberration. PVCs, on the other hand, usually have one or two fixed morphology patterns.
3. Variation of the coupling interval. PVCs usually have fixed coupling.
4. No attempt at a compensatory pause. PVCs may be followed by a compensatory pause.

In practice, it may be quite difficult to distinguish between PVCs and aberrant conduction of atrial flutter or atrial fibrillation on the surface ECG (Fig. 14–9). With intracardiac electrophysiologic study, differentiation is less difficult: aberrantly conducted beats are preceded by a His electrogram with a normal or prolonged HV interval, and PVCs are either preceded by a His bundle electrogram with a short HV interval or, more commonly, not preceded by a His bundle electrogram at all. We have resorted to such study in two patients and found that each patient had both aberrantly conducted beats and PVCs.

Premature Junctional Contractions With Aberration. If a QRS complex with a different morphology from the regular QRS is premature and has no preceding premature P wave, it could be either a premature junctional contraction with aberrancy or a PVC. This distinction is only possible in children with the use of intracardiac recordings: in a premature junctional contraction, the HV interval is normal or prolonged; in a PVC, either the HV interval is short or, more commonly, there is no His bundle electrogram preceding the ventricular electrogram. If only a surface ECG is available, we have chosen to identify all such complexes as PVCs. There is only one possible exception: the patient who clearly has premature junctional contractions (i.e., premature beats not preceded by a premature P wave with a normal QRS complex). If, on the same electrocardiogram, this patient has premature junctional contractions and other beats with a wide QRS complex that occur at a shorter coupling interval (and therefore could be premature junctional beats with aberration), it is permissible to interpret the wide beats as "either premature junctional beats with aberration, or PVCs."

Intermittent Antegrade Conduction Through a Kent Bundle. This arrhythmia is also known as intermittent Wolff-Parkinson-White syndrome. Many PVCs that occur late in ventricular diastole actually begin after the inscription of the next sinus P wave (Fig. 14–10). The distinction between this arrhythmia and a premature atrial contraction with aber-

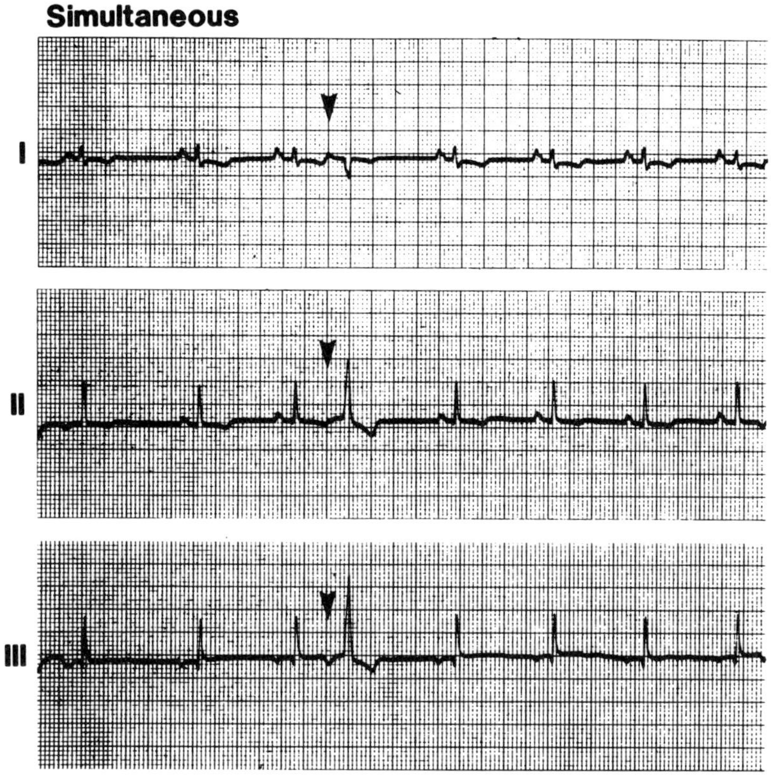

FIGURE 14–5
Premature atrial contraction with aberration. The axis of the normal sinus P waves is 0°, while the axis of the premature P wave *(arrow)* is −15°.

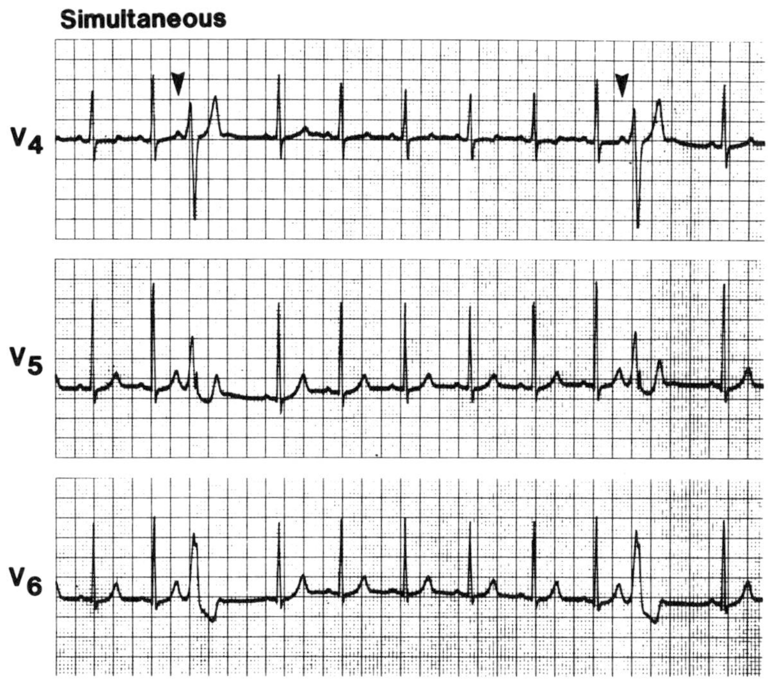

FIGURE 14–6
Premature atrial contractions with aberration. Note that the premature P waves (*arrows*) occur on the T waves of the preceding sinus QRS. In lead V_4, the sinus T wave begins with a negative deflection, while the P wave begins with a positive deflection. This record also illustrates the value of simultaneous recordings of different leads. In leads V_5 and V_6, the P wave is much more difficult to distinguish from the preceding T wave.

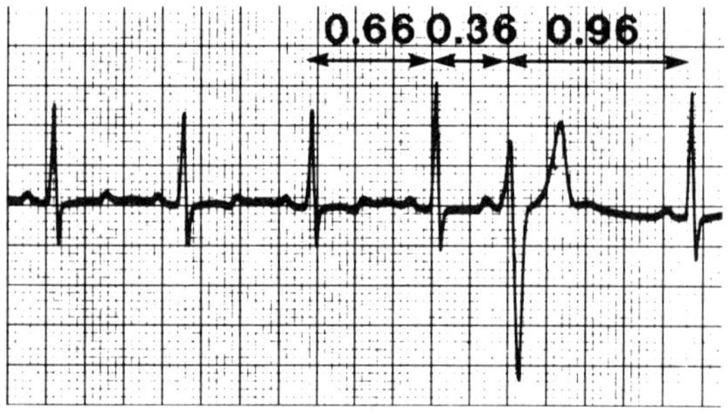

A

Lead V_4

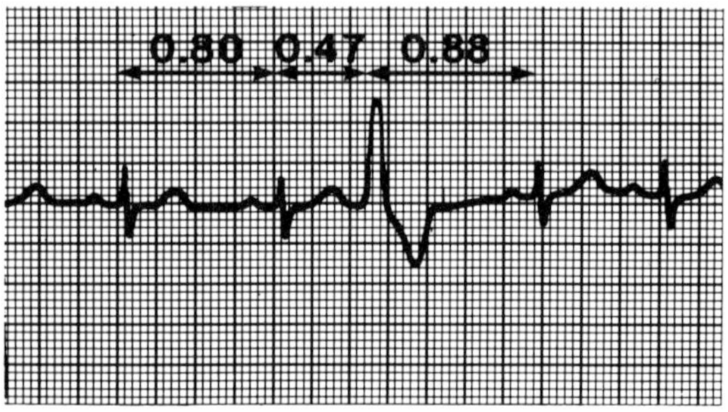

B

Lead II

FIGURE 14–7
Premature atrial contraction with fully compensatory pause.

rancy is not difficult, since the P wave is not premature, and the P wave has the same axis and morphology as the sinus P wave. However, the distinction between such a late diastolic PVC and intermittent conduction over a Kent bundle with a short PR interval and aberrant QRS may be more difficult. The transition to Kent bundle conduction may occur gradually over several beats, showing several intermittent fusion QRS morphologies between the normal QRS and the preexcited QRS. The widest QRS should occur at the end of the sequence. The change to Kent bundle conduction usually accompanies a change in the rate of the prevailing rhythm, either an increase or a decrease. Inspection of prior electrocardiograms in sinus rhythm with obvious Wolff-Parkinson-White conduction may reveal a similar morphology. On the other hand, PVCs tend to occur singly or in pairs, and a rate change may not accompany the appearance of PVCs. In a tracing where there is such a question, it is most helpful to scan the entire record for a wide QRS beat that is not preceded by a P wave. This makes the diagnosis of a PVC. It is likely that other beats of similar morphology are also PVCs. If it is not possible to find a wide QRS beat without a preceding P wave, then the diagnosis is still in question.

Similar or Different Morphology: Uniform and Multiform PVC

PVCs that have the same shape in the same surface electrocardiographic leads are said to be uniform, and those that have different shape are multiform (Fig. 14–11). Fusion complexes must not be mistaken for multiform PVCs. If a complex is not preceded by a P wave, fusion cannot have occurred between a normally conducted sinus QRS and another PVC, because atrial depolarization has not yet begun when the ventricles are

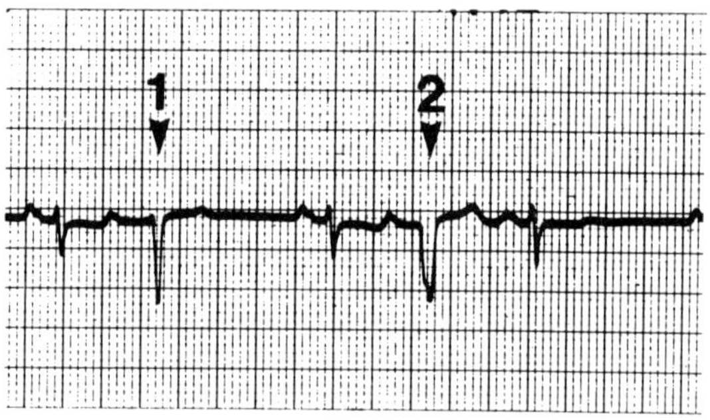

A

Lead AVL

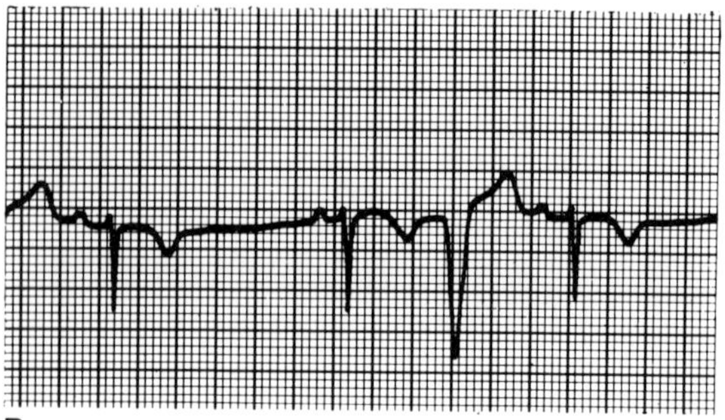

B

Lead V_1

FIGURE 14–8
Interpolated premature atrial contraction. The first PAC (1) resets the sinus node and causes a pause, but the second premature atrial contraction (2) does not disturb sinus rhythm and is therefore interpolated.

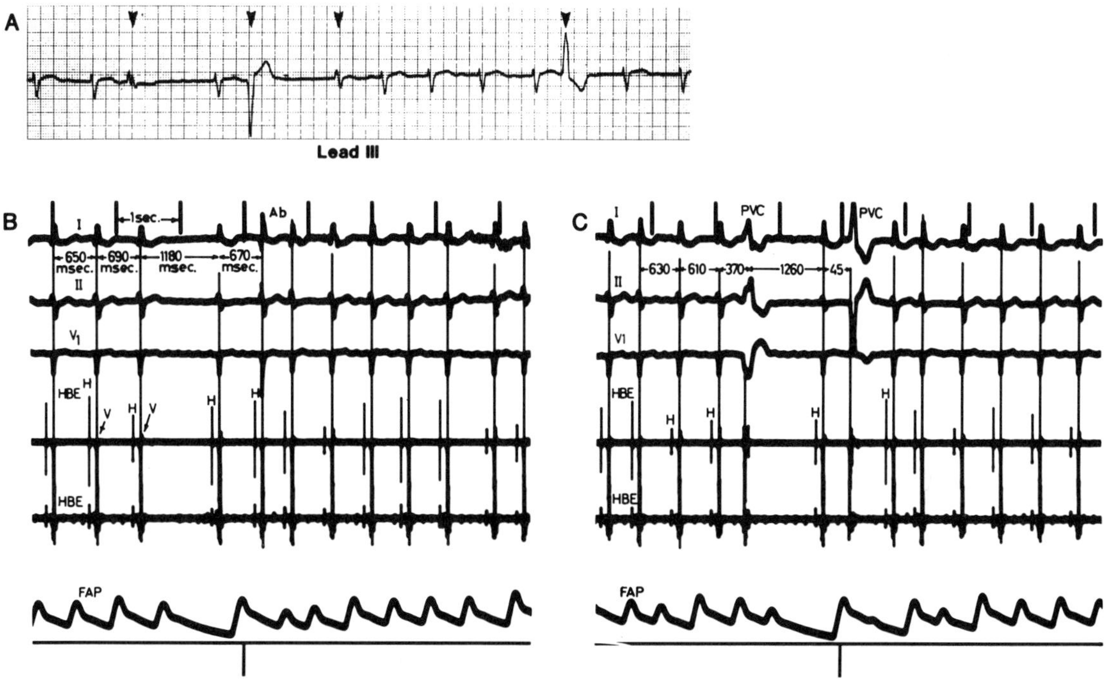

FIGURE 14–9
Surface electrocardiogram of atrial flutter-fibrillation. There are four QRS complexes (*arrows*) that differ in contour from the regular QRS. It is difficult to determine with certainty from this electrocardiogram which complexes are caused by aberrant conduction and which are PVCs.

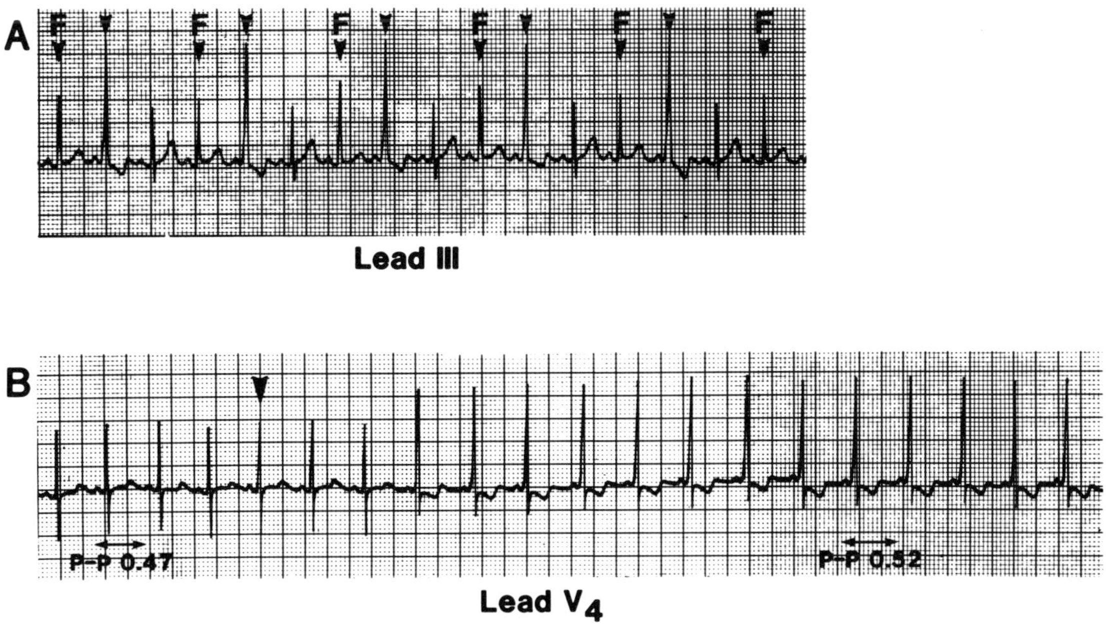

FIGURE 14–10
Late diastolic premature ventricular contractions. Each arrow marks a PVC. The sinus rate remains unchanged. This 11-month-old infant underwent intracardiac electrophysiologic evaluation to prove that the complexes were PVCs and not conduction via a Kent bundle as in Wolff-Parkinson-White syndrome. F = fusion complexes between PVCs and sinus beats.

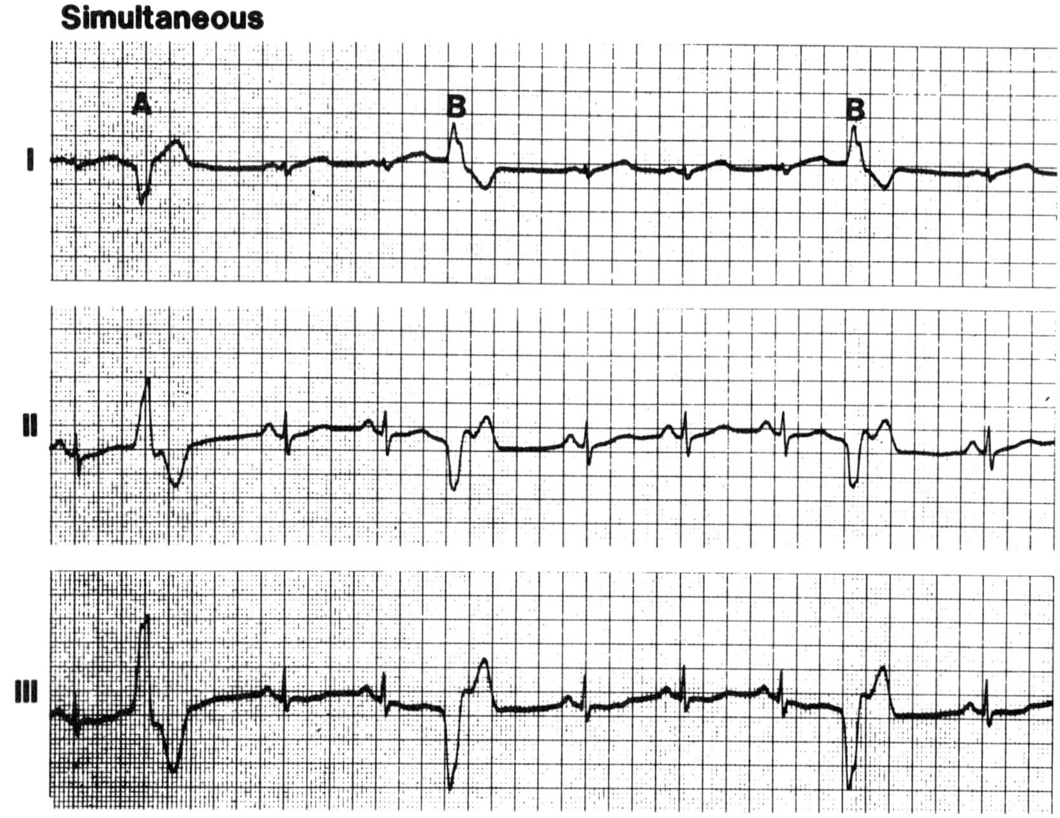

FIGURE 14–11
Multiform premature ventricular contractions. Two different morphologies (A and B) of premature ventricular contractions are found in each simultaneous lead. Uniform PVC may be found in Figure 14–12.

activated. Therefore, two dissimilar complexes may be called multiform, even though their major deflections are in the same direction, as long as neither is immediately preceded by a sinus P wave. If one of the complexes has a preceding sinus P wave, this may be a fusion complex. Two PVCs with major deflections in the opposite directions are usually multiform, but fusion must be sought in each case.[4] Fusion may also occur between two morphologies of multiform PVCs.

Until recently, the terms "unifocal" and "multifocal" have been used, implying that if PVCs have the same morphology, they originate in the same place in the heart every time, and if PVCs have different morphologies, they originate from different sites. It has become customary to label all PVCs with a left bundle-branch block pattern as "right ventricular" and those with a right bundle-branch block pattern as "left ventricular."[5] However, using intracardiac electrophysiologic studies, it has been demonstrated that (1) PVCs with the same morphology may originate at different sites, (2) PVCs with different morphologies may originate from the same site and use different exit pathways, and (3) the morphology of the surface ECG may be misleading as to the site of origin.[6] This is especially true in adults. In children who have a relatively normal heart without conduction delay, we have found relatively good correlation between the QRS morphology and the site of origin. We consider it important to characterize PVCs as either uniform or multiform, and to further classify them by their morphology, recognizing some of the possible inherent inaccuracies.

Coupling Interval: Ventricular Parasystole

The coupling interval of the PVC is defined as the time between the onset of the preceding QRS and the onset of the PVC (Fig. 14–12). The shorter the coupling inter-

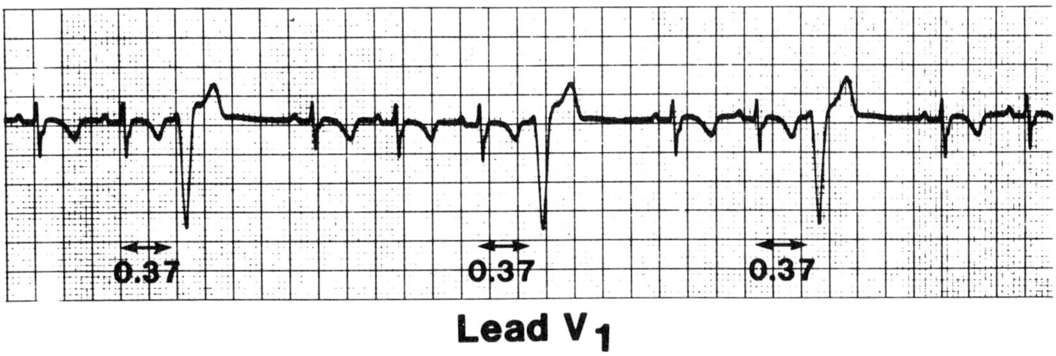

FIGURE 14–12
Uniform premature ventricular contractions with fixed coupling interval. The interval from the sinus QRS to the premature ventricular contraction is 0.37 s for each premature ventricular contraction.

val, the closer the PVC is to the apex of the preceding T wave. The period of 10 ms to 50 ms following the apex of the T wave constitutes the "ventricular vulnerable period."[4, 7] This is so called because ventricular extrastimuli applied during this period ("R on T") have been reported to result in ventricular tachycardia and ventricular fibrillation in adults. In recent studies of sudden death in adults, many episodes of sudden death recorded with a Holter monitor reveal the initiating PVC to be one with a long coupling interval (not "R on T"); therefore, this entire concept has been questioned. One situation in which "R on T" may have disastrous consequences is in the application of a DC shock. If the shock is applied at the apex of the T wave, it may result in ventricular fibrillation, even in children.

For each morphology of PVC, the coupling interval may be fixed or variable. Variable coupling is defined as a difference in coupling interval of more than 0.08 s. With multiform PVCs, each different morphology may have a coupling interval that differs from the other morphologies, but if the coupling interval is the same for all beats with the same morphology, then this is fixed coupling.

The vast majority of children have fixed coupling. If there is variable coupling with the same morphology of PVC, the inter-ectopic intervals (time between each PVC) should be measured. If the inter-ectopic intervals can be factored so that each interval is a multiple of a single basic interval (within 0.08 s), then ventricular parasystole is diagnosed. Assume a patient with variable coupling had inter-ectopic intervals of 2.99 s, 4.37 s, 2.92 s, and 2.98 s (Fig. 14–13); the common factor is 1.47 s. We infer that a small area of the ventricle is depolarizing every 1.47 s (41 times per minute) and that there is variable entrance block and exit block in the area so that, for example, if the inter-ectopic interval is 4.37 s, then there is 3:1 exit block from the area. Entrance block must be theorized because parasystole, in the classic sense, is unaffected by any other rhythm; for example, sinus impulses do not invade the area and cause reset. This is the classic explanation of parasystole. More recent data, however, indicate that it may be possible for the sinus rhythm to partially invade an area, thus "modulating" the parasystolic area. Since the newer criteria make it possible for almost any rhythm to be defined as parasystolic, it is best to stay with the more classic definition in diagnosis of parasystole in children. Random, nonparasystolic coupling (in which the inter-ectopic intervals are not multiples of a basic interval) is the rarest type of coupling in children and adults (Fig. 14–14).[8] This may represent a form of modulated parasystole.

Patterns of PVCs: Bigeminy, Trigeminy, and Couplets

Ventricular bigeminy is a regular alternation of PVCs with the underlying normal QRS complexes, in which every other beat is a PVC (Fig. 14–15). Bigeminy tends to be a very stable and self-sustaining rhythm.[4] The reason for this is given in Langendorf, Pick, and Winternitz's "rule of bigeminy,"[9] which

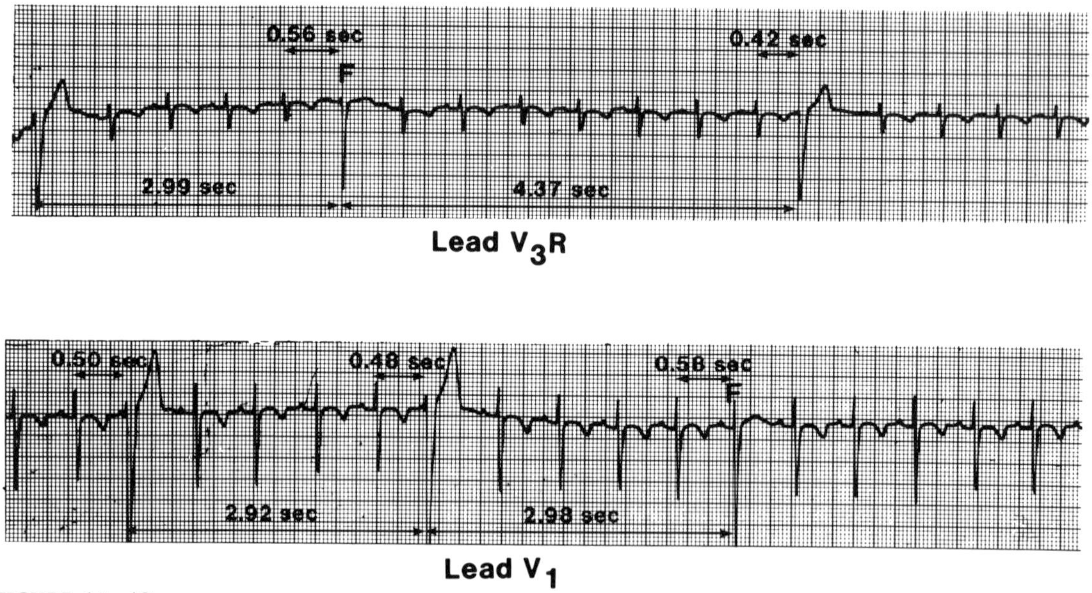

FIGURE 14–13
Uniform premature ventricular contractions with variable coupling intervals (shown above the electrocardiograms). These leads were recorded in close succession from the same patient. Note the variation in coupling interval from 0.42 s to 0.58 s. The inter-ectopic intervals are shown beneath the electrocardiograms. The inter-ectopic intervals are each a multiple of 1.47 s, indicating a diagnosis of ventricular parasystole. F = fusion complexes.

begins with the observation that PVCs are common with slow heart rates (long cycle lengths). If a PVC (which, by definition, has a shorter cycle length than the sinus beat) is followed by a compensatory pause (longer cycle length than the sinus beat), the long cycle length of the compensatory pause will favor a PVC (Fig. 14–15). This PVC then generates another compensatory pause, and the rhythm continues as bigeminy. Ventricular trigeminy is a regular alternation of PVCs and QRS complexes, with every third beat being a PVC (Fig. 14–16). A couplet is defined as two PVCs in a row without an intervening normal QRS complex. Couplets are also referred to as "paired PVCs" (Fig. 14–17).[10] Bigeminy, trigeminy, and couplets may occur with uniform PVCs or multiform PVCs. For example, bigeminy with multiform PVCs is termed "multiform bigeminy" (Figs. 18 and 19).

VENTRICULAR TACHYCARDIA

ECG Characteristics

Ventricular tachycardia is a series of three or more repetitive excitations that originate

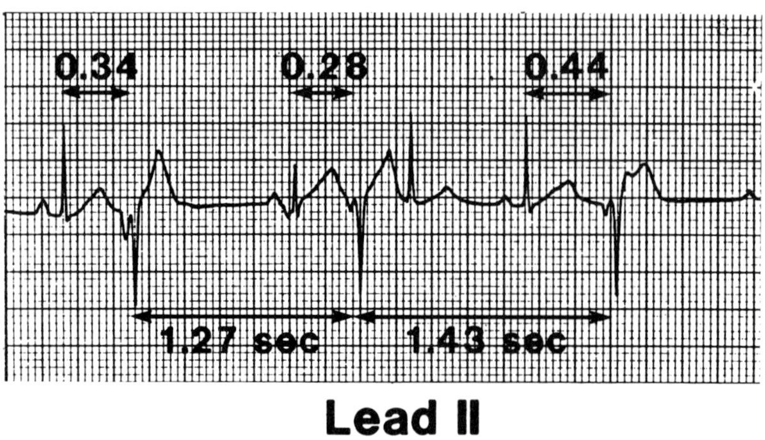

FIGURE 14–14
Uniform premature ventricular contractions with non-parasystolic variable coupling intervals. The coupling intervals are shown above the ECG, and the inter-ectopic intervals are shown below the ECG.

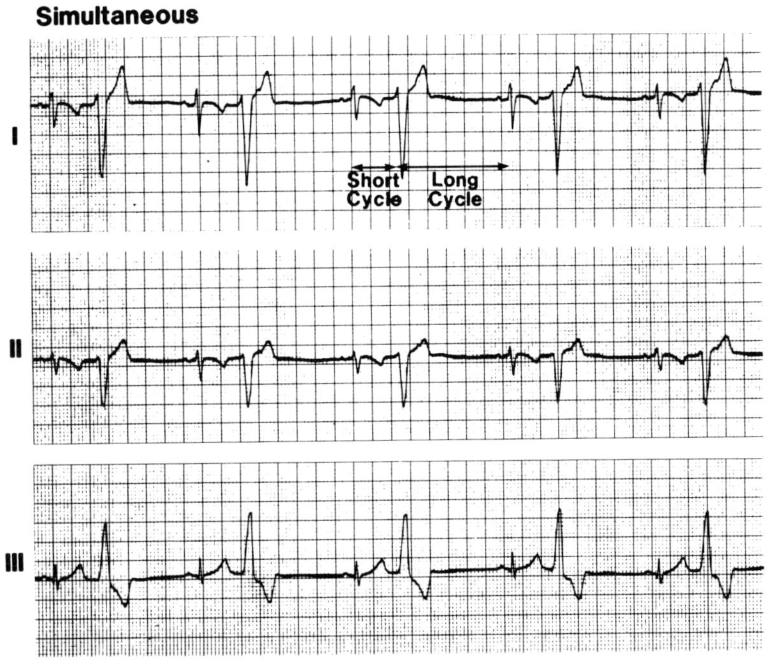

FIGURE 14–15
Ventricular bigeminy. Uniform premature ventricular contractions alternate with sinus beats. Premature ventricular contractions tend to occur following long cycles.

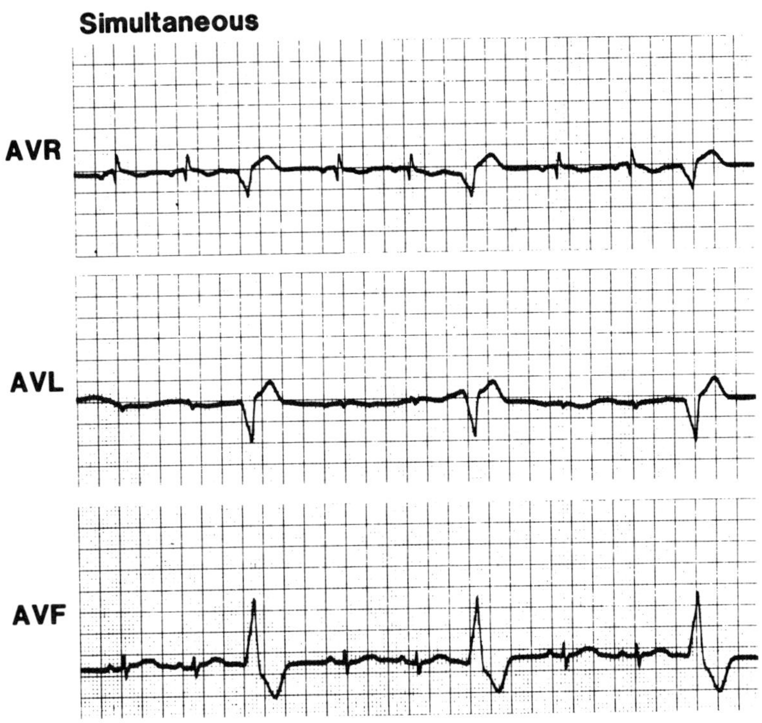

FIGURE 14–16
Ventricular trigeminy. Uniform PVCs occur after every two sinus beats.

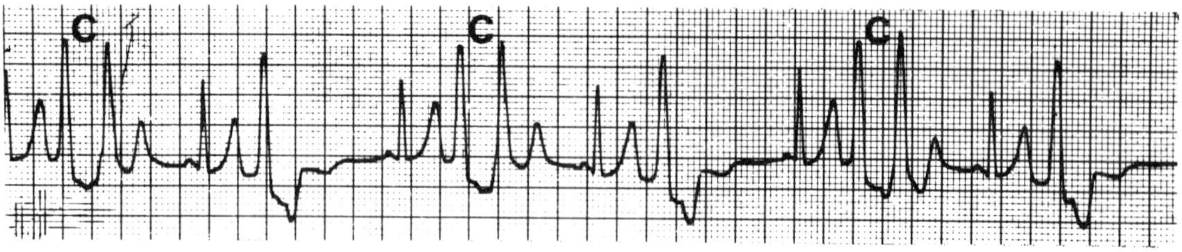

Lead II

FIGURE 14–17
Pairs of uniform premature ventricular contractions (couplets), marked with a "C."

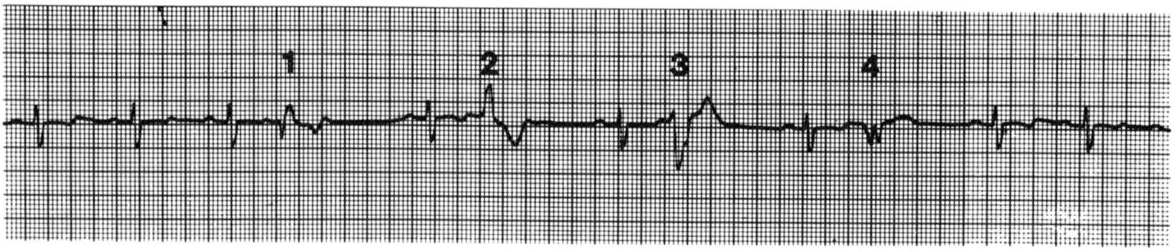

Lead I

FIGURE 14–18
Multiform bigeminy. Multiform premature ventricular contractions alternate with sinus beats. There are four different morphologies of PVCs. None is a fusion complex.

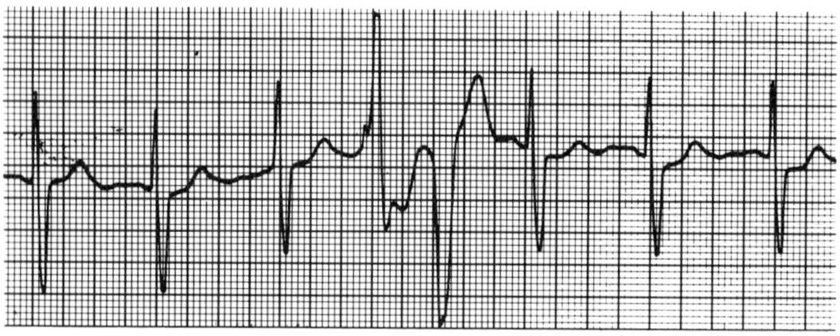

Lead V_5

FIGURE 14–19
Multiform couplet (two consecutive premature ventricular contractions). Neither is a fusion or a sinus capture beat with aberration.

FIGURE 14–20
Ventricular tachycardia in a young infant at a rate of 350/min. Note the QRS duration is only 0.045 s. There is AV dissociation (P waves marked by arrows), with an atrial rate of 140/min.

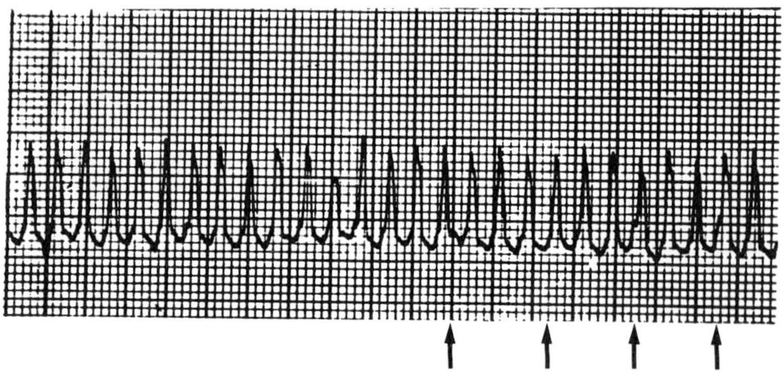

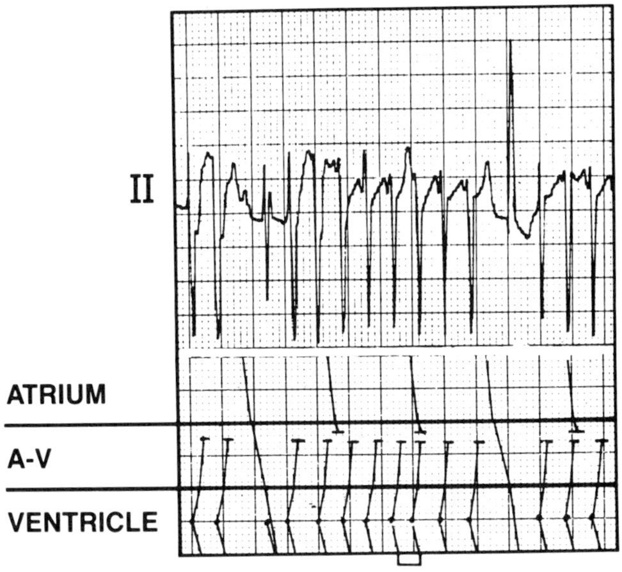

FIGURE 14–21
Ventricular tachycardia at 440/min. All the characteristics of ventricular tachycardia are satisfied. The fourth beat from the right is a sinus capture beat; the third beat from the left is a fusion complex. The ventricular tachycardia beats have a narrow QRS that has a completely different morphology from the sinus capture beat, despite being approximately the same duration.

from the ventricle. Ventricular tachycardia is also defined as a rate faster than 120 beats per minute (bpm) in children. On the surface ECG, each QRS is different from the underlying sinus rhythm. This is the most important consideration, since the QRS complex may not be absolutely "wide" for the age of the patient. This is especially true in infants in whom the QRS duration in ventricular tachycardia ranges from 0.06 s to 0.11 s[11] (Figs. 14–20 and 14–21). In older children, the QRS complex is more often prolonged as age increases >0.09 s in those older than 3 years) (Figs. 14–22 and 14–23). In infants, the most common QRS morphology during ventricular tachycardia is right bundle-branch block with left axis deviation;[11] however, in Pederson et al's study in older children, 10 of 17 patients (59%) had a complete left bundle-branch block pattern during ventricular tachycardia, four of 17 had a complete right bundle-branch block pattern, and two of 17 had both right and left bundle-branch block patterns in the same tracing.[12]

Ventricular tachycardia must be differentiated from tachycardias with a "different

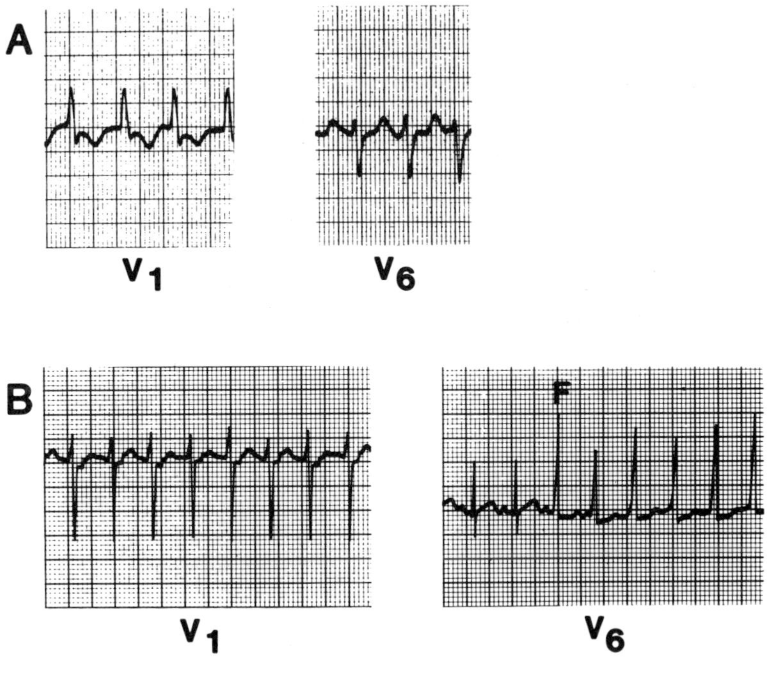

FIGURE 14–22
(A) Ventricular tachycardia with complete right bundle branch block pattern in a 10-year-old. The QRS duration is 0.15 s, and the QRS rate is 140/min. *(B)* Ventricular tachycardia with complete left bundle branch block pattern in a 10-day-old infant. Ventricular tachycardia is shown beginning in lead V_6. Note the fusion complex (F). The QRS duration is 0.09 s, which is longer than the sinus QRS duration of 0.06 s. The ventricular tachycardia rate is 200/min.

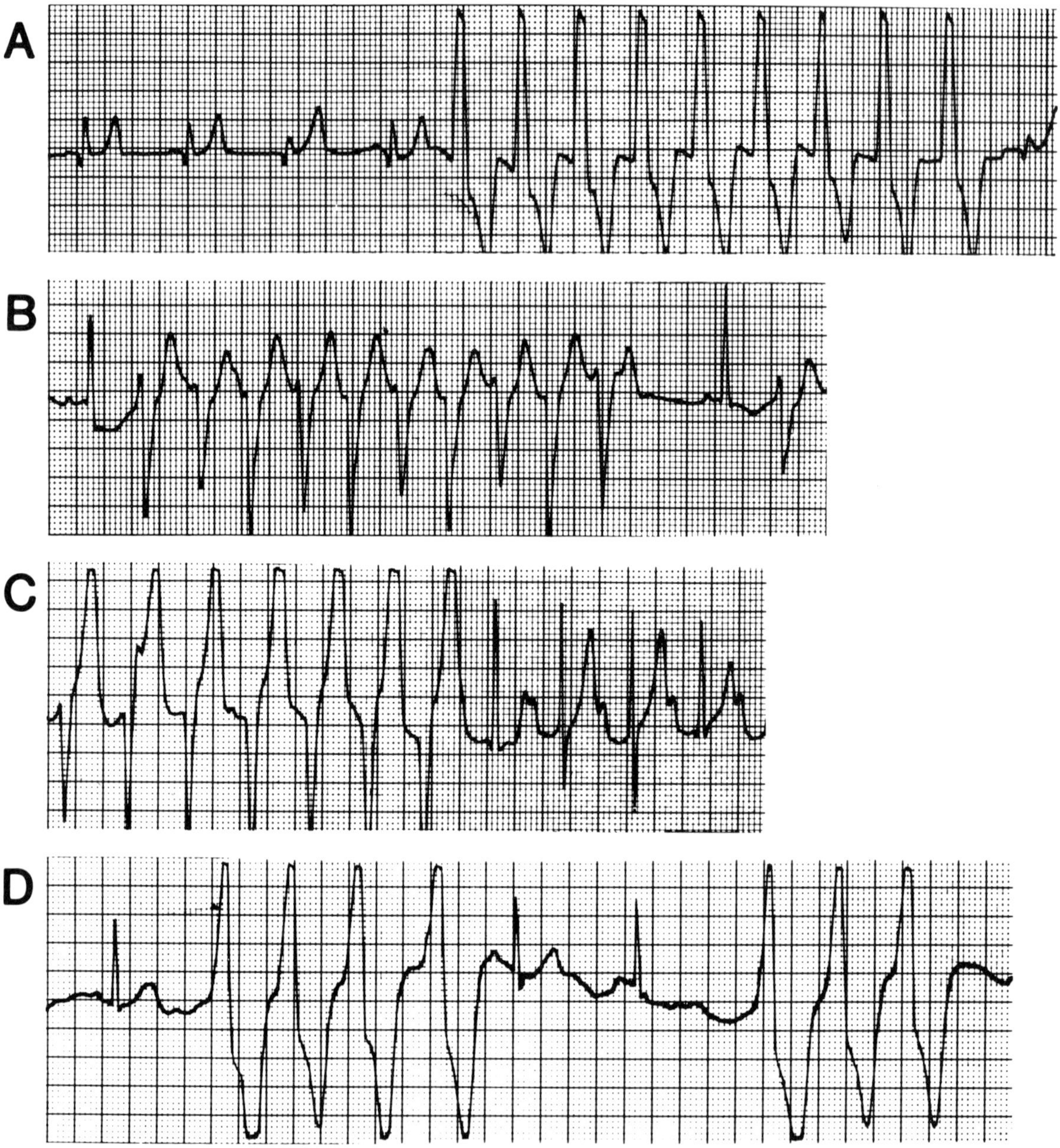

FIGURE 14–23

Different morphologies of ventricular tachycardia as recorded by 24-hour electrocardiographic tape monitoring. All tracings are a modified lead II. Sinus beats are shown for comparison. *(A)* 8-year-old child; QRS duration 0.13 s, QRS rate 140/min. *(B)* 12-year-old child; QRS duration 0.11 s, QRS rate 200/min. *(C)* 4-year-old child; QRS duration 0.11 s, QRS rate 140/min. *(D)* 15-year-old child; QRS duration 0.17 s, QRS rate 130/min.

QRS" (note that the term "wide QRS" should not be used, since frequently the QRS is not wide). Therefore, the differential diagnosis consists of supraventricular tachycardia (SVT) or atrial flutter with aberration. Aberration of supraventricular tachycardia is very rare in children: only 10 of 120 patients with SVT (8%) had a wide QRS during tachycardia (see chapter 13). Only one of our 10 patients with SVT had a morphology of complete left bundle-branch block during supraventricular tachycardia. This was the result of antegrade conduction through a bundle of Kent during tachycardia. This morphology had also been present during sinus rhythm and was caused by the Wolff-Parkinson-White syndrome. No patient had complete left bundle-branch block during SVT that was not present during sinus rhythm. No patient had a completely normal QRS in sinus rhythm and a QRS with prolonged duration or abnormal bundle-branch morphology during SVT. Therefore, if a child has a tachycardia with a bundle-branch morphology, the chances are greater than 90% that it is of ventricular origin.

Other points that favor the diagnosis of ventricular tachycardia are:

1. AV dissociation (Fig. 14–24). This was present in 16 of 17 children in Pederson et al's[12] study of pediatric ventricular tachycardia and in 7 of 11 patients reported by Videbaek et al.[13] If AV dissociation is present with a wide QRS tachycardia, the diagnosis of ventricular tachycardia (with the very rare exception of supraventricular tachycardia resulting from a Mahaim fiber) is practically assured. The absence of AV dissociation is not helpful, however, because ventricular tachycardia in children may occur with 1:1 retrograde capture of the atria.
2. Intermittent fusion or sinus capture beats (Fig. 14–25).
3. Morphology of ventricular tachycardia similar to single PVCs. If the patient had other electrocardiograms and PVCs were noted, the morphology of ventricular tachycardia should be compared with that of PVCs. This is only helpful if the morphology is similar. If the morphology is not identical, it could still be ventricular tachycardia.
4. Rate. In children, it is rare for ventricular tachycardia to have a rate of 300 bpm or more. In our series of ventricular tachycardia in infants,[11] the rate ranged from 167 bpm to 440 bpm (mean, 252 bpm), with only three patients having a rate of 300 bpm or more. The most rapid ventricular tachycardia ever recorded was 500 bpm (see Fig. 14–20).

Bidirectional Tachycardia and Torsades de Pointes

Bidirectional tachycardia is a type of ventricular tachycardia in which the QRS morphologies alternate. In general, there is constant right bundle-branch block during the tachycardia, with alternating right axis deviation and left axis deviation of the QRS complex (Fig. 14–26). This must be distinguished from ventricular bigeminy. In bidirectional tachycardia, the interval between RR intervals is absolutely constant, whereas in bigeminy, there is an alternating long-short pattern to the RR intervals.

Torsades de pointes was first described by Dessertenne[14] and translates as "twisting of the peaks." In this arrhythmia, the QRS gradually changes from one morphology to another morphology. As the QRS undergoes this transition, there is usually a narrow QRS that is a balance between the two wider morphologies (Fig. 14–27). Each "torsades" covers several "pointes" and so the QRS morphology usually changes completely every five to 10 beats.[15] Because this type of arrhythmia generally occurs in patients with a prolonged QT interval, it has been suggested that torsades de pointes should be diagnosed only if the patient has a prolonged QT interval in sinus rhythm. This is most difficult to do, since frequently a diagnosis must be made on the basis of an electrocardiogram recorded during a tachyarrhythmia without an electrocardiographic pattern in sinus rhythm.

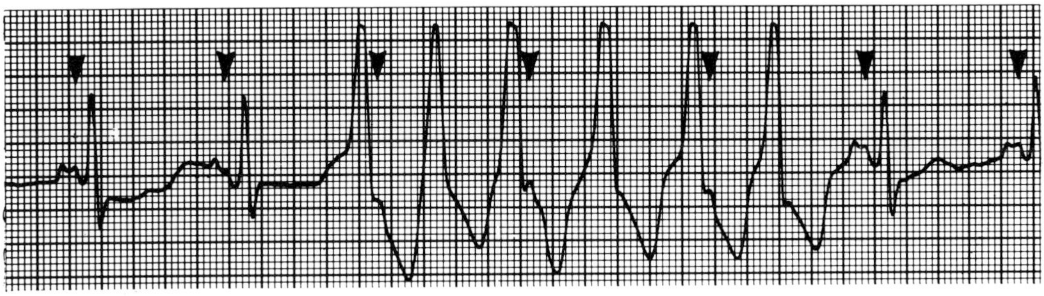

FIGURE 14–24
Ventricular tachycardia with AV dissociation. Note that the P waves (*arrows*) continue undisturbed through the episode of ventricular tachycardia.

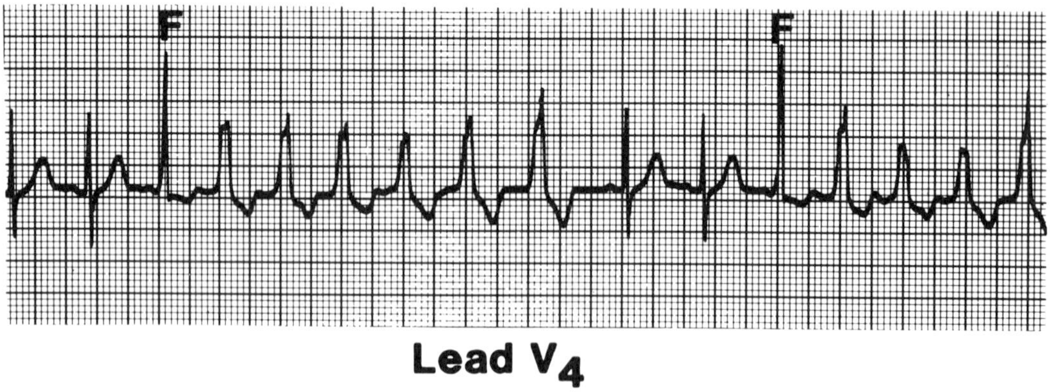

FIGURE 14–25
Ventricular tachycardia with fusion beats (F).

In children, if a tachyarrhythmia with the characteristics of torsades de pointes occurs, then this should be the diagnosis regardless of the pattern in sinus rhythm.

Accelerated Ventricular Rhythm

Davidson[16] has defined accelerated ventricular rhythm as a rhythm "about the same rate of the underlying sinus rhythm and therefore faster than the expected rate of an idioventricular focus but slower than the usual rate of ventricular tachycardia." There is disagreement as to whether accelerated ventricular rhythm should be separated from ventricular tachycardia, and if these two rhythms are to be separated, where to draw the line of separation.[13, 16–18] It seems reasonable to separate them, since accelerated ventricular rhythm is benign.[18] Accelerated ventricular rhythm is defined, in infants and children, as a rhythm with all the characteristics of ventricular tachycardia, but with a rate approximately the same as the prevailing sinus rhythm (usually less than 120 bpm) (Fig. 14–28).

NONINVASIVE EVALUATION OF PVCs AND VENTRICULAR TACHYCARDIA

Since there is a difference in prognosis between PVCs in children with normal hearts

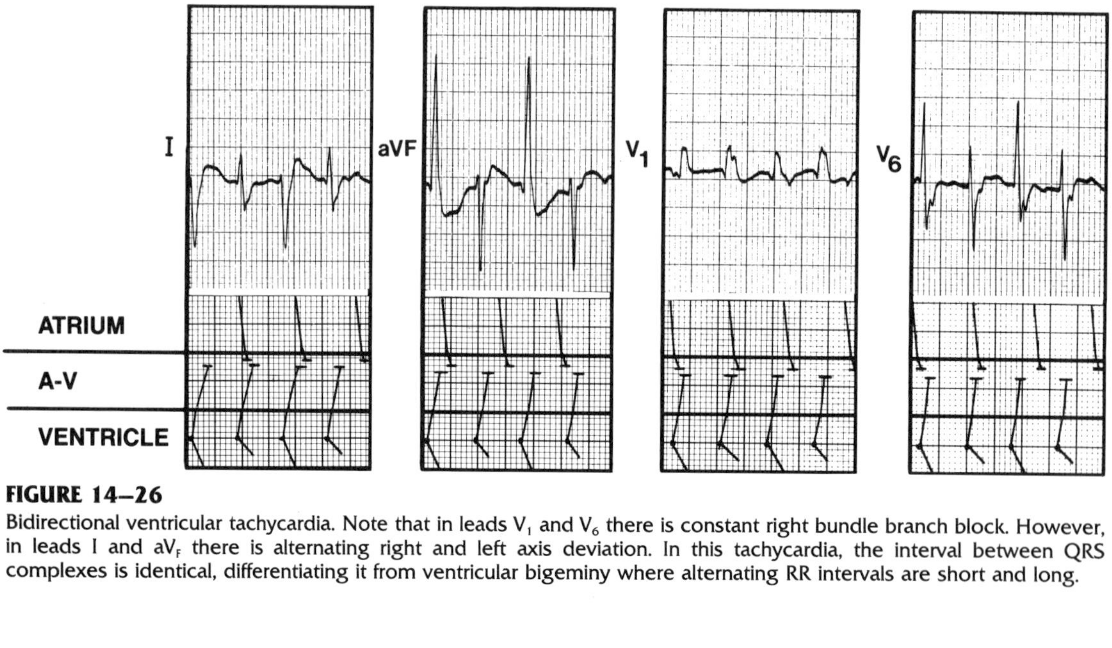

FIGURE 14–26
Bidirectional ventricular tachycardia. Note that in leads V_1 and V_6 there is constant right bundle branch block. However, in leads I and aV_F there is alternating right and left axis deviation. In this tachycardia, the interval between QRS complexes is identical, differentiating it from ventricular bigeminy where alternating RR intervals are short and long.

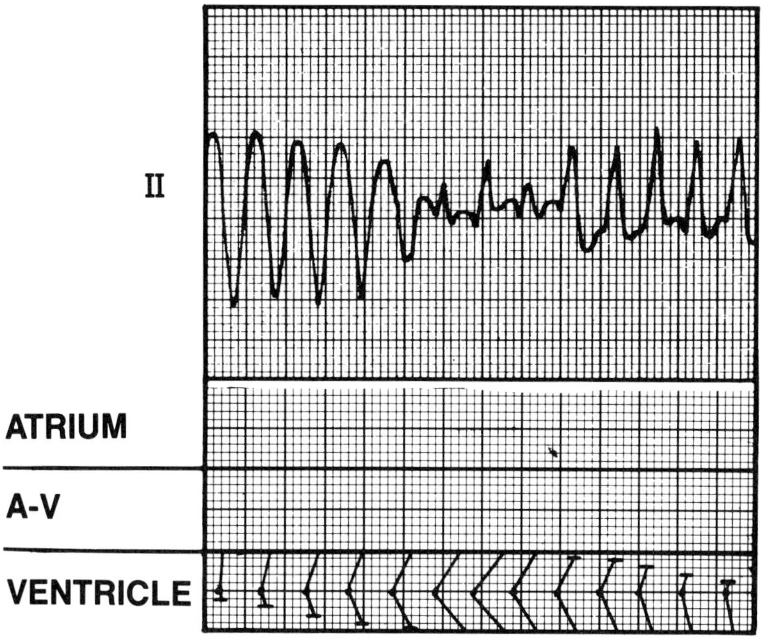

FIGURE 14–27
Torsades de pointes. Note that the QRS morphology gradually shifts from negative to positive with a narrow QRS complex between the two morphologies.

and those in children with abnormal hearts, it is important to determine the presence of any acute or chronic causative factor. Clues may be apparent from the history: drugs (especially drinks and decongestants containing caffeine), previous myocarditis, or predisposition to electrolyte imbalance (e.g., hyperkalemia in the adrenogenital syndrome).[19] Unfortunately, a history of palpitations is not usually helpful in the diagnosis of ventricular arrhythmias. In a study in adults, Reiffel, Schulhof, and Joseph found that only 50% of the patients with palpitations had any arrhythmia and in less than 20% was there an arrhythmia that required treatment.[20] Physical examination may reveal the findings of mitral valve prolapse or evidence of unsuspected congenital or acquired heart disease.

The echocardiogram is essential in this evaluation, not only to demonstrate mitral valve prolapse (which should be detected on physical examination), but also to search for occult hypertrophic or congestive cardiomyopathy or arrhythmogenic right ventricular dysplasia. Unfortunately, in children it is possible to have arrhythmogenic right ventricular dysplasia with an entirely normal noninvasive evaluation, including two-dimensional echocardiography, and it is for this reason that cardiac catheterization is sometimes necessary in patients with ventricular tachycardia to rule out arrhythmogenic right ventricular dysplasia. A chest radiograph is rarely obtained, since cardiomyopathy may exist even in the presence of a normal size cardiac silhouette on chest radiograph.

The routine electrocardiogram should be examined carefully for the QT interval. Measurement of the QT interval in children can be difficult for three reasons:

1. Children have larger U waves than adults. It is difficult to know whether to include the U wave in the measurement of the QT interval. In the original article describing the prolonged QT interval syn-

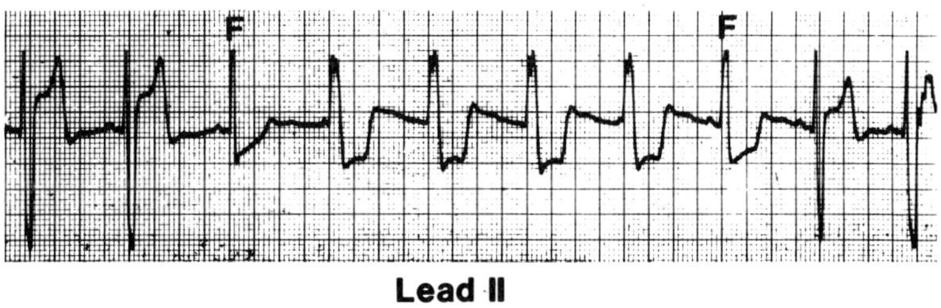

FIGURE 14–28
Accelerated ventricular rhythm. The sinus rate is 73/min, and the ventricular rate is 75/min. Note fusion complexes (F), which mark the beginning and the end of the accelerated ventricular rhythm.

drome, Jervell and Lange-Nielsen[21] advocated including the U wave "if it was large." The definition of "large" has been quite varied. In children, we recommend including a notched T wave or U wave in the measurement of the QT interval if that portion of the wave is more than 50% of the amplitude of the initial portion of the T wave (Fig. 14–29).

2. The QT interval is not the same in all leads. At the present time, the only normal values available are for lead II, and this should be the usual lead measured. However, if there is an excessively large U wave in leads V_4 through V_6, then lead II should be measured and the U wave included.

3. The QT interval must be corrected for heart rate. In 1922, Bazett[22] described the relationship:

$$\text{corrected QT (QTc)} = \frac{\text{measured QT}}{\sqrt{\text{RR}}}$$

This was done in awake adults using only lead II; the normal corrected QT was less than 0.44 s. Since that time, numerous problems with this method of correction have been found. First, the normal corrected QT depends on the state of sympathetic or parasympathetic tone (e.g., the QTc increases with sleep.[23] In addition, infants and children have considerable sinus arrhythmia. Over several beats, the QT interval generally stays the same, while the RR interval may change drastically, thus changing the QTc. In practice, the longest RR interval can be measured; the QT applied to this RR should be the QT of the beat immediately following the RR interval. The same process can be repeated for the shortest RR interval, and an average QT can be calculated. In sinus arrhythmia, if only the shortest RR interval is taken (thus resulting in the longest possible corrected QT interval), falsely prolonged QT intervals may result. In the study by Anderson,[24] falsely prolonged QT intervals would have caused 14 of 42 patients to have a QTc greater than

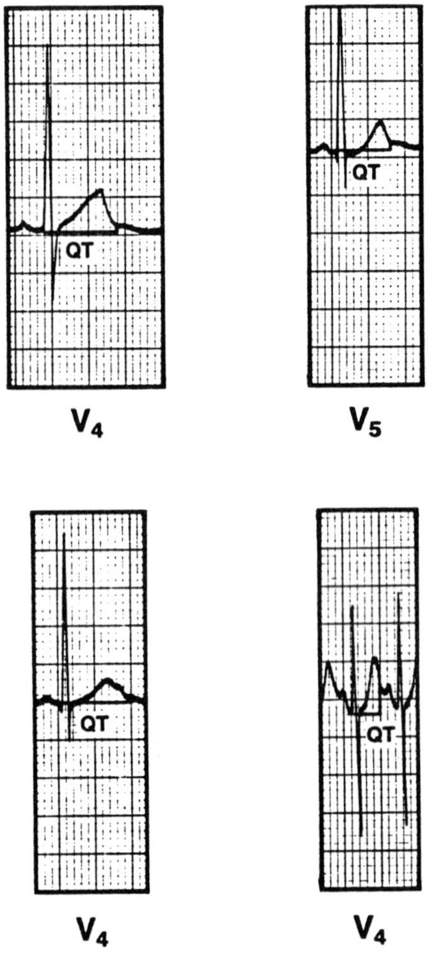

FIGURE 14–29
Measurement of the QT interval. *Top left:* With a notched T wave followed by a U wave, the down slope of the T wave is extrapolated to the baseline. *Top right:* With a notch < 50% of the peak of the T wave, the early segment is extrapolated to the baseline. *Bottom left:* With a notch > 50% of the peak of the T wave, the second portion of the wave is extrapolated to the baseline. *Bottom right:* With superimposed P waves, the downslope of the T wave is extrapolated to the baseline.

0.44 s, with the longest being 0.53 s. Even in the absence of sinus arrhythmia, the corrected QT in many infants may be slightly longer than 0.44 s. In the study by Leistner et al,[25] the upper limit of normal QTc at 1 month of age is 0.453 s; at 2 months, 0.468 s; at 3 months, 0.470 s; and at 4 months, 0.468 s; these are somewhat longer than those reported by Schwartz,[26] in which the QTc did not exceed 0.44 s throughout infancy. Since the data are conflicting, it is wise to be suspicious of any infant or child with a QTc greater than 0.44 s, but this finding should not be used in isolation (see section on prolonged QT interval syndromes).

In addition to measuring the QT interval, the shape of the T waves (and U waves) should be noted. Jervell and Lange-Nielsen[21] admitted that they did not know whether to call the prominent wave found in their patients a T wave or a U wave. This is especially complicated in children since it is difficult to distinguish a U wave from a biphasic T wave at rapid rates. A wave should be called a U wave only if the T wave returns to the baseline before the beginning of the next wave; otherwise, it is a notched T wave. If either the second component of the notched T wave or the U wave is greater than 50% of the amplitude of the initial component, this should be noted, since it is abnormal (Fig. 14–30).

The coupling interval, the constancy of coupling, and the specific morphology (right or left bundle-branch block) should be recorded. In addition, multiform PVCs or couplets should be distinguished from single uniform PVCs.

All patients with suspected ventricular arrhythmias should undergo exercise testing. In our laboratory, children as young as 4 years of age have been able to undergo successful treadmill exercise testing. It has been said that the QT interval should shorten with exercise.[27] In our experience, it is difficult to measure the QT interval during exercise, and the characteristic response in children has not been determined. According to Schwartz,[28] the QTc measured 1 minute after exercise (which can be easily done) may be a sensitive indicator for patients with the prolonged QT interval syndrome; it should not be greater than 0.44 s. In children with a normal heart, PVCs are suppressed in response to exercise and return in the immediate post-exercise period. Although normal children may not completely suppress PVCs with exercise, the exercise test is used in normals to be sure ventricular tachycardia does not develop. In children with an abnormal heart, there is no characteristic response; the arrhythmia may worsen or improve with exercise. In fact, we have encountered two children who had undergone repair of tetralogy of Fallot whose PVCs completely disappeared with exercise; these children later died suddenly.[12, 29] Therefore, in patients with an abnormal heart, the exercise test is used simply to screen for the presence of PVCs.

Twenty-four–hour continuous electrocardiographic tape monitoring (Holter monitoring) is an important part of the noninvasive evaluation, since most children with PVCs and even ventricular tachycardia are asymptomatic. However, we usually do not perform Holter monitoring on patients with a normal heart and uniform PVCs. While the greatest variability is usually from day to night (with the larger amount of PVCs and ventricular tachycardia during the day), there is also considerable variability from day to day in an individual patient. For this reason, in order to assess a patient fully, especially before beginning drug therapy, it is recommended that two consecutive 24-hour Holter electrocardiograms be obtained.[30, 31] The child's arrhythmia should then be categorized by the most severe form observed. Even if a patient has 10 beats of ventricular tachycardia only once, he is classified as a ventricular tachycardia patient. Also on the 24-hour electrocardiogram, the QT interval should be measured at several different points while the patient is awake. At the present time, normal values are not available for the QTc while the child is asleep, but it is certainly possible to measure the QTc on the Holter. The filter settings on Holter recorders are such that it is conceivable for the QT to be artifactually short (filtering out the end of the T wave), but it should not be artifactually long. In patients with a possible prolonged QT interval syndrome, Holter monitoring may reveal the presence of T wave alternans. This diagnosis is made when successive T waves alternately change in polarity from upright to inverted every other beat.

The quantitative assessment of "frequent PVCs" is arbitrary. The Lown classification for ventricular arrhythmias (developed for adults) considers more than 30 per hour to be "frequent." Since the heart rate of a child

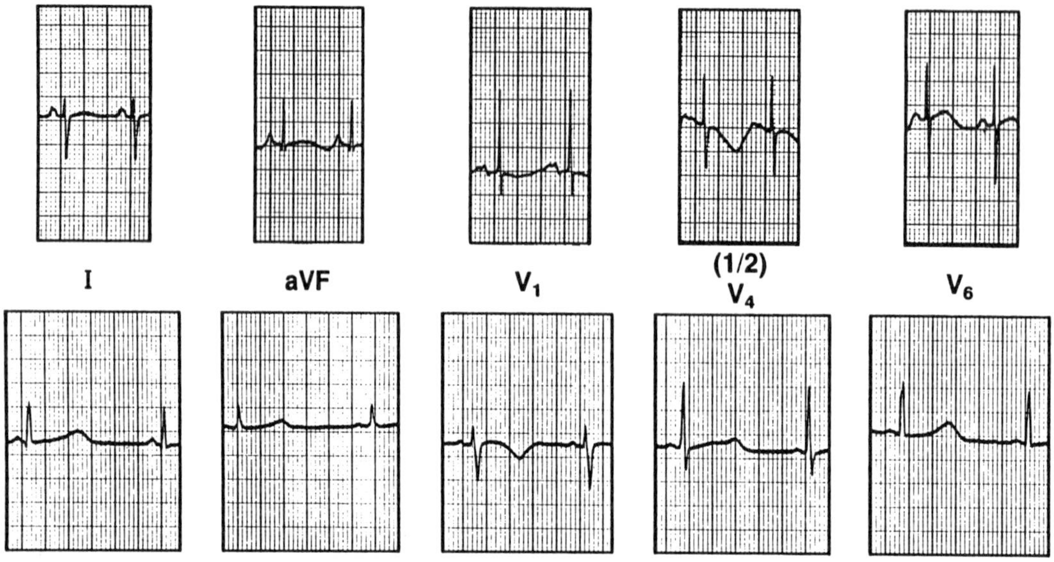

FIGURE 14–30
Congenital prolongation of the QT interval. Top tracings are from a 9-day-old infant with a history of ventricular tachycardia and ventricular fibrillation from the age of 4 days. All the T waves are abnormal; the T waves in lead V_4 (at half standard) are especially unusual. Bottom tracings are from a 12-year-old boy who had his first episode of syncope at 10 years of age. He was being treated for a "familial seizure disorder," although the actual cause of the "seizures" was probably ventricular tachycardia. Note that the terminal portion of the T wave in lead V_4 is greater in amplitude than the initial portion.

can be considered to be almost double that of an adult, it would seem reasonable that 60 per hour, or one per minute, could be considered "frequent" in a child. This represents 1440 PVCs per day. On the low end of the scale, adults with coronary disease who have fewer than 10 PVCs per hour are at no greater risk to die suddenly than those who have no PVCs. These data are not available in children; however, it seems reasonable that fewer than 10 to 20 PVCs per hour should be considered "infrequent."

The final method of noninvasive assessment in a child with a suspected ventricular arrhythmia is signal-averaged electrocardiography, discussed fully in chapter 5.

ELECTROPHYSIOLOGIC MECHANISMS OF PVCs AND VENTRICULAR TACHYCARDIA

The theorized electrophysiologic mechanisms for PVCs and ventricular tachycardias are the same as those for supraventricular arrhythmias: reentry, abnormal automaticity, and triggered activity (see chapters 3, 6, and 12). It is unknown, at present, if these mechanisms can be ascertained from the surface electrocardiogram of a patient with PVCs or ventricular tachycardia. For example, parasystole may result from either accelerated normal automaticity or abnormal automaticity. In the classic form of parasystole, there is complete entrance block into the ectopic focus (so that it is not reset) and variable exit block (the ectopic focus escapes to excite the surrounding myocardium whenever a PVC is seen). Moe et al[32] and Jalife and Moe[33] have shown that even fixed coupled PVCs (which have classically been thought of as resulting from reentry) can be caused by parasystole. Zimmermann et al[34] have suggested ways in which triggered activity may be inferred from the surface electrocardiogram, most notably if the PVCs or ventricular tachycardia occur at higher basal heart rates (shorter preceding RR intervals) and if the coupling intervals to the PVCs are directly related to the preceding cycle length. However, until more data become available from direct recordings, attempting to infer the mechanism of ventricular arrhythmias from the surface electrocardiogram should be approached with a great deal of caution.

Even assessment of the true electrophysiologic mechanism of a ventricular arrhythmia from intracardiac electrophysiologic study is difficult, because the criteria are still in evolution. One "mechanism" for ventricular arrhythmias that can be elucidated is "bundle-branch reentry" or "macro-reentry." This is a phenomenon that has been noticed with the wide use of the ventricular extrastimulus technique and appears to be a benign consequence of method.[35] Bundle-branch reentry may be demonstrated when, during a ventricular extrastimulus study, the premature ventricular stimulus (S_2) is followed by not one, but two ventricular responses (V_2, V_3) that are similar in morphology and activation sequence (Fig. 14–31). The mechanism is based on the fact that the bundle branches have the longest refractory periods of any of the parts of the ventricle. Therefore, a PVC delivered into the right ventricular apex at a relatively short coupling interval is likely to find the right bundle branch in its effective refractory period. As a result, the premature stimulus cannot propagate in the retrograde manner through the right bundle branch, but must travel slowly through the septal muscle to reach the left ventricle (see Fig. 14–31). When the impulse arrives at the left ventricle, the left bundle branch may no longer be refractory, and the impulse may travel retrogradely through the left bundle branch. It is then possible that when the impulse arrives at the proximal end of the left bundle branch, the bundle of His and the right bundle branch may no longer be refractory. In this case, the impulse will travel retrograde through the bundle of His (inscribing a His bundle electrogram) and at the same time antegrade through the right bundle branch, to excite the ventricle a short time later from the same point at which V_2 began. For this reason, V_3 usually has a similar morphology to V_2. It is said that V_3 must be preceded by a His electrogram, but we believe that there could be more conduction delay in the His bundle than in the right bundle branch and the His bundle could be depolarized after the right ventricular myocardium, thereby masking the His bundle electrogram. For this reason, the diagnosis of macro-reentry may be difficult. This phenomenon occurs in normal children and is not related to prior history of ventricular tachycardia, prior surgical ventriculotomy, or right bundle-branch block on the surface electrocardiogram. The importance of macro-reentry is that it be distinguished from the pathologic ventricular arrhythmias that have different names for the same problem: "micro-reentry," "intra-ventricular reentry (IVR)," and "non–bundle-branch reentry (NBBR)." In these situations, the morphology of V_3 is different from V_2, and a His bundle electrogram does not precede V_3 (Fig. 14–32).

The distinction among micro-reentry, abnormal automaticity, and triggered activity in the cardiac catheterization laboratory follows the same principles as those used for supraventricular tachycardia (see chapters 2, 6, and 11). The most difficult distinction is between reentry and triggered activity. Both may be induced and terminated by premature beats or rapid pacing. It appears that triggered activity may be more easily induced by trains of extrastimuli (10 or more beats), whereas reentry is more easily induced by two or three extrastimuli.[36] The next criterion is that, in general, the interval from the last initiating beat to the first spontaneous beat of the tachycardia is shorter at more rapid inducing cycle lengths with triggered activity (i.e., there is a direct relationship between coupling interval and inducing cycle length) whereas with reentry, this relationship is inverse. Finally, triggered activity tends to have decreasing cycle lengths at the beginning of the tachycardia ("warm-up"), whereas reentry may have alternating long and short cycle lengths ("oscillation"). These latter two "rules" are less definite.[37, 38]

The only positive diagnostic criterion for abnormal automaticity is the spontaneous initiation of a rhythm with progressively shortening cycle lengths ("warm-up"). The other major criterion is negative: rhythms caused by abnormal automaticity cannot be initiated or terminated by premature stimuli or overdrive pacing. The problem with this definition is that if a rhythm cannot be induced by pacing or terminated by pacing, it could be any of the three mechanisms. The final criterion that has been used for abnormal automaticity is the "reset" phenomenon, in which premature beats introduced at progressively shorter cycle lengths result in less than a fully compensatory pause with an equal return cycle length. This has recently been found in reentrant rhythms with entrainment as well as in triggered activity, indicating that this is not a specific response.[6, 36, 39] Therefore, with few exceptions, it is not possible at present to assess with certainty the mechanism of a ventricular tachyarrhythmia.

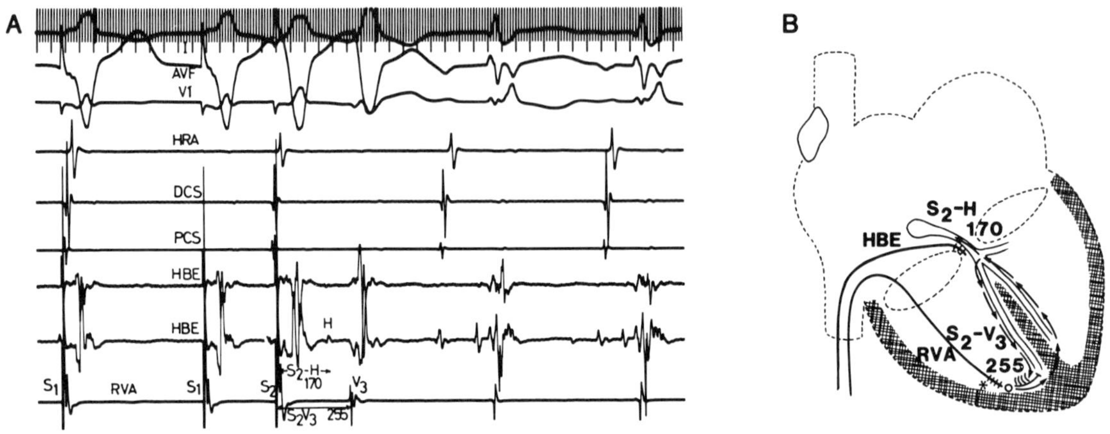

FIGURE 14–31

(A) Intracardiac recordings showing a V_3 phenomenon. The tracing begins with the last two beats of paced ventricular rhythm at a cycle length (S_1S_1) of 480 ms. A premature ventricular stimulus is introduced at an S_1S_2 interval of 250 ms. After V_2 there is a nonstimulated ventricular complex that is identical in morphology on the surface electrocardiogram leads to the paced complexes. Note that the earliest activation of V_3 is in the right ventricular apex at the same point at which the premature ventricular stimulus was introduced. V_3 occurs 255 ms after the premature ventricular stimulus. A His bundle electrogram (H) is inscribed 170 ms after the premature ventricular stimulus. *(B)* Diagram explaining the intracardiac electrophysiologic recordings shown in A. Two catheters are diagrammed, one in the right ventricular apex (RVA) and one in the area of the His bundle (HBE). The numbers are times in milliseconds after the premature stimulus has been delivered through the RVA catheter. The impulse blocks in the right bundle branch but conducts through the septal musculature retrograde through the left bundle branch. The impulse then continues retrograde to depolarize the His bundle 170 ms after the stimulus (S_2-H), and the impulse spreads antegradely through the right bundle branch, beginning to excite the right ventricle at the point where S_2 originally blocked. V_3 is detected first with the right ventricular apex catheter 255 ms after S_2.

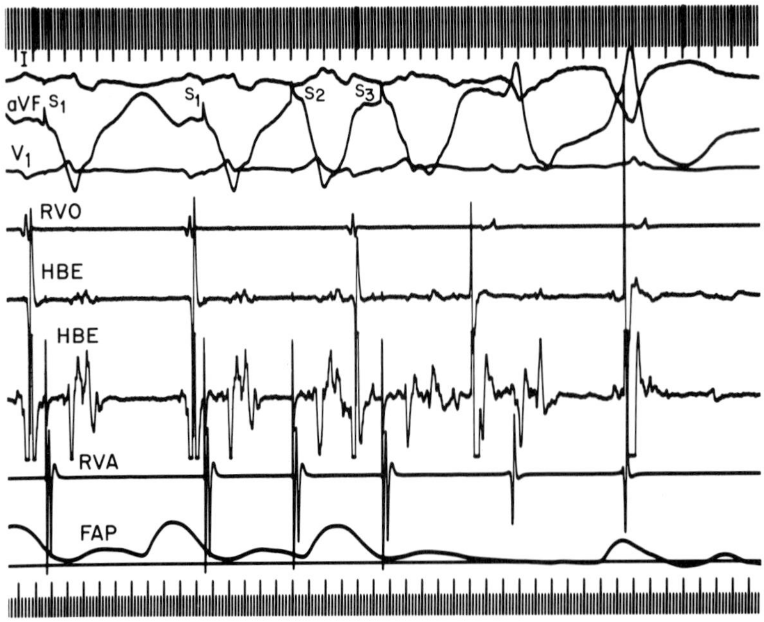

FIGURE 14–32

The tracings have the general organization as those in Figure 14–31. In this patient, after two ventricular premature beats (S_2 and S_3), there are two "micro-reentry" or "nonbundle branch reentry" beats. These beats have a different morphology from the paced beats.

Hopefully, in the future, with monophasic action potential recordings or even more advanced techniques, we will be better able to assess the electrophysiologic mechanisms of these arrhythmias.

INTRACARDIAC ELECTROPHYSIOLOGY STUDY FOR VENTRICULAR ARRHYTHMIAS

Indications

The indications for electrophysiology study continue to change as studies reporting the relative worth of this procedure in different situations become available. At the present time, there are two unequivocal indications for electrophysiology study. The first is to establish a diagnosis in a patient with an undiagnosed "wide QRS" (or "different QRS") tachycardia. While ventricular tachycardia is the most likely diagnosis in such a patient, it is possible that this could be antidromic Wolff-Parkinson-White syndrome or tachycardia utilizing a Mahaim fiber (see chapters 10 and 11). The second unequivocal reason for performing an electrophysiology study is for intracardiac mapping in a patient who is going to have surgical ablation of ventricular tachycardia. This technique will be discussed in the next section.

All the remaining indications are relative. For example, in many centers, electrophysiology studies are done to attempt prediction of the effectiveness of antiarrhythmic drug therapy. The concept is to induce sustained ventricular tachycardia first in the baseline state; the patient is then started on chronic oral drug therapy, and after the drug has reached steady state with a therapeutic serum concentration, the patient is returned to the electrophysiology laboratory and attempts are again made to induce ventricular tachycardia. This technique is used relatively infrequently in children, since it is not common to induce sustained ventricular tachycardia in a child. We largely reserve chronic drug electrophysiology studies for patients who are symptomatic and who have recurrent sustained ventricular tachycardia. It is an extremely invasive procedure and involves repeated trips to the catheterization laboratory. In addition, chronic drug studies may not be useful, particularly if the ventricular arrhythmia is being treated with phenytoin.[40] Some data suggest that phenytoin may be protective from sudden death and may eliminate large numbers of premature ventricular contractions from the Holter electrocardiogram; however, the patient may still have inducible ventricular tachycardia while being treated with the drug.[41] Recent findings also show that sudden death can be prevented in patients after repair of tetralogy of Fallot, with treatment of ventricular arrhythmias based on virtual elimination of any ventricular arrhythmias from the Holter electrocardiogram. This raises the question as to the necessity of invasive assessment of drug efficacy in asymptomatic patients.[42] Nonetheless, in patients with very low levels of ambient ectopy who have inducible sustained ventricular tachycardia, chronic drug testing with electrophysiology studies is a necessity.

In certain groups of patients, there is a known association between ventricular arrhythmias and later sudden death (e.g., postoperative tetralogy of Fallot).[43] If such a patient had syncopal or presyncopal episodes on the Holter monitor without obvious cause (neither bradyarrhythmias nor "significant" ventricular arrhythmias), electrophysiology study should be considered along with attempts to induce ventricular tachycardia. The data on intracardiac electrophysiology studies in patients after repair of tetralogy of Fallot will be discussed in a subsequent section.

Finally, between 50% and 75% of children who are thought to have a "normal" heart and ventricular tachycardia will be found to have a hemodynamic or angiographic abnormality at cardiac catheterization.[44] Children with ventricular tachycardia, therefore, require hemodynamic and angiographic assessment. In general, since children with a truly normal heart and clinical ventricular tachycardia do not usually have inducible ventricular tachycardia in the electrophysiology laboratory, tachycardia induction may also be a test for determining if the heart is truly normal.[45] If the heart is truly normal, sustained ventricular tachycardia will not be induced; alternatively, if sustained ventricular tachycardia is induced, the heart is probably abnormal. The data are small in number, and further studies are required to clarify this point. In these patients, myocardial biopsies should be performed at the same time as the angiographic and electrophysiology study.

Clearly, there needs to be a provocative test created with appropriate sensitivity and specificity to identify patients at risk of sudden death. It is likely that the tests will be some combination of electrical and pharmacologic stimulation. At the present time, despite Holter electrocardiograms and electrophysiology studies showing normal results, patients with certain conditions continue to die suddenly. These conditions include postoperative tetralogy of Fallot, prolonged QT interval, congestive cardiomyopathy, and hypertrophic cardiomyopathy. Our predictive ability must be improved.

In the area of research, several problems remain to be investigated. The role of electrophysiology study as a prognostic test in asymptomatic patients with ventricular arrhythmias is not known. In general, the findings at electrophysiology study have paralleled the clinical arrhythmias. The majority of patients after repair of tetralogy of Fallot who have ventricular tachycardia on the Holter electrocardiogram also have inducible nonsustained or sustained ventricular tachycardia in the electrophysiology laboratory.[46] However, it is not yet known whether the patient who has no clinical ventricular arrhythmias and who has inducible ventricular tachycardia in the electrophysiology laboratory is at risk for sudden death; similarly, the prognosis is unknown for the patient with numerous multiform premature ventricular contractions and couplets who has no inducible ventricular arrhythmia at electrophysiology study. These questions need to be answered with prospective randomized studies.

Another area of research is in the diagnosis of the prolonged QT interval syndrome. We frequently encounter children who have had one or two syncopal episodes and whose corrected QT intervals are at the upper limits of normal. It is not yet possible to stimulate ventricular arrhythmias in the electrophysiology laboratory in such patients. A likely reason for this is that the mechanisms may not be reentrant. Techniques for studying these patients in the electrophysiology laboratory need to be developed.

Attempts to ascertain a truer mechanism for many of the ventricular arrhythmias also need to be made. For example, patients with an otherwise normal heart may have ventricular tachycardia that is completely suppressed by verapamil. These arrhythmias could be caused by triggered activity.[38] Catheter recording techniques or pacing protocols need to be developed to make it possible to define the mechanism for ventricular tachycardia with more specificity.

One additional area of research is concerned with direct treatment of arrhythmias in the electrophysiology laboratory. Thus far, attempts have been confined to the use of electrical ablative techniques using a defibrillator. It is likely that over the next several years, newer, safer, and more accurate techniques will be developed (e.g., laser, cooling, ultrasound, etc.) and electrophysiology will be expanded into another area of therapeutics.

Technique

The overall plan for electrophysiologic study of ventricular tachycardia is shown in Table 14–1. Basic measurements are made with the patient in sinus rhythm. After tachy-

TABLE 14–1
OUTLINE OF ELECTROPHYSIOLOGY STUDY OF VENTRICULAR TACHYCARDIA*

Basic measurements
- Conduction dispersion
- Effective refractory period dispersion
- Late potentials

Induce VT
- Rapid atrial pacing
- Rapid ventricular pacing
- Single or double premature ventricular stimuli into paced atrial rhythm
- Single or double premature ventricular stimuli into paced ventricular rhythm
- "Burst" ventricular pacing

If VT is noninducible, repeat the above five steps at different sites or with patient receiving infusion of isoproterenol

Characterize VT
- Is it ventricular tachycardia?
- Ventricular activation sequence; presence of late potentials or continuous activity
- Ventricular cycle length
- Introduction of premature ventricular stimuli

Terminate VT
- Asynchronous slow ventricular pacing ("underdrive")
- Single or double premature ventricular stimuli into ventricular tachycardia
- "Overdrive" ventricular pacing
- "Burst" ventricular pacing
- Cardioversion

Drug studies
- Drug success: inability to induce sustained ventricular tachycardia

*Reprinted from Gillette PC, Garson A Jr: Pediatric Cardiac Dysrhythmias. New York, Grune & Stratton, 1981, p 334.

cardia is induced and a ventricular origin confirmed, the ventricular tachycardia is characterized by basic measurements, and if the patient's hemodynamic status permits, the response of ventricular tachycardia to certain perturbations is analyzed. Then the tachycardia is terminated by whatever means possible. Finally, drugs may be administered while attempting to reinduce ventricular tachycardia and the resulting response measured.

BASIC MEASUREMENTS

In most children, four catheters are used. One catheter is positioned in the coronary sinus to record from the base of the left ventricle, and another is placed across the tricuspid valve to record atrial septal activation, a His bundle electrogram, and ventricular septal activation. The other catheters may be moved to different sites to record ventricular activation (for example, from the right ventricular apex and right ventricular infundibulum). In most ventricular tachycardia studies, it is essential to have a catheter in the atrium to record an atrial electrogram. Otherwise it is difficult to tell, especially with the initiation of a nonsustained arrhythmia, which beats are supraventricular capture beats. Using the technique of Mullins,[47] in which a long sheath is introduced transseptally into the left atrium or left ventricle, an electrode catheter may be placed into the left ventricle if the child does not have a patent foramen ovale. It is also possible to use the retrograde arterial approach to position the catheter in the left ventricle. It is an electrophysiologic principle that reentrant arrhythmias are more easily induced with a stimulus site close to the reentry circuit. Since, in children, the majority of the circuits lie in the right ventricle, right ventricular stimulation usually achieves this goal. This is in contrast to adults, where most circuits lie in the left ventricle or left side of the septum where left ventricular stimulation may occasionally be necessary. Since the induced arrhythmias in children can be extremely rapid and lead to hemodynamic deterioration, all patients undergoing such a study should have systemic arterial blood pressure continuously monitored by a plastic cannula inserted into the femoral artery.

In studying a patient with ventricular arrhythmias who may undergo drug treatment that could potentially suppress the sinus node or AV conduction, both sinus node function and AV conduction system function should be assessed. Unfortunately, assessment of the sinus node and AV conduction system by current intracardiac electrophysiologic techniques is only helpful if the two functions are grossly abnormal. Nonetheless, assessment of these parameters has been recommended recently by a consensus panel to standardize intracardiac electrophysiologic studies.[48]

Each of the intracardiac recordings made from various sites should be examined for the presence of "late potentials."[49] These are discrete, high-frequency depolarizations that occur after the end of the QRS complex. They are thought to be the manifestations of delayed activation in a group of fibers and the result of a severe, although localized, conduction disturbance. Late potentials may occur near the site of origin of ventricular tachycardia. Therefore, even if it is impossible to induce ventricular tachycardia, the findings of late potentials in sinus rhythm may indicate the possible site of an arrhythmia in a patient known to have clinical episodes of ventricular tachycardia. This has been shown by Deanfield, McKenna, and Rowland in patients who had undergone surgery for tetralogy of Fallot.[50] Patients with induced ventricular tachycardia had significantly more delayed and fragmented electrograms than did those without ventricular tachycardia.

Recently, the recording of monophasic action potentials on the endocardial surface has been employed as a possible means of assessing action potential duration as well as the presence of early and late afterdepolarizations and automaticity.[51] It is possible that in the future these measurements will provide information about specific mechanisms of arrhythmias and drug actions in individual patients.

INDUCED VENTRICULAR ARRHYTHMIAS

Several methods are available to induce ventricular arrhythmias. Since rapid atrial pacing and the introduction of premature atrial beats into sinus rhythm can induce ventricular arrhythmias, the "ventricular induction" protocol actually begins with the assessment of sinus node and AV conduction system function. Some patients who were thought to have triggered activity as the basis for their arrhythmias had ventricular tachycardia induced by atrial pacing.[37, 38] The reason for this is that the cycle length change was probably sufficient to induce the arrhythmia, instead of the complex interaction involving conduction delay of successive ventricular extrastimuli that might be necessary for induction of a reentrant arrhythmia.

In the past, the ventricular extrastimulus protocol began with the introduction of single and paired premature ventricular extrastimuli into sinus rhythm. This was based on the data from Greene, Reid, and Schaeffer,[52] who found that the induction of even a single micro-reentrant beat implied a high chance of sudden death in adults with coronary disease. This has proved to be a rare and nonspecific finding in both adults and children, and so we now begin our ventricular extrastimulus protocol with the introduction of single premature ventricular extrastimuli delivered after eight ventricular paced beats at a constant cycle length (Figs. 14–31 and 14–32). The first cycle length used is usually 500 ms (S_1S_1), and the premature ventricular extrastimulus is delivered 480 ms after the last ventricular paced beat (S_1S_2). The S_1S_2 interval is decreased sequentially by 10 ms until the ventricular extrastimulus fails to capture. This S_1S_2 interval is the effective refractory period at that site and at that cycle length. The effective refractory period may change with decreasing cycle length (usually with a shorter refractory period), and may change with a different site in the ventricle. The measurement of the absolute refractory period, the "dispersion" of refractory periods between different sites in the ventricles, and the change in refractory period with different cycle lengths have all been examined as possible predictors of ventricular arrhythmias. Thus far, none of these parameters has shown any significant predictive power. This technique may be extended, and double premature ventricular extrastimuli may be introduced into ventricular paced rhythm (Fig. 14–33). Once the effective refractory period of S_1S_2 has been reached (e.g., 200 ms), the S_1S_2 interval is increased by 50 ms (e.g., 250 milliseconds), and the interval between the first and second premature extrastimulus (S_2S_3) is set equal to the S_1S_2 (e.g., 250 ms) (Fig. 14–34). The S_2S_3 interval is progressively shortened by 10 ms each time, until S_3 fails to capture. Then the S_1S_2 interval is shortened by 10 ms. Since the refractory period of S_2S_3 is dependent on the S_1S_2 cycle length, with the shorter S_1S_2, the previously refractory S_3 will now capture. The S_2S_3 is again progressively shortened until S_3 fails to capture, then S_1S_2 is shortened again. This sequence is followed until S_2 fails to capture. A similar sequence is followed for the introduction of triple ventricular extrastimuli, where initially the S_1S_2, S_2S_3, and S_3S_4 are set equal. The S_3S_4 is then progressively shortened until S_4 fails to capture, and then the S_2S_3 is shortened by 10 ms, etc. After triple ventricular extrastimuli are delivered at one cycle length at the right ventricular apex, a second drive cycle length (usually 400 ms) is used. If sustained ventricular tachycardia is not induced, then "burst" ventricular pacing is employed (see Fig. 14–34): the ventricle is paced for eight beats at a cycle length of 300 ms (200 per minute). The cycle length is progressively decreased in 20-ms steps until every other stimulus fails to capture (usually at approximately 180 ms). If none of these maneuvers is successful in inducing sustained ventricular tachycardia from the right ventricular apex, then the catheter is moved to the right ventricular outflow tract and the same protocol is followed. If ventricular tachycardia still cannot be induced, then infusion of isoproterenol (0.1 μg/kg/min) may be instituted and the maneuvers tried again.

Sensitivity and Specificity of Electrophysiology Protocols

In general, there are two distinct reasons for attempting induction of ventricular tachycardia in a child, and the induction protocols need to be tailored appropriately. The first reason is to reproduce a known clinical arrhythmia in a patient with documented sustained ventricular tachycardia. This can be done prior to an ablation attempt so that intracardiac mapping can be performed with localization of the site of earliest endocardial activation. Alternatively, it can be important to induce sustained ventricular tachycardia so that drugs to suppress the arrhythmia can be investigated. These indications are similar to the ones used for electrophysiology study in adults with ventricular arrhythmias, and a similar philosophy is used in devising the induction protocol. The most aggressive protocol possible that does not result in a nonclinical arrhythmia should be used. In these patients, since the clinical arrhythmia is pre-

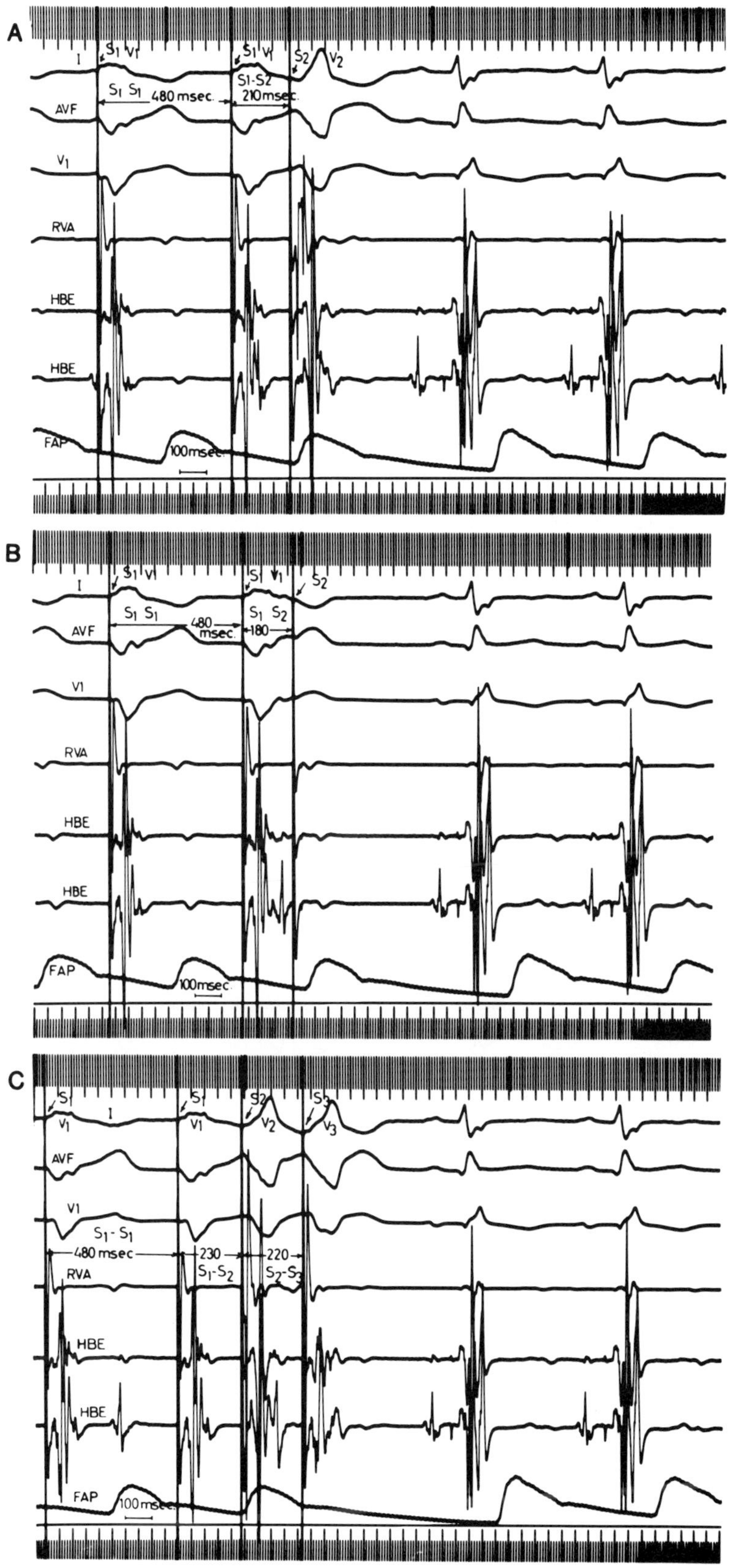

FIGURE 14–33

Intracardiac recordings during premature ventricular stimulation into paced ventricular rhythm in a single patient. Shown in each part of this figure are the last two of eight paced ventricular beats at a cycle length of 480 ms. These are followed by premature ventricular stimuli. *(A)* Single premature ventricular stimulus is delivered at a coupling interval (S_1S_2) of 210 ms. This is followed by a single ventricular response (V_2), and sinus rhythm resumes. *(B)* Cycle length of the premature ventricular stimulus has been shortened to 180 ms. There is no ventricular response. Therefore, 180 ms is the effective refractory period of the right ventricular apex at the paced cycle length of 480 ms. *(C)* S_1S_2 interval has been lengthened to 230 ms, and a second premature stimulus (S_3) has been introduced 220 ms after S_2. Both S_2 and S_3 are followed by single ventricular responses. No unstimulated extrasystoles are induced.

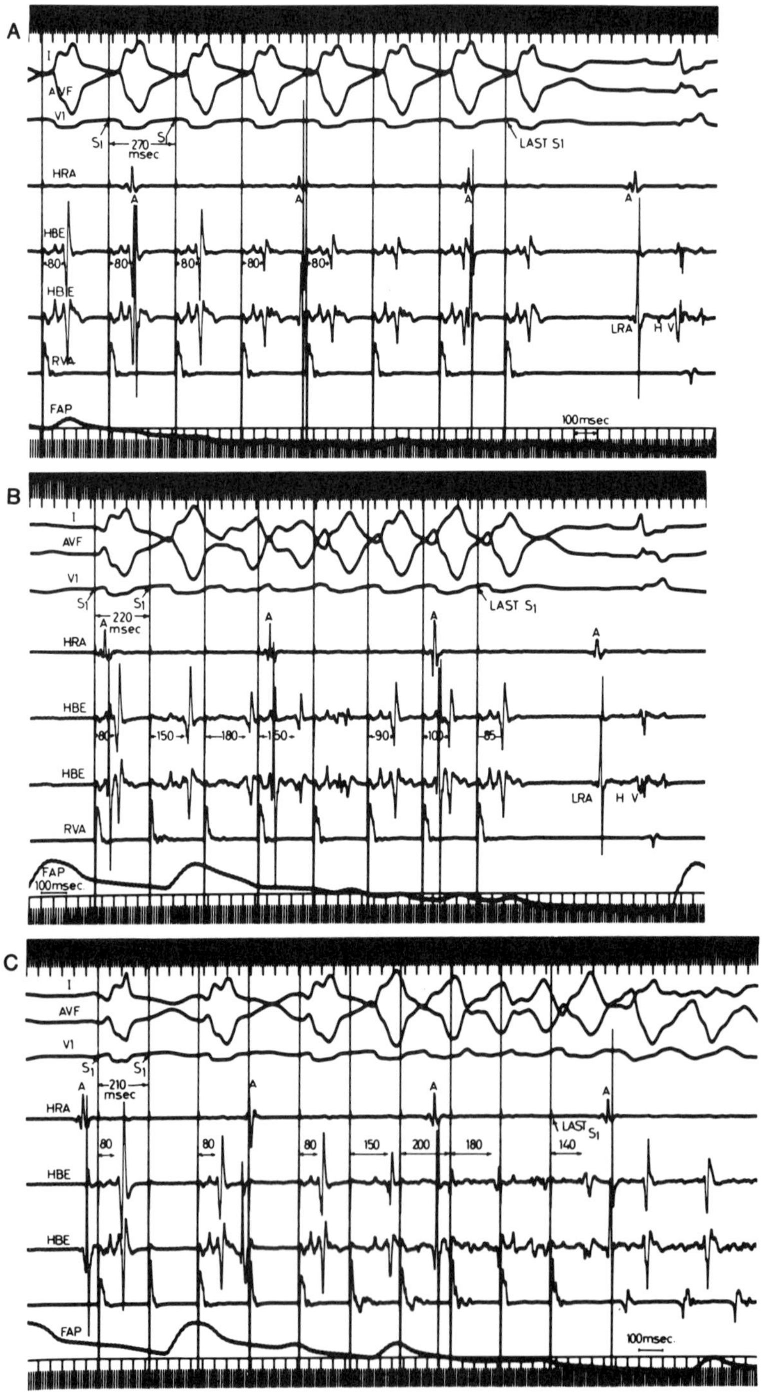

FIGURE 14–34
Intracardiac recordings during burst ventricular pacing of the right ventricular apex in a single patient. *(A)* At a cycle length of 270 ms (equivalent to a heart rate of 222 bpm), there is 1:1 capture of the ventricle, and the interval from the stimulus that originates in the right ventricular apex to the right ventricular septal electrogram (recorded on the HBE lead) is constant at 80 ms. An isoelectric period follows each ventricular electrogram in the HBE lead. No unstimulated extrasystoles are induced. *(B)* At a pacing cycle length of 220 ms (equivalent to a heart rate of 272 bpm), there is progressive increase in conduction time from the right ventricular apex to the right ventricular septal electrogram (from 80 ms to 180 ms). This is accompanied by a disorganization of the ventricular complexes as seen on the surface ECG leads. Then constant conduction resumes on the last three beats. The isoelectric area after the ventricular electrogram (HBE lead) is shortened but still present after every beat with cessation of pacing, and sinus rhythm resumes without nonstimulated extrasystoles. *(C)* At a pacing cycle length of 210 ms (equivalent to a heart rate of 286 bpm), there is 2:1 block of the stimulus to the ventricle seen on the first four paced beats. Then 1:1 stimulus to ventricular conduction begins, and there is progressive conduction delay from the stimulus in the right ventricular apex to the right ventricular septal electrogram, similar to that shown in Figure 14–34(B). However, after the eighth paced beat, continuous activity without an isoelectric period is recorded on the HBE lead, and ventricular tachycardia is induced. With cessation of pacing, ventricular tachycardia continues.

sumably available for comparison, and since it is essential to induce sustained ventricular tachycardia, it would seem reasonable to deliver triple, or even quadruple, ventricular extrastimuli in the right ventricle and in the left ventricle at several cycle lengths, with augmentation by isoproterenol if necessary. If a ventricular tachycardia is induced with a different morphology than the known ventricular tachycardia, or ventricular fibrillation is induced with very aggressive parts of the protocol (triple or quadruple ventricular extrastimuli), it is not likely that these arrhythmias have clinical significance, but it is important to attempt to be as aggressive as possible to reproduce the clinical arrhythmia.

The philosophy is entirely different in many children, in whom the electrophysiology study is being used in an attempt at prognostication. For example, in patients who have undergone repair of tetralogy of Fallot, it would be helpful to know which patients are at risk for the later development of ventricular tachycardia. For this indication, the induction protocol must be aggressive enough that the test is sufficiently sensitive to identify patients at risk, but not so aggressive that the specificity is lost, and a large number of patients who are not at risk have arrhythmias induced. In order to tailor these studies, it is important to understand the response of normal children. We have studied 77 children with an otherwise normal heart and supraventricular tachycardia using ventricular extrastimulus testing.[45] We found that with double ventricular extrastimuli delivered into paced ventricular rhythm at a cycle length of 500 ms and with burst ventricular pacing (all performed at the right ventricular apex), none of these children developed even a single micro-reentrant beat. Therefore, when using this extrastimulus protocol in the child with a normal heart, it is abnormal to have even a single micro-reentrant beat induced. We performed the same extrastimulus protocol on an equal number of patients with an abnormal heart (e.g., unoperated congenital heart disease, mitral valve prolapse, hypotrophic cardiomyopathy, and postoperative congenital heart disease). We found a reasonably good correlation between the presence of ventricular arrhythmias on the Holter electrocardiogram and inducibility in the catheterization laboratory, although 5% of patients without any ventricular arrhythmia on the Holter recording had micro-reentrant beats induced, and 7% had nonsustained ventricular tachycardia induced. On the other hand, of those with ventricular tachycardia on the Holter recording, 93% had an arrhythmia induced, including 13% with nonsustained ventricular tachycardia and 53% with sustained ventricular tachycardia. The results of this study demonstrate that paired ventricular extrastimuli and burst pacing is, in general, an adequate protocol. Recently, Benson and Anderson[53] have found the use of triple ventricular extrastimuli to be an important adjunct in inducing ventricular tachycardia in children with previous cardiac arrest. Had the triple ventricular extrastimuli not been used, the electrophysiology study would have failed to identify ventricular tachycardia as the cause of the cardiac arrest (i.e., the study would not have been sensitive enough). Therefore, it may be that triple ventricular extrastimuli should be included in most prognostic protocols in children. As in adults,[54] this may result in the initiation of nonclinical arrhythmias, but in our brief experience the introduction of triple ventricular extrastimuli in normal patients rarely results in even a single micro-reentrant beat. While it may be possible to induce several micro-reentrant beats in patients with an abnormal heart who are not at risk for ventricular arrhythmias, it is likely that the induction of sustained monomorphic ventricular tachycardia with triple ventricular extrastimuli is a warning signal. It is important to point out, however, that it has not yet been demonstrated that the induction of sustained monomorphic ventricular tachycardia in asymptomatic children and young adults with a normal Holter electrocardiogram has any prognostic significance. Additional follow-up studies will be necessary in a larger number of patients to determine the specific value of intracardiac electrophysiologic studies in predicting which patients are likely to develop clinical arrhythmias.

CHARACTERIZE VENTRICULAR TACHYCARDIA

Is It Ventricular Tachycardia?

The intracardiac electrophysiologic definition of ventricular tachycardia is a tachycardia in which the His bundle electrogram occurs after the onset of the QRS complex, or in which no His bundle electrogram precedes the QRS complex (Figs. 14–35 and 14–36). It is understood that a stable His bundle electrogram must have been present prior to the onset of tachycardia. It must also be certain that the reason for the loss of the His bundle electrogram is not movement of the catheter. The best proof of this is reappearance of the His bundle electrogram with resumption of sinus rhythm. By strict definition, ventricular tachycardia is also present if a His bundle precedes the QRS complex during tachycardia, but the HV interval is shorter than the HV interval in sinus rhythm. This has been correlated with tachycardia occurring in a bundle branch (so-called "fascicular tachycardia"). The reason for the short HV interval is explained as follows. If it is assumed that an area in the proximal part of the right bundle branch is causing the tachycardia and that approximately 35 ms are required for the impulse to travel down the right bundle branch to begin ventricular excitation, but at the same time the impulse travels retrogradely to excite the bundle of His, (for example, only requiring 10 ms), then the interval between the observed His deflection (actually a retrograde His deflection) and the onset of ventricular activation is 25 ms. In the same patient, in sinus rhythm, it is assumed that the interval between an antegrade His deflection and ventricular activation is 35 ms.

Certain definitions are necessary in the description of ventricular tachycardia. "Sustained" refers to a tachycardia that lasts for at least 30 s or requires intervention before that time because of hemodynamic collapse. "Nonsustained" refers to an arrhythmia that lasts from three beats to 30 s. "Monomorphic" is defined as a uniform morphology of the ventricular tachycardia, whereas "polymorphic" refers to a continuously changing morphology. If after several beats of one morphology, the tachycardia changes to a different morphology and remains in that morphology, it should still be referred to as monomorphic tachycardia.

Using these criteria, there are two types of tachycardia with which ventricular tachycardia may be confused. The first is the rare antidromic type of reciprocating tachycardia caused by Wolff-Parkinson-White syndrome in which the reentry circuit uses the Kent bundle as the antegrade limb and the AV node as the retrograde limb. In this type of tachycardia, the His bundle electrogram may occur after the end of the QRS, or the His bundle electrogram may be obscured by the ventricular electrogram. The following three points are helpful in distinguishing between these two types of tachycardia:

1. If there is AV dissociation, it must be ventricular tachycardia, since in Wolff-Parkinson-White, the atria form part of the reentry circuit and AV dissociation cannot occur.
2. In Wolff-Parkinson-White, the QRS morphology during tachycardia can be reproduced by pacing the atria at the proximal end of the Kent bundle. Pacing the atria will not reproduce the morphology of ventricular tachycardias.
3. A properly timed premature atrial extrastimulus can shorten the VV interval even when the bundle of His is refractory, thus suggesting that the antegrade limb of the tachycardia does not involve the His bundle.

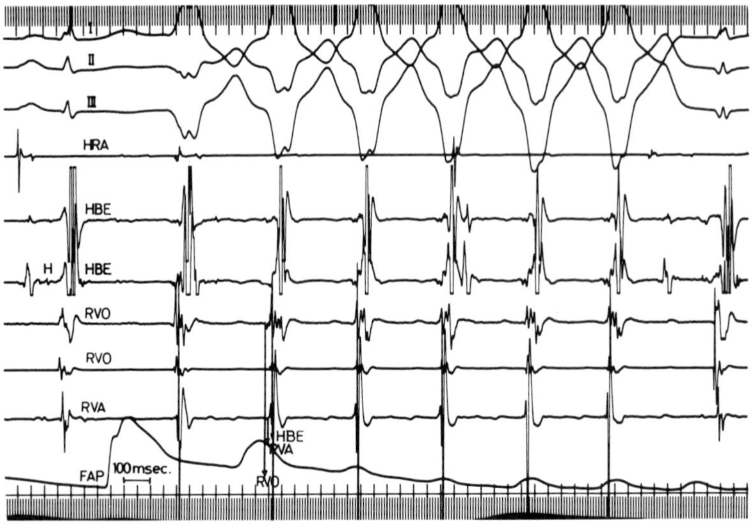

FIGURE 14–35
Intracardiac recordings during ventricular tachycardia.

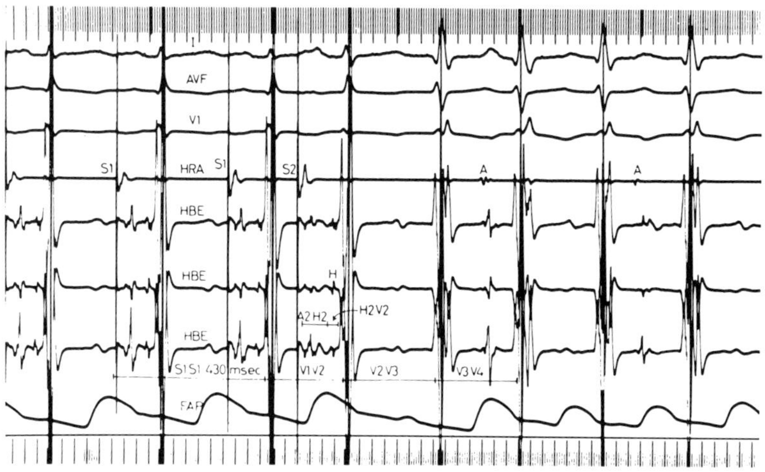

FIGURE 14–36
Induction of ventricular tachycardia by atrial pacing. The last two atrial paced beats (S_1S_1, 430 ms) of a train of eight beats are shown, followed by an atrial premature extrastimulus (S_2) that conducts to the ventricle. Note that there is a His bundle electrogram (H) preceding each ventricular complex of the first four beats to the left of the tracing. The last four beats are slightly wider, have no His bundle electrogram preceding them, and represent ventricular tachycardia. Note that there is AV dissociation on the right of the tracing.

The second type of tachycardia that can be confused with ventricular tachycardia is tachycardia resulting from a Mahaim fiber that connects the His bundle directly to the right ventricular myocardium. In this type of tachycardia, there may be AV dissociation, but pacing the atria will reproduce the morphology of the QRS complex during tachycardia. These concepts are more fully described in chapters 12 and 13 on preexcitation and supraventricular tachycardia.

We may also use atrial pacing to distinguish between supraventricular tachycardia with aberration and ventricular tachycardia. If atrial pacing at a more rapid rate than the tachycardia results in normalization of the QRS complex, the diagnosis is ventricular tachycardia.[55] If the QRS does not change with rapid atrial pacing or becomes more aberrant, then the diagnosis is supraventricular tachycardia. Also helpful in making the diagnosis of ventricular tachycardia is the presence of fusion and capture beats during atrial pacing.

Ventricular Activation Sequence

When ventricular tachycardia is initiated, catheters should be moved to several sites in the ventricles and the ventricular activation sequence determined. The earliest site of endocardial activation can be determined by identifying the earliest local ventricular electrogram (Figs. 14–37, 14–38, and 14–39). The finding of continuous electrical activity throughout the cardiac cycle most likely identifies an area of slow conduction (see Fig. 14–34).[6] An area of slow conduction may correlate with the site of onset of tachycardia as determined at surgery; however, there may be areas of slow conduction in the ventricle that are unrelated to the primary site of origin of tachycardia.

Ventricular Cycle Length

At the start of ventricular tachycardia (whether spontaneous or induced), it is important to observe the changes in ventricular cycle lengths that occur in the first few beats and correlate these with the initiating cycle lengths, since there may be a relationship of these parameters to the cellular mechanism (see section on electrophysiologic mechanisms).

TERMINATION OF VENTRICULAR TACHYCARDIA

Using programmed stimulation, single, double, or triple premature ventricular extrastimuli may be introduced into the tachycardia in an effort to terminate the arrhythmia. The same procedure is followed as that used for induction of ventricular tachycardia by premature ventricular extrastimuli, except that the pacemaker is set to sense the QRS complex of ventricular tachycardia, and premature beats are brought progressively closer to the preceding QRS of the tachycardia. The ventricle may be paced at a rate of 10 to 20 beats per minute faster than the tachycardia ("overdrive" pacing), or "burst" ventricular pacing may be used to terminate ventricular tachycardia in the same way that it was used to initiate the arrhythmia. If the tachycardia stops in response to any of these

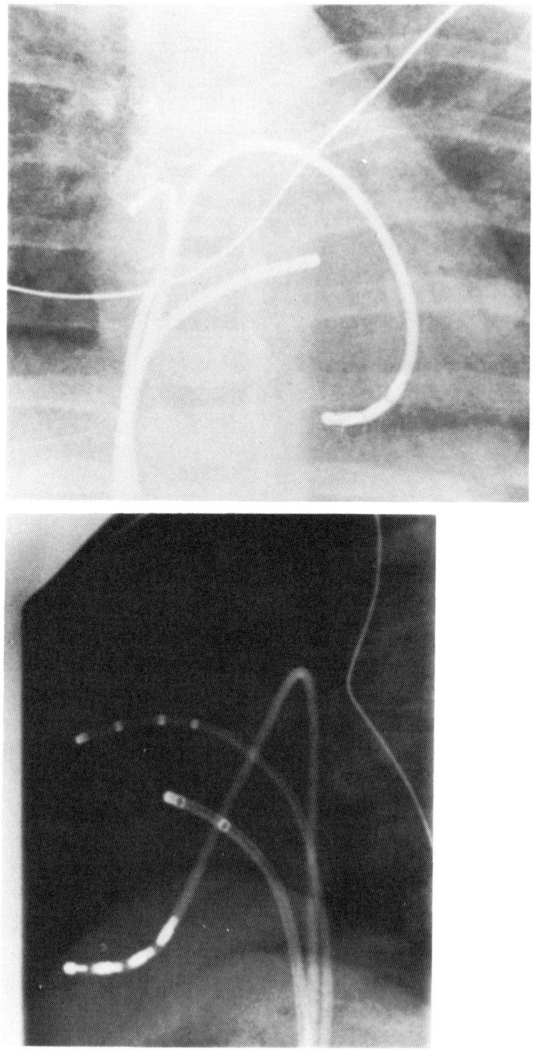

FIGURE 14–37
Anteroposterior (top) and lateral (bottom) radiographs taken showing catheter positions for the tracings shown in Figure 14–38. One catheter is in the superior right ventricle, one is in the His bundle region, and the most inferior catheter has been placed transseptally into the left ventricle, with the tip pointing anteriorly.

maneuvers, it is likely to be a result of reentry or triggered activity and not abnormal automaticity. Synchronized DC electrocardioversion (0.5–1.5 J/kg) may be used both diagnostically and therapeutically. If the patient becomes symptomatic from ventricular tachycardia, or if none of the other measures used to terminate the tachycardia have been successful, cardioversion should be performed. It can also be used as a diagnostic tool, since cardioversion will not stop ventricular tachycardia caused by automaticity, but in the majority of cases is successful in stopping ventricular tachycardia caused by reentry or triggered activity. If none of these measures is successful, the tachycardia could still be caused by reentry or triggered activity with "concealed perpetuation" (i.e., the tachycardia continues despite the fact that the majority of the heart is depolarized by the cardioversion).[6]

Drug Studies

The performance of electrophysiologic studies in the patient who has been treated with an antiarrhythmic drug may be helpful in choosing a long-term agent. The studies rely on two assumptions: (1) The ventricular tachycardia induced by electrophysiologic study is the same tachycardia that was demonstrated clinically in the patient. This has been discussed previously. (2) The response to the drug in the electrophysiology laboratory predicts the long-term clinical response.

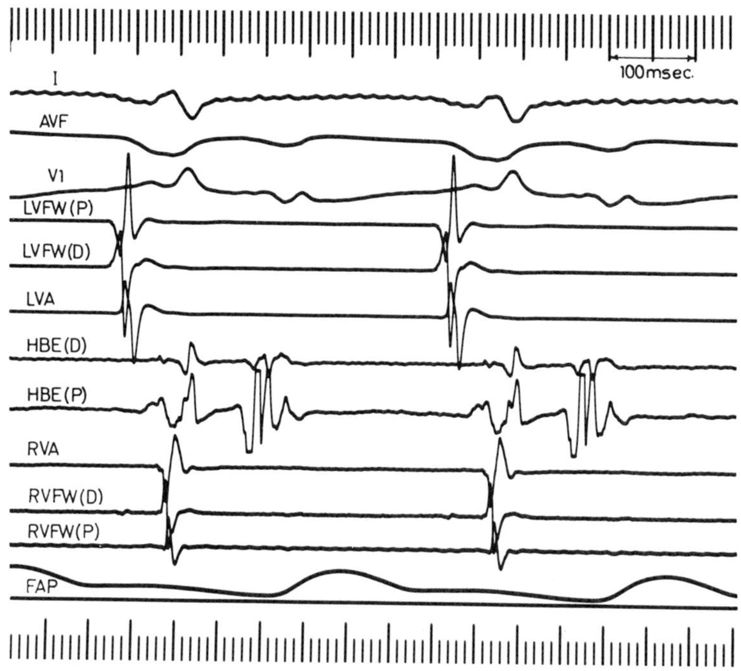

FIGURE 14–38
Tracings recorded with the catheter positions noted in Figure 14–37. At the top of the tracing are the three surface ECG leads, followed by three from the left ventricular catheter (LVFW = left ventricular free wall, proximal and distal; LVA = left ventricular apex). The next two tracings are in the His bundle region (HBE, distal and proximal) followed by the right ventricular tracings (RVA = right ventricular apex; RVFW = right ventricular free wall, distal and proximal). Note that the earliest site of endocardial activation is in the distal left ventricular free wall pair of electrodes. This occurs approximately 20 ms before the onset of the surface QRS complex.

For certain drugs, this has been shown to be true in both adults and children.[39, 41, 56–58]

At present, the only agents used clinically for acute intravenous infusion are procainamide (10–15 mg/kg over 30 min) and propranolol (0.2 mg/kg over 15 min). The acute intravenous effects of these drugs appear to be similar to the long-term oral effects. In fact, the acute intravenous effects of procainamide in general correlate with the long-term oral effects of any of the type Ia drugs (procainamide, quinidine, disopyramide), although individual variations do occur, with success of one and failure of another. The acute intravenous effects of propranolol correlate somewhat with its long-term oral effect. Either drug can be given after the initiation of ventricular tachycardia during the baseline study and the effect measured. Drug success in the catheterization laboratory is defined as an inability to induce sustained ventricular tachycardia by any means of stimulation. Drug proarrhythmia is defined as (1) a resultant paradoxic increase in the rate of induced ventricular tachycardia, (2) the finding that ventricular tachycardia is easier to induce, or (3) the fact that once ventricular tachycardia is induced, it is incessant.[39] Other indicators of drug proarrhythmia are the degeneration to ventricular fibrillation or the

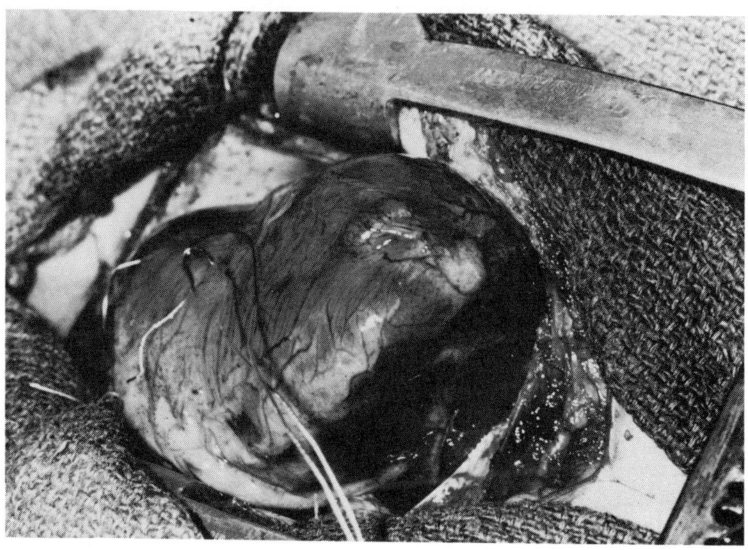

FIGURE 14–39
Operative photograph of the heart from the same patient studied in Figures 14–37 and 14–38. The heart is viewed from the apex. At the site of earliest endocardial activation, slightly posterior to the apex, was a lobulated tumor measuring 8 mm.

presence of hemodynamic compromise during ventricular tachycardia that had previously been well tolerated.

Drugs other than procainamide and propranolol are given orally, and the patient is returned to the electrophysiology laboratory after he or she has reached steady state (at least five half-lives). It has recently become apparent that for certain drugs, the electrophysiologic response does not necessarily predict the clinical response. For phenytoin, mexiletine, encainide, flecainide, propafenone, and amiodarone, the induction of ventricular tachycardia does not necessarily imply that ventricular tachycardia will recur clinically. On the other hand, the lack of induction while taking the drug doses generally correlates with the lack of appearance clinically.[41, 57]

A limited number of children have undergone chronic drug electrophysiologic testing. In eight patients who had undergone surgery to repair tetralogy of Fallot, Kugler et al[56] were able to find drugs that suppressed the inducibility of ventricular tachycardia in 100% of them: four with phenytoin and four with propranolol. Deal et al were less successful, reporting one success in 12 patients with type Ia drugs, one in three with propranolol, and one in four with phenytoin. While these studies are clearly of value in selected patients, we have found that other methods (e.g., Holter monitor or treadmill) may be equally effective in selecting an acceptable drug. On the other hand, if a patient has recurrent, symptomatic, sustained ventricular tachycardia, a drug must be found that prevents the induction of ventricular tachycardia by electrophysiology study before the patient leaves the hospital.

PVCs AND VENTRICULAR TACHYCARDIA: CLINICAL SITUATIONS AND MANAGEMENT

Acute Ventricular Arrhythmias

There are numerous acute clinical situations in which children may develop PVCs or ventricular tachycardia. Some of the more common causes are listed in Table 14–2. They fall into several categories. The first is disturbances in ventilation or electrolytes. The second consists of ventricular arrhythmias that can be induced by temperature change, such as diving into cold water.[59] This can create complex interaction with sinus bradycardia from facial immersion and ventricular arrhythmias potentiated by the sinus bradycardia and by sympathetic stimulation for the remainder of the body entering the cold water. The third class is drugs. The most likely drugs to induce ventricular arrhythmias are the sympathomimetics, especially drugs used for intravenous augmentation of contractility, and the oral decongestants.[60] "Recreational" amphetamines, hallucinogens, and marijuana release norepinephrine and may cause ventricular arrhythmias in patients with an underlying abnormal heart. Almost all of the antiarrhythmic drugs, particularly quinidine, can cause ventricular arrhythmias.[15, 61–64] There have also been recent reports of amiodarone-induced torsades de pointes.[65, 66] Some of the rarer causes include ventricular tachycardia secondary to hyperkalemia from large doses of potassium penicillin,[67] torsades de pointes from organophosphate poisoning (organophosphates have usually been associated with bradycardia),[68] and the statistical increase of premature ventricular contractions in women taking oral contraceptives.[69]

The last category of acute causes of ventricular arrhythmias involves the myocardium directly. The most obvious cause is the intracardiac catheter. Certainly, myocardial damage from infarction (commonly) or cardiac surgery (rarely) may cause acute ventricular arrhythmias. Ventricular arrhythmias may also occur for the first time during bacterial endocarditis.[70] The majority of these conditions are readily diagnosed. However, myocarditis deserves special comment, since it may be difficult to diagnose. Not all patients with myocarditis present with the characteristic appearance of chest pain, congestive heart failure, and electrocardiographic changes. In fact, 5% to 10% of children dying suddenly have active myocarditis at the time of their death,[71, 72] and as much as 50% of adults have autopsy evidence of previous myocarditis. Therefore, it is possible that myocarditis could present in an otherwise asymptomatic patient with ventricular tachycardia. Rocchini, Chun, and Dick reported that 10% of their children who presented

TABLE 14–2
ACUTE CAUSES OF PVCs AND VENTRICULAR TACHYCARDIA IN CHILDREN*

Hypoxia	Intracardiac catheters	Digitalis
Acidosis	Myocardial damage (immediately after cardiac surgery)	Quinidine, procainamide
Hypoglycemia	Myocardial infarction	Phenothiazines
Hypokalemia	Anesthetics (cyclopropane and Fluothane)	Sympathomimetics
Hyperkalemia		Caffeine
Myocarditis (including rheumatic fever)		Nicotine

*Reprinted from Gillette PC, Garson A Jr (eds): Pediatric Cardiac Dysrhythmias. New York, Grune & Stratton, 1981, p 321.

with ventricular tachycardia also had an occult myocarditis found by ventricular biopsy.[73] Chronic myocarditis has been reported in 50% of adults with "idiopathic" ventricular tachycardia.[74] However, the incidence of myocarditis on biopsy during cardiac catheterization depends not only on the number of biopsy specimens, but also on the criteria used by the pathologist for the diagnosis, and these criteria are currently not well standardized. Nonetheless, it is important to identify patients with flagrant acute myocarditis, since specific treatment with anti-inflammatory drugs may influence the course of the myocarditis and the arrhythmia (see section on treatment).[74]

In most cases, the prognosis for the patient depends on how quickly the disorder can be normalized (e.g., the type of inhalation anesthesia can be quickly changed, whereas myocardial infarction evolves slowly), and the likelihood that hemodynamics will deteriorate as a result of ventricular arrhythmia. Arrhythmias that might be well tolerated on a chronic basis are often poorly tolerated in an acutely ill patient. Single uniform PVCs are generally well tolerated in children in any situation. The length and constancy of the coupling interval and the morphology and frequency of the PVCs does not affect the prognosis in the acute situation. Even ventricular bigeminy is frequently well tolerated as long as the number of effective beats per minute is approximately normal for age. For example, if a patient with bigeminy has late diastolic PVCs (long coupling interval) so that the ventricle fills almost completely before each PVC, then each PVC may result in an almost normal stroke volume. In this case, if there are 45 sinus beats per minute alternating with 45 PVCs, the number of effective beats may be 90 per minute. However, if the PVCs have a short coupling interval, there may be little or no ventricular filling before each PVC, so that the number of effective beats may be 45 per minute. Therefore the prognosis for uniform PVCs depends on the hemodynamic status of the patient. On the other hand, the patient with multiform PVCs, couplets, or ventricular tachycardia may develop ventricular fibrillation in the acute situation; therefore these arrhythmias have a poor prognosis on the basis of potential electrical instability and should be treated regardless of the hemodynamic perturbation.

CHRONIC VENTRICULAR ARRHYTHMIAS

Single, uniform premature ventricular contractions may occur either in children with an otherwise normal heart or in children with an abnormal heart. However, as the ventricular arrhythmia becomes more serious, it is less likely to occur in a child with a perfectly normal heart. In fact, ventricular tachycardia can be said to be a "marker" for an abnormal heart. Among 38 children with ventricular tachycardia, Rocchini, Chun, and Dick found 21 with obvious heart disease: five with mitral valve prolapse, three with myocarditis, three with prolonged QT, four who had undergone surgery for tetralogy of Fallot, four with unoperated aortic valve disease, and two who had undergone valve replacement surgery. Eleven patients were thought to be "normal" on the basis of chest roentgenograms and M-mode echocardiograms. Recently, Garson,[75] Deal et al,[58] and Dunnigan et al[76] have demonstrated that when cardiac catheterization is performed in children with ventricular tachycardia who were thought to have an otherwise normal heart, occult cardiomyopathy or arrhythmogenic right ventricular dysplasia may be diagnosed. In children and young adults with symptomatic ventricular tachycardia or ventricular fibrillation, 85% have an abnormal heart.[77, 78]

In general, the age of the patient is a relevant factor in the diagnosis and treatment of ventricular arrhythmias. In children younger than 3 years, ventricular arrhythmias are rare. Among those with ventricular tachycardia, by far the most common diagnosis is "incessant idiopathic" ventricular tachycardia. In the childhood and young adult age group, the majority are thought to have a "normal" heart, although, as we have seen, many do not. Also in this age group, there are an increasing number of patients with ventricular arrhythmias and congenital heart disease, usually occurring after intracardiac repair of their defects. There are also increasing numbers of patients with a prolonged QT interval recognized as the cause of ventricular tachycardia. In adults, on the other hand, by far the most common cause is coronary artery disease.

Infants

In the first week of life, premature ventricular contractions are found in 33% of newborns on a screening electrocardiogram.[79] In our experience, premature ventricular contractions in newborns are much less common than premature atrial contractions. In most infants with premature, wide QRS complexes, a P wave can be found if the preceding T wave is searched very carefully. This is especially true in infants who also have obvious premature atrial beats with a narrow QRS complex following the premature P wave. It is extremely rare for a normal newborn infant to have both premature atrial contractions and premature ventricular contractions. Even in those who have only premature ventricular contractions in the newborn period, the prognosis is benign, whether the PVCs are fixed coupled or parasystolic;[80] they generally disappear within the first 4 to 8 weeks of life.[79] In such an infant, it is important to examine the electrocardiogram carefully for the presence of a prolonged QT interval or signs of myocarditis. If the PVCs persist beyond 1 or 2 months of age, it is worthwhile to obtain an echocardiogram to be sure there is no evidence of cardiomyopathy or other structural abnormality of the heart, such as an obvious tumor. Accelerated ventricular rhythm in infancy also has a benign prognosis.[81]

Of 14 newborns who presented with paroxysmal ventricular tachycardia, Stevens et al[82] found a medical reason for the tachycardia in 43% (in the mother: mepivacaine toxicity and heroin overdose; in the infant: congenital heart disease, hyperkalemia caused by the adrenogenital syndrome, or myocarditis). It is interesting to note that three of these 14 cases presented with fetal ventricular tachycardia. These were diagnosed only retrospectively after the ventricular tachycardia was diagnosed postnatally. Digoxin had not been successful in converting the intrauterine tachycardia in any of these infants. It may be possible to diagnose ventricular tachycardia by timing ventricular contraction with a combination of echo and Doppler techniques. The diagnosis could certainly be made if AV dissociation was present. However, in the presence of 1:1 retrograde conduction of ventricular tachycardia, the diagnosis cannot be made on the basis of AV dissociation, and other criteria must be sought.

Stevens et al[82] found that among the 14 infants with paroxysmal episodes of ventricular tachycardia only three persisted beyond the newborn period. In other series, an infant with paroxysmal episodes of ventricular tachycardia lasting from three beats to several hours has a good prognosis, assuming that the QT interval is normal.[81, 83] Since long episodes of ventricular tachycardia may lead to hemodynamic compromise, these infants should be treated for 6 months. The most likely drug to be absorbed and to be effective in newborns and young infants is propranolol; phenytoin is not absorbed well in the first year of life. If propranolol is not effective, either mexiletine or quinidine may be used.

Infants with occasional paroxysmal episodes of ventricular tachycardia need to be distinguished from those with "incessant" ventricular tachycardia, defined as presence of the arrhythmia for more than 10% of any day. In most of these infants, tachycardia is present throughout the day and night. Our first case was most instructive. At 6 months of age, the infant was noted by her pediatrician to have a "rapid heart rate." The rate had returned to normal by the time an electrocardiogram was obtained. She was entirely asymptomatic and remained asymptomatic until the age of 15 months, when she was taken to the local emergency room for lethargy, pallor, and shortness of breath. Her heart rate was found to be 300 bpm. The diagnosis was made of "supraventricular tachycardia with aberration." She was given intravenous digoxin for this arrhythmia and within minutes had ventricular fibrillation. She was defibrillated but remained in this tachycardia throughout most of the day and night for 3 weeks. The tachycardia was not responsive to conventional antiarrhythmic drugs. At the age of 18 months, she was transferred to Texas Children's Hospital, and the diagnosis of ventricular tachycardia was made (see Fig. 14–21). On echocardiography and cineangiography, she had reduced left ventricular function but no anatomic abnormality was seen. At the age of 19 months, she underwent electrophysiology study. The diagnosis of ventricular tachycardia was confirmed, with the earliest site of endocardial activation at the left ventricular apex. The tachycardia could be terminated with premature ventricular extrastimuli, but it returned after several sinus beats. Because of continued tachycardia and low cardiac output, she was taken to the operating room with the idea of ablating that area of the heart. To our surprise, a small (5 mm × 12 mm) gray lesion was found on the epicardial surface at the left ventricular apex (Fig. 14–40). Removal of this lesion resulted in sinus rhythm. On pathologic examination, the gray area was entirely made up of large, pale staining cells with the general characteristics of Purkinje cells (Fig. 14–41).[84] At last follow-up (7.5 years after surgery), the patient remained in sinus rhythm without medication.

Incessant idiopathic ventricular tachycardia is a disease of infancy. We have encountered 20 patients, all younger than 26 months (mean age, 10 months) when first presenting with a tachyarrhythmia. There were significantly more females (13) than males (7). Of the 20 patients, six had undergone an episode of cardiopulmonary arrest (four of whom had ventricular fibrillation when given digitalis for the incorrect diagnosis of supraventricular tachycardia with aberration), nine presented with congestive heart failure resulting from the incessant tachycardia, and only five were asymptomatic but were found to have a rapid heart rate on a routine physical examination. The rate of the ventricular tachycardia ranged from 170 bpm to 440 bpm (mean, 260 bpm). The most common QRS morphology was that of right bundle-branch block with left axis deviation (nine of 20 patients), but all the different morphologies of bundle-branch block were seen in individual patients. In 18 of the 20, the tachycardia morphology remained the same from day to day; in two patients, there was more than one morphology of different sustained monomorphic ventricular tachycardias.

At electrophysiology study, the morphology of the QRS complex generally corresponded to the site of earliest endocardial activation. The most common single location was the posterior left ventricular free wall (six of 20), followed by the left ventricular septum. Overall, 13 of 20 were in the left ventricle, four were in the right ventricle, and three spread throughout the endocardium of both the right and left ventricles. In 17 of the 20 patients, premature stimuli and rapid pacing were performed; in 13 of the 17, the tachycardia could be terminated briefly by premature stimuli.

All 20 patients had received multiple conventional antiarrhythmic drugs (mean, 3.2 drugs per patient), and 12 had received amiodarone. All drugs had failed to appreciably affect either the rate of the tachycardia or the percentage of the day the patient spent in tachycardia. Accordingly, all 20 patients underwent surgery. At surgery, epicardial and endocardial mapping were again repeated, and the earliest endocardial activation was found to be the same as in the catheterization laboratory. At the site of earliest activation, 15 of the 20 were found to have a tumor (13 Purkinje cell tumors, two rhabdomyomas). One patient had no visible findings, but on biopsying the site of earliest activation, chronic myocarditis was found. Two patients were found to have only nonspecific fibrosis, and two patients (early in the series) had no biopsy performed. All patients had excision of the site of earliest activation as well as cryoablation of the surrounding tissue.

Immediately after surgery, all 20 patients were in sinus rhythm. Two patients died early in the postoperative period, one from a severe neurologic insult that had occurred before surgery at the time of a cardiopulmonary arrest resulting from the ventricular tachycardia; the other had removal of an extensive tumor in the endocardium of both the right and left ventricles and died postoperatively of low cardiac output. There was one late death from congestive heart failure

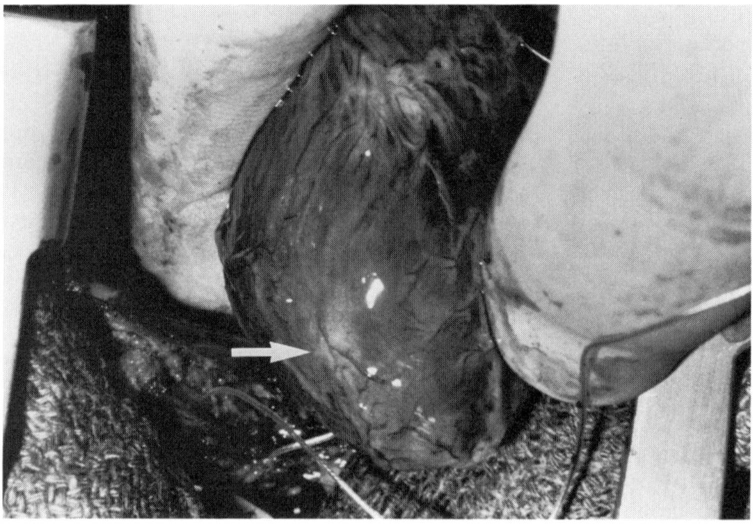

FIGURE 14–40
The left ventricle is held between the thumb (right) and forefinger (left). The arrow demonstrates an area of gray-white discoloration. Pathologic investigation (see Fig. 14–41), revealed a Purkinje hamartoma.

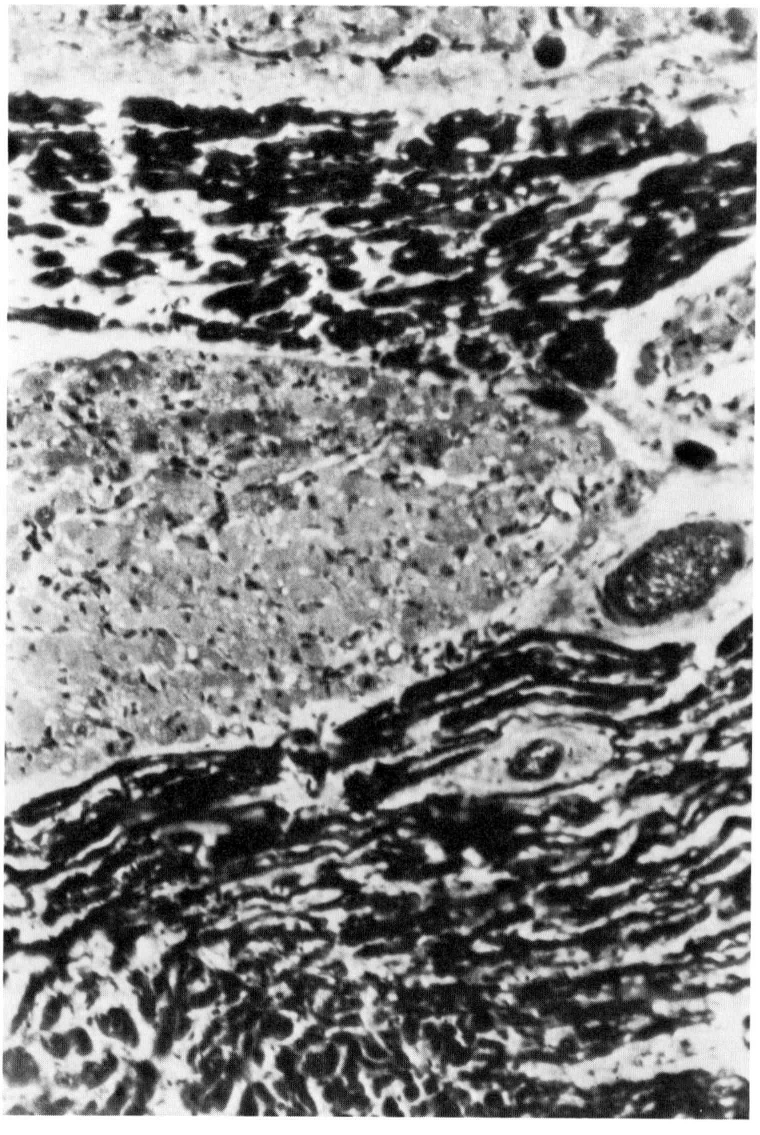

FIGURE 14–41
Microscopic view of a Purkinje hamartoma. Normal myocardium is above and below. In the middle of the section is an area of large, pale-staining cells, the Purkinje hamartoma. (Original magnification, × 100.)

in another patient with extensive tumor resection. The other 17 patients are alive and in sinus rhythm in follow-up from 14 months to 7 years (mean, 2.2 years). Only two are on antiarrhythmic drugs. The reduced ventricular function that had been present preoperatively resolved in 13 of the 14 patients. Therefore, we have found that incessant ventricular tachycardia in infants younger than three years is likely to be caused by a tumor, despite a normal echocardiogram and angiogram. The most common type of tumor was the Purkinje cell tumor, which has previously been reported only in pathologic series involving sudden death in children.[85, 86] Since incessant ventricular tachycardia did not respond to medical therapy and was treated successfully with surgery, we recommend that surgery be considered early in the course of these patients.

Children With an Otherwise Normal Heart

Single uniform PVCs may be detected on a routine resting ECG in 0.3% to 2.2% of children with an otherwise normal heart.[3, 87, 88] Jacobsen et al[3] performed a long-term follow-up study in 17 children (eight boys and nine girls) with a normal heart. All were asymptomatic and had single uniform PVCs on routine ECG taken at rest. Parasystole was present in one. The other 16 patients had fixed coupled PVCs without evidence of parasystole. Four patients had ventricular bigeminy, and three had trigeminy. The mean age at first detection of the PVCs was 6.6 years. The PVCs were abolished in each patient with light exercise. These 17 patients were recalled for repeat examination a mean of 7.2 years after the first examination. The mean age at second examination was 13.8 years. In nine of the 17, PVCs were not detected on follow-up. The nine patients without PVCs were compared to the eight who still had PVCs. There was no difference in sex, presence of bigeminy or trigeminy on initial tracings, coupling interval, age at onset, or age at follow-up. All patients continued to be asymptomatic. These conclusions have been substantiated in two other studies,[89, 90] except that in two of the 19 patients in the study by Rosanski, Steinfeld, and Kupersmith,[89] the PVCs were not suppressed by exercise but did not increase. We consider the normal response to exercise in children to be suppression of PVCs. We have performed intracardiac electrophysiology studies on five patients with an otherwise normal heart whose PVCs were not suppressed by exercise. None had any inducible ventricular arrhythmia. Therefore, in children with an otherwise normal heart, single uniform PVCs are benign. This appears to be true even if the PVCs occur in a bigeminal or trigeminal pattern. Parasystole does not appear to have any consequence in children.[90] The "R on T" phenomenon also does not appear to have any prognostic significance, except possibly in patients with a prolonged QT interval. The evaluation of the patient who presents with single uniform premature ventricular contractions and an otherwise normal heart is controversial. We obtain an echocardiogram to be sure there is not an underlying left ventricular cardiomyopathy, hypertrophic cardiomyopathy, or dilation of the right ventricle suggesting arrhythmogenic right ventricular dysplasia. However, even in patients with uniform PVCs by history and physical examination, it is rare to find any evidence on the echocardiogram. In addition, the treadmill exercise test should be performed, because occasionally a patient with single uniform PVCs will develop ventricular tachycardia during the test, which places the patient in a completely different category (see later discussion). However, if the echocardiogram is normal and the treadmill exercise test does not reveal ventricular tachycardia, we do not recommend any additional follow-up or treatment of patients with single uniform PVCs.

Multiform premature ventricular contractions are very rare in children with a normal heart. Of the four patients with multiform premature ventricular contractions and a normal heart reported by Jacobsen et al,[3] one died suddenly. None of the patients had undergone cardiac catheterization or had an echocardiogram, and it is possible that they did not really have a normal heart. There are also few reports on couplets in children with a normal heart. In the study by Schubert and Epstein,[91] the majority of children with couplets had an abnormal heart. Since there are so few reports of multiform premature ventricular contractions or couplets in children with a normal heart, it is important to assess these children carefully for the presence of a cardiac abnormality. This involves careful measurement of the QT interval, detailed echocardiography, and the treadmill exercise test. It is possible that these patients are similar to children with ventricular tachycardia and will be found to have an underlying cardiac abnormality. At the present time, if the heart is entirely normal and the patient is asymptomatic, we do not recommend treatment for multiform PVCs or couplets, but would recommend follow-up to be sure ventricular tachycardia did not develop.

It is important to distinguish accelerated ventricular rhythm from ventricular tachycardia, because accelerated ventricular rhythm in children appears to be benign.[18,92] One of our patients with accelerated ventricular rhythm remained asymptomatic but developed progressive cardiac enlargement. This seemed to be caused by the continued AV dissociation and increased mean ventricular rate. When the arrhythmia was treated, the cardiac size returned to normal. It is uncertain how often this will occur, and patients with accelerated ventricular rhythm should be followed yearly with echocardiography to be sure that the cardiac size is not increasing. Otherwise, if the heart is entirely normal and the patient is asymptomatic, treatment is not necessary.

The findings in children thought to have an otherwise normal heart and ventricular tachycardia are different from those in previously discussed arrhythmias. Deal et al[58] recently reported 24 children, aged 6 to 21 years old, with ventricular tachycardia. All were thought to have a normal heart. Symptoms, most often syncope or presyncope, occurred in 14 of the patients (67%); in 9, these symptoms were related to exercise. The most common morphology was left bundle-branch block (18 of 24 patients), and the rate ranged from 130 bpm to 300 bpm. During electrophysiology study, sustained monomorphic ventricular tachycardia could be induced in 11 of 18 patients. Only two of seven patients who received isoproterenol had tachycardia appear during the infusion. The site of earliest activation was in the right ventricle in 15 of 17 patients.

While all the patients were initially thought to have a normal heart, 26% were found on echocardiography to have an abnormality in either the right or left ventricle with either dilation, reduced ejection fraction, or both. During cardiac catheterization, 70% of the patients were found to have an abnormality; half had arrhythmogenic right ventricular dysplasia, and the other half had left ventricular congestive cardiomyopathy. Similar findings were reported by Fauchier et al:[93] the majority of those thought to have a normal heart had arrhythmogenic right ventricular dysplasia found only at cardiac catheterization. Therefore, the echocardiogram was not sensitive enough to detect these abnormalities in children.

Dunnigan et al[76] found that of six children who presented with sustained monomorphic ventricular tachycardia, three had evidence at cardiac catheterization of congestive cardiomyopathy, and the other three had evidence of restrictive cardiomyopathy. In four of the six patients, the cardiac muscle biopsy was abnormal, with increased areas of fibrous tissue. While none of these patients had myocarditis, myocardial inflammation has been reported in 50% of adults who had "idiopathic ventricular tachycardia" and who were thought to have an otherwise normal heart.[74] In children, we have found myocarditis in 2 of 11 "normals" with ventricular tachycardia and in 1 of 6 thought to have an idiopathic dilated cardiomyopathy and ventricular tachycardia.[94] Similar findings have recently been reported in adults.[95, 96] It appears that ventricular tachycardia is a marker for a patient with an abnormal heart; the patient should be investigated thoroughly, and a positive diagnosis attempted.

The prognosis for ventricular tachycardia in children with a normal heart depends entirely on whether the heart is found to be truly normal at cardiac catheterization. In an average follow-up of 5 years in a series of 15 children with ventricular tachycardia who had a normal heart proven at cardiac catheterization, there were no deaths, and only two patients had symptoms, both with palpitations.[75] Rocchini, Chun, and Dick found significantly fewer symptoms in children with ventricular tachycardia who had a normal heart compared with those who had an abnormal heart.[73] In addition, all those who had symptoms had a heart rate during ventricular tachycardia greater than 150 bpm. Deal et al[58] found that two of their 23 patients previously thought to have a normal heart and ventricular tachycardia died suddenly. However, both had been symptomatic, both had had exercise-related ventricular tachycardia, both had had ventricular tachycardia induced during electrophysiology study, and neither had had a normal heart at cardiac catheterization.

Garson reviewed 106 published cases of ventricular tachycardia in children thought to have a normal heart.[97] Of these 106, only 31 had had cardiac catheterization.[73, 98, 99] There were three deaths; none had had prior cardiac catheterization, one had been known to have syncopal episodes, and one had had arrhythmogenic right ventricular dysplasia as disclosed at autopsy. There was no information about the third patient.[100–102] In the 103 survivors, two findings emerged: ventricular tachycardia in patients with a truly normal heart was resistant to treatment with traditional antiarrhythmic drugs,[98] and the arrhythmia was also persistent throughout follow-up, disappearing in only approximately 20% of the patients.

The mechanisms of ventricular tachycardia in patients with a truly normal heart are not known. From the surface electrocardiogram, it appears to be consistent with either triggered activity[34] or reentry.[103] One explanation of the common morphology of right bundle-branch block with left axis deviation in older children and young adults with ventricular tachycardia has been bundle-branch reentry involving the left posterior fascicle.[37] Regardless of the mechanism, it appears that verapamil (which could be successful in either mechanism) is effective in a large number of these patients.[103, 104]

In summary, children with ventricular tachycardia thought to have an otherwise normal heart should have anatomic and hemodynamic cardiac catheterization with myocardial biopsy. In addition, according to the data of Deal et al,[58] it may be worthwhile to perform intracardiac electrophysiology studies. If the heart is entirely normal (including biopsy), the patient is asymptomatic, there is no ventricular tachycardia induced during electrophysiology study, and the tachycardia is not related to exercise (see next section), the prognosis for the patient is likely to be benign, the arrhythmia is exceedingly difficult to treat, and therefore the patient may be left untreated. On the other hand, if this is not the case, the patient should probably receive treatment, beginning with either verapamil or a β-blocker. It is possible that the newer antiarrhythmic drugs, especially the class Ic agents (encainide and flecainide), may be especially effective in this group of patients. Vignola, Rozanski, and Lister[74] found that if the patient has active myocarditis on the biopsy, treatment with prednisone and azathioprine resulted in disappearance of the myocarditis and disappearance of the ventricular arrhythmia within 6 months. This was an uncontrolled study. Therefore, in an individual patient, the risk-benefit ratio should be assessed by weighing the specific ventricular arrhythmia against treatment with immunosuppressive and cytotoxic drugs.

EXERCISE-RELATED VENTRICULAR TACHYCARDIA

Exercise-related ventricular tachycardia is defined as the occurrence of the arrhythmia in association with exercise by history or on an exercise test, whether the arrhythmia appears during or after the exercise test. Like other types of ventricular tachycardia, exercise-related ventricular tachycardia is a marker for an abnormal heart; arrhythmogenic ventricular dysplasia is found in 50% to 75% of these patients at cardiac catheterization.[102, 105–109] In fact, among children with exercise-related syncope, the most common diagnosis is ventricular tachycardia.[76, 110–112] In a study by Ryujin et al[113] on syncope in athletes, 10 of 19 (53%) had exercise-related ventricular tachycardia (nine of the 10 had mitral valve prolapse); interestingly, an additional five patients had Wolff-Parkinson-White on the resting electrocardiogram. While it is clear that either supraventricular tachycardia or atrial flutter with a rapid ventricular response could lead to exercise-related syncope, ventricular tachycardia was more common. Between 10% and 45% of patients with exercise-related ventricular tachycardia have died.[58, 99, 110, 113] The prognosis appears especially poor if the patients have exercise-related syncope as well as exercise-related ventricular tachycardia.

There appear to be two different mechanisms for exercise-related ventricular tachycardia. In the first type (comprising about 70% of patients), ventricular tachycardia can usually be reproduced at cardiac catheterization by the infusion of isoproterenol. It cannot be induced by electrical stimulation. Coumel, Leclerq, and Lucet believe this is a variant of the prolonged QT syndrome.[15] Palileo et al[105] have suggested an alternate explanation: this could be a catecholamine-induced cardiomyopathy in athletes with large stroke volumes, causing mechanical trauma of the right ventricular outflow tract against the sternum. In this type of patient, treatment with β-blockers appears to be effective.

In the second type of exercise-related ventricular tachycardia (found in the remaining 30% of patients), ventricular tachycardia can be induced in the catheterization laboratory.[38] The underlying mechanism may be triggered activity; this has been supported by the observation that inducible ventricular tachycardia in the catheterization laboratory is suppressed by both adenosine and verapamil.[114, 115]

Since there is a high incidence of cardiac abnormality, especially arrhythmogenic right ventricular dysplasia, in exercise-related ventricular tachycardia, all patients should have cardiac catheterization. Electrophysiology studies should be performed at the same time to determine if the tachycardia is inducible or if it can be reproduced by the infusion of isoproterenol. This will help in guiding therapy. All patients should be treated chronically. If the tachycardia was reproduced by isoproterenol infusion, chronic treatment should begin with a β-blocker. If the tachycardia was inducible during electrophysiology study, treatment should begin with verapamil. It is likely (especially if it is possible that this is a variant of the long QT syndrome) that drugs that could prolong the QT (e.g., quinidine, procainamide, disopyramide, amiodarone) should be avoided. Furthermore, it has been recommended that athletes be restricted from participating in sports for at least 6 months after initiation of therapy for ventricular tachycardia to be sure that there is no clinical recurrence.[116] They should also have treadmill exercise testing to be sure the arrhythmia is suppressed before being allowed to participate in sports.

LONG QT SYNDROMES

Idiopathic Long QT Syndrome

In 1957, Jervell and Lange-Neilsen[21] described a disease complex with (1) syncope or sudden death, (2) prolongation of the QT interval, (3) congenital nerve deafness, and (4) hereditary transmission in an autosomal recessive pattern. Romano, Gemme, and Pongigliono[117] in 1963 and Ward[118] in 1964 reported a syndrome with similar characteristics, except the hearing was normal, and the hereditary pattern was more consistent with autosomal dominant transmission.[26, 27]

Since then, a great deal more information has become available. There appears to be a syndrome affecting patients with cardiac electrical instability and a propensity to sudden death from this electrical instability. Most (but not all) of these patients have a long QT interval; few have abnormal hearing and about half have hereditary transmission.[15, 26] In fact, not all people with a prolonged QT have the syndrome and therefore are not at risk for sudden death; conversely, rare patients with a normal QT may have the syndrome. Therefore, the QT interval is only a marker. This is demonstrated when patients with a prolonged QT interval take propranolol; the QT interval does not shorten, but they are protected from sudden death. Thus, it is of the utmost importance to attempt to diagnose which individuals have the syndrome and are therefore likely to suffer sudden death. Schwartz[26] has proposed certain "major" and "minor" criteria for the diagnosis of the syndrome. The major criteria are (1) a corrected QT interval (Bazett's formula[22]) greater than 0.44 (see section on noninvasive evaluation in this chapter); (2) family members with the long QT syndrome; (3) syncope related to noise or anger. The minor criteria are (1) congenital deafness; (2) bradycardia (Vincent[119] has found that in children with the prolonged QT syndrome, the heart rate is lower than normal for those younger than 3 years and then normalizes); (3) large, bizarre, notched T waves (Fig. 14–30; the second component of the T wave [or U wave] may be larger than the first component; in many cases, the T waves are frankly inverted in the lateral precordial leads); (4) T wave alternans (Fig. 14–31). Schwartz requires two major criteria, or one major and two minor criteria, for the diagnosis of the syndrome. In children, we modify the requirement to allow the diagnosis of the syndrome in any patient with a prolonged corrected QT interval and one minor criterion. Certain tests, (such as exercise testing, epinephrine infusion, monophasic action potential recordings, and ventricular extrastimulus studies) may also be helpful in diagnosing the syndrome.

1. *Exercise Testing*. It has been stated that in patients with the long QT syndrome, the QT does not shorten appropriately with exercise, and these patients fail to achieve a

normal maximum heart rate. In our experience, exact measurement of the QT interval during exercise is frought with difficulties and inter-observer variation. Yu et al[120] have published values for the QTc in exercise in adults. The baseline measurement was 0.420 s. During exercise, the QTc ranged from 0.440 s to 0.443 s. One minute after exercise, the QTc had returned to baseline at 0.422 s. In the second minute after exercise, it was 0.408 s and then gradually returned back to 0.420 s by the tenth minute after exercise. This would agree with Schwartz's suggestion that measurement of the QTc 1 minute after exercise is a sensitive indicator of patients with the prolonged QT interval syndrome.[26] Presumably, a QTc greater than 0.440 s is suggestive of the syndrome, but further research is required to confirm these observations. Coumel, Leclerq, and Lucet have suggested that patients with exercise-related ventricular tachycardia have a variant of the long QT syndrome.[15] However, Von-Bernuth et al[110] reported on exercise testing in 23 children and young adults with the idiopathic long QT syndrome and found only exercise-related ventricular tachycardia in one of these patients; five of them later died suddenly. Therefore, the absence of exercise-related ventricular tachycardia in patients with the long QT syndrome is not helpful.

2. *Epinephrine Infusion.* In patients with known long QT syndrome, epinephrine infusion may increase the U wave amplitude and cause ventricular arrhythmias.[121] We have found during electrophysiology study that when these patients undergo epinephrine infusion and then have programmed electrical stimulation, ventricular fibrillation may result. While this is a somewhat disturbing test, it may provide a positive diagnosis of the syndrome, since other patients with a structurally normal heart do not have ventricular fibrillation with epinephrine infusion.

3. *Monophasic Action Potential Recordings.* Bonatti, Rolli, and Botti have reported monophasic action potential recordings in patients with the long QT syndrome.[51] There were marked differences in monophasic action potential duration in different areas of the right ventricle. The normal difference among monophasic action potential duration is 38 ms, but in patients with the long QT interval, the difference was 100 ms or more). They also found undulations during the repolarization phase of some of the action potentials that were suggestive of early afterdepolarizations.

4. *Ventricular Extrastimulus Studies.* At present, classical ventricular extrastimulus testing has not been helpful in inducing ventricular arrhythmias in patients with the long QT interval syndrome. However, it may be possible in the future to devise protocols in which ventricular arrhythmias could be produced (e.g., protocols attempting to reproduce the bigeminal pattern that usually initiates torsades de pointes may be effective).

We have recently reported 26 children with a corrected QT interval greater than 0.44 s. These were not necessarily patients with the true syndrome, but instead represented the spectrum of children who have abnormally prolonged QT on the electrocardiogram.[122] The age at diagnosis of the prolonged QT interval ranged from 1 week to 27 years, with a mean of 12 years. The initial presentation was a cardiac arrest in two patients, syncope in 12 patients, and palpitations in four patients. Eight patients were asymptomatic; three had the diagnosis made on an electrocardiogram obtained for bradycardia, and five had the diagnosis made on an electrocardiogram obtained because another family member had a prolonged QT interval. On the electrocardiogram, 15 of the 26 children had a corrected QT interval greater than 0.50 s. Each of these 15 patients had syncope (nine of 15), a positive family history (nine of 15), or both (six of 15). In comparison, 11 patients had a corrected QT interval less than 0.50 s. Syncope occurred in four, a positive family history in five, and both syncope and a positive family history in two patients. In follow-up of our 26 children, there were four sudden deaths. All of these patients had a corrected QT interval greater than 0.50 s. Only one of the four was known to be taking a β-blocker at the time of treatment. Conversely, the majority of the patients were taking either β-blockers or phenytoin. After beginning this treatment, six of the seven patients with prior episodes of syncope had a cessation in syncopal episodes; the seventh required a pacemaker and left stellate ganglionectomy for elimination of symptoms. The major conclusion from this study was that children with a corrected QT interval of 0.50 s or greater are likely to have the syndrome, whereas those with a corrected QT interval less than 0.50 s may or may not have the syndrome.

There are two special situations in children

with idiopathic prolonged QT intervals. First, we have observed three children in whom the corrected QT interval was markedly prolonged immediately after birth (without any other obvious cause), and these children had either ventricular tachycardia or cardiac arrest. By 1 year of age, the QT interval had completely normalized, and there were no ventricular arrhythmias. DiSegni et al[123] reported a case of an infant with severe bradycardia in a prolonged QT interval with recurrent ventricular tachycardia who required a permanent pacemaker in the first weeks of life. The bradycardia, the prolonged QT interval, and the ventricular arrhythmias all disappeared by 1 year of age. It is difficult to know whether these represent transient sympathetic imbalance or transient electrical instability that may occur in the first year of life and then disappear. This would corroborate Schwartz's[26] hypothesis that some cases of the sudden infant death syndrome may be a result of sympathetic imbalance and electrical instability marked by a prolonged QT interval. Because a change in sympathetic innervation is postulated to occur in the first year of life, this hypothesis may explain our three cases as well as a small proportion of cases of sudden infant death syndrome. It is difficult to know how to manage the patient with previous symptoms and a prolonged QT interval who completely normalizes by 1 year of age. In two of our patients who have reached the age of 3 years with a continued normal QT interval and without recurrent symptoms, we have discontinued β-blockade, with no resulting lengthening of the QT interval and no reappearance of symptoms or arrhythmia.

The second special situation concerns the association of a prolonged QT interval with high grade (usually complete) AV block. Esscher[124] reviewed 273 cases with congenital complete AV block and found that 59 (22%) had a prolonged QT interval when corrected for heart rate. It could be said that this was simply an artifact of the correction caused by extreme bradycardia, except that 50 of these 59 patients had syncopal episodes. It is not known whether the syncope was the result of tachyarrhythmias or bradycardia. We have had one patient, who was previously thought to be completely normal, present with a syncopal episode at the age of 4 years. His electrocardiogram revealed complete AV block with a ventricular escape rate of 45 beats per minute and a corrected QT of 0.53 s. His history indicated that when he arrived in the emergency room unconscious, he had a heart rate of more than 200 bpm. Therefore, it is possible that the syncope was caused by ventricular tachycardia rather than paroxysmal AV block. In all children with congenital complete AV block, the QT interval should be measured carefully. Batisse, Belloy, and Fermont[125] reported five infants with congenital complete AV block and a prolonged QT interval in the first year of life. One of these infants died suddenly. In another, the QT interval shortened by 1 year of age, and AV conduction returned to normal. Nickolic, Arnold, and Coles[126] reported an infant with the same combination of problems; a long period of asystole was recorded, and the patient underwent a permanent pacemaker implantation without complications. Therefore, it appears that in infants and children with the combination of prolonged QT interval and complete AV block, the prognosis may be poor, because of either extreme bradycardia or ventricular tachycardia. These children should probably be managed relatively aggressively with a combination of a permanent pacemaker and β-blockade. The cause of this combination remains speculative. If the primary problem is the prolonged QT interval with long action potential durations, the bundle of His or both bundle branches could have extremely long action potentials, leading to functional block. This theory is supported in a report by Takamizawa, Takao, and Ohta,[127] in which an infant with a prolonged QT interval and 2:1 AV block was given mexiletine. The QT interval shortened, and 1:1 conduction returned. Alternatively, it is possible that endocardial fibrosis resulting from the cardiac dilation associated with the large stroke volume necessitated by the complete AV block could cause the QT interval to prolong. This hypothesis is less attractive, since it does not explain the dynamic nature of the AV conduction.

POSSIBLE MECHANISMS

The most popular theory for the idiopathic long QT syndrome has been proposed by Schwartz.[26, 27] This states that the primary abnormality is one of cardiac sympathetic innervation with an underactive right stellate ganglion leading to compensatory hyperfunction of the left stellate ganglion. Experimentally, if the right stellate ganglion of an animal is ablated, the QT interval prolongs. One observation supporting such a hypothesis was made by James and MacLean,[128] who found neuritis in the sympathetic nerves in patients with a prolonged QT interval. The clinical effect of an underactive right stellate ganglion would be sinus bradycardia, and the clinical effect of an overactive left stellate ganglion could be ventricular electrical instability with marked disparity in the length of the refractory periods among parts of the left and right ventricles that could lead to ventricular arrhythmias.

The Schwartz hypothesis must be reconciled with the observation that, in animals, a likely cellular eletrophysiologic mechanism of torsades de pointes involves early afterdepolarizations.[129, 130] Bonatti, Rolli, and Botti[51] have also found oscillations in monophasic action potentials preceding an episode of torsades de pointes in a patient with the idiopathic long QT syndrome. The cellular mechanism of early afterdepolarizations (rather than a reentrant mechanism) would fit the clinical observations that in patients with the long QT syndrome, it is not possible to induce ventricular arrhythmias with the usual forms of intracardiac electrical stimulation. Also, the morphology and usual spontaneous termination of torsades de pointes could be explained by early afterdepolarizations. If the membrane potential is continually depolarized because of a very long action potential, it is conceivable that this single area could be almost continually depolarized, and instead of successive activation of a wave front (a "pebble" effect, likely to produce monomorphic ventricular tachycardia), there could be progressive exit block, with the ventricle depolarized in a circular pattern such that the morphology of the torsades de pointes changes continually, returning to the same morphology when the area of depolarization returns to the top of the circle.

It is possible to relate the Schwartz hypothesis of sympathetic imbalance to early afterdepolarizations, since it is known that norepinephrine prolongs action potential duration. An excessive secretion of norepinephrine related to the hyperactive left stellate ganglion could prolong action potential duration and produce early afterdepolarizations. It may be that there is a basic, genetic abnormality of the potassium channel, thus allowing for early afterdepolarizations and torsades de pointes in response to sympathetic stimulation.

RECOMMENDATIONS

Children with the prolonged QT interval syndrome can present with a cardiac arrest or sudden death without preceding symptoms. In general, resuscitation from cardiac arrest is much less successful in children than in adults.[131] One possible reason for this is that the adult ventricle is more likely to fibrillate than is the ventricle in a child, and therefore the degree of insult necessary to fibrillate the ventricle of a child could be greater than that in an adult. Furthermore, an adult with long QT syndrome is selected: he or she has survived childhood. Therefore, while sudden death rarely occurs in adults without preceding symptoms, we have seen that this is not true in children, whose first symptom may be sudden death. Therefore we recommend that in children with the diagnosis of the prolonged QT syndrome (meeting the modified Schwartz[26] criteria), treatment should be instituted, regardless of the presence or absence of symptoms. We would begin treatment with a β-blocking agent. Although there are few reports of patients taking long-acting β-blockers, we have maintained five such patients on atenolol; there have been no symptoms and no sudden deaths in these patients. Additionally, the class Ib agents, (phenytoin, mexiletine, and tocainide) have all been reported to be effective in treating this syndrome.[127, 132] If symptoms continue while taking medication, then the next step is implantation of a pacemaker, especially if the child has bradycardia. A great number of patients with a prolonged QT interval develop torsades de pointes following a bigeminal cycle. It is thought that the compensatory pause following the premature beat is part of the pathophysiology of the rapid tachyarrhythmia that follows. Therefore if a pacemaker is implanted and the long pause is prevented following a premature beat, episodes of torsades de pointes may be eliminated or reduced.[133] The next possible treatment for such patients is left stellate ganglionectomy, proposed by Locati et al to eliminate the hyperactive left stellate output.[134] There has been controversy over the success of this operation.[135] In children, it has not been performed frequently enough to make any conclusions. Most patients continue to take β-blockers even after surgery. The final treatment for this syndrome is the use of the automatic implantable defibrillator first described by Mirowski et al.[136] This device has the same appearance as an implantable pacemaker, although present models of the defibrillator are larger. Epicardial implantation of the electrodes is necessary. The device senses ventricular fibrillation and after confirming the diagnosis by a number of algorithms, delivers shocks of up to 30 joules. The automatic debrillator has been implanted into a child with the long QT syndrome and has functioned well.[137]

Acquired Long QT Syndromes

The following four general categories of conditions can cause an acquired long QT syndrome:

1. Electrolyte imbalances caused by hypocalcemia, hypomagnesemia, liquid protein diets, or malnutrition with anorexia nervosa.[138] Hypocalcemia appears to be the most common cause of acquired long QT syndrome.

2. Drug-induced long QT, caused by phenothiazines, tricyclic antidepressants, vasodilators (lidoflazine), organophosphates, procainamide, disopyramide, and quinidine, with quinidine being the most common cause. It is difficult to predict which patient will develop the "idiosyncratic" reaction of torsades de pointes as a result of quinidine treatment. This reaction generally occurs early in the course of treatment as the serum concentration is increasing, and usually occurs with subtherapeutic plasma concentrations. If, in a patient taking any such drug (especially quinidine), the corrected QT interval prolongs by greater than 33%, or the absolute QTU interval is greater than 600 ms, then the patient is more likely to have torsades de pointes.[61, 64, 138] Although amiodarone prolongs the QT interval in almost all patients, it is rare for this drug to produce torsades de pointes, although it does occur.[65]

3. Central nervous system trauma and injury (especially subarachnoid hemorrhage), which can lengthen the QT interval. Such trauma has been associated with cardiac subendocardial lesions that can prolong the QT; alternatively, this may be a reflection of sympathetic imbalance on a central nervous system basis.

4. Primary myocardial problems. Myocarditis, ischemia, and prolapse may also cause the QT interval to prolong.

BRADYARRHYTHMIAS

Patients with sick sinus syndrome and bradycardia or those with complete AV block have in common a slow ventricular rate. This slow ventricular rate with its accompanying long repolarization process predisposes the patient to premature ventricular contractions.[9, 139, 140] Winkler, Freed, and Nadas[141] have reported that 68% of children with complete AV block have at least single uniform premature ventricular contractions with exercise testing. Sudden deaths occurred in those patients who had congenital complete AV block and complex ventricular arrhythmias such as multiform premature ventricular contractions, couplets, or ventricular tachycardia. It is not yet known if pacemaker implantation eliminates the ventricular arrhythmias, since it is possible that although the rate may predispose to the arrhythmias, there may also be endocardial fibrosis that is a fixed anatomic substrate, and pacing would not remove the fixed substrate.[124]

UNOPERATED CONGENITAL HEART DISEASE

Mitral Prolapse

While mitral prolapse appears to be a relatively common incidental finding, the incidence of ventricular arrhythmias and sudden death in patients with mitral prolapse is clearly higher than that in the general population. Therefore mitral prolapse will be treated in this chapter as a form of congenital heart disease. The overall incidence of ventricular arrhythmias in children with mitral prolapse is 39% on 24-hour electrocardiogram, demonstrating that there are significantly more ventricular arrhythmias in children with mitral prolapse than in normal children.[142] "High grade" ventricular arrhythmias (multiform PVCs, couplets, or ventricular tachycardia) were found in 4% of children with mitral prolapse who underwent an exercise test and in 8% who had Holter monitoring. Conversely, of those children who had ventricular tachycardia, 13% to 16% had mitral prolapse.[73, 78] Despite the high prevalence of mitral valve prolapse and ventricular arrhythmias in childhood, sudden death is extremely rare in the true pediatric age group. In the two largest studies, using more than 200 children, there were no reported sudden deaths in children younger than 16 years.[142, 143] However, children with Marfan's syndrome and mitral valve prolapse are an exception. Chen et al[144] reported 24 children with Marfan's syndrome; six of these patients had mitral valve prolapse. All of the patients with mitral prolapse had ventricular arrhythmias (three had ventricular tachycardia), and five had accompanying long QT syndrome.[144] Sudden death occurred in two patients with Marfan's syndrome and mitral valve prolapse, both at the age of 16 years. The overall experience seems to be that in late adolescence and early adulthood, patients with mitral valve prolapse may die suddenly. Anderson[145] reported 50 children with mitral valve prolapse whom he had been following. In two of the patients (both seen initially at the age of 7 years with mitral prolapse and without ventricular arrhythmias), sudden death occurred at the ages of 20 and 21 years. Mitral prolapse has also been reported in 3% to 25% of athletes dying suddenly in their teenage or young adult years.[146, 147]

The mechanism of ventricular arrhythmias in mitral prolapse remains speculative. Rosenthal, Hamer, and Gang[148] found that among patients with mitral valve prolapse and ventricular arrhythmias, 45% had inducible ventricular tachycardia, compared with inducible ventricular tachycardia in only 8% of patients with a structurally normal heart and ventricular arrhythmias. In the three young adults reported by Zipes et al[37] to have ventricular tachycardia caused by triggered activity, two had mitral valve prolapse. Therefore it is possible that at least some of these arrhythmias are caused by triggered activity and the others are probably caused by reentry. The pathophysiology of these arrhythmias is unknown. Bharati and Lev[149] reported three teenagers who died suddenly and at autopsy had sclerosis of the left and right side of the ventricular septum, with fatty infiltration of the approaches to the AV node. Two of these three patients had mitral valve prolapse. It has been speculated that increased tension in the papillary muscles could create stretch and fibrosis with conditions appropriate for arrhythmogenesis. Finally, there has been speculation of the connection between mitral valve prolapse and long QT syndromes. Mitral valve prolapse can be part of a larger syndrome that is thought to involve sympathetic imbalance similar to that found in the long QT syndrome. There have not been sufficiently large studies to resolve this question. However, when treating ventricular arrhythmias in patients with mitral prolapse, drugs that prolong repolarization (e.g., quinidine, procainamide, disopyramide, and amiodarone) should be avoided, even if the QT interval is normal in a patient with mitral valve prolapse.

Since sudden death is exceedingly rare in the pediatric age group, the majority of patients with mitral valve prolapse and ventricular arrhythmias should not be treated. However, if the patient is symptomatic from severe palpitations or has presyncope or syncope with high grade ventricular ectopy, treatment is indicated. Complex ventricular ectopy (multiform premature ventricular contractions, couplets, or ventricular tachycardia) is rare in children with mitral prolapse who are younger than 16 years (0% incidence in Bissett, Schwartz, and Mayer's study[143] and 8% incidence in Kavey et al's study[142]); patients with complex ventricular ectopy should be considered for treatment, especially as they approach their late teens and especially if they have ventricular tachycardia.

Aortic Valve Disease

In unoperated patients with aortic stenosis or aortic regurgitation, ventricular arrhythmias are relatively common. In adults, ventricular arrhythmias were found in 84% of those who underwent Holter monitoring; 16% of the patients had frequent premature ventricular contractions (more than one per minute), 51% had multiform premature ventricular contractions, 34% had couplets, and 18% had ventricular tachycardia. The arrhythmias were significantly related to reduced ejection fraction but were not related to gradient or degree of aortic regurgitation. Similar Holter studies have not been done in children. In our study of sudden death in a pediatric cardiology population, however, five of the 101 sudden deaths were in patients with unoperated aortic stenosis or aortic regurgitation, a number equal to those with a prolonged QT interval.[150]

In our experience, the development of ventricular arrhythmias in children with aortic stenosis or aortic regurgitation may accompany a change in hemodynamic status, either a worsening in gradient or degree of regurgitation. Therefore the development of arrhythmias is a possible indication for operation in borderline cases. In cases where operation is otherwise not indicated, complex ventricular arrhythmias should be treated.

Tetralogy of Fallot

Sullivan et al[151] performed Holter monitoring on 40 patients before repair of tetralogy of Fallot. They found that none of the 22 patients younger than 5 years had PVCs, but eight of the 18 patients older than 5 years had ventricular arrhythmias before repair, with all of them starting during adolescence. This has also been our experience. Despite the presence of ventricular arrhythmias, sudden death is rare in these patients before repair. Surgical treatment should be performed in these individuals with the hope of improving oxygenation and correcting the hemodynamics, thus possibly eliminating the ventricular arrhythmias. However, it has not been demonstrated that operation will eliminate the arrhythmias if they have occurred before operation.

Ebstein's Anomaly

The association of Ebstein's anomaly (i.e., malformation of the tricuspid valve) with Wolff-Parkinson-White syndrome is well known. However, it is less well known that 25% of unoperated patients with Ebstein's anomaly have ventricular arrhythmias.[152] In the study by Lambert, Menon, and Wagner[153] on sudden death in children, 6% of the patients who died suddenly had Ebstein's anomaly. It is not known whether they had Wolff-Parkinson-White syndrome or ventricular arrhythmias. In our experience, two patients with Ebstein's anomaly who died suddenly both had ventricular arrhythmias that were very difficult to treat. Since sudden death appears to be a relatively high risk in these patients, complex ventricular arrhythmia should be treated. Perhaps consideration should also be given to treatment of very frequent uniform premature contractions.

Pulmonary Vascular Obstructive Disease (Eisenmenger's Complex)

In Garson and McNamara's study of children and young adults who died suddenly,[150] Eisenmenger's complex was the most common diagnosis. In fact, between 14% and 47% of those with Eisenmenger's complex are reported to die suddenly.[72] However, when we examined the electrocardiograms of seven patients who died suddenly, only one had ventricular arrhythmias and the other six had no known arrhythmia. We have studied the Holter recordings of two patients with Eisenmenger's complex who died while wearing the Holter. In both, there was progressive sinus bradycardia and asystole without any ventricular arrhythmia. The pertinent question, however, is whether a patient with Eisenmenger's complex and ventricular arrhythmias should be treated with antiarrhythmic drugs. It seems reasonable that a patient with marked hypoxemia, ventricular hypertrophy, and pressure overload of the right ventricle should have ventricular arrhythmias treated, but there are no data to support this concept. We recommend treatment of such patients who have complex ventricular arrhythmias, but avoid treatment in patients with lesser grades of arrhythmia.

Ventricular Tumors

In older children, ventricular tumors are a rare cause of ventricular arrhythmias. Unlike in infants younger than 3 years, incessant idiopathic ventricular tachycardia does not seem to occur in older children, and we have not operated on older children with idiopathic ventricular tachycardia. Therefore there is no information on the likelihood of a microscopic tumor causing ventricular tachycardia. On the other hand, tumors visible by either echocardiography or angiocardiography may cause ventricular arrhythmias in older children, and for this reason (especially in patients with ventricular tachycardia) angiocardiography should be performed. In older children, the most common ventricular tumor is rhabdomyoma.[154]

CARDIOMYOPATHY

Hypertrophic Cardiomyopathy

In a study recently completed by the members of the Pediatric Electrophysiology Society on 135 children with hypertrophic cardiomyopathy, 53 (39%) had an arrhythmia on routine ECG. These consisted of atrial fibrillation and atrial flutter, AV conduction disease, supraventricular tachycardia, and sinus node disease, with 10% of the patients having ventricular arrhythmias on routine electrocardiogram. On Holter electrocardiograms, 31% of the patients had uniform premature ventricular contractions, 7% had multiform premature ventricular contractions, 7% had couplets, and 7% had ventricular tachycardia. Similar types of arrhythmias are found in adults.[155–157]

In the study by Frank, Watkins, and Prisant,[156] six out of 50 patients had syncopal episodes, but only one of the patients had ventricular tachycardia causing syncope. Atrial flutter, supraventricular tachycardia, and sinus bradycardia were each present in one patient, and two patients had slow junctional rhythm following spontaneous conversion of atrial flutter-fibrillation. Therefore it is not reasonable to assume that a syncopal patient with hypertrophic cardiomyopathy necessarily has a ventricular arrhythmia.

In terms of risk of sudden death, the Pediatric Electrophysiology Society reported a 13% incidence of sudden death with a follow-up of 7 years. On routine ECG, none of the patients who died suddenly had premature ventricular contractions (three had atrial flutter-fibrillation, two had sinus bradycardia, one had AV block, and one had PACs). Of the 11 patients who had Holter recordings before their sudden death, five had uniform premature ventricular contractions, one had multiform premature ventricular contractions, three had couplets, and two had ventricular tachycardia. McKenna et al[155] reported a 30% incidence of sudden death with an average follow-up of 9 years. The average age at death was 14 years. The presence of arrhythmias was not a predictor of sudden death. This has been the case in studies on adults as well.[155, 158, 159] McKenna et al found that 50% of the patients with sudden death had prior syncopal episodes, and only one of these seven patients with syncope was alive in follow-up.

Hypertrophic cardiomyopathy is well known to cause sudden death in the general population. In a study of all sudden deaths involving children in Rochester, New York, by Harris, Alexson, and Manning,[71] hypertrophic cardiomyopathy was found in 16% of those who died suddenly, whereas 48% of the athletes reported by Maron[147] who died suddenly had hypertrophic cardiomyopathy. In all patients with hypertrophic cardiomyopathy, there is a problem in identifying the patient at risk for sudden death; neither the Holter electrocardiogram nor the electrophysiology study appears to be predictive.[159] In the pediatric electrophysiology study data, the major predictor of sudden death was a family history of hypertrophic cardiomyopathy; the risk was even higher if the family members with hypertrophic cardiomyopathy had arrhythmias or had died suddenly.

It appears that all patients with hypertrophic cardiomyopathy are at risk of sudden death. Unfortunately, patients with entirely negative results on the Holter electrocardiogram are still at risk. However, it may be possible to identify from the preceding data a low risk patient who does not require treatment: one who is asymptomatic, has no arrhythmia on the Holter recording, and has a completely negative family history. The remainder of patients appear to be at risk and perhaps should be treated prophylactically. This should only be done if treatment of ventricular arrhythmias will prevent sudden death. The data on β-blocking treatment have not consistently demonstrated prevention of sudden death. In the pediatric electrophysiology study data, β-blockade did not prevent sudden death since 11 of the 17 patients with sudden death were being treated with a β-blocker (albeit at a low dose, with a mean of 1.7 mg/kg). Enough patients have not been treated with verapamil to know whether this will prevent sudden death. Spicer et al[160] used verapamil to successfully treat exercise-related ventricular tachycardia in three patients with hypertrophic cardiomyopathy. Finally, data in adults suggest that the use of amiodarone does prevent sudden death in patients with hypertrophic cardiomyopathy. McKenna et al[161] gave amiodarone to 53 young adults with hypertrophic cardiomyopathy. The majority had ventricular arrhythmias; however, supraventricular tachycardia and atrial flutter-fibrillation occurred frequently in these patients as well. With a median follow-up of 18 months, there were no sudden deaths in these patients, compared with an incidence of 8% per year in a comparable series of patients treated with conventional drugs. If further study shows that amiodarone does indeed prevent sudden death, then the mode of death may be related to a tachyarrhythmia in the majority of patients, rather than to sinus bradycardia or AV block. In a child with the risk factors of syncope and a positive family history, treatment with amiodarone should be seriously considered.

The mechanism of ventricular arrhythmias in hypertrophic cardiomyopathy remains speculative. Bharati and Lev[149] have reported the "helter-skelter" organization of cells throughout the involved areas of myocardium in hypertrophic cardiomyopathy. Spach, Kootsey, and Mosher[162] have demonstrated that anisotropic conduction through areas of cells with opposing orientation may be sufficient to initiate reentry circuits simply on the basis of slowed conduction and block in areas of the tissue with different properties. Alternatively, the hypertrophic cells could have an arrhythmogenic potential on their own (e.g., being calcium overloaded, which could lead to triggered activity).

Congestive Cardiomyopathy

Friedman et al[163] reported that 11 of 63 children with congestive cardiomyopathy had arrhythmias on routine electrocardiogram. While ventricular arrhythmias were common (13 of 63), they made up less than half of the overall arrhythmia profile (atrial flutter, four; atrial fibrillation, four; supraventricular tachycardia, three; sinus bradycardia, two; atrial premature beats, one). Interestingly, similar to those with hypertrophic cardiomyopathy, few patients with known arrhythmias die suddenly. The only two sudden deaths (3%) in a mean follow-up of 4 years, were in patients without known preceding arrhythmias. Therefore in children, although sudden death is rare, the prediction of sudden death based on preceding arrhythmia has thus far not been possible.

In adults with congestive cardiomyopathy, both ventricular arrhythmias and a markedly reduced ejection fraction seem to be poor predictors.[164, 165] Although it is possible to place a patient in a statistically high risk category on the basis of these noninvasive tests, the risk for an individual patient is still difficult to assess. Even when using electrophysiology studies in congestive cardiomyopathy, the presence or absence of inducible ventricular tachycardia does not predict outcome.[166]

The mechanism for the ventricular arrhythmias in congestive cardiomyopathy is unknown, but is likely not the same as that in hypertrophic cardiomyopathy, since the cellular architecture as well as the intracellular pathology are probably different. It is known that the ventricular tachycardia maps to the mid myocardium or epicardium frequently in these patients, and therefore it is likely that ischemia, which is primarily an endocardial process, may not be an important factor in these arrhythmias. In our own experience, we have found in transplanted hearts that the most electrophysiologically abnormal cells do not necessarily correlate with areas of fibrosis. Therefore, the arrhythmias may result from an underlying cellular abnormality, although they could also be the result of reentry around large fibrotic areas, such as those seen following myocardial infarction.

In both adults and children, ventricular arrhythmias in congestive cardiomyopathy are difficult to eliminate. Even when using amiodarone in adults, Josephson[167] found persistent ventricular arrhythmias and sudden death. For the patient with ventricular arrhythmias and congestive cardiomyopathy, treatment is definitely indicated. On the other hand, since sinus bradycardia may occur in these patients, prophylactic treatment of patients without arrhythmias, especially with drugs such as amiodarone that could suppress the sinus node, does not appear warranted.

Arrhythmogenic Right Ventricular Dysplasia

While hypertrophic cardiomyopathy and congestive cardiomyopathy are well recognized entities, arrhythmogenic right ventricular dysplasia requires further definition. In flagrant cases, the diagnosis of arrhythmogenic right ventricular dysplasia is relatively straightforward: the patient has a left bundle-branch block ventricular tachycardia; the right ventricle is large, dilated, and poorly functioning, with dyskinetic areas primarily in the right ventricular outflow tract, diaphragmatic surface, and septum; and there is right ventricular conduction delay on the electrocardiogram. However, the more subtle forms (much more common in children) may be difficult to diagnose. In our experience, the patient may have only ventricular tachycardia that originates in the right ventricle and a dilated right ventricular outflow tract.[108] In cases such as these, the subtle dilation may be missed, even when using the most sensitive noninvasive techniques currently available, including high resolution two-dimensional echocardiography. Therefore, in order to make the diagnosis of mild arrhythmogenic right ventricular dysplasia, cardiac catheterization is usually necessary. It is also possible for the process to extend into the left ventricle, and these patients may have left ventricular tachycardia. Fortunately, in cases where the left ventricle is involved, the right ventricular abnormality still predominates, and the diagnosis can be made on this basis.

The pathology of arrhythmogenic right ventricular dysplasia involves replacement of myocardium by adipose tissue, beginning in the epicardium and extending to the endocardium. The subepicardial layer appears as a plexiform structure with partially degenerated myocardial fibers that may be the site of slowing necessary for reentrant arrhythmias. Arrhythmogenic right ventricular dysplasia has been likened to Uhl's anomaly ("parchment right ventricle"). Uhl's anomaly is a congenital anomaly with an almost complete absence of right ventricular muscle fibers. Uhl's anomaly does not have the epicardial-to-endocardial distribution, but instead has only a few scattered zones of myocardial fibers. Because of the primarily epicardial process, it may be possible to miss the diagnosis of arrhythmogenic right ventricular dysplasia by endocardial biopsy during cardiac catheterization. While it is true that both Uhl's anomaly and arrhythmogenic right ventricular dysplasia result in loss of right ventricular myocardial fibers, the differences otherwise outweigh the similarities. If arrhythmogenic right ventricular dysplasia were a milder form of Uhl's anomaly, we would see many more intermediate forms between arrhythmogenic right ventricular dysplasia and Uhl's anomaly in childhood. On the other hand, arrhythmogenic right ventricular dysplasia almost never occurs in the flagrant, dilated form in patients younger than 10 years. Rather, it most often presents in childhood in a mild form with subtle, pronounced trabeculation or outflow tract dilation. The more severe forms occur in adulthood. There has not been enough follow-up to determine whether arrhythmogenic right ventricular dysplasia that initially presents in a mild form in childhood progresses to a severe form in that same patient as the child becomes an adult.[168] In certain families, arrhythmogenic right ventricular dysplasia has been inherited as an autosomal dominant trait with incomplete penetrance.[102]

The incidence of arrhythmogenic right ventricular dysplasia in the general population is unknown. Fauchier et al[93] found an arrhythmogenic right ventricle in 14 of 20 young adults with ventricular tachycardia who were thought to have an otherwise normal heart. Deal et al[58] found that 35% of the children with ventricular tachycardia and a normal echocardiogram had arrhythmogenic right ventricular dysplasia. Among children and young adults with exercise-induced ventricular tachycardia, arrhythmogenic right ventricular dysplasia is the most common diagnosis.[107, 132]

It is important to make the diagnosis of arrhythmogenic right ventricular dysplasia, because it may cause sudden death without previous symptoms. Arrhythmogenic right ventricular dysplasia is now being diagnosed at autopsy in children with ventricular tachycardia who were thought to have an otherwise normal heart. These children had not had cardiac catheterization, but at autopsy, the right ventricle was typical for arrhythmogenic right ventricular dysplasia.[100, 101] The same pathology has been found recently in several cases of athletes dying suddenly during sports.[106, 146] Since it appears possible to diagnose arrhythmogenic right ventricular dysplasia at cardiac catheterization, we recommend complete anatomic cardiac catheterization, including right ventricular angiography, in all children with ventricular tachycardia who are thought to have an otherwise normal heart.

Because the natural history of arrhythmogenic right ventricular dysplasia is unknown, it is difficult to assess which patients require treatment. It is likely that asymptomatic children with single premature ventricular contractions do not require treatment and that patients with symptoms or ventricular tachycardia (especially if it is exercise-induced) do require treatment. In our experience, it has been difficult to suppress ventricular arrhythmias in patients with arrhythmogenic right ventricular dysplasia. Class Ib agents (phenytoin and mexiletine) have been successful in only 25% of children with arrhythmogenic right ventricular dysplasia.[169] The use of β-blockers has been equally unsuccessful. Preliminary experience with d-sotolol has been encouraging. Surgical therapy directed at ablating the area of ventricular tachycardia may be successful in temporarily suppressing the arrhythmia; however, since the process involves many areas of the ventricle, it is possible that another area may cause a new arrhythmia. In an attempt to deal with this problem, Guiraudon and Klein[170] performed total right ventricular disconnection for patients with right ventricular dysplasia. This allows ventricular tachycardia to occur in the segment that has been removed, but it does not conduct to the remainder of the heart. While this procedure has been effective in a few patients, in our experience there have been serious hemodynamic consequences, and ventricular tachycardia has recurred in the nonresected septum. For these reasons, we recommend any surgical attempt at treatment of ventricular arrhythmias in arrhythmogenic right ventricular dysplasia only as a last resort.

POSTOPERATIVE CONGENITAL HEART DISEASE

In the 1960s, intracardiac repair of congenital cardiac defects became routine. There was a great deal of enthusiasm as children who had previously been cyanotic began to enjoy completely normal life-styles. However, in the 1970s it became apparent that some of these children were dying suddenly late after the operation. Many of the sudden deaths occurred in patients whose repair involved incision or suturing in the ventricle. The more complex the lesion, the higher the incidence of late sudden death. For example, in lesions involving a right ventriculotomy, sudden death occurs in 1% to 2% of patients following ventricular septal defect repair, in approximately 5% of patients following tetralogy of Fallot repair, and in 31% of patients with truncus arteriosus with single pulmonary artery.[43, 171, 172] In lesions involving the left side of the heart, approximately 3% of children die suddenly after aortic valvotomy or aortic replacement.[75, 150]

Tetralogy of Fallot

Of all the types of postoperative congenital heart disease, the largest body of information has been collected about postoperative tetralogy of Fallot. It is the most common single cause of sudden death in children between 1 and 16 years of age.[71, 150]

On routine electrocardiogram, 10% of the patients have premature ventricular contractions; 30% have ventricular arrhythmias occurring in association with a treadmill exercise test. In children with an otherwise normal heart, the routine response of premature ventricular contractions is to disappear with exercise. However, there have been four sudden deaths reported following exercise tests in patients who had repair of defects with tetralogy physiology. In two of these patients, the ventricular arrhythmias were completely suppressed by exercise, and in the other two, ventricular tachycardia developed during exercise.[29, 132] Therefore, in these patients, suppression of premature ventricular contractions by exercise does not appear to be a benign response. Exercise testing should be carried out in these patients to determine if any ventricular arrhythmias develop, not to determine if they are suppressed by exercise.

On Holter electrocardiograms, the incidence of ventricular arrhythmias in postoperative tetralogy patients is 50%, with 9% of the patients having nonsustained ventricular tachycardia.[29, 43, 173–176] During electrophysiology study using a protocol with paired premature ventricular extrastimuli and burst pacing at two sites in the right ventricle, 26% of the patients had nonsustained ventricular tachycardia and 10% had sustained ventricular tachycardia.[46] The ventricular arrhythmias can originate from any area in the ventricle associated with a large amount of scarring. Ventricular arrhythmias have been reported to originate in relation to the anterior right ventriculotomy; however, ventricular arrhythmias have also been mapped to the posterior right ventricular infundibulum in the area of the infundibular resection and from the ventricular septum in the area of scarring related to the ventricular septal defect patch.[57]

There is a general correlation between patients who have syncope, a high grade of ventricular arrhythmias on the Holter monitor, and inducible nonsustained or sustained ventricular tachycardia at electrophysiology study. Deal et al[177] found that six of seven patients with clinical ventricular tachycardia had inducible ventricular tachycardia at electrophysiology study. However, in a specific patient, there may be discordance among all three tests. For example, Cloez et al[178] found that only three of six patients with clinical ventricular tachycardia had inducible ventricular tachycardia. On the other hand, asymptomatic patients with no arrhythmia on the Holter electrocardiogram may have inducible sustained ventricular tachycardia, or a syncopal patient with only infrequent single uniform premature ventricular contractions on the Holter electrocardiogram may have absolutely no arrhythmia induced during electrophysiology study. Clearly, further studies will be necessary to determine specifically which patients are at risk of sudden death.

Both spontaneous and inducible ventricular arrhythmias are related to abnormal hemodynamics. Among our 484 patients, the prevalence of premature ventricular contractions on routine electrocardiogram was 8% in patients with a right ventricular systolic pressure less than 40 mm Hg, but increased to 30% in patients with a right ventricular systolic pressure greater than 90 mm Hg.[42] Other authors have found clinical ventricular arrhythmias on the routine electrocardiogram or Holter recording associated with increased right ventricular systolic pressure,[179–182] increased right ventricular end-diastolic pressure and decreased right ventricular ejection fraction,[179, 181, 183] decreased cardiac output,[183] and decreased left ventricular ejection fraction.[182,183] In the study by Deanfield, McKenna, and Hallidie-Smith,[174] there was no relationship found between clinical ventricular arrhythmias and abnormal hemodynamics.

A general correlation between abnormal hemodynamics and inducible nonsustained or sustained ventricular tachycardia at electrophysiology study has also been found.[46] However, in a specific patient, ventricular arrhythmias may exist in the presence of excellent hemodynamic repair. Other factors related to the presence of inducible ventricular arrhythmias include age at operation and length of time following surgery.[179, 181] These two factors are not independent, because many more operations were done on older children 20 years ago than they are now. Mathematical analysis reveals that the more significant factor is the duration since surgery; as children who have had repair of tetralogy of Fallot enter adulthood, the incidence of ventricular arrhythmias will continue to rise.[42]

Sudden death is related to preceding ventricular arrhythmias. In Garson et al's series,[43] 38% of those patients with premature ventricular contractions on routine electrocardiogram died suddenly between 1 and 10 years after the operation. The relationship of sudden death to abnormal hemodynamics is evident: 100% of our patients who died suddenly had both right ventricular systolic pressure greater than 60 mm Hg and right ventricular end-diastolic pressure greater than 8 mm Hg. In the mid 1970s, it was suggested that late complete AV block was responsible for these sudden deaths and that the pattern of right bundle-branch block–left anterior hemiblock indicated a high risk.[184] In retrospect, all the patients with sudden death in that study also had ventricular arrhythmias, and more recent reports have demonstrated that the majority of patients who later died suddenly did not have preceding right bundle-branch block–left anterior hemiblock, but instead had ventricular arrhythmias.[185] The final demonstration of the relationship between sudden death and ventricular arrhythmias is that treatment of the ventricular arrhythmias abolishes sudden death.[42] Since 1978, we have treated all patients after repair of tetralogy of Fallot who had frequent uniform premature ventricular contractions or complex arrhythmias on the Holter electrocardiogram. Our goal of treatment has been an absolute reduction of premature ventricular contractions to fewer than 10 uniform premature ventricular contractions per hour, regardless of the frequency or type of ventricular arrhythmia before treatment. Of our 484 patients who had repair of tetralogy, we have treated 44. In 42 of the 44, a successful drug was found by our criteria, and none of these patients died. Both of the patients without successful treatment died, as did seven of the 21 who were untreated.[42] While this suggests that ventricular arrhythmias are an important cause of sudden death, late complete AV block does occur and may also be a cause of sudden death.

The drugs that have been found to be effective in treating ventricular arrhythmias in these patients have largely been the class Ib agents, phenytoin and mexiletine.[40, 41, 169, 186, 187] In our treated patients, phenytoin was successful in 88%, mexiletine in 89%, and quinidine in only 14% of the patients. We have chosen to manage patients based on the Holter electrocardiogram, not only because this management has been shown to be effective, but also because the patient population is different from the usual adult patient population. Very few of our patients present with symptomatic, sustained ventricular tachycardia, and so there is not the urgency for treatment required in the adult population, many of whom have been resuscitated from a sudden cardiac arrest. If there is a great deal of ambient ectopy in any of our patients who have symptomatic episodes, they are treated based on the Holter results, with the intent of reducing ventricular arrhythmia. In a symptomatic patient with very little ambient ectopy, we perform repeated electrophysiology studies while the patient is taking different antiarrhythmic drugs orally. In drug-electrophysiology studies done in 20 postoperative tetralogy patients,[41, 56] a drug that eliminated the induction of sustained ventricular tachycardia could only be found in 11 patients: quinidine or procainamide were successful in one of 12, propranolol in five of 11, and phenytoin in five of 12 (despite nine of 12 without ventricular arrhythmia recorded on the Holter while taking phenytoin). Since it is likely that phenytoin is an effective agent that suppresses ventricular arrhythmias on the Holter electrocardiogram in many patients and may also prevent sudden death, the observation that patients taking phenytoin still have inducible arrhythmias in the catheterization laboratory may place phenytoin in a category similar to that of amiodarone, in which the clinical findings and the electrophysiology findings are not necessarily similar.

If medical treatment fails, it is possible to perform primary surgery to ablate the ventricular tachycardia. Harken, Horowitz, and Josephson[188] reported a postoperative tetralogy patient with ventricular tachycardia that was found to be caused by a macroreentry circuit around the ventriculotomy incision. Simple excision of the scar cured the ventricular tachycardia. In our experience, it is a rare case in which the ventriculotomy incision is used as a macro-reentry circuit. We have found that ventricular tachycardia more commonly originates from any area adjacent to a large scar (including posterior infundibulum and ventricular septum adjacent to the ventricular septal defect repair, where the circuit did not use a large amount of tissue as a macro-reentry circuit). We have operated on five such patients; in four of the five, tachycardia was ameliorated (abolished in three of five, and responsive to previously ineffective drugs in one of five). Using present techniques, it is extremely difficult to map the infundibulum in the catheterization laboratory to be certain whether the tachycardia is originating from the anterior or posterior wall of the infundibulum. Inability to induce the tachycardia in the operating room presents a major problem in surgical ablation. Catheter ablation with high energy shocks has been attempted in several patients. We are aware of one patient in whom electromechanical dissociation ensued immediately after the shock, and the patient died. Ablation of arrhythmogenic areas in the right ventricle by a catheter technique should eventually be an important part of our armamentarium, but at present, the method by which it is achieved with high energy shocks has the potential for early and late death.[189] We do not recommend this procedure as it is currently performed. In the future, more controllable methods (e.g., laser or cryoablation) may make the procedure more feasible.

A final possible surgical treatment for ventricular arrhythmias is related to improvement in hemodynamics. Since ventricular arrhythmias are, in general, related to abnormal hemodynamics, it is theoretically possible, for example, that by reducing the right ventricular systolic pressure by operating on pulmonary stenosis, hemodynamics could be directly improved, with a resulting indirect improvement in ventricular arrhythmias. We have attempted this in four patients. In two, the arrhythmias improved; in one, they were unchanged; and in one, they worsened. In this latter patient, the hemodynamics could not be improved with reoperation. More data will be necessary before we can determine the likelihood of success. However, since it is extremely likely that abnormal hemodynamics are related to sudden death, it seems reasonable to perform reoperation on a patient with residual pulmonary stenosis if the stenosis can be relieved. Even though the ventricular arrhythmias may not disappear, the chance of sudden death would appear to be less, perhaps because ventricular tachycardia would be better tolerated.

Aortic Valve Surgery

While there are somewhat less data available for patients who have aortic valve surgery (either valve replacement or aortic valvotomy) than for patients following tetralogy of Fallot, the two groups appear to have a similar course. In fact, conditions on the left side in the patient who has aortic valvotomy and aortic regurgitation (i.e., a scar at the annulus and systolic and diastolic pressure overload) are similar to those on the right side in postoperative tetralogy of Fallot. This is discussed in further detail in the section on nonischemic ventricular arrhythmias. Von-Olshausen et al[190] studied 51 adults an average of 14 months after aortic valve replacement. They found that ventricular arrhythmias were present in 70% of these patients and that couplets and ventricular tachycardia were related to an ejection fraction of less than 55% postoperatively. In these patients, sudden death was also related to ventricular arrhythmias. Santinga et al[191] found that premature ventricular contractions were present on routine electrocardiogram in 44% of those patients who died suddenly, while PVCs were only present in 10% of those who remained alive ($p < 0.05$). In a Holter study, Konishi et al[192] found that all patients who died suddenly after aortic valve replacement had more than three PVCs per hour. All of the patients who died suddenly also had worse ventricular function than those who did not die suddenly.

It seems to be a recurrent theme that ventricular arrhythmias, abnormal hemodynamics, and sudden death are related. The same criteria should be used for treatment of these patients as is used for patients after repair of tetralogy of Fallot. In the Von-Olshausen study, surgical treatment (i.e., aortic valve replacement to improve the hemodynamics) improved the ejection fraction, and the ventricular arrhythmias improved.[190] In our own experience, we have had several teenagers with aortic stenosis and aortic regurgitation who had ventricular tachycardia prior to aortic valve replacement. After the operation, they had only single uniform premature ventricular contractions. Therefore, the indications for surgery in this group of patients might also include improvement of hemodynamics in order to reduce ventricular arrhythmias.

Ventriculomyotomy for Hypertrophic Cardiomyopathy

In the study by Borggrefe et al in which 31 adult patients with hypertrophic cardiomyopathy were studied before and after ventriculomyotomy, 6 of the 31 had ventricular couplets or ventricular tachycardia both before and after surgery; 5 had these arrhythmias only before, and 7 only after; therefore there is no real effect of this operation on the incidence of ventricular arrhythmias. There have not been sufficient studies to determine if this operation has an effect on sudden death.

Ebstein's anomaly

Oh et al[152] reported that in the immediate postoperative period following repair of Ebstein's anomaly, 8 of 52 patients had ventricular tachycardia or ventricular fibrillation. In the ensuing months, 5 of the 52 died suddenly; 4 of these 5 had perioperative ventricular tachycardia or ventricular fibrillation. Oh et al recommended prophylactic treatment with procainamide for the first 3 months after surgery for all patients who have had repair of Ebstein's anomaly. A possible exception is the patient who never had any arrhythmia either before or immediately after surgery. This group of patients appears to be at high enough risk for sudden death that frequent or complex ventricular arrhythmias late postoperatively should be treated aggressively.

Conclusions

In patients following repair of tetralogy of Fallot and other similar lesions, ventricular arrhythmias and sudden death are related. The risk of sudden death is likely to be higher than that indicated in early reports, since it is now known that the incidence of ventricular arrhythmias increases with each succeeding year after surgery. The actual data will be difficult to obtain, since a large number of these patients are now being treated for their ventricular arrhythmias. One difference between pediatric patients and their adult counterparts is that in children, at least in this particular problem, sudden death may be preventable by treatment with antiarrhythmic drugs.

Therefore it is apparent that some patients with ventricular arrhythmias require drug treatment. It is not yet established which particular patients require treatment. Using the criterion of treating those with frequent or complex ventricular arrhythmias clearly results in overtreatment. More specific criteria are needed. At some institutions, only those with inducible, sustained ventricular tachycardia during electrophysiology study are treated.[193] Because the prognostic ability of a positive or negative electrophysiology study has not yet been demonstrated, treatment based on the electrophysiology study may be premature. Finally, it has been suggested that only symptomatic patients be treated.[175] This is also unlikely to solve the problem, since many patients with palpitations have no arrhythmia, and more than half the patients with sudden death after tetralogy of Fallot repair are completely asymptomatic before death.[194] Hopefully, with further prospective study, the relative value of the Holter electrocardiogram and the electrophysiology study will be ascertained, and a rational plan for treatment of specific patients can be devised. At present, suppression of ventricular arrhythmias on the Holter recording appears to be an adequate way of assessing treatment in these patients. Further follow-up will be necessary to determine if chronic electrophysiologic drug testing is preferable. Finally, the agents that are successful in suppression of ventricular arrhythmias in these patients are different from those traditionally used in adult patients with ischemic heart disease and ventricular arrhythmias. This observation forms the basis for the hypothesis discussed in the section that follows.

NONISCHEMIC VENTRICULAR ARRHYTHMIAS IN CHILDREN AND ADULTS: A UNIFYING HYPOTHESIS

The observation that the class Ib agents (phenytoin and mexiletine) are effective in treating arrhythmias in children following surgery for congenital heart disease, and that the class Ia agents (quinidine and procainamide) are not effective, has led to a great deal of discussion. The adult with ischemic heart disease and ventricular arrhythmias generally has the opposite findings, with a good response to quinidine and a poor response to phenytoin. The explanation for these findings may have important implications. Three possibilities are that (1) the ages of the patients are different, (2) the drugs act differently, and (3) the diseases produce different mechanisms of ventricular arrhythmias in the two groups.

In attempting to explain the difference in drug response on the basis of the age of the patient, it is important to recognize that the majority of the patients being treated for ventricular arrhythmias after repair of congenital heart disease are not children. Most of them are older than 15 years, and many are older than 30 years. Therefore it is difficult to ascribe the success of phenytoin to the fact that it is more effective in children. Furthermore, it has recently been shown that both phenytoin and quinidine have similar cellular electrophysiologic effects on both neonatal and adult Purkinje fibers.[195]

Certainly, the class Ia and class Ib agents are different in electrophysiologic effects. While both quinidine and phenytoin block the sodium channel, quinidine increases the action potential duration, and phenytoin has either no effect or may decrease the action potential duration. However, the most interesting difference between the two classes of drugs is with respect to delayed afterdepolarizations and triggered activity. Both phenytoin and mexiletine have been shown to decrease delayed afterdepolarizations, while quinidine may actually cause an increase in delayed afterdepolarizations and lead to sustained triggered activity.[196–198] Therefore if the ventricular arrhythmias in patients after repair of congenital heart disease were initiated by delayed afterdepolarizations, the observation that phenytoin is effective and quinidine is not effective in treatment could be consistent with the mechanism of delayed afterdepolarizations as the cause of the arrhythmias.

A final possibility for the explanation of the differential drug effect is that the underlying substrate of postoperative congenital heart disease is electrophysiologically different from that of myocardial infarction. The features of postoperative tetralogy of Fallot are hypertrophy, cellular disarray (in the region of the infundibulum), a large ventriculotomy incision, and (in the majority of patients) right ventricular dilation as a result of postoperative pulmonary insufficiency. This is potentially different from the patient with coronary disease who suffers a myocardial infarction and has ventricular tachycardia related to the infarct scar.

In order to examine the possible cellular mechanisms involved in arrhythmias after repair of tetralogy of Fallot, we have created a canine model. Creation of a "pre-op" tetralogy for the first part of the animal's life was accomplished by banding the pulmonary artery (causing increased right ventricular pressure) and performing a pulmonary artery to the left atrium anastomosis (causing cyanosis). After approximately 4 months, the animal is "corrected" on cardiopulmonary bypass and undergoes de-banding, closure of the anastomosis, and right ventriculotomy. The animal is then observed for the next 6 months, with repeated 24-hour electrocardiograms and electrophysiology studies.

In preliminary experiments done on animals with continued elevated right ventricular systolic pressure after repair, we have found ventricular arrhythmias. On 24-hour electrocardiograms in three animals, the coupling interval of the premature beat was directly related to the preceding cycle length, suggesting a possible mechanism of triggered activity.[199] In one animal during electrophysiology study, the inducing cycle length was directly related to the rate of the induced ventricular tachycardia, another possible suggestion of triggered activity.[200]

Therefore our early animal studies suggest that delayed afterdepolarizations could be involved in the initiation of ventricular arrhythmias in patients after repair of tetralogy of Fallot. This finding is strengthened by the recent report of delayed afterdepolarizations in patients after repair of tetralogy of Fallot. Benito et al[201] performed monophasic action potential recordings in 10 patients after intracardiac repair of tetralogy of Fallot. All had ventricular arrhythmias greater than Lown grade 2 on the Holter electrocardiogram. In 6 of the 10, delayed afterdepolarizations were found and initiated spontaneous ventricular arrhythmias in the electrophysiology laboratory.

In attempting to explain the observation that the class Ib drugs are effective in treatment of ventricular arrhythmias after repair of tetralogy of Fallot, we arrive at the hypothesis that the reason for the difference in drug response is that the cellular mechanism for the initiation of the ventricular arrhythmias may be different in patients after repair of tetralogy than in those with myocardial infarction. However, this hypothesis does not apply only to patients after repair of tetralogy of Fallot. There are other diseases that have in common the features of ventricular arrhythmia, sudden death, hypertrophy, and cellular disarray. Additional features include the presence of areas of fibrosis (either native or surgically induced) and, possibly, cardiac dilation. Diseases that fit these general criteria include aortic stenosis/aortic insufficiency (both pre- and postoperative), hypertrophic cardiomyopathy (both unoperated and after septal myotomy/myectomy), and systemic hypertension. There is additional evidence that delayed afterdepolarizations are involved in the initiation of arrhythmias in these patients as well. First, in both pre- and postoperative patients with aortic stenosis/aortic insufficiency, phenytoin and mexiletine are effective in treating ventricular arrhythmias.[40, 169, 202] Also, in children with hypertrophic cardiomyopathy, both phenytoin and verapamil have been shown to be effective in the treatment of ventricular arrhythmias.[71, 203] Finally, the patient reported by Zipes et al who was thought on the basis of intracardiac electrophysiology study to have ventricular tachycardia caused by delayed afterdepolarizations and triggered activity, had systemic hypertension.[37] Moreover, delayed afterdepolarizations have been found by cellular electrophysiologic studies to be the likely cause of ventricular arrhythmias in rats with experimentally induced systemic hypertension.[204]

The unifying hypothesis is that patients with hypertrophy, cellular disarray, and areas of scarring have a different cellular mechanism for ventricular arrhythmias (i.e., delayed afterdepolarizations and triggered activity) than do patients with ischemic heart disease and myocardial infarction (i.e., reentry), regardless of age. This difference in mechanism, rather than the difference in age, explains the differential effect of certain drugs in children and adults with ventricular arrhythmias.

While this hypothesis accounts for the electrophysiologic observations, we must go further to explain how the disease process leads to the initiating ventricular arrhythmia that then ends in irreversible ventricular fibrillation and sudden death.

Returning to the situation after repair of tetralogy of Fallot, it has been found that ventricular tachycardia originates in areas adjacent to large areas of scar. This may not necessarily be in the right ventricular outflow tract in the area of the ventriculotomy, but may also be in fibrotic areas surrounding the ventricular septal defect patch or the infundibular resection.[57] In one patient, the reentrant ventricular tachycardia was mapped and found to progress around the entire area of the ventriculotomy incision as a macroreentrant circuit.[188] In our experimental animals, we found ventricular tachycardia related to the ventriculotomy, but the findings are more consistent with a micro-reentrant circuit at the edge of the ventriculotomy than with macro-reentry involving the entire incision.

Regardless, in certain situations there are ventricular arrhythmias that have their site of origin near large fibrous areas. If the fibrous areas are reduced (as in patients with no right ventriculotomy), the ventricular arrhythmias have been found to be reduced.[205] In our experimental model, we have also found that a simple ventriculotomy is not likely to lead to ventricular arrhythmias.[206] However, with the addition of persistently elevated right ventricular systolic and/or diastolic pressure to the ventriculotomy, ventricular arrhythmias do occur in these animals.[207] On pathologic examination, the ventriculotomy incision in animals with normal right ventricular hemodynamics had microscopically straight and smooth borders with little irregularity. On the other hand, animals with a ventriculotomy that healed in the presence of elevated right ventricular systolic and end-diastolic pressure had a much more irregular appearance, with fibrous tissue extending at right angles like "fingers" into the surrounding myocardium. It is possible that a more irregular scar is the genesis of the ventricular arrhythmias. It might be that, electrophysiologically, the cells in the region of these fibrous extensions could be altered and lead to triggered activity. This is currently under investigation in our animal model.

The initiating premature ventricular beat must become ventricular tachycardia. It is known that postoperative tetralogy patients with ventricular tachycardia have areas of slow conduction in the right ventricle. This has been demonstrated both during intracardiac electrophysiologic study (where the electrograms in the region of the right ventricular outflow tract and the summit of the ventricular septum are wide and fragmented[50] and by the presence of "late potentials" recorded by signal-averaged electrocardiography in postoperative tetralogy patients who have ventricular tachycardia. There are significantly more late potentials in postoperative tetralogy patients with ventricular tachycardia than in those with single premature beats or those without any ventricular arrhythmias. If a single premature beat that was originated by a delayed afterdepolarization encountered such an area of slow conduction, this could then lead to a reentrant ventricular tachycardia. It is also possible that fibrosis in the outflow tract and summit of the ventricular septum, similar to that found in myocardial infarction, leads to denervation of distal (inferior) parts of the ventricles. This could further create inhomogenous areas leading to reentry.

Once the reentry circuit is begun, it is likely that a hypertrophied, enlarged right ventricle will continue to sustain the ventricular tachycardia. It has been shown that with a decrease in volume, caused by Valsalva maneuver, termination of ventricular tachycardia may occur.[208] It is likely that the opposite could occur with an enlarged, dilated right ventricle, leading to continuation of the arrhythmia.

Next it is important to account for the progression from sustained ventricular tachycardia to ventricular fibrillation. As discussed previously, it is unlikely that a patient with a completely normal heart and ventricular tachycardia will have ventricular fibrillation or sudden death. On the other hand, the patient who has undergone repair of tetralogy of Fallot, especially one with abnormal hemodynamics, is at a markedly increased risk of ventricular fibrillation and sudden death. There are three possible explanations for this finding. First there is a primary electrical reason. It has been demonstrated that patients with ventricular tachycardia are more likely to have ventricular fibrillation in the presence of large areas of delayed conduction.[209] The second explanation is hemodynamic. In our experimental model, we have found that in dogs with pulmonary stenosis and elevated right ventricular pressure, the *left* ventricle became ischemic in response to rapid ventricular pacing at 300 bpm (simulating ventricular tachycardia). It is known that ischemia is a potent stimulus to ventricular fibrillation.[210] In addition, it has been reported that animals with hypertrophy like that found in tetralogy of Fallot are more likely to have ventricular fibrillation with ischemia than are animals without hypertrophy.[211] Palik, Graham, and Burger[212] have reported that in patients with high right ventricular pressures after repair of defects similar to tetralogy of Fallot, there is both right and left ventricular dysfunction. It is possible that the cause of this dysfunction is intermittent ischemia. The third possible cause of degeneration of ventricular tachycardia to ventricular fibrillation is elevated serum catecholamines. In our experimental model, we have found that in the animals with a pulmonary artery band, the serum norepinephrine increases markedly during rapid ventricular pacing. This does not occur in normal animals. The elevated norepinephrine could be of cardiac origin (i.e., released in association with ischemia) or of adrenal origin (i.e., in response to reduced cardiac output). Nonetheless, the increase in norepinephrine in the presence of ventricular tachycardia could certainly predispose to ventricular fibrillation.[213]

Finally, we must account for the observation that some postoperative tetralogy patients who are found to be in ventricular fibrillation are very difficult to defibrillate. It is known that in the presence of ventricular hypertrophy, the ventricular defibrillation threshold is increased, and successful eventual defibrillation is less common than in the non-hypertrophied heart.[214] This is certainly the case in postoperative tetralogy of Fallot, where right ventricular hypertrophy rarely, if ever, regresses.[215]

In summary, if a patient has a disease characterized by hypertrophy, cellular disarray, areas of scarring, and abnormal hemodynamics, it is likely that cells in the irregular border zone surrounding a scar will have delayed afterdepolarizations and triggered activity. This can cause single premature ventricular beats or sustained ventricular tachycardia. Areas of slow conduction and inhomogeneity could then allow the single premature beat to become a reentrant ventricular tachycardia. In the presence of a large right ventricle, the first few beats of ventricular tachycardia are likely to sustain. Sustained ventricular tachycardia may then undergo degeneration to ventricular fibrillation because of fragmented conduction, or ischemia, or increased serum norepinephrine. In the presence of hypertrophy, the fibrillating heart is difficult to defibrillate, and sudden death may result.

This hypothesis applies to diseases in patients of all ages, not just children. Perhaps an understanding of this process will lead to improved survival for children as well as for adults with nonischemic ventricular arrhythmias.

PVCs AND VENTRICULAR TACHYCARDIA TREATMENT

Acute Treatment

Almost all types of ventricular arrhythmias should be treated in patients with acute onset of arrhythmia who are otherwise seriously ill. We do not recommend treatment of uniform PVCs, even those in the bigeminal pattern, unless the arrhythmia causes a deterioration in hemodynamics. Multiform PVCs, couplets, and ventricular tachycardia should be treated immediately.

PVCs AND COUPLETS

1. Treat possible acute causes. The acute causes of ventricular arrhythmias are listed in Table 14–2. Because abnormalities in many of the electrolytes and blood gases can cause ventricular arrhythmias, values of these parameters should be obtained immediately following the acute appearance of ventricular arrhythmias. The abnormality detected

should be corrected at once. Also, an intracardiac catheter should be repositioned. If drugs are to be administered intravenously, a decision must be reached as to the risk/benefit ratio. For example, if a patient receiving isoproterenol for asthma has a few uniform PVCs and the isoproterenol is crucial to the antiasthmatic treatment, then the isoproterenol should be continued. Certainly if higher grades of ventricular ectopy develop, the drug must be reduced or discontinued.

The treatment of ventricular arrhythmias caused by three particular drugs needs to be emphasized. The first is digitalis. It is rare for children to develop ventricular arrhythmias in digitalis intoxication. When they occur, they generally are accompanied by AV block. The specific treatment for digitalis intoxication is Fab antidigoxin antibodies. These are becoming increasingly available. If they are not available, the specific treatment for digitalis intoxication is intravenous phenytoin. The total dose of 15 mg/kg is given over 1 hour. Because intravenous phenytoin is unstable and precipitates if diluted, the undiluted phenytoin must be kept in a syringe, and 1/12 of the total dose should be rapidly injected every 5 minutes, followed by a flush of normal saline to be sure there is no phenytoin left in the plastic tubing. Phenytoin cannot be given by intravenous drip. For the first four to five injections, patients report a burning at the injection site. Approximately 30 to 40 minutes after the first dose, most patients become lightheaded. There may also be transient hypotension, which responds to a lengthening of the intervals between phenytoin injections. Because of the hypotension, we do not recommend intravenous phenytoin for patients with severely abnormal hemodynamics. We have found in some patients a lag between the increase in serum phenytoin concentration and the effect, lasting up to 2 hours after the completion of the loading dose protocol. Following intravenous loading, it is then possible to begin maintenance therapy with either oral or intravenous phenytoin. We have used the phenytoin serum concentration extensively to monitor treatment. There are numerous laboratory methods for determination of phenytoin serum concentration, and it is important to be aware of the therapeutic range for the laboratory reporting the results. It is possible to have the effective range differ by more than 50% among the different methods. In general, the therapeutic range is between 10 μg/mL and 20 μg/mL.

The second drug to be discussed is quinidine. For patients with PVCs or couplets caused by quinidine intoxication (torsades de pointes will be discussed under ventricular tachycardia), it has been advocated to give sodium to reverse the effects of quinidine, which is a sodium channel blocker. The simplest method is to give 1–2 mEq/kg of sodium bicarbonate to see if this has an effect on the arrhythmia. In a patient with relatively stable hemodynamics, 3% saline may also be used. Lidocaine or magnesium sulfate may also be used (see following discussion).

The final drug to be considered is amiodarone. It is rare for amiodarone to result in ventricular arrhythmias, but effective treatments have been mexiletine[65] and magnesium sulfate.[66]

If treatment of the "reversible" causes of PVCs and couplets has not been effective, the remaining steps in the treatment regimen may be used.

2. Lidocaine, 1 mg/kg IV push. This may be repeated once every 5 minutes for a total of three doses. This may be followed by an intravenous drip of 0.5–1.5 mg/kg/h.

3. Procainamide, 10–15 mg/kg IV drip over 1 hour. This should not be used in cases of drug intoxication with type Ia drugs (such as quinidine) or amiodarone, or in patients with long QT syndromes.

4. Atropine, 0.01 mg/kg IV push. This should be used only if the sinus rate is slow or normal. The increase in rate caused by atropine may suppress the PVCs.

5. Temporary atrial or ventricular pacing. If the sinus rate is slow or normal, the increase in ventricular rate by pacing at a rate faster than the sinus rate may suppress the PVCs. If AV conduction is intact, atrial pacing provides for more uniform activation of the ventricles, improved cardiac output, and possibly more effective suppression of the PVCs.

VENTRICULAR TACHYCARDIA

1. If the patient's hemodynamic status is acceptable, steps one through four listed for PVCs and couplets may be followed in rapid succession. The acute treatment of torsades de pointes can begin with lidocaine and should not include procainamide. The next step is to insert a temporary transvenous pacemaker and pace either the atrium or the ventricle (assuming AV conduction is intact)

at a relatively rapid rate (150 per minute for infants and 120 per minute for older children). This has been effective in suppressing torsades de pointes. Finally, especially in cases of drug-induced torsades de pointes, magnesium sulfate may be used. This has not been reported in children; the adult dose is 1–2 g IV push, followed by 1 g/min IV infusion; this calculates to 15–30 mg/kg IV push, followed by 15 mg/kg/min IV infusion.[66] If the patient is capable of taking oral drugs, mexiletine 3–5 mg/kg every 8 hours can be used as well.

2. If the patient's hemodynamic status is unacceptable, then synchronized DC electrical cardioversion should be performed with 0.5 to 1.5 watt-seconds/kg.[216]

3. Overdrive ventricular pacing may also be used to terminate ventricular tachycardia. Pacing may need to be attempted at a rate 30 bpm to 50 bpm faster than the tachycardia for an interval of 5 to 10 minutes, and then stopped. This may stop the ventricular tachycardia, but may also accelerate the tachycardia or cause ventricular fibrillation. If this method is attempted, the team should be prepared to use immediate cardioversion/defibrillation.

4. Propranolol, 0.025 mg/kg IV push may be repeated once every 5 to 10 minutes for a total of four doses. Intravenous propranolol should only be used if the team is prepared to initiate emergency ventricular pacing if bradycardia should result.

5. There are a number of investigational agents, including amiodarone, flecainide, and propafenone, that will soon be available for intravenous use. All of these drugs may acutely depress myocardial contractility, and it is important to be prepared to support the circulation if these drugs are used. The use of intravenous verapamil for ventricular tachycardia is not likely to be effective. In adults and children, when verapamil was used mistakenly for ventricular tachycardia (thinking the patient had supraventricular tachycardia with aberration), the majority of patients developed acute hemodynamic deterioration; some experienced cardiac arrest. The ventricular tachycardia rarely converted. However, verapamil may be a reasonable choice for advanced ventricular fibrillation, since one of the possible pathophysiologies of ventricular fibrillation is intracellular calcium overload. Similarly, bretylium is not a drug for ventricular tachycardia, because it releases norepinephrine from the nerve endings and could precipitate ventricular fibrillation in a patient with ventricular tachycardia. Therefore the use of bretylium should be limited to patients with ventricular fibrillation.

Chronic Treatment

In the previous sections on the specific causes of chronic arrhythmias, the discussion centered around which patients to treat. This section is concerned with how to treat these patients and will begin with drug treatment, followed by catheter ablation, surgery, and electronic devices.

DRUG TREATMENT

In practically all situations in children, treatment of chronic ventricular arrhythmias should begin with antiarrhythmic drugs. We usually assess treatment efficacy with the Holter monitor, although in certain situations, especially with symptomatic sustained ventricular tachycardia, chronic drug electrophysiology studies may be used. Because there is a great deal of baseline variability in children with ventricular arrhythmias,[31] it is most helpful to obtain two baseline Holter recordings before treatment. We generally define "treatment success" as the virtual elimination of any ventricular arrhythmia from the Holter electrocardiogram, (i.e., fewer than 10 uniform premature ventricular contractions per hour). In some patients this may not be possible; elimination of the highest grade of ventricular arrhythmia is always required. For example, in the patient with nonsustained ventricular tachycardia, this must be completely eliminated from two successive Holter recordings. Recent evidence has suggested that the dosage for the newer antiarrhythmic drugs is more accurate when calculated on the basis of body surface area rather than body weight.[217–220] Because the dosage range is only approximate, we generally increase a drug until there are symptomatic side effects, unacceptable effects on the electrocardiogram (such as accessive QRS prolongation), or the serum concentration (always obtained at the trough level, immediately before a dose) is obviously in the toxic range established for adults. Since many of these drugs must be given three or four times a day, we attempt to make the schedule as convenient as possible, such as "with meals" for drugs taken three times a day or "with meals and at bedtime" for drugs taken four times per day. Unless the patient demonstrates symptoms from ventricular tachycardia associated with a slightly longer dosage interval at night, it does not seem reasonable to ask the patient and parents to awaken during the night for a dose. The following discussion of drug therapy will begin with a brief review of who should be treated, as well as some of the drug doses and drug side effects. A full discussion of these drugs, including their doses, is given in Chapter 3. In this discussion, the major effects and side effects will be given.

Type Ia Agents

Type Ia drugs (quinidine, procainamide, disopyramide) have been the mainstay of treatment in adults. Many pediatric cardiologists have used these drugs with varying amounts of success, but we have experienced problems with each of them. For this reason, we have reserved the use of the type Ia drugs for ventricular arrhythmias only after other drugs have failed. There are certain patients in whom these drugs should not be used, such as patients with long QT syndromes and possibly patients with mitral valve prolapse, since there has been an association made between mitral prolapse and some of the long QT syndromes. These drugs should be used cautiously in patients with depressed left ventricular function. Disopyramide has especially been associated with a marked reduction in left ventricular function and should not be used in patients with abnormal ventricular function; quinidine and procainamide are safer in these patients. Patients with infranodal conduction system disease (especially with a prolonged HV interval) may have a worsening in conduction and develop AV block with the use of these agents. Unless the status of the conduction system is known, they should be used cautiously in patients who have had repair of congenital heart disease. Also, patients with sinus bradycardia may develop sinus node exit block with the use of these drugs. For this reason, the joint American College of Cardiology/American Heart Association Committee on Pacing has recommended that a pacemaker be implanted in patients following the Mustard or Senning operation who may potentially require sinus node suppressant drugs (including the type Ia drugs). Since ventricular arrhythmias are known to be a problem in patients who have had the Mustard operation as well as in those who have undergone ventricular septal defect repair, this recommendation is also applicable to these patients.[221]

Despite all these concerns, the type Ia drugs may be extremely effective in certain patients with ventricular arrhythmias. The major side effects of quinidine are nausea and diarrhea. Torsades de pointes has been reported in children (mostly those with an abnormal heart) receiving quinidine within the first 2 weeks of beginning therapy.[61] For this reason, we recommend beginning quinidine in the hospital, with close observation for the first 2 weeks. In those with an abnormal heart, superimposed hypokalemia exacerbates quinidine intoxication, and the serum potassium concentration as well as the quinidine serum concentration should be monitored closely, at least every 6 months. The major side effect of procainamide appears to be the development of drug-induced lupus. In addition, procainamide is rapidly metabolized in children, requiring at least four doses per day. Disopyramide appears to have fewer gastrointestinal side effects than quinidine, but the depression of ventricular function can be severe; since the majority of children treated with ventricular arrhythmias do not have a normal heart, we have not found it necessary to use disopyramide in children.

Type Ib Agents

Type Ib agents (phenytoin, mexiletine, and tocainide) are primarily used in patients with postoperative congenital heart disease, especially those with abnormal hemodynamics.[222] They seem to be less effective in postoperative congenital heart disease patients with more normal hemodynamics. These drugs are also effective in patients with the long QT syndromes and possibly in patients with mitral valve prolapse. In patients with arrhythmogenic right ventricular dysplasia and congestive cardiomyopathy, they are approximately 50% effective, and in those with a normal heart, they are about 25% effective. They are valuable primarily because they do not depress ventricular function when given orally. Similar to the type Ia agents, these drugs are not mutually exclusive, and success or failure with one does not necessarily imply success or failure with another. As a result, each of them may be tried in a given situation. The major limiting side effect of phenytoin has been the development of a rash in 10% to 20% of patients. This occurs within the first 10 days of use of the drug. Despite reports that phenytoin use may result in the Stevens-Johnson syndrome, we have only observed this once. We have not seen exacerbation of ventricular arrhythmias with phenytoin or the other type Ib drugs. The major side effects of mexiletine are nausea and headaches; the side effects of tocainide are similar, with the addition of isolated reports of agranulocytosis. Ataxia and confusion are the only side effects of overdosage with these agents.

Type Ic Agents

Type Ic agents (encainide and flecainide) have been dubbed the "PVC killers." While there has been little experience with the use of these drugs for the treatment of ventricular arrhythmias in children, it is likely that they will be effective in almost all situations, especially in those patients with more normal hemodynamics. Since they do prolong intraventricular conduction, they need to be used cautiously in patients with prolonged HV intervals (e.g., those with postoperative congenital heart disease). Their use in prolonged QT syndromes has been unproven. They do not directly affect repolarization and may find a use in patients with frequent ventricular arrhythmias in these syndromes. In children, encainide has largely been used in supraventricular arrhythmias.[217] There have been no negative inotropic effects. In general, encainide effect (not toxicity) is marked by QRS prolongation. Rarely, encainide causes ventricular arrhythmias (a "proarrhythmic" effect). This is seen early in treatment, and therefore patients should be hospitalized for the initiation of encainide. The effects of flecainide are likely to be similar, with the addition that flecainide may depress ventricular function and have sinus node suppressive effects. The magnitude of these effects in children remain to be investigated.

Type II Agents

The major indication for the use of type II agents (β-blockers) is in children with the long QT syndromes. They may also be effective for exercise-related ventricular tachycardia. In patients with relatively normal hemodynamics (mild cardiomyopathy or mild arrhythmogenic right ventricular dysplasia), they seem to be the best agents for initial treatment, but are still only approximately 60% effective.[222] They are approximately 50% effective in postoperative congenital heart disease patients, and may also be effective as an adjunct to another antiarrhythmic drug, especially if the ventricular arrhythmia tends to be more prevalent with activity. The major drawback to these drugs are their tendency to cause ventricular dysfunction, sinus bradycardia, and AV block. They must be used cautiously in patients with a propensity to these problems. One side effect that has received an increasing amount of attention in the adult literature has been the production of depression and a decreased attention span. We have observed this in children, although the incidence is not known. Among the β-blockers, we have had the greatest experience with propranolol, which must be given three or four times a day. Atenolol, which must be given only once per day, is currently the long-acting β-blocker of choice. It appears to have the fewest side effects, since it crosses the blood–brain barrier the least of any of these agents. Nonetheless, even with this drug, the previously mentioned side effects may occur.

Type III Agents

The primary type III agent used is amiodarone, which is used to treat patients with "life-threatening" arrhythmias. This includes those patients with ventricular arrhythmias who have paroxysmal symptoms such as syncope, or those patients known to be at a high risk for sudden death (e.g., patients after repair of congenital heart disease who have extremely abnormal hemodynamics). Since these drugs cause marked QT interval prolongation, they should probably not be used in patients with long QT syndrome and possibly not in patients with mitral valve prolapse. Because of the marked sinus suppressant effects, they should not be used in patients with known sick sinus syndrome unless absolutely necessary, and then probably only with prophylactic implantation of a pacemaker. These drugs are also known to cause AV block and so a dual-chambered pacemaker should be implanted in a patient with sick sinus syndrome who is being treated with amiodarone.

The major side effects of amiodarone in children are sun sensitivity, nausea and headaches (occasionally), and very rarely hypothyroidism or hyperthyroidism. Microdeposits are rare in children younger than 10 years. Hepatitis and peripheral neuropathy have been reported in a few patients. Pulmonary toxicity has not yet been reported in a child. The use of sotalol, another type III agent, in children has not yet been widespread enough to determine its effectiveness or side effects.

Type IV Agents

Type IV agents (calcium channel blockers such as Verapamil) are not traditionally thought to be useful in patients with ventricular arrhythmias. However, there are certain patients in whom they may be effective. They are likely to be most effective in patients with a relatively normal heart (e.g., in those with mild arrhythmogenic right ventricle or mild congestive cardiomyopathy) or in those with an entirely normal heart and idiopathic ventricular tachycardia. They may also be effective in a subgroup of patients with exercise-related ventricular tachycardia or hypertrophic cardiomyopathy. It is speculated that these drugs may be effective in certain patients with postoperative congenital heart disease or unoperated congenital heart disease. They are probably not effective in patients with long QT syndromes. The major side effects of verapamil are peripheral vasodilation, decreased myocardial contractility, sinus bradycardia, and AV block and should therefore be used cautiously in patients prone to these problems. Intravenous verapamil has not been reported to convert ventricular tachycardia, and it probably should not be used for this purpose.

CATHETER ABLATION

Catheter ablation has been discussed in the section on postoperative congenital heart disease. In the future, ablation of arrhythmogenic areas of the heart during cardiac catheterization may be an important part of therapy. However, the way it is currently performed with high energy shocks appears to produce more risk than benefit.

SURGERY

Indications for surgical treatment of ventricular arrhythmias are as follows:

1. Tumor removal. In the infant with incessant ventricular tachycardia, there almost always appears to be a small area of the ventricle that, when removed, results in sinus rhythm. The majority of these patients appear to have microscopic ventricular tumors as the cause of the tachycardia. We have not observed rapid incessant ventricular tachycardia in children older than 3 years, and so there is no information on the likelihood of finding a microscopic tumor as the cause of ventricular arrhythmias in older children. Certainly, tumors visible either echocardiographically or by angiography can cause ventricular arrhythmias, and their removal can cure the ventricular arrhythmias.[223–225]
2. Primary surgery for ventricular tachycardia ablation in older children. We have performed surgery to ablate ventricular tachycardia in postoperative tetralogy of Fallot, and this procedure may be successful in eliminating the arrhythmia. Harken, Horowitz, and Josephson[188] have reported similar results.
3. Reduction in ventricular arrhythmia by improvement in hemodynamics. In certain patients after the operation to improve hemodynamics in tetralogy of Fallot or after aortic valve replacement in aortic stenosis, ventricular arrhythmias may improve because of improved hemodynamics.
4. Left stellectomy for idiopathic long QT syndrome. This is discussed in the section on long QT syndrome. There have been both positive and negative reports as to the success of this operation. It is not likely to be harmful, and even Horner's syndrome with noticeable ptosis usually resolves. It should probably be attempted in patients with prolonged QT syndrome who continue to have symptomatic episodes of torsades de pointes in spite of medical and pacing therapy.[134, 135] In general, β-blocking therapy is continued after this operation.

ELECTRICAL DEVICES

Antitachycardia pacemakers that introduce either premature ventricular extrastimuli or burst ventricular pacing have been implanted in a few children for resistant ventricular arrhythmias. The obvious risk is acceleration of the ventricular tachycardia to a more rapid rate or the induction of ventricular fibrillation. Implantation of such a device is indicated in a patient whose ventricular arrhythmias are not responsive to amiodarone in combination with other antiarrhythmic drugs and in whom the ventricular arrhythmia can be terminated repeatedly in the cardiac catheterization laboratory with a pacing protocol that can be reproduced by the antitachycardia pacemaker. It is also important to demonstrate that this pacing protocol does not produce hemodynamic or electrical instability, such as acceleration of the arrhythmia or ventricular fibrillation. Another type of device currently available is the automatic implantable defibrillator.[136] This has been implanted in a child with the long QT syndrome.[137] The indications are similar to those for the antitachycardia pacemaker, except that the patient should lose consciousness with the arrhythmia, since the administration of the defibrillating shock is painful. In the future, combination implantable devices will be available that will be capable of performing pacing protocols, cardioversion, and defibrillation.

VENTRICULAR FIBRILLATION

Ventricular fibrillation is a series of incoordinated ventricular depolarizations associated with no cardiac output.[1] Ventricular fibrillation is quite rare in children. Walsh and Krongrad[226] reviewed the terminal electrical activity of 100 children younger than 18 years. In only six (6%) was the terminal event ventricular fibrillation. In all others, the terminal event was bradycardia followed by asystole.

ECG Characteristics

On the surface ECG, ventricular fibrillation is a series of low amplitude, rapid, irregular depolarizations without identifiable QRS complexes (Fig. 14–42).[44] In ventricular fibrillation, two types of onset are observed: type A is characterized by rapid initiation of fibrillation with one or two premature beats; in type B, the excitation process becomes gradually disorganized after relatively long periods of ventricular tachycardia.[4] The morphology of ventricular fibrillation is not unlike that of electrical interference or that observed when an ECG electrode has lost contact with the patient. Therefore when ventricular fibrillation is suspected, the ECG electrodes should be rapidly checked for patient contact, and loss of pulse in the patient should be confirmed. Ventricular fibrillation may be of such low amplitude ("fine ventricular fibrillation") that it appears similar to asystole.[227] For this reason, multiple ECG leads should also be rapidly examined.

Clinical Situations and Prognosis

Although spontaneous conversion from ventricular fibrillation to sinus rhythm has been reported,[4] ventricular fibrillation is almost always permanent and fatal if not treated. While hypoxia, electric shock, chest trauma, hypothermia, and any of the other situations listed in Table 14–2 may cause ventricular fibrillation in children with a normal heart, the vast majority of children with ventricular fibrillation have an abnormal heart.[12, 228] There are predominantly three groups of children who are vulnerable to ventricular fibrillation. The first group consists of patients with a prolonged QT interval.[213, 228] The second group comprises those with severe myocardial hypertrophy or underlying myocardial disease (e.g., the newborn with very severe aortic stenosis or pulmonary stenosis and massive ventricular hypertrophy, or the child with congestive cardiomyopathy or uncorrected congenital heart disease).[12] The third group consists of those patients with Wolff-Parkinson-White syndrome who have a short antegrade refractory period of the bundle of Kent, allowing for transmission of supraventricular impulses early during repolarization of the ventricles.[45] It is not known whether ventricular fibrillation is caused by the rapid ventricular rate or by the superimposition of successive beats on the preceding T wave during the vulnerable period.[7] Since atrial fibrillation is more likely in children with Wolff-Parkinson-White syndrome beginning in the early teenage years,[229] ventricular fi-

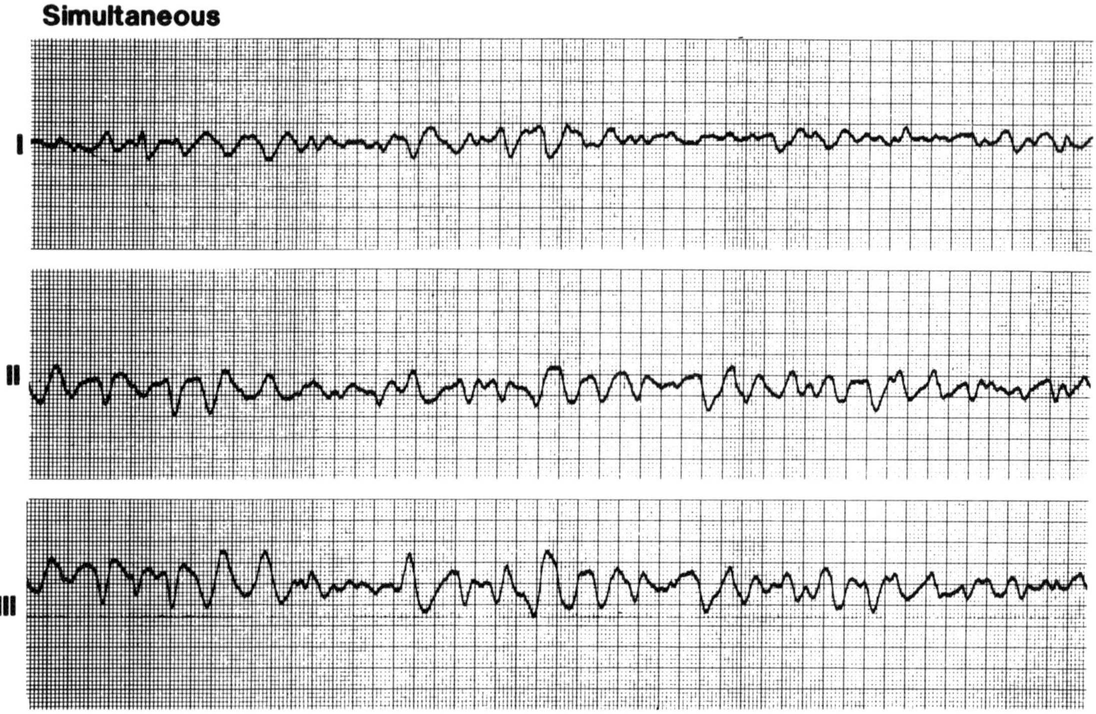

FIGURE 14–42
Surface electrocardiogram from a patient with ventricular fibrillation. The depolarizations are disorganized and resemble electrical interference or loss of electrode contact with the patient.

brillation is also most likely to occur at that time in patients with Wolff-Parkinson-White syndrome. It is difficult to predict from an electrophysiology study which patients are likely to develop ventricular fibrillation. In adults, it appears that if the antegrade functional refractory period of the Kent bundle is greater than 300 ms, it is very unlikely for the patient to develop ventricular fibrillation. In those with shorter refractory periods, ventricular fibrillation may or may not occur.[230]

Mechanisms

Non-uniform electrical recovery of the ventricles appears to be necessary for ventricular fibrillation.[4, 213] In patients with a prolonged QT interval, asymmetric effects of sympathetic tone can cause differential alterations in ventricular refractoriness.[27] Patients with myocardial disease have numerous areas of patchy fibrosis allowing for non-uniform conduction and repolarization. Finally, the effect of the shortened refractory period of the Kent bundle may allow for a supraventricular impulse to conduct to the ventricles early in repolarization, when parts of the myocardium are fully repolarized and other areas may still be relatively or absolutely refractory (Fig. 14–43).[231]

Classically, the onset of ventricular fibrillation has been explained by either unifocal impulse formation, multifocal impulse formation, or reentry.[4] The experimental and clinical data favor reentry as at least part of the underlying mechanism. The reason that ventricular fibrillation appears to be so rare in children is best explained by the observation that a critical mass of myocardium is necessary for either atrial or ventricular fibrillation,[232] and children generally have a small heart. In children with an abnormal heart, it is possible that different electrical properties effectively isolate certain areas of the myocardium and allow for ventricular fibrillation. In these children, the cellular milieu (e.g., calcium overload) may make it more likely for ventricular fibrillation to occur.

Management

All management of ventricular fibrillation is acute. The treatment is basically the same

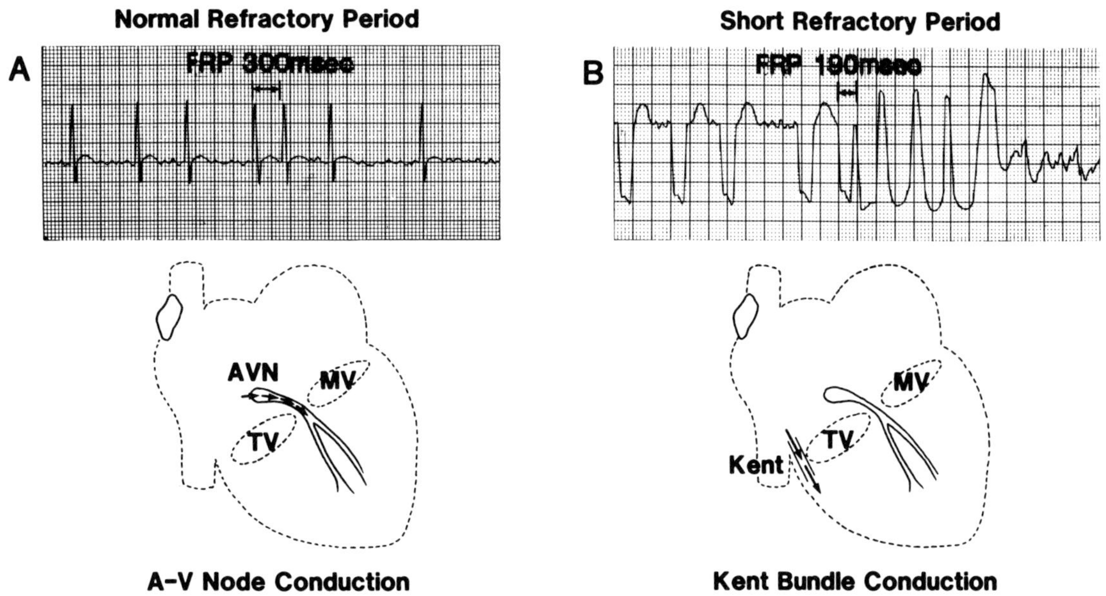

FIGURE 14–43
Possible mechanism for ventricular fibrillation in patients with atrial fibrillation and Wolff-Parkinson-White syndrome. *(A)* Normal conduction. The drawing of the surface electrocardiogram shows the shortest possible RR interval as 300 ms. This is the functional refractory period (FRP) of the AV node. The diagram shows that the AV node is protective and allows only consecutive conducted atrial impulses to excite the ventricles after the T wave of the previous beat. *(B)* Antegrade conduction through a bundle of Kent. The drawing of the surface electrocardiogram shows the functional refractory period of the bundle of Kent to be 190 ms, which is much shorter than that of the AV node, allowing for conduction of atrial impulses to the ventricles during the T wave of the preceding ventricular beat and possibly inducing ventricular tachycardia and ventricular fibrillation.

as that outlined for symptomatic ventricular tachycardia. If ventricular fibrillation either does not respond to the first attempt at defibrillation or is recurrent, bretylium tosylate may be administered. This drug is discussed completely in chapter 3. It is important to note that the onset of action of bretylium takes from 3 to 6 minutes and that the half-life is quite long; therefore, the time of administration of bretylium should be noted carefully, and successive defibrillations planned accordingly. In addition, multiple doses of bretylium are probably not necessary. The administration of isoproterenol may be effective in that it reduces ventricular action potential duration and causes more uniform electrical excitation and repolarization; however, the increase in catecholamines may make ventricular fibrillation more resistant. Therefore, isoproterenol should be reserved for patients with truly refractory ventricular fibrillation. The same situation holds for the administration of intravenous verapamil. We have seen, in a few patients with ventricular fibrillation and markedly hypertrophied hearts, that the acute administration of calcium channel blockers allowed for electrical defibrillation that had previously been unsuccessful. Certainly these drugs may alter myocardial contractility, but in refractory ventricular fibrillation, this side effect may be more reversible than the arrhythmia.[214] One technique used in refractory ventricular fibrillation has been to insert a catheter into the right ventricle and perform internal defibrillation with 360 joules in a configuration similar to that for catheter ablation.[233] However, if this is attempted in a child, the dosage of energy should be 1–2 watt-seconds/kg. The final treatment for ventricular fibrillation, especially if it occurs in a child with a potentially reversible myocardial problem, is to initiate emergency cardiopulmonary bypass.

After restoration of sinus rhythm, management is directed at finding an underlying abnormality. If the patient was previously thought to be normal, then the QT interval should be measured very carefully, since this may represent the underlying abnormality. If the patient has the Wolff-Parkinson-White syndrome, electrophysiologic studies should be undertaken with the goal of mapping the Kent bundle and performing surgical ablation. Ventricular fibrillation in a patient with Wolff-Parkinson-White syndrome is an absolute indication for surgery. Children who have ventricular fibrillation without any underlying reason should undergo extensive evaluation for detection of congenital or acquired heart disease. This evaluation should include anatomic and electrophysiologic cardiac catheterization.

If an underlying cause cannot be demonstrated, it should be assumed that the patient has an underlying abnormality similar to the long QT syndrome, and the patient should be treated chronically with propranolol or phenytoin. Quinidine and procainamide should be avoided because of their tendency to prolong the QT interval. If the patient has recurrent ventricular fibrillation, an automatic defibrillator or similar device can be implanted.[234]

Ventricular fibrillation is the rarest of cardiac arrhythmias found in children and also the most dangerous. The majority of children who have ventricular fibrillation have either a structurally abnormal heart, a prolonged QT interval, or Wolff-Parkinson-White syndrome. These abnormalities may be detected with a routine electrocardiogram and echocardiogram. It is therefore imperative that patients with syncope or patients who are resuscitated from cardiac arrest have these tests as part of their initial diagnostic examination.

Acknowledgments

This research was supported in part by grants HL24916, HL07190, and RR00188 from the National Institutes of Health, Bethesda, Maryland, and by a grant from the J. S. Abercrombie Foundation.

References

1. Schamroth L: The Disorders of Cardiac Rhythm. Oxford, Blackwell, 85–94, 1970.
2. Garson A: The Electrocardiogram in Infants and Children: A Systematic Approach. Philadelphia, Lea & Febiger, 1983, pp 95–98.
3. Jacobsen J, Garson A, Gillette P, et al: Premature ventricular contractions in normal children. J Pediatr 92:36, 1978.
4. Watanabe T, Dreifus LS: Cardiac Arrhythmias: Electrophysiologic Basis for Clinical Interpretation. New York, Grune & Stratton, 217–267, 1977.
5. Lewis S, Kanakis C, Rosen K, et al: Significance of site of origin of premature ventricular contractions. Am Heart J 97:159, 1979.
6. Josephson M, Horowitz L, Farshidi A, et al: Recurrent sustained ventricular tachycardia. 1. Mechanisms. Circulation 57:431, 1978.
7. Han J: Ventricular vulnerability to fibrillation. In Dreifus LS, Likoff W (eds): Cardiac Arrhythmias. New York, Grune & Stratton, 1973, pp 87–95.
8. Talbot S, Dreifus L: Characteristics of ventricular extrasystoles and their prognostic importance. Chest 67:665, 1975.
9. Langendorf R, Pick A, Winternitz M: Mechanisms of intermittent ventricular bigeminy. I. Appearance of ectopic beats dependent upon length of the ventricular cycle, the "rule of bigeminy." Circulation 11:422, 1955.
10. Kuo C, Surawicz B: Coexistence of ventricular parasystole and ventricular couplets: Mechanism and clinical significance. Am J Cardiol 44:435, 1979.
11. Garson A, Smith R, Moak J, et al: Incessant ventricular tachycardia in infants: Purkinje cell tumors and surgical cure. Circulation 74(suppl II):119, 1986.
12. Pederson D, Foster P, Troup P, et al: Ventricular tachycardia and ventricular fibrillation in a young population. Circulation 60:988, 1979.
13. Videbaek J, Andersen E, Jacobsen J, et al: Paroxysmal tachycardia in infancy and childhood, II. Paroxysmal ventricular tachycardia and fibrillation. Acta Paediatr Scand, 62:349, 1973.
14. Dessertenne, F. La tachycardie ventriculaire a deux foyers opposes variables. Arch Mal Coeur 59:263–272, 1966.
15. Coumel P, Leclerq J, Lucet V: Possible mechanisms of the arrhythmias in the long QT syndrome. Eur Heart J 6(suppl D):115–129, 1985.
16. Davidson RM: Chronic accelerated ventricular rhythm. J Electrocardiography 9:249, 1976.
17. Vetter VL, Horowitz LN, Josephson ME: Recurrent sustained ventricular tachycardia in pediatric patients. Circulation 57,58(suppl II):II–196, 1978.
18. Gaum W, Biancamello T, Kaplan S: Accelerated ventricular rhythm in childhood. Am J Cardiol 43:162, 1979.
19. Addy D, Littlewood J: Ventricular tachycardia associated with hyperkalemia. Am J Dis Child 117:705, 1969.
20. Reiffel JA, Schulhof E, Joseph B: Palpitations and dizziness: Arrhythmia frequency determined by transtelephonic monitoring. Circulation 72(suppl III):476, 1985.
21. Jervell A, Lange-Nielsen F: Congenital deaf-mutism, functional heart disease with prolongation of the QT interval and sudden death. Am Heart J 54:59, 1957.
22. Bazett HC: An analysis of the time relations of electrocardiograms. Heart 7:353–370, 1918.
23. Browne KF, Prystowsky EN, Zipes DP: Diurnal variation of QT interval in man. Circulation 66:II–128, 1982.
24. Anderson RC: Q-T interval in sinus arrhythmia. J Electrocardiol 14(4):407–408, 1981.
25. Leistner H, Haddad G, Lai T, et al: Heart rate pattern during sleep in an infant with congenital prolongation of the Q-T interval (Romano-Ward syndrome). Chest 84(2):191–194, 1983.
26. Schwartz PJ: The sudden infant death syndrome. In Reviews in Perinatal Medicine, vol 4. New York, Raven Press, 1981, pp 475–524.
27. Schwartz P, Periti M, Malliani A: The long QT syndrome. Am Heart J 89:378, 1975.

28. Schwartz PJ: The idiopathic long QT syndrome: Progress and questions. Am Heart J 109(2):399–411, 1985.
29. Garson A, Gillette P, Gutgesell H, et al: Stress-induced ventricular ectopy after tetralogy of Fallot repair. Am J Cardiol 46:1006–1012, 1980.
30. Morganroth J, Michelson EL, Horowitz LN: Limitations of routine long-term electrocardiographic monitoring to assess ventricular ectopic frequency. Circulation 58:408–413, 1978.
31. Hordof A, Steeg C, Garofano G, et al: Ambulatory electrocardiography for the evaluation of ventricular arrhythmias in children. In Proceedings of the Second World Congress of Pediatric Cardiology. New York, 1985, p 105.
32. Moe GK, Jalife J, Mueller WJ, et al: A mathematical model of parasystole and its application to clinical arrhythmias. Circulation 56:968, 1977.
33. Jalife J, Moe GK: A biologic model of parasystole. Am J Cardiol 43:761, 1979.
34. Zimmermann M, Maisonblanche P, Cauchemez B, et al: Determinants of the spontaneous ectopic activity in repetitive monomorphic ventricular tachycardia. J Am Coll Cardiol I:1219–1227, 1986.
35. Akhtar M, Damato A, Batsford W, et al: Demonstration of reentry within the His-Purkinje system in man. Circulation 50:1150, 1974.
36. Johnson N, Danilo P, Wit A, et al: Response to pacing of triggered activity occurring in catecholamine-treated canine coronary sinus. Circulation 72:III–381, 1985.
37. Zipes D, Foster P, Troup P, et al: Atrial induction of ventricular tachycardia: Reentry versus triggered automaticity. Am J Cardiol 44(1):1–8, 1979.
38. Sung R, Shapiro W, Shen E, et al: Effects of verapamil on ventricular tachycardias possibly caused by reentry, automaticity, and triggered activity. J Clin Invest 72(1):350–360, 1983.
39. Josephson M, Horowitz L: Electrophysiologic approach to therapy of recurrent sustained ventricular tachycardia. Am J Cardiol 43:631, 1979.
40. Garson A, Kugler J, Gillette A, et al: Control of late postoperative ventricular arrhythmias with phenytoin in young patients. Am J Cardiol 46:290–294, 1980.
41. Mehta AV, Sanchez GR, O'Riordan AC: Amiodarone therapy in children with refractory tachydysrhythmias. In Proceedings of the Second World Congress of Pediatric Cardiology. New York, 1985, p 108.
42. Garson A, Randall DG, McVey P, et al: Prevention of sudden death after repair of tetralogy of Fallot: Treatment of ventricular arrhythmias. J Am Coll Cardiol 6:221–227, 1985.
43. Garson A, Nihill M, McNamara D, et al: Status of the adult and adolescent after repair of tetralogy of Fallot. Circulation 59:1232, 1979.
44. Garson A, Gillette P, Porter C, et al: Ventricular tachycardia in children with a normal heart. Circulation 66(suppl II):170, 1982.
45. Garson A, Gillette P, Porter C: Electrophysiologic induction of ventricular dysrhythmias in 152 children with normal or abnormal heart. J Am Coll Cardiol 1:614, 1983.
46. Garson A, Porter J, Gillette P, et al: Induction of ventricular tachycardia during electrophysiologic study after repair of tetralogy of Fallot. J Am Coll Cardiol 1:1493–1502, 1983.
47. Mullins C: New catheter technique for transseptal left heart catheterization in infants and children. Circulation 59,60(suppl II):II–251, 1979.
48. Waldo AL, Akhtar M, Wellens HJ: The minimally appropriate electrophysiologic study for the initial assessment of patients with documented sustained monomorphic ventricular tachycardia. J Am Coll Cardiol 6:1174–1177, 1985.
49. Fontaine G, Guiraudon G, Frank R, et al: Arrhythmogenic right ventricular dysplasia: A previously unrecognized syndrome. Circulation 59,60(suppl II):II–75, 1979.
50. Deanfield J, McKenna W, Rowland E: Local abnormalities of right ventricular depolarization after repair of tetralogy of Fallot: A basis for ventricular arrhythmia. Am J Cardiol 55(5):522–525, 1985.
51. Bonatti V, Rolli A, Botti G: Recording of monophasic action potentials of the right ventricle in long Q-T syndromes complicated by severe ventricular arrhythmias. Eur Heart J 4(3):168–79, 1983.
52. Greene H, Reid P, Schaeffer A: The repetitive ventricular response in man. N Engl J Med 299:729, 1978.
53. Benson D, Anderson R: Cardiac arrest in young, ostensibly healthy patients: Clinical hemodynamic and electrophysiologic findings. Am J Cardiol 52:65–69, 1983.
54. Herre J, Mann D, Luck J, et al: Effect of increased current, multiple pacing sites and number of extrastimuli on induction of ventricular tachycardia. Am J Cardiol 57(1):102–107, 1986.
55. Easley RM, Goldstein S: Differentiation of ventricular tachycardia from junctional tachycardia with aberrant conduction: The use of competitive atrial pacing. Circulation 37:1015, 1968.
56. Kugler J, Cheatham J, Gumbiner C, et al: Results of phenytoin and propranolol drug electrophysiology studies for ventricular tachycardia in patients having repaired lesions with tetralogy of Fallot physiology. Circulation 72(suppl III):341, 1985.
57. Kugler J, Pinsky W, Cheatham J, et al: Sustained ventricular tachycardia after repair of tetralogy of Fallot: New electrophysiologic findings. Am J Cardiol 51(7):1137–1143, 1983.
58. Deal B, Miller S, Scagliotti D, et al: Ventricular tachycardia in the young without overt heart disease. Circulation 72(suppl III):340, 1985.
59. Keatinge W, Hayward M: Sudden death in cold water and ventricular arrhythmia. J Forensic Sci 26(3):459–461, 1981.
60. Prieto J, Quevedo M, Kutz M, et al: Vagal influence in experimental arrhythmias caused by dopamine. Arch Inst Cardiol Mex 55(5):395–398, 1985.
61. Barton CW, Dick M, Rosenthal A: Quinidine syncope in children. J Am Coll Cardiol 5:429–433, 1985.
62. Seger JJ, Nguyen T, Ruder M, et al: Drug related polymorphous ventricular tachycardia. Circulation 72(suppl III):442, 1985.
63. Roden D, Woosley R: QT prolongation and arrhythmia suppression. Am Heart J 109:411–415, 1985.
64. Itoh J, Munemura S, Satoh H: A study of the inheritance pattern of Romano-Ward syndrome. Clin Pediatr 21:20, 1982.
65. Kugler JD: Control of torsades de pointes by tocainide in children with congenital and acquired prolonged QT interval. In Proceedings of the Second World Congress of Pediatric Cardiology. New York, 1985, p 107.
66. Tzivoni D, Keren A, Cohen A, et al: Magnesium sulfate—a new therapy for torsade-de-pointes. Circulation 68(suppl III):427, 1983.

67. Debrand M, Tsueda K: Ventricular tachycardia due to hyperkalemia induced by potassium penicillin G overdose. Acta Anaesthesiol Belg 31(1):35–37, 1980.
68. Ludomirsky A, Klein H, Sarelli P, et al: Q-T prolongation and polymorphous ("torsade de pointes") ventricular arrhythmias associated with organophosphorus insecticide poisoning. Am J Cardiol 49(7):1654–1658, 1982.
69. Romhilt DW, Chaffin C, Choi SC, et al: Arrhythmia on ambulatory ECG monitoring in women without apparent heart disease. Am J Cardiol 54:582–586, 1984.
70. Garson A, Gillette PC: Treatment of chronic ventricular dysrhythmias in the young. PACE 4:658–669, 1981.
71. Harris P, Alexson C, Manning J: Sudden unexpected death in adolescence. In Proceedings of the Second World Congress of Pediatric Cardiology. New York, 1985, p 58.
72. Vetter VL: Sudden death in children and adolescents. In Morganroth J, Horowitz LN (eds): Sudden Cardiac Death. New York, Grune & Stratton, 1985, pp 33–46.
73. Rocchini AP, Chun P, Dick M: Ventricular tachycardia in children. Am J Cardiol 47:1091–1097, 1981.
74. Vignola PA, Rozanski JJ, Lister JW: Lymphocytic myocarditis presenting as unexplained ventricular arrhythmias: Diagnosis with endomyocardial biopsy and response to immunosuppression. J Am Coll Cardiol 4:812–819, 1984.
75. Garson A: Chronic dysrhythmias in ambulatory children. Appl Cardiol 12(5):15–25, 1984.
76. Dunnigan A, Pierpont M, Smith S, et al: Cardiac and skeletal myopathy associated with cardiac dysrhythmias. Am J Cardiol 53(6):731–737, 1984.
77. Liberthson R, Brian A, McGovern M, et al: Electrophysiologic observations and survival analysis in children and young adults with symptomatic ventricular tachycardia or fibrillation. Circulation 72(suppl III):197, 1985.
78. Morady F, Scheinman M, Hess D, et al: Clinical characteristics and results of electrophysiologic testing in young adults with ventricular tachycardia or ventricular fibrillation. Am Heart J 106(6):1306–1314, 1983.
79. Southall DP, Richards J, Mitchell P: Study of cardiac rhythm in healthy newborn infants. Br Heart J 43:14–20, 1980.
80. Blanchard W, Bucciarelli R, Miller B: Ventricular parasystole in a newborn infant. J Electrocardiol 12(4):427–429, 1979.
81. Bisset GS, Janos GG, Gaum WE: Accelerated ventricular rhythm in the newborn infant. J Pediatr 104:247–249, 1984.
82. Stevens D, Schriener R, Hurwitz R, et al: Fetal and neonatal ventricular arrhythmia. Pediatrics 63(5):771–777, 1979.
83. Bergdahl DM, Stevenson JG, Guntheroth WG: Prognosis in primary ventricular tachycardia in the pediatric patient. Circulation 62:897, 1980.
84. Garson A, Gillette P, Titus J, et al: Surgical treatment of ventricular tachycardia in infants. N Engl J Med 310:1443–1445, 1984.
85. James T, Beeson C, Sherman E, et al: De subitaneis mortibus: XIII multifocal Purkinje cell tumors of the heart. Circulation 52:333–344, 1975.
86. Ferrans V, McAllister H, Haese W: Infantile cardiomyopathy with histiocytoid change in cardiac muscle cells: Report of six patients. Circulation 53:708–719, 1976.
87. Ishihara H, Hosaki J, Tsuchiya S, et al: Arrhythmias in healthy school children. In Proceedings of the Second World Congress on Pediatric Cardiology. New York, 1985, p 101.
88. Lang D, Kupferschmid C, Von Bernuth G: Long term observation of ventricular extrasystole in children with normal hearts. Deutsch Med Wochenschr 111(3):7–10, 1986.
89. Rozanski J, Steinfeld L, Kupersmith J: Maximal stress testing in evaluation of arrhythmias in children: Results and reproducibility. Am J Cardiol 43:951, 1979.
90. Oetgen W, Galioto F, Scott L: Cardiac arrhythmias due to ventricular parasystole in a 12-year-old child. South Med J 76(5):660–662, 1983.
91. Schubert CJ, Epstein ML: Significance of ventricular couplets and triplets in children and young adults. In Proceedings of the Section on Cardiology Scientific Sessions. American Academy of Pediatrics, 1984, p 31.
92. Coeurderoy A, Almange C, Laurent M, et al: Accelerated idioventricular rhythm. 2 new cases in children. Arch Mal Coeur 78(5):777–780, 1985.
93. Fauchier J, Desveaux B, Cosnay P, et al: Complex ventricular arrhythmia in apparently healthy young subjects. Arch Mal Coeur 78(9):1333–1343, 1985.
94. Nihill M: Endomyocardial biopsy in children. In Proceedings of the Second World Congress on Pediatric Cardiology. New York, 1985, p 54.
95. Sugrue D, Holmes D, Gersh B, et al: Cardiac histologic findings in patients with life-threatening ventricular arrhythmias of unknown origin. 4(5):952–957, 1984.
96. Strain J, Grose R, Factor S, et al: Results of endomyocardial biopsy in patients with spontaneous ventricular tachycardia but without apparent structural heart disease. Circulation 68(6):1171–1181, 1983.
97. Garson A: Experimental and clinical findings in ventricular arrhythmias in the young. In Aliot E, Lazzara R. (eds): Ventricular Tachycardias. Boston, Martinus Nijhoff, (in press).
98. Fulton D, Chung K, Tabakin B, et al: Ventricular tachycardia in children without heart disease. Am J Cardiol 55(11):1328–1331.
99. Matsushima M, Nagashima M, Ogawa A, et al: Clinical characteristics of ventricular tachycardia in children. In Proceedings of the Second World Congress Pediatric Cardiology. New York, 1985, p 41.
100. Rowland T, Schweiger M: Repetitive paroxysmal ventricular tachycardia and sudden death in a child. Am J Cardiol 53(11):1729, 1984.
101. Belhassen B: Sudden death in a child with ventricular tachycardia. Am J Cardiol 54(8):1172, 1984.
102. Ruder M, Wonston S, Davis J, et al: Arrhythmogenic right ventricular dysplasia in a family. Am J Cardiol 56:799–800, 1985.
103. Delise P, Raviele A, Di-Pede F, et al: Idiopathic ventricular tachycardia responsive to verapamil. G Ital Cardiol 15(1):54–62, 1985.
104. Ohe T, Shimomura K, Aihara N, et al: Idiopathic sustained ventricular tachycardia: Results of electrophysiological studies. Circulation 72(suppl III):159, 1985.
105. Palileo E, Ashley W, Swiryn S, et al: Exercise provocable right ventricular outflow tract tachycardia. Am Heart J 104(2):185–193, 1982.

106. Panidis I, Greenspan A, Mintz G, et al: Inducible ventricular fibrillation in arrhythmogenic right ventricular dysplasia. 110(5):1067–1069, 1985.
107. Soloman S, Osdol V, Massumi A, et al: Exercise induced ventricular tachycardia and arrhythmogenic right ventricular dysplasia: Electrophysiologic and therapeutic considerations. Texas Heart Inst J 10:351–357, 1983.
108. Dungan W, Garson A, Gillette A: Arrhythmogenic right ventricular dysplasia: A cause for ventricular tachycardia in children with apparently normal hearts. Am Heart J 102:745–750, 1981.
109. Bricker J, Traweek M, Smith R, et al: Supraventricular tachycardia during exercise testing in children. In Proceedings of the Second World Congress on Pediatric Cardiology. New York, 1985, p 107.
110. Von-Bernuth G, Bernsau U, Gutheil H, et al: Tachyarrhythmic syncopes in children with structurally normal hearts with and without Q-T prolongation in the electrocardiogram. Eur J Pediatr 138(3):206–210, 1982.
111. Benson D, Gallagher J, Sterba R, et al: Catecholamine induced double tachycardia: Case report in a child. PACE 3(1):96–103, 1980.
112. Burton A, Kuehl K: Ventricular tachycardia in previously healthy children. Circulation 72(suppl III):196, 1985.
113. Ryujin Y, Arakaki Y, Takahashi O, et al: Ventricular arrhythmias in children: The validity of exercise stress tests for their diagnosis and management. Jpn Circ J 48(12):1393–1398, 1984.
114. Lerman B, Belardinelli L, DiMarco J: Adenosine sensitive ventricular tachycardia: Evidence suggesting cyclic AMP mediated triggered activity. J Am Coll Cardiol 7(2):155A, 1986.
115. Keung E, Huycke E, Sung R: Exercise-induced ventricular tachycardia: Catecholamine sensitivity versus cycle-length dependency. J Am Coll Cardiol 7(2):155A, 1986.
116. Sixteenth Bethesda Conference. Cardiovascular abnormalities in the athlete: Recommendations regarding eligibility for competition. J Am Coll Cardiol 6:1186–1232, 1985.
117. Romano C, Gemme G, Pongiglione R: Aritmie cardiache rare delle'eta pediatrica. Clin Pediatr 45:565, 1963.
118. Ward O: A new familial cardiac syndrome in children. J Irish Med Assoc 54:103, 1964.
119. Vincent G: The heart rate of Romano-Ward long Q-T syndrome patients. Circulation 72(suppl III), 1985.
120. Yu P, Bruce R, Lovejoy F, et al: Observations on the change of ventricular systole (Q-T interval) during exercise. J Clin Invest 29:279–289, 1950.
121. Schechter E, Anderson J, Prabhu S, et al: Epinephrine infusion in the congenital long-QT syndrome. J Am Coll Cardiol 7(2):155A, 1986.
122. Ross B, Garson A, McNamara D: Factors affecting outcome in children with long Q-T syndrome. Circulation 70(suppl II):320, 1984.
123. Di-Segni E, David D, Katzenstein M, et al: Permanent overdrive pacing for the suppression of recurrent ventricular tachycardia in a newborn with long QT syndrome. J Electrocardiol 13(2):189–192, 1980.
124. Esscher E: Congenital complete heart block in adolescence and adult life. A follow-up study. Eur Heart J 2(4):281–288, 1981.
125. Batisse A, Belloy C, Fermont L: Prolonged Q-T interval with functional AV block in neonates and young infants. Arch Fr Pediatr 38(9):657:62, 1981.
126. Nikolic G, Arnold J, Coles D: Torsade de pointes and asystole in a child with complete heart block and prolonged Q-T interval. Aust Paediatr J 19(3):187–191, 1983.
127. Takamizawa K, Takao A, Ohta F: Mexiletine for successful treatment of the long Q-T syndrome. In Proceedings of the Second World Congress on Pediatric Cardiology. New York, 1985, p 101.
128. James T, MacLean W: Paroxysmal ventricular arrhythmias and familial sudden death associated with neural lesions in the heart. Chest 78(1):22–23, 1980.
129. Levine J, Spear J, Guarnieri T, et al: Cesium chloride-induced long Q-T syndrome: Demonstration of after depolarizations and triggered activity in vivo. Circulation 72(5):1092–1093, 1985.
130. Craelius W, Chen V, Zeiler R, et al: In vivo recording of early afterdepolarizations preceding torsades de pointes. J Am Coll Cardiol 7(2):124A, 1986.
131. Friesen R, Duncan P, Tweed W, et al: Appraisal of pediatric cardiopulmonary resuscitation. Can Med Assoc J 126(9):1055–1058, 1982.
132. Bricker T, Garson A, Gillette P: A history of seizures in the family associated with sudden cardiac deaths. Am J Dis Child 138:866–868.
133. Kay G, Plumb V, Arciniegas J, et al: Torsade-de-pointes: The long–short initiating sequence and other clinical features. J Am Coll Cardiol 2:806–817.
134. Locati E, Schwartz PJ, Moss AJ, et al: Long-term survival after left cervico-thoracic sympathectomy in high risk long Q-T syndrome patients with refractory ventricular arrhythmias. J Am Coll Cardiol 7:235, 1985.
135. Packer D, Coltori F, Smith M, et al: Sudden death after left stellectomy in the long Q-T syndrome. Am J Cardiol 54(10):1365–1366, 1984.
136. Mirowski M, Reid P, Mower M, et al: Termination of malignant ventricular arrhythmias with an implanted automotive defibrillator in human beings. N Engl J Med 303:322–324, 1980.
137. Platia E, Griffith L, Watkins L, et al: Management of the prolonged Q-T syndrome and recurrent ventricular fibrillation with an implantable automatic cardioverter-defibrillator. Clin Cardiol 8(9):490–493, 1985.
138. Clark M, Lazzaraza R, Jackman W: Torsade de pointes: Serum drug levels and electrocardiographic warning signs. Circulation 66:II–71, 1982.
139. Von Bernuth G, Belz G, Evertz W, et al: QTU abnormalities, sinus bradycardia and Adams-Stokes attacks due to ventricular tachyarrhythmia. Acta Paediatr Scand 62:675, 1973.
140. Levy A, Camm A, Keane J: Multiple arrhythmias detected during nocturnal monitoring in patients with congenital complete heart block. Circulation 55:247, 1977.
141. Winkler R, Freed M, Nadas A: Exercise induced ventricular ectopy in children and young adults with complete heart block. Am Heart J 99:87–92, 1980.
142. Kavey R, Blackman M, Sondheimer H, et al: Ventricular arrhythmias and mitral valve prolapse in childhood. J Pediatr 105(6):885–890, 1984.
143. Bissett GS, Schwartz DC, Meyer RA: Clinical spectrum and long-term follow-up of isolated mitral valve prolapse in 119 children. Circulation 62:423–428, 1980.

144. Chen S, Fagan L, Nouri S, et al: Ventricular dysrhythmias in children with Marfan's syndrome. Am J Dis Child 139(3):273–276, 1985.
145. Anderson R: Idiopathic mitral prolapse and sudden death. Am Heart J 100:941–942, 1980.
146. Topaz O, Edwards JE: Pathologic features of sudden death in children, adolescents and young adults. Chest 87:476–482, 1985.
147. Maron B: Sudden death in athletes. Am J Cardiol 41:803, 1978.
148. Rosenthal M, Hamer A, Gang E: The yield of programmed ventricular stimulation in mitral valve prolapse patients with ventricular arrhythmias. Am Heart J 110(5):970–976, 1985.
149. Bharati S, Lev M: Arrhythmogenic ventricles. PACE 6(5):1035–1049, 1983.
150. Garson A, McNamara D: Sudden death in a pediatric cardiology population: Relationship to prior arrhythmias. J Am Coll Cardiol 5:134B–138B, 1985.
151. Sullivan I, Presbitero P, Gooch V, et al: The influence of surgery on ventricular arrhythmias in tetralogy of Fallot: a prospective study. Circulation 72(suppl III):197, 1985.
152. Oh J, Holmes D, Hayes D, et al: Cardiac arrhythmias in patients with surgical repair of Ebstein's anomaly. J Am Coll Cardiol 6(6):1351–1357, 1985.
153. Lambert EC, Menon VA, Wagner HR: Sudden unexpected death from cardiovascular disease in children. Am J Cardiol 34:89–96, 1974.
154. Ludomirsky A, Bricker JT, Garson A, et al: Cardiac tumors in children: Clinical and diagnostic evaluation. In Proceedings of the Tenth World Congress of Cardiology. 1986, p 168.
155. McKenna W, Deanfield J, Franklin R, et al: Arrhythmia in children and adolescents with hypertrophic cardiomyopathy: Incidence and relation to prognosis. J Am Coll Cardiol 7(2):204A, 1986.
156. Frank M, Watkins L, Prisant L: Potentially lethal arrhythmias and their management in hypertrophic cardiomyopathy. Am J Cardiol 53(11):1608–1613, 1984.
157. Borggrefe M, Kuhn H, Koniger H: Arrhythmias in hypertrophic obstructive and non-obstructive cardiomyopathy. Eur Heart J (suppl 4):245–251, 1983.
158. Maron B, Henry W, Clark C, et al: Asymmetric septal hypertrophy in childhood. Circulation 53:9–19, 1976.
159. Kuck K, Kunze K, Dernedde J: Value and limitations of programmed electrical stimulation in hypertrophic cardiomyopathy. Circulation 72(suppl III):631, 1985.
160. Spicer R, Rocchini A, Crowley D, et al: Chronic verapamil therapy in pediatric and young adult patients with hypertrophic cardiomyopathy. Am J Cardiol 53:1614–1619, 1984.
161. McKenna W, Harris L, Rowland E, et al: Amiodarone for long-term management of patients with hypertrophic cardiomyopathy. Am J Cardiol 54(7):802–810, 1984.
162. Spach MS, Kootsey JM, Mosher CE: The functional role of structural complexities in the propagation of depolarization in the atrium of the dog. Circ Res 50:175–191, 1982.
163. Friedman R, Moak J, Smith R, et al: Prognostic implications of dysrhythmias in children with congestive cardiomyopathy. Circulation 72(suppl III):341, 1985.
164. Haussaguerre M, Bonnet J, LeGoff G: Prevalence and significance and prognosis of ventricular arrhythmia in 236 cases of dilated myocardiopathy. Arch Mal Coeur 79:32–38, 1986.
165. Von-Olshausen K, Schafer A, Mehmel H, et al: Ventricular arrhythmias in idiopathic dilated cardiomyopathy. Br Heart J 51(2):195–201, 1984.
166. Guarnieri E, Reid P, Grunwald L, et al: Failure of electrophysiologic testing to predict death in congestive cardiomyopathy. Circulation 72(suppl III):159, 1985.
167. Josephson ME: Sustained ventricular tachycardia in patients with idiopathic dilated cardiomyopathy: Electrophysiologic testing and lack of response to antiarrhythmic drug therapy. Circulation 70:451–456, 1984.
168. Fontaine G, Guiraudon G, Frank R, et al: Arrhythmogenic right ventricular dysplasia and Uhl's disease. Arch Mal Coeur 75(4):P361–P372, 1982.
169. Moak J, Gillette P, Garson A: Mexiletine: An alternative to dilantin in pediatric ventricular arrhythmias: Circulation 70(suppl II):207, 1984.
170. Guyraudon G, Klein GJ: Total disconnection of the right ventricular free wall. Circulation 67:463–470, 1983.
171. Moller J, Patton C, Varco R: Postoperative ventricular septal defect: 24–30 years follow-up of 232 patients. In Proceedings of the Second World Congress on Pediatric Cardiology. New York, 1985, p 20.
172. Fyfe D, Driscoll DJ, Danielson G, et al: Truncus arteriosus with single pulmonary artery: Influence of pulmonary vascular obstructive disease on early and late operative results. J Am Coll Cardiol 5:1168–1172, 1985.
173. Kavey R, Blackman M, Sondheimer H: Incidence and severity of chronic ventricular dysrhythmias after repair of tetralogy of Fallot. Am Heart J 103(3):342–350, 1982.
174. Deanfield JE, McKenna WJ, Hallidie-Smith K: Ventricular arrhythmia in unrepaired and repaired tetralogy of Fallot. Relation to age, timing of repair and hemodynamic status. Br Heart J 52:77–81, 1984.
175. Deanfield JE, Gersony WE, Hallidie-Smith K: Prognostic significance of ventricular arrhythmias after repair of tetralogy of Fallot: A prospective study. In Proceedings of the Second World Congress on Pediatric Cardiology. New York, 1985, p 14.
176. Matina D, Mouly A, Massol J, et al: Troubles du rhythme ventriculare apres reparation de tetralogie de Fallot. Arch Mal Couer 78:103–110, 1985.
177. Deal B, Miller S, Scagliotti D, et al: Electrophysiologic drug testing in ventricular arrhythmias following tetralogy of Fallot repair. Circulation 72(suppl III):197, 1985.
178. Cloez J, Khalife K, Weber J, et al: Late ventricular tachycardia after surgical correction of congenital cardiopathy: Impact, severity and predictive factors. Arch Mal Coeur 77(5):534–542, 1984.
179. Kobayashi J, Hirose H, Nakano S, et al: Ambulatory electrocardiographic study of the frequency and cause of ventricular arrhythmia after correction of tetralogy of Fallot. Am J Cardiol 54(10):1310–1313, 1984.
180. Wessel H, Bastanier C, Paul M, et al: Prognostic significance of arrhythmias in tetralogy of Fallot after cardiac arrest. Am J Cardiol 46:843–848, 1980.
181. Katz N, Blackstone E, Kirklin J, et al: Late survival

and symptoms after repair of tetralogy of Fallot. Circulation 65(2):403–410, 1982.
182. Burns R, Liu P, Druck M: Analysis of adults with and without complex ventricular arrhythmias after repair of tetralogy of Fallot. J Am Coll Cardiol 4(2):226–233, 1984.
183. Kavey RE, Byrum CJ, Blackman, MS: Ventricular arrhythmias and biventricular dysfunction after repair of tetralogy of Fallot. J Am Coll Cardiol 4:126–131, 1984.
184. Wolff G, Rowland T, Ellison R: Surgically induced right bundle branch block with left anterior hemiblock. Circulation 45:587–593, 1972.
185. Fuster V, McGoon D, Kennedy M: Long-term evaluation (12–22 years) of open heart surgery for tetralogy of Fallot. Am J Cardiol 46:635–640, 1980.
186. Kavey R, Blackman M, Sondheimer H: Phenytoin therapy for ventricular arrhythmias occurring late after surgery for congenital heart disease. Am Heart J 104(4):794–798, 1982.
187. Malcolm I, Stubington D, Gibbons J: Mexiletine for ventricular arrhythmia after repair of tetralogy of Fallot. Can Med Assoc J 123(6):530–532, 1980.
188. Harken A, Horowitz L, Josephson M: Surgical correction of recurrent sustained ventricular tachycardia following complete repair of tetralogy of Fallot. J Thorac Cardiovasc Surg 80(5):779–781, 1980.
189. Moak J, Friedman R, Garson A, et al: Therapeutiques electrophysiologiques en pediatrie. In Kachaner J, Batisse A (eds): Progres en Pediatrie: Phythmologie Pediatrique. Paris, France, Doin (in press).
190. von-Olshausen K, Amann E, Hofmann BF, et al: Ventricular arrhythmias before and late after aortic valve replacement. Am J Cardiol 54(1):142–146, 1984.
191. Santinga J, Kirch M, Fiora J, et al: Factors relating to late sudden death in patients having aortic valve replacement. Ann Thorac Surg 29:249–253, 1980.
192. Konishi Y, Matsuda K, Nishiwaki N, et al: Ventricular arrhythmias late after aortic and/or mitral valve replacement. Jpn Circ J 49(6):576–583, 1985.
193. Byrum C, Sondheimer H, Kavey R, et al: Ventricular arrhythmia non-therapy guided by electrophysiologic testing. Am Heart J 110:707, 1985.
194. Deanfield J, McKenna W, Hallidie-Smith K: Detection of late arrhythmia and conduction disturbance after correction of tetralogy of Fallot. Br Heart J 44(3):248–253, 1980.
195. Spinelli W, Rosen M: Developmental and use-dependent effects of phenytoin on neonatal and adult Purkinje Fibers. J Am Coll Cardiol 7:123, 1986.
196. Rosen M, Gelband H, Merker C, et al: Mechanisms of digitalis toxicity: Effects of ouabain on phase four of canine Purkinje fibers transmembrane potential. Circulation 47:681–686, 1973.
197. Amerini S, Cardonin P, Cerbai E, et al: Electrophysiological mechanisms for the antiarrhythmic action of mexiletine on digitalis, reperfusion and reoxygenation-induced arrhythmias. Br J Pharmacol 86(4):805–815, 1985.
198. Tseng G, Wit A: Arrhythmogenic effects of quinidine on triggered activity in atrial muscle. Circulation 72(suppl III):380, 1985.
199. Moak J, Rosen M: The effects of pacing on ouabain-induced sustained rhythmic activity. Circulation 66(suppl II):79, 1982.
200. Johnson N, Danilo P, Wit A, et al: Response to pacing of triggered activity occurring in catecholamine-treated canine coronary sinus. Circulation 72(suppl III):381, 1985.
201. Benito F, Aguado A, Fernandez A, et al: Delayed after depolarizations in patients post-repair of tetralogy of Fallot: Could be considered a mechanism in the genesis of ventricular arrhythmias? In Proceedings of the Second World Congress on Pediatric Cardiology. New York, 1985, p 111.
202. Garson A, Smith R, Moak J, et al: Sudden death in children related to ventricular arrhythmias. J Am Coll Cardiol 5:130B–134B, 1985.
203. Gillette P, Garson A: Electrophysiologic and pharmacologic characteristics of automatic ectopic supraventricular tachycardia. Circulation 56:571–575, 1977.
204. Aronson R: Afterpotentials and triggered activity in hypertrophied myocardium from rats with renal hypertension. Circ Res 48:720–728, 1981.
205. Kawashima Y, Matsude H, Kobayashi J, et al: Ninety consecutive corrective operations for tetralogy of Fallot with or without minimal right ventriculotomy. J Thorac Cardiovasc Surg 90(6):856–863, 1985.
206. Moak J, Garson A: Late electrophysiologic effects of experimental right ventriculotomy. J Am Coll Cardiol 7:49, 1986.
207. Garson A: Ventricular arrhythmias after congenital heart surgery: A canine model. Pediatr Res 18:1112–1120, 1984.
208. Waxman M, Wald R, Finley J, et al: Valsalva termination of ventricular tachycardia. Circulation 62(4):843–851, 1980.
209. Cassidy D, Vassallo J, Miller J, et al: 1985. Differences in endocardial electrophysiologic characteristics in coronary artery disease patients with ventricular tachycardias versus cardiac arrest. Circulation 72(suppl III):160, 1985.
210. Benchimol A, Matsuo S, Wang TF: Phasic coronary arterial flow velocity during arrhythmias in man. Am J Cardiol 29:604–615, 1972.
211. Tepper D, Sarda M, Capasso J, et al: Does hypertensive hypertrophy cause myocardial electrical instability? J Am Coll Cardiol 7:111A, 1986.
212. Palik I, Graham T, Burger J: Ventricular function in patients with obstructed right ventricular pulmonary artery conduits. J Am Coll Cardiol 7:201A, 1986.
213. McRae J, Wagner G, Rogers M: Paroxysmal familial ventricular fibrillation. J Pediatr 84:151–120, 1974.
214. Fyke F, Vlietstra R, Danielson G, et al: Verapamil for refractory ventricular fibrillation during cardiac operations in patients with cardiac hypertrophy. J Thorac Cardiovasc Surg 86(1):108–111, 1983.
215. Reduto L, Berger H, Johnstone D: Radionuclide assessment of exercise right and left ventricular performance following total correction of tetralogy of Fallot. Circulation 58:145–150, 1978.
216. Gutgesell H, Tacker W, Geddes L, et al: Energy dose for ventricular defibrillation of children. Pediatrics 58:898, 1976.
217. Strasburger J, Garson A: Encainide treatment of refractory supraventricular tachycardia in children. Am J Cardiol 58:49C–54C, 1986.
218. Evans V, Garson A: Ethmozine: A promising drug for atrial automatic ectopic tachycardia. Am J Cardiol (in press).

219. Garson A, Gillette P, McVey P, et al: Amiodarone treatment of critical arrhythmias in children and young adults. J Am Coll Cardiol 4:749–755, 1984.
220. Garson A: Dosing the newer antiarrhythmic drugs in children: Considerations in pediatric pharmacology. (Editorial) Am J Cardiol 57:1405–1407, 1986.
221. Frye RL, Collins JJ, DeSanctis RW: Guidelines for permanent cardiac pacemaker implantation, May 1984. Circulation 70:331A–339A, 1984.
222. Garson A: Evaluation and treatment of chronic ventricular dysrhythmias in the young. Cardiovasc Rev 2:1164–1196, 1981.
223. Iwa T, Kamata E, Misaki T, et al: Successful surgical ablation of reentrant ventricular tachycardia caused by myocardial fibroma. J Thorac Cardiovasc Surg 87(3):469–473, 1984.
224. Narumi J, Takeuchi Y, Tsuji T, et al: The successful operative treatment of a patient with a cardiac lipoma causing frequent tachyarrhythmia. 27(10):1471–1475, 1979.
225. Engle MA, Ebert PA, Redo SF: Recurrent ventricular tachycardia due to resectable cardiac tumor. Circulation 50:1052–1057, 1974.
226. Walsh C, Krongrad E: Terminal cardiac electrical activity in pediatric patients. Am J Cardiol 43:421, 1979.
227. Ornato JP, Gonzales ER, Beck CL: Treatment of presumed asystole during pre-hospital cardiac arrest: Superiority of electrical countershock. Am J Emerg Med 3:395–399, 1985.
228. Wennevold A, Sandoe E: Paroxysmal ventricular fibrillation in children. Acta Med Scand 202:425, 1977.
229. Sterba R, Maloney JD: Atrial fibrillation in adolescents with Wolff-Parkinson-White syndrome. In Proceedings of the Second World Congress on Pediatric Cardiology. New York, 1985, p 42.
230. Klein G, Bashore T, Sellers T, et al: Ventricular fibrillation in the Wolff-Parkinson-White syndrome. N Engl J Med 301(20):1080–1085, 1979.
231. Dreifus L, Watanabe Y, Reitman N, et al: Ventricular fibrillation: A possible mechanism of sudden death in patients with Wolff-Parkinson-White syndrome. Circulation 43:520, 1971.
232. Greenspan K: Mechanisms of ventricular fibrillation. In Dreifus LS, Likoff W (eds): Cardiac Arrhythmias. New York, Grune & Stratton, 1973, pp 195–202.
233. Mann E, Inouye I, Sakun V, et al: Emergency defibrillation using a temporary pacing electrode catheter. PACE 8(5):753–756, 1985.
234. Veltri EP, Mirowski M, Reid P: Clinical efficacy of the automatic implantable defibrillator: 6 year clinical experience. Circulation 74:II–109, 1986.

CHAPTER 15

HEMODYNAMIC FUNCTION IN ARRHYTHMIAS

Derek A. Fyfe, James E. Lowe, Ralph J. Damiano & Thomas D. Christopher

The hemodynamic impact of cardiac arrhythmias is dependent on many complex and interrelated factors. This is illustrated by the observation that supraventricular tachyarrhythmias may cause decreased cardiac output at heart rates identical to those achieved during exercise, in which normal sinus rhythm is maintained and cardiac output is increased.[1, 2] The presence of intrinsic heart disease also significantly accentuates the impact of the arrhythmia.[3] Abnormalities in the synchrony of contraction of the atria and ventricles may result in the loss of the transport function of the atria,[4, 5] and thus the electrophysiologic mechanism of the arrhythmia may alter the hemodynamic performance of the heart. Finally, prolonged duration of an arrhythmia may eventually lead to myocardial dysfunction, which may only be reversed by restoration of a more normal rate or sinus rhythm.

BRADYCARDIA

Changing heart rate is an important physiologic compensatory mechanism of the cardiovascular system.[6] At constant stroke volume, cardiac output increases linearly with heart rate. During bradycardia the stroke volume increases, and cardiac output is maintained. The success of this compensation depends on the compliance of the heart and may be limited in the fetus or newborn in whom ventricular compliance may be low.[7] The fetus and newborn have a limited ability to respond to stimuli that increase resting fiber length; therefore, heart rate being the principal determinant of cardiac output, bradycardia is poorly tolerated. Lack of atrioventricular synchrony may further reduce cardiac output in patients with congenital atrioventricular block with slow ventricular rates. Neonates with ventricular rates less than 55 bpm and atrial rates more than 140 bpm are at increased risk of dying in the first year of life.[8] Resting heart rates of less than 50 bpm in older children with complete atrioventricular block are more frequently seen in those who have experienced Adams-Stokes attacks. This may be an indication that this is the lowest limit at which adequate cardiac output can be maintained.[9] The additional presence of congenital heart disease and/or atrioventricular valve regurgitation, either of which imposes an obligatory volume load on the heart, is commonly associated with heart failure when complete atrioventricular block is present.[10] Acute bradycardia may not allow time for a compensatory response in vascular tone to occur, and therefore cardiac decompensation may occur at rates at which chronic bradycardia may be tolerable.

SINUS TACHYCARDIA

Rapid sinus tachycardia with rates of more than 200 bpm and as high as 230 bpm has been reported and most often occurs in small infants under extreme stress (e.g., during infections).[11] Normal atrioventricular synchrony is maintained, and no prolongation of conduction through the atrioventricular nodes occurs. This tachycardia is gradual in onset and is probably mediated by excessive circulating catecholamines stimulated by illness or by pharmacologic agents. Rapid sinus tachycardia does not usually result in acute hemodynamic compromise, although hypotension has been reported to occur in patients with concurrent septicemia.[11]

Sinus tachycardia may, however, be associated with evidence of left ventricular dysfunction when the tachycardia is sustained for prolonged periods of time. Engel, Bush, and Schaal reported the occurrence of ventricular dysfunction in a young woman after 9 years of sustained sinoatrial tachycardia.[12] Administration of propranolol diminished the heart rate, and after 3 months of treatment, cardiac function returned to normal. Sobczyk et al reported the case of a child with congenital atrioventricular block in whom sinus rates were consistently elevated to 100 bpm at rest and 150 bpm while awake following placement of an atrial sensing pacemaker.[13] Left ventricular fractional shortening measured by M-mode echocardiography dropped from 37% at the time of pacemaker implantation to 13% 18 months later. Invasive electrophysiologic testing confirmed the site of the tachycardia focus to be in the usual location of the sinus node. Following the addition of β-blocker therapy and reprogramming of the pacemaker to a slower rate of ventricular pacing, the left ventricular function subsequently returned to normal.

ATRIAL FIBRILLATION

The circulatory abnormalities caused by atrial fibrillation vary greatly between individual patients, and their severity is markedly influenced by coexistent heart disease such as mitral stenosis or hypertrophic cardiomyopathy. In patients with organic heart disease, the development of atrial fibrillation is associated with significantly increased mortality. Atrial fibrillation may be paroxysmal or sustained and is most frequently a sequelae of hypertensive cardiovascular disease in adults, although it may also occur in patients with normal hearts. In patients with normal hearts, prolonged atrial fibrillation may lead to cardiac enlargement and congestive heart failure. The development of heart failure appears to depend on the ventricular rate occurring during the arrhythmia. Rates from 122 bpm to 170 bpm (mean, 146 bpm) were most frequently associated with heart failure, compared to rates averaging 100 bpm in patients without failure.[14] Patients who developed heart failure tended to do so in the first weeks to months of the sustained arrhythmia. Few patients developed heart failure after the first year of the arrhythmia. One case of sustained atrial fibrillation for 44 years without the development of heart failure has been reported.[14]

Lemery et al reported the presence of severe dilated cardiomyopathy in a patient following 11 years of atrial fibrillation.[15] In this case, drugs had been ineffective in maintaining ventricular rates below 200 bpm. Following catheter ablation the ventricular rate decreased to between 100 bpm and 120 bpm. The echocardiographic shortening fraction improved from 18% to 38% at follow-up exam.

Atrial fibrillation in children is uncommon and most often occurs in patients following surgery for congenital heart disease.[16] The hemodynamic effects of atrial fibrillation are usually studied by comparing data taken during the arrhythmia to data taken following cardioversion to normal sinus rhythm. After an extensive review of such studies, McIntosh and Morris concluded that in most patients cardiac output is reduced during atrial fibrillation and returns to normal when sinus rhythm is restored.[17] Reale studied 12 patients in this way and noted a reduction in pulmonary arterial systolic, right ventricular systolic, end-diastolic, and left and right atrial pressures following conversion from atrial fibrillation to sinus rhythm.[18] If mitral stenosis was present, left atrial pressures increased as a result of the large A wave during atrial contraction.

The irregularly irregular atrial depolarization during atrial fibrillation frequently leads to rapid ventricular rates. Diastolic filling times are therefore shortened and extremely variable. Consequently, left ventricular and aortic systolic pressure, pulse pressure, and ejection times are likewise highly variable.[17] The loss of augmentation of ventricular filling because of ineffective atrial contraction further compromises cardiac output. In patients with mitral stenosis, atrial fibrillation impairs the ability of the atria to fill the left ventricle. Because of the short diastolic filling period during rapid ventricular rates, insufficient time may be available to equalize the pressure on either side of the stenosed mitral valve. This results in prolongation of the period of left ventricular isometric contraction and means that left ventricular pressure has to rise to increased levels in order to close the mitral valve.[19]

ATRIAL FLUTTER

Atrial flutter is an infrequent cardiac arrhythmia in children. Only 8% of cases occur in patients with normal hearts. In Garson et al's collaborative study of 380 patients, atrial flutter most frequently occurred in those with previously operated congenital heart disease (e.g., atrial palliation of transposition of the great vessels or other atrial surgery).[20] Atrial flutter is associated with a fourfold increase in the incidence of sudden death in such patients.

Following the onset of atrial flutter, 30% of patients were asymptomatic, 28% had symptoms of congestive heart failure, 24% reported palpitations, and 19% had either syncope or dizziness. In three cases, atrial flutter was found during attempted resuscitation from sudden death. Syncope was more common in patients with normal hearts or in those with Wolff-Parkinson-White syndrome.[20]

The hemodynamics of atrial flutter in patients with otherwise normal hearts may be different in impact than, for example, in a patient with poor right ventricular function after atrial repair of transposition of the great vessels where sequential atrial contractions may be beneficial. The ventricular rate during atrial flutter is usually increased above that during sinus rhythm and depends on the degree of atrioventricular conduction block present. Harvey et al demonstrated that cardiac output was lower during atrial flutter than during either atrial fibrillation or sinus rhythm in 11 of 12 patients.[21] It has been postulated that the continuous atrial contractions impede venous inflow.[22]

SUPRAVENTRICULAR TACHYCARDIA

Acute Effects

The acute hemodynamic effects of supraventricular tachycardia are numerous and appear to be not only a result of rapid rates, but also a consequence of alterations in atrioventricular synchrony that drastically reduce diastolic filling of the ventricles. Goldreyer, Kastor, and Kerschbaum performed hemodynamic monitoring during electrophysiologic catheterization in eight patients in whom paroxysms of supraventricular tachycardia provoked severe symptoms.[23] Following initiation of supraventricular tachycardia, systemic blood pressure dropped rapidly, with no pulsatile flow for several beats. Stroke volume during tachycardia decreased inversely as heart rate increased and led to a disproportionately large decrease in the diastolic interval compared to systole. The reduced ventricular filling was not immediately augmented by increased atrial filling, as atrial pressures remained low at the beginning of supraventricular tachycardia. At this time many patients reported symptoms of dizziness and near syncope. Following several beats of supraventricular tachycardia, pulmonary artery diastolic pressures and atrial pressures increased with the appearance of a tall "AV" wave. As the tachycardia continued, atrial pressures of more than 30 mm Hg occurred. Reflexly increased systemic vascular resistance also allowed subsequent partial blood pressure compensation. Cardiac output was decreased by more than 35% during supraventricular tachycardia in highly symptomatic patients.

In another study in which patients were not selected by symptom severity, similar decreases in systemic arterial pressure, dp/dt_{max}, and cardiac index occurred during supraventricular tachycardia. With time these parameters improved but did not return to normal until the tachycardia was interrupted. Interestingly in this study, verapamil used to terminate supraventricular tachycardia had no appreciable negative inotropic effects.[24]

Atrioventricular Synchrony During Supraventricular Tachycardia

Alterations in the synchronization of atrial and ventricular contractions characterize many different types of arrhythmia. The beneficial hemodynamic contribution of atrioventricular synchrony to ventricular filling and cardiac output during normal sinus rhythm has been well established.[25, 26] Atrial contraction augments left ventricular end-diastolic (filling) pressure (LVEDP) without increasing mean left atrial pressure. This increases left ventricular end-diastolic fiber length and improves contractility in accordance with Starling's law of the heart.[25, 26] This is particularly beneficial in patients with left ventricular dysfunction in whom LVEDP and left atrial pressure may already be elevated. Atrial contraction enables LVEDP to be optimized, avoiding the pulmonary venous congestion that might ensue if left atrial mean pressure was similarly increased.

During supraventricular tachycardia, normal atrioventricular synchrony is usually lost as a result of the abnormally long PR interval during the tachyarrhythmia, causing abnormal elevations of atrial pressure and contributing to poor ventricular diastolic filling. During re-entrant tachycardia, atrial depolarization occurs very shortly after ventricular depolarization. As a result, the atrial contraction occurs while the atrioventricular valves are held closed by ventricular systole, resulting in a combined A and V wave in the atria. Because of the resultant poor atrial emptying, a gradually increasing atrial pressure occurs that leads to pulmonary and systemic venous congestion. As a result of the decremental conduction properties of the atrioventricular node during orthodromic tachycardia, when the tachycardia rate is faster, the PR interval is longer, and the atrioventricular asynchrony will become worse. Prolongation of atrioventricular conduction does not occur during exercise, presumably because conduction is enhanced by elevated circulating catecholamines.

Ventricular Function in Acute Supraventricular Tachycardia

During acute episodes of supraventricular tachycardia, the diastolic interval and therefore the duration of coronary artery perfusion are severely reduced. This occurs at a time when myocardial oxygen consumption is increased. It has been speculated that myocardial ischemia may occur during supraventricular tachycardia, but evidence for this in patients with normal hearts is lacking.[23]

Studies using radionuclide angiography have demonstrated that the effects of supraventricular tachycardia and rapid atrial pacing are similar to each other but differ from those of exercise-induced tachycardia.[3, 27, 28] During rapid atrial pacing, as the heart rate increases, the end-diastolic and end-systolic volumes decrease while the ejection fractions remain constant. Cardiac outputs remain unchanged at pacing rates from 80 bpm to 160 bpm.[29] Atrial pacing therefore differs significantly from exercise, during which oxygen uptake, cardiac output, and ejection fraction increase.[27, 28] In studies on patients with supraventricular tachycardia, radionuclide angiography showed a marked decrease in left ventricular end-diastolic volume (LVEDV) and stroke volume, but an increase in cardiac output and ejection rate. Left ventricular ejection fractions were unchanged or decreased in some patients, particularly if heart disease was present. If very rapid rates were used, ejection fractions decreased.[3]

Sustained Chronic Supraventricular Tachycardia

Whereas significant hemodynamic embarrassment may accompany acute tachycardia, symptoms of chronic congestive heart failure may gradually occur if the supraventricular tachycardia is sustained. In young children with supraventricular tachycardia, 24% presented with heart failure.[30] Heart failure was more frequent in the younger child and with faster heart rates or if congenital heart disease was present. Chronic tachycardia characterized by slower rates and fewer symptoms has often been considered benign.[31–34] However, certain patients with chronic supraventricular tachycardia have been found to have severe cardiomyopathy as evidenced clinically by cardiomegaly, congestive heart failure, and left ventricular dysfunction.[35–45] Moreover, various tachyarrhythmias have been observed in patients with dilated cardiomyopathy.[46–51] In this group, it has not been clear whether this was a primary phenomenon, with the tachycardia inducing the cardiomyopathy, or a secondary phenomenon, with the dysrhythmia occurring as a result of the diseased atrial or ventricular myocardium.[52] Kugler et al[41] reported five children with chronic tachycardia and left ventricular dysfunction manifested by decreased ejection fraction, cardiomegaly, and symptoms of congestive heart failure. After antidysrhythmic therapy, there was resolution of signs and symptoms of congestive heart failure, cardiomegaly, and improvement in ejection fraction. These findings suggest that chronic tachycardia could cause reversible left ventricular dysfunction in children and should be considered as an etiology in patients with dilated cardiomyopathy. Gillette et al[42] reported two cases of congestive cardiomyopathy caused by tachycardia secondary to an automatic atrial focus. Both patients showed dramatic improvement of symptoms and resolution of cardiomegaly following surgical cryoablation of the ectopic focus. Packer et al[43] reported eight patients with chronic uncontrolled supraventricular tachycardia and significant left ventricular dysfunction in the absence of any other underlying disease. Following control of the tachycardia, there was a documented improvement in left ventricular dysfunction at rest in six of eight patients and during exercise in one additional patient. Several patients also have recently been reported with objective evidence of left ventricular dysfunction following prolonged supraventricular tachycardia and with documented improvement in myocardial performance following treatment.[44, 45]

EXPERIMENTAL STUDIES

Despite these clinical reports, there has been little experimental work that accurately defines the functional or metabolic effects of chronic supraventricular tachycardia. Therefore a series of studies was designed to determine the consequences of prolonged supraventricular tachycardia on myocardial function, energy compound stores, and tolerance to ischemia.

Twelve adult foxhounds underwent implantation of atrial pacemakers programmed to pace asynchronously at a rate of 190 ± 5 bpm using epicardial leads sewn into the right atria.[53] Weekly electrocardiograms documented pacemaker capture and ventricular response. Serial radionuclide angiograms were performed at regular intervals for 3 months during continuous atrial pacing. In five dogs, the pacemakers were removed after 3 months of chronic tachycardia, and the animals allowed to recover for 3 months. Cardiac performance was monitored during this recovery period with serial radionuclide angiograms.

No dogs developed clinical symptoms or signs of heart failure, and all animals showed normal exercise tolerance. Two animals were excluded from the study; one developed atrial fibrillation at 10 weeks, and one had ventricular response of less than 170 bpm during atrial pacing.

Functional Results

Chronic supraventricular tachycardia resulted in dramatic changes in the measured functional indices. Two radionuclide angiograms from a representative animal are shown in Figure 15–1. Following 2 months of chronic tachycardia, this dog displayed marked cardiac enlargement, with end-diastolic volume increased from 67 mL to 222 mL. Concomitantly, left ventricular ejection fraction dropped from 34% to 24%.

All animals exhibited similar derangements in hemodynamic measurements. Ejection fraction dropped progressively and significantly during chronic supraventricular tachycardia (Fig. 15–2) and was depressed in every animal studied. Ejection fraction was significantly depressed at 1 week. After 4 weeks there was no further decline, but by 12 weeks ejection fraction had dropped from a mean control value of $49 \pm 3\%$ to $29 \pm 3\%$ ($p < 0.0005$).[54] These decreases in ejection frac-

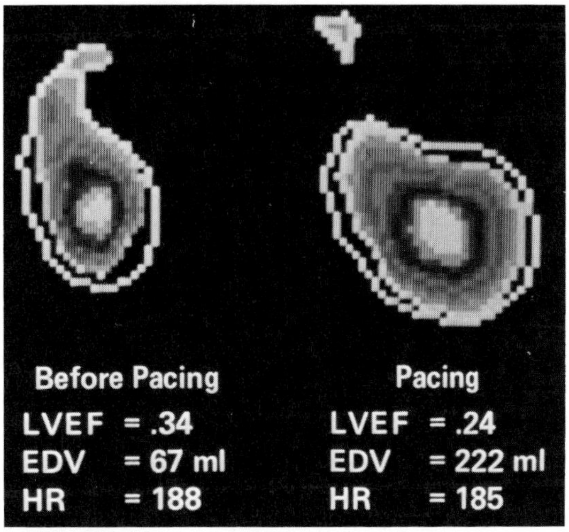

FIGURE 15–1
Radionuclide angiograms from one animal at control (left) and following two months of chronic atrial tachycardia (right). LVEF, Left ventricular ejection fraction; EDV, end-diastolic volume; HR, heart rate.

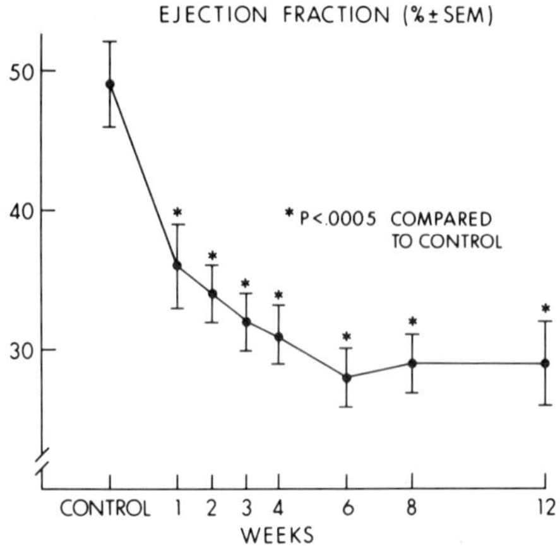

FIGURE 15–2

Changes in ejection fraction during chronic supraventricular tachycardia, shown as mean ± SEM. Ejection fraction was significantly depressed following 1 week of continuous tachycardia, and remained so throughout the entire study period, as determined by both multiple paired *t* tests and a repeated measures analysis of variance.

tion resulting from chronic tachycardia did not occur during acute increases in heart rates from 120 bpm to 190 bpm.

End-diastolic volume increased progressively during the study (Fig. 15–3), beginning 2 weeks following the onset of pacing. At the twelfth week of pacing, end-diastolic volume

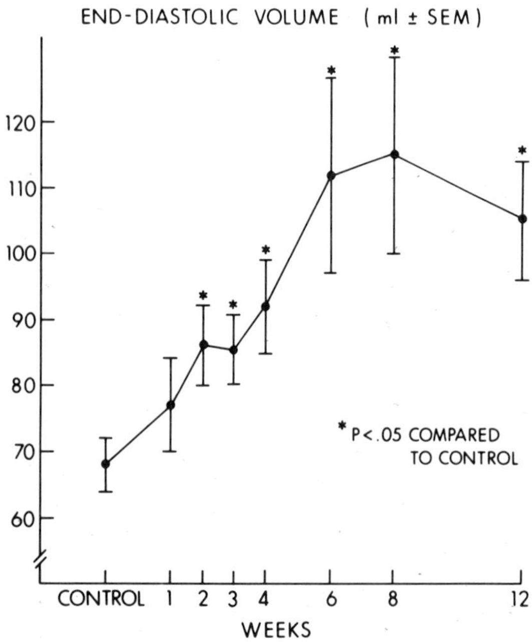

FIGURE 15–3

Changes in end-diastolic volume, expressed as mean ± SEM, during chronic tachycardia. Using a repeated measures analysis of variance, this change in end-diastolic volume over time was highly significant ($P < 0.001$).

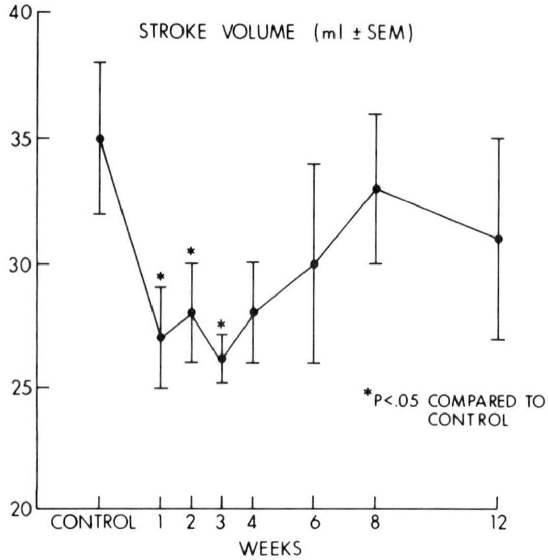

FIGURE 15–4

Changes in stroke volume, expressed as mean ± SEM, during chronic supraventricular tachycardia. The *P* values were determined using multiple paired *t* tests. There was no significant change over time utilizing a repeated measures analysis of variance.

increased from a control value of 69 ± 4 mL to 105 ± 9 mL ($p < 0.0005$). Unlike in chronic tachycardia, end-diastolic volume did not change significantly during acute tachycardia. Elevation of the end-diastolic volume partially compensated for the decrease in ejection fraction as can be seen in the resulting changes in stroke volume.

Initially, stroke volume was significantly depressed (Fig. 15–4); after 3 weeks of tachycardia, stroke volume had decreased from 34 ± 3 mL to 26 ± 1 mL ($p < 0.0005$). Although never returning to control levels, stroke volume improved and was no longer significantly different from control after 4 weeks of tachycardia.

These functional changes during chronic supraventricular tachycardia were very different from those seen during acute tachycardia. An acute increase in heart rate from 120 bpm to 190 bpm resulted in no significant change in ejection fraction (49 ± 2% to 49 ± 3%; p = NS* (Fig. 15–5). Chronic atrial tachycardia, on the other hand, resulted in a dramatic and significant decrease in ejection fraction.

End-diastolic volume was also affected differently by acute and chronic tachycardia. Acute tachycardia resulted in a small, nonsig-

*NS = no significant difference.

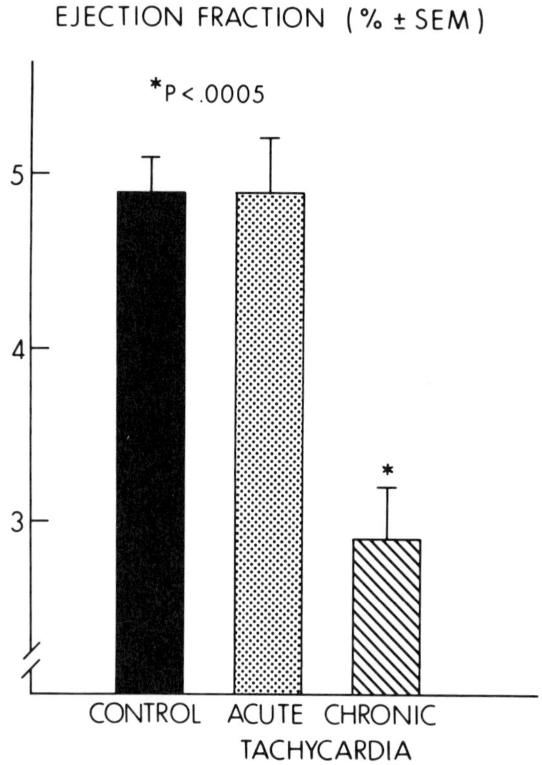

FIGURE 15–5
Changes in ejection fraction, expressed as mean ± SEM, during acute and chronic tachycardia. Control data were obtained at 120 bpm; acute and chronic tachycardia data were obtained at 190 bpm.

nificant decrease in end-diastolic volume (75 ± 6 mL to 69 ± 4 mL). Conversely, chronic tachycardia resulted in a large and significant increase in end-diastolic volume (Fig. 15–6).

As expected from the diverse effects on end-diastolic volume and ejection fraction, acute and chronic tachycardia had varying influences on cardiac output (Fig. 15–7). Acute tachycardia increased cardiac output from 4.6 ± 0.3 L/min to 6.1 ± 0.5 L/min ($p <$ 0.0005). Following chronic tachycardia, cardiac output was not significantly increased. Thus acute and chronic tachycardia have distinctly different effects on cardiac function.

Reversibility of Functional Alterations

In order to examine the reversibility of the functional alterations documented, five animals were allowed to recover for 12 weeks and followed with serial radionuclide angiograms (Fig. 15–8). End-diastolic volume, which was increased significantly following 12 weeks of pacing, remained elevated and when examined at the end of the recovery period was 91 ± 6 mL, compared to a control value of 67 ± 5 mL ($p < 0.05$). Ejection fraction, although markedly decreased following 12 weeks of chronic tachycardia, returned to control levels after only 2 weeks of recovery. Stroke volume was initially insignificantly increased during the recovery period and remained elevated compared to control levels ($p < 0.05$) (Fig. 15–9). This dramatic increase in stroke volume was a result of the ejection fraction returning to normal while the end-diastolic volume remained chronically elevated.

These experimental data document for the first time the functional consequences of prolonged supraventricular tachycardia in the canine model. Three months of sustained supraventricular tachycardia resulted in severe left ventricular dysfunction characterized by markedly decreased ejection fraction and progressive left ventricular dilatation with an increase in left ventricular end-dia-

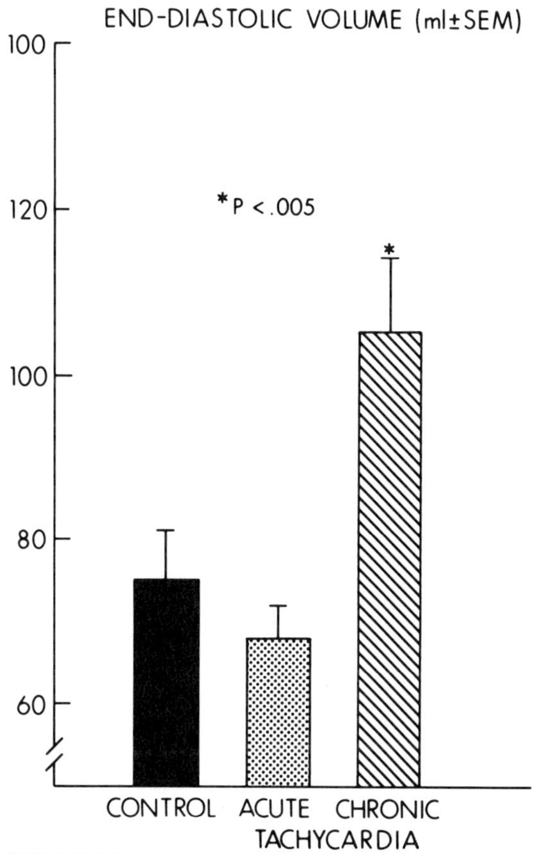

FIGURE 15–6
Changes in end-diastolic volume, expressed as mean ± SEM, during acute and chronic tachycardia.

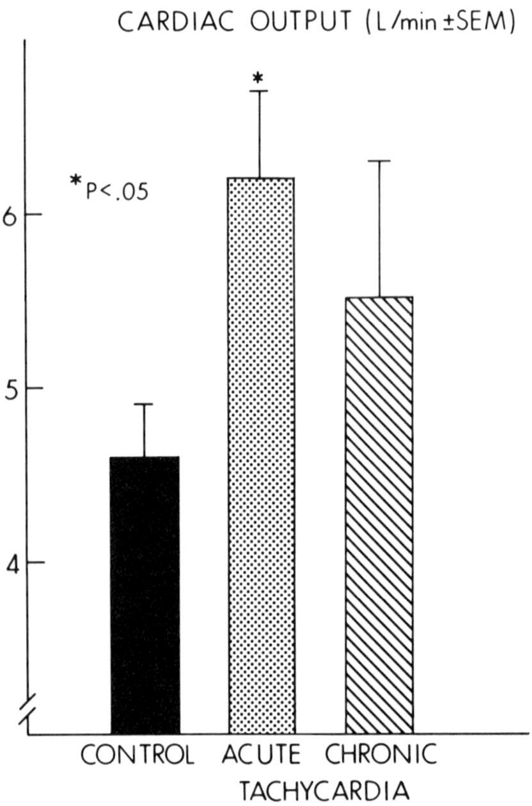

FIGURE 15–7
Changes in cardiac output in L/min, expressed as mean ± SEM, during acute and chronic tachycardia.

stolic volumes. Although stroke volume was initially depressed, it eventually returned to normal as a consequence of the elevation of left ventricular end-diastolic volume. Thus chronic tachycardia caused significant left ventricular dysfunction, and increases in left ventricular end-diastolic volume helped to restore cardiac output and stroke volume to near normal levels by the Frank-Starling mechanism.

The physiologic effects of chronic and acute tachycardia in the same animals were very different. Acute increases in heart rate from 120 bpm to 190 bpm resulted in a marked increase in cardiac output, a small decrease in end-diastolic volume, and no change in ejection fraction. There was no documented detrimental effect of acute tachycardia on myocardial performance. These findings are in agreement with the findings of other investigators who have demonstrated no appreciable changes in ejection fraction during acute supraventricular tachycardia in normal subjects.[3, 29] Thus the chronic left ventricular dysfunction observed in this study was not secondary to an acute hemodynamic deterioration but was instead a long-term effect of incessant tachycardia.

In the animals allowed to recover from sustained tachycardia, rapid restoration of myocardial function was evidenced by the return of ejection fraction to normal 2 weeks following the cessation of pacing. However, the left ventricular dilatation, as manifested by the increased end-diastolic volume, persisted throughout the recovery period and maintained cardiac output at levels above that recorded prior to the initiation of tachycardia.

These findings of supraventricular tachycardia–induced left ventricular dysfunction and myocardial dilatation are in agreement

FIGURE 15–8
Changes in end-diastolic volume and ejection fraction following 12 weeks of chronic supraventricular tachycardia and during 12 weeks of recovery. End-diastolic volume, however, remained significantly elevated during the entire recovery period as determined both by paired *t* tests and a repeated measures analysis of variance.

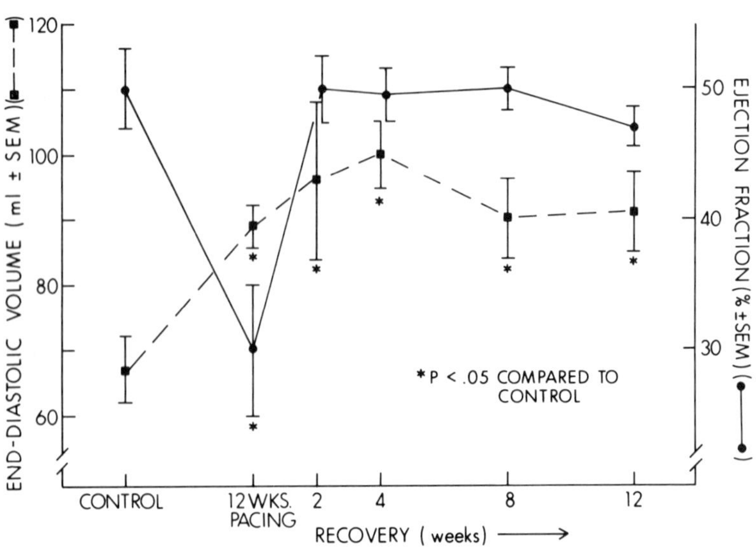

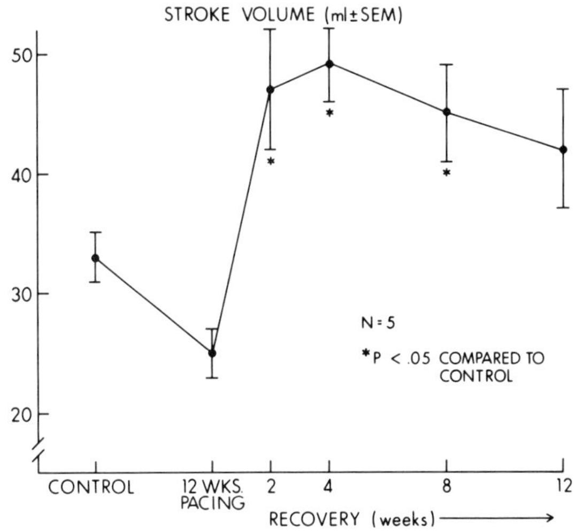

FIGURE 15–9

Changes in stroke volume, in milliliters, expressed as mean ± SEM, are shown following 12 weeks of pacing and during the recovery period. Stroke volume was significantly increased during the recovery period when utilizing a repeated measures analysis of variance.

with previous experimental and clinical reports.[35, 38, 41–43, 55] However, no experimental work has been previously done investigating the chronic functional effects of atrial tachycardia. Coleman et al[55] produced congestive heart failure in six dogs following 13 to 29 days of chronic pacemaker-induced ventricular tachycardia at rates of 280 bpm. Aortic pressure, heart rate, and the ratio of stroke volume to end-diastolic volume were decreased, while cardiac output was actually increased, presumably secondary to hypervolemia and an elevated end-diastolic volume. This study documents similar results in a model employing slower and more physiologic rates over a longer period of time. The model used in the present study utilized atrial pacing and avoided acute peripheral hemodynamic changes, and therefore more closely simulated the clinical setting of chronic supraventricular tachycardia.

The present experimental study strongly supports the conclusion that chronic tachycardia may cause left ventricular dysfunction and dilated cardiomyopathy that is clinically reversible. The reason for the left ventricular dysfunction and dilatation seen with chronic tachycardia remains unknown. From these data, it does not appear to be secondary to acute hemodynamic compromise, since acute tachycardia at the same rate resulted in an increase in cardiac output with no change in ejection fraction. In order to rule out valvular dysfunction as a possible contributing factor, cardiac catheterization data was obtained on the two dogs with the largest end-diastolic volume following 3 months of pacing. These studies revealed no evidence of aortic or mitral valve regurgitation. Thus chronic tachycardia and the resultant left ventricular dilatation caused no significant impairment of aortic or mitral valve function.

Progressive left ventricular dysfunction resulting from sustained tachycardia may be caused by depletion of myocardial high energy phosphates. The chronic tachycardia can be assumed to result in increased energy demands through an increased contractile effort per unit of myocardial mass. The metabolic regulatory mechanisms appear to be able to compensate acutely. It has been shown that 60 minutes of acute tachycardia at rates of 250 bpm does not significantly deplete high energy phosphates.[56] However, these same regulatory mechanisms may not be able to maintain high energy phosphate stores over a long period of time, as high energy phosphate depletion occurs following chronic ventricular tachycardia.[55] Depression of both atrial and ventricular high energy phosphates occurs following chronic supraventricular tachycardia (Lowe et al, work in progress).

Following cessation of tachycardia, a rapid recovery of ventricular function and ejection fraction occurs. Further investigation is needed to elucidate the physiologic mechanism responsible for this recovery. It is possible that the high energy phosphate pool may be restored, with resultant resolution of the left ventricular dysfunction.

Left ventricular dilatation persisted for 3 months following termination of pacing and appears to be a more chronic sequela of persistant tachycardia in the canine experiments reported here. With the rapid recovery of ejection fraction and the chronically elevated end-diastolic volume, all dogs had supra-normal cardiac outputs. Thus the 3 months of tachycardia actually resulted in a type of "training," in which the hearts enlarged and could generate large cardiac outputs once pacing was stopped and ejection fraction was restored to normal. The time course of further changes in end-diastolic volume is unknown and requires further investigation.

Tachycardia at slow rates and not accompanied by symptoms or hemodynamic compromise has long been considered benign. However, these experimental results clearly document that chronic supraventricular tachycardia can lead to left ventricular dysfunction. Since the chronic tachycardia may be the primary problem leading to secondary left ventricular dysfunction, evaluation of all patients with left ventricular dysfunction or dilated cardiomyopathy should include assessment of heart rate and rhythm. The cessation of tachycardia in this study resulted in a rapid improvement of ventricular function. Both these experimental data and clinical reports suggest that appropriate treatment of the tachyarrhythmia can lead to dramatic functional and clinical improvement. In summary, these results support the recommendation that chronic supraventricular tachycardia should be aggressively treated because of its eventual detrimental effect on left ventricular function.

ACCELERATED JUNCTIONAL ECTOPIC TACHYCARDIA

Accelerated junctional ectopic tachycardia (JET) is an automatic tachycardia arising in the atrioventricular junction with very rapid ventricular rates, often of more than 200 bpm. In pediatric patients this arrhythmia has been associated with 50% mortality[57, 58] despite aggressive medical management.

The sustained presence of atrioventricular dissociation with rapid ventricular rate usually occurring in a young patient recovering from open heart surgery makes JET perhaps the most hemodynamically malignant of all supraventricular arrhythmias. Hypotension is a constant accompanying feature in postoperative patients.[59] Infants without associated congenital heart disease have been reported in whom sustained JET had been present for several months despite multiple drug treatments.[60] Left ventricular dysfunction has also been present in these cases.

VENTRICULAR ECTOPIC BEATS AND TACHYCARDIA

The impact of frequent nonsustained premature ventricular contractions on the myocardium is largely unknown. It may be, however, that with increasingly frequent ectopic ventricular contractions, subtle deleterious effects on myocardial performance may occur. Kennedy et al have reported such abnormalities in patients without clinically apparent heart disease who had frequent premature ventricular contractions.[61] More than half the patients studied had abnormalities of end-systolic and end-diastolic volume indices, end-diastolic pressure, and echocardiographic circumferential fiber shortening. Abnormalities were more prevalent among patients with higher frequencies of premature ventricular contractions.

Ventricular tachycardia is usually associated with rapid hemodynamic deterioration caused by inadequate cardiac output. However, as in chronic supraventricular tachycardia, some patients may tolerate sustained ventricular tachycardia at slower rates, and these are then amenable to hemodynamic study. Huang and Baron have assessed cardiac performance in six patients with inducible sustained ventricular tachycardia.[62] When compared to sinus rhythm, the cardiac index and stroke volume index during ventricular tachycardia were reduced, and mean pulmonary capillary wedge, pulmonary artery, and right atrial pressures were all significantly increased. Although aortic systolic pressure fell, mean aortic pressure was unchanged.

CHRONIC VENTRICULAR TACHYCARDIA

Several recent reports have demonstrated the occurrence of myocardial dysfunction in patients with prolonged ventricular tachycardia. One notable case was that of a 60-year-old man with documented ventricular tachycardia persisting for 70 days at rates of 120 bpm to 160 bpm and culminating in congestive heart failure with radiographic findings of cardiomegaly.[63] Congestive heart failure associated with chronic ventricular tachycardia may be ameliorated by controlling the rate of the tachycardia. Bergdahl et al reported five children with chronic ventricular tachycardia, three of whom presented with congestive symptoms.[64] In each case, slowing the tachycardia with pharmacologic agents was sufficient to result in clinical improvement of symptoms. This may be the only

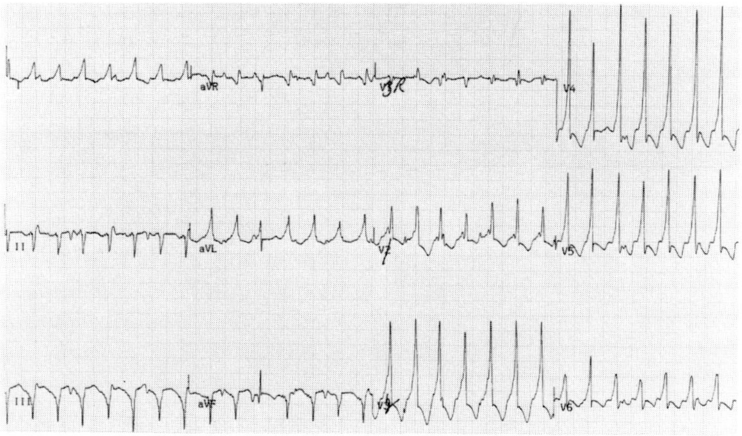

FIGURE 15–10
Surface electrocardiogram obtained on admission to this hospital before electrophysiologic study showing ventricular tachycardia with atrioventricular dissociation. The ventricular rate is 180 bpm to 215 bpm; the atrial rate is approximately 172 bpm.

achievable goal, as complete suppression of the arrhythmia is frequently difficult or impossible to achieve. Rocchini, Chun, and MacDonald likewise noted in a study of 38 children that only patients with rates of more than 150 bpm became symptomatic, and asymptomatic patients had rates less than this.[65] Rates were frequently more rapid in patients in whom coexistent heart disease was present.

Subtle findings of myocardial dysfunction were found at catheterization in 67% of patients studied by Deal et al. The most frequent abnormalities were elevated left ventricular end-diastolic volumes and regional wall motion abnormalities.[66]

Histologic evidence of myocardial abnormalities may be present in some patients with serious ventricular arrhythmias who were otherwise considered normal.[67] The occurrence of cardiomyopathy with tachycardia in patients thought to have structurally normal hearts has led to the question of which came first, the tachycardia or the cardiomyopathy.[52] The occcurrence of sustained ventricular tachycardia in children with apparently normal hearts suggests that the cardiomyopathic features may be secondary. This view is bolstered by the reversibility of serious functional abnormalities once the tachycardia is controlled.

Kugler et al described a 14-year-old patient with sustained ventricular tachycardia at a rate of 150 bpm whose echocardiographic left ventricular shortening fraction was 25% prior to treatment with antiarrhythmic drugs and improved to 31% with conversion to sinus rhythm.[41]

Our own experience likewise suggests that multiple functional cardiac abnormalities caused by ventricular tachycardia are reversible. In a recent case, a 13-month-old boy presented with severe congestive heart failure and ventricular tachycardia for 10 days

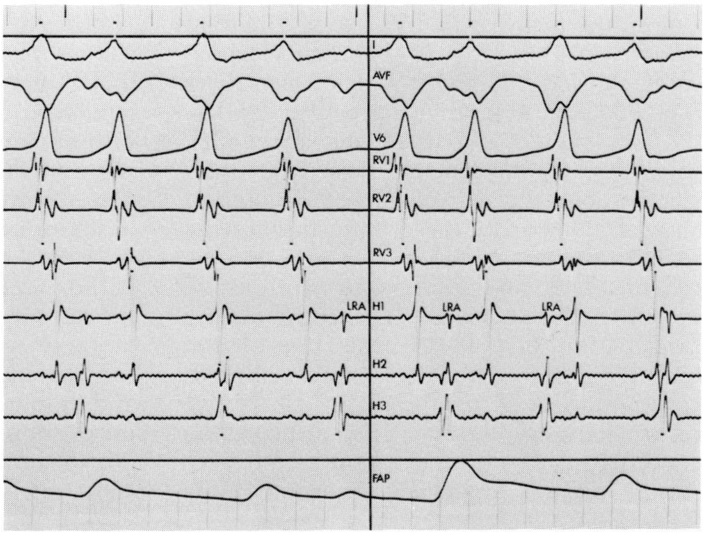

FIGURE 15–11
Electrophysiologic recording during ventricular tachycardia with atrioventricular dissociation. The ventricular rate is 224 bpm; the atrial rate is 160 bpm. From top to bottom: electrocardiographic leads I, aVF, and V_6; right ventricular electrograms RV_1, RV_2, and RV_3; high left atrial electrogram (LRA Hi); His bundle electrograms (H_2, H_3); and femoral artery pulse tracing (FAP).

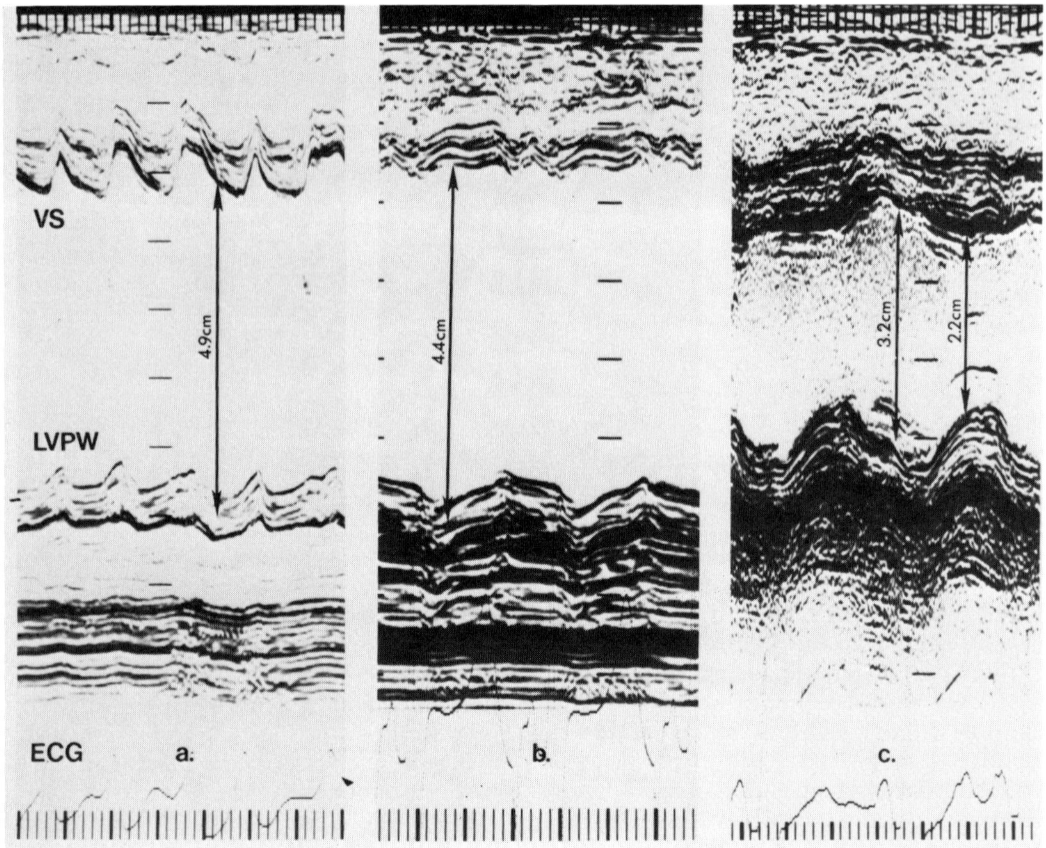

FIGURE 15–12
M-mode echocardiograms. *(A)* Preoperative echocardiogram during ventricular tachycardia (190 bpm), showing severe cardiac dilation with poor contractility and paradoxic ventricular septal (VS) motion. Diastolic dimension of the left ventricle (LV) is 4.9 cm (normal range, 2.5 cm to 3.1 cm). *(B)* Echocardiogram recorded 2 hours after cryoablation during atrial pacing (100 bpm) showing persistent ventricular dilation and dysfunction. Left ventricular diastolic dimension = 4.4 cm. *(C)* Echocardiogram recorded 2 weeks after cryoablation during sinus rhythm (95 bpm) showing normalization of cardiac dimensions and contractility. Left ventricular diastolic dimension is 3.2 cm; shortening fraction is 31%. LVPW = left ventricular posterior wall.

in the hospital following a 2-week illness (Fig. 15–10).[68] Electrophysiologic catheterization showed the tachycardia focus to originate in the left ventricle (Fig. 15–11). Echocardiography showed both right and left ventricles to be dilated and poorly contractile (Fig. 15–12). The presence of severe mitral regurgitation was confirmed by pulsed Doppler echocardiography. Immediately following surgical ablation of the ectopic tachycardia focus in the left ventricle, the left ventricle was still dilated and poorly contractile despite normal atrioventricular synchrony during atrial pacing at a slower heart rate of 100 bpm (see Fig. 15–12). After 2 weeks of medical therapy and resolution of congestive heart failure, repeat echocardiography showed complete normalization of left ventricular diastolic diameter and contractility (see Fig. 15–12). Mitral regurgitation was likewise resolved.

Subsequently we have treated a 3-year-old child with sustained ventricular tachycardia for a month prior to hospital admission. Similar cardiac dilatation and dysfunction were present, with severe mitral and tricuspid regurgitation and a shortening fraction of 15%. Treatment in this case was with high dose infusions of both procainamide and lidocaine, which restored sinus rhythm within 12 hours of treatment. Interestingly, despite the known myocardial depressant properties of these agents, complete normalization of cardiac chamber dimensions and function and resolution of atrioventricular valve regurgitation was documented by the eighth day of sinus rhythm. The presence of severe atrioventricular valve regurgitation at the initial presentation of both of the previously described patients indicates that the valvular dysfunction was causally related to either the tachycardia or to the ventricular dilatation and dysfunction. The complete reversibility of the valve dysfunction following control of the arrhythmia clearly suggests that the tachyarrhythmia was the cause of the mitral regurgitation.

References

1. Schlant RC: Normal Physiology of the Cardiovascular System. In Hurst JW, Logue RB, Schlant RC, et al (eds): The Heart and Veins. New York, McGraw-Hill, pp 79–109, 1974.
2. Kristensson BE, Arnman K, Ryden L: The haemodynamic importance of atrioventricular synchrony and rate increase at rest and during exercise. Eur Heart J 6:773–778, 1985.
3. Swiryn S, Pavel D, Byrom E, et al: Assessment of left ventricular function by radionuclide angiography during induced supraventricular tachycardia. Am J Cardiol 47:555–561, 1981.
4. Rahimtoola SH, Ehsani A, Sinno MZ, et al: Left atrial transport function in myocardial infarction: Importance of its booster pump function. Am J Med 59:686–694, 1975.
5. Leman RB, Kratz JM: Radionuclide evaluation of dual chamber pacing: Comparison between variable A-V intervals and ventricular pacing. PACE 8(1):408–414, 1985.
6. Braunwald E (ed): Heart Disease: A Textbook of Cardiovascular Medicine, ed 2. Philadelphia, WB Saunders Company, 1984, p 438.
7. Rudolph AB: Congenital Diseases of the Heart. Chicago, Year Book Medical Publishers, 1974, p 12.
8. Michaelsson M, Engle MA: Congenital complete heart block: An international study of the natural history. Cardiovas Clin 4(3):86–101, 1972.
9. Karpawich PP, Gillette PC, Garson A, et al: Congenital complete atrioventricular block: Clinical and electrophysiologic predictors of need for pacemaker insertion. Am J Cardiol 48:1098–1102, 1981.
10. Silverman NH, Kleinman CS, Rudolph AM, et al: Fetal atrioventricular valve insufficiency associated with nonimmune hydrops: A two-dimensional echocardiographic and pulsed Doppler ultrasound study. Circulation 72(4):825–832, 1985.
11. Fisher DJ, Gross DM, Garson A: Rapid sinus tachycardia: Differentiation from supraventricular tachycardia. Am J Dis Child 137:164–166, 1983.
12. Engel TR, Bush CA, Schaal SF: Tachycardia-aggravated heart disease. Ann Intern Med 80(3):384–388, 1974.
13. Sobczyk WL, Kugler JD, Latson LA, et al: Sinus tachycardia-induced left ventricular dysfunction after VDD pacemaker implantatioin in a patient with congenital complete atrioventricular block. Am Heart J 112(5):1102–1105, 1986.
14. Phillips E, Levine SA: Auricular fibrillation without other evidence of heart disease: A cause of reversible heart failure. Am J Med 7(2):478–489, 1949.
15. Lemery R, Brugada P, Cheriex E, et al: Reversibility of tachycardia-induced left ventricular dysfunction after closed chest catheter ablation of the atrioventricular junction for intractable atrial fibrillation. Am J Cardiol 60(16):1406–1408, 1987.
16. Radford DJ, Izukawa T: Atrial fibrillation in children. Pediatrics 59(2):250–256, 1977.
17. McIntosh HD, Morris JJ: The hemodynamic consequences of arrhythmias. Prog Cardiovasc Dis 8(4):330–363, 1966.
18. Reale A: Acute effects of countershock conversion of atrial fibrillation upon right and left heart hemodynamics. Circulation 32:214–222, 1965.
19. Tavel ME, Feignenbaum H, Campbell RW: A study of the Q-1 interval in atrial fibrillation with and without mitral stenosis. Circulation 31:429–435, 1965.
20. Garson A, Bink-Boelkens M, Hesslein PS, et al: Atrial flutter in the young: A collaborative study of 380 cases. J Am Coll Cardiol 6(4):871–878, 1985.
21. Harvey RM, Ferrer MI, Richards DW, et al: Cardiocirculatory performance in atrial flutter. Circulation 12(4):507–519, 1955.
22. Ferrer MI, Harvey RM: Some hemodynamic aspects of cardiac arrhythmias in man. A clinico-physiologic correlation. Am Heart J 68(2):153–165, 1964.
23. Goldreyer B, Kastor JA, Kerschbaum KL: Hemodynamic effects of induced supraventricular tachycardia in man. Circulation 54(5):783–789, 1976.
24. Schlepper M, Weppner HG, Merle H: Haemodynamic effects of supraventricular tachycardias and their alterations by electrically and verapamil induced termination. Cardiovasc Res 12:28–33, 1978.
25. Braunwald E, Frahm CJ: Studies on Starling's law of the heart, IV: Observations on the hemodynamic functions of the left atrium in man. Circulation 24:633–641, 1961.
26. Braunwald E: The control of ventricular function in man. Br Heart J 27(1):1–6, 1965.
27. Slutsky R, Karliner J, Ricci D, et al: Response of left ventricular volume to exercise in man assessed by radionuclide equilibrium angiography. Circulation 60:565–571, 1979.
28. Sorensen SG, Ritchie JL, Caldwell JH, et al: Serial exercise radionuclide angiography. Circulation 61:600–609, 1980.
29. Rozenman Y, Weiss AT, Atlant H, et al: Left ventricular function during atrial pacing: A radionuclide angiographic study. Clin Cardiol 7:349–355, 1984.
30. Garson A Jr, Gillette PC, McNamara DG: Supraventricular tachycardia in children: Clinical features, response to treatment and long-term follow-up in 217 patients. J Pediatr 98:875–882, 1981.
31. Shachnow N, Spellman S, Robin I: Persistent supraventricular tachycardia: Case report and review of literature. Circulation 10:232–236, 1959.
32. Epstein ML, Benditt DG: Long-term evaluation of persistent supraventricular tachycardia in children: Clinical and electrocardiographic features. Am Heart J 102:80–89, 1981.
33. Hay JD, Keidan SE: Persistent ectopic auricular tachycardia in children. Br Heart J 14:345–349, 1952.
34. Weiss HB, McGuire J: Ectopic tachycardia, auricular in origin of unusual duration. Am Heart J 12:585–591, 1936.
35. Gallagher JJ, Sealy WC: The permanent form of junctional reciprocating tachycardia: Further elucidation of the underlying mechanism. Eur J Cardiol 8:413–430, 1978.

36. Levine HD, Smith C Jr: Repetitive paroxysmal tachycardia in adults. Prognosis-relationship to nervous systems and to classical tachycardia. Cardiology 55:2–21, 1970.
37. Sung RJ, Chang MS, Chiang BN: Clinical electrophysiology of supraventricular tachycardia. Cardiol Clin 1:225–238, 1983.
38. Engel TR, Bush CA, Schaal SF: Tachycardia-aggravated heart disease. Ann Intern Med 80:384–388, 1974.
39. Keane JF, Plauth WH Jr, Nadas AS: Chronic ectopic tachycardia in infancy and childhood. Am Heart J 84:748–757, 1972.
40. Morgan CL, Nadas AS: Chronic ectopic tachycardia in infancy and childhood. Am Heart J 67:617–627, 1964.
41. Kugler JD, Baisch SD, Cheatham JP, et al: Improvement of LV dysfunction after control of persistent tachycardia. J Pediatr 105:543–548, 1984.
42. Gillette PC, Smith RT, Garson A Jr, et al: Chronic supraventricular tachycardia: A curable cause of congestive cardiomyopathy. JAMA 253:391–392, 1985.
43. Packer DL, Bardy GH, Worley SJ, et al: Tachycardia induced cardiomyopathy: A reversible form of left ventricular dysfunction. Am J Cardiol 57:563–570, 1986.
44. McLaren CJ, Gersh BT, Sugrue DD, et al: Tachycardia induced myocardial dysfunction, a reversible phenomenon? Br Heart J 53:323–327, 1985.
45. Giorgi LV, Hartzler GO, Harnaker WR: Incessant focal atrial tachycardia: A surgically remediable cause of cardiomyopathy. J Thorac Cardiovasc Surg 87:466–473, 1984.
46. Greenwood RD, Nadas AS, Fyler DC: The clinical course of primary myocardial disease in infants and children. Am Heart J 92:549–560, 1976.
47. Bharati S, Lev M, Denes P, et al: Infiltrative cardiomyopathy with conduction disease and ventricular arrhythmia: Electrophysiologic and pathologic correlation. Am J Cardiol 45:163–173, 1980.
48. Johnson RA, Palacios I: Dilated cardiomyopathies of the adult, I. N Engl J Med 307:1051–1058, 1982.
49. Johnson RA, Palacios I: Dilated cardiomyopathies of the adult, II. N Engl J Med 307:1119–1126, 1982.
50. Huang SK, Messer JV, Denes P: Significance of ventricular tachycardia in idiopathic dilated cardiomyopathy: Observations in 35 patients. Am J Cardiol 51:507–512, 1983.
51. Shabetai R: Cardiomyopathy: How far have we come in 25 years, how far yet to go? J Am Coll Cardiol 1:252–263, 1983.
52. Gallagher JJ: Tachycardia and cardiomyopathy: The chicken-egg dilemma revisited. J Am Coll Cardiol 6:1172–1173, 1985.
53. Damiano RJ, Tripp HF Jr, Asano T, et al: Left ventricular dysfunction and dilatation resulting from chronic supraventricular tachycardia. J Thorac Cardiovasc Surg 94:135–143, 1987.
54. SAS Institute, Inc: SAS User's Guide: Statistics, version 5 edition. Cary, NC, SAS Institute Inc, 1985, p 956.
55. Coleman HN, Taylor RR, Pool PO, et al: Congestive heart failure following chronic tachycardia. Am Heart J 81:790–798, 1971.
56. Tripp HF, Lewis W, Veronee C, et al: Effects of acute tachycardia on left ventricular adenine nucleotide levels and subsequent tolerance to ischemia. J Thorac Cardiovasc Surg 92:931–935, 1986.
57. Garson A Jr, Gillette PC: Electrophysiologic studies of supraventricular tachycardia in children, 1. Clinical electrophysiologic correlations. Am Heart J 102:233, 1981.
58. Garson A Jr, Gillette PC: Junctional ectopic tachycardia in children: Electrocardiography, electrophysiology and pharmacologic response. Am J Cardiol 44:298, 1979.
59. Bash SE, Shah JJ, Albers WH, et al: Hypothermia for the treatment of postsurgical greatly accelerated junctional ectopic tachycardia. J Am Coll Cardiol 10(5):1095–1099, 1987.
60. Gillette PC, Garson A, Porter CJ, et al: Junctional automatic ectopic tachycardia: New proposed treatment by transcatheter His bundle ablation. Am Heart J 106(4):619–623, 1983.
61. Kennedy HL, Pescarmona JE, Bouchard RJ, et al: Objective evidence of occult myocardial dysfunction in patients with frequent ventricular ectopy without clinically apparent heart disease. Am Heart J 104(1):57–65, 1982.
62. Huang SK, Baron SB: Hemodynamic and 2D/Doppler echocardiographic assessment during sustained ventricular tachycardia. Circ Res 35(1):107A, 1987.
63. Papadopoulos C, Blazer CJ: Ventricular tachycardia of 70 days' duration with survival. Am J Cardiology 11(1):107–111, 1963.
64. Bergdahl DM, Stevenson JG, Kawabori I, et al: Prognosis in primary ventricular tachycardia in the pediatric patient. Circulation 62(4):897–901, 1980.
65. Rocchini AP, Chun PO, MacDonald D: Ventricular tachycardia in children. Am J Cardiol 47:1091–1097, 1981.
66. Deal BJ, Miller SC, Scagliotti D, et al: Ventricular tachycardia in young population without overt heart disease. Circulation 73(6):1111–1118, 1986.
67. Hosenpud JD, McAnulty JH, Nelson RN: Unexpected myocardial disease in patients with life threatening arrhythmias. Br Heart J 56:55–61, 1986.
68. Fyfe DA, Gillette PC, Crawford FA, et al: Resolution of dilated cardiomyopathy after surgical ablation of ventricular tachycardia in a child. J Am Coll Cardiol 9(1):231–234, 1987.

SECTION IV
TREATMENT

CHAPTER 16

ACUTE NONPHARMACOLOGIC TREATMENT OF TACHYARRHYTHMIAS AND BRADYARRHYTHMIAS

Jeffrey P. Moak

Nonpharmacologic techniques for acute arrhythmia management have gained in popularity during the past 5 years. Interest in the use of electrical techniques to convert tachyarrhythmias back to a normal rate and rhythm has burgeoned because (1) electrical therapy is highly effective, (2) the response to its effect is immediate, (3) side effects are few, and (4) it can be applied repetitively (over minutes to hours) with little concern regarding cumulative effects becoming additive and producing toxicity. While moderately effective, the acute control of tachycardia with antiarrhythmic drugs is frequently delayed in onset (minutes to hours) and can be accompanied by significant side effects. Furthermore, electrical conversion of tachyarrhythmias using electrode catheter techniques provides added therapeutic safety: backup pacing for postconversion bradycardia.

In this chapter we will discuss the use of electrical techniques for recording atrial activity to facilitate arrhythmia diagnosis, stimulation techniques for conversion of tachyarrhythmias originating in the atrium, transthoracic cardioversion and defibrillation, and external transthoracic pacing.

ARRHYTHMIA DIAGNOSIS: TECHNIQUES FOR RECORDING ATRIAL ACTIVITY

The correct diagnosis of any arrhythmia requires knowledge of the relationship between atrial and ventricular activity. Not infrequently, atrial activity may be difficult to discern on the surface electrocardiogram during tachyarrhythmias, either because atrial activity (P wave) is observed in the previous QRS complex or T wave, or the P wave voltage is diminutive. Transesophageal recording techniques have been used since the late 1950s for diagnosing complex arrhythmias.[1, 2] With the use of an esophageal electrogram, not only can the presence or absence of atrial activity be discerned, but also the relationship between atrial and ventricular activity can be analyzed. The diagnosis of many complex arrhythmias can thereby be simplified.[3]

The use of the transesophageal technique for arrhythmia diagnosis is illustrated in Figure 16–1. This figure presents an electrocardiogram (lead II) recorded from a 3-year-old child in the recovery room following repair of tetralogy of Fallot. Four hours following surgery, the patient had the rhythm displayed in Figure 16–1(A). P wave activity is occasionally evident but appears to be inverted, suggesting junctional bigeminy with retrograde atrial capture. A rhythm strip obtained using an esophageal electrogram is demonstrated in Figure 16–1(B). Atrial activity is apparent at a rate of 167 bpm. The relationship between atrial and ventricular activity suggests sinus tachycardia and 3:2 atrioventricular Wenckebach conduction.

Esophageal electrocardiography has been found helpful in the intraoperative diagnosis of arrhythmias. Investigators have compared the diagnostic utility of esophageal electrocardiography with limb lead surface electrocardiograms in patients undergoing intracardiac repair of congenital heart defects. Arrhythmia analysis using the esophageal electrogram facilitated correct arrhythmia diagnoses and appropriate therapeutic management. Diagnostic information necessary for therapeutic decisions was obtainable from 67% of esophageal tracings, in contrast to only 22% of recorded surface electrocardiograms.

Dunnigan, Benson, and Benditt pointed out the difficulty in diagnosing atrial flutter on the surface electrocardiogram in infants in the absence of classic flutter waves.[4] Only two of eight patients studied had classic flutter waves. However, with the use of transesophageal electrocardiography, atrial flutter with 2:1 atrioventricular conduction was easily diagnosed in the other six patients in their study. This observation is particularly relevant to patients who have undergone Mustard or Senning repair. Atrial flutter frequently occurs in these patients (20%) and may be difficult to diagnose on the surface electrocardiogram.[5, 6] Flutter waves are frequently atypical and low in voltage. Atrial flutter should be the presumed diagnosis in any postoperative Mustard or Senning patient whose heart rate is in the 140 bpm to 160 bpm range. This diagnosis can subsequently be easily confirmed using transesophageal electrocardiography.

Several other investigators have reported on the diagnostic usefulness of 24-hour ambulatory esophageal recordings.[7, 8] Good-to-excellent quality recordings with limited noise can be achieved in 76% of patients. Esophageal electrocardiography facilitated electrocardiographic diagnosis of wide complex QRS tachycardias and was particularly helpful in differentiating supraventricular tachycardia with aberrant ventricular conduction from ventricular tachycardia.

The placement of atrial epicardial electrodes at the conclusion of intracardiac surgery has also been reported to be useful for

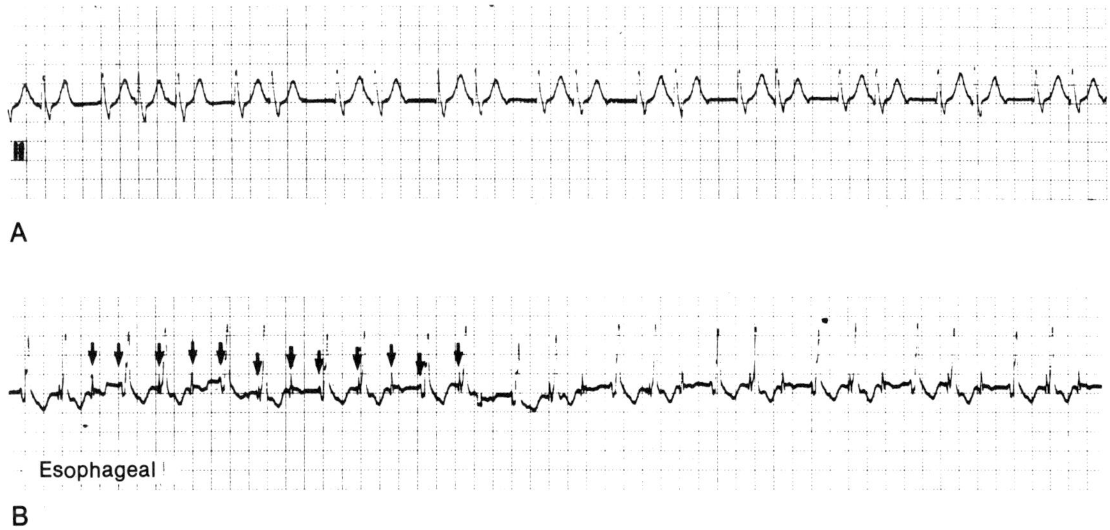

FIGURE 16–1

Transesophageal electrocardiography. *(A)* Electrocardiographic lead II. *(B)* Esophageal recording. Arrows demonstrate atrial electrograms recorded from esophageal electrode catheter. An atrial rhythm (cycle length = 360 ms) with 3:2 AV conduction was apparent.

arrythmia diagnosis and treatment. Yabek et al have described their experience with atrial epicardial electrodes in more than 100 patients ranging in age from 1 day to 17 years.[9] Recording of atrial activity was helpful in (1) determining sinus or sinus-like rhythm in patients following Mustard repair in whom the surface electrocardiogram failed to demonstrate P waves; (2) diagnosing atrial tachyarrhythmias (supraventricular tachycardia, atrial fluttter, or atrial fibrillation); and (3) differentiating aberrant atrial from ventricular ectopic complexes. Figure 16–2 illustrates the application of recording an atrial electrogram from epicardial atrial electrodes for diagnostic confirmation of an arrhythmia in a 1-day-old patient after surgery for critical aortic stenosis. Atrial fibrillation was suspected from the surface electrocardiogram (Fig. 16–2[*A*]). The diagnosis was confirmed by recording atrial activity from the atrial epicardial electrodes placed during surgery. (Fig. 16–2[*B*]).

The placement and use of atrial epicardial electrodes has proven safe in postoperative patients. Waldo and MacLean have reported their experience in the use of epicardial electrodes in more than 9000 patients.[10] No arrhythmias have been precipitated from the inadvertent delivery of electrical current through the electrode wires. No infectious complications were reported. In only two instances did bleeding occur following removal of the electrode wires.

Our experience in using atrial epicardial electrodes in the postoperative management of children following cardiac surgery has been similar. We recommend placing two separate atrial electrodes on the right atrium in an area free from previous atrial injury. Because of occasional difficulty in using these electrodes for sensing and pacing, they are tested in the operating room prior to closure of the thorax. The major limitation of this technique is the obvious requirement that the patient undergo a thoracotomy.

Signal averaging techniques have been utilized for identifying atrial activation and determining the mechanism of atrial tachyarrhythmias. Kuchar, Kelly, and Thornburn reported using the signal-averaged electrocardiogram to successfully identify atrial activation in 23 of 24 patients (95%) with atrial tachyarrhythmias.[11] The arrhythmias studied included atrioventricular reciprocating tachycardia, atrioventricular nodal reentrant tachycardia, atrial flutter, and primary atrial tachycardia. Definition of the mechanism of the supraventricular arrhythmia was easily accomplished once the atrial cycle length, RP-PR relationship, and pattern of atrioventricular conduction were known. The major limitation of the signal-averaged technique is its dependence on a fixed temporal relationship

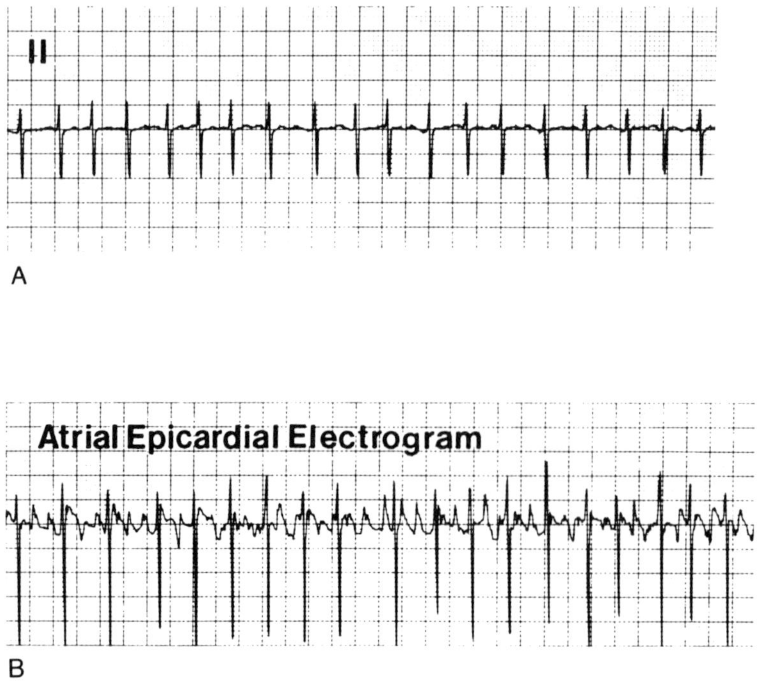

A

B

FIGURE 16–2
Atrial epicardial electrocardiography. *(A)* Electrocardiographic lead II. No definite P wave activity was evident on the surface electrocardiogram. *(B)* Atrial epicardial electrogram showed an atrial tachyarrhythmia with a cycle length of 500 ms. Constantly changing morphology of the atrial electrograms suggested the arrhythmia to be atrial fibrillation.

between the P wave and the QRS complex. Any fluctuations of the P-QRS relationship will lead to distortion of the atrial waveform. Because of variable timing of atrial activity throughout the cardiac cycle, the averaging process regards this as noise and cancels out the atrial signal. Therefore the applicability of signal-averaged electrocardiography is limited to arrhythmias that are regular.

ACUTE NONPHARMACOLOGIC TREATMENT OF TACHYARRHYTHMIAS

Transesophageal Pacing

INDICATIONS

Transesophageal pacing can be useful for termination of supraventricular tachycardia or atrial flutter, assessing the effects of antiarrhythmic agents in patients with inducible supraventricular tachycardia, and evaluation of palpitations in children (Table 16–1). However, transesophageal pacing is most effective in converting supraventricular tachycardia to normal sinus rhythm. Benson et al reported successful acute conversion of supraventricular tachycardia in 12 of 14 infants and in seven of seven children ranging in age from 1 to 9 years.[12, 13] Gallagher et al similarly found overdrive pacing from the esophagus successful in restoring sinus rhythm in 33 of 38 patients (87%) whose mean age was 35 years.[14] Conversion of supraventricular tachycardia in older children with dilated and poorly functioning hearts has been less successful in our experience.

TABLE 16–1
INDICATIONS FOR TRANSESOPHAGEAL PACING

1. Termination of atrial tachyarrhythmias
   a. Supraventricular tachycardia
   b. Atrial flutter
2. Assessment of antiarrhythmic drug efficacy
3. Diagnostic evaluation of palpitations
4. Noninvasive determination of accessory pathway properties in the Wolff-Parkinson-White syndrome
   a. Accessory pathway ERP
   b. Functional refractory period during atrial fibrillation
5. Emergency atrial pacing for bradycardia
6. Diagnosis of electrophysiologic mechanism of supraventricular tachycardia

Repeated antitachycardia pacing is a useful technique for controlling recurrent paroxysmal supraventricular tachycardia until therapeutic antiarrhythmic drug concentrations can safely be achieved or effective drug combinations identified. Sugrue et al have reported the use of intracardiac antitachycardia pacing techniques to terminate frequent paroxysms of supraventricular tachycardia in infants.[15] We have found this method for achieving short-term arrhythmia control similarly effective in the rare patient in whom rapid arrhythmia suppression is difficult. In order to avoid the complications attendant with indwelling venous catheters, we have instead used the transesophageal technique. Overdrive transesophageal atrial pacing can successfully convert atrial flutter to sinus rhythm. Figure 16–3(A) shows the surface electrocardiogram of a 12-hour-old neonate who presented with intrauterine tachycardia at 36 weeks gestational age. The differential diagnosis of the rhythm was atrial flutter with 2:1 atrioventricular conduction, or supraventricular tachycardia. An esophageal electrogram revealed an atrial rate of 350 bpm and 2:1 atrioventricular conduction. Overdrive atrial pacing at a cycle length of 160 ms was performed (Fig. 16–3[*B*]). After atrial pacing for 30 s, atrial flutter converted to sinus rhythm.

Campbell et al have compared the effectiveness of overdrive pacing for atrial flutter conversion using intracardiac and transesophageal techniques during 33 episodes of atrial flutter (30 patients).[16] Ten of 16 episodes (63%) and eight of 17 episodes (47%) were successfully converted using the intracardiac and transesophageal techniques, respectively. No clinical, hemodynamic, or electrophysiologic variable differentiated those patients who were most likely to respond. The transient development of atrial fibrillation was not an infrequent occurrence in their study (7 of 30 patients, or 23%). Dunnigan, Benson, and Benditt have successfully used the transesophageal technique to convert four of five infants (80%) with atrial flutter to sinus rhythm.[4] Our experience is concordant with previous investigators (six of eight patients, or 75%).

Butto et al have reported the efficacy of transesophageal pacing for termination of the atrial tachycardias (e.g., atrial flutter or atrial muscle reentry) that commonly occur in patients who have had baffle operations for complete transposition of the great ves-

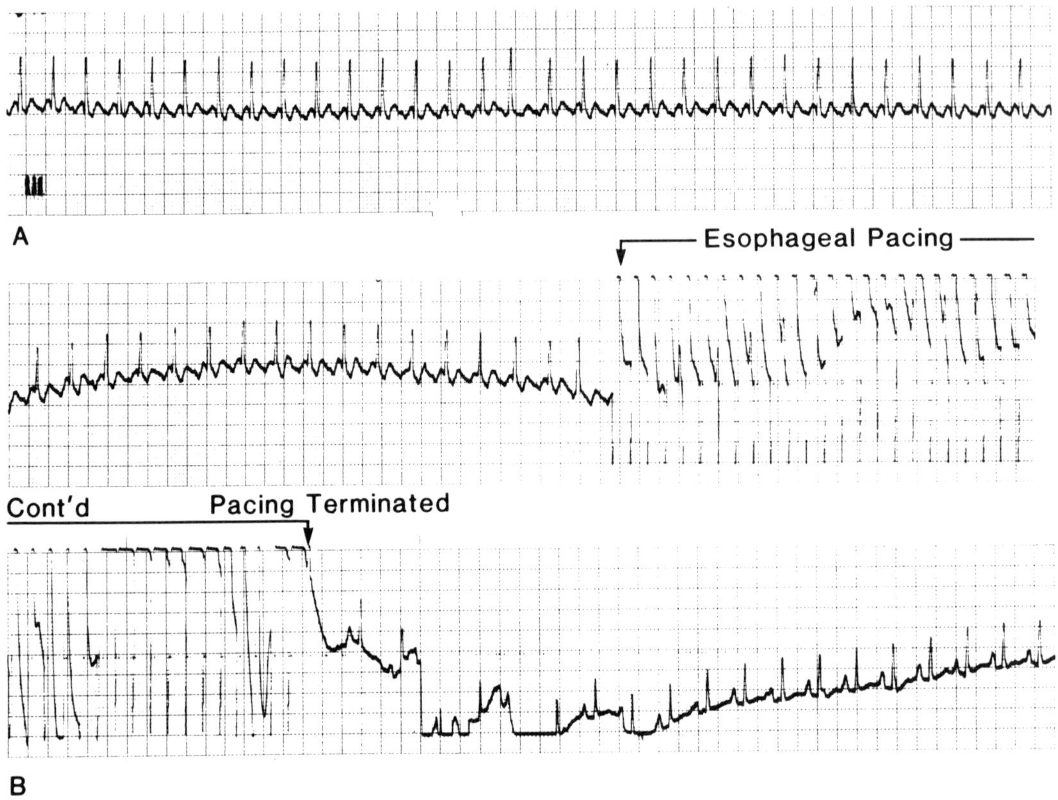

FIGURE 16–3
Transesophageal pacing. *(A)* Lead III of the electrocardiogram demonstrated atrial flutter with predominantly 2:1 AV conduction. *(B)* Transesophageal pacing. Atrial pacing was initiated at a cycle length of 160 ms and continued for 30 s. Sinus rhythm ensued following termination of pacing.

sels.[6] Short bursts of rapid pacing (four to 10 beats) converted 48 of 51 tachycardia episodes (94%). Twenty percent of tachycardia episodes were transiently converted to atrial fibrillation. Acceleration of the ventricular rate necessitated DC cardioversion on one occasion.

Atrial pacing has the following advantages over DC cardioversion:

1. Prolonged bradycardic episodes may follow DC cardioversion of atrial tachyarrhythmias. Significant postconversion bradycardia has been reported to occur in 10% to 24% of countershocked patients.[17] The length of the postconversion pause is related to multiple factors such as countershock intensity, type of wave form, whether the patient is concomitantly taking antiarrhythmic agents with sinus node suppressant activity, and whether the arrhythmia occurs in the setting of sick sinus syndrome. Atrial pacing offers additional safety. In the event of prolonged bradycardia, atrial pacing can be instituted immediately, avoiding any adverse hemodynamic sequela.
2. Atrial pacing can be performed safely in patients receiving digitalis, whereas there is an increased risk of postconversion ventricular arrhythmias in DC cardioversion patients who are receiving digitalis.[17]
3. Atrial pacing does not require general anesthesia, which is frequently used for DC cardioversion.

However, there are disadvantages to the transesophageal pacing technique. Patients frequently complain of chest discomfort during the procedure. Esophageal discomfort is the most common side effect observed during performance of this technique. The sensation of heartburn commonly occurs when electrical stimulation is performed with current strengths >15 mA.[14, 18] Esophageal mucosal erythema has been observed by esophagoscopy following transesophageal electrical stimulation. No long-term complications of esophageal stricture or erosion have been reported. The intensity of pain is directly related to the current amplitude and duration of pacing. Overdrive pacing of atrial flutter to sinus rhythm frequently requires high current amplitudes (24 mA to 28 mA) and prolonged pacing durations (15 s to 30 s). Rarely, atrial flutter with 2:1 atrioventricular block will be conducted 1:1 if conversion is unsuccessful. Rapid atrial pacing may accelerate the rate of atrial flutter or convert atrial flutter to atrial fibrillation. We have observed diaphragmatic stimulation when high current strengths were needed in order to capture the atrium. Benson et al reported two unusual and rare complications: brachial plexus stimulation and ventricular capture, in one patient each.[12] Inadvertent ventricular pacing has not been observed in our experience, even when stimulating with extremely high current strengths.

Several groups of investigators have used the transesophageal pacing technique to predict drug efficacy in patients with recurrent supraventricular tachycardia. Benson et al have used the transesophageal atrial pacing technique to predict long-term effectiveness of digoxin in 18 infants with recurrent supraventricular tachycardia.[19] None of the infants whose supraventricular tachycardia was noninducible while receiving digoxin therapy had a recurrence on chronic therapy. In contrast, 10 of the 15 patients (67%) with inducible tachycardia on chronic digoxin therapy had recurrences of their arrhythmia. In a similar manner, Gonzalez et al studied the effect of amiodarone in 10 patients with recurrent atrial fibrillation and the Wolff-Parkinson-White syndrome.[20] Using this method, these investigators were able to demonstrate a prolongation of the effective refractory period of the accessory pathway and an increase in the shortest RR interval during atrial fibrillation. Our experience in performing drug testing with the transesophageal stimulation technique has been limited to three patients. Two patients were diagnosed with reciprocating atrioventricular tachycardia, and one patient had ventricular tachycardia that could be induced during atrial pacing. Electrophysiologic testing has been helpful in predicting long-term therapy in two of these patients.

The noninvasive diagnostic evaluation of the patient who presents with occasional episodes of palpitations is frequently disappointing. Twenty-four–hour ambulatory electrocardiograms and treadmill exercise tests are normal in the vast majority of patients studied, thus not allowing the physician to make a specific arrhythmia diagnosis. Dunningan et al have used transesophageal atrial pacing to diagnose the origin of recurrent palpitations in 12 of 17 children whose noninvasive work-up was normal.[21] Supraventricular tachycardia was initiated in 11 patients, and atrial flutter in one patient. In five patients, no arrhythmia was induced, although ventricular tachycardia was later documented in one patient.

METHOD

After the decision is made to perform transesophageal recording or stimulation, consideration should be given to sedation. In general, it has not been necessary to administer premedication to newborns or young infants. To allay anxiety in older children and adolescents, a verbal description of the procedure is given first. Sedation, based on our experience, is best achieved in young children with either (1) a combination of meperidine hydrochloride (1 mg/kg) and promethazine hydrochloride (0.5 mg/kg) or (2) ketamine (1 mg/kg). Satisfactory comfort and cooperation is achieved in adolescent and young adult patients sedated with diazepam (0.1–0.2 mg/kg) and morphine sulfate (0.1 mg/kg) intravenously.

The catheters we prefer to use for transesophageal pacing are silicone rubber–coated bipolar electrode catheters: Medtronic 6992A coronary sinus pacing lead (15 mm interelectrode spacing) for infants, and Medtronic 6992 coronary sinus pacing lead (28 mm interelectrode spacing) for older children.* Our overall success rate has been enhanced with the use of these catheters. Previously, we had used standard 4 or 5 French tripolar electrode pacing catheters. Several investigators have reported using the Arzco Medical Electronics "pill" electrode.†[22] Satisfactory atrial recordings and low stimulation thresholds have been observed using this electrode system. The pill electrode may provide slightly more comfort for the patient.

For each patient, an estimate of the depth of insertion is made by externally measuring the distance from the external nares to the xiphisternum. The pacing catheter is inserted through the nares in a fashion similar to

*Medtronic, Minneapolis, Minnesota.
†Arzco, Chicago, Illinois.

nasogastric cannulation. Older patients are given some liquids to swallow when the catheter tip has passed through the posterior pharynx. Once the catheter has been inserted to the estimated depth, a bipolar electrogram is recorded. Using an electrocardiographic recorder that transcribes three ECG leads simultaneously, the electrode poles from the esophageal catheter are attached to the right arm and left arm inputs, respectively. The electrocardiographic recorder is turned on, and leads I, II, and III are visualized. The esophageal electrogram will be evident on lead I. If the electrogram is not seen or has a low amplitude, the electrode catheter is slowly pulled back until the largest atrial electrogram is recorded. Noise from diaphragmatic activity or esophageal motility infrequently interferes with esophageal recording. To filter out any unwanted signals, a preamplifier (Arzco esophageal ECG preamplifier) can be used to connect the esophageal catheter to the ECG recorder.[22]

Transesophageal stimulation is performed with a Medtronic model 2346 programmable stimulator. This stimulator is capable of delivering constant current, square wave pulses. Benson et al have studied many of the determinants of the transesophageal pacing threshold.[23] In their study, they found no significant differences in pacing threshold when electrode pole spacings of 15 mm, 22 mm, or 28 mm were used. Stimulation with a pulse width greater than 10 ms rarely lowered current threshold requirements. In contrast, stimulation with pulse widths less than 10 mA increased current requirements exponentially. The most critical determinant of pacing threshold was finding an optimal catheter insertion depth. We begin stimulation at a pulse width of 10 ms and a current strength of 10 mA to 12 mA. If atrial capture does not occur, the current strength is slowly increased by 2-mA increments. Patients begin to complain of chest discomfort when paced at current strengths greater than 15 mA to 18 mA. The catheter position is adjusted and stimulation repeated using a lower current intensity when the the patient begins to complain of esophageal burning and atrial capture is not evident.

Antitachycardia Pacing

The basic pacing techniques available for termination of tachycardia are competitive underdrive pacing, programmed extrastimulation, and burst or overdrive pacing.[24] Competitive underdrive pacing refers to asynchronous pacing at a rate below the tachycardia. This technique works well when the tachycardia termination zone is large enough to ensure that a single randomly placed pacing stimulus can terminate the arrhythmia. Programmed electrical stimulation terminates tachycardia in much the same way as underdrive pacing. However, this pacing method involves the precise delivery of extrastimuli during tachycardia, in contrast to the random delivery of underdrive pacing. Furthermore, single, double, or triple pulses may be applied during programmed electrical stimulation. Burst pacing provides four to 10 beats of rapid stimulation at a rate 30 bpm faster than the tachycardia. Prolonged stimulation (more than 3 s) at a rate less than 30 bpm faster than the tachycardia is referred to as overdrive pacing.

For termination of supraventricular tachycardia, rapid atrial pacing has proved more effective than programmed electrical stimulation.[24–28] In the experience of German and Strauss, burst atrial pacing terminated 93% of tachycardia episodes, in contrast to 73% of episodes terminated with atrial extrasystoles.[25] Ward, Camm, and Spurrel reported that underdrive atrial pacing was the least successful pacing mode for tachycardia termination.[26] Although burst atrial pacing appears to be the most effective pacing mode for supraventricular tachycardia termination, its use may be complicated by the development of atrial fibrillation or tachycardia acceleration.[27] Rapid atrial pacing is known to stimulate the release of endogenous catecholamines. Sympathetic stimulation may either increase the rate of the tachycardia or facilitate atrioventricular conduction if the underlying arrhythmia is atrial tachycardia associated with atrioventricular block. Atrial fibrillation has been reported to be induced in 16% to 37% of patients undergoing burst atrial pacing.[25–28] All previously discussed reports have used intracardiac techniques for stimulation. Little data are available to suggest the optimal pacing mode for supraventricular tachycardia termination using the transesophageal technique.

Induction of atrial fibrillation during rapid transesophageal atrial pacing for supraventricular tachycardia termination has been rare in our experience. Furthermore, although we recognize that programmed electrical stimulation is moderately effective and associated with less patient discomfort, we prefer overdrive atrial pacing because of its higher success rate.

For termination of atrial flutter, rapid atrial pacing is clearly the preferred pacing mode.[10, 29] Termination of atrial flutter episodes has been reported in 67% to 100% of trials. Only rarely have single or double atrial extrastimuli been effective in converting atrial flutter to sinus rhythm. Atrial pacing at rates 110% to 129% faster than the flutter rate and at durations between 20 s and 30 s has been most successful. The faster the atrial paced rate, the more likely is the induction of atrial fibrillation. Atrial fibrillation generally occurs following atrial pacing at rates greater than 135% of the flutter rate. Termination of flutter usually requires 10 s to 30 s of pacing; rarely will it terminate with shorter periods of stimulation.

Cardioversion and Defibrillation

The transthoracic application of high electrical energy currents can effectively convert either supraventricular or ventricular tachyarrhythmias to sinus rhythm in pediatric patients. Cardioversion differs from defibrillation in that the electrical discharge is synchronized with the R wave to avoid inducing ventricular fibrillation by accidental discharge during the ventricular vulnerable period. During ventricular fibrillation, R wave synchronization is impossible, because ventricular depolarization is continuous.

Restoration of sinus rhythm by cardioversion or defibrillation is most successful for reentrant arrhythmias but is ineffective for terminating automatic tachycardias. The arrhythmias responsive to electrical countershock include supraventricular tachycardia, atrial flutter, atrial fibrillation, ventricular tachycardia, and ventricular fibrillation. Digitalis toxic arrhythmias are a relative contraindication for the use of this method of arrhythmia management.[17]

DOSAGE

Based on available information for 13 human subjects ranging in weight (W) from 3.2 kg to 126 kg, Tacker et al[30] were able to construct the following defibrillation threshold curve:

$$E\ (J/kg) = 1.88\ W\ (kg)^{1.16}$$

Gutgesell et al further extended these observations by successfully terminating 63 of 71 episodes (89%) of ventricular fibrillation in 27 children, using an energy dose of 2 J/kg.[31] In every case, defibrillation was ultimately aborted by countershock with 4 J/kg or less. Whether an energy dose <2 J would be adequate for successful defibrillation was not addressed. However, Gutgesell et al pointed out that many variables other than body weight may also affect the defibrillation threshold.[31]

COMPLICATIONS

Arrhythmias After DC Shock

A variety of arrhythmias and conduction disturbances have been described following DC countershock (Table 16–2). The occurrence and frequency of arrhythmias and conduction abnormalities are dependent on the presence and type of pre-countershock arrhythmias, cardiac disease, metabolic derangements, digitalis toxicity, and shock strength.[17]

Digitalis intoxication can greatly sensitize the heart to electrical discharge.[32–34] Electrical countershock in patients with digitalis toxicity is frequently accompanied by the induction of ventricular tachycardia and ventricular fibrillation. Furthermore, once initiated, these arrhythmias may be difficult to terminate. Clinical and experimental evidence suggests that the incidence of post-shock arrhythmias is related to the degree of digitalis excess as well as the strength of the delivered current.[32, 33] However, the incidence of post-

TABLE 16–2
ARRHYTHMIAS OCCURRING AFTER DC COUNTERSHOCK

Tachyarrhythmias:
Atrial fibrillation
Supraventricular tachycardia
Ventricular tachycardia
Ventricular fibrillation
Bradycardia and AV conduction abnormalities:
Sinus bradycardia
AV block
Right bundle-branch block
Left bundle-branch block

cardioversion arrhythmias in patients with digoxin levels within the therapeutic range is not significantly increased.[34] The withholding of digitalis therapy for 24 hours prior to the cardioversion procedure or the prophylactic administration of local anesthetic antiarrhythmic agents is rarely indicated in this setting. For the patient suspected of having digitalis toxicity, however, an alternate course of management must be pursued. Options include either discontinuing digitalis therapy until signs and symptoms of toxicity have disappeared or prophylactically administering lidocaine and cardioverting the patient with the lowest effective energy dose.

Morphologic and Functional Damage

The occurrence of myocardial damage after DC countershock in human patients has been suggested by electrocardiographic (ST segment) changes, release of cardiac enzymes into plasma (CPK), and scintigraphic techniques.[35, 36] Furthermore, several case reports commenting on the pathologic findings following frequent delivery of high energy shocks to patients with refractory arrhythmias, underscore the hazards of the countershock procedure.[37] However, data available suggest that when countershock is properly performed using moderate energy doses, histologic injury is rare in human subjects.

In addition to morphologic damage, functional impairment of myocardial contractility may result from electrical countershock. Animal studies have demonstrated depression of left ventricular dp/dt, increases in diastolic stiffness, and increases in left ventricular diastolic pressure.[38]

Embolism

Although systemic and pulmonary emboli have been encountered in 1% to 2% of adult patients cardioverted from atrial fibrillation, this complication is rare in the pediatric age group undergoing electrical countershock.[17] Anticoagulation prior to electrical reversion of atrial arrhythmias has been recommended for adult patients. None of the 100 subjects anticoagulated by Lown, Kleiger, and Williams experienced embolism following reversion to sinus rhythm.[32] In the pediatric age group, the risk/benefit ratio for anticoagulation prior to cardioversion is low. Our policy has been to perform two-dimensional echocardiography prior to cardioversion. When atrial thrombi are apparent, anticoagulation is instituted.

How do these considerations affect the technique of cardioversion and defibrillation in children? The energy levels utilized for cardioversion and defibrillation are based on body weight. The doses will be described in the following sections for each specific arrhythmia. An anterior lateral paddle position is universally used for cardioversion. The paddles chosen are those with the largest diameter allowing contact with the chest wall. A generous amount of electrode paste is applied to the undersurface of the electrode paddles and firm pressure is applied during the procedure. If the first shock is unsuccessful, a second shock at double the energy level of the first shock is then applied.

SPECIAL PRECAUTIONS FOR PACEMAKER PATIENTS

Cardioversion or defibrillation of the pacemaker patient is not more complex than in non-pacemaker patients. Attention to detail and a few simple rules will avoid unnecessary problems. Electrical countershock directly over the pacemaker should be avoided. The electrode paddles should be placed distant from the pulse generator. Programming the sensing circuit to low sensitivity is unnecessary and will not protect its circuitry. Immediately after the procedure the sensing and pacing circuits of the pulse generator should be assessed. Furthermore, the programmed mode should be reviewed. Reprogramming to an alternate pacing mode may occasionally occur during DC countershock.

METHOD OF CARDIOVERSION

Cardioversion is performed following a 4- to 8-hour fast. Digoxin therapy is withheld for 2 to 4 hours prior to cardioversion. The procedure is performed in an intensive care unit or the cardiac catheterization laboratory. An intravenous line is started for drug administration. Blood pressure is monitored prior to administration of sedatives and following cardioversion.

Our technique of anesthesia involves the intravenous administration of ketamine (0.5–

1.0 mg/kg intravenously) and/or diazepam (0.1 mg/kg). Prior to being anesthetized, the patient is connected to an electrocardiographic monitor capable of R wave synchronization. An energy level is decided for the first shock and set on the defibrillator. The anesthesia is given while the heart rate and blood pressure are monitored. After ensuring that the patient is completely anesthetized, the first shock is applied with R wave synchronization. The patient's rhythm is monitored for several minutes to assess the effectiveness of the shock. If successful, the procedure is terminated, and the patient's vital signs and rhythm are monitored for 2 hours prior to the patient's return to his or her room. If unsuccessful, a second shock is applied at double the energy level utilized for the first shock. Each shock should be separated by 2 to 3 minutes, for two reasons. First, the risk of producing myocardial injury will be lower, and second, delayed reversion of the arrhythmia can occur up to 2 minutes after electrical shock.

Termination of Specific Arrhythmias

Atrial Flutter. Atrial flutter is the most common supraventricular arrhythmia requiring elective cardioversion. This arrhythmia may develop any time from fetal life through childhood. The atrial rate ranges from 280 bpm to 450 bpm, and the AV conduction ratio ranges from 1:1 to high degrees of block. Of 380 patients studied by Garson et al, 8% had normal hearts, 6% had cardiomyopathy, and 81% had congenital heart disease.[5] Of the patients with congenital heart disease, atrial flutter developed after a surgical procedure in almost all of these patients. Abnormal sinus node function is commonly present in these postoperative patients. For this reason, cardioversion of atrial flutter in any patient with possible sick sinus syndrome should be performed in the cardiac catheterization laboratory with a pacing catheter present in the right ventricle.

In our experience, many adolescent patients prefer to attempt conversion of their atrial flutter to sinus rhythm with rapid overdrive pacing rather than with DC cardioversion. Under light anesthesia, a pacing catheter can be inserted through the femoral venous approach and placed in the right atrium, or the transesophageal technique can be employed. Atrial overdrive pacing is started at a rate 20 bpm faster than the flutter rate and continued for a duration of 30 s. Atrial pacing is then terminated, and the underlying atrial rhythm analyzed. This technique has been successful in 80% to 90% of pediatric patients with atrial flutter.[22]

If atrial overdrive pacing is unsuccessful, electrical DC cardioversion is then performed. In our experience, DC cardioversion converted all patients with atrial flutter to sinus rhythm. An energy level of 0.5 J/kg is usually successful in converting atrial flutter to sinus rhythm, but we have had a rare experience with a single patient requiring an energy level of 5 J/kg to convert to sinus rhythm.

Atrial Fibrillation. Atrial fibrillation is rare in infants and children and commonly occurs in patients with underlying heart disease. The cardiac conditions associated with atrial fibrillation in children are severe rheumatic heart disease, congenital heart disease (Ebstein's anomaly, tricuspid atresia, and atrial septal defect), cardiomyopathy, atrial tumor, and the Wolff-Parkinson-White syndrome. Rarely, atrial fibrillation may occur in children with no underlying heart disease. Consideration is given to the following factors prior to performing DC cardioversion: presence and degree of atrial dilatation, chronicity of atrial fibrillation, echocardiographic presence of atrial thrombi, prior and concurrent antiarrhythmic medications, and the possibility of digoxin toxicity. If atrial fibrillation is of recent onset in a patient with mild atrial dilatation and no echocardiographic evidence of atrial thrombi, elective cardioversion is performed without any anticoagulation. Usually an attempt at medical cardioversion with digoxin and quinidine is done prior to DC electrical cardioversion. If this fails and there is no suspicion of sinus node dysfunction, cardioversion is performed in the ICU. If there is any suspicion of abnormal sinus node function, cardioversion is performed in the cardiac catheterization laboratory with a pacing catheter placed in the right ventricle. In those patients with recurrent chronic atrial fibrillation being treated with digoxin and local anesthetics, an attempt at restoration of sinus rhythm is made with amiodarone. If sinus rhythm has not been restored after 7 to 10 days of amiodarone loading, elective DC cardioversion is performed in the catheterization laboratory with a pacing catheter present in the right ventricle. We feel this is crucially important because of the marked sinus node depressant effects of amiodarone.

Supraventricular Tachycardia. The majority of supraventricular tachycardias do not require cardioversion, as they usually respond to vagal maneuvers or esophageal atrial pacing. For those patients with supraventricular tachycardia and hypotension or congestive heart failure, we recommend immediate elective cardioversion using an energy level of 0.25–0.5 J/kg. This may be increased to 1 J/kg if needed. In a multicenter investigation of the Wolff-Parkinson-White syndrome and supraventricular tachycardia presenting in the first 4 months of life, elective cardioversion was successful in 73% of the 59 patients who underwent this procedure.[36]

Ventricular Tachycardia. Ventricular tachycardia unresponsive to intravenous lidocaine or procainamide infusion can be successfully terminated with synchronized DC cardioversion performed with 0.5–1.0 J/kg. We have used the self-adhesive electrode pads for cardioversion of ventricular tachycardia.[39] Prior to attempting ventricular tachycardia induction by programmed electrical stimulation, these electrode pads are applied in an anteroposterior position. They are connected to the defibrillator through a connector (manufactured by the R2 Corporation). Cardioversion has been uniformly successful and expeditiously performed in the setting of induction of a hemodynamically unstable ventricular tachycardia.

No attempt to assess the efficacy and safety of transvenous cardioversion of ventricular tachycardia in pediatric patients has been made. This technique has been shown to have an overall efficacy for termination of ventricular tachycardia ranging from 62% to 100% in adult patients.[40] Transvenous cardioversion of ventricular tachycardia can be performed with extremely low energy levels, barely perceived by the patient. The use of this new technology, however, has limited application in the pediatric population.

Ventricular Fibrillation. Ventricular fibrillation is rare in children. In a review by Walsh and Krongrad, the terminal electrical activity of 100 children younger than 18 years was analyzed.[41] In only 6% was the terminal event ventricular fibrillation. In all others, the terminal event was bradycardia followed by asystole. Although spontaneous cardioversion from ventricular fibrillation to sinus rhythm can occur, ventricular fibrillation is almost always permanent and fatal if not treated. For defibrillation, we use an energy dose of 2 J/kg; R wave synchronization is not possible. If this attempt is unsuccessful, the energy dose should be doubled. For ventricular fibrillation unresponsive to electrical countershock, consideration should be given to factors such as hypoxia, acidosis, or hypoglycemia, which are known to interfere with successful defibrillation.

TRANSTHORACIC PACING FOR BRADYARRHYTHMIAS

In 1952, Zoll introduced transthoracic external pacing for treatment of bradycardia.[42] As originally designed, this technique had limited applicability, because the associated stimulation of skin and muscle was extremely painful. However, refinements in the technique have reduced the threshold for cardiac stimulation, making the procedure more tolerable.[43] Its advantages include ease of application, immediate availability, and low complication rate. However, transvenous endocardial pacing requires considerable technical skill and time for electrode insertion.

The indications for transthoracic pacing are several. Sharkey, Chaffee, and Kapsner have found the technique useful for treatment of bradycardia after cardioversion of atrial tachyarrhythmias.[44] Transthoracic pacing may be prophylactically applied in the operating room to patients at high risk for bradycardia as a result of either sick sinus syndrome or atrioventricular conduction abnormalities.[45] Rosenthal et al have successfully performed underdrive pacing for termination of sustained ventricular tachycardia.[46] Noninvasive pacing can stabilize a patient until temporary transvenous endocardial pacing can be established. Emergency external pacing may improve survival in patients during cardiac arrest associated with asystole or significant bradycardia.

Noninvasive transcutaneous pacing has received little attention in the pediatric age group. Beland et al studied the energy threshold requirements and transthoracic impedance in 21 pediatric patients.[47] They found that chest impedance and energy requirements did not vary with age, weight, or chest size, and transcutaneous pacing was easily accomplished without any complications. Although initially promising, further study is required for determining the therapeutic value of this technique for arrhythmia management in children.

References

1. Butterworth S, Poindexter CA: The esophageal electrocardiogram in arrhythmias and tachycardia. Am Heart J 32:681–688, 1946.
2. Enselberg CD: The esophageal electrocardiogram in the study of atrial activity and cardiac arrhythmias. Am Heart J 41:382–409, 1951.
3. Garson A, Gillette PC, McNamara DG: A Guide to Cardiac Dysrhythmias in Children. New York, Grune & Stratton, 1980, pp 3–105.
4. Dunnigan A, Benson DW, Benditt DG: Atrial flutter in infancy: Diagnosis, clinical features, and treatment. Pediatrics 75:725–729, 1985.
5. Garson A, Bink-Boelkens M, Hesslein PS, et al: Atrial flutter in the young: A collaborative study of 380 cases. J Am Coll Cardiol 6:871–878, 1985.
6. Butto F, Dunnigan A, Overholt ED, et al: Transesophageal study of recurrent atrial tachycardia after atrial baffle procedures for complete transposition of the great arteries. Am J Cardiol 57:1356–1362, 1986.
7. Schuchard GH, Tristani FE: A new use of the esophageal lead: Continuous telemetry monitoring. Am Heart J 111:1007–1009, 1986.
8. Schnittger I, Rodriguez I, Winkle RA: Esophageal electrocardiography: A new technology revives an old technique. Am J Cardiol 57:604–607, 1986.
9. Yabek SM, Bechara FA, Berman W, et al: Use of atrial epicardial electrodes to diagnose and treat postoperative arrhythmias in children. Am J Cardiol 46:285–289, 1980.
10. Waldo AL, MacLean WAH: Diagnosis and Treatment of Cardiac Arrhythmias Following Open Heart Surgery. Mount Kisco, NY, Futura, 1980.
11. Kuchar DL, Kelly RP, Thornburn OW: High-frequency analysis of the surface electrocardiograms of patients with supraventricular tachycardia: Accurate identification of atrial activation and determination of the mechanism of tachycardia. Circulation 74:1016–1026, 1986.
12. Benson DW, Dunnigan A, Sterba R, et al: Atrial pacing from the esophagus in the diagnosis and management of tachycardia and palpitations. J Pediatr 102:40–46, 1983.
13. Benson DW, Dunnigan A, Benditt DG, et al: Transesophageal study of infant supraventricular tachycardia: Electrophysiologic characteristics. Am J Cardiol 52:1002–1006, 1983.
14. Gallagher JJ, Smith WM, Kerr CR, et al: Esophageal pacing: A diagnostic and therapeutic tool. Circulation 65:336–341, 1982.
15. Sugrue DD, McLaran C, Hammill SC, et al: Refractory supraventricular tachycardia in the neonate: Treatment with temporary antitachycardia pacing. Mayo Clin Proc 60:169–172, 1985.
16. Campbell R, Dick M, Jenkins J, et al: Atrial overdrive pacing for conversion of atrial flutter in children. Pediatrics 75:730–736, 1985.
17. DeSilva RA, Grayboys TB, Podrid PJ, et al: Cardioversion and defibrillation. Am Heart J 100:881–895, 1980.
18. Nishimura M, Katoph T, Hanai S, et al: Optimal mode of transesophageal atrial pacing. Am J Cardiol 57:791–796, 1986.
19. Benson DW, Dunnigan A, Benditt DG, et al: Prediction of digoxin treatment failure in infants with supraventricular tachycardia: Role of transesophageal pacing. Pediatrics 75:288–293, 1985.
20. Gonzalez MD, Guillen RH, Pellizzon OA, et al: Study of Wolff-Parkinson-White syndrome by transesophageal pacing and assessment of long term amiodarone therapy. Am J Cardiol 55:852–856, 1985.
21. Dunnigan A, Overholt ED, Zales VR, et al: Transesophageal atrial pacing for evaluation of palpitations in children. Am Heart J 110:708, 1985.
22. Jenkins JM, Dick M, Collins S, et al: Use of the pill electrode for transesophageal atrial pacing. PACE 8:512–527, 1985.
23. Benson DW, Sanford M, Dunnigan A, et al: Transesophageal atrial pacing threshold: Role of interelectrode spacing, pulse width and catheter insertion depth. Am J Cardiol 53:63–76, 1984.
24. Osborn MJ, Holmes DR: Antitachycardia pacing. Clin Prog Electrophysiol Pacing 4:239–267, 1985.
25. German LD, Strauss HC: Electrical termination of tachyarrhythmias by discrete pulses. PACE 7:514–521, 1984.
26. Ward DE, Camm AJ, Spurrell RAJ: The response of regular re-entrant supraventricular tachycardia to right heart stimulation. PACE 2:586–595, 1979.
27. Greenberg ML, Kelly TA, Lerman BB, et al: Atrial pacing for conversion of atrial flutter. Am J Cardiol 58:95–99, 1986.
28. Holt P, Crick JCP, Sowton E: Antitachycardia pacing: A comparison of burst overdrive, self-searching and adaptive table scanning programs. PACE 9:490–497, 1986.
29. Watson RM, Josephson ME: Atrial flutter. 1. Electrophysiologic substrates and modes of initiation and termination. Am J Cardiol 45:732–741, 1980.
30. Tacker WA, Galioto FM, Giuliani E, et al: Energy dosage for human chest electrical ventricular defibrillation. N Engl J Med 290:214–215, 1974.
31. Gutgesell HP, Tacker WA, Geddes LA, et al: Energy dose for ventricular defibrillation of children. Pediatrics 58:898–901, 1976.
32. Lown B, Kleiger R, Williams BJ: Cardioversion and digitalis drugs: Changed threshold to electric shock in digitalized animals. Circ Res 17:519–531, 1965.
33. Leja FS, Euler DE, Scanlon PJ: Digoxin and susceptibility of the canine heart to countershock-induced arrhythmia. Am J Cardiol 55:1070–1075, 1985.
34. Mann DL, Maisel AS, Atwood E, et al: Absence of cardioversion-induced ventricular arrhythmias in patients with therapeutic digoxin levels. J Am Coll Cardiol 5:882–890, 1985.
35. Eysmann SB, Marchlinski FE, Buxton AE, et al: Electrocardiographic changes after cardioversion of ventricular arrhythmias. Circulation 73:73–81, 1986.
36. Pauletto P, Scannapieco G, Compostella L, et al: Myocardial damage after d.c. countershock: Myoglobin and ck-mb radioimmunoassay evaluation. Acta Cardiologica 39:115–120, 1984.
37. Karch SB, Billingham ME: Morphologic effects of defibrillation: A preliminary report. Crit Care Med 12:920–921, 1984.
38. Geddes LA, Niebauer MJ, Babbs CF: Fundamental criteria underlying the efficacy and safety of defibrillating current waveforms. Med Biol Eng Comput 23:122–130, 1985.

39. Kerber RE, Martins JB, Kelly KJ, et al: Self-adhesive preapplied electrode pads for defibrillation and cardioversion. J Am Coll Cardiol 3:815–820, 1984.
40. Ciccone JM, Saksena S, Shah Y, et al: A prospective randomized study of the clinical efficacy and safety of transvenous cardioversion for termination of ventricular tachycardia. Circulation 71:571–578, 1985.
41. Walsh CK, Krongrad E: Terminal cardiac electrical activity in pediatric patients. Am J Cardiol 51:557–561, 1983.
42. Zoll PM: Resuscitation of the heart in ventricular standstill by external electrical stimulation. N Engl J Med 248:768–771, 1952.
43. Falk RH, Zoll PM, Zoll RH: Safety and efficacy of noninvasive cardiac pacing: A preliminary report. N Engl J Med 309:1166–1168, 1983.
44. Sharkey SW, Chaffee V, Kapsner S: Prophylactic external pacing during cardioversion of atrial tachyarrhythmias. Am J Cardiol 55:1632–1634, 1985.
45. Berliner D, Okun M, Peters RW, et al: Transcutaneous temporary pacing in the operating room. JAMA 254:84–86, 1985.
46. Rosenthal ME, Stamato NJ, Marchlinski FE, et al: Noninvasive cardiac pacing for termination of sustained, uniform ventricular tachycardia. Am J Cardiol 58:561–562, 1986.
47. Beland MJ, Hesslein PS, Finlay CD, et al: Transcutaneous cardiac pacing in children. Circulation 74(suppl 2):176, 1986.

CHAPTER 17

CATHETER ABLATION OF DYSRHYTHMIAS

Paul C. Gillette

Five techniques are currently available for the treatment of tachyarrhythmias. Pharmacologic treatment is both the oldest and the most frequently used and has the advantages of being relatively inexpensive and easy to start. Some medical treatments have been in use for many years. Medical treatment of tachyarrhythmias has the disadvantages of being unpredictably ineffective, requiring the patient to remember to take the medicine, having largely unpredictable side effects, and being noncurative.

In recent decades, four new techniques for treating tachyarrhythmias have been developed. They are pacing, defibrillation, direct surgery, and catheter ablation. Pacing and defibrillation have the disadvantages of not being curative, of periodically reminding the patient that he or she is ill, and of being expensive. Surgery is curative and very effective. It is, however, expensive and requires a major procedure. Therefore, catheter ablation was investigated in order to provide a onetime curative procedure with less expense and less risk.

We define catheter ablation as any technique intended to ablate cardiac tissue using a catheter. Several energy forms have been used, including defibrillator discharges,[1–3] lasers,[4] and radio-frequency energy.[5] Virtually every part of the heart has been ablated for every type of arrhythmia. Both reentry circuits and automatic foci have been ablated.

The bundle of His was the first structure to be ablated by catheter.[2, 3] This procedure is not curative, since a pacemaker is required because of the complete AV block produced. Ablation of atrial muscle, accessory connection, and ventricular muscle do not require pacemakers and are possibly curative.

TECHNIQUE

The most widely used technique is that of discharging a defibrillator through an electrode catheter to a large receiving electrode on the skin.[5] The current density is great at the small intracardiac electrode and small at the large skin electrode. The discharge creates a lightning ball (fulguration) inside the heart.[6] Gas is released, and metal is vaporized on the electrode; a large pressure wave is formed. Ablation occurs as a result of thermal, electrical, and barotrauma. An endocardial or transmural scar is formed.

The patient undergoing catheter ablation is sedated as usual for cardiac catheterization.[7] He or she is monitored with electrocardiogram (ECG), arterial pressure, and pulse oximetry. Blood gases should be measured before and after ablation. Echocardiography should be immediately available. Standard emergency equipment should also be available as well as equipment for percutaneous and tube pericardiocentesis. Just before ablation the patient is further sedated with ketamine (1–2 mg/kg intravenously) and a very mild dose of diazepam (0.05–0.1 mg/kg).

The ablation catheter is positioned percutaneously from a femoral or brachial vein depending on the structure to be ablated. Standard woven Dacron electrode catheters are used. A ventricular pacing catheter should always be in place, with a pacemaker connected and capture verified. This is true even when AV block is not anticipated, as in atrial automatic focus ablation.

Mapping is of critical importance in ablation. The site to be ablated must be within 0.5 to 1 cm of the ablation electrode. The bundle of His is the easiest site to map; the largest unipolar His deflection is chosen. When His bundle ablation is done for atrial arrhythmias, the proximal His bundle should be sought by obtaining a large atrial deflection as well as a large His deflection. If a His bundle lesion (such as occurs in junctional automatic tachycardia) is to be ablated, then a more distal lesion may be preferable. Mapping of other arrhythmias (such as atrial automatic foci) involves finding the earliest point of endocardial activation. It is assumed that this is close to the true site of origin of the arrhythmia. It is impossible to be absolutely sure when the earliest site has been found. A reference catheter is left in a stable position, and an exploring catheter is moved until earlier and earlier sites are found. The earliest site will usually be considerably before the beginning of the surface P wave or QRS.

It is generally considered that ablation should not be carried out near a large coronary artery such as the circumflex or right coronary arteries. Spasm has occurred, and permanent damage might result. The coronary sinus is a dangerous place to perform ablation.[8] The circumflex artery is nearby, and the coronary sinus is a thin structure that can be ruptured by catheter ablation. The mouth of the coronary sinus may be safer. The right atrial free wall and right atrial appendage have been successfully and safely ablated with <100 watt-seconds. The atrial and ventricular septae and ventricular free walls seem to be the safest structures for ablation, but even ventricular ablation is not without problems. Deaths have occurred after ventricular catheter ablation not only as a result of cardiac perforation, but also as a result of a sudden decrease in myocardial performance.

Ablation is carried out using the catheter electrode as the cathode and the skin electrode as the anode. Three to five watt-seconds/kg are used for the His bundle or ventricle and 1–2 watt-seconds/kg for the right atrium or mouth of the coronary sinus. A dual unipolar electrode has been successful for the coronary sinus.[9] Care must be taken so that patients do not injure themselves when their muscles contract. A muscle relaxant is given, and laboratory personnel may hold the patient using rubber gloves. Some patients have had brief apnea immediately after ablation, so a bag and mask should be available.

The exact brand of defibrillator does not seem to be important, but the discharge should be synchronized to the R wave of the electrocardiogram. The external pacemaker should be set to non-demand mode, since the defibrillator discharge leaves a large after-potential on each catheter. The pacemaker should be turned off during the discharge. Internal pacemakers may be left in demand mode and a magnet applied if the pacemaker is temporarily inhibited after defibrillator discharges. The skin pad should be kept as far from an internal pacer as possible.

After the ablative discharge, the patient should be closely monitored. Auscultation of the chest should be done to detect pericardial friction rubs or distant heart sounds. Arterial blood pressure and pulse oximetry should also be closely observed. The patient should be observed in the catheterization laboratory for 1 hour for signs of decompensation or return of activity of the ablated structure. Additional shocks may be given if necessary. It is much more difficult to map for second shocks because of tissue damage from the first shock.

TYPES OF ARRHYTHMIAS AND RESULTS

We have performed catheter ablation for several different types of arrhythmias.[10, 11] Junctional automatic ectopic tachycardia, a frequently fatal arrhythmia, has been catheter ablated successfully four times.[10, 12] Each of the four patients had some junctional irritability, but it decreased after several days. Each patient has an atrial synchronous pacemaker. One patient takes atenolol to decrease her junctional escape rate to less than the sinus rate. One patient is in sinus rhythm with normal AV conduction, indicating that we destroyed the focus without completely destroying the bundle of His. In one 1-day-old infant we were unable to localize the bundle of His. Catheter His bundle ablation remains the technique of choice for junctional automatic tachycardia.

AV node reentry tachycardia is usually controllable with drugs or surgery. In the unusual case in which it is not controlled by drugs, catheter ablation of the bundle of His has been successful. This requires a permanent pacemaker. We have been unsuccessful in attempting to injure the AV node just enough to disrupt the reentry circuit without destroying AV conduction. We have recently successfully performed surgical modification of the AV node to cure AV node re-entry SVT. We prefer this approach, which does not require a pacemaker, over catheter ablation, despite the fact that it requires cardiopulmonary bypass.

Ablation of accessory connections has been difficult. We have been able to temporarily ablate posterior septal accessory connections in several patients but have only been able to permanently ablate them in one.[13] We have not attempted a left free wall pathway and have failed on one right free wall pathway. Two days after the failed attempt, the patient was found during surgical ablation to have blood in the pericardium and a 1-cm square ecchymosis at the site of ablation. Because of the excellent results of surgery for ablation of accessory connections, we prefer surgery over catheter ablation. However, a current use for catheter ablation is in patients who have had a failed surgery for an accessory connection. Several months after surgery, a dense scarring of the pericardium is present in such patients. Use of a large amount of energy and/or ablation is possible in sites not usually considered acceptable because of the danger of rupture. We have been successful in four of five patients in whom this was attempted, without any detectable sequelae.

Atrial automatic tachycardias are a small but important part of supraventricular tachycardia in children, representing about 5% of all supraventricular tachycardias. We have been successful in two of five atrial automatic foci attempted. Surgical success rates are greater than 90%. As a result, we currently favor surgery over catheter ablation for this mechanism.

We have little experience with ventricular tachycardia. Results in adult patients are variable, and this technique is probably not appropriate for pediatric patients.

No deaths or serious complications occurred in our series of catheter ablations. The success rate for areas other than the His bundle was disappointing. This, together with the excellent results of surgery and the complications reported by others, have led us to temporarily abandon the technique except for use in the His bundle. As other energy sources become available (e.g., cryothermia, radio-frequency), we believe the technique will be used again.

Cryoablation of the bundle of His has been reproducibly performed in swine.

References

1. Fontaine G, Cansell A, Lampe L, et al: Endocavitary fulguration (electrode catheter ablation): Equipment-related problems. In Fontaine G, Scheinman MM (eds): Ablation in Cardiac Arrhythmias. Mt. Kisco, NY, Futura Publishing, 1987, pp 85–100.
2. Scheinman MM, Morady F, Hess D, et al: Catheter-induced ablation of the technique for His bundle ablation in dogs. Am J Physiol 241:H283, 1981.
3. Gallagher JJ, Svenson RH, Kasell JH, et al: Catheter technique for closed-chest ablation of the atrioventricular conduction system. A therapeutic alternative for the treatment of refractory supraventricular tachycardia. N Engl J Med 306:194, 1982.
4. Narula OS: Laser catheter technique for induction of AV nodal delays: Possible applications for management of supraventricular tachyarrhythmias. In Fontaine G, Scheinman MM (eds): Ablation in Cardiac Arrhythmias. Mt. Kisco, NY, Futura Publishing, 1987, pp 405–417.
5. Fontaine G, Lechat Ph, Cansel GG, et al: Advances in the treatment of cardiac arrhythmias in the last decade: Definition and role of ablative techniques. In Fontaine G, Scheinman MM (eds): Ablation in Cardiac Arrhythmias. Mt. Kisco, NY, Futura Publishing, 1987, pp 5–20.
6. Fontaine G, Volmer W, Nienaltowska E: Approach to the physics of fulguration. In Fontaine G, Scheinman MM (eds): Ablation in Cardiac Arrhythmias. Mt. Kisco, NY, Futura Publishing, 1987, pp 101–116.
7. Gillette PC, Zinner A: The use of fulguration in the treatment of tachydysrhythmias in children. In Fontaine G, Scheinman MM (eds): Ablation in Cardiac Arrhythmias. Mt. Kisco, NY, Futura Publishing, 1987, pp 269–276.
8. Fisher JD, Brodman R: Fulguration of left-sided accessory pathways through the coronary sinus. In Fontaine G, Scheinman MM (eds): Ablation in Cardiac Arrhythmias. Mt. Kisco, NY, Futura Publishing, 1987, pp 223–241.
9. Morady F, Scheinman MM, Winston SA, et al: Transcatheter ablation of posteroseptal accessory ablation. In Fontaine G, Scheinman MM (eds): Ablation in Cardiac Arrhythmias. Mt. Kisco, NY, Futura Publishing, 1987, pp 191–196.
10. Gillette PC, Garson A, Porter CJ, et al: Junctional automatic ectopic tachycardia: A new proposed treatment by transcatheter His bundle ablation. Am Heart J 106:619, 1983.
11. Silka MJ, Gillette PC, Garson A, et al: Transvenous catheter ablation of a right atrial automatic ectopic tachycardia. J Am Coll Cardiol 5:999, 1985.
12. Garson A Jr, Gillette PC: Junctional ectopic tachycardia in children: Electrocardiography, electrophysiology and pharmacologic response. Am J Cardiol 44:298–302, 1979.
13. Critelli G, Gallagher JJ, Monda V, et al: Transvenous catheter ablation of the atrioventricular conduction in permanent junctional reciprocating tachycardia. In Fontaine G, Scheinman MM (eds): Ablation in Cardiac Arrhythmias. Mt. Kisco, NY, Futura Publishing, 1987, pp 207–221.

CHAPTER 18

PACEMAKERS FOR CHILDREN

Richard T. Smith, Jr.

The field of cardiac pacing has undergone an amazing evolution since the first devices were implanted in 1959. At that time, the idea of implanting a pacemaker in a child seemed an almost impossible undertaking even without considering the problems inherent in maintaining the pacing system on a long-term basis. The early pulse generators were large and the battery longevity minimal by current standards. Problems requiring surgical revision or replacement of the pulse generator or pacing leads were frequent. However, improvements in techniques and devices followed quickly, and children became candidates for pacing for problems that left untreated would result in certain death. By the late 1960s and early 1970s, rapidly accelerating technical capabilities sparked by the need for more and better devices for adults had led to more frequent implantation of pacemakers in children. The beginning of the 1980s brought further improvements, allowing implantation of devices in infants and children not only as a lifesaving measure but to control symptoms as well. At present, pediatric pacing has become a recognized subspecialty with an interest in achieving further improvements in pacemaker therapy for children.

With the improving reliability of pacing systems and increasing physician experience, the indications and ideal methods for pacing in children are continuously changing. Considerable attention is now directed toward better defining current indications for pacing in the variety of clinical situations encountered in children. Many new and different pacemakers are available, including those capable of closely mimicking normal cardiac rhythm (physiologic pacemakers); many of them are small enough for implantation in children of any size.

Only 1% to 2% of pacemaker recipients are children. Most commonly, bradycardia requiring pacing is the result of surgical treatment of congenital heart disease. A significant minority of pediatric pacemaker recipients have congenital complete AV block. The majority of adult patients require pacing as a result of degenerative or ischemic cardiovascular disease. Pacing in children and adults differs in many other obvious ways, including patient size, anticipated duration of pacing, potential somatic growth, activity level, and sometimes the importance of the cosmetic result. Therefore, pacing in children requires a somewhat different approach and specific expertise to deal with the problems encountered. With modern pacemaker therapy now available for children, the time has come for greater involvement by pediatric cardiologists and thoracic surgeons with special interest in children. For physicians less frequently involved in the care of children, the unique facets of pediatric pacing must be emphasized.

This chapter reviews the indications for pacemaker implantation, current technology, the selection of a pacing system, and appropriate follow-up for infants and children. Pacing results, complications, and problems specific to the pediatric age group are also reviewed. Special attention is given to the important differences between adults and children. For a more complete review of the terminology and technical aspects of pacing, several up-to date sources are available.[1–5]

INDICATIONS

The indications for pacemaker implantation in children are in continuing evolution related to rapid advances in technology, increased knowledge, and experience. By necessity, even the most experienced clinical investigators formulate recommendations based on little published data and limited patient experience. Not surprisingly, indications for pacing, especially for children, are often controversial. As pacing-related morbidity has declined and pulse generator and pacing lead longevity has increased, a shift toward more aggressive use of pacemakers has occurred. In certain cases, pacemakers are implanted primarily to improve cardiac output and exercise capability rather than to prevent sudden death, although this is often a secondary reason.

This section will discuss current guidelines for pacemaker implantation in children and review the origins of these recommendations.

ACC/AHA Pacing Guidelines

Recently, the subcommittee on pacemaker implantation for the joint American College of Cardiology/American Heart Association task force on assessment of cardiovascular procedures attempted to identify consensus among experts on indications for pacemaker implantation.[6] The goal was to identify acceptable and prudent guidelines for use by physicians and the regulating and reviewing organizations overseeing pacing practices. The need for these guidelines has been underlined by the increasing number of physicians involved with pacemakers and by public suspicion that pacemakers were being implanted in some cases without justification. The report outlines basic principles and specific indications for pacemaker implantation in adults and children.

The specific recommendations for children are similar to those for adults. However, there are clinical situations occurring in the pediatric population but not often encountered in adult pacing that warrant review. A list of indications similar to those appearing in the ACC/AHA report is presented in Figure 18–1. They are divided into indications usually agreed on by most implanting physicians, indications considered controversial, and rhythm disturbances not considered either an indication or a precursor to the need for a pacemaker.[7–13]

Congenital Complete Atrioventricular Block and Conduction Defects

Congenital complete atrioventricular block (AVB) is the most common cause of chronic bradycardia in unoperated young patients, often occurring without structural congenital heart disease. The diagnosis of congenital AVB is often made during the newborn period, but may go undetected until later in life. At the time when pacemakers were first implanted in children, the decision to implant a pacemaker was straightforward: if an event clearly predictive of the possibility of sudden death (e.g., syncope or near syncope) occurred, a pacemaker was implanted. This approach is supported by an abundance of indirect and anecdotal evidence as well as a smaller body of published data.[8, 11, 12] As pacing has become more reliable and less troublesome, many physicians have expanded the indications to include patients who may derive potential hemodynamic benefit from pacing, but who may not be at high risk for sudden death (see Fig. 18–1, class 1b). An example would be the adolescent with congenital AVB and limited exercise tolerance without other manifest symptoms. The patient might well benefit from the improved exercise tolerance and cardiac output provided by a "physiologic" type pacemaker.

Age-related heart rate criteria for pacemaker implantation have been advocated by some experts for children without symptoms.[9, 14, 15] The most frequently cited age-related heart rates are listed in Table 18–1. Infants with rates less than 55 bpm and children with rates less than 45 bpm should receive a pacemaker regardless of symptoms. Rates below those listed are thought to predict the development of congestive heart failure and are assumed to be associated with an increased risk of sudden death. Because of the small size of the population at risk and the only recent availability of pacemakers, few studies since early natural history studies have been performed to support these judgments.

Infants and children with significant structural congenital heart disease and AVB are considered differently than those with structurally normal hearts. They are less able to increase cardiac output with exercise and may have limited cardiac reserve. Therefore,

CLASS 1: PACEMAKER INDICATIONS (NONCONTROVERSIAL)

A. Second or third degree AV block with symptomatic bradycardia.
B. Advanced second or third degree AV block with moderate to marked exercise intolerance (i.e., inability to keep up with peers).
C. Second or third degree AV block, or sinus node dysfunction and congestive heart failure not responsive to medical management.
D. External ophthalmoplegia with bifascicular block (Kernes-Sayer syndrome).[7]
E. Sinus node dysfunction with symptomatic bradycardia.
F. Bradycardia-tachycardia syndrome in a child with the need for antiarrhythmic drugs other than digitalis.
G. An asymptomatic neonate with congenital atrioventricular block and a ventricular rate less than 55.[12]
H. Asymptomatic children with second or third degree AV block and a ventricular rate less than 45.[11]
I. Congenital AV block with wide QRS escape rhythm.[8]
J. Asymptomatic patients after cardiac surgery with advanced second or third degree AV block.[18, 19]
K. Asymptomatic infra-His second or third degree AV block.[9]
L. Complex ventricular arrhythmias associated with second or third degree AV block.[13]

CLASS 2: PACEMAKER INDICATIONS (CONTROVERSIAL)

A. Second or third degree AV block within the bundle of His in an asymptomatic patient.[9]
B. Prolonged pacemaker recovery time.[10]
C. Transient surgical second or third degree AV block that reverts to bifascicular block.

CLASS 3: CONDUCTION DISTURBANCES NOT REQUIRING PACING

A. Postoperative bifascicular block in the asymptomatic patient.
B. Postoperative bifascicular block with first degree AV block in the asymptomatic patient.
C. Transient surgical AV block that returns to normal conduction during the early postoperative period (1–2 weeks).

FIGURE 18–1

Pacing indications based on those published by the ACC/AHA task force. The indications have been modified somewhat to account for further evolution. Classes 1F through 1L may still be considered controversial by certain physicians. The published justifications for these recommendations appear in the references indicated.

a slightly different set of standards applies. For example, a pacemaker might be recommended for an infant with a structural heart defect and a heart rate of 65 bpm or less when an infant with the same heart rate but without an associated structural heart defect would not be considered for a pacemaker. In this case, it is presumed that AV synchrony and a more rapid paced heart rate would be advantageous to the infant with a structural defect; if possible, a physiologic pacemaker should be implanted. Heart rate criteria should only be used as a guideline and should not be used to the exclusion of good medical judgment.

TABLE 18–1

ASYMPTOMATIC BRADYCARDIA IN COMPLETE ATRIOVENTRICULAR BLOCK: PACEMAKER IMPLANTATION GUIDELINES (>6-s ECG recording while awake)*

	NORMAL HEART RATE (bpm)	STRUCTURAL HEART DEFECT HEART RATE (bpm)
Infants	<55	<65
Children	<45–50	<55–60
Adolescents	<40	<50

*The heart rates listed are felt by some experts to warrant concern and lead to consideration for pacemaker treatment even in the asymptomatic patient. Although the exact rates are arbitrary, they are felt to be the dividing point between higher and lower risk.

Other factors considered important include the presence of congestive heart failure,[9, 11, 14, 15] ventricular ectopy,[13] rapid atrial rate,[14] the anatomic location of the block,[16, 17] intrinsic pacemaker recovery time,[10] and the presence of a prolonged QT interval.

Other forms of congenital AV conduction system disease such as type II second degree AVB and intermittent complete AVB are considered identical to complete AVB. Bifascicular and trifascicular block are not necessarily indications for pacemaker implantation, but if present in a patient complaining of paroxysmal symptoms, intermittent AVB should be suspected and pacemaker implantation considered.

In summary, a pacemaker should be implanted in anyone with symptomatic complete AVB with or without structural heart disease. A pacemaker should be strongly considered in asymptomatic newborns with heart rates less than 55 bpm and for infants with heart rates of less than 65 bpm accompanied by significant structural heart disease. For older asymptomatic children, a pacemaker should be strongly considered for waking heart rates of less than 45 bpm (less than 55 bpm in the presence of structural heart disease). The decision to recommend pacemaker implantation is usually multifactorial, especially in older children and adults, and should be influenced by the technical capabilities of the care facility involved and the experience of the implanting cardiologist or surgeon.

Surgically Acquired Complete Atrioventricular Block and Conduction Defects

Surgically acquired AVB is an infrequent but important complication of intracardiac surgery for congenital heart disease. It is the most common cause of acquired complete AVB during childhood. The risk of sudden death with acquired complete AVB is greater than with congenital AVB. Several retrospective studies have suggested that the risk of death from surgically acquired AVB may be as high as 35% in unpaced patients and even higher when significant residual defects are present.[8, 16, 18, 19] Similar high risk is not present when immediate postoperative AVB resolves during the early postoperative period.[7, 12] Most patients with surgical AVB that is not permanent will have return of normal or near normal conduction within 2 weeks of the procedure. Although later return of normal conduction sometimes occurs (as long as 1 month or more after surgery), it is unusual. Waiting more than 2 weeks after surgery to implant a permanent pacemaker prolongs hospitalization and increases the difficulties and hazards associated with temporary pacing systems. In anticipation of possible transient postoperative block, both atrial and ventricular epicardial temporary pacing wires should be placed at the time of most, if not all, intracardiac operations. These wires are usually adequate to protect the patient until either conduction returns or a permanent pacemaker is implanted.

In the past, localization of the site of block by intracardiac electrophysiologic evaluation has been recommended.[17] If block was located within or above the His bundle, a pacemaker was not implanted in an asymptomatic patient. If block was below the bundle, a pacemaker was thought to be indicated. The prognostic importance of the site of block has not been demonstrated, and current consensus is that a pacemaker should be inserted regardless of the site of AV block. This approach eliminates the need for invasive electrophysiologic testing in patients with postsurgical AVB.

AVB can also be acquired from other causes, most of them very rare. These include bacterial endocarditis, meningitis, Lenegre's disease, mesothelioma of the AV node, progressive external ophthalmoplegia, myocarditis, bacterial sepsis, myotonic dystrophy, severe combined immune deficiency, and long QT syndrome. The diagnosis of acquired AVB may be serendipitous or the result of dramatic symptoms such as syncope. When children are symptomatic or have severe bradycardia, immediate temporary pacing is required.[10] With acquired (nonsurgical) AVB, asymptomatic presentation is uncommon. As with surgically acquired AVB, permanent pacing should be delayed for 10 days to 2 weeks pending possible return of AV nodal or His bundle function. The delay offers the opportunity to establish and possibly treat the cause. A permanent pacemaker should be implanted if conduction does not return. The management of acquired type II second degree AVB is the same as complete AVB.

Sinus Node Dysfunction

The establishment of the need for a pacemaker may be difficult in patients with sinus bradycardia with or without associated tachycardia. Clinically, significant sinus node dysfunction commonly follows surgical repair or palliation of a structural congenital heart defect, especially when the atria have been involved in the surgical repair. Important sinus node dysfunction in a child with a structurally normal heart is uncommon. Manifestations of sinus node dysfunction (usually bradycardia) may appear only intermittently and therefore are difficult to document. Additionally, episodic tachycardia may be associated with bradycardia and incorrectly assumed to be responsible for the patient's symptoms. Specifically, episodes of either supraventricular tachycardia (SVT) or ventricular tachycardia (VT) may result in long periods of asystole following spontaneous tachycardia interruption, causing syncope. An example of this phenomenon appears in Figure 18–2. This patient no longer has symptoms after implantation of a pacemaker. Also, SVT or VT may be the direct

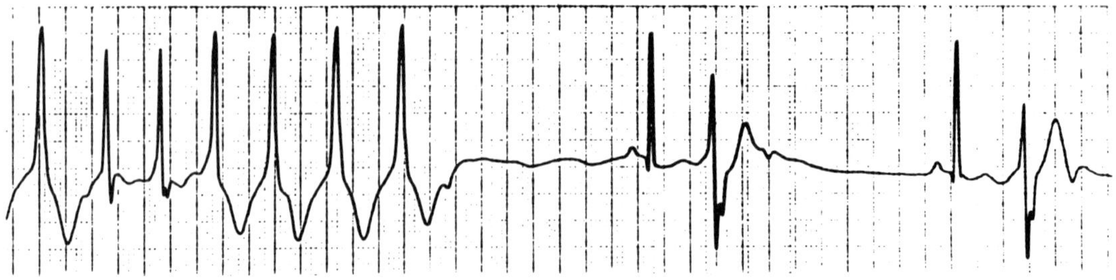

FIGURE 18–2
Electrocardiogram from a 12-year-old girl with complex ventricular ectopy and frequent syncopal and near-syncopal episodes. The rhythm strip was recorded during ambulatory monitoring at the time of a near-syncopal episode. These episodes were eliminated following pacemaker implantation.

cause of syncope, and bradycardia may be an "innocent bystander." Treatment of either tachyarrhythmia with medications that inhibit sinus node function may result in previously asymptomatic bradycardia becoming symptomatic. There are other causes of syncope clearly not prevented by implantation of a pacemaker. Therefore, proof of association between bradycardia and symptoms is essential. Documentation of symptomatic bradycardia often requires persistence because of its often intermittent nature. Transtelephonic and ambulatory ECG monitoring or event detection systems may be required for long periods and may still require "luck" to record bradycardia during symptoms. Invasive electrophysiologic studies lack sensitivity in documenting sinus node abnormalities and are only performed in selected cases after other less invasive efforts have failed.

Documenting the association between sinus node dysfunction and symptoms, although frequently difficult, is imperative for the reasons previously stated. There are no generally accepted low-rate criteria for pacemaker implantation in patients without symptoms. However, heart rates below certain levels or periods of asystole longer than a few seconds will cause most prudent physicians to recommend pacemaker implantation even in the absence of symptoms. For neonates and infants, heart rates similar to those used in complete AVB are reasonable. (See Table 18–1). The occurrence of sinus bradycardia in infants is very rare, and a meticulous search for transient or treatable causes is mandatory. For older children and adolescents, a waking heart rate of less than 40 bpm should be considered carefully. Not uncommonly, however, a well conditioned teenager may have a normal awake resting heart rate in the 40s and at times a sleeping heart rate less than 30 bpm. This child does not need a pacemaker. There is general acceptance that sinus pauses longer than 3.5 to 4.0 s are abnormal and warrant concern regardless of when they occur. Heart rates and long pauses in the range cited above should not be used as absolute criteria for pacemaker implantation in asymptomatic patients with sinus node dysfunction. Fortunately for the physician making the decision to implant a pacemaker, infants and children with potentially dangerous bradycardia without symptoms are rare. Sudden death caused by bradycardia without mitigating factors such as hemodynamically significant structural heart disease is very uncommon.

Following cardiac surgical procedures involving the atrium (such as the Mustard or Senning repairs for transposition of the great arteries, atrial septal defect closure, correction of total anomalous pulmonary return, the Blalock-Hanlon procedure, the Fontan procedure, and others), sinus node dysfunction is relatively common and is often associated with tachyarrhythmias. These patients may be completely asymptomatic until the tachyarrhythmias are treated with one of the commonly used antiarrhythmic medications (usually an agent other than digitalis). Antiarrhythmic drugs such as quinidine, procainamide, disopyramide, flecainide, encainide, propanolol, and amiodarone may markedly suppress sinus node function. When given to patients with preexistent sinus node dysfunction, the risk of syncope (and therefore sudden death) increases. Sinus node dysfunction is presumed following one of these procedures, and many experts feel a pacemaker is indicated prior to administration of one of these drugs, even in the asymptomatic patient. However, the decision to implant a pacemaker prophylactically in an asymptomatic patient is a difficult one. Although there are many anecdotal reports of sudden death in such patients, there are little or no published data for guidance. Prophylactic pacemaker implantation in the case of mild or clinically nonapparent sinus node dysfunction before treatment of tachycardia with a medication likely to suppress the sinus node is controversial.

Summary

The following axioms are crucial in the decision to implant a pacemaker in a young patient:

1. Pacemaker implantation is always indicated when a significant chance exists of sudden death as a result of bradycardia without a pacemaker. Syncope or near syncope associated with bradycardia are absolute indications of pacing to prevent sudden death.
2. The association between syncope (or less dramatic symptoms such as fatigue or palpitations) and bradycardia should be established before pacemaker implantation in patients with sinus node disease. Proof of association between symptoms and chronic bradycardia may be difficult, but if the relationship is established, the benefits of a permanent pacemaker are assured.
3. Rarely is the first syncopal spell fatal in patients with a structurally normal heart and a predisposition for syncope as a result of bradycardia. Patients with structural congenital heart disease in addition to bradycardia are at higher risk for sudden death than patients without congenital heart disease and may require pacing before dramatic symptoms become manifest.
4. Pacemaker implantation criteria are age dependent. The lower limit of normal for ventricular rate is higher for the newborn than for the adolescent.
5. Clinical judgment is important. Regardless of the specific implantation criteria, the decision to implant a pacemaker must be individualized.

NASPE/BPG CODE

With the development of pacing came a proliferation of confusing pacing terminology that left all but the most experienced physician unsure of the various functions of the pacemaker in question. Clearly, a system for standard description of pacemaker type and function was needed. In 1974, the Intersociety Commission for Heart Disease Resources created the first version of this descriptive system: the ICHD code. In 1981, the same committee extended the code to five letters to account for new technology. In 1987, the North American Society of Pacing and Electrophysiology (NASPE) and the British Pacing Group (BPG) further revised the code. Each position in the code describes an aspect of pacemaker function.

The first letter of the code identifies the chamber or chambers where pacing occurs. There are three choices: the atrium (A), the ventricle (V), or both the atrium and ventricle (D, for dual). When the ICHD code is used to describe an unimplanted single-chambered system that may be used for either atrial or ventricular pacing, the letter S (single) may be used instead of A or V.

The second position describes the pacemaker sensing characteristics. The character used may also be A for atrial, V for ventricular, D for dual, or O for the absence of sensing (usually only a temporary pacing mode). S may also be used as previously noted for the first position.

The third position describes the pacemaker response to sensed endogenous atrial or ventricular cardiac activity. The response may be inhibition (I) or triggering (T) of paced output. In dual-chambered pacing, a combination of these responses occurs. In this case, a D (for dual responses) is used (either inhibited or triggered output).

Using this code, a pacemaker capable of pacing the ventricle, sensing endogenous ventricular activity, and inhibiting paced output (if endogenous activity occurs, and pacing the ventricle if not) is designated VVI. Similarly, a single-chambered atrial pacemaker that can pace and sense the atrium and be inhibited by atrial activity is designated AAI. A dual-chambered pacemaker that is capable of pacing either chamber, sensing activity in either chamber, and either triggering or inhibiting paced output (with resulting atrioventricular synchrony) is a

DDD pacemaker. Other commonly encountered permanent pacing modes are VDD and DVI. Many different temporary pacing modes such as AOO, VOO, and DOO are used in the pacemaker clinic during diagnostic testing. All five position designations are summarized in Figure 18–3.

The last two code positions as amended by NASPE in 1987 refer to the special features such as programmability, telemetry, rate modulation, and antitachycardia pacing capability. Specifically, the fourth position describes device programmability and may be P, M, C, R, or O. Pacing rate and output programmability only are designated by P. If, in addition to rate and output, other parameters such as mode, sensitivity, AV interval, and refractory periods are programmable, then M (multiprogrammable) would occupy the fourth position. C (for communications) is used to refer to devices with telemetry functions in addition to programmability. Rate modulation by a signal other than the atrium is designated by R. Nonprogrammable pacemakers are described by the letter O in the fourth position.

The fifth position refers to the type of antitachycardia response, if any. The response may be pacing (P), shock (S), or both (D). Revisions of all letters of the code more specifically describing dual-chamber pacing modes, programmability, rate modulation, and tachycardia response have been proposed and are gaining acceptance.[20–22]

PACEMAKER OPERATIONS

Pacemakers operate by delivering a small amount of electrical energy to cardiac muscle, stimulating contraction. Modern pacemakers stimulate only in the absence of endogenous cardiac activity. When endogenous cardiac activity is detected (sensed) by the pacemaker, pacing is inhibited. Therefore pacing occurs only when needed. The capacity to stimulate the heart and sense endogenous cardiac activity are the cornerstones of modern pacemaker therapy.

During the past few years, pacemakers have been developed with a variety of capabilities appropriate for specific groups of pacing problems. With the new capabilities has come an increasing complexity of pacemaker operations. The reward is the capacity to select a pacemaker with capabilities specific to the particular rhythm abnormality. To understand these increasingly complex operations, an understanding of more basic function is required. This section reviews selected basic concepts related to pacing and pacemaker operations.

Electrical Principles

Stimulation of the heart muscle occurs when the negative pole (anode) and the positive pole (cathode) of the pacemaker battery are briefly connected, allowing current flow. If the energy delivered exceeds the minimum required for cardiac muscle stimulation, contraction occurs. The completed circuit is made up of the two poles of the battery, pacing lead wires, and electrodes as well as the intervening cardiac and body tissues. Pacing systems employ one of two possible electrode configurations: unipolar or bipolar

REVISED NASPE/BPG PACEMAKER CODE

POSITION	I	II	III	IV	V
Category	Chamber(s) paced	Chamber(s) sensed	Response to sensing	Programmability rate modulation	Antitachyarrhythmia function
	O = None A = Atrium V = Ventricle D = Dual (A+V)	O = None A = Atrium V = Ventricle D = Dual (A+V)	O = None T = Triggered I = Inhibited D = Dual (T+I)	O = None P = Simple Programmable M = Multiprogrammable C = Communicating R = Rate modulation	O = None P = Pacing (antitachyarrhythmia) S = Shock D = Dual (P+S)
Manufacturers' designation only	S = single (A or V)	S = single (A or V)			

Note: Positions I through III are used exclusively for antibradyarrhythmia function.

FIGURE 18–3

The North American Society of Pacing and Electrophysiology (NASPE) in conjunction with the British Pacing and Electrophysiology Group (BPG) revised the pacemaker function code originally proposed by the Intercommission on Heart Disease to provide a standardized method of description of pacemaker function. This revised version appears above. (Adapted from the NASPE/BPG Generic (NBG) Pacemaker Code.)

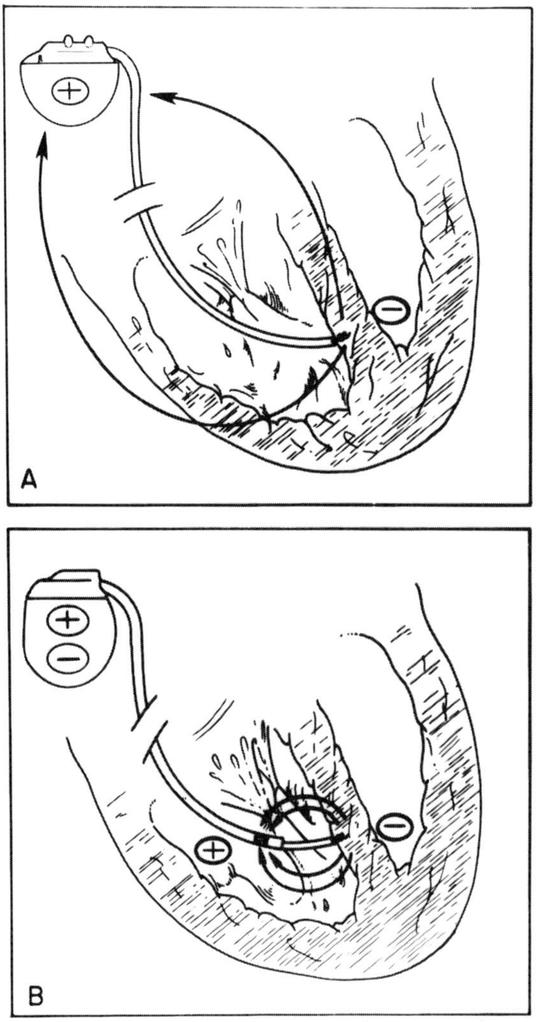

FIGURE 18–4
(A) Unipolar pacing system. With unipolar pacing, the electrical circuit is formed by the tip electrode fixed to the right ventricular endocardium, which is the uninsulated surface of the pulse generator housing. *(B)* Bipolar pacing system. A smaller, more discrete circuit is formed by the tip electrode fixed to the right ventricular endocardium and a ring electrode located proximal to the tip electrode.

(Fig. 18–4). With unipolar pacing, there is a single electrode at the cardiac end of the pacing lead and the pulse generator housing serves as a larger "indifferent" electrode. During a paced impulse, current flows through the large circuit formed by the components of the pacing system and the body tissue. With bipolar pacing, there is a small ring electrode located on the pacing lead just proximal to the tip electrode. Current flows between these two electrodes. The advantages and disadvantages of each configuration will be reviewed in a later section.

Although each electrical circuit formed by battery, body, and pacing lead is unique, the relationship between current flow, voltage, and resistance for all circuits is the same and is described by this simplified expression of Ohms law:

$$V \text{ (voltage)} = I \text{ (current)} \cdot R \text{ (resistance)}$$

Voltage is a measure of the force resulting in the flow of electricity. The current (which is the rate at which the charge moves, quantitated in milliamperes) varies directly with the voltage; the greater the voltage, the greater the current flow, assuming resistance is constant. Resistance is the opposition to flow of electrons inherent in a particular conductive material. The term "impedance" is used to describe combined resistance of specific circuits and is appropriately applied to pacing systems. The impedance of a given pacing lead system is usually stable and should not change significantly after implantation. The rate at which energy is consumed by a pacing system is dependent on the frequency of stimulation (paced rate), the duration of each stimulation (pulse width), the battery voltage, and the system impedance. Maintaining circuitry functions such as sensing requires relatively little energy but is important over the life of the pacemaker.

Pacing Thresholds

The pacing threshold is the minimum energy required to stimulate contraction of cardiac muscle. Many factors affect threshold, and marked fluctuations may occur. The pacing threshold is lowest immediately following implantation of the pacing electrode. Gradually, cardiac tissue reacts to the presence of the electrode first with an inflammatory response and subsequently with formation of fibrous tissue. This reaction is associated with an increasing pacing threshold, reaching its highest level between 1 and 3 months after initial lead implantation. Following the threshold peak, a gradual drop occurs to an intermediate chronic level. Once established, the threshold usually remains relatively stable indefinitely. Variations in autonomic tone, medications, electrolyte balance, lead position, and lead type, illness, and other causes affect thresholds. There may be as much as a 50% daily variability in measured threshold, and therefore a "safety margin" in the pacemaker output is required to account for these changes. The "safety margin" is the degree to which the pacemaker output exceeds the pacing threshold.

Most pacemakers allow noninvasive variation of either voltage or pulse width (and commonly both) for establishing a safety margin. However, changes in the voltage and pulse width are not equivalent with respect to the safety margin. The relationship between voltage, pulse width, and threshold is depicted by the strength-duration curve, demonstrated in Figure 18–5. An asymptomatic curve depicts the pacing threshold at different combinations of voltage and pulse width. The morphology of the measured strength-duration curve among patients is usually similar; however, the actual voltage and pulse width threshold may vary considerably for different lead systems. Establishing a safety margin will be discussed further in a later section.

Sensing

Sensing, or detection by the pacemaker of endogenous cardiac activity, is one of the most important advances in the development of modern pacemakers. The ability to sense cardiac activity is important for two reasons. First, accurate sensing of cardiac depolarization allows unnecessary pacing to be safely inhibited and therefore conserves battery energy. Second, a pacing spike occurring inappropriately during repolarization may induce dangerous arrhythmias. Sensing allows the inhibition of pacing during either atrial or ventricular repolarization, thereby preventing arrhythmia induction (Fig. 18–6). Additionally, dual-chambered pacemakers may utilize sensed atrial activity to trigger ventricular pacing. The result is atrioventricular synchrony; the heart rate is then dictated by the sinus node and changes with metabolic need.

The amplitude of the usual sensed cardiac event is approximately 1/250 to 1/1600 that of the amplitude of a single pacemaker output (3–20 mV, compared to 5 V). Importantly, noncardiac muscular or other electrical activity and cardiac muscular repolarization (the T wave) should not be confused with the electrical signal of depolarization (the QRS complex). If sensing of activity other than cardiac depolarization does occur, pacing is inappropriately inhibited, resulting in no cardiac contraction and, therefore, no cardiac output. When inappropriate inhibition occurs, it is called "oversensing." The converse is "undersensing" and occurs when the amplitude or other detectable characteristics of a normal depolarization are not sufficient to meet the pacemaker's minimum criteria for classification as a P wave or R wave. Fortu-

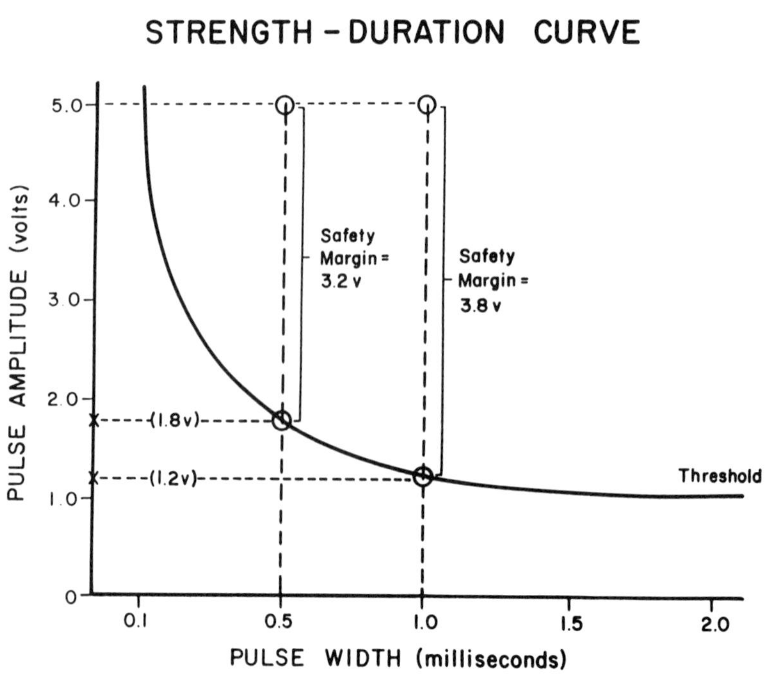

FIGURE 18–5
The strength-duration curve. This theoretical curve depicts the relationship of pulse amplitude and pulse width to pacing threshold. The safety margin (defined as the amount by which the programmed pacing amplitude exceeds the threshold at a specific pulse width) is also plotted. Note that there is minimal improvement in safety margin with an increase in pulse width from 0.5 to 1.0

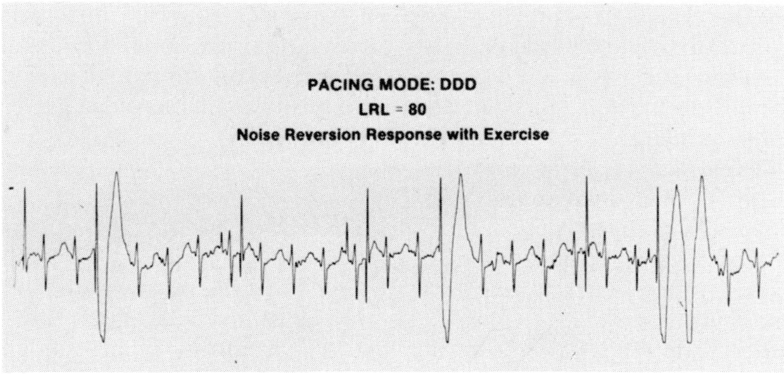

FIGURE 18–6
The rhythm strip was recorded during exercise. A normal protective feature of the pacemaker, "the noise reversion response" occurs. This response is characterized by intermittent asynchronous pacing when the pacemaker senses excessive electrical activity. The intention is to prevent loss of pacing when cardiac contraction cannot be verified by the device. In this example, a repetitive ventricular response is induced by the asynchronous pacemaker spike, illustrating the potential for arrhythmia induction resulting from loss of sensing and resultant pacing during the vulnerable period.

nately, most noncardiac electrical events and T waves have amplitude and frequency differences allowing differentiation from normal cardiac repolarization.

Pulse Generator Components

The pulse generator or pacemaker includes a number of components: housing, battery, electrical circuitry, and lead connector. Each component has been designed with specific purposes and requirements in mind and will be discussed independently. Pacing leads will be considered separately and are not part of the pulse generator.

PACEMAKER HOUSING

Several important physical requirements must be met by a pacemaker housing. The housing must be light, strong, resistant to corrosion, biologically inert, preferably nonmagnetic, and allow hermetic (airtight) sealing. Today's pacemaker housings are made most commonly of titanium and meet the given requirements.

BATTERY

The ideal pacemaker battery is small, has a long life expectancy, a low rate of self-discharge and does not produce gas as a by-product of its chemical reaction and therefore may be hermetically sealed within the titanium housing. Many different types of batteries with differing chemical composition have been used for pacemakers. The first batteries were zinc mercuric oxide. Because the inherent voltage of these batteries is only 1.35 V, it was necessary to connect five or six batteries in series to achieve sufficient voltage output to dependably result in cardiac pacing. Furthermore, because the chemical reaction occurring in the battery created gas, hermetic sealing was not possible, making protection of the device against degradation by the body difficult. The overall result was a large pulse generator, a short battery life expectancy, and a potential for sudden failure. Pulse generator size alone precluded implantation in small patients.

The zinc mercuric oxide batteries were followed by a variety of battery types, including rechargeable (cadmium nickel oxide) and nuclear (plutonium or promethium) batteries, and finally by a large family of batteries with lithium as the anodal substance. The rechargeable batteries were large and required recharging every 1 to 2 weeks. The inconvenience, in addition to large size, precluded extensive use. Nuclear power sources offered longevity, with the expected service life considerably longer than the average adult patient's life expectancy. However, the cost of the pulse generator and close control by the Nuclear Regulatory Commission (NRC) also inhibited extensive use.

Lithium anode batteries, now used almost

exclusively, come the closest to achieving the current goals for an optimal pacemaker battery. The most widely used type of lithium battery is lithium iodide. Lithium iodide batteries generate approximately 2.8 V and with more recently developed circuitry may be increased in multiples of approximately 2.8 V to voltage outputs as high as 10 V. There is a low rate of self-discharge, and because no gas is produced in the chemical reaction, they may be hermetically sealed.

Battery longevity is dependent on several factors. The most important are battery size, stimulation frequency, and the output per stimulation. Prospective estimates of battery life span vary from 3 years for a dual-chambered pacemaker used in a small child to 15 years for a large single-chambered device needed infrequently.

Other types of lithium batteries still in use include lithium silver chromate, lithium thionyl chloride, and lithium copper sulfide. There have been few recent advances in battery technology. Lithium iodide batteries have become smaller, but only at the expense of longevity. Currently the major developmental thrust is not toward development of new power sources, but rather toward improvement of longevity by improving the efficiency of energy delivery. The smallest currently available pulse generator weighs 22 g (Fig. 18–7).

CIRCUITRY

Perhaps the most significant advance in the pacing industry has been the use of microcircuitry. Spinoffs from the rapidly growing computer industry not only have allowed miniaturization, but have also markedly increased pulse generator versatility. The complimentary metal oxide semiconductor (CMOS) is the type of integrated miniaturized circuit used in most modern pacemakers and incorporates most of the electrical components necessary for complex pacing functions. Advantages of the CMOS-based circuitry include the lack of welded or soldered connectors prone to malfunction, minimal heat production, and minimal energy required to maintain the circuit function. The greatest advantage, however, is versatility. Some currently available devices are capable

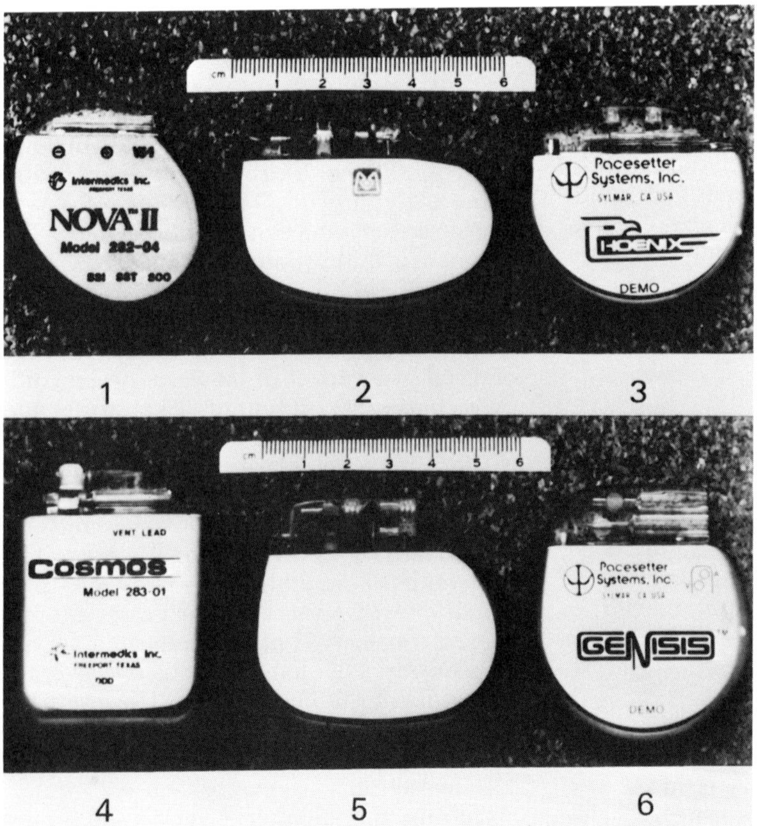

FIGURE 18–7
Top: The pacemakers pictured are examples of small single-chambered pacemakers currently available. Bottom: These three pacemakers are examples of currently available dual-chambered physiologic pacemakers.

of storing and managing 15 to 20 different functions. Pacemakers capable of performing sophisticated electrophysiologic testing controlled noninvasively are now undergoing clinical trials. Clearly, the ability to adjust multiple parameters in response to clinical changes has been expedient in reducing pacing problems requiring revision of the pacing system.

CONNECTORS

Another component of the pulse generator is the lead connector or connector block. This component deserves mention because differences between manufacturers in design of the lead connector pin and the pacemaker's connector block may result in incompatibility. At the time of pulse generator replacement, care should be taken to confirm compatibility between the new pulse generator and the existing pacemaker leads. This is particularly true of in-line bipolar leads.

Recent changes in connector block design have decreased both the functional and actual size of many pulse generators.

Programmability

Programmability is defined as "noninvasive, user-produced, stable but reversible change in pacemaker function."[23, 24] Some degree of programmability is present in all modern pacemakers. Programmability offers several important advantages. First, pacing characteristics may be tailored to each child. Variability of parameters such as pacing rate is especially important in young patients whose normal rates differ significantly according to age. Second, with the use of programmability, reoperation for many pacing problems may be delayed or prevented. For example, increasing energy output may compensate for elevated pacing thresholds, or reprogramming the pacing mode to VVI mode from DDD may eliminate potential problems of a malfunctioning atrial lead. Third, decreasing energy output in response to decreasing pacing threshold allows battery longevity to be maximized. Finally, programmability may be used to accomplish therapeutic goals. In the pediatric pacemaker clinic, the most commonly used programmable therapeutic function is temporary overdrive pacing for treatment of supraventricular tachycardia, most commonly atrial flutter. An example of this function appears in Figure 18–8.

There are dangers to programmability, especially in the hands of inadequately trained individuals. Pacemaker-dependent patients may be at significant risk if either pulse width or voltage output are inadvertently programmed to subthreshold or near threshold level. For this reason, familiarity with programming equipment is essential.

Telemetry

Telemetry refers to an ability to transmit information between the programmer and pacemaker. When both are possible, the pacemaker has bidirectional telemetry. This information may include the type, model, and serial number of the pacemaker, and the previously programmed parameters. "Real time" refers to the actual measurement by the pacemaker of various intervals, lead resistance, or battery functions. The recent introduction of the many diagnostic telemetry functions such as continuous event recording (numbers of paced, sensed, and premature events occurring since the counting circuits were last cleared), electrograms, and direct battery characteristic measurement have added useful tools to the task of patient and pacemaker evaluation.

Timing Cycles

The timing of ventricular output in the early nonsensing pacemakers was simple. Electrical stimuli were emitted by the pacemaker at a constant rate. The development of pacemakers with sensing capability increased the complexity of the timing of cardiac stimulation. Dual-chambered pacemakers with sensing in both atrium and ventricle have more complex timing cycles than any previous devices. Understanding the behavior of the pacemaker depends on knowledge of the timing cycles specific to the device in use and is necessary to differentiate normal and expected pacemaker behavior from malfunction. There are many, often subtle, differences in response to sensed events among the devices of different man-

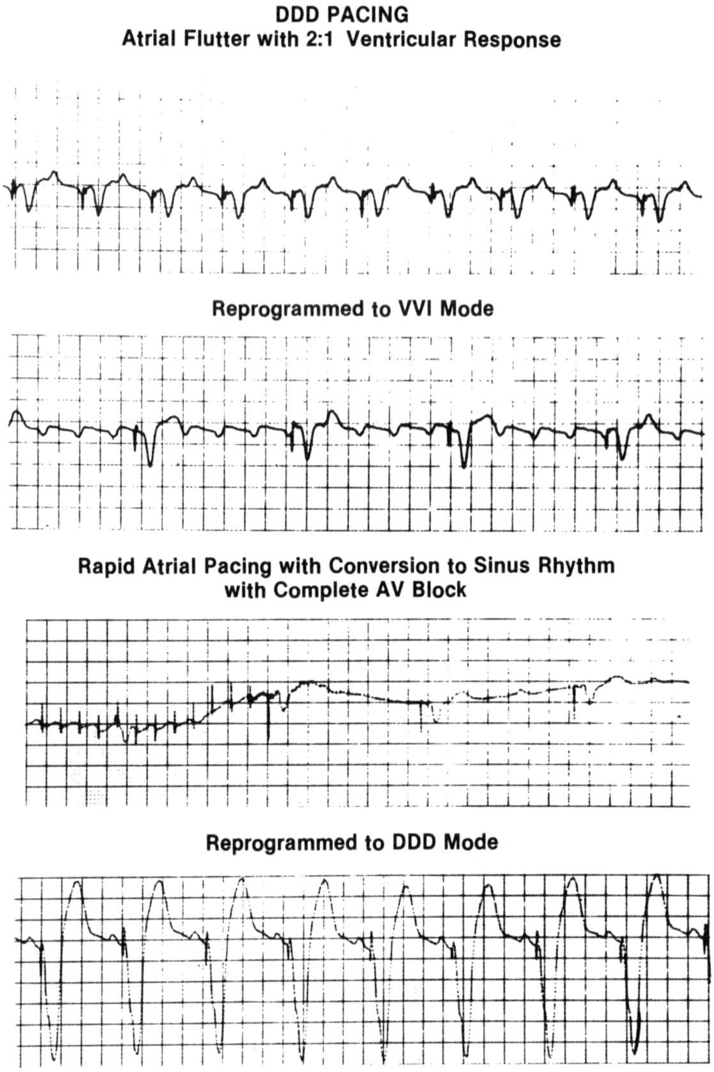

FIGURE 18–8
These electrocardiographic recordings illustrate a therapeutic use of an implanted DDD pacemaker. The patient has surgery-induced complete AV block. The top panel shows atrial flutter with 2:1 ventricular paced response. In the second panel, the device has been reprogrammed to VVI mode. Flutter waves are obvious. The third panel demonstrates temporary physician-activated rapid atrial pacing at 310 bpm. When temporary pacing is discontinued, the atrial flutter has been converted to sinus rhythm. In the last panel, the device has been reprogrammed to DDD mode with resultant atrial sensing and ventricular pacing.

ufacturers. Each manufacturer employs different methods to protect against pacing pitfalls such as cross talk, pacemaker-mediated tachycardia, oversensing, and PVCs.

Figure 18–9 presents schematically the timing cycles of a typical DDD pacemaker. There are two timing circuits, one atrial and one ventricular. The labeled intervals may be subdivided into three types: timing intervals, refractory periods, and blanking periods. The timing intervals include the lower rate limit, the AV interval, and the upper tracking limit (or upper rate limit). Knowledge of these intervals is especially important to orderly electrocardiographic evaluation of any atrial tracking pacemakers (VDD or DDD). The refractory periods are the intervals during which the pacemaker is inhibited from responding to endogenous activity. Sensed endogenous cardiac events occurring during the refractory periods, however, may trigger a response at the end of the refractory period. This characteristic distinguishes refractory periods from blanking periods. During the latter, the sensing circuit is completely off and the pacing circuits are "blinded" to endogenous activity.

Depending on the device, many of these intervals are externally programmable. Generally, the purpose of programmable pacing intervals, refractory periods, and blanking periods is to allow tailoring of the device characteristics to specific patients. Most pacemakers have detailed manuals that describe the specific timing circuit behavior. When choosing a pacemaker for implantation or

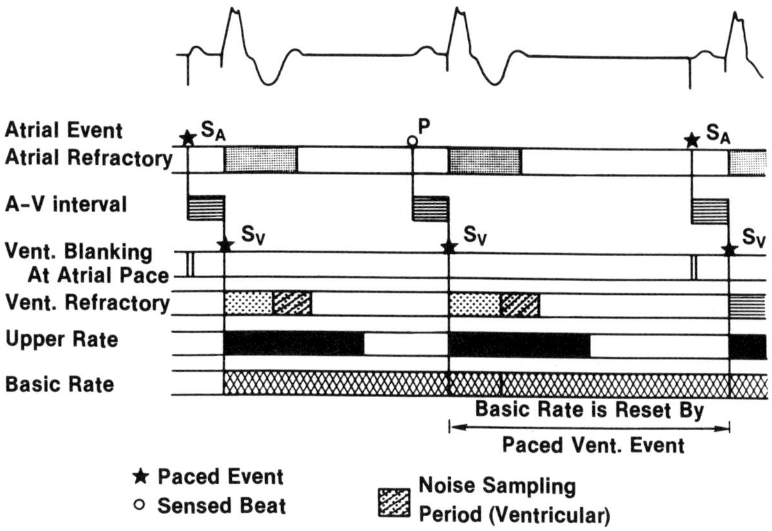

FIGURE 18–9
DDD timing diagram. Similar diagrams are used to describe pacemaker behavior under varying conditions. Initially, this diagram demonstrates the pacemaker's response when endogenous cardiac rhythm is absent [atrial (SA) followed by ventricular (SV) pacing]. An endogenous P wave then occurs and is sensed (P) by the pacemaker. The ventricle is paced following the programmed AV interval. Again, no endogenous cardiac rhythm occurs and atrial followed by ventricular pacing spikes are again delivered. A more detailed description may be found in the Medtronic "Symbios" technical manual. (Adapted from Medtronic, Inc., Minneapolis, MN).

evaluating an electrocardiogram of a pacemaker patient, familiarity with both the programmed settings and the specific circuitry characteristics is essential for accurate conclusions. Pseudopacemaker malfunction is far more common than actual circuitry malfunction. If a circuitry malfunction is suspected, careful review of the technical manual or discussion with the technical support personnel of the manufacturer is advisable.

PHYSIOLOGIC PACING

The designation "physiologic" pacing has been used for most nontemporary pacing modes other than VVI. The modes most commonly referred to as physiologic are AAI, VAT, DVI, VDD, DDD, and the new single-chamber pacing modes that increase pacing rate in response to some measure of increasing metabolic demand. The intention of the term "physiologic" is to describe pacing modes that mimic the sequence of electrical (and therefore hemodynamic) events that occur in the normal heart, therefore maximizing hemodynamic efficiency. True physiologic pacing, however, is not possible with currently available pacing systems. The following requirements are necessary for true physiologic pacing:

1. The paced cardiac rate should be dictated by the normal sinus node or by an accurate predictor of the changing metabolic requirement.

2. The ventricular paced event should follow atrial contraction at an interval that optimizes cardiac output. Presumably, this interval should change in response to changing autonomic tone.

3. The ventricular activation sequence should be similar to that in the normal heart.

4. A true "physiologic" pacemaker should allow ventricular rate to vary in the same range as a normal individual, which in the case of a child may be as high as 220 bpm.

One of the first pacing modes referred to as "physiologic" was "AV synchronous," or DVI. With DVI pacing, an atrial stimulus is inserted before each ventricular pacing stimulus at the lower pacing limits, resulting in synchronous atrioventricular contraction. This pacing mode falls short of achieving a hemodynamically normal rhythm in several ways. The most important is failure to increase ventricular rate with increasing metabolic demand. However, the main impetus for development of DVI pacemakers was elimination of "pacemaker syndrome" in adult patients. Pacemaker syndrome is broadly defined as the development of symptoms such as fatigue or palpitation at times of AV dissociation or 1:1 VA conduction. Pacing in the DVI mode is usually effective at preventing the pacemaker syndrome. Figure 18–10 compares the blood pressure response occurring when DVI pacing is changed to VVI. This response underlines the important contribution of AV synchrony.

The development of dependable methods of atrial sensing led to the atrial synchronous (VDD) pacing mode. Atrial-sensed, ventric-

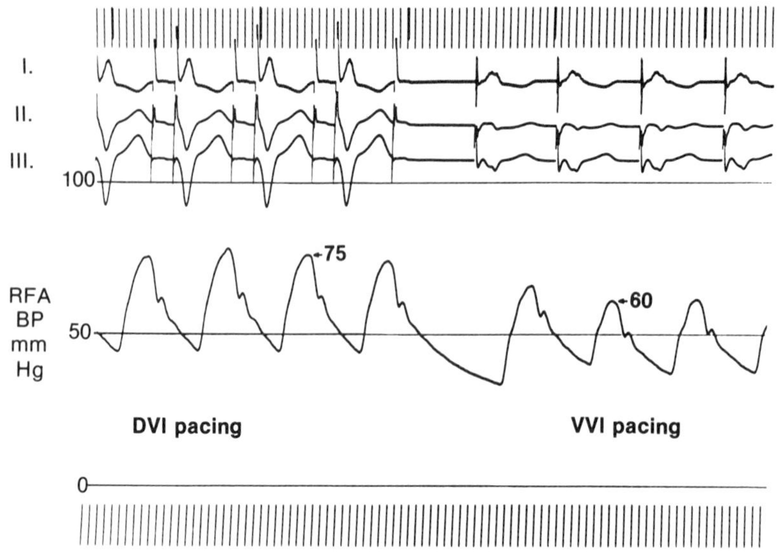

FIGURE 18–10
Tracings recorded during a pacemaker revision. Electrocardiographic leads I, II, and III appear at top. Continuous blood pressure recording from an indwelling arterial line appears at bottom. Initially, AV sequential pacing results in a peak systolic pressure of 75 mmHg. A change to ventricular pacing results in a sustained decrease in systolic pressure. RFA, right femoral artery; BP, blood pressure; mmHg, millimeters of mercury.

ular-paced rhythm still falls short of true physiologic pacing because of loss of AV synchrony at the lower rate limit, the lack of variability of the AV interval, and the lack of a normal ventricular activation sequence. However, the VDD mode was a large step toward more physiologic pacing and does provide both rate responsiveness (the sinus node dictates the ventricular paced rate) and AV synchrony (except at the lower rate limit). The DDD mode provides only the additional advantage of ensuring AV synchrony at the lower rate limit.

Recently, new sensor-driven pacing systems have been referred to as physiologic. These devices sense changing metabolic demand by methods other than sensing sinus node activity. The only method of sensing metabolic demand currently approved by the FDA for use in patients utilizes a piezoelectric crystal that senses body movement. The crystal is located within the pulse generator. As body movement increases, the crystal is deformed, creating an electrical signal proportional to the level of exercise. The paced rate then increases gradually to the upper rate limit, assuming exercise continues. Other methods of sensing metabolic demand either currently in use or under development include sensing of changes in the QT interval, blood temperature, oxygen saturation, stroke volume, and respiratory rate. These methods are especially advantageous for patients with sinus node dysfunction or chronic atrial arrhythmias because dependable exercise heart rate responsiveness is often not possible or is unsafe with other methods. If an atrial sensing ventricular pacing system were used in patients with atrial arrhythmias, rapid, inappropriate, potentially dangerous ventricular pacing might result. Another advantage of sensor-driven pacemakers is the requirement of only one lead for pacing.

All current possible pacing modes fall short of being truly physiologic, except possibly sensor-driven atrial pacing in patients with normal atrioventricular conduction. Extensive worldwide investigations are being directed at analyzing the importance of each component of heart rhythm at rest and with exercise. Specifically, the contributions of atrioventricular synchrony, both at rest and with exercise, and the importance of rate responsiveness alone are being examined extensively. The role of the AV interval and the effect of the ventricular activation sequence on cardiac output are also being considered. There have been no studies directed at comparing cardiac output during different modes of pacing at higher paced rates. Such studies will be necessary to objectively evaluate the overall importance of physiologic pacing in children.

Atrioventricular Synchrony

Atrioventricular (AV) synchrony may be provided by the AAI, VDD, DVI, and DDD modes of pacing. The contribution of AV synchrony to cardiac output at rest has been clearly demonstrated.[25–27] Estimates of the contribution range from a 15% to a 30%

increase in cardiac output when compared with AV dissociation. The relative importance of AV synchrony probably decreases somewhat as the heart rate increases.[27–29] Another advantage of AV association is the prevention of pacemaker syndrome. Pacemaker syndrome is uncommon in children, but when symptoms are related to AV dissociation, reestablishment of AV association results in elimination of symptoms. Although pediatric patients with nonsurgical AV block can compensate for the loss of AV synchrony when at rest, significant benefits of AV synchrony are experienced with exercise (unpublished data).

Rate Responsiveness

Increasing the cardiac rate in response to exercise has been clearly shown to be of great importance in increasing cardiac output.[27–32] In normal children, cardiac output increases from the resting level as much as three- to fivefold with exercise. Although other mechanisms play important roles in exercise adaptation, heart rate is the most important. We have found increases in cardiac output in response to exercise following implantation of a rate-responsive pacemaker in children (unpublished data). These differences are manifested both by detectable increases in measured cardiac output and by increases in exercise duration when compared to VVI pacing. In adults, there is no clearly demonstrable difference between AV synchronous, rate-responsive pacing and rate-responsive pacing alone.[27] Similar studies have not been done in children.

Other Factors

Other factors important to the cardiac response to varying metabolic needs include variations in the AV interval and ventricular activation sequence. Little clinical information analyzing the hemodynamic importance of varying AV intervals is yet available. Certainly, the benefits of mimicking the changing AV interval and normal ventricular activation are not as important as achieving synchrony and rate responsiveness.

CHOOSING A PACING SYSTEM FOR CHILDREN

Devices, leads, and implantation techniques appropriate for adults may be inappropriate for children. Important factors such as patient size and expected somatic growth have significant impact on the choice of pacemaker and pacing leads. The decisions required in selecting an appropriate pacing system may be subdivided into (1) endocardial or epicardial implantation technique; (2) unipolar or bipolar electrical configuration; (3) the type of device and pacing mode; and (4) the type of pacing leads. These choices are considered below.

Endocardial vs Epicardial Implantation

The method of implantation is influenced by several factors. Children weighing less than 10 kg and children with right to left shunts may be considered for the epicardial approach. In rare instances, the epicardial approach is chosen because of the desire to avoid the small infraclavicular scar and bulge created by implantation of the pulse generator in the endocardial technique. However, development of the subpectoral implantation technique for children has improved the potential cosmetic result, and the implant approach is less often affected by cosmetic concerns. Figure 18–11 presents the chest radiographs of a newborn infant immediately following epicardial DDD pacemaker implantation and 1 year later.

Children not excluded for the reasons listed previously are candidates for endocardial pacing. Endocardial pacing has several technical advantages. First, both atrial and ventricular capture thresholds are generally lower, both at implant and chronically. More importantly, the incidence of pacing problems is significantly lower and the pacing system longevity greater with the endocardial technique.[33] Problems not requiring surgical intervention, most commonly atrial undersensing, occur with relative frequency with epicardial pacing and only rarely with endocardial pacing. Additionally, relocating the electrode or removing certain types of endocardial pacing leads (active fixation type)

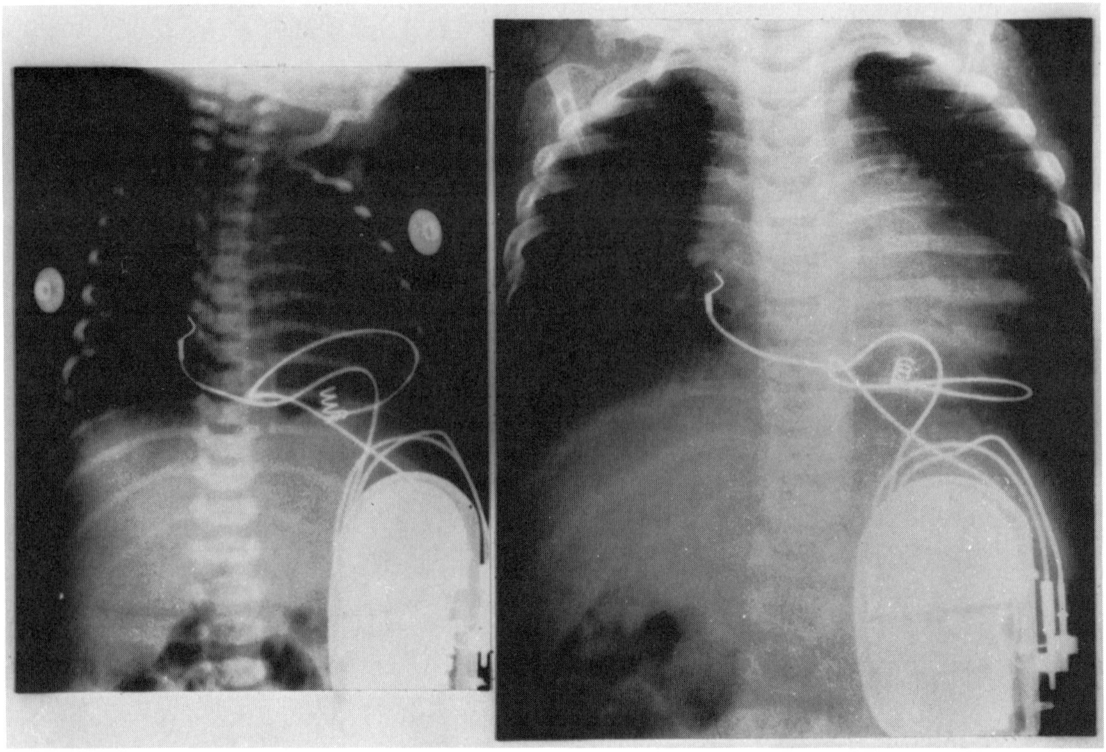

FIGURE 18–11
Two roentgenograms taken of the same patient. The roentgenogram on the left was taken at 3 days of age, one day after pacemaker implantation. The roentgenogram on the right was taken 1 year later. The pulse generator required replacement at 3 years, 9 months after implant for battery depletion. The original atrial and ventricular pacing leads continue to function normally. This patient is now 4 years old.

is possible and may be relatively simple. With epicardial systems, replacement is the only possible reparable response to a lead malfunction and requires thoracotomy. Lead splicing is difficult, unreliable, and no longer recommended. Procedures performed in the catheterization laboratory usually require only local anesthesia and sedation, obviating the need for general anesthesia and the attendant inconvenience and risk.

Based on these considerations, the implant method of choice is the endocardial approach unless contraindicated by patient size or cardiac anatomy.

Unipolar vs Bipolar Configuration

Unipolar pacing systems have been used more frequently for pacing in children primarily because of the limited availability of acceptable bipolar leads. Most unipolar leads have smaller diameter and are more flexible than the thicker and more rigid currently available bipolar leads.

There are no bipolar epicardial leads. Also, there are few available active fixation bipolar leads with uniform diameter, which enhances removability. Although the importance of removability is not generally accepted, its importance in the pediatric population is self-evident. To establish a bipolar epicardial system, two leads must be implanted for each chamber paced. This approach has not often been used, mostly because the possibilities for malfunction are increased.

The advantages of bipolar endocardial pacing include less vulnerability to myopotential inhibition (skeletal muscle activity sensed by the pacemaker as cardiac activity, resulting in appropriate inhibition of pacing stimuli) and less frequent pectoral muscle stimulation. Far field R wave sensing is less of a problem with bipolar pacing. In children, myopotential inhibition and pectoral muscle stimulation are relatively common but rarely cause clinically significant problems. When these problems do occur, adjustments of output or sensitivity often result in their elimination. As smaller, more flexible bipolar endocardial active fixation leads become available, bipolar pacing in children will be used frequently.

Pacing Mode and Type of Device

One of four permanent pacing modes should be considered for treatment of bradycardia in infants, children, and adolescents: AV universal (DDD), atrial demand (AAI), ventricular demand (VVI), and either atrial or ventricular activity responsive pacing. In children with complete AVB, sinus node function is usually normal. Therefore, rate-variable AV synchrony is readily achieved with DDD pacing. This "physiologic" pacing mode most closely approximates normal and is the mode of choice for children with complete AVB. Patients with sinus node disease and/or intermittent or subclinical abnormalities of AV node function may also benefit from implantation of an atrial synchronous ventricular pacing device (DDD). The implanting physician should demonstrate normal or near normal AV conduction before implanting an atrial demand (AAI) or atrial activity responsive (AAI-activity) pacemaker. The criteria for adequate AV nodal function is intact AV conduction at an atrial paced rate of greater than 100/minute.[34] Normal or near normal AV nodal refractory periods also support the decision to implant an atrial device. Usually, AV nodal testing is performed at the time of planned pacemaker implantation. If the AV node is not found to be adequate, a DDD device is instead implanted.

For children with isolated sinus node dysfunction (as may occur following the Mustard or Senning procedure), an AAI or AAI-activity pacemaker is implanted, assuming the preceding criteria are met. These children, unlike their adult counterparts with sinus node dysfunction, often have normal or near normal chronotropic sinus node responsiveness to exercise. Therefore, rate-responsive atrial pacemakers are less likely to be of benefit. The advantages of AAI pacing are AV synchrony at rest, simplicity, and pulse generator size. The major disadvantage is failure to protect the patient from the effects in intermittent, progressive, or rate-related loss of AV conduction. Because rapidly progressive AV nodal dysfunction is rare in children, atrial pacing is safe and effective in patients with normal or near normal AV nodal function as documented in the catheterization laboratory.[34]

Dual-chambered devices without both sensing and pacing in the atrium (DVI or VDD) offer no advantages. Dual-chambered DDD devices are now available in sizes and shapes that allow implantation even in neonates. When implanting a dual-chambered pacemaker in any age group, only DDD devices should be considered.

For children with symptomatic episodic bradycardia caused by intermittent failure of AV conduction or associated with cardioinhibitory vagal reactions, a ventricular demand (VVI) pacemaker may be appropriate. Individualization is important. Some patients with vasovagal syncope benefit from AV synchrony as well as bradycardia control. For example, patients with vasovagal syncope may be prevented from fainting by a VVI pacemaker, but will continue to have symptoms of dizziness in situations that were previously associated with syncope. Ventricular pacing alone without AV synchrony may be insufficient to eliminate symptoms completely. However, with a "physiologic" pacemaker all symptoms may be prevented.

Using the general approch outlined, the majority of pacemakers implanted in children are "physiologic" dual-chambered systems. The minority are single-chambered (AAI or VVI) systems.

Leads

A wide variety of pacing leads are currently available. These leads are generally dependable and theoretically long lasting (10 to 20 years). When implanted properly, adequate pacing thresholds persist for extended periods. The current thrust in development of new pacing leads is toward improving the pacing electrode to provide lower pacing thresholds, thereby increasing battery longevity. A major problem in pediatric patients with most newly available leads has been that most are passive fixation "tined" leads (Fig. 18–12). Tined leads have several small blunt flanges at the lead tip that anchor the lead

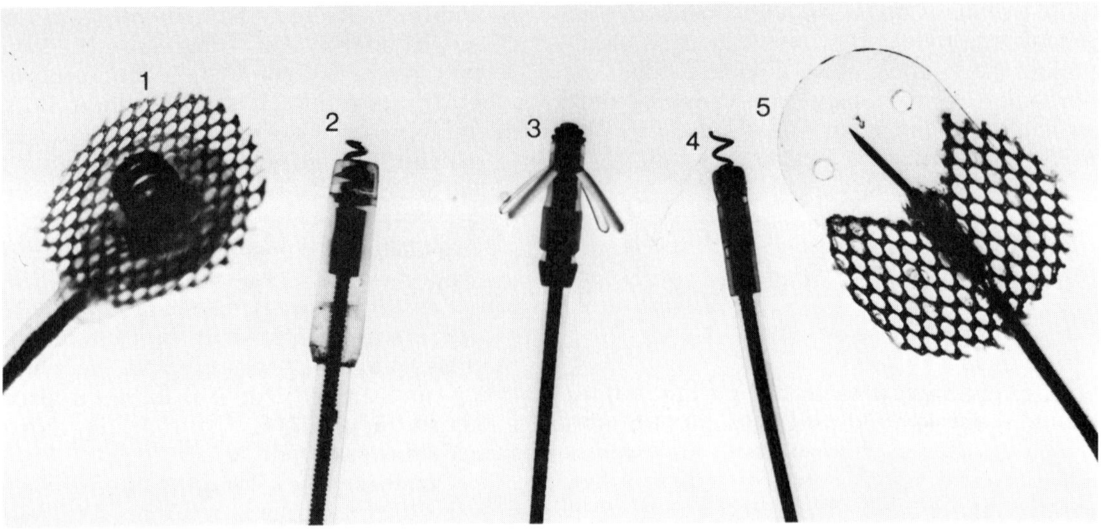

FIGURE 18–12
Examples of epicardial (1 and 5) and endocardial (2–4) pacing leads appear above. Lead 1 is a typical example of a myocardial lead used for epicardial ventricular pacing in pediatric patients. Lead 5 is one of the few available atrial epicardial pacing leads, the "stab-on" lead. Leads 2–4 are commonly used endocardial leads; leads 2 and 4 are active fixation leads and 3 is a passive fixation lead.

by becoming entrapped by the cardiac trabeculi. Once placed, these leads are difficult to remove. Removal may be necessitated by bacterial endocarditis, lead fracture, or development of a superior pacing lead or new types of pacing systems. Therefore in children, because many years of pacing are anticipated, endocardial active fixation (screw-in) leads are preferred. The removal or repositioning of screw-in leads is relatively simple in many instances, although they should be removed only by experienced physicians.

A limited variety of epicardial pacing leads are available. All are unipolar and most are designed only for ventricular use. The most commonly used epicardial atrial lead is the Medtronic 4951 stab-on lead. This lead may be implanted from the subxiphoid approach in most patients with reasonable results. However, the incidence of late atrial sensing and pacing problems is high regardless of the method of implantation.

There are many different ventricular epicardial pacing leads available from many manufacturers. There are no good comparative studies to assist in the selection of an epicardial ventricular pacing lead.

FOLLOW-UP

The decision to implant a pacemaker in a child carries a commitment to long-term follow-up, which is essential for optimal results. Preferably, the implanting center should have a pacemaker clinic managed by personnel specially trained in pediatric pacing. In a pacemaker clinic accustomed to caring for adults, the occasional clinical visits of children may be surrounded by anxiety and uncertainty. As is true of pacemaker clinics caring for adults, commitment to the details of appropriate surveillance is essential for the best results. The responsibility of the pacemaker follow-up system has expanded beyond the limited task of identifying impending battery depletion to include more extensive evaluation of the hemodynamic benefit and identification of more subtle abnormalities that suggest impending pacemaker system failure. Figure 18–13 outlines one system for early and long-term follow-up. The goals of a follow-up system should be to (1) identify or predict impending pacemaker or lead malfunction; (2) identify approaching battery depletion; (3) offer support and guidance through education and personnel available to the patients and their families; and (4) maintain an up-to-date knowledge of the new methods and equipment available in pacing.

As noted, the system begins with education immediately following implantation. While the child remains in the hospital, common concerns and misconceptions should be reviewed. Specifically, sports participation, fol-

FOLLOW-UP PROTOCOL FOR PACEMAKER PATIENTS
Immediate Postimplant (ICU):
1. CXR: rule out pneumothorax, confirm lead placement.
2. ECG, ECG, and magnet application: confirm proper function.

Recovery Period:
1. Telemetry for 48 hours.
2. Broad spectrum antibiotics IV for 48 hours.
3. Complete noninvasive pacing system testing.
4. 24-hour Holter monitor before discharge.
5. Practice transtelephonic transmission.
6. Patient and family teaching: wound care, acceptable activities, dispel myths.

Intermediate Follow-up:
1. Transtelephonic practice tracing from home.
2. Clinic visit 1 month to 6 weeks after discharge.
   a. CXR.
   b. ECG.
   c. Complete noninvasive pacing system testing.
   d. Reprogramming to account for chronic thresholds.

Long-Term Follow-up:
1. Transtelephonic transmissions monthly for 12 months, then every third month until the approach of battery depletion.
2. Clinic visits every 6 to 12 months—initial clinic evaluation repeated.
3. Treadmill stress test 1 year postimplant, if possible.
4. 24-hour Holter monitor if there is suspicion of malfunction.

FIGURE 18–13
General methods of testing and follow-up during the early, intermediate, and late post-implantation periods. Using these methods, problems are effectively identified and/or diverted. ICU, intensive care unit; CXR, chest x-ray; ECG, electrocardiogram; IV, intravenous.

low-up schedules, need for future battery replacement, and the methods of identification of battery depletion should be reviewed. Also at this time, a transtelephonic monitoring device is provided, and its use is reviewed.

Specific recommendations for recreational participation depend on the reason for pacing and the degree of pacemaker dependence. All patients are directed away from activities likely to involve collisions such as organized football, contact karate, boxing, and motorcycle riding. Activities such as tennis, golf, and running are encouraged as possible, taking into account associated cardiac defects. Other commonly encountered sports such as baseball, basketball, and soccer are considered on an individual basis. In our experience, injuries to the pacing system related to the latter activities have not occurred.

The second area of concern to pacemaker patients with newly implanted pacemakers is related to environmental hazards such as microwave ovens. Environmentally related damage or disruption of pacing and pacing circuitry is now very uncommon. The patients are cautioned to avoid high-energy electrical fields, arc welders, high-output radio transmitters, and nuclear magnetic imagers or other intense magnetic fields. Because of the very low incidence of environmentally related problems, the relative resistance of pacemakers to these problems should be stressed.

Following discharge, the pacemaker clinic personnel will frequently receive calls from the patient or patient's family with questions. The manner in which initial contacts are handled by the pacemaker clinic personnel is very important to the development of rapport and will directly affect the willingness of patients for future contact.

Extensive noninvasive pacemaker testing is performed in the clinic before discharge, 6 weeks after discharge, and routinely once each year. This evaluation seeks to demonstrate all aspects of normal pacemaker functioning.

Noninvasive Pacemaker Clinic Evaluation

Initially, resting rhythm is recorded with the patient connected to an electrocardiographic recording device. A sample of this and each subsequent test is saved for later review and documentation.

The Magnet Mode. Next, a magnet is placed over the pulse generator and the rhythm recorded. The result of placing a magnet over the pacemaker in most cases is asynchronous pacing. The sensing circuit is inactivated, and pacing rate may be the programmed rate or a standard rate that may or may not be programmable. There are a number of possible diagnostic benefits of the magnet mode. If endogenous rhythm is inhibiting paced rhythm, the ability of the pacemaker to capture the heart may be unknown. By applying the magnet, capture may be documented. With many devices, especially the older ones, the pacing rate during magnet operation is designed to indicate remaining battery life: the pacing rate decreases or increases proportional to the remaining battery life. There are many possible magnet responses, and therefore the specific characteristics of the device being tested should be known or reviewed prior to testing.

Capture Threshold. The pacing capture threshold is then determined for each chamber. The methods of measuring the threshold also vary among devices. Most pacemaker interrogation and programming devices have methods for avoiding or immediately reacting to inadvertent programming to subthreshold output levels. An example is a temporary "auto-threshold" mode that progressively decreases the output until noncapture is noted by the operator. Removal of the programming device from the proximity of the pulse generator immediately returns the pacemaker to the previously programmed values. The purpose of measuring thresholds is to detect unexpected changes and to allow adjustment of the device output to avoid wasting energy while ensuring adequate energy to successfully pace the heart, regardless of usual threshold fluctuations.

Pacemaker Dependence Evaluation. Pacemaker dependence is loosely defined as the presence of symptoms during inhibition or absence of pacemaker output. Pacemaker dependence is assumed if there is a period of asystole of greater than 3 to 4 seconds following sudden inhibition of pacemaker output. A past history of syncope or near syncope should also suggest pacemaker dependence. There may be considerable variability in the results of testing for pacemaker dependence, and therefore the test should be used only for adjunctive information. Absolute pacemaker dependence is rare, and death resulting from loss of output following damage to the device, even in patients with pacemaker dependence as defined by these criteria, is unlikely. However, the degree to which activities are restricted should depend somewhat on this determination. Although there is a general consensus that collision-oriented athletic activities such as football and contact karate should be prohibited, participation in other less violent sports is controversial and perhaps should be considered in non-pacemaker–dependent patients in whom the consequences of pacemaker damage are only the need for repair of the system. To allow participation by these lower risk patients is consistent with the goal of promoting reasonable normalcy in children with pacemakers. As with every other fact of pacing in pediatrics, the recommendations for activity should be individualized, and sports participation mutually agreed on by the physician and the family.

Pacemaker Programming. Once the pacing threshold and pacemaker dependence have been established, the pacemaker output may be programmed (set) to provide a pacing output safety margin to account for daily fluctuations in threshold. How much above the capture threshold the pacemaker should be set depends on several factors. Because thresholds may vary as much as 50%, the energy output should be at least 100% above the measured threshold. Accomplishing this depends on the particular method of varying pacemaker output allowed by the device in use. The possibilities are (1) varying pulse width, (2) varying voltage, or (3) varying current. The relationships between energy consumption and safety margin depend on the type of changes made. For example, when the voltage output is doubled, the energy consumption is squared. However, if the pulse width is doubled, energy consumption will only double. In the latter case, an understanding of the strength-duration curve is especially important. As described earlier in this chapter, the strength-duration curve is asymptotic, and changes in pulse width to values greater than 0.3 to 0.4 may have little effect on safety margin considering the lack of significant slope at this portion of the curve. Many newer devices allow adjustment of more than one output parameter, which in turn allows construction of an individual strength-duration curve (see Fig. 18–5). Once constructed, pacemaker output may be more accurately chosen to allow an adequate safety margin while minimizing energy consumption.

Sensing Threshold. The majority of pacemaker patients in pediatrics have atrial sensing pacemakers and atrial sensing abnormalities are the most common pacing system malfunction. Therefore, performing sensing thresholds, especially the atrium, should be a routine part of the evaluation. Following implant, sensing function changes little in the absence of a pacing lead malfunction. To evaluate sensing, programming the pacemaker to a slower pacing rate may be required to allow underlying rhythm to occur and sensing to be demonstrated. Some of the newer pulse generators will record and quantify the intracardiac electrogram allowing direct evaluation for the electrogram amplitude. With this information, the sensing characteristics of the pulse generator may be adjusted to insure sensing of endogenous cardiac activity and avoid "oversensing" of electrical activity other than that desired.

Pacemaker Telemetry. Pacemaker telemetry refers to the capability of the pacemaker to communicate a broad range of information back to the programmer. The type of information communicated varies widely between manufacturers and specific devices and may include the following:

1. The programmed values
2. The measured pacing parameters (when the information is measured by the device, as opposed to relaying stored information, telemetry is referred to as real time)
3. Electrograms (some with superimposed timing diagrams)
4. Lead impedance
5. Battery life information
6. Cumulative pacing and spontaneous event recording
7. Identifying information such as the type of device, leads, and serial numbers.

Other Procedures. Perhaps most important to the pacemaker clinic evaluation is the patient's interval history. The patient and the family are carefully questioned concerning palpitations, syncope or near syncope, new drug treatment, and recent illnesses or accidents. The physical examination infrequently provides clues to pacemaker problems. The pacemaker site should always be carefully examined for impending erosion, erythema, swelling, or pacemaker movement or migration. Finally, a chest roentgenogram is routinely obtained. The leads are carefully examined for fractures or changes in electrode position. The chest roentgenogram is also an important method of evaluating the effects of growth on the position of the pacing lead. However, only rarely has growth created a clinical problem involving the pacing lead. Therefore, the pacing lead appearance alone should not be used as a criteria for an interventional procedure. Increases in cardiac size may reflect the need for a more hemodynamically supportive pacing mode.

Long-term Follow-up. Yearly clinical visits and more regular transtelephonic pacemaker evaluations make up the majority of subsequent pacemaker follow-up. Transtelephonic tracings are requested each month for the first year following implantation of new pacing leads. For the subsequent 2 to 3 years, the tracings are requested only every 3 months. As the time for expected battery depletion approaches, monthly transmissions are again requested. Optimally, the pacemaker clinic should have a system for keeping track of the transmission and clinic visit schedule. Many adult pacemaker clinics take the initiative to contact patients by phone at the time of scheduled transmissions, but with children the time of transmission may be better determined by the parents. However, the pediatric pacemaker clinic has a responsibility to minimize the number of patients becoming lost to follow-up and thereby limiting the children receiving inadequate care.

RESULTS

A meaningful summary of published pediatric pacing experience is difficult. Because the need for cardiac pacing is unusual, no single center has a large enough patient population from which to draw important conclusions. Several other factors have also contributed to the difficulty of establishing appropriate expectations, including the rapid changes in available technology, the variety of techniques, and the heterogeneous nature of problems requiring pacing. Comparing previous pacing experience with current experience has little validity. However, certain problems have remained in spite of improvement in equipment and methods. Pacing leads remain the "Achilles' heel" of pacemaker therapy. Lead dislodgements, fractures, time-related deterioration, difficulty in lead removal, rising or high thresholds, and patient growth resulting in lead stress remain the most important theoretic and common problems in pediatric pacing. Difficulties associated with a lifetime of cardiac pacing perhaps remain to be discovered.

Many small series with reasonably prolonged follow-ups are available. An excellent brief summary of the published pacing experience prior to 1981 was compiled by Young.[35] A total of 448 patient reports in 14 separate series was summarized. Surgical complete AVB was the pacing indication in 60%, and congenital AVB unassociated with surgery was the pacing indication in 30%. The remaining patients underwent pacing for sinus node dysfunction. The average follow-up duration was 44 months, with a maximum of 168 months (14 years). In these groups there were 78 deaths, 32 of which were thought possibly related to pacemaker failure. In each series, the pacemakers were implanted almost exclusively by the epicardial approach and were single chambered (mostly ventricular). The overall outcome reflected a marked but unquantifiable improvement in survival as compared to children with similar problems prior to the availability of pacemakers. Since 1981, a number of additional series have been published.[33, 36–46] Most of these published reports include patients seen prior to 1981. Several important advances occurring around 1981 had an important impact on the pacing practices in pediatrics. Almost simultaneously, atrial sensing pacemakers, transvenous pacing, and improved methods for implantation of dual-chambered epicardial pacing systems became available. During the subsequent years, the techniques have been revised and improved, and the appropriate use of each has become clearer.

These new techniques and pacemakers have had a significant effect on pacing results. Clearly, factors affecting pacemaker longevity such as improved pacemaker leads and small pulse generator size have changed the outcome to some degree. The new techniques applied beginning in 1981 mark a clear breaking point in pacing practice and therefore serve as the beginning point for a review of a single large center experience.[33] We reviewed the indications, methods, complications, and pacing system longevity related to method and type of pacing systems implanted at Texas Children's Hospital between January, 1981, and August, 1986. During this period, 247 pacing systems were implanted or revised in 207 children and adults younger than 30 years. The pacing systems were implanted for AVB in 73%, for sinus node dysfunction in 24%, and for other reasons in 3% of patients. Surgical damage to the conduction system was the cause of AVB in approximately 50% of patients with pacemakers for AVB. Sinus node dysfunction was mostly related to atrial surgery for congenital heart disease. The few remaining patients received pacemakers for treatment of idiopathic sick sinus syndrome, vasovagal syncope, supraventricular tachycardia, or the prolonged QT syndrome. The guidelines for implantation reviewed in a previous section were followed without exception.

The epicardial implantation technique was used for 130 pacing systems, and 117 were implanted by the endocardial technique. The pacing systems implanted through 1985 are presented by pacing mode method and the year implanted in Figure 18–14. Note that the majority of the pacing systems (59%) were atrial sensing ventricular pacing systems (VDD or DDD). Early in the series the more common method of implantation was epicardial, but the endocardial technique predominated later. During the years of 1981 and 1982, 62% of systems were epicardial, while in 1984 and 1985, 36% of systems were epicardial. Barring unexpected changes in available technology, the ratio of epicardial vs endocardial and single- vs dual-chamber systems should remain fairly constant.

The pacing system problems occurring in all pacing systems implanted at Texas Children's Hospital after 1981 were reviewed. A total of 281 pacing systems were included, and 46 pacing system problems were serious enough to warrant surgical intervention. The specific categories of problems and their frequency, categorized by implantation approach, are presented in Table 18–2. The only significant differences in the frequency of pacing problems related to the method of implantation were the leads developing exit block, the number of "premature" battery depletions, and the occurrence of pocket erosion. Exit block and premature battery depletions were more common in the epicardial group. Pocket erosion was more common in the endocardial group. Since this review, the incidence of pocket erosion seems to have decreased because of the smaller sizes and better shapes of available devices. No change in the frequency of exit block is apparent. The difference between the endocardial and epicardial groups in frequency of premature battery depletions has increased in the epicardial group, primarily because of two fac-

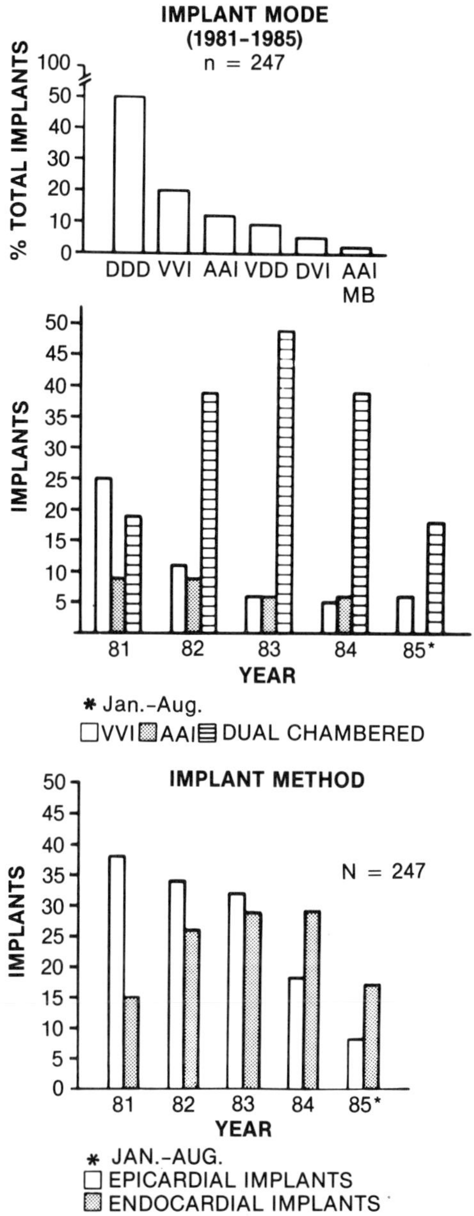

FIGURE 18–14
The mode and methods of pacemaker implantation between 1981 and 1985 appear in the above graphs. The relative frequency of the different pacing modes used for all implants appears at the top. The middle graph demonstrates the changes in pacing mode and type of approach during the course of the study. The number of dual-chambered implants increased between 1981 and 1985 and then stabilized. The bottom graph demonstrates the change in preference between endocardial and epicardial pacing that has occurred.

tors: (1) the patients in the epicardial group are younger, usually requiring higher pacing rates; and (2) the thresholds are higher both at implant and chronically, requiring higher output to achieve adequate safety margins.

The overall incidence of problems was low and was comparable to the incidence reported for adult pacemaker patients.[47] With the exception of atrial undersensing, there was no appreciable difference among implantation techniques and between patients with and without structural defects. Atrial undersensing, however, was a problem almost exclusively in patients with leads implanted by the epicardial approach. Inadequate sensing was related to more difficult atrial exposure at surgery, more complicated cardiac anatomy, and limitations inherent in the atrial epicardial lead. Even in this active young patient population, observing only the previously discussed physical limitations, the incidence of traumatic pacemaker lead damage was extremely low (two occurrences, both epicardial systems).

The cumulative "survival" life of the pacing systems implanted beetween January 1981 and August 1986 at Texas Children's Hospital is presented in Figure 18–15. Survival of a pacing system is defined as the absence of any abnormality requiring surgical revision. The likelihood of a pacing system functioning 5 years after implant is greatest for single-chambered endocardial systems. Epicardial systems have been more prone to problems requiring revision. The difference in results between these approaches is related to the particular problems mentioned above. Since this review was completed, a significant number of epicardial systems have become depleted between 3 and 4 years after implant. If these systems were now included, further discrepancies in longevity between endocardial and epicardial implantation approaches would be apparent. The pacing system survival probability has certainly increased since the beginning of this series, with the greater number of problems clustered during the first few years of the study.

SUMMARY

This chapter has attempted review of pacing in pediatric patients. The most important message is that care, special skill, interest, and judgment, and not dogma, are critically important to pacing of children. Based on the decreasing frequency of problems and improvements in reliability, patients and their families should expect even fewer pac-

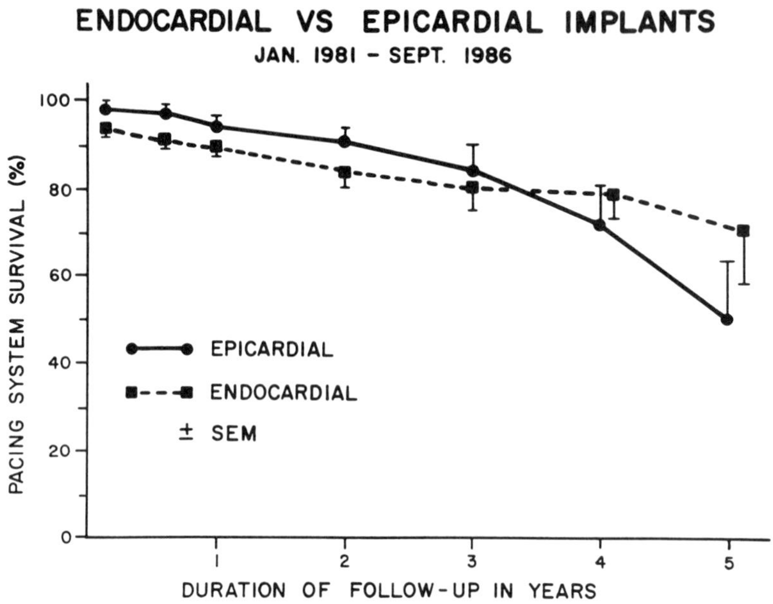

FIGURE 18–15
A cumulative life table analysis of pacing system survival for pacing systems implanted between 1981 and 1986. The systems were divided by method of implantation. The graph relates the likelihood of not requiring any form of surgical revision of a pacing system following its initial implantation. Revision for any reason was considered a failure whether caused by battery depletion, lead failure, or other problems. Significant improvements in pacing techniques and equipment are expected to improve these results.

ing problems in the future. In light of the success with physiologic pacing and the absence of discernible increased morbidity, aggressive pursuit of rate responsiveness and AV synchrony is justified. The ability to establish single- or dual-chambered pacing systems, either endocardially or epicardially, with low morbidity allows the choice of pacemaker and implant method best suited for the patient.

A commitment to achieving and maintaining optimal results requires special expertise and is essential for pacing of children. This commitment involves a follow-up system that incorporates knowledge of potential problems, their treatment, and prevention. Suc-

TABLE 18–2
PACING SYSTEM PROBLEMS REQUIRING SURGICAL REVISION (N=281)*

	ENDOCARDIAL (N=149)	EPICARDIAL (N=132)	TOTAL REVISED (N=46)
Technical			
Lead dislodgement	2	3	5
Sensing failure	2	1	3
Diaphragm pacing	2	0	2
Perforation	1	0	1
Total	7	4	11
Lead related			
Exit block	1	5	6
Fracture	3	1	4
Other	2	1	3
Total	6	7	13
Premature Depletion	3	7	10
Infection			
Erosion	6	0	6
Primary infection	1	2	3
Total	7	2	9
Pulse Generator			
Loss of output	1	0	1
Loss of sensing	2	0	2
Total	3	0	3

*Between 1981 and 1986, 281 pacing systems were implanted and reviewed for the occurrence of problems requiring surgical revision. The problems were classified as "technical" (potentially avoided by variations in technique or lead positioning), lead related, "premature" depletion (considered "premature" because depletion occurred during the usual warranty period but not truly a malfunction), infection, and problems related to pulse generator circuitry. These problems were further subdivided by method of implantation.

cessful pacing of children also requires technical skill on the part of the physician. The child is best served by the physician who adheres closely to prudent implant indication and individualizes the choice of pacing techniques and equipment.

In providing pacing support for children, a long-ranged view must be taken, and the possible conversion of any system to a radically new system should be considered. Based on the advances of the past 25 years, pacing in the future will continue to move toward development of pacing systems that are increasingly dependable, last longer, and more closely approximate the normal cardiac conduction system function.

References

1. Furman S, Hayes DL, Holmes DR Jr: A Practice of Cardiac Pacing. Mount Kisco, NY, Futura, 1986.
2. Chung, EK: Artificial Cardiac Pacing: A Practical Approach, ed 2. Baltimore, Williams & Wilkins, 1984.
3. Gillette PC, Griffin JC: Practical Cardiac Pacing. Baltimore, Williams & Wilkins, 1986.
4. Samet P, El-Sherif N: Cardiac Pacing, ed 2. Clinical Cardiology Monographs. New York, Grune & Stratton, 1980.
5. Moses HW, Taylor GW, Schneider JA, et al: A Practical Guide to Cardiac Pacing. Little, Brown, 1983.
6. Frye RL, et al: Guidelines for permanent cardiac implantation, May 1984: A report of the Joint American College of Cardiology/American Heart Association Task Force on Assessment of Cardiovascular Procedures (Subcommittee on Pacemaker Implantation). Circulation 70:331a–339a, 1984.
7. Krongrad E: Prognosis for patients with congenital heart disease and postoperative intraventricular conduction defects. Circulation 57:867–870, 1978.
8. Daicoff GR, Aslami A, Tobias JA, et al: Management of postoperative complete heart block in infants and children. Chest 66:639–641, 1974.
9. Gillette PC: Recent advances in mechanisms, evaluation, and pacemaker treatment of chronic bradydysrrhythmias in children. Am Heart J 102:920–929, 1981.
10. Mahoney LT, et al: Pacemaker management for acute onset of heart block in childhood. J Pediatr 107:207–211, 1985.
11. Karpawich PP, et al: Congenital complete atrioventricular block: Clinical and electrophysiological predictors of need for pacemaker insertion. Am J Cardiol 48:1098–1102, 1981.
12. Squarcia U, Merideth J, McGoon DC, et al: Prognosis of transient atrioventricular conduction disturbances complicating open heart surgery for congenital heart defects. Am J Cardiol 28:648–652, 1971.
13. Hurwitz RA, Riemenschneider TA, Moss AJ: Chronic postoperative heart block in children. Am J Cardiol 21:185–189, 1968.
14. Morriss JH, Eugster GS, Nora JJ, et al: His bundle recording in progressive external ophthalmoplegia. J Pediatr 81:1167–1170, 1972.
15. Gillette PC: Indications for permanent cardiac pacing. In Gillette C, Griffin J (eds): Practical Cardiac Pacing. Baltimore, Williams & Wilkins, 1986.
16. Driscoll PJ, et al: Management of surgical complete AV block in children. Am J Cardiol 43:1175–1180, 1979.
17. Morriss JH, et al: Pacemakers—Indicators, implantation and followup in pediatric cardiac dysrhythmias. In Gillette PC, Garson A Jr (eds): Pediatric Cardiac Dysrhythmias. New York, Grune & Stratton, 1981.
18. Murphy DA, Tynan M, Graham GR, et al: Prognosis of complete atrioventricular dissociation in children after open-heart surgery. Lancet 750–752, 1970.
19. Hofschire PJ, Nicoloff DM, Moller JH: Postoperative complete heart block in 64 children treated with and without cardiac pacing. Am J Cardiol 39:559–562, 1977.
20. Parsonnet V, Furman S, Smyth NPD: A revised code for pacemaker identification. Five position pacemaker code (ICHD). PACE 4:400–403, 1981.
21. Parsonnet V, et al: Optimal resources for implantable cardiac pacemakers. Report of Inter-Society Commission for Heart Disease Resources. Circulation 68:226a–244a, 1983.
22. Berstein, et al: Report of the NASPE Code Committee. PACE 7:400, 1984.
23. Mulch HFW, Pahstan P, Ilda M: Programmable cardiac pacemakers: First experience with the Ommicor system. J Cardiovasc Surg 15:522, 1974.
24. Furman S: Pacemaker programmability in artificial cardiac pacing vs practical approach. In Chung E (ed): Artificial Cardiac Pacing. 2nd ed. Baltimore, Williams & Wilkins, 1983.
25. Ogawa S, et al: Hemodynamic consequences of atrioventricular and ventriculoatrial pacing. PACE 1:8–15, 1978.
26. Iwase M, et al: Evaluation by pulsed Doppler echocardiography of the atrial contribution to left ventricular filling in patients with DDD pacemakers. Am J Cardiol 58:301–306, 1986.
27. Kristensson B, Arnman K, Smedgard P, et al: Physiologic versus single rate ventricular pacing. PACE 8:73–84, 1985.
28. Fananapazir L, Bennett DH, Monks P: Atrial synchronized ventricular pacing: Contribution of the chronotropic response to improved exercise performance. PACE 6:601–608, 1983.
29. Pehrsson SK: Influence of heart rate and atrioventricular synchronization of maximal work tolerance in patients treated with artificial pacemakers. Acta Med Scand 214:311–316, 1983.
30. Segel N, et al: The circulation effects of electrically induced changes in ventricular rate at rest and during exercise in complete heart block. J Clin Invest 43:1541, 1964.
31. Kristensson BE, Arnman K, Ryden L: The haemodynamic importance of atrioventricular synchrony and rate increase at rest and during exercise. Eur Heart J 6:773–778, 1985.
32. Pehrsson SK: Influence of heart rate and atrioventricular synchronization of maximal work tolerance in patients treated with artificial pacemakers. Acta Med Scand 214:311–315, 1983.
33. Smith RT Jr, et al: Actuarial analysis of pacing system survival in young patients. Circulation 74(suppl II):120, 1986. Abstract.
34. Gillette PC, Wampler DG, Shannon C, et al: Use of

atrial pacing in a young population. PACE 8:94–100, 1985.
35. Young D: Permanent pacemaker implantation in children: Current status and future considerations. PACE 4:61–67, 1981.
36. Taliercio CP, et al: Permanent cardiac pacing after the Fontan procedure. J Thorac Cardiovasc Surg 90:414–419, 1985.
37. Venetti A, et al: Cardiac stimulation in children. A multicenter study of 241 patients. Arch-Mal-Coeur Dec 77(13):1510–1516, 1984.
38. Gillette PC, et al: Pacemaker treatment of sick sinus syndrome in children. J Am Coll Cardiol 1:1325–1329, 1983.
39. Ector H, et al: Pacing in children. Br Heart J 53:541–546, 1985.
40. Gillette PC, et al: Transvenous pacing in pediatric patients. Am Heart J 105:843–847, 1983.
41. Gillette PC, Ott DA, Shannon C: Cardiac pacing in children and young adults. Clin Prog Pacing Electrophysiol 1:156–165, 1983.
42. Ruschewski W, et al: Pacemaker implantation in children. J Cardiovasc Surg 22:278, 1981.
43. Simon AB, et al: Ventricular pacing in children. PACE 5:836–844, 1982.
44. Goldman BS, Williams WG, Hill T, et al: Permanent cardiac pacing after open heart surgery: Congenital heart disease. PACE 8:732–739, 1985.
45. Ward DE, et al: Cardiac pacing in children. Arch Dis Child 57:514–520, 1982.
46. Hafez A, et al: Pacemakers in infants and young children; comparative study of pleural and lumbar modes of implantation. Arch-Mal-Coeur 76(10): 1140–1144, 1983.
47. Phibbs R, Marriott H: Complications of permanent transvenous pacing. N Engl J Med 312:1428–1432, 1985.

CHAPTER 19

TRANSVENOUS IMPLANTATION TECHNIQUE

Paul C. Gillette & Vicki Zeigler

Most pacemakers are implanted in adults by the transvenous approach which was pioneered in 1959 by Furman, Schwedel, and Escher.[1] Venous access is obtained by either venesection or puncture of a major vein, and the implantation may be carried out either in an operating room or a cardiac catheterization laboratory. The procedure may be done by a cardiologist or a surgeon, either one with or without assistance of the other. Currently, more and more pediatric pacemakers are being implanted by the transvenous approach.

There are pros and cons for each site for implantation. The operating room may have an advantage in sterility, but catheterization laboratories tend to have better x-ray and electrical equipment. As the techniques of implantation have changed (e.g., subclavian vein puncture) and the complexities of pulse generators have increased (e.g., having DDD and antitachycardia capabilities), pacemaker implantation has fallen more and more in the province of the cardiologist.

Transvenous pacing is contraindicated in patients with a right to left shunt. Careful consideration must be given to the risk-benefit ratio in patients with even a potential right to left shunt. In general, all shunts should be closed before a transvenous pacemaker is implanted.

THE IMPLANTING PHYSICIAN

Although teams of cardiologists and surgeons are frequently used, this seems unnecessary and may add to the implant cost. The physician performing the implant should have specific training in pacemaker implantation. The Intersociety Commission on Heart Disease (ICHD) report suggests prior performance of 25 implants and 10 reoperations.[2] The implanting physician must also maintain his or her expertise by performing at least 25 implants each year.[2] Expertise in cardiac catheterization techniques and cardiac electrophysiology is also useful. The physician must maintain his or her knowledge of the most recent developments in cardiac pacing. The design of pulse generators and leads is changing so rapidly that this takes a major time commitment. If the implanting physician is also the follow-up physician, the knowledge used in each area is complementary. The implanting physician's intimate knowledge of the implant in each patient may also help in planning follow-up for individual patients.

The implanting physician should be well trained in cardiopulmonary resuscitation, intubation, and emergency thoracentesis. A cardiovascular surgeon should be available in the case of an intrathoracic complication such as cardiac perforation.

THE PROCEDURE ROOM

The procedure room should meet operating room sterility requirements. There should be an alternate location in close proximity in case major equipment malfunctions. Electrical safety practices should be strictly adhered to and the equipment frequently tested for electrical leakage currents.

Equipment present in the implant room should include (1) high quality fluoroscopy with the ability for both anteroposterior and lateral images (either biplane or rotating tube or table); (2) television viewing; (3) an electrically isolated oscilloscopic multichannel recorder; (4) a pacing system analyzer for threshold determination, measurement of intrinsic signals, and pulse generator testing; (5) a programmer for the particular pacemaker being implanted and for the one to be removed if it is different; (6) a wide selection of pacing kits with extra stylets, screwdrivers, splicing equipment, boots, etc.; (7) a full set of surgical instruments; and (8) an electrocautery for use before the lead is implanted. Emergency equipment should include an external pacemaker, a defibrillator, suction equipment, emergency drugs, intubation equipment and an Ambu bag, oxygen, and trays for tube thoracotomy, pericardiocentesis, and thoracentesis. A second piece of each equipment should be available in the hospital should the need arise to use it.

SUPPORT PERSONNEL

In addition to the implanting physician, at least three other people should be present. The first is a nurse or technician who works primarily with pacemaker patients (preferably the nurse who will be responsible for this patient's follow-up, as the follow-up of a patient is initiated at the time of implant). The second person is usually a nurse who works in or is in charge of the procedure room and who will function as a floating nurse. The third person should be familiar with and in charge of the x-ray equipment. One of these three, usually the pacemaker nurse, must be familiar with the pacing systems analyzer, the pulse generator being implanted, and that pacemaker's programmer. This person should also be responsible for ensuring that the appropriate pulse generator and leads are available for each particular patient's needs. It is considered best practice not to be dependent on an industry representative to deliver the pacemaker and perform the active testing.

IMPLANTATION

Preparation for implantation should begin the day before implantation when the patient is admitted to the hospital. A complete history and physical examination are performed. The procedure is explained in detail to the patient and family and informed consent is obtained in writing. The handedness of the patient is determined, and the side of implantation is discussed. Laboratory work (e.g., complete blood count, prothrombin time, partial thromboplastin time, platelet count, and two-dimensional echocardiogram to look for venous anomalies) is ordered. A unit of packed red blood cells is cross-matched.

The patient is given nothing by mouth for at least 4 hours before implantation and is bathed in antibacterial soap the night prior to implantation. Before premedication, the patient is asked to empty his or her bladder. Sedation is accomplished with meperidine (2 mg/kg intramuscularly, up to 60 mg) and promethazine (1 mg/kg intramuscularly in the same syringe, up to 30 mg), which tend to increase heart rate.

When the patient arrives in the procedure room, a stable intravenous line is placed in the side opposite to the side the pacemaker is to be implanted in, and electrocardiographic monitoring is established. Transcutaneous oxygen saturation is measured continuously by pulse oximetry. An indwelling arterial line is placed for continuous pressure monitoring and blood gas determination. An antibiotic is given through the intravenous line before the procedure is begun (we use cefazolin, 12.5 mg/kg, up to 1 g).[3]

Each person in the room should completely cover his or her hair and should wear a mask and shoe covers. Traffic in and out of the room should be forbidden. The side of the chest, neck, and upper abdomen to be used should be cleansed with 70% ethyl alcohol. The area is draped with an iodophor-impregnated plastic sheet. If subclavian puncture is to be used, a vertical roll should be placed under the patient's spine to cause the shoulders to fall back. One percent lidocaine is used to infiltrate the area of the incision and pulse generator pocket.[4] In children younger than 15 years, we routinely use intravenous ketamine (1 mg/kg) repeatedly to obtain heavy sedation. An incision large enough to accept the pulse generator is made 1 cm below and parallel to the clavicle. If the cephalic vein is to be used, the lateral one-third of the incision should be lateral to the deltopectoral groove. If the subclavian puncture is to be used, the incision is more medial.

Some physicians who use the subclavian approach enter the vein by percutaneous puncture before the incision is made.

The subcutaneous tissue is cut using the coagulation channel of an electrocautery. The greater pectoral muscle is then divided by a blunt spreading incision (Fig. 19–1). A fascial plane is found between the pectoral and the intercostal muscles (Fig. 19–2). The pocket is formed by blunt dissection and any bleeding stopped with electrocautery before lead insertion is begun (Fig. 19–3). Care is taken not to disrupt the nerve to the pectoral muscle.

Cephalic Vein Isolation

The cephalic vein lies in a triangle formed by the clavicular head of the pectoralis major muscle medially, the deltoid muscle laterally, and the clavicle superiorly.[5, 6] The cephalic vein has been the standard site for lead introduction until recently, when the subclavian vein has gained popularity. The cephalic vein is found by dissecting in the fat between the pectoralis and the deltoid muscles. In the rare instance that the cephalic vein is unsuitable, there may be another vein slightly deeper in the triangle that is suitable. Alternately, the subclavian vein may be used.

When the vein is located, 1 cm or more of length should be dissected free, the distal end ligated, and a proximal controlling ligature placed. It is wise to start somewhat distally in case the vein tears during lead introduction. A small transverse incision is made with iris scissors. The implanting physician should ensure that the intima has been incised by loosening the proximal tie and observing bleeding. A catheter introducer or iris forceps is used to open the vein for introduction of the lead, which is previously straightened by full introduction of the stylet. Care must be taken that the proximal tie is

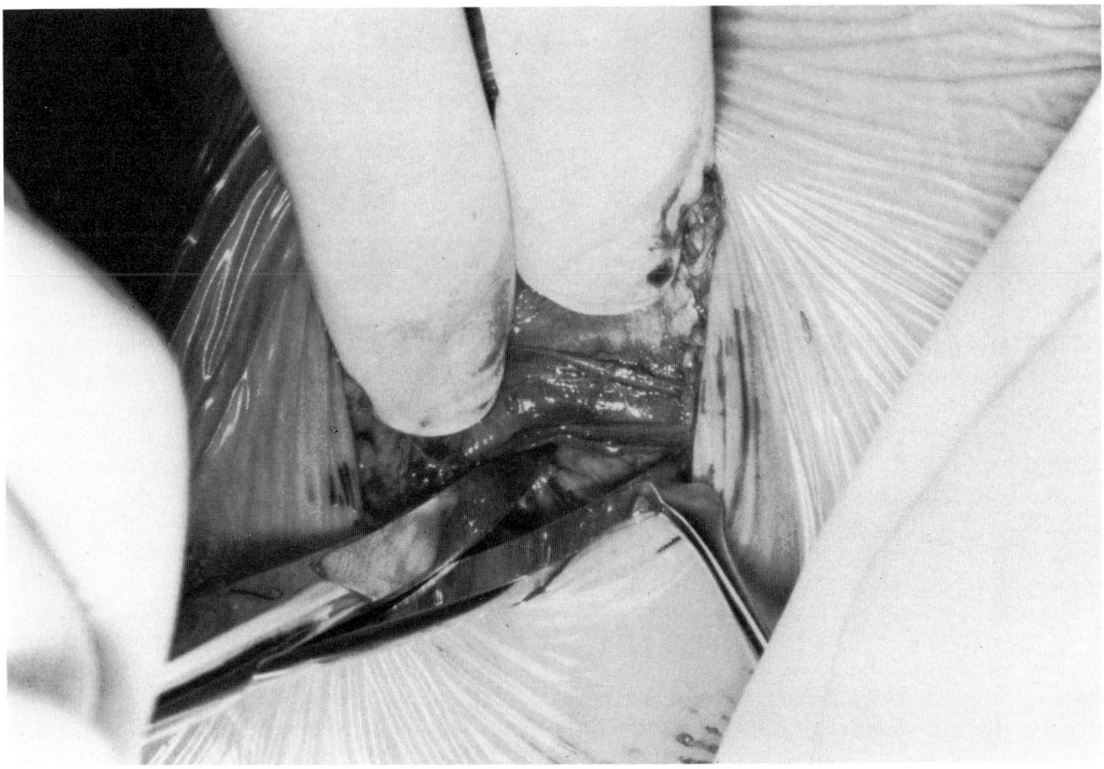

FIGURE 19–1
View from left shoulder in an 18-month-old child undergoing transvenous pacemaker implantation. The skin has been opened parallel to the clavicle. Subcutaneous tissue has been opened with electrocautery, and the tips of curved scissors are being used to spread a plane through the pectoralis major muscle. Fat and fascia can be seen just below the muscle between the tips of the scissors. This patient had undergone Senning repair of transposition of the great arteries and had preoperative and postoperative atrial flutter and postoperative severe sinus bradycardia.

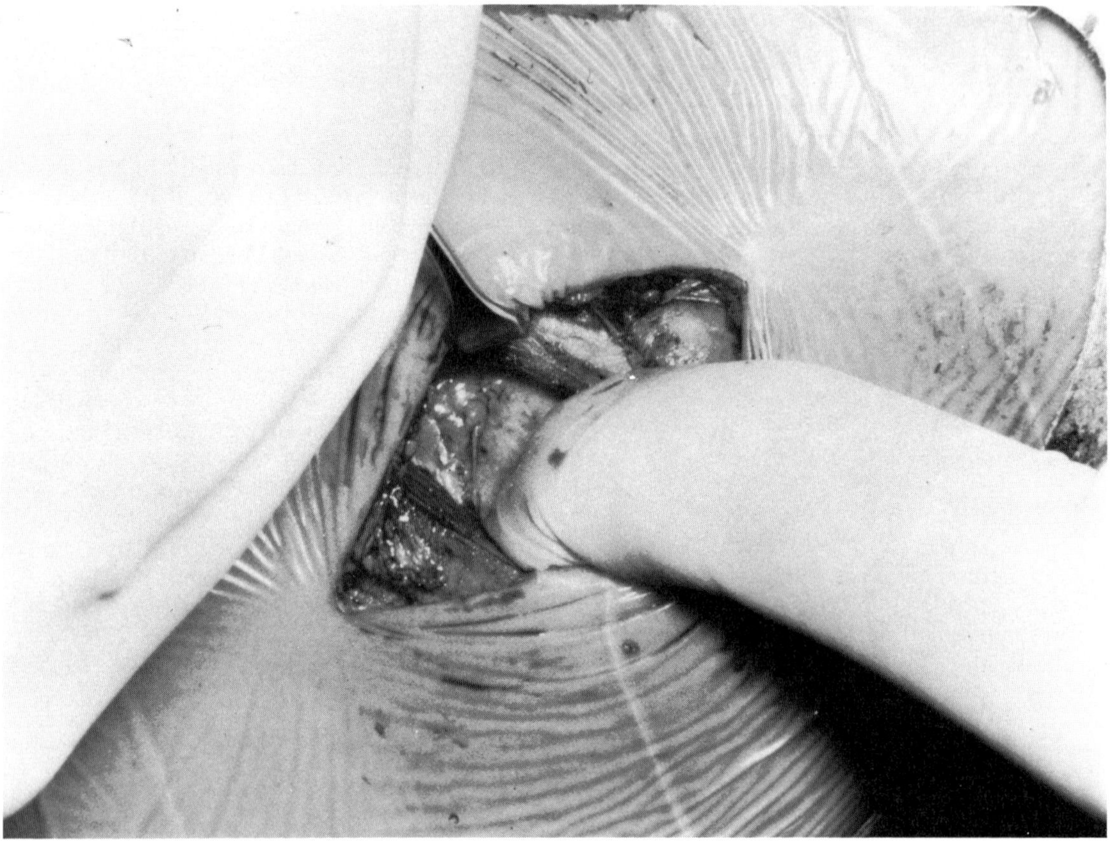

FIGURE 19–2
Demonstration of the fascial plane beneath the pectoralis major muscle in which the pacemaker pocket is built.

loosened as the lead is introduced. Rotation of the lead may facilitate entry. The cephalic-subclavian vein junction forms a nearly 90° angle. Traction on the cephalic vein or the whole shoulder will decrease the angle and may allow the lead to enter the subclavian vein. Withdrawal of the stylet may also facilitate this maneuver by softening the lead tip. If the lead still cannot be maneuvered, the possibility that it is not in the lumen of the vein should be considered. Usually, once the lead is in the subclavian vein, it can easily be positioned to the right atrium.

If the cephalic vein cannot be used or if a second entry site is necessary, other veins in the anterior chest wall may be used.[7] Alternately, the external or internal jugular veins can be located through a second incision. Much more frequently, direct puncture of the subclavian vein is used as a secondary site. Sometimes two leads can be introduced into the cephalic vein.

Subclavian Vein Approach

A pacing lead introduction kit is used to introduce leads into the subclavian vein.[8–10] The same adult needle, wire, and introducer size is used for patients weighing more than 15 kg. For patients weighing less than 15 kg, a 19 gauge percutaneous needle is used with a 0.025 gauge "J"-tipped spring guide. A 0.038 wire is exchanged through a plastic cannula. The standard tear-away introducer is then used. The subclavian vein is entered from the subpectoral pocket with the needle attached to a syringe (which is partially filled with dilute saline solution) by directing the tip of the needle under the clavicle above the first rib at about the middle of the clavicle. The needle is directed upward to a point 1 to 2 cm above the suprasternal notch.[11] The needle is aspirated gently as it is advanced. If the vein is not entered or if the artery is entered inadvertently, the needle is removed,

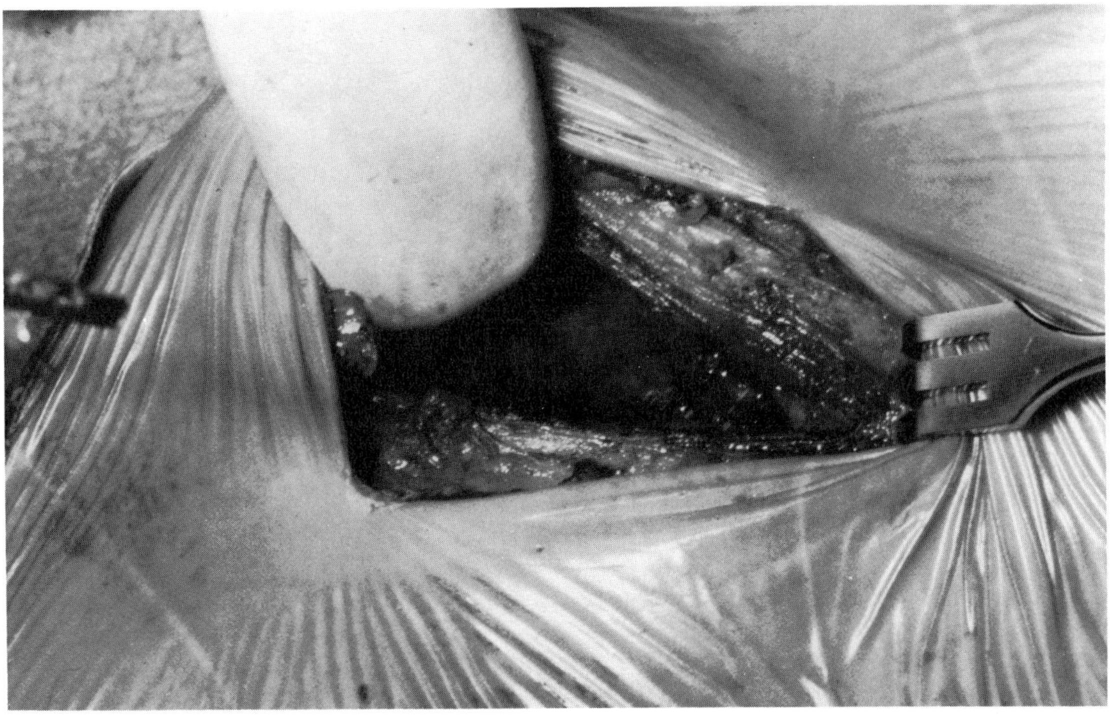

FIGURE 19–3
Demonstration of the technique of using a digit to create a pacemaker pocket beneath the pectoralis major muscle.

pressure applied, and the needle inserted in a slightly different direction. A catheter may be positioned in the subclavian vein from the femoral vein. Fluoroscopy can then be used to aim the needle at the catheter. This allows a more lateral puncture of the vein, to avoid having the leads pinched by the clavicle and the first rib.

The patients are well hydrated before the procedure, and intravenous fluids are run at a rapid rate until the subclavian vein has been entered. As a further precaution to prevent air from entering the venous system, uncooperative patients are sedated so they do not gasp or take sudden deep breaths during this part of the procedure. When a good blood return is obtained, the "J"-tipped guidewire is passed through the needle into the vein and advanced to the right atrium. After the guidewire is observed in the right atrium or inferior vena cava, the sheath dilator set is introduced through the fascia into the subclavian vein. If difficulty is encountered in positioning the sheath dilator into the superior vena cava, a slight backward movement of the guidewire will facilitate this maneuver.

After the dilator is removed, the lead is positioned through the sheath into the right heart, and the sheath is removed and pressure applied while the sheath is torn in half. The guidewire is left in the vascular system so that either a second sheath dilator set may be inserted to position a second lead or a different lead can be chosen if the first one proves to be unsatisfactory for any reason.[12] After one or two leads are inserted, pressure is applied over the area for 5 minutes, or until bleeding has ceased. If a large sheath is used, two leads can be introduced through one sheath, but this seems less preferable than the retained guidewire technique.[13]

One of the most important factors in obtaining subclavian vein puncture is proper positioning of the patient. A vertical roll should be placed between the shoulder blades to cause the shoulders to fall back. The ipsilateral arm is at the patient's side. If the wire or a lead enters the jugular vein, it can be withdrawn and repositioned with the patient's head turned toward the implanting physician.

In 100 attempts at subclavian vein puncture, we encountered five instances in which the subclavian vein could not be entered; in these five instances, two alternatives were used. If a single lead system was to be used, the cephalic vein was dissected. If two leads were needed, the femoral vein was entered by the percutaneous technique, and a sheath introducer set was used to position a catheter in the venous system. This catheter was then placed in the subclavian vein and used for aiming the introducing needle using the biplane fluoroscope. In each case the patient's heavy weight was a factor, and it was necessary to enter the chest at almost a 90° angle to puncture the vein. This technique was successful in each case, and no problems resulted.

In two cases when a lead change was necessary 2 weeks and 5 weeks after an initial implant, the sheath of a standard pacemaker introducer set was advanced over the old lead, which had been stiffened with a stylet. This technique was unsuccessful in one case 9 months after primary implant.

Positioning the Ventricular Lead

Bipolar leads are used exclusively. The leads are then positioned, first in the right ventricle, either using a curved guidewire to direct the lead through the tricuspid valve or by withdrawing a straight wire and forming a loop with the lead in the right atrium that can then be advanced into the right ventricle and straightened using a straight guidewire. These techniques appear to be equally successful. Positioning the right ventricular lead in the apex may cause diaphragmatic stimulation. Positioning the lead approximately one-third to halfway superior on the ventricular septum prevents this problem. It is helpful to allow the ventricular lead to float out into a distal pulmonary artery to confirm that it is not in the coronary sinus before finally positioning it. Transvenous pacing is possible, although more difficult, in patients with systemic venous abnormalities.[14]

Positioning the Atrial Lead

Adult-sized patients (over 50 kg), who have a normal or near normal sized right atrial appendage receive a J-tined lead. The J-tined lead is positioned in the right atrial appendage by retracting the straight stylet, which is used to position it in the mid right atrium. The tip of the J lead usually advances easily into the right atrial appendage. Care is taken that the J lead does not position itself in the ventricular outflow tract, where it may mimic the typical atrial to-and-fro sway on fluoroscopy. A typical lateral rotating motion on anteroposterior fluoroscopy is observed in patients who have not had previous open heart surgery. On lateral fluoroscopy an extreme anterior position is noted (Figs. 19–4 and 19–5). Since the patients are sedated and cannot be asked to take a deep breath, judgment is required in leaving enough extra lead to result in a proper position in both upright and reclining posture. In general, as much lead is introduced as possible to allow for growth in children.

Screw-in leads are positioned using a J-shaped stylet. It is often necessary to tighten

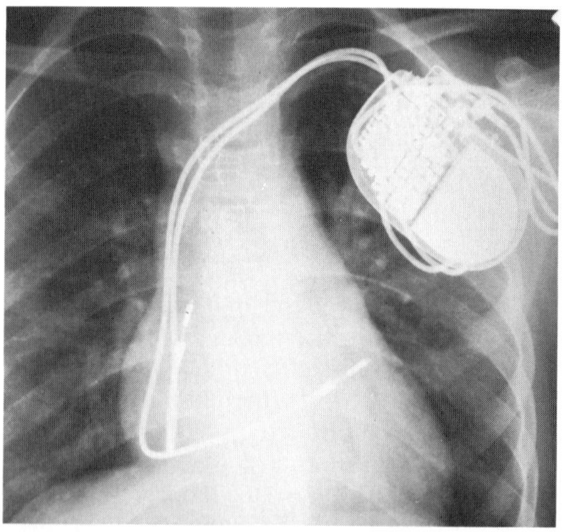

FIGURE 19–4
Demonstration of the position of atrial and ventricular leads in a typical DDD pacemaker implant. The atrial lead has been screwed in to the stump of the right atrial appendage with a generous loop left for growth. The ventricular lead has been screwed in to the mid portion of the ventricular septum, again with room left for growth by pushing the ventricular lead down against the right atrial lateral border. The positioning of the ventricular lead at the right ventricular apex will often lead to diaphragmatic pacing.

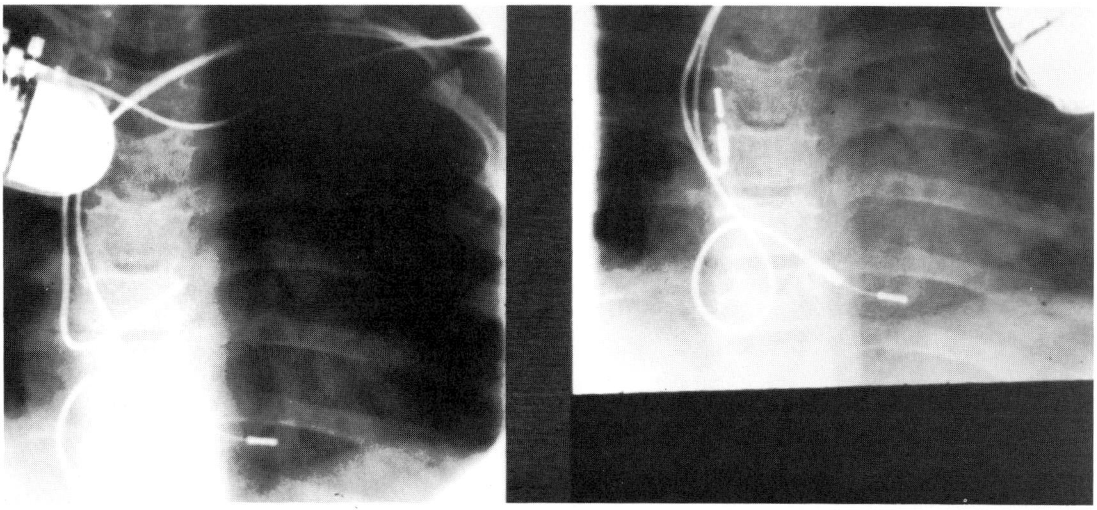

FIGURE 19–5

Incorrect (left) and correct (right) position of an atrial lead. In the figure on the left, the atrial lead has passed through the tricuspid valve and is in the right ventricular outflow tract. In the figure on the right, the ventricular lead has been placed on the bottom third of the ventricular septum with a loop left for growth. The atrial lead is in the correct position in the right atrial appendage. Note that the correct position is higher almost at the superior vena cava, whereas the right ventricular outflow tract position is almost to the ventricular lead.

the stylet in small children. In patients who have had previous open heart surgery, very little rocking motion is seen, probably because the heart is fixed in the pericardium by adhesions. Screw-in leads are also used in patients who have had Mustard or Senning repair for transposition of the great arteries. In these patients, the lead is passed through the superior vena cava–right atrial junction to the anatomic left atrium, which is the functional right atrium in postoperative transposition of the great arteries (Fig. 19–6). The lead is positioned against the roof of the left atrium by gentle traction on the lead and then screwed in. Care must be taken not to position the lead too laterally toward the

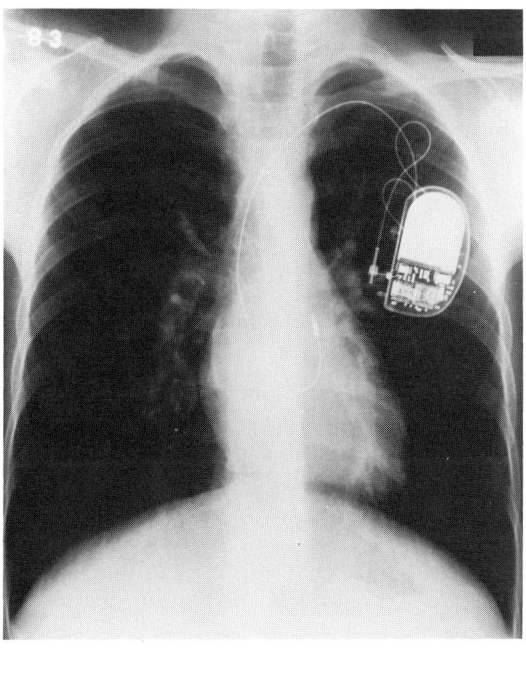

FIGURE 19–6

Demonstration of the correct position of an atrial lead in a patient after Mustard repair of transposition of the great arteries. The lead has been passed through the SVC right atrial junction and screwed into the roof of the left atrium. The tip of the lead is well away from the left heart border where the phrenic nerve runs.

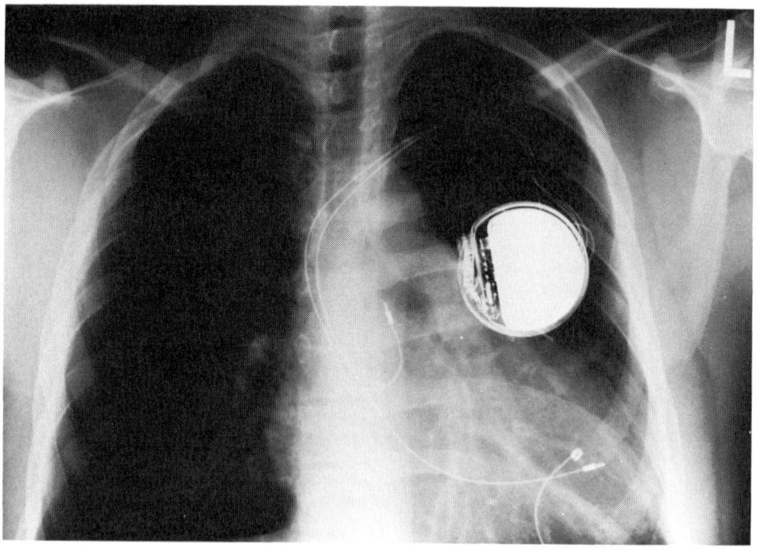

FIGURE 19–7
Demonstration of typical lead positioned in a DDD implant in a patient following repair of transposition of the great arteries. The leads have been passed through the left subclavian vein and positioned in the roof of the left atrium and in the mid third of the left ventricle. An old epicardial lead is seen crossing the endocardial ventricular lead.

base of the left appendage, because one instance of phrenic nerve pacing from this position has occurred. Two patients who had had the Mustard operation were found to have near total obstruction of the superior vena cava–right atrial junction without any residual right atrial appendage; they were not considered to be candidates for transvenous atrial pacing. One patient with partial superior vena cava–right atrial obstruction had angioplasty of this area and was then able to have the lead placed. In patients who have had a Mustard or Senning operation, a catheter is first inserted percutaneously from the groin or from the arm opposite that in which the pacemaker is intended to be implanted in order to search for an appropriate passageway between the superior vena cava and the right atrium. This is done in case it is found that transvenous pacing is unsuitable for this patient, thus avoiding an unnecessary incision.

Dual-chamber pacing may also be used in post Mustard or Senning patients (Fig. 19–7). Screw-in leads are used for both the atrium and ventricle. Two unipolar atrial leads may be used to form a bipolar system (Fig. 19–8).

Atrial pacing is also performed with screw-in electrodes in patients who have undergone the Fontan operation (Fig. 19–9). Often several positions must be tested until one with an adequate P wave and a sufficiently low threshold is found. Transvenous ventricular pacing is not possible after a Fontan operation. Some variations of the Fontan operation also make atrial pacing impossible when a direct end-to-end superior vena cava to pulmonary artery anastomosis is made.

Intraoperative Testing

When the lead is positioned in what is considered to be the optimal position, it is tested for stimulation, threshold, and intrinsic deflection (Figs. 19–10 and 19–11). In some patients (e.g., patients with complete

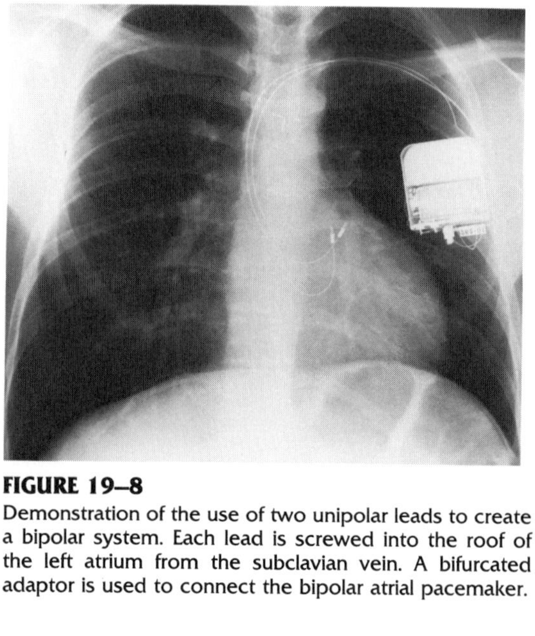

FIGURE 19–8
Demonstration of the use of two unipolar leads to create a bipolar system. Each lead is screwed into the roof of the left atrium from the subclavian vein. A bifurcated adaptor is used to connect the bipolar atrial pacemaker.

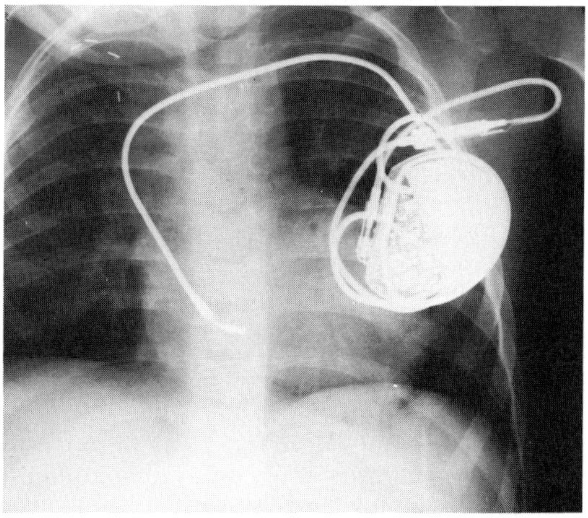

FIGURE 19–9
Demonstration of implant technique in an 18-month-old patient after Fontan repair. The lead has been positioned in the bottom of the right atrium near the usual position of the tricuspid valve. This is a bipolar screw-in lead positioned from the left subclavian vein.

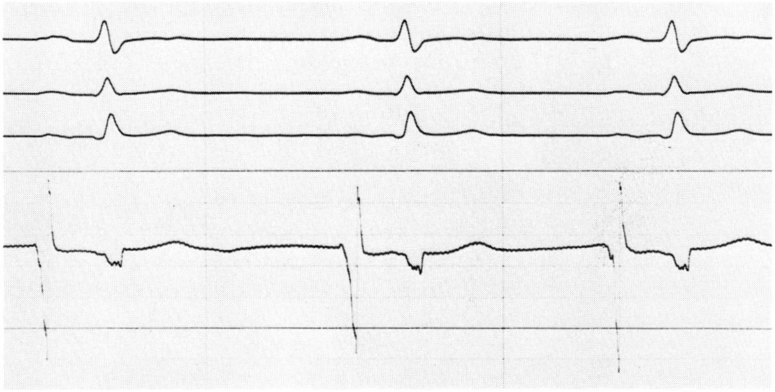

FIGURE 19–10
Surface leads I, II, and III recorded simultaneously with a bipolar atrial electrogram and 1-s time lines. The atrial electrogram is approximately five times larger than the ventricular fire field electrogram recorded from the same lead. This will allow sensitivity settings to sense the atrial depolarization without sensing ventricular depolarization.

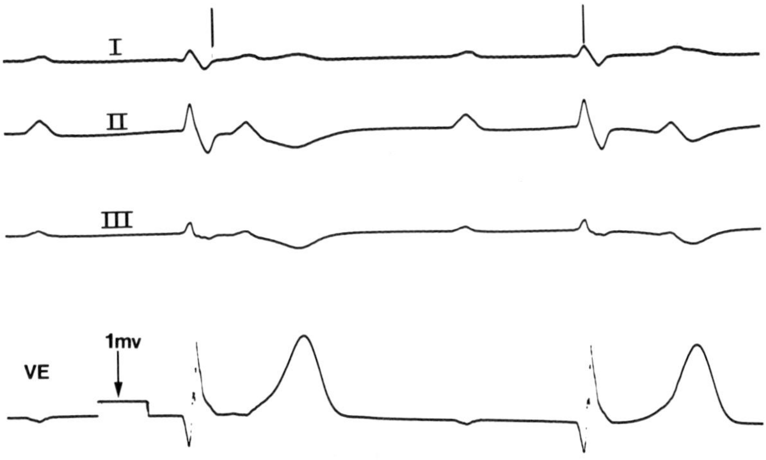

FIGURE 19–11
Surface leads I, II, and III are recorded together with a bipolar ventricular electrogram (1 mV calibration) and 1-s time lines. Ventricular electrogram is approximately 8 mV. Note that the T wave recorded on the ventricular electrogram is as large as the ventricular electrogram itself. The refractory period of the pacemaker will prevent it from sensing the T wave artifact.

atrioventricular (AV) block and sick sinus syndrome) it is difficult to tell if atrial capture is being obtained. In patients with intact AV conduction, atrial capture can be assumed even if P waves cannot be seen, if intrinsic AV conduction results in an increase in QRS rate. The insertion of a temporary atrial electrode catheter from the brachial or femoral vein will enable recording of an atrial electrogram, which then allows determination of the atrial threshold. If it is satisfactory, the lead is sutured into position using absorbable suture around the anchoring sleeve (Fig. 19–12). The pulse generator is tested using the pacing systems analyzer or telemetric programmer and, if satisfactory, is attached to the lead and implanted. The electrocardiogram should then be observed for proper function and the magnet applied if this would show additional function (i.e., for stimulation if the pulse generator is continuously sensing).

The incision is then closed using 2-0 absorbable suture for the muscle and subcutaneous layer and a 4-0 absorbable subcuticular suture for the skin with the knots buried (Fig. 19–13). The skin edges are then further approximated using sterile adhesive strips over benzoin. A nonadhesive pad is then positioned over the sterile adhesive strips, and sterile 4 × 4 gauze dressing and tape are applied.

POSTOPERATIVE CARE

The patient should be monitored in the intensive care unit or telemetry unit for several hours while a chest roentgenogram, ECG, and complete blood count are performed. The prophylactic antibiotic should be continued for 48 hours intravenously. The dressing is removed after 48 hours, and the wound is inspected. The adhesive strips are left in place for 2+ weeks (until they virtually fall off) to obtain the best cosmetic result. The patient is asked to keep the area dry until complete healing has occurred and to report any redness or drainage. The patient may be ambulated and fed on the same day that implantation is performed and dis-

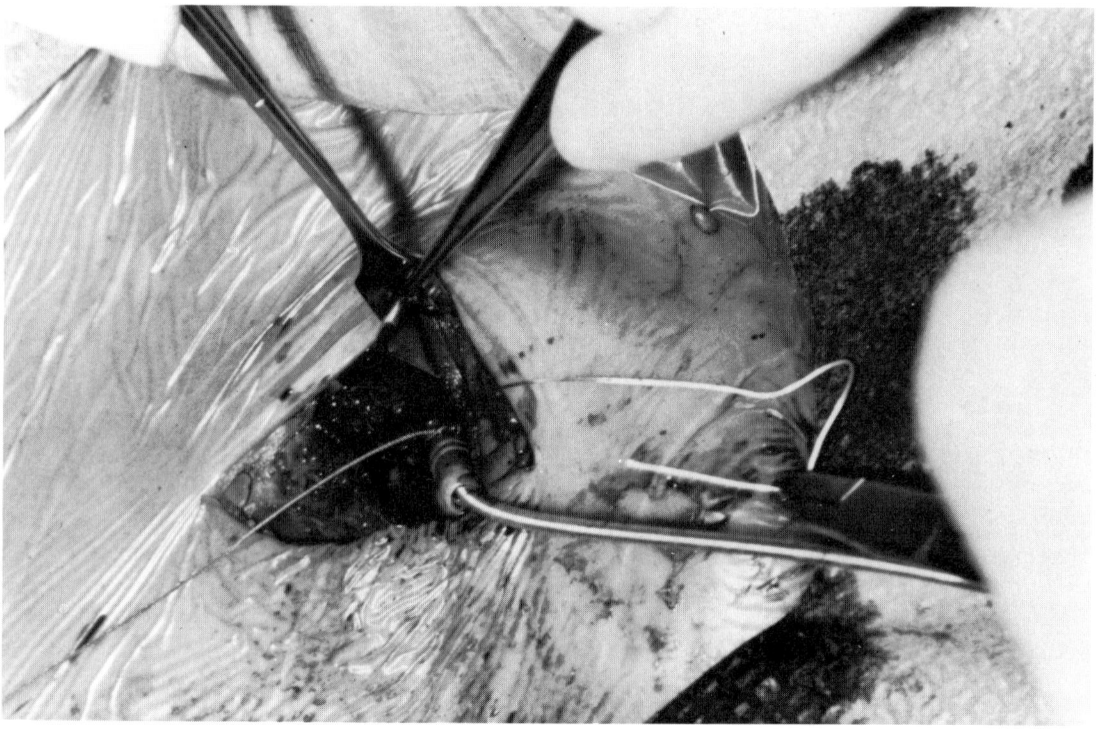

FIGURE 19–12

Demonstration of the technique for tie-down of a single lead that has punctured the subclavian vein under the pectoralis major muscle. The tie-down sleeve can be seen inside the muscle, and a 2-0 absorbable suture has been used to tie the sleeve around the lead to hold the lead in position during the first weeks of implant.

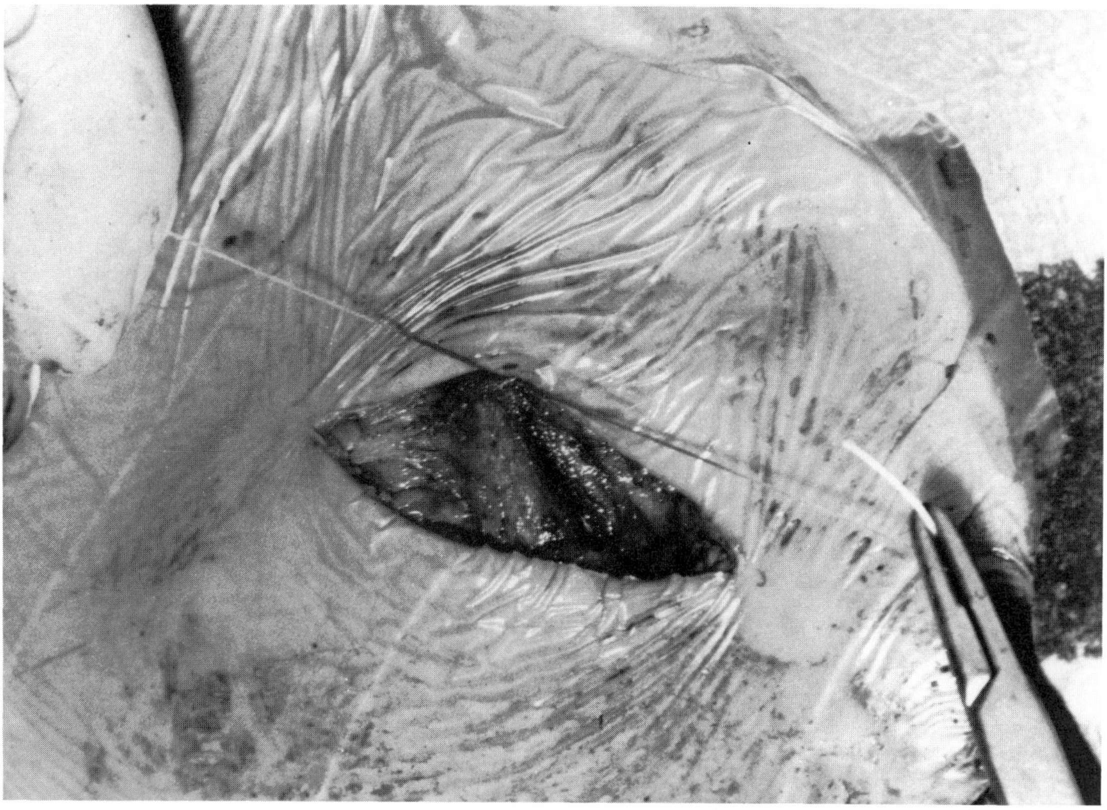

FIGURE 19–13
Demonstration of technique of resuturing the pectoralis major muscle after the pacemaker has been implanted. A running stitch of 2-0 absorbable sutures was used for the pectoralis muscle and for the subcutaneous tissue, whereas a 4-0 absorbable suture on a cutting needle is used to close the skin.

charged in 3 days to be reevaluated in 4 to 6 weeks.

PULSE GENERATORS AND LEADS

Major advances have been made in pulse generator and lead technology. Dual-chamber pulse generators are now smaller than single-chamber pacemakers of several years ago (Fig. 19–14). Thinness has improved markedly (Fig. 19–15), and single-chamber pulse generators have also shrunk markedly (Fig. 19–16). Leads have undergone major improvements in electrode configuration, stabilizing apparatus, insulation, and size. Tines (Fig. 19–17), screws (Fig. 19–18), fins (Fig. 19–18), and other devices are used to hold the leads in place. Various electrode configurations such as grooved and porous tips improve thresholds. Steroids also prevent threshold rise. If a steroid-releasing lead cannot be used, parenteral steroids can be used instead. Bipolar in-line connectors have helped to decrease overall pacemaker size (Fig. 19–19).

COMPLICATIONS

Complications are more likely with the subclavian puncture technique. Hemothorax or hemopericardium have been reported but are rare. Perforation of the right ventricle is less frequent with new lead designs, and when it does occur, it rarely results in cardiac tamponade. Perforation and deformation of the tricuspid valve have been reported but have not seemed to be hemodynamically important.[15] Thrombosis of veins occurs but is only rarely symptomatic.[16, 17] Endocarditis can occur on pacemaker leads, and the lead

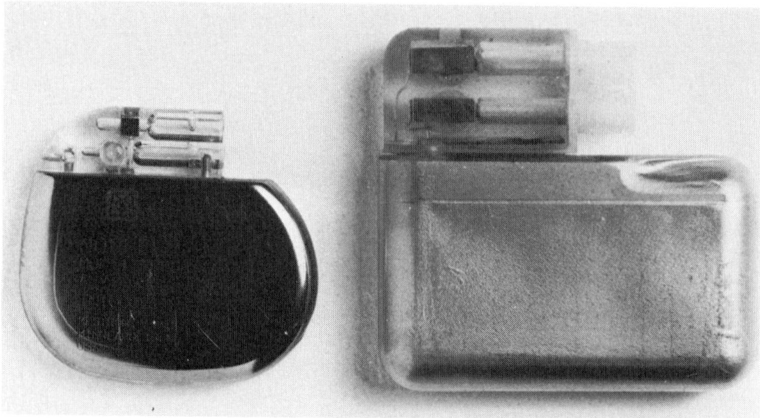

FIGURE 19–14
On the left is a 1980s model dual-chamber DDD pacemaker. On the right is a 1970s model single-chamber rechargeable pacemaker. Note the difference in size, height, and length.

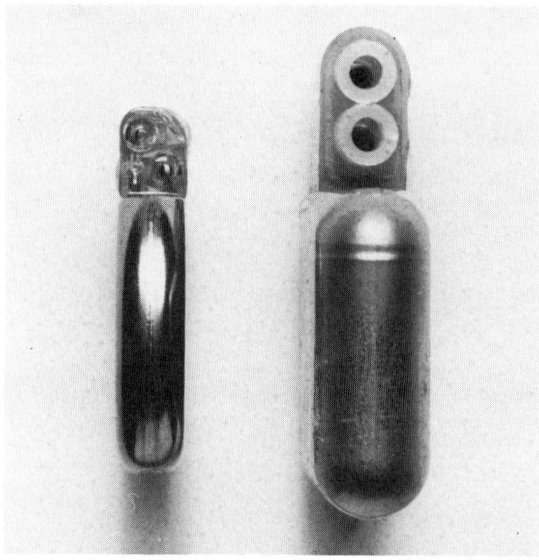

FIGURE 19–15
Demonstration of the thickness of a 1980s model dual-chambered pacemaker and a 1970s model single-chamber bipolar rechargeable pacemaker.

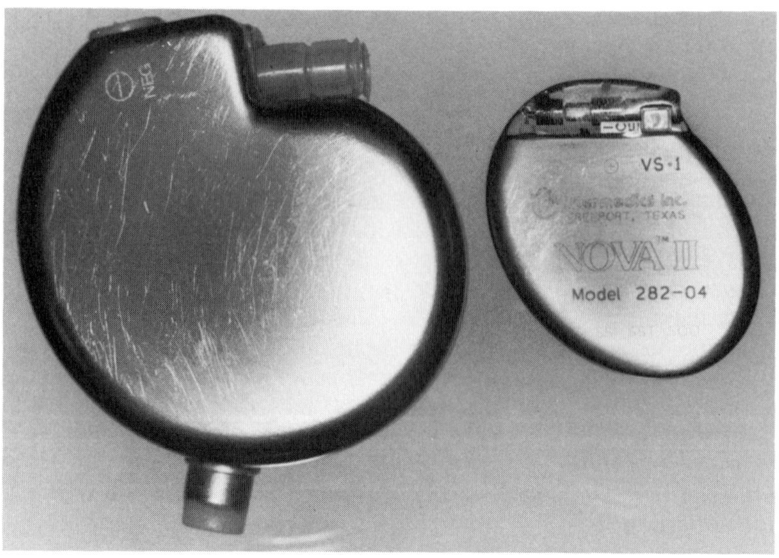

FIGURE 19–16
On the left is a 1960s model bipolar single-chamber pacemaker that is programmable by inserting a Keith needle into the adaptor on the bottom. On the right is a 1980s model single-chamber, multiprogrammable, telemetric bipolar pacemaker.

FIGURE 19–17
Shown is a tined target-tip platinized low-threshold pacing lead manufactured in the 1980s. The dislodgement rate with this lead is extremely low, and thresholds are also almost universally very low.

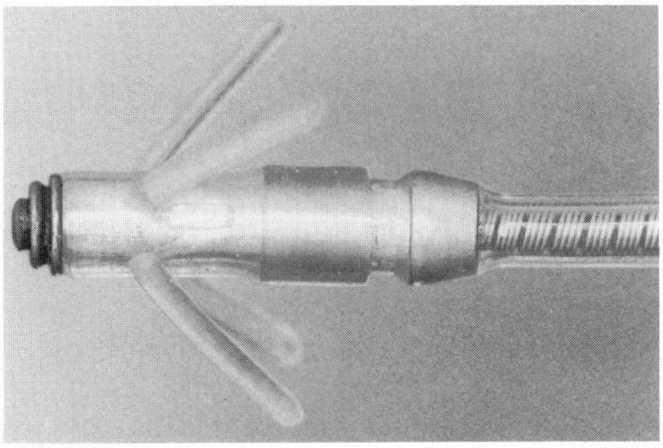

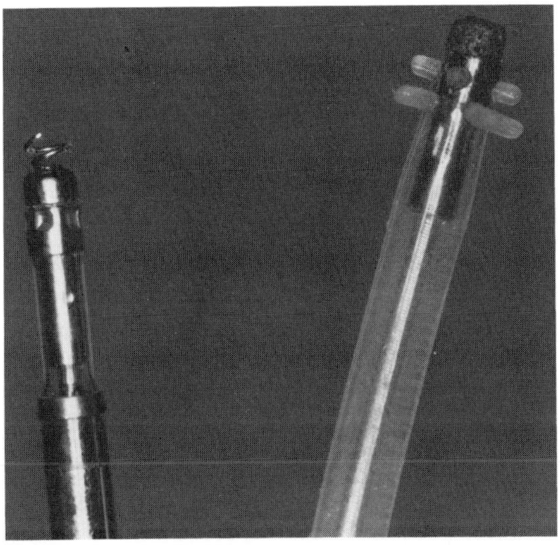

FIGURE 19–18
Left: A bipolar screw-in lead with a fixed screw. Right: A porous-tipped low-threshold lead with short, stubby fixation devices.

FIGURE 19–19
Demonstration of two types of bipolar in-line connectors that are incompatible with each other. Each has functioned very satisfactorily and has resulted in considerably smaller pacemaker headers and pulse generator systems.

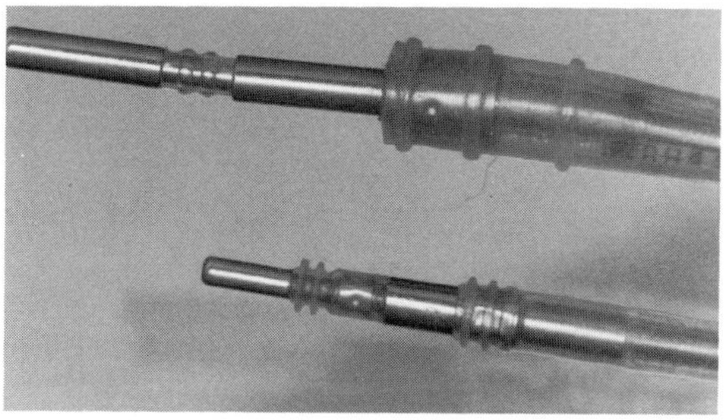

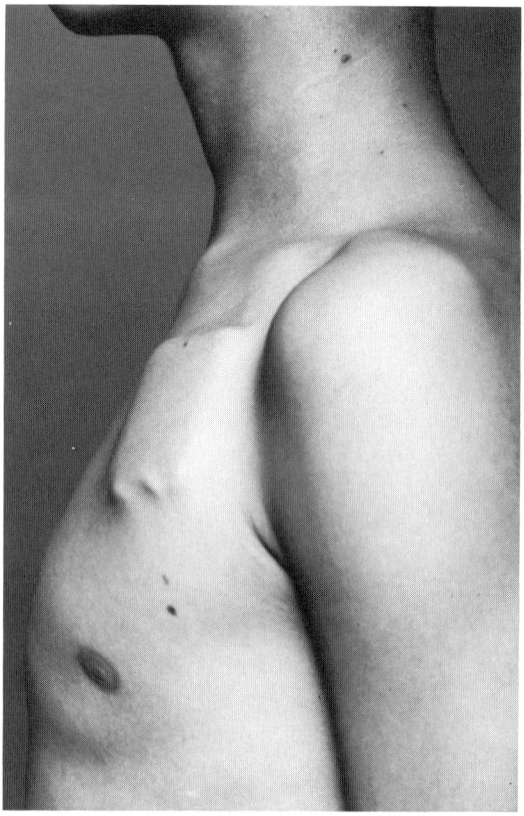

FIGURE 19–20
Demonstration of the cosmetic appearance of a dual-chamber pacemaker implanted in a subcutaneous pocket in a thin 15-year-old boy.

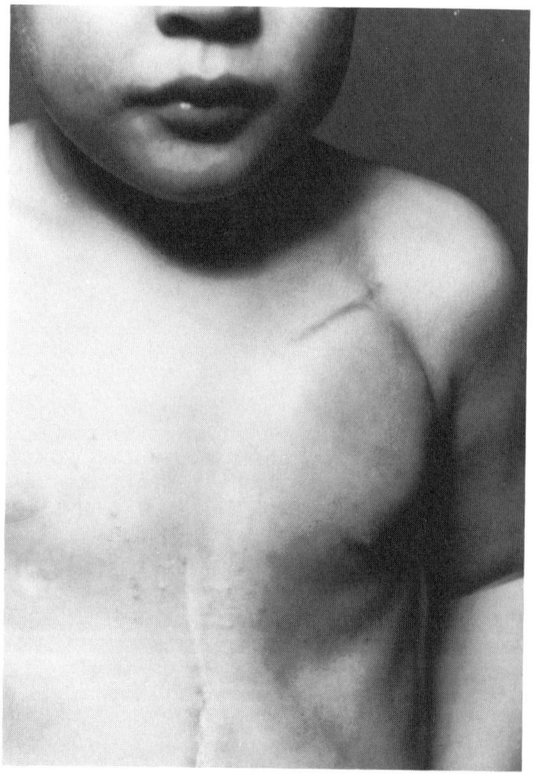

FIGURE 19–21
Demonstration of the cosmetic appearance of a dual-chamber DDD pacemaker implanted in a subpectoral pocket in a 2-year-old child.

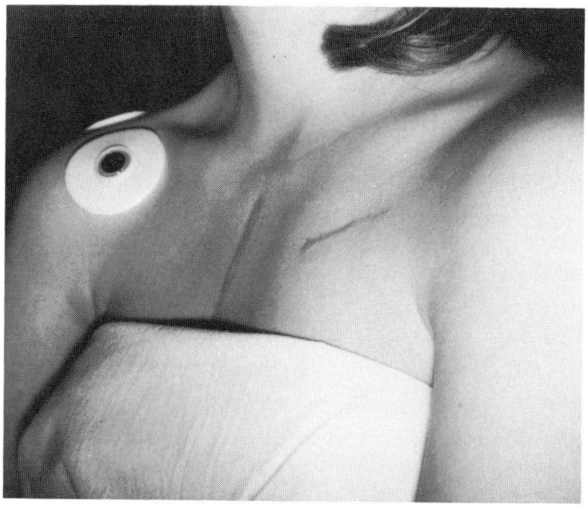

FIGURE 19–22
Demonstration of the cosmetic appearance of a DDD pacemaker implanted in a subpectoral pocket in a 15-year-old girl.

must then be removed to effect a cure.[18] The removal of tined leads is difficult, and open heart surgery may sometimes be necessary. Erosion or frank infection of the pacemaker pocket occurs in a small percentage of patients, and again, the pacemaker must be removed to cure the infection. Constrictive pericarditis has been reported once after transvenous pacemaker implant.[19]

COSMETIC APPEARANCE

Great care must be taken to maximize the cosmetic result. Teenagers are particularly aware of their appearance. Formerly, large, square subcutaneous pulse generators were unsightly and easily suffered erosion (Fig. 19–20). The use of a subpectoral pocket has improved the cosmetic result and further protected the pulse generator from trauma and infection. This is particularly true in toddlers (Fig. 19–21) but is also important in teenagers (Fig. 19–22).

RESULTS

The results of transvenous and epicardial pacemakers are discussed in chapter 18. Two

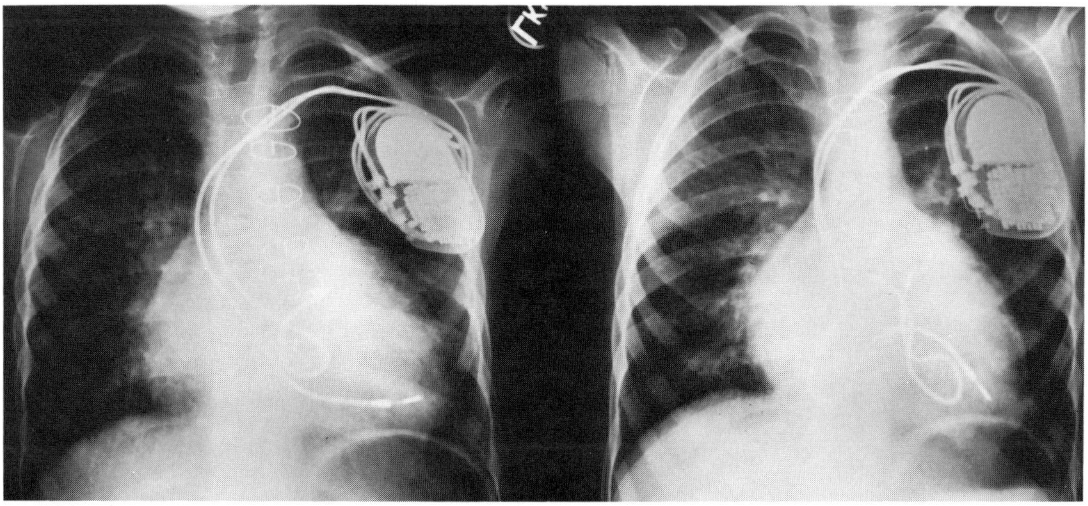

FIGURE 19–23
Inward lead migration in a patient who had implantation of a DDD pacemaker at age 4 years after tricuspid valve replacement following repair of D-transposition of the great arteries. Both atrial and ventricular leads have migrated significantly inward without causing any clinical problems over a 2-year period.

points deserve discussion here: venous thrombosis and growth. Using venous plethysmography, two-dimensional echocardiography, Doppler ultrasound, and venous angiography, we found no evidence of subclinical thrombosis in 20 children studied. Most patients had two bipolar leads. Lead stretching and dislodgment seem to be minimal problems with growth. Using absorbable suture for the tie down, we have not had to advance a lead; in fact, some leads seem to advance themselves (Fig. 19–23). Transvenous pacing continues to be the approach of choice in infants and children weighing more than 10 kg.

References

1. Furman S, Schwedel JB, Escher DJW: Use of an intracardiac pacemaker for Stokes-Adams seizures. N Engl J Med 261:943, 1959.
2. Parsonnet V, Furman S, Smyth NPD, et al: Optimal resources for implantable cardiac pacemakers. Circulation 68:227A–244A, 1983.
3. Muers MF, Arnold AG, Sleight P: Prophylactic antibiotics for cardiac pacemaker implantation. Br Heart J 46:539–544, 1981.
4. Kosowsky BD, Mufti SI, Grewal GS, et al: Effect of local lidocaine anesthesia on ventricular escape intervals during permanent pacemaker implantation in patients with complete heart block. Am J Cardiol 51:101–104, 1983.
5. Furman S, Fisher JD: Appraisal and reappraisal of cardiac therapy. Am Heart J 94:250–259, 1977.
6. Hawthrone WJ, Austen WG, Corning H, et al: Permanent endocardial pacing in complete heart block. Ann Intern Med 66:831, 1967.
7. Arnold AG: Permanent cardiac pacing using anterior pectoral veins. Br Heart J 43:321–324, 1980.
8. Littleford PO, Parsonnet V, Spector SD: Method for the rapid and atraumatic insertion of permanent endocardial pacemaker electrodes through the subclavian vein. Am J Cardiol 43:980–982, 1979.
9. Miller FA, Holmes DR, Gersh BJ, et al: Permanent transvenous pacemaker implantation via the subclavian vein. Mayo Clin Proc 55:309–314, 1980.
10. Damos DA, Mucha P Jr, van Heerdan JA: Subclavian vein. Mayo Clin Proc 55:315–321, 1980.
11. McGoon MD, Maloney JD, McGoon DC, et al: Long-term endocardial atrial pacing in children with postoperative bradycardia-tachycardia syndrome and limited ventricular access. Am J Cardiol 49:1750–1757, 1982.
12. Belott PH: Retaining guidewire, introducer technique for unlimited access to the central circulation: A review. Clin Prog Pacing Electrophysiol 1:59–69, 1983.
13. Bognolo DA, Vihayanagar R, Eckstein PF, et al: Two leads in one introducer technique for AV sequential implantation. PACE 5:217–221, 1982.
14. Ronnevik PK, Abrahamsen AM, Tollefsen I: Transvenous pacemaker implantation via a unilateral left superior vena cava. PACE 5:808–813, 1982.
15. Isnr JM: The pathology of pacemakers. Intell Rep Cardiac Pacing Electrophysiol 2:2–6, 1983.
16. Deanfield JE, Fox KM, Allison DJ: Facial swelling: A complication of transvenous pacing. Clin Cardiol 5:308–309, 1982.
17. Kenney EL, Allen RP, Weidner WA, et al: Recurrent pulmonary emboli secondary to right thrombus around a permanent pacing catheter: A case report and review of the literature. PACE 2:196–202, 1979.
18. Bichhorn EJ, Winters WL, Crawford ES, et al: Bacterial endocarditis and right atrial vegetation. JAMA 246:2724–2725, 1981.
19. Foster CJ: Constrictive pericarditis complicating an endocardial pacemaker. Br Heart J 47:497–499, 1982.

CHAPTER 20

EPICARDIAL PACEMAKER IMPLANTATION

David A. Ott

Artificial pacing via the so-called epicardial approach (actually myocardial) is preferable in some children for a variety of reasons.[1, 2] Patients weighing less than 30 to 40 pounds in general are not good candidates for pervenous pacing because of size limitations. In addition, locating the pacemaker pulse generator in a pocket beneath the left rectus abdominus muscle via the subxyphoid approach is cosmetically superior and allows unencumbered motion of the torso, whereas a pacemaker in the subclavicular location may be cumbersome, depending on individual activity levels. The primary disadvantage of epicardial pacing is that it requires general anesthesia for initial placement and is associated with a small but significant incidence of post-pericardiotomy syndrome. Conversely, epicardial pacing avoids the small but potential risk of endocarditis, embolization, or perforation inherent with endocardial pacing. Originally epicardial pacing was accomplished through a thoracotomy incision, which is described herein.[3–18] This technique is generally of historic interest only. Since beginning the subxyphoid technique of dual-chamber physiologic DDD pacing, we rarely have occasion to require thoracotomy for pacemaker implantation.[19–23]

ELECTRODES AND MODE OF PACING

Both unipolar and bipolar systems are available. At the current state of pacemaker technology, however, bipolar pacing offers no real advantages over simple unipolar pacing. Both systems provide cathode (negative terminal) pacing, because this provides slightly lower pacing thresholds and electrolytic corrosion is less at the cathode. Experimentally there is slightly less possibility of inducing ventricular tachycardia or fibrillation with cathode terminal pacing.

In unipolar pacing systems the body of the pulse generator functions as the indifferent electrode, and only one lead is placed on the heart. The unit itself is smaller, a fact of some significance in small children.

The unipolar configuration can sense smaller electrical potentials; thus it has the advantage of increased sensitivity, but the disadvantage of being more susceptible to external electrical interference. This problem has been circumvented by an encapsulated design that provides additional interference shielding. Current state-of-the-art pacemakers are not susceptible to interference from microwave ovens, electric razors, or other sources of interference. Unipolar lead configurations generate large pacing spikes owing to the greater distance between electrodes; this is advantageous for transtelephonic monitoring, but may confuse other monitoring systems and interfere with electrocardiographic interpretation. Spike size can be reduced for monitoring purposes by choosing electrocardiographic electrode sites at right angles to the pacemaker electrode field (generally lead I).

Neither epicardial nor endocardial pacing is clearly superior for ventricular pacing and sensing thresholds. Pervenous endocardial pacing, however, is slightly superior in providing long-term dependable sensing at the atrial level, particularly in postoperative patients who have some element of epicardial fibrosis.[24–29] The Medtronic 4951 fishhook-type lead* has proven to be an efficient lead for atrial pacing and may be implanted high on the right atrium via the subxyphoid approach, thus eliminating the need for thoracotomy (Fig. 20–1). Newly developed variations of this lead impregnated with steroids may result in resolution of atrial lead sensing problems. Ventricular pacing is efficiently accomplished with screw-in leads, which have a corkscrew configuration penetrating either 5.5 mm (three-turn model) or 3.5 mm (two-turn model) into the ventricular myocardium.[30–32]

THORACOTOMY TECHNIQUE

The thoracotomy approach requires entry into the pleural cavity through a short anterior incision in the fourth, fifth, or sixth interspace, dividing the serratus anterior muscle but sparing the more posteriorly located latissimus dorsi muscle (Fig. 20–2). The pericardium is opened longitudinally anterior to the phrenic nerve, and a screw-in lead is implanted in the anterolateral or posterolateral surface of the left ventricle, avoiding areas of epicardial fat and blood vessels. Care must be taken to avoid placement of the lead near the course of the phrenic nerve in order to preclude troublesome diaphragmatic pacing. In some cases it may be necessary to displace the nerve posteriorly or anteriorly to prevent this complication. If a bipolar system is desired, the leads should be placed 2.5 cm to 3 cm apart to ensure satisfactory myocardial stimulation. The lead is tunneled through the costophrenic angle anteriorly and connected to the generator through a separate short subcostal incision, placing the unit beneath the rectus abdominus muscle or more laterally between the external and internal oblique muscles. Sufficient slack must be maintained in the lead to avoid tension and allow for growth.

The thoracotomy approach may also be used for implantation of epicardial atrial pacemaker leads. This can be accomplished from either the left or right sides. If bipolar leads are used for atrial pacing, they should be placed 1 cm to 2 cm apart near the base of the right atrial appendage in the area of the sinus node or at the base of the left atrial appendage just above the circumflex coronary artery.

*Medtronic, Minneapolis, Minnesota.

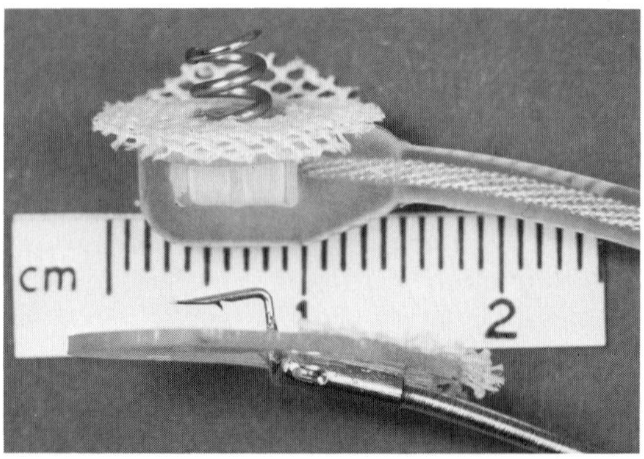

FIGURE 20–1
Electrodes used for implantation on the epicardial surface of the heart. Fishhook-type lead (Medtronic 4951) is used for atrial or ventricular pacing. Two- or three-turn screw-in leads (various manufacturers) are used for ventricular pacing.

SUBXYPHOID TECHNIQUE

The subxyphoid approach to the ventricle provides a rapid, safe, and efficient means of implanting a lead directly on the epicardial surface of the right or left ventricle or right atrium with minimal postoperative morbidity and a significant cosmetic advantage (Fig. 20–3). One small incision is required, no muscle fibers are cut, and entrance into the pleural cavity is avoided. We therefore prefer this approach for all epicardial unipolar ventricular and atrial pacemaker configurations.

A short upper midline or left subcostal incision is made, and the anterior fascia of the left rectus muscle is isolated immediately below the costal margin. This fascia is divided transversely or longitudinally near the midline. The upper rectus muscle is split in the direction of its fibers, or it may be retracted laterally, exposing the origin of the posterior rectus fascia at the left costal margin and xyphoid process of the sternum. The division of this fascia at the costal margin exposes the prepericardial fat immediately above the diaphragm. A transverse incision in the pericardium at its junction with the diaphragm exposes the marginal portion of the right ventricle. Retraction of the costal margin by the surgical assistant and of the heart by the surgeon using ring forceps or another device exposes the inferior surface of the left ven-

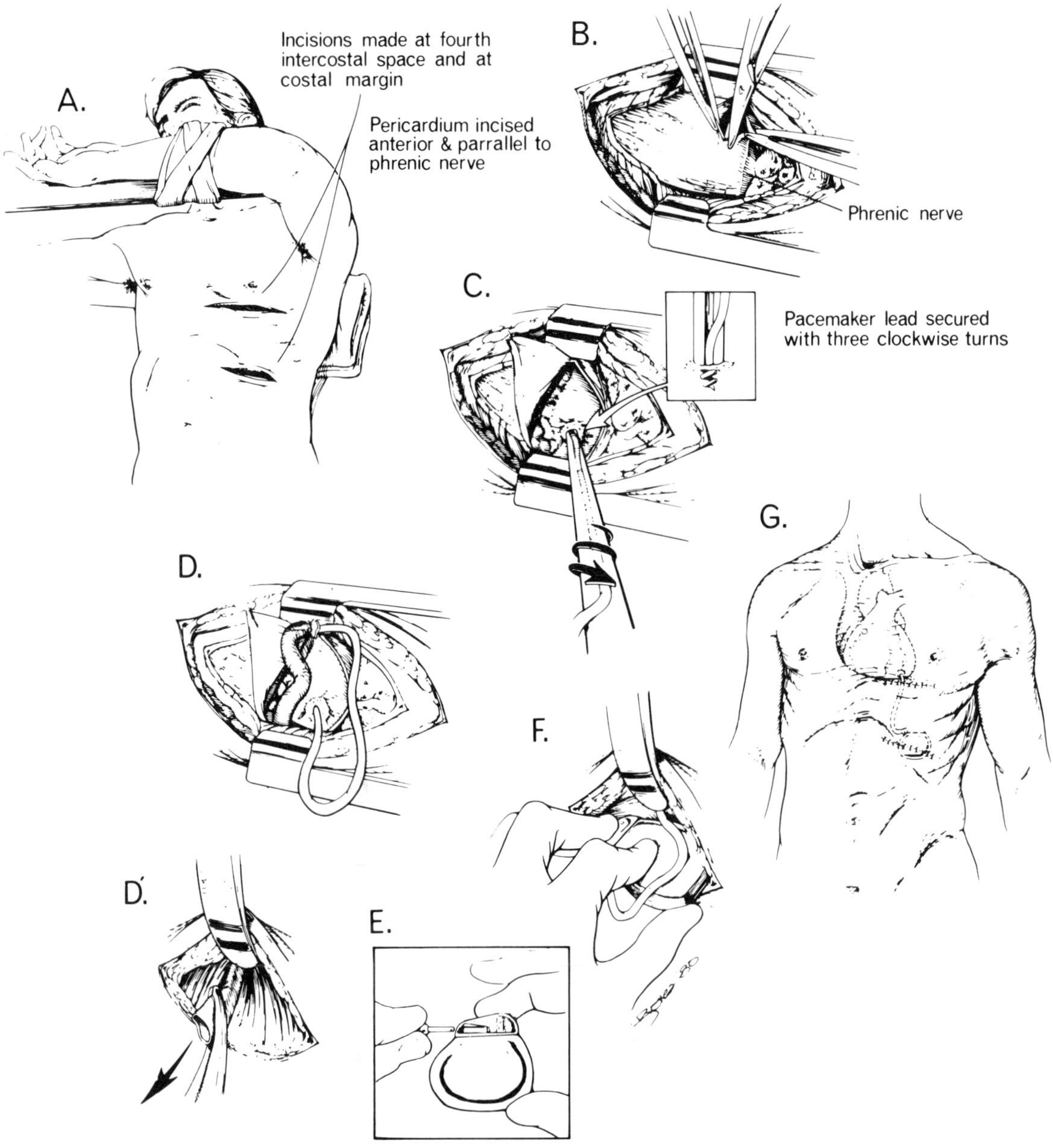

FIGURE 20–2
Thoracotomy approach for pacemaker insertion. *(A)* Incision. *(B)* Pericardium incised. *(C)* Lead implantation. *(D)* Lead tunneled to abdomen. *(E)* Attachment of lead to pulse generator. *(F)* Placement of generator into pocket. *(G)* System in place.

tricle lateral to the posterior descending vein. A headlight with focused illumination and surgical magnifying loops are useful at this point. A standard two-turn or three-turn electrode is implanted on the diaphragmatic surface of the left ventricle away from the phrenic nerve. The thin apex of the left ventricle should be avoided, since it is prone to perforation. An atrial lead can also be placed on the lateral wall of the right atrium if indicated. For this purpose, the fishhook-type, self-retaining lead is required because of the difficulty in exposure and the thin wall of the atrium. Anchoring the lead with suture is indicated, if possible. Following placement of the leads, the lead wire is looped gently and connected to the pulse generator, which is placed in a pocket posterior to the upper rectus muscle fibers but anterior to the posterior rectus fascia. Migration of the generator is thus prevented, and the pacemaker is usually not visible from the surface.

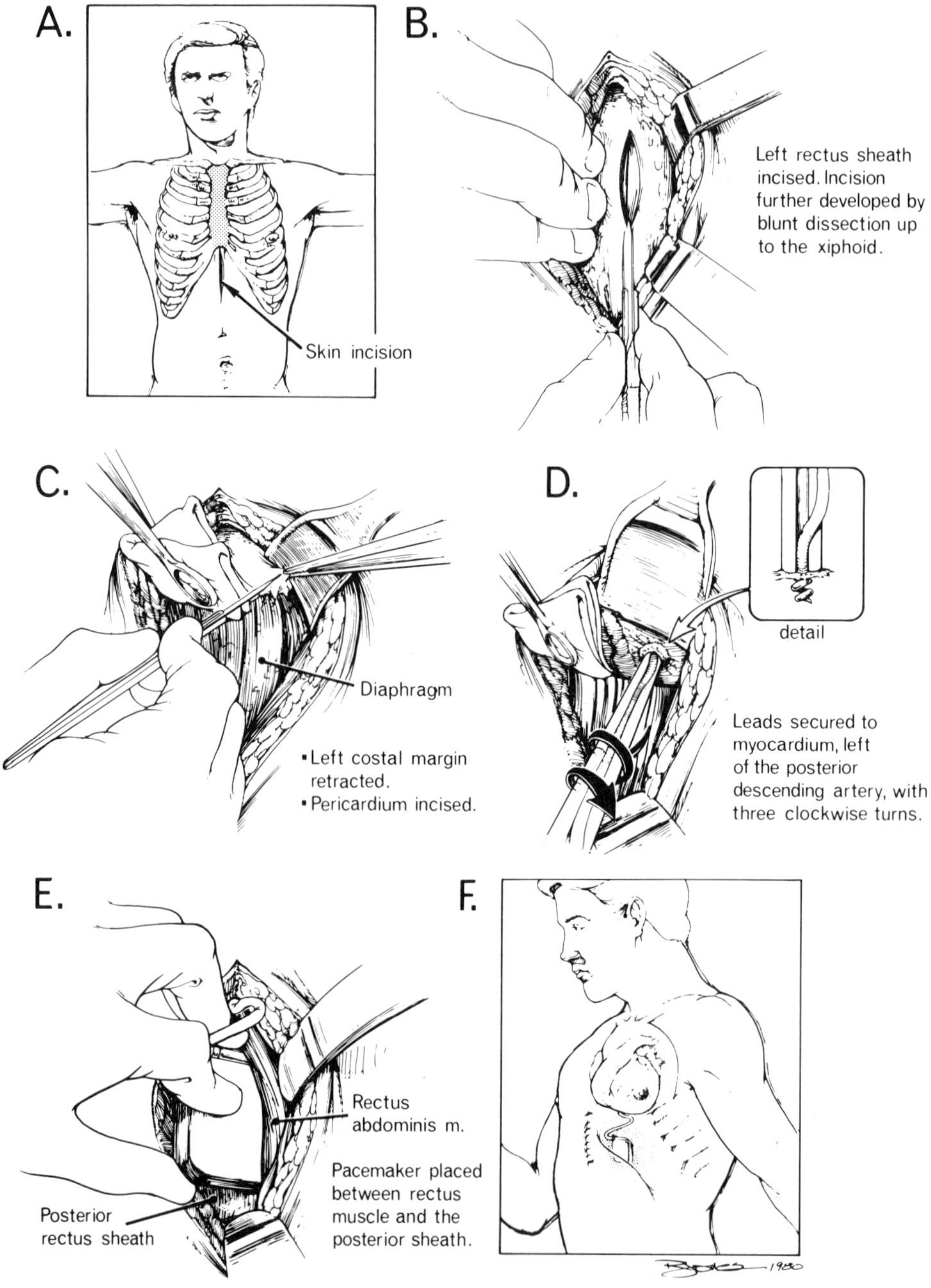

FIGURE 20–3

Subxiphoid approach for pacemaker implantation. Both atrial and ventricular leads may be implanted by this method. *(A)* Incision. *(B)* Division of rectus sheath. *(C)* Retraction of rectus with exposure and incision of pericardium. *(D)* Lead insertion. *(E)* Pulse generator placed into pocket. *(F)* System in place.

References

1. Meyer JA, Miller K: Perforation of the right ventricle by electrode catheters: A review and report of nine cases. Ann Surg 168:1048–1060, 1968.
2. Kaulbach MG, Krukonis EE: Pacemaker electrode-induced thrombosis in the superior vena cava with pulmonary embolization: A complication of pervenous pacing. Am J Cardiol 26:205–207, 1970.
3. Chardack WM, Gage AA, Greatbatch W: A transistorized, self-contained, implantable pacemaker for the long term correction of complete heart block. Surgery 48:643, 1960.
4. Weirich WL, Gott V, Lillehei CW: Treatment of complete heartblock by combined use of myocardial electrode and artificial pacemaker. Surg Forum 3(360), 1957.
5. Amato JJ, Payne DD, Rheinlander HF, et al; Intermuscular abdominal implantation of permanent pacemakers in infants and children. Ann Thorac Surg 25:243, 1978.
6. Culliford AT, Isom OW, Doyle E: Pacemaker implantation in the extremely young: A safe and cosmetic approach. J Thorac Cardiovasc Surg 75:763, 1978.
7. Donahoo JS, Haller JA, Zonnebelt S, et al: Permanent cardiac pacemakers in children: Technical considerations. Ann Thorac Surg 22:584, 1976.
8. Idriss FS, Otto R, Nikaidoh H, et al: Implantation of permanent pacemakers in the first month of life for congenital heart block. J Thorac Cardiovasc Surg 65:851, 1973.
9. Lynch MF, Jensen NK, Urdaneta L: Permanent cardiac pacemakers implanted in the pleural space. J Thorac Cardiovasc Surg 76:101, 1979.
10. Salama FD: A suggested site for the implantation of myocardial pacemakers in infants and young children. Thorax 31:346, 1976.
11. Shearin RPN, Fleming WH: Fourteen years of implanted pacemakers in children. Ann Thorac Surg 25:144, 1978.
12. Williams GD, Campbell GS: Pacemaker installation in the pediatric patient: an improved technique. Surgery 66:412, 1969.
13. Lajos TZ, Wanka J: Epicardial atrial pacing. Ann Thorac Surg 25:64, 1978.
14. Mulder DG, Frank CG: Epicardial pacemaker implantation for complete heart block. Ann Thorac Surg 6:424, 1968.
15. Chardack WM, Gage AA, Federico AJ, et al: The long-term treatment of heart block. Progr Cardiovasc Dis 9:105, 1966.
16. Furman S, Escher DJ, Solomon N: Experiences with myocardial and transvenous implanted cardiac pacemakers. Am J Cardiol 23:66, 1969.
17. Tyers GFO, Hughes HC Jr, Torman HA, et al: The advantages of transthoracic placement of permanent cardiac pacemaker electrodes. J Thorac Cardiovasc Surg 69:8, 1975.
18. Harthorne JW, DeSanctis RW, Sulit YQ, et al: Epicardial versus endocardial pacemakers: Analysis of 109 cases. Ann Thorac Surg 6:417, 1968.
19. Ott DA, Gillette PC, Cooley DA: Atrial pacing via the subxyphoid approach. Texas Heart Inst J 9:149–152, 1982.
20. Ott DA, Gillette PC: Epicardial approach to cardiac pacing. In Gillette PC, Griffin J (eds): A Practical Guide to Cardiac Pacing. Baltimore, Williams & Wilkins, 1986.
21. Stewart S: Placement of the sutureless epicardial pacemaker lead by the subxyphoid approach. Ann Thorac Surg 18:308, 1974.
22. Parsonnet V, Gilbert L, Zucker IR, et al: Subcostal, transdiaphragmatic insertion of a cardiac pacemaker. J Thorac Cardiovasc Surg 49:739, 1965.
23. DeLeon SY, Llbawi MN, Idriss FS: Pacemaker implantation in infants and children: A simplified approach. Ann Thorac Surg 30:599–601, 1980.
24. Overdijk AD, Dekker E: Comparison of thresholds in epicardial and endocardial stimulation of the human heart by chronically implanted pacemaker electrodes. Am Heart J 77:172, 1969.
25. Mansour KA, Dorney ER, Tyras DH, et al: Cardiac pacemakers: Comparing epicardial and pervenous pacing. Geriatrics 3:151–155, 1973.
26. Gillette PC, Garson A, Shannon C: Cardiac pacing in children and young adults. Clin Prog Pacing Electrophysiol 1(2):156–165, 1983.
27. Gillette PC, Garson A, Burns G, et al: Permanent pacemaker treatment of the sick sinus syndrome in pediatric patients (Abstract). Proc N Am Soc Pacing Electrophysiol 2:105, 1980.
28. Henglein D, Gillette PC, Shannon C, et al: Long-term follow-up of pulse width threshold of transvenous and myo-epicardial leads. PACE 7:203–214, 1984.
29. Gillette PC, Shannon C, Garson A, et al: Pacemaker treatment of sick sinus syndrome in children. J Am Coll Cardiol 1(5):1325-1329, 1983.
30. Mansour KA, Fleming WH, Hatcher CR Jr; Initial experience with a sutureless screw-in electrode for cardiac pacing. Ann Thorac Surg 16:127–135, 1973.
31. Mansour KA, Miller JI, Symbas PN, et al: Further evaluation of the sutureless, screw-in electrode for cardiac pacing: Experience with 300 implantations. J Thorac Cardiovasc Surg 77:858, 1979.
32. Hoitsma HFW, Defeyter PJ, Van Mourik JC, et al: First results obtained with an epicardial screw-in electrode. Ach Chirurg Neerland 29:47–54, 1977.

CHAPTER 21

SURGICAL TREATMENT OF TACHYARRHYTHMIAS

David A. Ott, Denton A. Cooley & Fred A. Crawford

Rapid advances in technology, including electrophysiologic mapping and open heart surgical techniques, have made possible the precise diagnosis, anatomic localization and surgical correction of cardiac arrhythmias.[1–9] Definitive surgical ablative procedures have been developed that can effect a cure of most types of cardiac tachyarrhythmias. Common to each of the procedures is intraoperative electrophysiologic confirmation of preoperative studies and surgical division or cryoablation of accessory pathways or ectopic foci. Surgical experience in the treatment of tachyarrhythmias in children has been limited to a few institutions, where it has been demonstrated that some types of tachyarrhythmias are relatively more common in infants and children; these include atrial ectopic tachycardias, ventricular tachycardia after repair of congenital heart defects, arrhythmogenic right ventricular dysplasia, and an unusual form of lethal ventricular tachycardia occurring exclusively in infants and associated with microscopic hamartomatous changes.[10–13]

Discussion of the various forms of surgically treatable tachyarrhythmias is conveniently approached in a combined anatomic and electrophysiologic manner.

SUPRAVENTRICULAR TACHYCARDIA CAUSED BY ACCESSORY PATHWAYS

Historical Aspects

In 1893, Kent, who was a pathologist, first described an unusual histologic structure that resembled a right anterior atrioventricular node.[4] In 1930, Wolff, Parkinson, and White described the clinical syndrome of supraventricular tachycardia associated with a delta wave on surface electrocardiogram in sinus rhythm.[4] Two years later, Holzman and Scherf suggested the possible connection between Kent bundles and Wolff-Parkinson-White syndrome,[4] and in 1943, Wood demonstrated histologically the presence of a Kent bundle in a patient with Wolff-Parkinson-White syndrome.[4] Burchell et al in 1967 made the first surgical attempt to ablate a Kent bundle pathway by injecting procaine into an area of myocardium localized by electrophysiologic mapping.[14] In 1968 Cobb et al first succeeded in isolating and dividing a Kent bundle surgically, resulting in a cure of the patient's tachycardia.[15] This historic operation was performed by mobilizing the right coronary artery and dividing the bundle by incision on the epicardial surface of the heart below the tricuspid annulus. Further experience by Sealy et al and others demonstrated that the most precise and predictable division of accessory pathways was achieved by making an endocardial incision immediately above the tricuspid or mitral value annulus.[16–24] The primary experience in the surgical treatment of tachyarrhythmias in the pediatric group has been reported by Ott, Cooley, Garson, Gillette, and others.[10, 11]

Indications for Surgical Intervention

Several types of patients may be considered candidates for surgical correction of tachycardia.[26–30] Those patients with recurrent, intractable, and incapacitating episodes of tachycardia despite an adequate medical regimen should be considered for surgical referral. The accessory pathway forms of tachycardia occurring after infancy generally do not resolve spontaneously, and thus these patients face a lifetime of medical treatment that may vary in effectiveness and is at best inconvenient in the pediatric age group and may be associated with significant side effects or problems with compliance. Therefore the prospect of a surgical cure is particularly appealing for children.

A second group of patients for whom referral for definitive surgery is appropriate are those with potentially life threatening supraventricular tachycardia, including those with a history of atrial fibrillation with a rapid ventricular response or those with cardiovascular collapse associated with the tachycardia. Patients who exhibit a rapid ventricular response (>250 bpm) to atrial pacing, atrial flutter, or atrial fibrillation, or in whom the effective refractory period of the anomalous pathway is short (<220 ms) have an increased risk of sudden death during tachycardia and should be considered for surgical treatment whether or not the arrhythmia is incapacitating.

Patients requiring surgical correction of other congenital heart defects and who also have accessory pathways of preexcitation should undergo operative mapping and division of the pathway at the time of intracardiac repair. Patients with Ebstein's anomaly of the tricuspid valve are the most common group in this category.[31–33] An unexplained but definite association exists between Ebstein's anomaly and Wolff-Parkinson-White syndrome, with 5% to 25% of patients with Ebstein's anomaly exhibiting the electrophysiologic abnormalities of the Wolff-Parkinson-White syndrome. Tachyarrhythmias in these patients may be life threatening.

Operative Mapping and Surgical Technique

Successful operative treatment of patients with accessory pathways requires close cooperation between surgeons, electrophysiologists, and technicians experienced in the electrophysiologic localization of the pathways and the technique for their safe and effective surgical ablation. A team effort between surgeon and cardiologist is extremely important in this area of cardiac surgery. By combining data for preoperative electrophysiologic studies performed in the cardiac catheterization laboratory with intraoperative epicardial and endocardial mapping, the surgeon and electrophysiologist can accurately locate one or more accessory pathways as they cross the atrioventricular groove. Intraoperative mapping confirms the results of preoperative studies, further localizes the precise location of the pathway, and finally, is used to assess the surgical result before termination of the procedure. Catheterization mapping is important, since evidence of Kent bundle conduction may occasionally be absent during operation, and supraventricular tachycardia may be difficult to induce. It is also important to do intraoperative mapping, because antegrade mapping of the ventricle is more accurate, and because multiple pathways may be more apparent in the operating room since mapping of the entire heart can be accomplished in a short period of time, thus making subtle pathways more obvious.

The operation is performed through a median sternotomy and requires cardiopulmonary bypass in most cases. Bipolar electrodes for both pacing and sensing are placed on the atrium and ventricles. Simplified clip-on leads have been developed for this purpose (Fig. 21–1). A mobile hand-held sensing probe is used to determine the site of earliest depolarization on the ventricular side of the annulus during atrial pacing and on the atrial side of the annulus during ventricular pacing

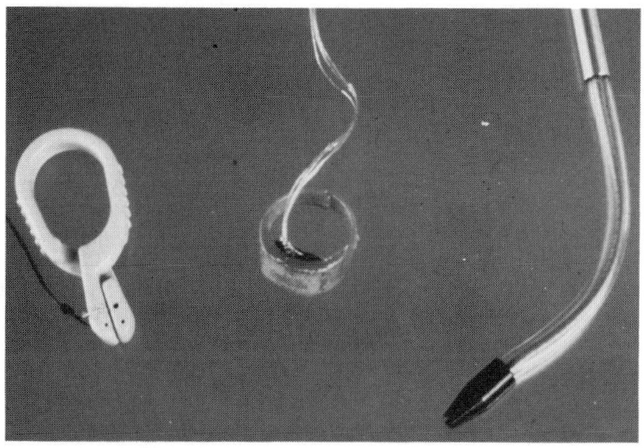

FIGURE 21–1
Pacing and sensing probes used for intraoperative mapping. Clip-on probe at left is used on the atrial appendage for both functions.

or during induced or spontaneous supraventricular tachycardia. Operative mapping in accessory pathway forms of tachycardia can be limited to the immediate area on either side of the atrioventricular groove, because only the precise point at which the pathway crosses the atrioventricular junction must be localized. Mapping is generally performed before cannulation and institution of cardiopulmonary bypass, but in some cases, mapping of the posterior wall of the heart may be more simply and safely performed during bypass because of the adverse effect that tachycardia and manipulation of the heart have on cardiac output.

Left-sided pathways localized to the area of the mitral valve annulus are divided during a period of induced cardioplegic cardiac standstill with the aorta cross-clamped (Fig. 21–2). The approach is similar to that used for mitral valve replacement, visualizing the supravalvular area through a left atriotomy incision. An endocardial incision is made just superior to the mitral annulus opposite the site of earliest epicardial depolarization, and the dissection is extended widely medially and laterally inferior to the coronary sinus and circumflex coronary artery until ventricular myocardium is exposed and epicardial fat dissected free (Fig. 21–3). During this dissection, fine filamentous fibers are divided that may contain the accessory pathways. Experience indicates that a similar dissection from the epicardial surface increases the chances for cure of the tachycardia. The endocardial and epicardial incisions are then closed with continuous suture.

Right-sided pathways cross the atrioventricular groove in the area of the tricuspid valve annulus near the main right coronary artery (Fig. 21–4). The dissection for the pathways is most effectively performed with the right atrium opened and the heart beating during cardiopulmonary bypass, although opening any cardiac chamber with the heart beating increases slightly the possibility of air entering the arterial system. We routinely stitch the foramen ovale (whether or not it is thought to be patent) immediately after opening the right atrium. In general, the opportunity for more precise mapping and surgical ablation outweigh the risk. Dissection is carried out above the tricuspid annulus until epicardium is exposed, with care being taken to avoid injury to the atrioventricular node and right coronary artery. Again a wide dissection is recommended to ensure division of all accessory pathways.

SEPTAL PATHWAYS

Accessory pathways located either anterior or posterior to the atrioventricular node present a somewhat different problem for the surgical team. Septal pathways represent approximately 20% of pathways in our series.[11] Epicardial mapping can localize the pathway to the area of the septum, but again, endocardial mapping with the heart beating provides the most precise means to localize the pathway as well as to isolate and prevent inadvertent damage to the atrioventricular node and His bundle pathway of normal conduction (Fig. 21–5). Sealy and Gallagher initially described a method of dissection of

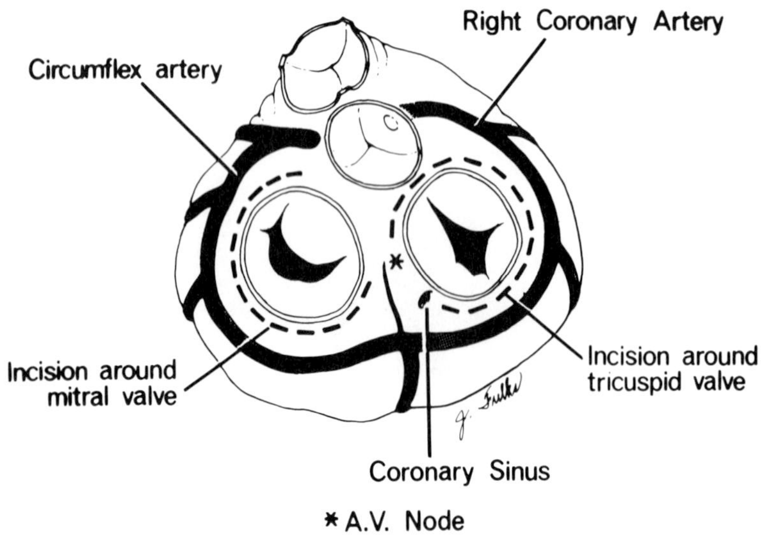

FIGURE 21–2
Cross-sectional diagrammatic representation of incisions (dashed lines) appropriate for right and left accessory pathways.

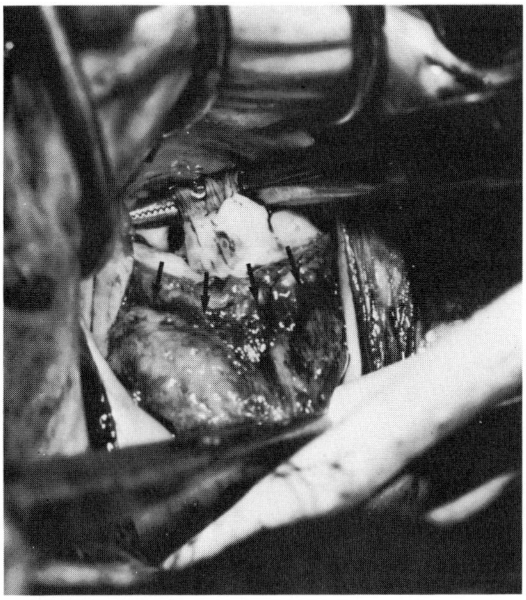

FIGURE 21–3
Surgical photo of dissection for left posterior Kent bundle demonstrating mitral valve posterior leaflet (retracted by clamp). Arrows indicate line of dissection posteriorly.

the septum to divide these pathways.[34] We have found that cryoablative techniques work very effectively in this area.[35] Often one application of the cryoprobe at −70° centigrade for 2 minutes to the endocardial area in question (usually near the mouth of the coronary sinus) will successfully ablate the pathway (Fig. 21–6).

CONCEALED ACCESSORY PATHWAYS

A subgroup of patients exists in whom reciprocating tachycardia occurs via an accessory pathway, and yet the delta wave of Wolff-Parkinson-White syndrome is not evident on surface EKG during sinus rhythm. Several authors have shown that these patients have an accessory pathway that conducts only in the retrograde fashion during tachycardia.[36–38] Antegrade conduction through the Kent bundle does not occur; during tachycardia, antegrade conduction follows the normal His bundle pathway, and the circuit is completed by retrograde conduction through the Kent bundle. This condition was noted in over one-third of our patients referred for surgical treatment of accessory pathway tachycardia. An estimated 50% to 60% of patients with supraventricular tachycardia but without the classical findings of Wolff-Parkinson-White syndrome may thus have accessory pathways amenable to surgical cure. Thus the primary care physician should consider the possibility of an accessory pathway in any patient exhibiting supraventricular tachycardia regardless of whether a delta wave is present on sinus rhythm EKG.

PERMANENT JUNCTIONAL RECIPROCATING TACHYCARDIA

Permanent junctional reciprocating tachycardia (PJRT), an incessant and refractory form of supraventricular tachycardia relatively more common in children than adults, has recently been elucidated.[39] This form of accessory pathway tachycardia is character-

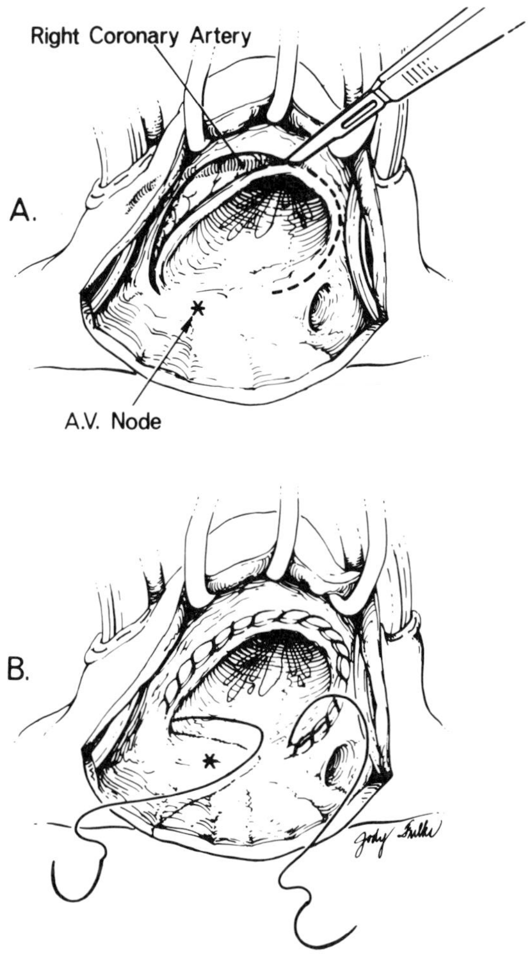

FIGURE 21–4
Surgeon's view of right atrial dissection. Note location of AV node in relation to incision.

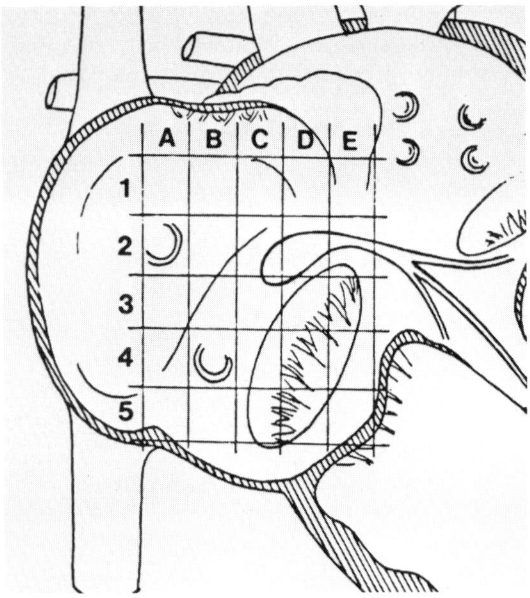

FIGURE 21–5
Map of right atrium showing AV node at C2 and coronary views at B4. Posterior septal pathways are cryoablated at the C3, C4, and B4 loci.

ized by retrograde P waves, a long RP interval, and normal PR interval (Table 21–1). It thus resembles sinus tachycardia with inverted P waves in leads II, III, and aVF. In this form of tachycardia, the accessory pathway represents the retrograde limb, is posterior septal in location, and demonstrates properties of decremental conduction. Because of the posterior septal location and possibility of complete heart block, few successful surgical cures have been reported until recently. We have demonstrated that this form of tachycardia can be cured predictably and relatively simply with a single application of the cryoprobe to the area inside the mouth of the coronary sinus.[35]

RESULTS

Surgical results in 79 patients younger than 18 years who underwent definitive surgery for supraventricular tachycardia caused by accessory pathways are summarized in Table 21–2; these include the earliest results of the series.[10–11] Increasing experience has resulted in improved cure rates so that surgery can now be recommended for accessory pathway forms of tachycardia with a greater than 95% expectation of cure. Left posterior pathways represent the most common type, accounting for 48.1% of patients referred for surgery. Posterior septal pathways account for 16.5% and are routinely treated by operative cryoablation of the accessory pathway. We have had experience in a large number of children, and our results are similar to those reported in other series.[25, 40–41]

ATRIAL ECTOPIC TACHYCARDIA

Supraventricular tachycardia secondary to an anatomic ectopic focus within the atrium is more frequently diagnosed in children

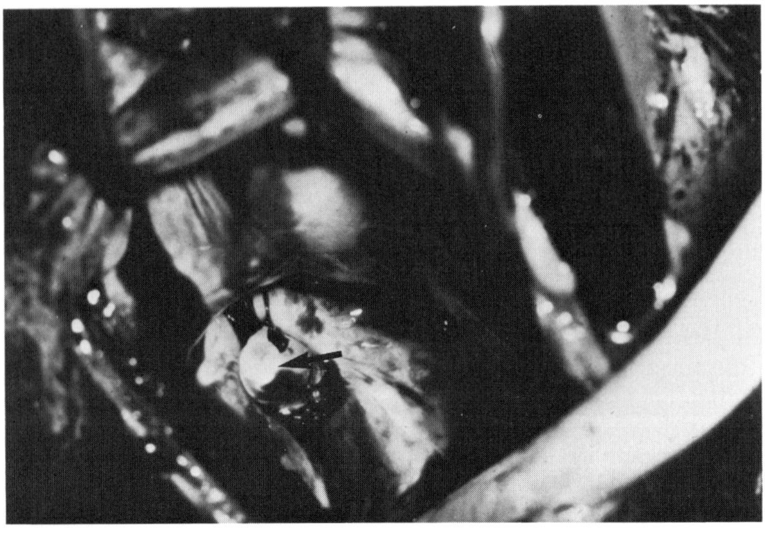

FIGURE 21–6
Crater left immediately after removal of cryoprobe from a posterior septal pathway (arrow). Thawing obliterates the crater in 1–2 min.

TABLE 21–1
ELECTROPHYSIOLOGIC CHARACTERISTICS OF AND SURGICAL TECHNIQUE FOR PERMANENT JUNCTIONAL RECIPROCATING TACHYCARDIA

Electrophysiologic characteristics
- Normal PR & AH interval
- Retrograde P wave occurring closer to succeeding QRS complex (long RP interval)
- Negative P wave in leads II, III, and aVF
- Posterior septal pathway with decremental conduction

Surgical technique
- Cryoablation in mouth of coronary sinus

than adults and is typically incessant or continuous and usually refractory to all forms of medication.[42–45] Cardiomyopathy may ensue as a result of long-standing tachycardia and may be misdiagnosed as primary cardiomyopathy with secondary tachycardia. We have had experience with patients referred for cardiac transplantation who were cured by definitive antitachycardia surgery, with a resulting return to normal cardiac size and function (Fig. 21–7). Thus surgery is usually recommended for patients with atrial ectopic tachycardia. Preoperative and intraoperative mapping are complicated in these patients by the broad atrial surface that must be mapped and by the frequent presence of multiple foci, some of which may not become manifest until after ablation of the primary or dominant focus. Accessory pathways need only be localized at the point of crossing the atrioventricular groove, whereas successful mapping for atrial ectopic tachycardia requires extensive mapping of the entire atrial surface. In addition, induction of tachycardia by programmed stimulation is usually not successful in these cases, resulting in an inability to map unless spontaneous tachycardia occurs. These factors combine to make precise mapping with surgery for atrial ectopic tachycardia somewhat more difficult. Despite these problems, however, successful surgical cure can be effected in approximately 90% of these patients (Tables 21–2 and 21–3). The ectopic focus is right atrial in location in two-thirds of patients, but multiple foci are present in as many as 40%. (Thus far, all reported multiple foci have been on the right.)

Surgical cure may be accomplished on rare occasion by simple excision of the atrial appendage when the focus is isolated to this area. More often, extensive cryoablation is required.[35] Generally this is accomplished without cardiopulmonary bypass, but if this is unsuccessful or if tachycardia recurs in the early postoperative period, cardiopulmonary bypass with or without cardioplegic cardiac standstill may be required. Forty-four percent of patients required cardiopulmonary bypass in our series.[42] Practical experience has demonstrated that cryoablation is most successful when performed on the atrium, which is emptied of blood presumably because of the elimination of the warming effect of circulating blood. In practice, surgical cure is attempted by beginning with simple excision of the atrial appendage if the focus maps to this area. If this is not successful, cryoablation is attempted first without cardiopulmonary bypass and then with cardiopulmonary bypass and an empty heart as indicated. Early recurrence of tachycardia can be expected in a small but definite percentage of patients with this difficult problem, usually within 24 hours of surgery; an aggressive policy of reoperation is warranted in view of the continuous, incessant, and ominous nature of this form of tachycardia. Partial or complete disconnection of the atria from the ventricles with reanastomosis may be success-

TABLE 21–2
SURGICAL RESULTS FOR VARIOUS FORMS OF TACHYDYSRHYTHMIAS IN CHILDREN

DIAGNOSIS	NUMBER	MEAN AGE (years)	MEAN FOLLOW-UP (months)	RESOLUTION OF TACHYCARDIA (%)
Supraventricular tachycardia secondary to accessory pathways	79	10.5	33.5	88.6*
Atrial ectopic tachycardia	18	8.6	28.1	88.9
Ventricular tachycardia in infancy	12	1.1	27.0	100.0
Ventricular tachycardia after tetralogy repair	3	17.0	20.0	100.0
Arrhythmogenic right ventricular dysplasia	2	14.5	14.0	50.0

*Currently, surgical cure is achievable in more than 95% of patients.

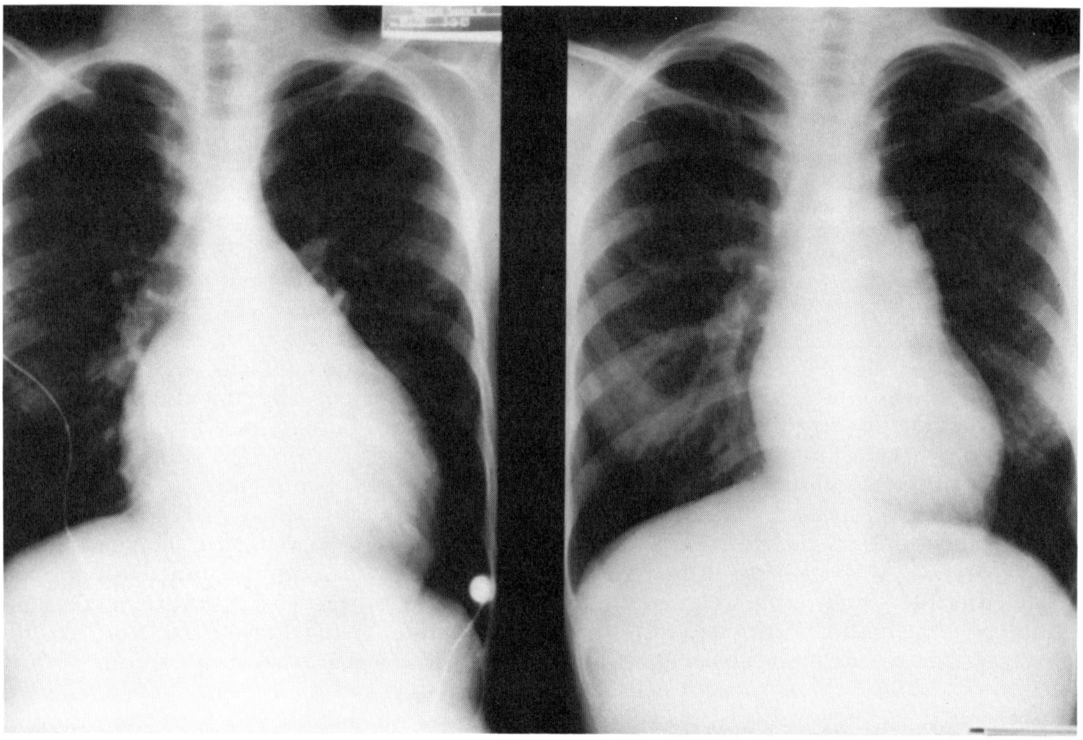

FIGURE 21–7
Preoperative and postoperative chest radiographs of an 11-year-old girl referred for cardiomyopathy and possible heart transplantation. Cryoablation of atrial ectopic tachycardia resulted in return to normal cardiac function.

ful if excision and cryoablation are unsuccessful in eliminating tachycardia.[11] However, we have had the experience of recurrence of tachycardia in a thin rim of atrial tissue left for reattaching the disconnected atrium.

VENTRICULAR ARRHYTHMIAS

Late Arrhythmias Following Congenital Heart Surgery

Clinically significant ventricular tachyarrhythmias are distinctly unusual in children. Ventricular tachycardia may occur as a late complication of the surgical repair of congenital heart defects, notably tetralogy of Fallot.[46–48] This may be associated with residual high right ventricular pressures or outflow tract aneurysm, or may simply be caused by an electrically abnormal area associated with a large area of scar [in the anterior right ventricular outflow tract (a result of ventriculotomy), the posterior infundibulum (from resection), or the ventricular septum (related to the ventricular septal defect patch)]. Surgical cure of these lesions can be affected by a combination of electrophysiologic mapping and either resection or cryoablation of arrhythmogenic areas in addition to surgical correction of any residual hemodynamic abnormalities (Table 21–2).[35]

Incessant Ventricular Tachycardia in Infancy

A potentially lethal form of ventricular tachycardia has been elucidated that occurs in infants younger than 2 years and that is associated with sudden death or cardiovascular collapse caused by incessant ventricular tachycardia and/or ventricular fibrillation.[49] Congestive heart failure and cardiomyopathy may ensue, since the tachycardia is generally resistant to medical treatment (including propranolol, lidocaine, phenytoin, quinidine, procainamide, amiodarone, and maxiletene). These infants require early surgical interven-

TABLE 21–3
CHARACTERISTICS OF AND SURGICAL RESULTS FOR ATRIAL ECTOPIC TACHYCARDIA IN 18 PATIENTS

	NUMBER	PRESENCE OF MULTIPLE FOCI	CARDIOPULMONARY BYPASS REQUIRED		RECURRENCE*	
			No.	*%*	*No.*	*%*
Location of ectopic focus						
Right atrium	13	6	NA		2	15.0
Left atrium	5	1	NA		0	0.0
Total	18	7			2	11.1
Surgical Technique						
Excision	1	NA	0	0.0	0	0.0
Cryoablation	9	NA	6	6.7	1	11.1
Excision and cryoablation	6	NA	0	0.0	0	0.0
Atrial disconnection	2	NA	2	0.0	1	50.0
Total	18		8	44.4	2	11.1

*All surgical failures occurred in patients with multiple foci.
NA = Not applicable.

tion because of the predictably lethal nature of this form of tachyarrhythmia. In a series of 19 infants (mean age, 13.7 months) presenting with the previously described clinical syndrome, only one had an angiographic or echocardiographic abnormality, that being a fibroma of the septum (Table 21–4).[35] Two others were noted at surgery to have previously undetected but grossly visible rhabdomyomas as the source of their tachyarrhythmias. Gross tumors are known to cause arrhythmias, but the majority of infants who die from this ventricular tachycardia syndrome without surgery are found to have only localized infiltrating abnormal areas of cellular proliferation of sparsely granulated, lipid-filled cells.[50–51] These areas have been variously described pathologically as histiocytoid cardiomyopathy or Purkinje cell tumors because of their cellular resemblance to the conduction system.[52–57] Electron microscopic studies in our lab suggest that these lesions represent a form of myocardial hamartoma (Fig. 21–8).[58] These areas can be electrophysiologically located with preoperative mapping and cured with a combination of excisional or cryoablative techniques.[35, 49]

TABLE 21–4
HISTOLOGY OF ABNORMAL FOCI IN 19 INFANTS OPERATED ON FOR MALIGNANT VENTRICULAR TACHYCARDIA

HISTOLOGY	NUMBER
Purkinje cell tumor (myocardial hamartoma)	11
Rhabdomyoma	2
Fibroma	1
Normal or nonspecific inflammation	3
No biopsy	2

The lesion is usually visible to the surgeon as a subtle flat area of greyish discoloration that superficially resembles myocardial scar or may even be mistaken for normal epicardial fat on initial inspection. In some cases, the lesion is not visible on the epicardial surface and becomes apparent only after incision into the myocardial wall at the area localized by operative mapping. In about 10% of cases, the tumor is diffusely infiltrative on the endocardial surface, involving the papillary muscles; in these cases definitive excision is impossible. In a few patients (about 20%), no visible lesion is found, but elimination of the tachycardia may still be accomplished by a judicious combination of cryoablation and excision of the suspected area.

Arrhythmogenic Right Ventricular Dysplasia

Life threatening ventricular tachycardia may also occur in association with a form of cardiomyopathy referred to as arrhythmogenic right ventricular dysplasia.[59–63] In this poorly understood and possibly genetic syndrome the entire right ventricular free wall may be infiltrated by patchy areas of fibrosis and fatty change. The right ventricle is dyskinetic and grossly abnormal in appearance. Recurrent and incessant ventricular tachycardia occurs, and sudden death may occur. Because arrhythmias may arise from multiple foci, definitive localized excision or cryoablation is usually not successful. More extensive procedures, including total disconnec-

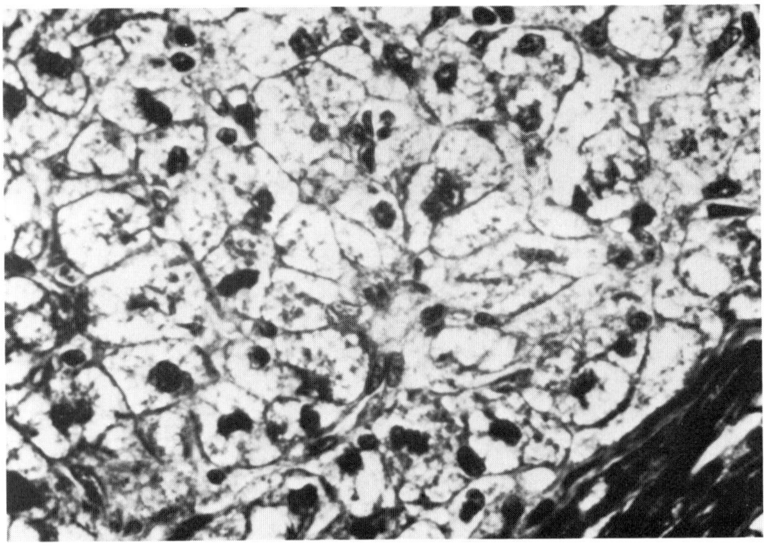

FIGURE 21–8
Histologic section of Purkinje cell tumor (myocardial hamartoma) from an infant with ventricular tachycardia. Normal myocardium is visible at lower right.

tion of the right ventricular free wall, can successfully eliminate tachycardia in most cases, but significant right heart dilatation and dysfunction result.[64] We have found disabling congestive heart failure following this operation. Therefore, extensive procedures designed to electrically isolate the entire right ventricular free wall should be limited to those patients with devastating arrhythmias that cannot be locally isolated with a less extensive procedure (Table 21–2).

CRYOABLATION

Reference has been made to the use of cryoablative methods in describing the surgical treatment of the various forms of tachyarrhythmias. In this technique, precise ablation of electrical activity without destruction of the fibrous matrix of the cardiac chamber wall is accomplished by freezing rapidly to −70° centigrade using decompressed nitrous oxide gas.[65–73] Cryoablative techniques are particularly useful in situations where excisional or incisional methods are not possible (e.g., atrial ectopic tachycardia) or are more likely to compromise other structures (e.g., normal AV node–His bundle pathways in patients with posterior septal Kent bundles).[35]

Cryoablative techniques have been used either alone or in combination with incisional methods in 30% of 175 children undergoing definitive electrophysiologically directed surgery for nonatherosclerotic tachyarrhythmias. Permanent elimination of the tachycardia was accomplished in more than 95% of patients (Table 21–5). Particularly in the infant heart, cryoablative methods provide the surgeon an alternative to purely incisional techniques.

TABLE 21–5
SUCCESS OF CRYOABLATION IN THE MANAGEMENT OF VARIOUS FORMS OF TACHYARRHYTHMIAS

TYPE OF TACHYARRHYTHMIA	NUMBER OF PATIENTS	MEAN AGE (yrs)	MEAN FOLLOW-UP (months)	RESOLUTION OF TACHYCARDIA (%)
Accessory pathway of Kent	16	11.3	22.2	93.7
Permanent junctional reciprocating tachycardia	6	10.5	6.3	100.0
Atrial ectopic tachycardia	18	8.6	28.1	88.9
Ventricular tachycardia	13	1.1	25.7	100.0

References

1. Garson A: The Electrocardiogram in Infants and Children; A Systematic Approach. Philadelphia, Lea & Febiger, 1983, pp 231–260.
2. Fisher DJ, Gross DM, Garson A: Rapid sinus tachycardia—differentiation from supraventricular tachycardia. Am J Dis Child 137:164–166, 1983.
3. Gillette PC, Garson A, Zinner A, et al: Continuous computer automated measurement of electrophysiologic data during cardiac catheterization. Comp Cardiol 324:391–393, 1981.
4. Gillette PC: Advances in the diagnosis and treatment of tachydysrhythmias in children. Am Heart J 102:111–120, 1981.
5. Garson A, Gillette PC: Electrophysiologic studies of supraventricular tachycardia in children, II. Prediction of specific mechanism by noninvasive features. Am Heart J 102:383–388, 1981.
6. Porter CJ, Gillette PC, McNamara DG: 24-hour ambulatory ECG's in the detection and management of cardiac dysrhythmias in infants and children. Pediatr Cardiol 1:203–208, 1980.
7. Garson A, Gillette PC: Electrophysiologic studies of supraventricular tachycardia in children, I. Clinical-electrophysiologic correlations. Am Heart J 102:233–250, 1981.
8. Porter C, Gillette PC, Garson A et al: Effects of verapamil on supraventricular tachycardia in children. Am J Cardiol 48:487–491, 1981.
9. Gillette PC, Garson A, Zinner A, et al: Automated on-line measurement of electrophysiologic characteristics. PACE 3:456–461, 1980.
10. Ott DA, Gillette PC, Garson A, et al: Surgical management of refractory supraventricular tachycardia in infants and children. J Am Coll Cardiol 5:124–129, 1985.
11. Ott DA, Garson A, Cooley DA, et al: Definitive operation for refractory cardiac tachyarrhythmias in children. J Thorac Cardiovasc Surg 90:681, 1985.
12. Ott DA, Cooley DA, Garson A, et al: Peremptory surgery for tachycardias. Cardio 32:34 (Nov/Dec), 1985.
13. Ott DA, Garson A, Gillette PC, et al: Surgery for refractory cardiac arrhythmias. Pract Cardiol 10:107–118, 1984.
14. Burchell HB, Frye RL, Anderson MW, et al: Atrioventricular and ventriculoatrial excitation in Wolff-Parkinson-White syndrome (type B). Circulation 36:663–672, 1967.
15. Cobb FR, Blumenschein SD, Sealy WC, et al: Successful surgical interruption of the bundle of Kent in a patient with Wolff-Parkinson-White syndrome. Circulation 38:1018–1029, 1968.
16. Sealy WC, Wallace AG, Ramming KP, et al: An improved operation for the definitive treatment of the Wolff-Parkinson-White syndrome. Ann Thorac Surg 17:107–113, 1974.
17. Coumel P, Waynberger M, Fabiato A, et al: Wolff-Parkinson-White syndrome. Problems in evaluation of multiple accessory pathways and surgical therapy. Circulation 45:1216–1230, 1972.
18. Meijne NG, Mellink HM, van Dam RT, et al: Surgical treatment of ventricular preexcitation. J Cardiovasc Surg 14:232–237, 1973.
19. Sealy WC, Boineau JP, Wallace AG: The identification and division of the bundle of Kent for premature ventricular excitation and supraventricular tachycardia. Surgery 68:1009–1017, 1970.
20. Iwa T: Surgery of supraventricular tachycardia. Circulation 42:287–293, 1978.
21. Wallace AG, Sealy WC, Gallagher JJ, et al: Surgical correction of anomalous left ventricular preexcitation: Wolff-Parkinson-White (type A). Circulation 49:206–213, 1974.
22. Sealy WC, Gallagher JJ, Wallace AG: The surgical treatment of the Wolff-Parkinson-White syndrome. Evaluation of the improved methods of identification and interruption of the Kent bundle. Ann Thorac Surg 22:443–457, 1976.
23. Wellens HJJ, Janse MJ, van Dam RT, et al: Epicardial mapping and surgical treatment in Wolff-Parkinson-White syndrome type A. Am Heart J 88:69–78, 1974.
24. Sealy WC, Gallagher JJ: Surgical treatment of left free wall accessory pathways of atrioventricular conduction of the Kent type. J Thorac Cardiovasc Surg 81:698–706, 1981.
25. Holmes DR, Danielson GK, Gersh BJ, et al: Surgical treatment of accessory atrioventricular pathways and symptomatic tachycardia in children and young adults. Am J Cardiol 55:1509–1512, 1985.
26. Gillette PC, Garson A Jr, Kugler JD, et al: Surgical treatment of supraventricular tachycardia in infants and children. Am J Cardiol 46:281–284, 1980.
27. Gillette PC, Garson A, Kugler JD: Wolff-Parkinson-White syndrome in children: electrophysiologic and pharmacologic characteristics. Circulation 60:1487–1495, 1979.
28. Gillette PC: The mechanisms of supraventricular tachycardia in children. Circulation 54:133–139, 1976.
29. Garson A, Gillette PC, McNamara DG: Supraventricular tachycardia in children. Clinical features, response to treatment, and long-term follow-up in 217 patients. J Pediatr 98:875–882, 1981.
30. Garson A, McNamara DG: Sudden death in a pediatric cardiology population. Relationship to prior arrhythmias. J Am Coll Cardiol 5:134B–138B, 1985.
31. Kugler JD, Gillette PC, Duff DE, et al: Elective mapping and surgical division of the bundle of Kent in a patient with Ebstein's anomaly who required tricuspid valve replacement. Am J Cardiol 41:602–605, 1978.
32. Kastor JD, Goldreyer BN, Josephson ME, et al: Electrophysiologic characteristics of Ebstein's anomaly of the tricuspid valve. Circulation 52:987–995, 1975.
33. McFaul RC, Davis Z, Guilliane ER, et al: Ebstein's malformation: Surgical experience at Mayo Clinic. J Thorac Cardiovasc Surg 72:910–915, 1976.
34. Sealy WC, Gallagher JJ: The surgical approach to the septal area of the heart based on experiences with 45 patients with Kent bundles. J Thorac Cardiovasc Surg 79:542–551, 1980.
35. Ott DA, Garson A, Cooley DA, et al: Cryoablative techniques in the treatment of cardiac tachyarrhythmias. Ann Thorac Surg 43:138–143 (Feb), 1987.
36. Gillette PC, Gallagher JJ, Sealy WC: Concealed anomalous cardiac conduction pathway: An operable cause of supraventricular tachycardia. J Pediatr 90:427–430, 1977.
37. Denes P, Wyndham CRC, Rosen KM: Intractable paroxysmal tachycardia caused by a concealed retrogradely conducting Kent bundle: Demonstration by epicardial mapping and cure of tachycardias by surgical interruption of the His bundle. Br Heart J 38:758–763, 1976.
38. Gillette PC: Concealed anomalous cardiac conduc-

tion pathways: A frequent cause of supraventricular tachycardia. Am J Cardiol 40:848–852, 1977.
39. Guarnieri T, Sealy WC, Kasell JH, et al: The nonpharmacologic management of the permanent form of junctional reciprocating tachycardia. Circulation 69(2):269, 1984.
40. Cox JL, Gallagher JJ, Cain ME: Experience with 118 consecutive patients undergoing operation for the Wolff-Parkinson-White syndrome. J Am Coll Cardiol 6(5):1167–1171, 1985.
41. Sealy WC, Anderson RW, Gallagher JJ: Surgical treatment of supraventricular tachyarrhythmias. J Thorac Cardiovasc Surg 73:511–521, 1977.
42. Gillette PC, Garson A, Cooley DA, et al: Definitive surgical treatment of atrial automatic ectopic focus tachycardias. Circulation 64(suppl 2):11, 1981. Abstract.
43. Gillette PC, Wampler DG, Garson A Jr, et al: Treatment of atrial automatic tachycardia by ablation procedures. J Am Coll Cardiol 6(2):1155–1162, 1985.
44. Gillette PC, Garson A, Hesslein PS, et al: Successful surgical treatment of atrial, junctional, and ventricular tachycardia unassociated with accessory connections in infants and children. Am Heart J 102:984–991, 1981.
45. Gillette PC, Garson A: Electrophysiologic and pharmacologic characteristics of automatic ectopic atrial tachycardia. Circulation 56:571–575, 1977.
46. Harken AU, Horowitz LN, Josephson ME: Surgical correction of recurrent sustained ventricular tachycardia following complete repair of tetralogy of Fallot. J Thorac Cardiovasc Surg 80(5):779–781, 1980.
47. Garson A, Gillette PC, Gutgesell HP, et al: Stress-induced ventricular arrhythmias after tetralogy of Fallot repair. Am J Cardiol 46:1006–1012, 1980.
48. Garson A, Randall DC, McVey P, et al: Prevention of sudden death after repair of tetralogy of Fallot. Treatment of ventricular arrhythmias. J Am Coll Cardiol 6:221–227, 1985.
49. Garson A, Gillette PC, Titus JL, et al: Surgical treatment of ventricular tachycardia in infants. N Engl J Med 310:1443–1445, 1984.
50. Engle MA, Ebert PA, Redo SF; Recurrent ventricular tachycardia due to resectable cardiac tumor. Circulation 50:1052–1057, 1974.
51. Bini RM, Westaby S, Bargeron LM, et al: Investigation and management of primary cardiac tumors in infants and children. J Am Coll Cardiol 2:351–357, 1983.
52. Ferrans VJ, McAllister HA Jr, Haese WH: Infantile cardiomyopathy with histiocytoid change in cardiac muscle cells: Report of six patients. Circulation 53:708–719, 1976.
53. James TN, Beeson CW II, Sherman EB, et al: DeSubitaneis Mortibus: XIII. Multifocal Purkinje cell tumors of the heart. Circulation 52:333–344, 1975.
54. Saffitz JE, Ferrans VJ, Rodriguez ER, et al: Histiocytoid cardiomyopathy: A cause of sudden death in apparently healthy infants. Am J Cardiol 52:215–217, 1983.
55. Haese WH, Maron BJ, Mirowski M, et al: Peculiar focal myocardial degeneration and fatal ventricular arrhythmias in a child. N Engl J Med 287:180–181, 1972.
56. Amini M, Bosman C, Marino B: Histiocytoid cardiomyopathy in infancy. A new hypothesis? Chest 77:556–558, 1980.
57. Rossi L, Piffer R, Turolla E, et al: Multifocal Purkinje-like tumor of the heart. Chest 87:340–345, 1985.
58. Kearney D, Titus JL, Hawkins E, et al: Pathological features of myocardial hamartomas causing childhood tachyarrhythmias. Circulation 75, No. 4, 705–710, 1987.
59. Guiraudon GM, Klein GJ, Gulamhusein SS, et al: Total disconnection of the right ventricular free wall: Surgical treatment of right ventricular tachycardia associated with right ventricular dysplasia. Circulation 2:463–470, 1983.
60. Marcus FI, Fontaine GH, Guiraudon G, et al: Right ventricular dysplasia. A report of 24 cases. Circulation 65:384, 1982.
61. Rossi P, Massumi A, Gillette P, et al: Arrhythmogenic right ventricular dysplasia. Clinical features, diagnostic techniques, and current management. Am Heart J 103:415, 1982.
62. Gaffney FA, Nicod P, Lin JC, et al: Non-invasive recognition of the parchment right ventricle (Uhl's anomaly arrhythmogenic right ventricular dysplasia) syndrome. Clin Cardiol 6:235, 1983.
63. Dungan WT, Garson A, Gillette PC: Arrhythmogenic right ventricular dysplasia. A cause of ventricular tachycardia in children with apparently normal hearts. Am Heart J 102:745–750, 1981.
64. Cox JL, Bardy GH, Damiano RJ Jr, et al: Right ventricular isolation procedures for nonischemic ventricular tachycardia. J Thorac Cardiovasc Surg 90(2):212–224, 1985.
65. Mikat EM, Hackel DB, Harrison L, et al: Reaction of the myocardium and coronary arteries to cryosurgery. J Lab Invest 37:632–641, 1977.
66. Taylor CB, Davis CB, Vawter GF, et al: Controlled myocardial injury produced by a hypothermal method. Circulation 3:239–253, 1951.
67. Misaki T, Allwork SP, Bentall HH: Longterm effects of cryosurgery in the sheep heart. Cardiovasc Res 17(2):61–69, 1983.
68. Wetstein L, Mark R, Kaplan A, et al: Nonarrhythmogenicity of therapeutic cryothermic lesions of the myocardium. J Surg Res 39(6):543–554, 1985.
69. Holman WL, Ikeshita M, Lease JG, et al: Alteration of antegrade atrioventricular conduction by cryoablation of peri-atrioventricular nodal tissue. Implications for the surgical treatment of atrioventricular nodal reentry tachycardia. J Thorac Cardiovasc Surg 88(1):67–75, 1984.
70. Klein GJ, Guiraudon GM, Perkins DG, et al: Controlled cryothermal injury to the AV node: Feasibility for AV nodal modification. PACE 8(5):630–638, 1985.
71. Holman WL, Ikeshita M, Douglas JM Jr, et al: Ventricular cryosurgery: Short-term effects on intramural electrophysiology. Ann Thorac Surg 35(4):386–393, 1983.
72. Ikeshita M, Holman WL, Lease JG, et al: The electrophysiologic effects of discrete cryosurgery for the treatment of supraventricular tachycardia due to AV nodal reentry. Jpn Circ J 48(2):127–135, 1984.
73. Camm J, Ward DE, Spurrel RA, et al: Cryothermal mapping and cryoablation in the treatment of refractory cardiac arrhythmias. Circulation 62:67, 1980.

CHAPTER 22

ACUTE PHARMACOLOGIC TREATMENT OF CARDIAC ARRHYTHMIAS

James C. Perry

The purpose of this chapter is twofold: (1) to provide management schemata for the acute therapy of supraventricular tachycardia, atrial flutter, complete atrioventricular block, and ventricular tachycardia; and (2) to present a drug formulary listing indications for use, dosage, mode of action, ECG changes, and side effects attributable to each agent. The reader is directed to the chapters on specific arrhythmias and pharmacology for more detail.

ACUTE MANAGEMENT OF ARRHYTHMIAS

Supraventricular Tachycardia

Supraventricular tachycardia (SVT) is defined as a narrow QRS tachycardia that virtually always has the same morphology and QRS axis (after the first 10 to 20 beats) as those seen in normal sinus rhythm. Formal electrocardiographic criteria are designed to include all potential causes of SVT and exclude the diagnoses of atrial flutter and atrial fibrillation. During SVT, the morphologies that may be seen are as follows:

1. No visible P waves, but QRS rate greater than normal.
2. Visible P waves, but abnormal P wave axis and a P rate greater than normal for age.
3. Visible P waves with a normal P wave axis, but a P rate greater than 230 bpm or greater than normal for age.
4. Visible P waves with normal P wave axis but with AV dissociation, with QRS rate greater than P wave rate.

Causes. Potential conditions that provide the substrate necessary for SVT include macroreentrant circuits secondary to accessory atrioventricular connections, microreentrant circuits possibly secondary to myocardial scarring or dishomogeneous impulse propagation, and ectopic foci. Congenital heart defects and their surgical repair can also provide the substrate for these conditions and the initiating factors for tachycardia (Table 22–1).

Acute Management. The flow diagram for acute management of SVT is presented in Figure 22–1. After a diagnosis of SVT has been established, it is crucial to determine if

TABLE 22–1
CAUSES OF SUPRAVENTRICULAR TACHYCARDIA

Congenital heart defects
Ebstein's anomaly
Postop Mustard, Senning, Fontan, and atrial and ventricular septal defect repair
AV canal defect
Mitral valve prolapse
Accessory connections
Drugs
Epinephrine
Methyphenidate
Ephedrine
Caffeine
Miscellaneous
Hyperthyroidism
Fever, sepsis
Myocarditis, cardiomyopathy

SVT*

- Ice bag
- Vagal maneuvers
- Transesophageal overdrive pacing
- Adenosine IV

Hemodynamic compromise?

YES

- DC cardioversion, 0.25–2 watt-seconds/kg
  Give lidocaine first if patient on digoxin
- Transvenous or transesophageal overdrive pacing

NO

- Verapamil IV, only if >1 year old, no CHF, no β-blockers
- Digoxin IV; discontinue if preexcitation present in NSR
- Procainamide IV

*If severe hemodynamic compromise, use DC cardioversion first, with lidocaine if indicated. After cardioversion to NSR, obtain 15-lead ECG to determine whether (a) preexcitation is present and (b) QRS axis and morphology in NSR is similar to that in tachycardia.

FIGURE 22–1
Acute management of supraventricular tachycardia.

AFL*

Postop patient with possible sinus node dysfunction (e.g., Mustard)?

YES

- Transesophageal or intracardiac overdrive atrial pacing with backup pacing ready for bradycardia/asystole
- DC cardioversion 1–2 watt-seconds/kg with sedation. Backup pacing available

NO

- Overdrive pacing or DC cardioversion

*If AFL recurs immediately, may use digoxin IV if no bypass tract; then procainamide IV (must already be on digoxin).

FIGURE 22–2
Acute management of atrial flutter.

Congenital (infants):

- Atropine
- Isoproterenol infusion
- Dopamine for BP support
- Pacing for ventricular rate < 50 bpm
- Pacing if CHD with ventricular rate < 55 bpm
- Temporary pacing for stressed infant

Surgical:

- Wait 14 days postop (AV conduction may return)
- Temporary pacing in interim if required for blood pressure support or symptoms
- Pacemaker implant if CAVB persists

Emergency:

- Balloon-tipped pacing catheter
- Transthoracic pacing

FIGURE 22–3
Acute management of complete atrioventricular block.

TABLE 22–2
CAUSES OF COMPLETE ATRIOVENTRICULAR BLOCK

- Congenital
  - L-transposition with ventricular inversion
  - Maternal lupus erythematosus
  - Single ventricle
  - AV canal defect
- Surgical
  - Postoperative AV canal, ventricular septal defect, tetralogy of Fallot, and aortic stenosis repair
- Acquired
  - Viral
  - Diphtheria
  - Rheumatic
  - Following balloon atrioseptostomy

TABLE 22–3
CAUSES OF VENTRICULAR TACHYCARDIA

- Metabolic/Electrolytic
  - Acidemia, hypoxemia, hyperkalemia, hypokalemia, hypercalcemia, hypoglycemia, hypothermia
- Drugs
  - Digoxin, quinidine
  - Sympathomimetics, phenothiazines, tricyclics
  - Caffeine, cocaine, nicotine
  - Halothane
- Congenital heart disease/Myocardial
  - Postop tetralogy of Fallot
  - Cardiomyopathy, myocarditis
  - Arrhythmogenic right ventricular dysplasia
  - Prolonged QT syndrome
  - Ventricular tumor
  - Muscular dystrophies
  - Bacterial endocarditis

the arrhythmia is causing hemodynamic compromise with symptoms of low cardiac output and congestive heart failure. If this is the case, then synchronized direct current cardioversion should be attempted first, with lidocaine given prophylactically if the patient is on digoxin. If it can be done expeditiously, either transvenous or transesophageal overdrive pacing can be performed.

Without signs of cardiac failure, use of the diving reflex, vagal maneuvers (not to include ocular pressure in children), or transesophageal pacing may convert tachycardia. As adenosine and ATP make their way into the pediatric antiarrhythmic armamentarium, these drugs may become primary agents in the therapy of acute SVT. Intravenous verapamil should not be used in children younger than 1 year and in those with congestive heart failure or who are currently taking β-adrenergic blocking agents.

Once normal sinus rhythm has been established, it is important to obtain a 15-lead electrocardiogram to determine whether preexcitation is present (and therefore discontinue digoxin) and whether the QRS morphology and axis in sinus rhythm are similar to those in tachycardia.

Atrial Flutter

Atrial flutter is classically defined by morphology and not by rate. Flutter waves are best seen in the inferior and right precordial leads; rates are commonly 300/min, but can range from 200/min to 500/min. Slow flutter rates (to 120/min) may be seen in some patients on amiodarone. AV conduction during flutter is variable and may be 1:1 in infants. In children with accessory connections, conduction of flutter down the bypass tract can give the appearance of ventricular tachycardia.

Causes. Atrial flutter can be seen in young infants with a normal heart and frequent

Text continued on page 598

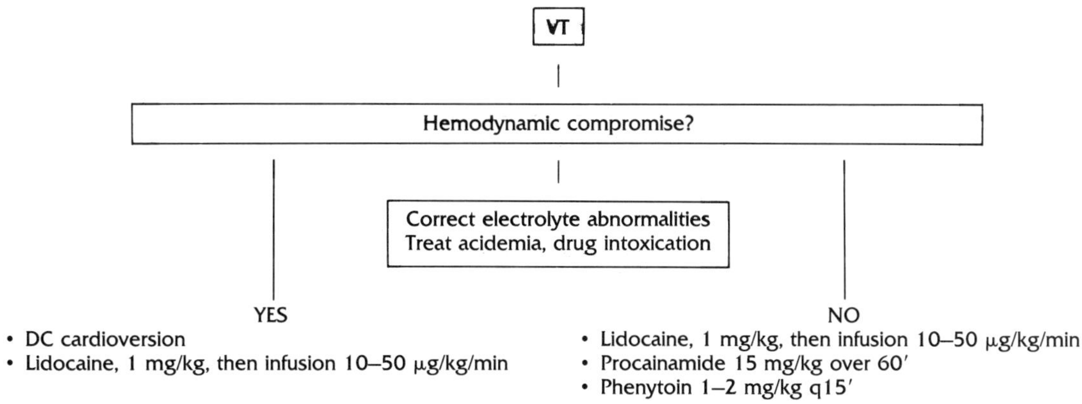

FIGURE 22–4
Acute management of ventricular tachycardia.

TABLE 22–4
ANTIARRHYTHMIC AGENTS

CLASS	DRUG	USES	DOSAGE (LEVEL)	MODE OF ACTION	ECG/EP CHANGES	SIDE EFFECTS
Ia Inhibit Na^+ fast channel Prolong repolarization Marked Na^+ channel inhibition with fast rate	Quinidine	AFL—with digoxin SVT-WPW with propranolol Resistant PVC/VT	PO only: 15–60 mg/kg/d; divided q6h for sulfate, q8h for gluconate (2–6 μg/mL)	Depress conduction and prolong refractoriness in A, HP, V; peripheral alpha block; vagolytic, negative inotrope; decrease phase 4 and automaticity (high dose)	Increased PR, QRS; ? Toxicity if QTc increases by 30% or QT 0.5 s Increased CSNRT, HRA-LSRA, HV, Kent ERP Decreased AH	Hypotension, SAN exit block, AV block (below His), VT, CHF, headache, rash, tinnitus, nausea, thrombocytopenia Digoxin—↑ dig level Phenytoin—↓ DPH $t^{1/2}$ Coumadin—↑ PT
	Procainamide	Conversion of AFL if on digoxin Conversion of SVT, multiform PVC, couplets, VT unresponsive to lidocaine Predict PO quinidine effect	IV: <1 yo = 7 mg/kg over 1 hr, then 3.5 mg/kg per dose q4h; >1 yo = 15 mg/kg over 1 hr, then 7 mg/kg per dose q4h If effect lasts <4 hr, infusion 1–4 mg/kg/hr PO = 15–50 mg/kg/d, divided q4h (PA = 5–10 μg/mL)	Similar to quinidine	Similar to quinidine	Similar to quinidine; lupus-like syndrome in slow acetylators Amiodarone—↑ PA
	Disopyramide	Similar to quinidine and procainamide	PO = 1–3 mg/kg/dose q6H (2–4 μg/mL)	Similar to quinidine Some Ca^{++} channel blockade, potent anticholinergic	Similar to quinidine, more PR than QRS prolongation	Similar to quinidine Electromechanical dissociation Anticholinergic
Ib Inhibit Na^+ fast channel Shorten repolarization Moderate Na^+ Inhibition with fast rate	Lidocaine	Multiform PVC, couplets, VT Precardioversion if on digoxin ? Predicts response to mexiletine, phenytoin	1 mg/kg IV q5min ×3, then infusion of 20–50 μg/kg/min (1–5 μg/mL)	Little effect on normal tissues; decreases Purkinje ERP, automaticity; increases VF threshold	Slight ↓ HP-ERP Slight ↓ QTc	Paresthesia, seizure; ↑ AV conduction in AFL, ↓ ventricular and junctional escape rates; may ↓ cardiac output
	Mexiletine	Chronic ventricular ectopy, useful in pts responsive to phenytoin but with side effects; useful in pts with decreased function and VA, especially postop	2.9–5.0 mg/kg/dose q8h PO (0.5–2.0 μg/mL) Serum concentration may not be predictive of effect	Structural analog of lidocaine; depresses conduction, especially at higher rates	None	Nausea (take food with drug), headache, paresthesia, rash, hepatitis (rare)

Class	Drug	Indications	Dosage	Mechanism	ECG effects	Side effects / interactions
	Phenytoin	Chronic ventricular arrhythmias, digitalis intoxication	PO = 4 mg/kg/dose q6h × 1 day, then 5–6 mg/kg/d divided q12h IV = bolus 15 mg/kg over 1 hr (q5min pushes) (15–20 μg/mL)	Similar to lidocaine; weak Ca^{++} channel blockade, suppresses digoxin-induced delayed afterdepolarizations; central sympathetic inhibition	Slight ↓ QTc; decreases V ERP; ↓ AH only in digoxin intoxication	Hypotension (IV), rash, gingival hyperplasia, ataxia Coumadin—↑ PT Verapamil—↑ verapamil effect (displaced from protein)
	Ethmozine	AET Ventricular ectopy AVN reentry?	200–600 mg/m²/d divided q8h	Phenothiazine derivative; suppresses abnormal automaticity; shortens repolarization	Slight ↑ PR, ↑ QRS; increases AH, HV	Headache, vertigo, paresthesia, tinnitus, nystagmus
	Tocainide	Similar to mexiletine		Structural analog of lidocaine	Minimal	Nausea, CNS disturbances, bone marrow, hepatitis
Ic Inhibit Na^+ fast channel Variable effect on repolarization Mild Na^+ Inhibition with fast rate	Encainide	PJRT AET/IAH SVT/WPW Ventricular arrhythmias	60–120 mg/m²/d divided q6–8h; max single dose 50 mg, max daily dose 200 mg Chronic therapy: two active metabolites	Depress abnormal automaticity; decrease conduction in AVN, accessory connections, ventricular myocardium; metabolites may increase refractoriness	Significant increase in PR, QRS; mild increase QTc	Headache, fatigue; proarrhythmic in high doses
	Flecainide	PJRT AET/IAH SVT PVCs/VT	100–225 mg/m²/d divided q8–12h (0.2–1.0 μg/mL) No active metabolites	Depress abnormal automaticity; slows conduction in AVN, accessory connection, ventricle	Mild increase in PR, mild increase in QRS at high doses; prolongs AH, HV, ERP-Kent	Blurred vision, nausea; use with caution in CHF (may decrease contractility); proarrhythmic—may change intermittent SVT-WPW to incessant at slower rate; may increase pacing threshold
	Propafenone	Postop JET	IV = 0.2 mg/kg q10 min (max 2 mg); when ventricular rate ≤ 150 bpm, begin infusion at 4–7 μg/kg per min and begin AV sequential pacing; use colloid during loading for BP support	Diffuse slowing of conduction; negative inotropism; mild beta and Ca^{++} blockade; prolongs both A and V refractoriness	Increases PR, QRS, QTc	Hypotension; decreases contractility; ? hepatic toxicity, paresthesia, headache

Table continued on following page

TABLE 22–4
ANTIARRHYTHMIC AGENTS *Continued*

CLASS	DRUG	USES	DOSAGE (LEVEL)	MODE OF ACTION	ECG/EP CHANGES	SIDE EFFECTS
II						
β-blockers	Propranolol	SVT-WPW: alone or with quinidine SVT-nonWPW: alone or with digoxin tetralogy spells; prolonged QT, VT; thyrotoxicosis	PO: 1–5 mg/kg/d, divided q6h (50–150 ng/mL) IV: 0.05–0.15 mg/kg Increase $t^1/_2$ if cyanotic	Non-selective beta blockade; some local anesthetic effect at high doses Suppress renin-aldosterone-angiotensin axis Non-polar, so crosses blood-brain barrier	Slows HR; may ↓ QT: ↑ CSNRT, SACT, AH, AVN ERP; no change in HV	Bronchospasm, depression, nightmares, sinus arrest, AV block, CHF, hypoglycemia; may ↑ LDL, VLDL; decreases contractility Contraindicated with verapamil
	Atenolol	SVT with or without WPW; hypertension; prolonged QTc; exercise-induced VT	12.5–50 mg PO qd approx. 1 mg/kg	More β_1 selective; no local anesthetic effect; central reduction of sympathetic output	Slows HR, may ↓ QT	Fewer CNS effects than propranolol; postural hypotension, CHF, diarrhea, nausea; may ↑ TG, VLDL Contraindicated with verapamil
III						
Prolong repolarization	Amiodarone	Life-threatening drug-resistant SVT (JET), AFL, VT: incessant drug-resistant SVT (WPW), IAH, ? PJRT, AET; drug of choice for congenital JET	PO: 10 mg/kg/d divided bid × 10 days, then 5 mg/kg qd; try to ↓ to < 5 mg/kg over 5/7 days IV: 1 mg/kg bolus q10min × 10, may repeat q12h; monitor effect by QTc (0.53 s), then decrease dose by 50%	Mild local anesthetic; α, β, and Ca^{++} blockade; at rapid stimulation rates, depresses conduction; smooth muscle vasodilator, depresses automaticity; "localized hypothyroidism" in all cardiac cells	↓ ↓ HR if SSS; ↑ QRS, ↓ QR ("effect" at 0.53 s); ↑ CSNRT, ↑ ERP in all cardiac tissues	Bradycardia—requires pacemaker (pts with AFL); corneal microdeposits, rash, nausea, ataxia; "effect"—rT3 > 50; "toxicity"—rT3 > 90; hypotension (IV); ↑ level of digoxin, quinidine, procainamide; Coumadin—↑ PT
	Bretylium	VF (digoxin toxicity) VT	5 mg/kg IV over 1 minute	Inhibits ME release, Epi reuptake; weak cholinergic effects and local anesthetic; increases VF threshold	No ECG changes	Transient ↑ BP and ↑ arrhythmia (if digoxin-induced); later ↓ BP from vasodilation; quinidine antagonizes bretylium
	D-sotolol	? WPW ? AFL ? ventricular ectopy	? 90–200 mg/m²/d divided bid	Prolongs repolarization and β-blocker (~ ⅓ as potent as propranolol)	May prolong QTc, HR	Orthostatic hypotension; torsades de pointes

IV						
Ca^{++} channel	Verapamil	SVT (acute, in pt > 1 yo and not on β-blockers) AVN reentry SVT Hypertrophic cardiomyopathy; some pts w/PVCs, VT	IV: 0.15 mg/kg over 3 min, may repeat once (have IV $CaCl_2$ ready) PO: 2–7 mg/kg/d divided tid, qid	Slow channel blockade; negative inotropism	Broad P wave, ↑ PR, increased AH; no change SACT, CSNRT; increased AVN ERP	Hypotension (IV); contraindicated with β-blockers; constipation, flushing; contraindicated in pulmonary hypertension, SSS, poor LV function Digoxin—↑ digoxin level Coumadin—↑ PT
Purinergic agonists	Adenosine ATP	Termination of reentry SVT; AV block to distinguish AFL ?	Adenosine: begin at 37.5 μg/kg IV, increase by 37.5 μg/kg q1min to effect (max 250 μg/kg) ATP: <1 yo: 2–5 mg IV >1 yo: 2–15 mg IV	Vagotonic, antiadrenergic, depress slow inward Ca^{++} current, increase K^+ conductance (hyperpolarization)	↑ AH	Sinus arrest, sinus bradycardia, flushing, nausea, headache, asthma
Digitalis glycosides	Digoxin	SVT (non-WPW) AV block in AF and AFL; ↓ rate AET, JET; Inotropic PACs	Total loading dose: Premature: 20 μg/kg PO NB–6 mo: 30 μg/kg PO > 6 mo: 50 μg/kg PO Total loading dose (TLD) is given as follows: ½ TLD, followed by ¼ TLD q8h × 2 Maintenance dose is 5–10 μg/kg/d, divided q12h IV dose = ¾ PO dose (1–2 ng/mL > 6 mo) (1.5–3 ng/mL < 6 mo)	Na-K ATPase inhibition, positive inotrope, vagotonic	Increases PR, depresses ST, decreases QT; SAN = ↓ HR, ↑ SACT Atr = ↓ ERP, ↑ auto AVN = ↑ ERP, ↑ AH Vent = ↓ ERP Toxicity: ↓ conduction, ↑ auto, delayed afterdepolarizations May ↑, no A or ↓ ERP of Kent bundle	AV block, SVT, PVCs (treat digoxin induced arrhythmias with phenytoin) Nausea, vomiting, FTT, lethargy, visual changes Quinidine, amiodarone, verapamil—↑ digoxin levels Worse with ↓ K^+, ↓ Ca^{++} Coumadin—↑ PT

A = atrium; AET = atrial ectopic tachycardia; AFL = atrial flutter; AH = atrial-His interval; AV = atrioventricular; AVN = atrioventricular node; BP = blood pressure; CHF = congestive heart failure; CSNRT = corrected sinus node recovery time; DPH = diphenylhydantoin; ERP = effective refractory period; FT = tetralogy of Fallot; FTT = failure to thrive; H = His bundle; HP = His-Purkinje; HR = heart rate; HV = His-ventricle interval; IAH = "idiopathic atrial hyperirritability" (chaotic atrial tachycardia); IV = intravenous; JET = junctional ectopic tachycardia; LDL = low-density lipoprotein; NB = newborn; NE = norepinephrine; PA = pulmonary artery; PJRT = permanent junctional reciprocating tachycardia; PO = by mouth; PT = prothrombin time; PVC = premature ventricular contractions; SACT = sinoatrial conduction time; SAN = sinoatrial node; SVT = supraventricular tachycardia; TG = triglyceride; V = ventricle; VA = ventricular arrhythmias; VF = ventricular fibrillation; VLDL = very low-density lipoprotein; VT = ventricular tachycardia; WPW = Wolff-Parkinson-White syndrome; yo = year old.

PACs, hydropic newborns who had intrauterine tachyarrhythmia, and many postoperative patients (e.g., following Mustard, Senning, atrial septal defect, Blalock-Hanlon, or Fontan procedures). It may also present in patients with dilated atria, rheumatic disease, mitral valve prolapse, pericarditis, myotonic dystrophy, and cardiomyopathy.

Acute Management. Atrial flutter infrequently converts with medical therapy alone. Overdrive pacing or synchronized direct current cardioversion (0.25–2.0 watt-seconds/kg) is therefore the mainstay of acute treatment. However, patients with sinus node dysfunction (typically the postoperative patient) often respond to these interventions with a resultant severe bradycardia or asystole. In these patients, provisions must be made for backup pacing—transesophageal (if reliable), transvenous, transcutaneous or using a previously implanted pacemaker (Fig. 22–2).

Complete Atrioventricular Block

Complete atrioventricular block (CAVB), or type II second degree AV block, consists of independent atrial and ventricular beats, without conduction of atrial impulses to the ventricles. Long rhythm strips need to be examined to be sure that CAVB exists. As a general rule, P waves that fall beyond the T wave and do not conduct to the ventricles should suggest CAVB; 20% to 25% of patients with congenital CAVB also have prolongation of the QTc interval and are at greater risk of sudden death.

Causes. CAVB may be either congenital, surgically acquired or result from infectious causes (Table 22–2). Approximately one-third of infants with congenital CAVB also have structural congenital heart disease, most commonly L-transposition of the great arteries with ventricular inversion.

Acute Management. Acute management is dependent upon patient age and underlying ventricular rate, presence of symptoms or congenital heart defect and etiology of CAVB (Fig. 22–3). Medical therapy is directed at attempts to increase the junctional or ventricular rate and support the systemic blood pressure. Generally accepted indications for implanting a permanent pacing system are reviewed in chapter 19. In the event of surgical CAVB, a waiting period of 14 days is warranted, as AV conduction may return. Temporary pacing using epicardial pacing wires placed at the time of surgery may be indicated. In an emergency setting, placement of either a balloon-tipped pacing catheter or a transthoracic pacing wire can be performed.

Ventricular Tachycardia

Ventricular tachycardia (VT) is defined as three or more consecutive ventricular beats, generally at a rate faster than 120 bpm. AV dissociation is usually present, although 1:1 retrograde ventriculoatrial conduction may occur. The QRS morphology is different from the morphology in normal sinus rhythm. Infant VT may present as a rapid, "narrow" QRS tachycardia with different QRS morphology.

Causes. VT can be secondary to metabolic and electrolyte abnormalities, drugs, or a variety of congenital heart defects and myocardial abnormalities (Table 22–3).

Acute Management. Any patient with VT and signs or symptoms of low cardiac output and/or congestive heart failure deserves an initial trial of synchronized direct current cardioversion. In all cases, it is important to examine the ECG immediately after cardioversion to assess resultant rhythm and QRS morphology. If the QRS in stable tachycardia is different from the sinus QRS, the diagnosis is VT. If the child is hemodynamically stable, medical conversion can be attempted as outlined in Figure 22–4. It is difficult, if not impossible, to maintain NSR unless underlying metabolic and drug abnormalities are corrected.

PHARMACOLOGIC THERAPY AND FORMULARY

Table 22–4 lists antiarrhythmic drugs in order of drug classification, their uses, dosages, modes of action, ECG and EP changes, and side effects. The cellular and clinical electrophysiologic properties of antiarrhythmic agents are covered in detail in chapter 2.

SECTION V
COMMON CLINICAL PROBLEMS

CHAPTER 23
SYNCOPE

Martin P. O'Laughlin

Syncope (from the Greek *synkoptein,* "to cut short")[1] remains an important and puzzling problem in pediatrics, as it is both a sign and a syndrome, an end result of many different causes. Syncope is a temporary loss of consciousness resulting from a reversible disturbance of cerebral function. It is a result of various pathophysiologies, some of which may progress to death. Specific characteristics of syncope include (1) loss of consciousness because of a lack of cerebral blood flow; (2) a rapid or sudden onset; (3) falling, if the patient is not supported, as a result of disruption of postural tone; and (4) transiency of the attack.[2, 3]

Noble has suggested that syncope may be caused by a decrease or loss of intrinsic cerebral circulation, a cardiac problem (i.e., a result of a transient decrease in cardiac output), a fall in systemic arterial pressure to values inadequate to perfuse the brain, or an inadequate supply of energy substrates in the blood delivered to the brain.[4]

In this chapter, a number of the common causes of syncope will be discussed, with particular reference to children. Cardiac, and especially arrhythmic, causes will be emphasized, and an approach to diagnosis by history, physical examination, and a logical sequence of laboratory tests will be suggested.

CLASSIFICATION

Various classifications have been proposed for syncope. The following general classification has been found useful:

I. Vasodepressor syncope ("vasovagal" or common faint)
II. Cardiovascular syncope
    A. Cardiac syncope
        1. Primary
        2. Secondary to arrhythmia
    B. Vascular syncope
III. Noncardiovascular syncope

Vasodepressor Syncope

Vasodepressor syncope, or fainting, is characterized by a sudden fall in blood pressure associated with dizziness, lightheadedness, or loss of consciousness and is accompanied by prominent symptoms of autonomic activity, such as pallor, perspiration, nausea, hyperventilation, and tachycardia followed by bradycardia.[5, 6] It is often initiated by environmental stimuli, such as anxiety, blood drawing (or even sight of a needle), or the sight of blood. Pathophysiology of the faint may involve interruption of a central vasomotor outflow pathway, leading to marked vasodilation, particularly in arteriolar resistance vessels. Cardiac output in general does not change. The heart rate changes are not thought to be mediated solely by the vagus nerve, as atropine has little or no effect.[7] The exact behavior of the venous capacitance vessels is not proven; vasodilation and pooling of venous blood have been assumed to occur. Some investigators have suggested that there is venoconstriction; because of the marked arteriolar dilation and bradycardia, there is almost certainly reduced venous return.[8]

The loss of consciousness in vasodepressor syncope results from a reduction in cerebral perfusion caused by hypotension. Hyperventilation secondary to anxiety that precedes the fall may further reduce cerebral perfusion by producing hypocapnia. A marked decrease in systemic arterial blood pressure must be present in order to reduce cerebral blood flow, which ordinarily is independent of blood pressure, except at very low arterial pressures. With normal or only slightly reduced cardiac output, peripheral vasodilation must be very great in order to reduce blood pressure to a point at which syncope results. This reflex vasomotor depression and extreme vasodilation may work in concert with a loss of baroreceptor reflexes that normally maintain cerebral perfusion pressure, and syncope ensues.[4]

When the patient, because of the fall, has lain on the floor, usually for less than 1 minute, there is a gradual return of cerebral perfusion and awakening. Only rarely does injury result from the fall. Syncope may recur if the person sits or stands too soon, and a recovery period of 10 to 30 minutes is often required. Sometimes, well-meaning observors contribute to recurrent syncope by helping the patient to his or her feet. Some relief may be obtained by elevation of the legs.

Though vasodepressor syncope is common and worrisome, it only infrequently requires intense therapy, and recurrence risk (given the same stimulus) is low. If treatment is indicated, measures to increase circulating blood volume (such as generous fluid intake or salt consumption) can be recommended in addition to support hose. The fainting spells are rarely so severe as to necessitate a pacemaker.[9]

Features in the history and examination help to differentiate the common faint from other forms of syncope (Table 23–1). In particular, the presence of warning signs and symptoms as described point to the likelihood of the simple faint as opposed to the more sudden, unheralded falls seen with some forms of cardiac syncope, which may result in injury to the patient.

Cardiovascular Syncope

CARDIAC SYNCOPE

Cardiac syncope may be primary (resulting from congenital or acquired cardiovascular disease) or secondary (resulting from disruptions in the cardiac rhythm). Certain features in the history give a clue to the possibility of cardiac syncope. Occurrence of syncope in the recumbent position suggests a cardiac cause. In addition, there is an absence of true premonitory symptoms or only a momentary warning by visual disturbances, faintness, or fullness or noises in the head.[2, 3] Provocation of syncope by exercise may point to arrhythmic or obstructive cardiac causes.

Primary

Hypercyanotic Spells. Primary cardiac causes of syncope include hypercyanotic spells, such as those seen in tetralogy of Fallot, tricuspid atresia, or transposition of the great arteries with left ventricular outflow tract obstruction (pulmonary or subpulmonary stenosis). Hypercyanotic spells are also encountered with Eisenmenger's syndrome.[10]

Syncope is the hallmark of a severe hypercyanotic episode or "tetralogy spell." This type of spell usually begins with crying, and quickly progresses to hyperpnea. The prolonged forced expiration of crying increases intrathoracic pressures and promotes a decrease in blood flow to the lungs and an increase in right-to-left shunting. This in turn causes more cyanosis and a decrease in the oxygen saturation and pH of the blood returning to the heart. In order to compensate for the hypoxemia and acidosis, the patient breathes harder and faster or cries more and more vigorously, and the cycle of the right-to-left shunting and hypoxemia worsens. With severe hypoxemia, loss of consciousness may occur. The spell may be broken in a number of ways, the most common of which involves calming the patient and bringing the knees to the chest in order to increase systemic vascular resistance and thus promote flow to the pulmonary bed. This history of crying hyperpnea and increasing cyanosis

TABLE 23–1
FEATURES THAT HELP DISTINGUISH THE SIMPLE FAINT FROM OTHER FORMS OF SYNCOPE

FEATURE	TYPICAL FAINT	ATYPICAL FAINT
Conditions	Crowds, hunger, heat, dehydration, pain (or perceived pain), emotion	During exercise, loud noises, extreme surprise, anger
Prior warning	Prodrome	No prodrome
Injury from fall	Rare	May occur
Duration	Less than 1 min	May be greater than 1 min
Recurrences	Rarely frequent	May occur frequently

should be obtained in order to invoke a "tetralogy spell" as the cause of syncope.

Low Cardiac Output. Other causes of cardiac syncope include those that produce low cardiac output, generally because of obstruction to blood flow. These include aortic valvular stenosis and subvalvular or supravalvular aortic stenosis.

Syncope in congenital or acquired calcific aortic stenosis has been recognized as a marker of severe obstruction and an indication to relieve that obstruction, either with valvotomy or valve replacement. Aortic stenosis is marked by well-known physical findings, including a precordial and carotid thrill and a systolic ejection murmur. Syncope characteristically occurs during exercise in patients with aortic stenosis.

Hypertrophic cardiomyopathy, or idiopathic hypertrophic subaortic stenosis, may present with syncope on a primary hemodynamic basis or secondary to arrhythmias. Patients may present with murmurs, chest pain, dyspnea, or palpitations. On the other hand, the first clue to the diagnosis might be syncope or sudden death. Fourteen of the 34 patients in the series of Canedo, Frank, and Abdulla[11] had at least one syncopal episode in the year prior to entry into the study. A family history of hypertrophic cardiomyopathy could identify other affected members.

Prosthetic valve malfunction can cause acute interruption of blood flow. Similarly, syncope sometimes results from obstruction to blood flow at the native mitral valve as a result of congenital or acquired mitral stenosis. Left atrial myxoma has been described as presenting with features of a triad of (1) constitutional complaints (including fever), (2) emboli, and (3) obstructive symptoms such as syncope or paroxysmal dizziness.[12]

Restriction in cardiac output may result in syncope from severe pulmonic stenosis or from primary pulmonary hypertension. Syncope with the syndrome of increased pulmonary vascular resistance results either from hypercyanotic spells as previously described or from marked acute increases in pulmonary vascular resistance that may depress cardiac output suddenly and lead to acute right ventricular failure. Indeed, it may be the cessation of blood flow resulting from an abrupt rise in pulmonary resistance that leads to sudden death in Eisenmenger's syndrome. Some patients without a right-to-left shunt (such as those with idiopathic primary pulmonary hypertension) apparently have benefited from the creation of an atrial-level communication by blade and balloon atrial septostomy (Fig. 23–1).[13, 14] The atrial septal defect created (Fig. 23–2) allows right-to-left shunting and preservation of cardiac output during exacerbations of pulmonary hypertension.

Cardiac syncope caused by low output can result from cardiac muscle disease such as endocardial fibroelastosis or myocarditis. Trauma, infection, or other causes may damage the heart directly and result in low output and loss of consciousness.

Myocardial Infarction. An important (but less common) cause of primary cardiac syncope is myocardial infarction. Myocardial infarction has occurred in children with congenital coronary artery anomalies, most notably anomalous origin of the left coronary artery from the pulmonary artery. In addition, certain malformations of the coronary artery system involve an anomalous course of the left coronary artery between the aortic and pulmonic trunks that has led to compression of this artery during exercise. Myocardial infarction has followed coronary arterial narrowing resulting from Kawasaki disease, as a sequela to obstruction. Other causes of myocardial infarction include aortic stenosis (particularly in combination with aortic insufficiency), shock, and myocarditis.

Secondary

Arrhythmic (Normal Heart). Syncope from arrhythmias is rare in the patient with a structurally normal heart.[15] However, certain arrhythmias can cause loss of cerebral perfusion because of decrease or interruption of blood flow. These include sinus or junctional bradycardia, atrioventricular block, atrial flutter or supraventricular tachycardia, and ventricular tachycardia. Complete atrioventricular block has been suggested to produce syncope either by decreased cardiac output or by the occurrence of associated ventricular tachycardia.[16]

Syncope with exercise or emotion in a patient with an otherwise structurally normal heart can result from long QT syndrome with "torsades de pointes" ventricular tachycardia (Fig. 23–3 and Fig. 23–4). Ventricular tachycardia is a cause of syncope associated with the long QT syndrome or "cardioauditory syndrome" as described by Jervell and Lange-Nielsen;[17] Romano, Gemme, and Pon-

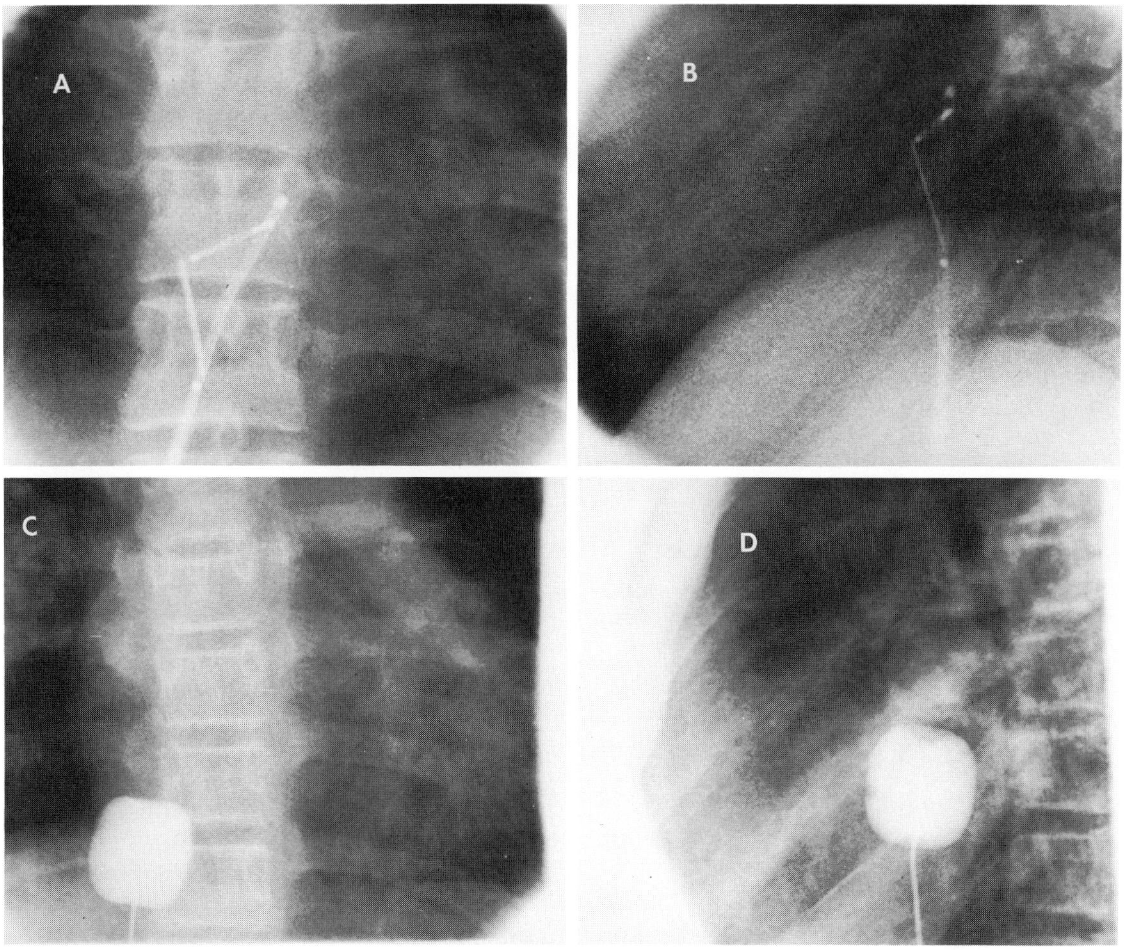

FIGURE 23–1

Blade and balloon atrial septostomy. Cineangiogram frames in the posteroanterior and lateral projections of a patient undergoing blade *(A* and *B)* and balloon *(C* and *D)* atrial septostomy. This patient was being treated for idiopathic primary pulmonary hypertension by creation of an atrial septal defect.

giglione;[18] and Ward.[19] The syncope related to ventricular tachycardia in long QT syndrome has been associated with fright or being awakened by a loud noise such as an alarm clock.[20] According to Schwartz and Moss, "Most of the affected patients become symptomatic in the first or second decade and, apart from the syncopal episodes, are completely normal; the events that trigger fatal syncopal attacks are abrupt physical or emotional stresses; an hereditable pattern is common, and tragic sudden deaths often occur in several members of an affected family."[21] Children have presented with syncope masquerading as seizures, with the syncope secondary to long QT syndrome. Four such children were described in one series, two of whom were deaf and two of whom were not. All were treated with β-blocking drugs by Horn et al.[22]

The long QT syndrome has been described and investigated as a paradigm of the link between cardiac and neural factors in the causation of syncope or sudden death.[23] It has been established that an imbalance between influence of the right and left stellate sympathetic ganglia produces electrocardiographic evidence of alterations in ventricular repolarization.[24] Specifically, hypoactive right or hyperactive left stellate sympathetic influence may be the cause of the long QT syndrome. In cases refractory to medical management (usually consisting of treatment with β-blockers), left stellate ganglionectomy has afforded some amelioration of syncopal attacks in some patients.[25, 26] Mortality in this

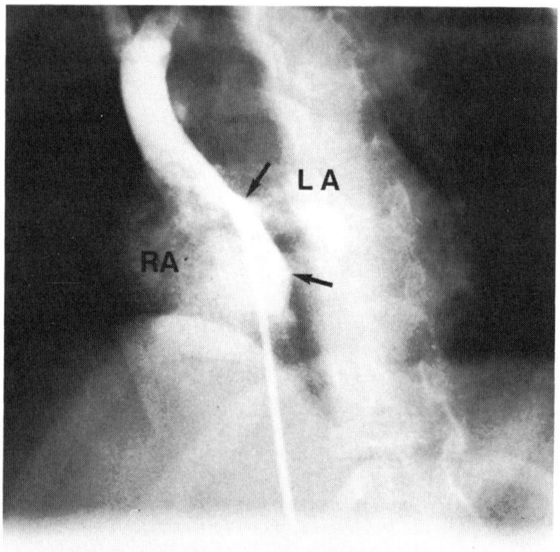

FIGURE 23–2
Angiographic four-chamber view of the atrial septal defect created by blade and balloon atrial septostomy. Injection has been in the superior vena cava. There is shunting of contrast from right atrium (RA) to left atrium (LA). The boundaries of the newly created atrial septal defect are shown by the arrows.

syndrome is high (71%) if patients are untreated. This mortality decreases to 7% if β-blocking drugs are used (with ganglionectomy reserved for refractory cases).[21, 27]

In an otherwise normal heart, arrhythmogenic right ventricular dysplasia has resulted in ventricular tachycardia and syncope. This disease should be suspected in any patient with ventricular tachycardia (especially exercise-induced) with a left bundle-branch block pattern. It is characterized by recurrent ventricular tachycardia with this morphology and a patchy right ventricular cardiomyopathy.[28] Generally, medical management of this disease is attempted before surgical isolation or cryoablation.[29]

Wolff-Parkinson-White syndrome may be associated with the development of atrial fibrillation or atrial flutter, and these dysrhythmias often present with breathlessness, near syncope, or syncope (Fig. 23–5). The diagnosis of Wolff-Parkinson-White syndrome is suggested by a history of palpitations and most often confirmed by electrocardiogram. Medical treatment may control the arrhythmias and syncope, but recurrent or severe symptoms may necessitate intracardiac mapping and incision or cryoablation of the accessory connection.

Special clinical circumstances produce arrhythmic syncope; these include metabolic derangements such as hypokalemia, hypoglycemia, or hypercalcemia. Sympathomimetic drugs have resulted in supraventricular or

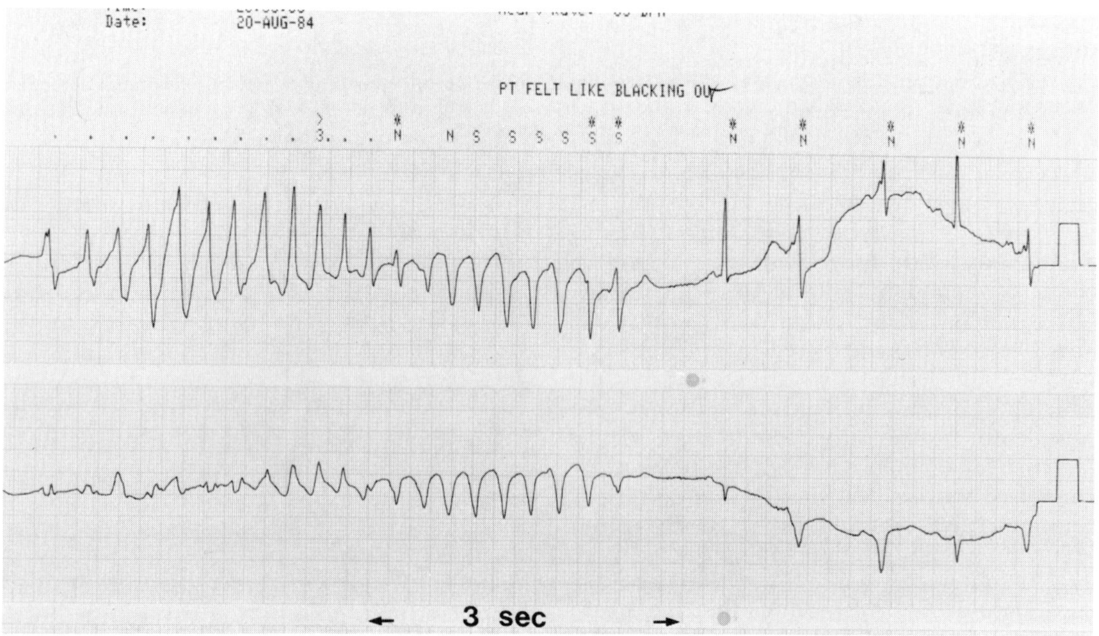

FIGURE 23–3
Two-channel cardioscan tracing from a 22-year-old woman with intermittent preexcitation and abnormalities of repolarization secondary to amiodarone. Multiform ventricular tachycardia (torsades de pointes) is seen. The comment at the top of the tracing was given in the patient's diary. The time scale is as marked.

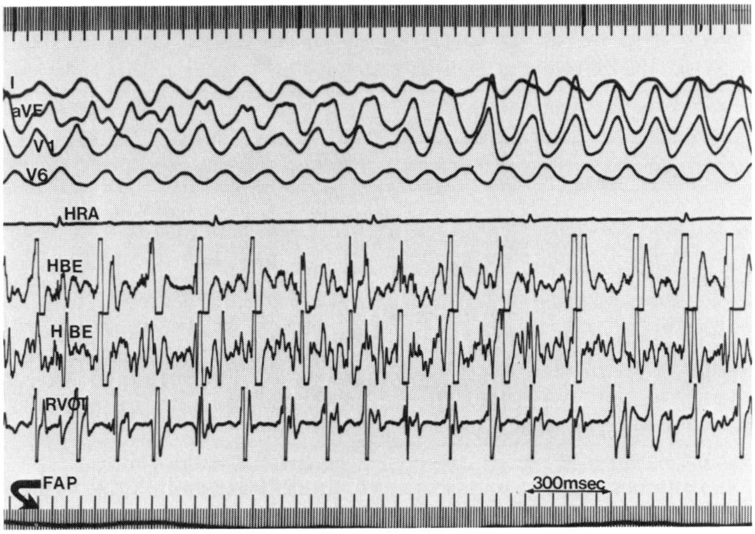

FIGURE 23–4
Tracing from electrophysiologic study of a patient with multiform ventricular tachycardia. The electrocardiogram channels are as marked. The other channels represent high right atrium (HRA), His bundle electrograms (HBE), right ventricular outflow tract (RVOT) catheter, and femoral arterial pressure (FAP), marked with the curved arrow. Time scale is as marked. Ventricular tachycardia with a changing axis is demonstrated. Atrioventricular dissociation is seen. The His bundle electrogram is not clearly discerned. Note the low and flat femoral arterial pressure curve. This patient required electrocardioversion shortly after this tracing was made.

ventricular tachycardias when used in doses that were too large or when they provoked idiosyncratic reactions.

Arrhythmic (Abnormal Heart). In children, congenital heart disease represents the most important source of arrhythmias leading to syncope. Table 23–2 shows a number of congenital and acquired heart conditions and the arrhythmias that have resulted in syncope in those diseases or conditions. Importantly, syncope with congenital heart disease, either pre- or postoperative, is much more common if the patient has abnormal hemodynamics or is receiving anti-arrhythmic drugs.

Sick Sinus Syndrome. Sick sinus syndrome has caused syncope and sudden death in patients with congenital heart disease, particularly patients who have undergone atrial surgery (Fig. 23–6). This syndrome has been defined in a number of different ways; one operational definition of sick sinus syndrome is sinus bradycardia or sinus arrest with or without supraventricular tachycardias. It is thought that the tachycardias may be the more likely cause of syncope, since some patients with pacemakers continue to have syncope and may die suddenly. Sick sinus syndrome has been described as including dizziness, seizures, paresis, and palpitations with chest pain during or after exertion. Syncope caused by sick sinus syndrome is sudden and brief, and places the patient at higher risk of sudden death.[30] Treatment of the syndrome with both anti-arrhythmic drugs and permanent pacemakers may decrease the risk of sudden death markedly.

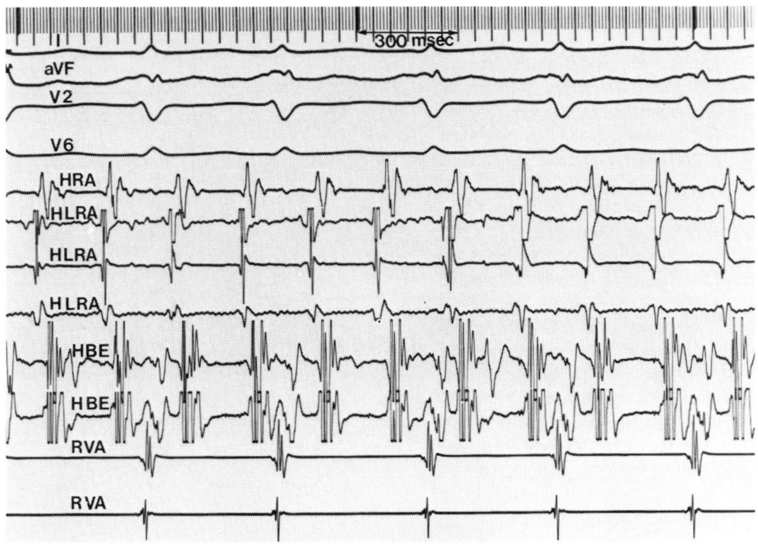

FIGURE 23–5
Atrial flutter with 2:1 block. Surface electrograms are as marked. Intercardiac recordings are from high right atrium (HRA), high lateral right atrium (HLRA), His bundle electrogram (HBE), and right ventricular apex (RVA). Time scale is marked. This patient was a 14-year-old boy with dilated cardiomyopathy and Wolff-Parkinson-White syndrome. Particularly with an accessory connection, there is danger of a change to 1:1 conduction and subsequent hypotension.

TABLE 23–2
CONGENITAL AND ACQUIRED HEART CONDITIONS AND ARRHYTHMIAS THAT HAVE RESULTED IN SYNCOPE IN THOSE CONDITIONS*

	ARRHYTHMIA				
DIAGNOSIS/CONDITION	*Sinus Bradycardia*	*AV Block*	*Atrial Flutter*	*SVT*	*VT*
PO TOF					×
PO Mustard	×		×		
PO AV canal/VSD		×			
Congestive CM	×		×		×
Myocarditis/endocarditis	×	×			×
HOCM		?			×
LTGA		×			
Ebstein's			×	×	
MS/MI			×		
Mitral prolapse					×

*An × indicates an important arrhythmia described in that diagnosis.
Abbreviations: AV = atrioventricular; CM = cardiomyopathy; HOCM = hypertrophic obstructive cardiomyopathy; LTGA = L-transposition of the great arteries (transposition with ventricular inversion); MI = mitral insufficiency; MS = mitral stenosis; PO = postoperative; SVT = supraventricular tachycardia; TOF = tetralogy of Fallot; VSD = ventricular septal defect; VT = ventricular tachycardia.

Atrial Arrhythmias. Atrial arrhythmias that cause syncope include atrial fibrillation, atrial flutter with rapid ventricular response, and sinus node disease. These appear more commonly in patients who have undergone atrial surgery (e.g., the Mustard and Senning operations, mitral valve annuloplasties or replacements, atrial septal defect repairs, atrioventricular canal repairs, or tricuspid annuloplasty for Ebstein's anomaly). As noted previously, atrial flutter with rapid ventricular response is a common problem in patients with accessory atrioventricular connections such as those with Wolff-Parkinson-White syndrome.

Atrioventricular Block. Another type of cardiac syncope resulting from arrhythmias is that caused by atrioventricular block. Second degree atrioventricular block is one cause of syncope. In most cases, Mobitz type I (Wenckebach) second degree atrioventricular block is very stable and requires no treatment, except for the underlying cause if it can be identified. On the other hand, Mobitz type II second degree atrioventricular block may be more ominous.

Classically, syncope from arrhythmias was caused by complete heart block, and has been known as the Adams-Stokes disease. These episodes are defined by Johannsen as "attacks

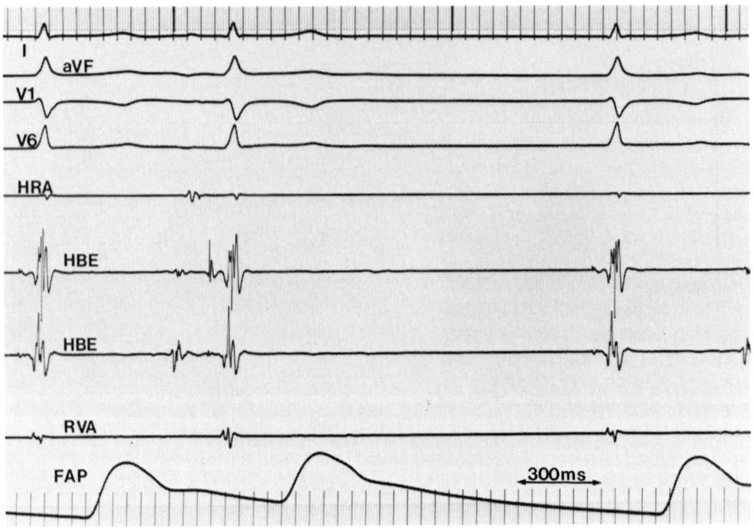

FIGURE 23–6
Intracardiac electrical study from a patient with sick sinus syndrome. Surface electrocardiograms are as marked. Intracardiac catheters include high right atrium (HRA), His bundle electrograms (HBE), and right ventricular apex (RVA). Femoral arterial pressure (FAP) is on the bottom tracing. Time scale is as marked. There is a low right atrial pacemaker as shown by the negative P wave in lead AVF. There is a 1390-ms pause after the middle beat, ending with a junctional escape beat. This patient is a 23-year-old woman 20 years status post-atrial septal defect repair. Her sick sinus syndrome was manifested by near-syncope in association with bradycardia, and transvenous dual-chamber pacing was instituted.

of acute cerebral ischemia in non-anesthetized patients on the basis of a sudden change in cardiac rhythm."[31]

Complete atrioventricular block may be congenital or acquired.[32, 33] The most common cause of acquired complete atrioventricular block is cardiac surgery. Patients with complete atrioventricular block following cardiac surgery are at high risk for syncope and sudden death, and pacemaker implantation is recommended. Congenital complete atrioventricular block in association with a normal heart may not require pacing (Fig. 23–7). In a study of 24 children with congenital complete atrioventricular block, Karpawich et al found that syncope was correlated with a persistent waking heart rate of fewer than 50 beats per minute. The authors recommended that pacemaker treatment be considered for patients who had heart rates lower than 50 bpm, who had experienced syncope, or who had developed congestive heart failure.[34]

Pacemaker therapy has prevented sudden death in patients with complete atrioventricular block, and syncope in such patients may be related to pacemaker failure or lead failure or fracture, which can cause disruption of the pacemaker circuit and reversion to the dangerous abnormal underlying rhythm.

Supraventricular Tachycardia and Atrial Flutter. Except for a few particular clinical circumstances, supraventricular tachycardia is not usually associated with syncope or sudden death.[35] Two such causes are junctional automatic focus tachycardia (in which sudden death occurs in up to 50% of patients) and Wolff-Parkinson-White syndrome, in which sudden death is less common (≤ 10%). Interestingly, patients with stable atrial ectopic supraventricular tachycardia may occasionally develop syncope with a sudden acceleration in rate. Atrial flutter, on the other hand, commonly causes near syncope or syncope with or without associated Wolff-Parkinson-White syndrome.[36]

Ventricular Tachycardia or Fibrillation. A clinical course characterized by syncope, dizziness, and palpitations was described by Rocchini, Chun, and Dick in 38 children with ventricular tachycardia.[37] Diagnoses in the 21 patients with underlying heart disease included mitral valve prolapse, myocarditis, prolonged QT syndrome, postoperative heart disease (particularly tetralogy of Fallot), and aortic or subaortic disease. There were 17 patients with no cardiac disease; 11 of these were asymptomatic, and only three of the 17 had frank syncope. The investigators found a relationship between the presence of underlying heart disease and the rate of ventricular tachycardia with symptoms. All symptomatic patients, with or without underlying cardiac disease, had a rate of ventricular tachycardia greater than 150 bpm. Exercise testing and Holter monitoring were used to follow these patients. Ventricular arrhythmias may represent the mechanism of syncope or death in hypertrophic cardiomyopathy and other types of left ventricular outflow tract obstruction. Ventricular tumors (i.e.,

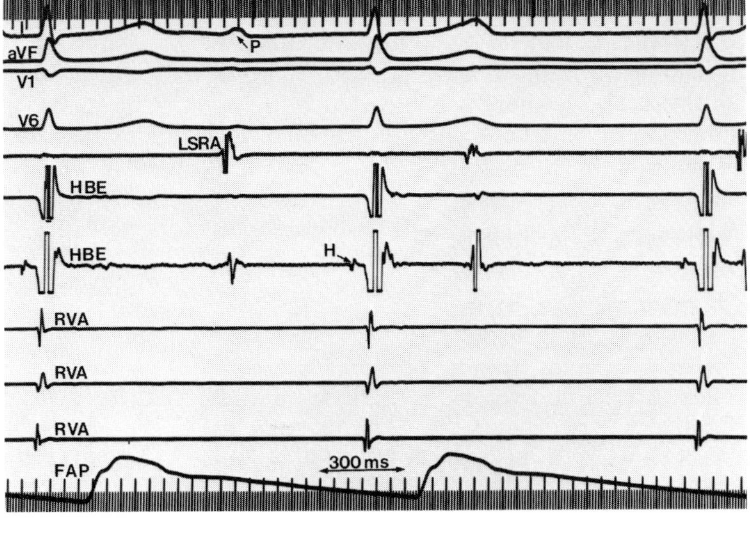

FIGURE 23–7
Intracardiac electrophysiologic study from an 8-year-old girl with congenital complete atrial ventricular block. Surface electrocardiograms are as marked. Intracardiac electrodes include low septal right atrium (LSRA), His bundle electrograms (HBE) and three electrodes in the right ventricular apical region (RVA). The femoral arterial pressure (FAP) is shown at the bottom of the tracing. Time scale is as marked. The P wave (P) and His bundle depolarization (H) are shown by the small arrows. Note the presence of atrioventricular dissociation and a P wave that does not conduct, although it is outside the expected refractory period of the atrioventricular conduction system. In this case, there is block above the His bundle, as demonstrated by the normal His-to-ventricle conduction time.

Purkinje cell tumors) are becoming recognized as an important cause of ventricular tachycardia, especially in infants.[38]

Syncope and near syncope have been reported in a minority of patients with the mitral valve prolapse syndrome. Patients with this syndrome often relate a history of fatigue, palpitations, chest pain, dyspnea, and exercise intolerance. Physical examination characteristically shows a thin, asthenic patient. Palpation of the precordium may reveal a bifid impulse, particularly in the left lateral decubitus position. Auscultation shows a midsystolic nonejection click and a late-systolic murmur.[39] Ventricular arrhythmias have been the cause of syncope or sudden death in patients with mitral valve prolapse.[40, 41] In one series of 20 patients, four had ventricular tachycardia or fibrillation on 24-hour electrocardiograms.[42]

Mitral valve prolapse syndrome has been investigated with a number of noninvasive tests in order to determine if dysfunction of the autonomic nervous system plays an important role in the symptoms. Gaffney et al found a decreased vagal responsiveness, an increased α-adrenergic response, and a normal β-adrenergic response in 19 women with mitral valve prolapse who were compared with 16 healthy controls.[43]

Boudoulas et al studied 20 symptomatic patients with mitral valve prolapse. Of these, six had experienced syncope or near syncope. The investigators found a greater level of excretion of epinephrine and norepinephrine in the patients with prolapse when they were compared to normal control patients. In addition, the time of electromechanical systole corrected for heart rate (an indicator of adrenergic state) was significantly shorter in patients with mitral valve prolapse than in controls. The authors concluded that these indices were consistent with abnormally high adrenergic tone in this syndrome.[44]

VASCULAR SYNCOPE

Orthostatic Syncope

When a person stands, normally there is reflex arterial and venous constriction and a slightly increased heart rate. The muscles in the legs act as a mechanical pump and, together with venous valves, favor preservation of venous return to the heart. In orthostatic syncope, one or more of the compensatory mechanisms fail, and there is a reduction in the blood pressure and perfusion of the brain, resulting in syncope. In contrast to vasodepressor syncope, there are fewer premonitory signs, with only a feeling of fullness in the head or lightheadedness. The time course is somewhat longer than that with the simple faint, and syncope may take seconds or even several minutes to develop after standing. Orthostatic syncope is predisposed to or precipitated by prolonged bedrest, prolonged standing, and conditions that decrease the circulating blood volume or impede venous return (e.g., bleeding, dehydration, adrenal insufficiency, or pregnancy).[45] Drugs that interfere with the sympathetic vasomotor response also predispose the patient to orthostatic syncope and include calcium channel blockers, vasodilators, and phenothiazines. Any antihypertensive drug has this effect. In addition, diuretics (which act to decrease sodium stores and circulating blood volume) may exacerbate orthostatic syncope.

There are a number of neurogenic causes of orthostatic syncope. These include any form of peripheral neuropathy, including diabetic neuropathy. Spinal cord or ganglion damage, tabes dorsalis, and syringomyelia may also interfere with the reflexes that preserve blood pressure on standing.

Cerebrovascular Syncope

Isolated syncope is rare as the only manifestation of cerebrovascular disease, but may occur with large or multiple vessel disease. In childhood, most forms of cerebrovascular syncope are embolic and result from endocarditis, complications of surgery or catheterization, or prosthetic valves. Intracardiac thrombus or tumor uncommonly causes cerebrovascular accidents and syncope. The "subclavian steal" syndrome may lead to dizziness or syncope with arm exercise in patients whose ipsilateral subclavian artery has been employed as a systemic-to-pulmonary arterial shunt.

Other Forms

Other relatively common types of vascular or autonomic syncope include vagovagal syncope, carotid sinus syncope, cough syncope, and post-micturition syncope. In vagovagal syncope, the entire reflex arc is comprised of the vagus nerve, and syncope results from severe bradycardia or atrioventricular block as a reflex result of vagal stimulation. The vagal afferent stimuli result from intubation, placement of a nasogastric tube, distention of viscera, or pleural or peritoneal effusion or irritation.

Carotid sinus syncope is caused by pressure on the baroreceptors in the carotid sinus. It often presents when pressure is placed inadvertently on the neck, such as when a patient is driving a car in reverse, shaving, or wearing a tight collar.[46] These are exaggerated cardioinhibitory and vasodepressor responses to carotid sinus massage or pressure. This type of response may be normal in a majority of patients older than 60 years, but it is not often seen in children. Vasodepressor syncope has been shown not to be responsive to pacing,[47] whereas cardioinhibitory carotid sinus syncope may improve with pacemaker placement.

Cough syncope or tussive syncope has been described in both children and adults. Cough itself produces reduced cardiac output through the Valsalva maneuver and peripheral vasodilation. In addition, there is increased spinal fluid pressure produced by the cough, which reduces the difference between arterial blood pressure and intracerebral pressure. Cerebral vascular resistance is increased reflexly by hypopcapnia as well. All these factors combine to cause syncope. This constellation has been seen particularly with patients with spasmodic cough such as in croup or asthma.

Post-micturition syncope comes after urination or drainage of a distended bladder or ascites. There are generally no premonitory signs. This is thought to be caused by the loss of intra-abdominal volume and reflexly decreased total peripheral resistance. A vasodepressor response from the Valsalva maneuver associated with voiding may also contribute.

Less common causes of syncope have been described, including swallowing syncope[48] and glossopharyngeal neuralgia.[2, 3]

Noncardiovascular Syncope

Noncardiovascular syncope can be caused by a deficiency in the energy substrates carried to the brain during hypoxia or hypoglycemia. Hypoxia can result from respiratory disease (particularly at high altitude), anemia, or breath-holding. Hypoglycemic syncope is characterized by the gradual onset of weakness, perspiration, and hunger. A history of diabetes is often obtained. There may be faintness or falling without complete loss of consciousness, and generally the heart rate and blood pressure remain normal. Other metabolic derangements such as hyperammonemia can produce a direct toxic effect on neural cells and a resulting loss of consciousness.

Hyperventilation syndrome is characterized by rapid, often deep breathing with a feeling of tightness in the chest, concern about the possibility of suffocation, and palpitations. When hypocapnia ensues, there may be circumoral and hand numbness and tingling. The episode lasts up to 30 minutes, with mildly increased heart rate and decreased blood pressure. The patient is able to reproduce the symptoms by hyperventilation, an important diagnostic clue.

Syncope resulting from seizures is suspected by repeated episodes of falling, sometimes with injury. The patient may describe an aura of auditory, visual, or olfactory sensations just before the seizure, though the aura is not always present. Signs associated with seizures include convulsion or tonic or clonic movements, incontinence, and prolonged loss of consciousness. Atonic seizures or "drop attacks" cause the patient to lose all skeletal muscular tone instantaneously, and fall suddenly to the floor. There may be head or face injury. The post-ictal state consists of drowsiness, headache, and confusion. During an attack, there is a normal blood pressure and tachycardia; an abnormal electroencephalogram is seen during or between attacks.[2, 3]

Vertigo presents generally in younger patients, aged 1 to 4 years. The patient may describe spinning of the room or environment. Often there is no true loss of consciousness. Blood pressure and heart rate remain normal during and after the event. Diagnosis is facilitated by oculocaloric testing.

Syncope resulting from hysteria is not associated with injury, and most often others are present. The hysteric syncopal episode may last up to 1 hour, during which there is normal heart rate and blood pressure. The condition, unlike orthostatic syncope or vasodepressor syncope, is not improved by the supine position. The patients characteristically provide an unemotional and unworried description of the event. In certain circumstances, there have been epidemics of hysterical fainting.[49]

Migraine headache may be severe enough to cause syncope. The vasospasm, when it affects the basal arterial system, is particularly prone to produce loss of consciousness. There is a premonitory aura of the migraine itself and loss of consciousness for some minutes. Heart rate and blood pressure are preserved, and the patient awakens with severe occipital or lateralizing headache. Other types of central nervous system disorders including post-traumatic disorders or trauma must be considered as well.

Drugs that do not produce orthostatic changes may nevertheless cause temporary loss of consciousness. These include hallucinogens, barbiturates, and narcotics. Cocaine, particularly in potent forms such as so-called "crack," causes syncope by producing ventricular arrhythmias, and has led to sudden death.

Antiarrhythmic drugs must always be a prime suspect in syncope in patients receiving them. In particular, quinidine has been associated with a sudden onset of loss of consciousness ("quinidine syncope"). This phenomenon is likely caused by prolongation of ventricular repolarization with effects on conduction that produce ventricular tachycardia or bradycardia.

EVALUATION OF THE PATIENT WITH SYNCOPE

History

A history of the syncopal episode is the most important diagnostic test. According to Wright and McIntosh, "Because (syncope) is a reversible state, the patient, as well as the observer, can describe the clinical events. Therefore, a careful analysis of the activities of the patient and the symptoms immediately preceding the loss of consciousness can and should be made."[50] A detailed description of the environment and events preceding the faint will give clues to the diagnosis.

Whether the loss of consciousness came suddenly, abruptly, and without warning, or whether there was lightheadedness, nausea, and sweating before the fall, helps to divide the causes into cardiac and vasodepressor. Whether there was loss of consciousness, and if so, for how long, should be sought. The presence of a fall and whether there was an injury sustained may separate hysteric fainting from that resulting from other causes. The past medical history of the patient will point to congenital heart disease, current drug treatment, or other predisposing factors. The clinician must search for a family history of syncope, deafness, seizures, or sudden death.

Physical Examination

During the physical examination, heart rate, blood pressure, and respiratory rate should be noted. The blood pressure should be obtained in the supine and sitting or standing position. Part of the evaluation for syncope should include taking the blood pressure after 10 minutes of standing. Normal children should not show a decrease in blood pressure after 10 minutes of standing. A thorough general physical examination with attention to the cardiovascular and nervous system is then performed. Features such as abnormalities in the heart rhythm, abnormal murmurs on cardiac examination, or focal neurologic signs may be found that point to a specific diagnosis. However, in most conditions, physical examination after the episode (or between episodes) is characteristically normal.

Laboratory Examination

Laboratory evaluation should be guided by the results of the history and physical examination. Tests that provide important information include electrocardiogram, hemoglobin, glucose, and calcium level. All patients with atypical syncope or recurrent typical syncope should have an electrocardiogram. The electrocardiogram must be inspected for sinus bradycardia, wandering atrial pacemaker, junctional rhythms, or premature ventricular extrasystoles. Measurements of the intervals must be made. A short or long PR interval may point to a conduction abnormality, and Wolff-Parkinson-White syndrome often is diagnosed on surface electrocardiograms. The QT interval measurements should be adjusted for heart rate by the method of Bazett, in which the QT interval in seconds is divided by the square root of the preceding RR interval in seconds.[51] The upper limit of normal is 0.44 s, and measurements longer than this in the presence of syncope are particularly suggestive of long QT syndrome. The morphology of the T waves should be inspected for consideration of this syndrome.[27] The voltage of the tracings from the precordial leads is examined for clues to ventricular hypertrophy.

Further Work-up

When certain features of the syncopal episode are suggested by history and physical and the diagnosis remains obscure after the initial laboratory work-up, specific referral or further testing may assist with diagnosis. A history consistent with seizure or an unexplained abnormal feature of the neurologic examination may prompt referral to a pediatric neurologist. Electroencephalogram, computerized axial tomography (CAT) scan, or caloric testing may then be performed by the consultant.

An abnormal electrocardiogram or a suspicion of arrhythmic or vascular cause of syncope should initiate additional evaluation, including graded treadmill exercise test. An exercise stress test may be particularly helpful in sorting out causes of exercise-induced syncope and will document the response of the patient to progressive exercise. These treadmill tests have been shown to be safe in children.[52] The exercise test has the added advantage of diminishing or abolishing benign premature ventricular extrasystoles in the majority of cases of children without heart disease.[37] In patients in whom long QT syndrome is suspected, it may be worthwhile to perform an exercise test in which the patient begins by running as fast as he or she can.

In cases in which a paroxysmal or intermittent dysrhythmia is suspected, 24-hour ambulatory monitoring is recommended. A continuous recording of the cardiac rhythm for 24 hours may disclose ventricular or supraventricular tachycardias, sinus bradycardia, sick sinus syndrome, or other possibly symptomatic dysrhythmias. This relatively simple test has been suggested by a number of authors for the investigation of syncope in children.[15, 53] With modern equipment, the continuous ambulatory recording of heart rhythm can be performed simply and without undue discomfort in children (Fig. 23–8).

Cardiac catheterization and electrophysiologic study have been described by Denes and Ezri[54] and Olshansky, Mazuz, and Martins[55] in the investigation of syncope. They chose adult patients in whom the etiologic diagnosis had remained unknown after a number of noninvasive tests. In these patients, the electrophysiologic studies proved very helpful in uncovering inducible sustained tachycardia, sinus node abnormalities, and supraventricular tachycardia. Olshansky, Mazuz, and Martins studied 105 patients with syncope of unknown cause. Of these, 37 (35%) were found to have inducible supraventricular tachycardia (9 patients) or ventricular tachycardia (24 patients) or both (four patients).[55] Treatment predicted to be effective by electrophysiologic study significantly reduced the incidence of recurrent syncope or cardiac arrest when compared to the incidence in patients who did not adhere to prescribed therapy or who received empirical treatment. Among 55 adult patients

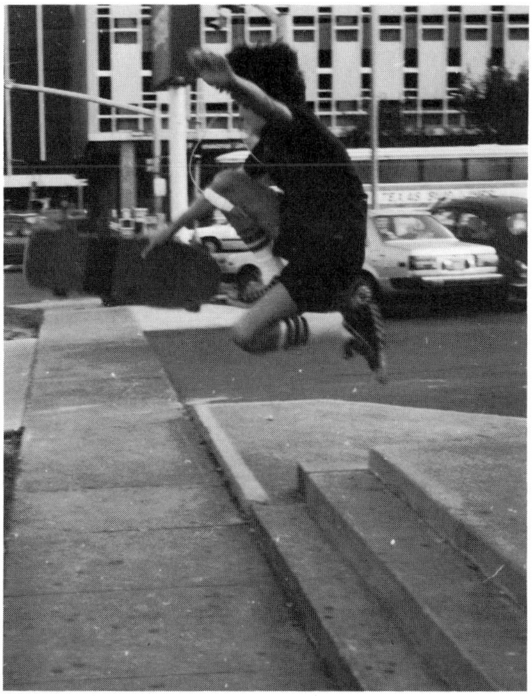

FIGURE 23–8
A patient performing a favorite activity (skateboarding) while undergoing continuous ambulatory electrocardiographic (Holter) monitoring. There is no confining or restraining influence of the monitoring device.

with unexplained syncope, Denes and Ezri discovered inducible supraventricular tachycardia in six and ventricular tachycardia or fibrillation in four (a total of 20%). A number of other electrophysiologic diagnoses were made, including sinus node abnormality, abnormal atrioventricular node function, and hypersensitive carotid sinus syndrome. In all, 74% of the patients had some abnormality on electrophysiologic study.[54] Carotid sinus massage during electrophysiologic study and the use of a tilt table to reproduce symptoms and signs of syncope may assist in electrophysiologic diagnosis.[47, 54]

In children, there have been mixed results with the use of electrophysiologic study. The usefulness of the test is related to the type of syncope (typical or atypical), to the type of rhythm thought to be the cause, and to the type of underlying heart disease. Table 23–3 shows a summary of the predictive value of several tests (routine electrocardiogram, treadmill test, Holter monitoring, and electrophysiologic study) based on our experience in patients with syncope and a number of possible causes thereof.

Long QT Syndrome. Long QT syndrome is usually present on routine electrocardiogram. Exercise study may provoke arrhythmias or may be normal. Holter monitoring will generally show the QT interval to be long at some point in the 24-hour period. Routine electrophysiologic study is no help.

Wolff-Parkinson-White Syndrome. Wolff-Parkinson-White syndrome is usually noted on the routine electrocardiogram and will be present on the 24-hour Holter monitor. Exercise test may be helpful in identifying a short effective refractory period of the accessory connection, and the electrophysiologic study is extremely helpful in prognosis and treatment.

Sinus Bradycardia. In sinus bradycardia, the routine electrocardiogram may not be helpful because of the intermittent nature of bradycardia. The Holter monitor will help, particularly if there are symptoms. Neither the treadmill nor electrophysiologic study has been helpful or sensitive in determining sinus node function.

Atrioventricular Block. Atrioventricular block may be present on routine electrocardiogram. Holter monitor may show the atrioventricular block as intermittent, particularly when associated with symptoms. Treadmill testing may show the development or worsening of atrioventricular block with exercise. Electrophysiologic study is usually not sensitive.

Atrial Flutter. Routine electrocardiogram, Holter monitor and treadmill test may help make the diagnosis of atrial flutter but will not exclude the possibility in a patient who is at high risk. Electrophysiologic induction of atrial flutter may be predictive.

Supraventricular Tachycardia. Unless the patient is in tachycardia, routine electrocardiogram and Holter monitor cannot confirm the diagnosis. Supraventricular tachycardia is not generally exercise related. Most forms of SVT can be induced at electrophysiologic study.

Ventricular Tachycardia. Ventricular tachycardia is usually not present on routine electrocardiogram. There may be many premature ventricular extrasystoles on Holter electrocardiogram that may point to a patient with ventricular arrhythmias. If there are no premature ventricular contractions on cardioscan, there will generally not be significant symptomatic ventricular arrhythmias as the cause of syncope. (In contrast, a normal Holter examination for suspected supraventricular tachycardia, atrial flutter, atrial ventricular block, or sick sinus syndrome is not conclusive.) Treadmill testing may increase

TABLE 23–3
GUIDE FOR EVALUATION OF A PATIENT WITH SYNCOPE AND SUSPECTED CONDITIONS*

SUSPECTED CONDITION OCCURRING WITH SYNCOPE	INVESTIGATIVE TOOL			
	Routine ECG	*Treadmill*	*Holter*	*EPS*
Long QT	±	±	+	−
WPW syndrome	±	±	+	+
Sinus bradycardia	−	−	+	−
Atrioventricular block	+	+	+	±
Atrial flutter	−	−	−	±
Supraventricular tachycardia	−	−	−	+
Ventricular tachycardia	−	+	+	+

*− = usually normal; + = usually abnormal; ± = unpredictable.
Abbreviations: ECG = electrocardiogram; EPS = electrophysiologic study; WPW = Wolff-Parkinson-White.

ventricular arrhythmias or provoke ventricular tachycardia. This will be helpful in making the diagnosis and in determining the success of treatment. Many patients with syncope and ventricular arrhythmias may have these arrhythmias induced and symptoms reproduced at electrophysiologic study.

Quantitative Evaluation of the Autonomic Nervous System

Specific investigation of the autonomic nervous system is performed in some laboratories. Syncope, as has been discussed, may result from a fall in heart rate or blood pressure caused by an abnormal response (or lack of a normal response) to a stimulus. The autonomic nervous system in general is responsible for physiologic adaptations to stress and in particular regulates heart rate, vascular impedance, and blood flow distribution. Malfunction or imbalances in this feedback system may cause syncope in prolonged QT syndrome, hypertrophic cardiomyopathy, and mitral valve prolapse, as well as in the simple faint, in vagovagal reaction, and in orthostatic hypotension. There has been renewed interest in the noninvasive quantitative evaluation of the autonomic nervous system, and a number of the techniques involved relate specifically to the investigation of syncope.

SUPINE AND STANDING HEMODYNAMICS AND CIRCULATING CATECHOLAMINE MEASUREMENTS

Normally, with a change from prone or supine to standing posture, there is a decrease in circulating blood volume because of venous pooling in the legs. This causes a fall in venous return and in blood pressure. The blood pressure drop activates baroreceptors that reflexly cause a prompt return of blood pressure to normal (or slightly elevated) levels by arteriolar vasoconstriction.

The increase in sympathetic nervous system tone is reflected by increased circulating norepinephrine and epinephrine. These chemicals approximately double in concentration after 5 minutes of standing in normal adults.[56] These catecholamines stimulate heart rate and support blood pressure with predominant stimulation of the α-adrenergic arteriolar receptors. Investigation of the heart rate and blood pressure responses to standing and the measurement of circulating catecholamines may provide clues to the pathophysiology and treatment of certain types of syncope such as orthostatic hypotension.

QUANTITATIVE VALSALVA MANEUVER

Analysis of the heart rate and blood pressure responses to the standardized Valsalva maneuver assists in assessment of a number of limbs of the autonomic nervous system. In this test, forced expiration is held in order to keep a mercury column at a determined height (e.g., 40 mm) for a certain period of time.

The normal response to the Valsalva maneuver has been divided into four phases.[57] In the first phase, increased intrathoracic pressure raises aortic pressure by mechanical compression and consequently decreases heart rate. The rate of fall of heart rate as compared with the rise in blood pressure offers an index of baroreceptor function and parasympathetic response. Phase two involves the decrease in venous return caused by the rise in intra-abdominal and intrathoracic pressure. This decreased return causes a fall in blood pressure and cardiac output, eliciting a compensatory rise in heart rate and peripheral vasoconstriction, evidence of sympathetic responsiveness. Phase three, release of the maneuver, results in a fall in blood presure because of relief of aortic compression. Phase four (recovery) occurs when venous return normalizes, and there is a characteristic overshoot of blood pressure related to residual vasoconstriction. This rise in pressure depends on an intact sympathetic nervous system, and the reflex bradycardia that follows gives an indication of parasympathetic function.

RESPONSES TO VASOACTIVE PHARMACOLOGIC AGENTS: PHENYLEPHRINE, ISOPROTERENOL, AND TYRAMINE

A normal response to infusion of phenylephrine (rise in blood pressure followed by a decrease in heart rate) relies on normal α-adrenergic receptors and baroreceptor sensitivity. Isoproterenol administration tests the β_1 receptors on the heart and the β_2 vascular smooth muscle receptors. Gradual infusion of this agent normally increases heart rate directly and decreases systemic vascular resistance by peripheral vasodilation. Tyramine has been implemented to test the integrity of the postganglionic sympathetic nervous system by stimulating release of norepinephrine from sympathetic nerve terminals. Specific deficits in one or more of these responses may be implicated in some patients with syncope of undetermined cause.

RECEPTOR MEASUREMENT

Recently it has become possible to measure sympathetic and parasympathetic autonomic receptors in experimental animals[58] and in man.[59] β-Adrenergic receptors on leukocytes and α-adrenergic receptors on platelets may be quantitated with ligand-binding techniques, in which radiolabeled catecholamine derivatives bound to those receptors are measured. Alterations in adrenergic receptors may prove to be important in certain subtypes of syncope such as that caused by orthostatic hypotension.[59]

CAROTID SINUS MASSAGE AND QUANTITATION OF SINUS ARRHYTHMIA

The variation in heart rate that normally occurs with respiration (sinus arrhythmia) is mediated mainly by the vagus nerve. In addition, the vagus nerve participates in the reflex bradycardic and hypotensive response caused by hypertension detected in the carotid bodies. Quantitative determination of the degree of sinus arrhythmia thus offers an indication of parasympathetic control of the heart,[60] and carotid massage tests the degree of vagal tone and responsiveness. These noninvasive tests may help in diagnosis of patients who have carotid sinus hypersensitivity or vagovagal reactions.

DIVING REFLEX

The diving reflex response, part of the assessment of the autonomic nervous system, may offer insight into both parasympathetic stimulation and sympathetic withdrawal. With immersion of the face into ice water, both responses occur. These result in a marked rapid drop in heart rate and usually mild peripheral vasoconstriction with preservation of blood pressure. Although the use of the diving reflex has been well established clinically for the treatment of supraventricular tachycardia,[61] its role in autonomic assessment of syncopal patients remains to be elucidated.

SUMMARY

Syncope in children is an important symptom of a system of diseases ranging from a simple faint to life-threatening cardiac arrhythmias. The history and examination will point to possible causes of syncope, and judicious use of laboratory evaluations and subspecialty referrals will most often lead to the correct diagnosis and effective treatment. The pathophysiology of these episodes remains intriguing and complex and is only recently beginning to be fully explored.

ACKNOWLEDGMENTS

The author would like to thank Ms. Candy Liedtke for expert secretarial assistance, Dr. Barry Marcus for ideas and information about the autonomic nervous system, and Dr. Arthur Garson, Jr., for assistance and guidance.

References

1. Webster's New Collegiate Dictionary. Springfield, MA, G & C Merriam, 1977.
2. Friedberg C: Syncope: Pathological physiology: Differential diagnosis and treatment (I). Mod Concepts Cardiovasc Dis XL:55–60, 1971.
3. Friedberg C: Syncope: Pathological physiology: Differential diagnosis and treatment (II). Mod Concepts Cardiovasc Dis XL:61–63, 1971.
4. Noble R: The patient with syncope. JAMA 237:1372–1376, 1977.
5. Weissler A, Warren J: Vasodepressor syncope. Am Heart J 57:786–794, 1959.
6. Goldstein D, Spanarkel M, Pitterman A, et al: Circulatory control mechanisms in vasodepressor syncope. Am Heart J 104:1071–1075, 1982.
7. Weissler A, Warren J, Estes E Jr, et al: Vasodepressor syncope: Factors influencing cardiac output. Circulation XV:875–882, 1957.
8. Epstein S, Stampfer M, Beiser G: Role of the capac-

itance and resistance vessels in vasovagal syncope. Circulation XXXVII:524–533, 1968.
9. Sapire D, Casta A, Safley W, et al: Vasovagal syncope in children requiring pacemaker implantation. Am Heart J 106:1406–1411, 1983.
10. Brammell H, Vogel J, Pryor R, et al: The Eisenmenger syndrome: A clinical and physiologic reappraisal. Am J Cardiol 28:679–692, 1971.
11. Canedo M, Frank M, Abdulla A: Rhythm disturbances in hypertrophic cardiomyopathy: Prevalence, relation to symptoms and management. Am J Cardiol 45:848–855, 1980.
12. Peters M, Hall R, Cooley D, et al: The clinical syndrome of atrial myxoma. JAMA 230:695–701, 1974
13. Rich S, Lam W: Atrial septostomy as palliative therapy for refractory primary pulmonary hypertension. Am J Cardiol 51:1560–1561, 1983.
14. Austen W, Morrow A, Berry W: Experimental studies of the surgical treatment of primary pulmonary hypertension. J Thorac Cardiovasc Surg 48:448–455, 1964.
15. Beder S, Cohen M, Riemenschneider T: Occult arrhythmias as the etiology of unexplained syncope in children with structurally normal hearts. Am Heart J 109:309–313, 1985.
16. Levy A, Camm A, Keane J: Multiple arrhythmias detected during nocturnal monitoring in patients with congenital complete heart block. Circulation 55:247–253, 1977.
17. Jervell A, Lange-Nielsen F: Congenital deaf-mutism, functional heart disease with prolongation of the Q-T interval, and sudden death. Am Heart J 54:59–68, 1957.
18. Romano C, Gemme G, Pongiglione R: Aritmie cardiache rare dell'eta' pediatrica. II. Accessi sincopali per fibrillazione ventricolare parossistica. Clin Pediatr 45:656–683, 1963.
19. Ward O: A new familial cardiac syndrome in children. J Irish Med Assoc LIV:103–106, 1964.
20. Wellens H, Vermeulen A, Durrer D: Ventricular fibrillation occurring on arousal from sleep by auditory stimuli. Circulation XLVI:661–665, 1972.
21. Schwartz P, Moss A: Prolonged Q-T interval: What does it mean? J Cardiovasc Med 7:1317–1330, 1982.
22. Horn C, Beekman R, Dick M, et al: The congenital long QT syndrome: An unusual cause of childhood seizures. Am J Dis Child 140:659–661, 1986.
23. Schwartz P: Sympathetic imbalance and cardiac arrhythmias. In Randall W (ed): Nervous Control of Cardiovascular Function. New York, Oxford University Press, 1984.
24. Yanowitz F, Preston J, Abildskov J: Functional distribution of right and left stellate innervation to the ventricles: Production of neurogenic electrocardiographic changes by unilateral alteration of sympathetic tone. Circ Res XVIII:416–428, 1966.
25. Moss A, McDonald J: Unilateral cervicothoracic sympathetic ganglionectomy for the treatment of long QT interval syndrome. N Engl J Med 285:903–904, 1971.
26. Schwartz P, Malliani A: Electrical alternation of the T-wave: Clinical and experimental evidence of its relationship with the sympathetic nervous system and with the long Q-T syndrome. Am Heart J 89:45–50, 1975.
27. Schwartz P: Idiopathic long QT syndrome: Progress and questions. Am Heart J 109:399–411, 1985.
28. Dungan W, Garson A Jr, Gillette P: Arrhythmogenic right ventricular dysplasia: A cause of ventricular tachycardia in children with apparently normal hearts. Am Heart J 102:745–750, 1981.
29. Rossi P, Massumi A, Gillette P, et al: Arrhythmogenic right ventricular dysplasia: Clinical features, diagnostic techniques, and current management. Am Heart J 103:415–420, 1982.
30. Yabek S, Dillon T, Berman W Jr, et al: Symptomatic sinus node dysfunction in children without structural heart disease. Pediatrics 69:590–593, 1982.
31. Johansson B: Adams-Stokes syndrome: A review and follow-up study of forty-two cases. Am J Cardiol 8:76–93, 1961.
32. Benson D Jr, Spach M, Edwards S, et al: Heart block in children: Evaluation of subsidiary ventricular pacemaker recovery times and ECG tape recordings. Pediatr Cardiol 2:39–45, 1982.
33. Pinsky W, Gillette P, Garson A Jr, et al: Diagnosis, management, and long-term results of patients with congenital complete atrioventricular block. Pediatrics 69:728–733, 1982.
34. Karpawich P, Gillette P, Garson A Jr, et al: Congenital complete atrioventricular block: Clinical and electrophysiologic predictors of need for pacemaker insertion. Am J Cardiol 48:1098–1102, 1981.
35. Gillette P: Supraventricular arrhythmias in children. J Am Coll Cardiol 5:122B–129B, 1985.
36. Rossi L, Thiene G: Mild Ebstein's anomaly associated with supraventricular tachycardia and sudden death: Clinicomorphologic features in 3 patients. Am J Cardiol 53:332–334, 1984.
37. Rocchini A, Chun P, Dick M: Ventricular tachycardia in children. Am J Cardiol 47:1091–1097, 1981.
38. James T, Beeson C II, Sherman E, et al: De subitaneis mortibus XIII. Multifocal Purkinje cell tumors of the heart. Circulation 52:333–344, 1975.
39. Devereux R, Perloff J, Reichek N, et al: Mitral valve prolapse. Circulation 54:3–14, 1976.
40. Jeresaty R: Sudden death in the mitral valve prolapse-click syndrome. Am J Cardiol 37:317–318, 1976.
41. Winkle R, Lopes M, Popp R, et al: Life-threatening arrhythmias in the mitral valve prolapse syndrome. Am J Med 60:961–967, 1976.
42. Campbell R, Godman M, Fiddler G, et al: Ventricular arrhythmias in syndrome of balloon deformity of mitral valve. Br Heart J 38:1053–1057, 1976.
43. Gaffney F, Karlsson E, Campbell W, et al: Autonomic dysfunction in women with mitral valve prolapse syndrome. Circulation 59:894–901, 1979.
44. Boudoulas H, Reynolds J, Mazzaferri E, et al: Metabolic studies in mitral valve prolapse syndrome. Circulation 61:1200–1205, 1980.
45. Barcroft H, Edholm O, McMichael J, et al: Posthaemorrhagic fainting: Study by cardiac output and forearm flow. Lancet 1:489–490, 1944.
46. Sugrue D, Wood D, McGoon M: Carotid sinus hypersensitivity and syncope. Mayo Clin Proc 59:637–640, 1984.
47. Hammill S, Holmes D Jr, Wood D, et al: Electrophysiologic testing in the upright position: Improved evaluation of patients with rhythm disturbances using a tilt table. J Am Coll Cardiol 4:65–71, 1984.
48. Woody R, Kiel E: Swallowing syncope in a child. Pediatrics 78:507–509, 1986.
49. Levine R: Epidemic faintness and syncope in a school marching band. JAMA 238:2373–2376, 1977.
50. Wright K Jr, McIntosh H: Syncope: A review of pathophysiological mechanisms. Prog Cardiovasc Dis XIII:580–594, 1971.

51. Bazett H: An analysis of the time relations of electrocardiograms. Heart 7:353–370, 1918.
52. Alpert B, Verrill D, Flood N, et al: Complications of ergometer exercise in children. Pediatr Cardiol 4:91–96, 1983.
53. Greenwood R, Rosenthal A, Sloss L, et al: Sick sinus syndrome after surgery for congenital heart disease. Circulation 52:208–213, 1975.
54. Denes P, Ezri M: The role of electrophysiologic studies in the management of patients with unexplained syncope. PACE 8:424–435, 1985.
55. Olshansky B, Mazuz M, Martins J: Significance of inducible tachycardia in patients with syncope of unknown origin: A long-term follow-up. J Am Coll Cardiol 5:216–223, 1985.
56. Robertson D, Johnson G, Robertson R, et al: Comparative assessment of stimuli that release neuronal and adrenomedullary catecholamines in man. Circulation 59:637–643, 1979.
57. Goldberg H, Elisberg E, Katz L: The effects of the Valsalva-like maneuver upon the circulation in normal individuals and patients with mitral stenosis. Circulation V:38–47, 1952.
58. Watanabe A, Jones L, Manalan A, et al: Cardiac autonomic receptors: Recent concepts from radiolabeled ligand-binding studies. Circ Res 50:161–174, 1982.
59. Motulsky H, Insel P: Adrenergic receptors in man: Direct identification, physiologic regulation, and clinical alterations. N Engl J Med 307:18–29, 1982.
60. Katona P, Jih F: Respiratory sinus arrhythmia: Noninvasive measure of parasympathetic cardiac control. J Appl Physiol 39:801–805, 1975.
61. Hamilton J, Moddie D, Levy J: The use of the diving reflex to terminate supraventricular tachycardia in a 2-week old infant. Am Heart J 97:371–374, 1979.

CHAPTER 24

ARRHYTHMIAS AND SPORTS

J. Timothy Bricker & Bertrand Ross

The request for recommendations or permission for sports participation is frequent in the arrhythmia clinic. The goal of parents and cardiologists is to provide both a risk-free situation for the patient and protection from unnecessary restrictions. Unfortunately precise information to assure this is unavailable and, in many instances, unobtainable. However, some useful generalizations may be made.

RISKS AND SPORTS

According to tradition, Pheidippedes died in 490 BC on the market square of Athens after bringing news of the defeat of Darius's forces of Persian invaders by Greek armies under the command of Mitiades. A literal translation of the Greek is that "his heart leapt from his chest." Concern about sudden death during athletic participation is the overriding consideration in advising individuals with arrhythmias about sports participation. Other potential risks for the athlete with an arrhythmia include injury (to self or others) from syncope during the sporting event and the possibility of deterioration of cardiac status as a result of training over a long term. These risks must be weighed against the benefits of athletic participation.

ARRHYTHMIAS AND RISKS OF SUDDEN DEATH

Most young athletes who die suddenly are not known to have a cardiac abnormality, and most young individuals with cardiac disease who die suddenly do not do so during exercise. Sudden death was demonstrated to be related to exercise or activity in approximately 10% of the cases of sudden unexpected cardiovascular death in children reported by Lambert et al in 1974.[1] Garson found a 0.004% incidence of sudden death in a large cardiac clinic during a 25-year period (101 of 23,402 patients); 22% of these were related to activity or exercise.[2] The overwhelming majority of these patients had had arrhythmias. It has become apparent that sudden death in children with structural cardiac defects may be related to an arrhythmia.[3–5] It has also been demonstrated that serious arrhythmias in this population are related to exercise.[6, 7] Drug therapy has been demonstrated to result in an improvement in exercise-related arrhythmias[6] and to be associated with a decline in sudden death in this relatively high-risk population.[8] Patients with poor hemodynamics and arrhythmias associated with operated congenital cardiac disease seem to be at highest risk for exercise-related sudden death.

Many of those who experience sudden cardiac death resulting from athletics have cardiac abnormalities that are inapparent prior to death. The leading cause of sudden cardiac death in young athletes is hypertrophic cardiomyopathy,[9, 10] which accounts for approximately one-half of the cases. Arrhythmias (both ventricular and supraventricular bradycardia and tachycardia) are probably a significant factor in the sudden death of athletes with hypertrophic cardiomyopathy.[11–13] There is no evidence that medical or surgical therapy can result in safe athletic participation for individuals with hypertrophic cardiomyopathy.[14]

Physiologic development of hypertrophy with training may be confused with pathologic hypertrophy. Exercise training of the adult cardiovascular system results in the development of significant left ventricular hypertrophy.[15–21] An increase in left ventricular thickness with training can also be seen in pre-adolescent children,[22] although this increase seems to be much less prominent than that which occurs in mature athletes. Isometric training will cause more hypertrophy than aerobic sports.[16, 17] Whether hypertrophy represents a cardiomyopathy or a response to training may be difficult to determine simply from echocardiographic measurements of left ventricular thickness in athletes who present for evaluation of arrhythmia. The pattern of hypertrophy and severity of hypertrophy is helpful in differentiating between these two situations.[23, 24] The "symmetry" of the hypertrophy and the relationship of wall thickness to ventricular chamber size are also of use.

Anomalies of the course or origin of the coronary arteries may result in sudden cardiac death during athletics.[25] Myocardial ischemia during intense exercise is thought to result from compression of the coronary artery and aorta. Typically there are no harbingers of sudden catastrophic events (other than the occasional patient with syncope) in these obstensibly healthy young individuals. Exercise-related arrhythmias, including exercise-related ventricular tachycardia, have been observed in individuals with coronary aneurysms[132] and with congenital coronary artery abnormalities.[26–28] Athletes with these rare anomalies may present for evaluation of an arrhythmia prior to death. If they do so, it is possible that a "benign" arrhythmia may be found and that a coronary abnormality may remain undetected.

Atherosclerotic cardiovascular disease of the coronary arteries may develop with unsuspected obstruction in the young athletes and result in sudden death.[9, 10, 29–33] These patients can obviously escape detection. However, it is again possible that such a case could present for evaluation of an arrhythmia that proves to be secondary to ischemia.

Myocarditis is diagnosed at autopsy of some cases of sudden cardiac death in athletes.[10] Arrhythmias may be a prominent feature of even mild cases of myocarditis.[34] This diagnosis should be considered in the athlete who presents with the recent onset of a symptomatic arrhythmia. Some have speculated that intense physical training can accelerate the deterioration with myocarditis and have suggested that athletes with a viral illness be held out of training for a month after onset of symptoms.[35] There is no definitive evidence that this is necessary, however, and most athletes promptly return to training after viral illnesses without adverse effects.

Sudden death occurring with exertion or excitement is a prominent feature of the hereditary syndromes of prolongation of the QT interval.[36–38] These syndromes seem to be more common than was previously recognized. The electrocardiographic findings are subtle, and affected families frequently escape detection for years. The importance of the family history in the diagnosis of the athlete referred for the evaluation of arrhythmia or symptoms possibly related to an arrhythmia must be emphasized. Careful measurement of the QT (or QTu) interval with calculation of a corrected QT interval on suspected cases is quite important.

Sudden death has been reported in patients with mitral valve prolapse.[29, 39–43] The prognosis of mitral valve prolapse is generally favorable; complications are infrequent and are unrelated to physical activity for the most part. In spite of the high prevalence of mitral valve prolapse,[44] cases of sudden death are extremely rare.[10] Mitral valve prolapse in children is common and, in the overwhelming majority of cases, quite benign.[45] However, serious arrhythmias, including arrhythmias during exercise, can occur in some children with mitral valve prolapse.[46] Although the finding of mitral valve prolapse increases the possibility that an arrhythmia is the cause of exercise-related symptoms, the risk of sudden death with exercise in young individuals with prolapse is not thought to be greatly increased compared to the general population.

Atrial flutter or fibrillation with a rapid ventricular response is one cause of sudden death[47] observed to occur with sports activity. Exercise may enhance atrioventricular conduction and result in sudden death in patients with chronic atrial flutter.[48]

Rapid atrioventricular conduction with atrial flutter or fibrillation may result in fibrillation of the ventricle of young individuals with ventricular preexcitation caused by an accessory pathway.[49, 50] This presumably is the mechanism of sudden death in athletes with Wolff-Parkinson-White syndrome.[50] Exercise may also precipitate orthodromic or antidromic supraventricular tachycardia with Wolff-Parkinson-White syndrome.[51] Athletes with preexcitation syndromes and exercise-related SVT who are hemodynamically unstable during tachycardia could be at risk for sudden death from SVT. An association between Wolff-Parkinson-White syndrome and hypertrophic cardiomyopathy has also been observed,[13] which could represent an additional unrecognized risk for athletes with Wolff-Parkinson-White syndrome, which is very rarely associated with sudden cardiac deaths in these patients.

Ventricular arrhythmias with exercise are a potential cause of death in individuals with arrhythmogenic right ventricular dysplasia.[10, 52] We have observed arrhythmogenic right ventricular dysplasia presenting with syncope in otherwise asymptomatic athletes.[16]

Young individuals with sports-related sudden death may be found at autopsy to have other structural cardiac abnormalities (Table 24–1).[53–62] Detection of these abnormalities in the apparently healthy young athlete, including the athlete with an arrhythmia, is unlikely to occur. Minor abnormalities of the conduction system in young athletes with sudden death might be incidental findings.[62]

Sudden death related to drug abuse in athletes has been a problem of great concern. Arrhythmias and myocardial infarction may occur with cocaine abuse.[63] Amphetamine abuse was found in seven of 198 cases of sudden death in athletes reviewed by Neimann.[64] While recreational drugs may be viewed as a public health or societal problem unrelated to the patient in the arrhythmia clinic, their abuse is a problem of such prevalence that it warrants special concern regarding the athlete presenting with an arrhythmia.

ARRHYTHMIAS AND RISKS OF INJURIES

Arrhythmias can occur in which the individual is only mildly symptomatic during the arrhythmia and is therefore thought to be at a low risk of sudden cardiac death. However, the possibility of lightheadedness occurring during a sport with resultant risk of injury to others or the individuals themselves should be considered with these athletes.[65] For example, it is easy to imagine how steeplechase, Grand Prix auto racing, or sky diving would each be a particular risk for an athlete in this category. In practice, individuals who seek out those sports with a high risk of traumatic injury seem to be the least likely to heed advice. However, it is important to address these issues with the athlete in the arrhythmia clinic.

TABLE 24–1
SUDDEN DEATH IN THE YOUNG ATHLETE: CARDIAC ASSOCIATIONS

Arrhythmias probably related to occurrence of sudden death
Postoperative cyanotic congenital cardiac disease; TOF, Mustard, Fontan procedures
Hypertrophic cardiomyopathy
Myocarditis
Aortic insufficiency
Mitral valve prolapse
Hereditary prolongation of the QT interval
Wolff-Parkinson-White syndrome
Arrhythmogenic right ventricular dysplasia
Primary ventricular arrhythmia
Primary atrial flutter
Sarcoidosis
Complete AV block
Cardiac tumor
Eisenmenger's syndrome
Ebstein's syndrome
Postoperative acyanotic congenital cardiac disease
Palliated cyanotic congenital cardiac disease
Primary pulmonary hypotension
Drug abuse
Conditions in which sudden death occurs, probably unrelated to arrhythmia
Aortic stenosis*
Cystic medial necrosis
Marfan's syndrome
Coarctation of aorta
Coronary abnormalities*
Anomalous left coronary from anterior sinus
Single coronary artery
Intramyocardial coronary artery
Coronary artery aneurysms
Exercise-induced coronary spasm
Atherosclerosis of coronary artery
Intussusception of coronary artery
Aneurysm of aortic cusp
Speculative association (incidental findings that may be unrelated to sudden death)
Narrowing of sinus node artery
Recent SA node hemorrhage
Abnormal course of SA node artery
Fatty infiltration of SA node
Ganglionitis and neuritis near SA node
Compression of AV node
Persisting fetal dispersion of AV node
Fibroma compressing His bundle
Hemorrhage in His bundle
Lipomatous infiltration of His bundle
Narrow AV node artery
Disrupted fibers of bundle branches
Fibrosis of the summit of the interventricular septum

*Ischemia-related arrhythmias possible.
Abbreviations: AV = atrioventricular; SA = sinoatrial; TOF = tetralogy of Fallot.

RISKS RESULTING FROM TRAINING

Athletic training results in structural and functional changes of the cardiovascular system. These changes may be detrimental to the status of the athlete with an arrhythmia. In addition, the physiologic changes that occur with training of the cardiovascular system can result in confusion as to whether disease or a normal adaptation is being observed. Incorrect classification of normal athletes as having heart disease may lead to needless dangerous interventions or investigations or psychologic trauma for the athlete, and possibly even financial loss if the athlete is a professional. Unfortunately, normal adaptational phenomena may also cause difficulty in the identification of those athletes who have cardiac abnormalities that subject them to danger during athletic performance.

Electrocardiographic changes in healthy athletes are common and can be so bizarre that it has been suggested that routine electrocardiography in athletes be avoided in order to prevent the needless labeling of large numbers of athletes as abnormal.[66] Cardiac dilation and ventricular hypertrophy are characteristic responses to intense athletic training.[67, 68] The hearts of athletes were first studied in an organized manner by electrocardiography, radiography, and stress testing during the 1928 Olympic games in Amsterdam.[69] Although cardiac enlargement was characteristic, the greatest degree of enlargement was found among athletes in endurance events. Highly aerobic or isotonic sports (such as distance running, dancing, and cross-country skiing) are analogous to a volume overload to the heart, and the ventricular dilation is prominent. Highly anaerobic or isometric sports (such as weight lifting) are analogous to a pressure overload and result in more hypertrophy than dilation.[16, 17, 70, 71] There is quite a bit of overlap in the degree of chamber hypertrophy and ventricular dilation among elite athletes in predominantly isometric sports.[68] These changes are reflected in the electrocardiogram.

Differentiation of cardiac disease from the athletic heart may be quite difficult. Physical findings include a slow pulse, an increased pulse volume, a laterally displaced and prolonged apex impulse,[71] mid-systolic murmur,[72–76] a third or fourth heart sound,[77] and a mid-diastolic filling rumble.[78, 79] Radiographic evidence of cardiomegaly and a globular heart shape may be associated with an increase in pulmonary vascular markings.[78]

Electrocardiographic evidence of left or right ventricular hypertrophy might be found.[70, 80, 87] An incomplete right bundle-branch block pattern of the QRS is extremely common among athletes, with prevalence from 50% to 80% reported.[70, 79, 87] Huston, Puffer, and Rodney have reviewed the reported incidences of various arrhythmias among athletes and compared them with the incidence in the general population.[78] Many, but not all, of the training-induced electrocardiographic changes are reversible with detraining. Training bradycardia is characteristic of the heart of the athlete;[81] heart rates in the 20s and 30s have been observed.[60, 70, 79, 82] Vagotonia[83–85] and intrinsic myocardial changes[86] have been implicated as the mechanism of training-induced bradycardia and of a decrease in sympathetic tone.[87] Total autonomic blockade or denervation will result in a lower intrinsic heart rate in the trained than in the untrained individual. Whether the bradycardia precedes or follows the structural cardiac adaptations is unknown.

Whether these structural changes are entirely reversible with detraining is unknown. Sinus bradycardia is the most common rhythm found; junctional or ventricular escape rhythms may be seen less frequently.[88, 89] Although the situation of the individual with a normal heart who "runs into a pacemaker" is extremely uncommon,[70] it is possible that training bradycardia is deleterious for some athletes with cardiac disease. For example, the patient in an untrained state with mild sinus node dysfunction after a Mustard operation might have a more dangerous if not at least a more difficult-to-evaluate arrhythmia after intense physical training.

Intracardiac electrophysiology studies are not known to be able to differentiate pathologic from physiologic bradycardia in the athlete. Ambulatory electrocardiography to correlate rate and symptoms in symptomatic individuals should be used as the basis for determining when intervention is required. Exercise testing will show a higher physical working capacity than average, with a normal or low-average peak exercise heart rate in patients with the athlete's heart syndrome. A test with a low or low-average physical working capacity, chronotropic impairment at peak exercise, and symptomatic post-exercise bradycardia is suggestive of pathologic rather than physiologic sinus bradycardia. Reevaluation after a 6-week period of enforced detraining should show enough resolution of training effect to allow differentiation in questionable cases.

Sinus arrhythmia is much more common in trained than in sedentary individuals.[79] This does not generally cause diagnostic confusion. Resting sinus arrhythmia in athletes disappears with exertion and has been attributed to a high resting vagal tone. Wandering atrial pacemaker and first degree atrioventricular conduction block are also found with greater frequency in trained than in sedentary individuals. Athletes with resting PR interval prolongation will demonstrate shortening of the PR interval with exercise.

Mobitz type I second degree atrioventricular conduction block is found in normal, highly trained athletes.[88, 89] Normal atrioventricular conduction is found after atropine is given or after cessation of training. Rare cases of Mobitz type II second degree block and third degree atrioventricular block have been observed.[79, 90] There have been well documented cases of development of advanced atrioventricular block with athletics that may be reversible with detraining. Patients demonstrating high levels of athletic performance have been found to have congenital complete atrioventricular block, and it is possible that a congenital case could escape detection until the patient becomes involved in sports as an adolescent. Demonstration of normal conduction with exercise, with sympathetic agonists, or with detraining supports the diagnosis of a training-related abnormality. Long-term follow-up of these individuals is required.

The incidence of premature ventricular contractions and ventricular tachycardia on ambulatory monitoring has not been shown to be greater in athletes than among controls, although training-induced bradycardia might produce conditions favorable to the development of ventricular ectopy and fibrillation.[91] There is no evidence that ventricular arrhythmias are part of the expected response to athletic training. Ventricular arrhythmias in the athlete should be approached in a manner similar to those occurring in the nonathletic individual.

Supraventricular tachycardia, atrial flutter, and atrial fibrillation may be seen in normal athletes.[92] It is not clear whether supraventricular tachycardias are more prevalent among athletes. Supraventricular arrhythmias occasionally occur in trained individuals at high intensity of exercise. Reevaluation of trained athletes with minimally symptomatic supraventricular tachycardia following a period of enforced detraining may be of interest, but otherwise the investigation and treatment of supraventricular tachycardia in the trained subject will be the same as for the sedentary subject.

Physiologic ST segment elevation or depression, J point elevation or depression, peaked T waves, and T wave inversion may be found in the athlete. Further investigation is not usually required. Bundle-branch block pattern of the QRS, a right or left deviation of the frontal plane QRS axis, an infarct pattern, and QT prolongation have been found in athletes who were subsequently determined to be normal.[79] However, none of these are considered routine findings for the athletic heart, and comprehensive evaluation is recommended. Reevaluation after enforced detraining may be a valuable part of the investigation of these athletes also. QT prolongation seen in athletes may represent hereditary prolongation with an associated risk of sudden death. Prolongation of the QT interval secondary to training in normal athletes has been postulated to result in an electrical instability of the heart of the normal athlete. QT prolongation should, in our opinion, result in termination of athletic participation. Although reevaluation after detraining could show normalization of QT interval, whether the individual with a training-induced QT prolongation is at low risk for sudden death when trained to a high level of fitness is unknown.

RISK/BENEFIT ANALYSIS

The assessment of a risk/benefit ratio is highly subjective. The risks are not precisely known, and perception of benefit varies greatly among athletes and physicians. It is our opinion that the responsibility for the decision about sports participation for the athlete with an arrhythmia must be shared with the athlete and the family. A risk-free environment cannot be assured, even for the athlete without heart disease. An extreme example is that of a professional athlete with syncope during sports that was diagnosed to be a result of torsades de pointes ventricular tachycardia. After successful treatment with amiodarone, he continued to play professional basketball.[93] The risk of catastrophic complications from this arrhythmia would be enough to make most cardiologists nervous. However, there is no question that the analysis of the benefits of sports for the athlete with a multimillion-dollar contract is different than that for the typical young athlete. Psychologic benefits of sports participation are acknowledged, and participation in athletics can improve the young individual's self-confidence and self-image. Psychologic benefits of being permitted to participate in athletics are particularly important to the adolescent whose self-image has been negatively affected by the presence of a cardiac defect or a scar from cardiac surgery. Paradoxically, more severe psychologic difficulty is sometimes seen in cases of mild physical disability.[94] Thus, the patients most likely to benefit from sports are often those for whom participation is quite feasible. Physical fitness has also been shown to improve academic performance.[95]

Physiologic benefits of sports include both cardiovascular and noncardiovascular aspects of conditioning. Benefits related to the pulmonary system, weight control, serum lipids, blood pressure, and the musculoskeletal system are well known.[96–108] Patterns of physical activity established in childhood should lead to a healthier life-style in the adult years. Physiologic adaptations to chronic physical activity are routinely employed in adult patients with coronary disease in a therapeutic manner. Cardiac rehabilitation programs have been attempted for children with cardiac disease and for patients after surgical repair of congenital cardiac lesions.[109–113] Potential benefits include an improved physical working capacity,[109, 110, 112] an improved systemic oxygen delivery during exercise,[112, 114] increased myocardial capillary density,[115] improved resting and working stroke volume,[115] improved oxygen extraction at maximal work,[115] and a raised threshold for ventricular fibrillation.[117, 118] Physiologic training effects are evident with prepubertal children involved in cardiovascular training programs.[22, 119] However, because cardiorespiratory fitness is not necessarily altered by participation of young children in sports,[119, 120] intense training in organized rehabilitation programs may be required to effect demonstrable changes in cardiorespiratory fitness.

Because of the subjective nature of the benefits of sports and the imprecise nature of risk assessment, most cases will require individualized sports recommendations. This is explained to the family, and after our best attempts to objectively assess the risks, the decision about sports participation is a shared one.

SPECIFIC RECOMMENDATIONS FOR ATHLETES WITH ARRHYTHMIAS

The recommendations of the 16th Bethesda Conference were an attempt to offer a standard of management for athletes with arrhythmias (Table 24–2).[121] Recommendations from the American Heart Association regarding sports for athletes with arrhythmias are also available and are similar to those of the Bethesda Conference.[122] Several generalizations may be made. Although the lack of symptoms alone should not lead to an automatic recommendation for athletic participation without careful consideration, the presence of symptomatic arrhythmia requires exclusion from sports until the arrhythmia is adequately controlled. Although formal exercise testing is of value in assessment of the individual prior to sports participation, graded ergometry protocols occasionally will poorly mimic the cardiovascular stress associated with the sport under consideration. Anaerobic or "sprint" cycle or treadmill protocols can identify arrhythmias missed on graded protocols. Ambulatory monitoring during activity similar to the individual's sport and training routine is of help. Reevaluation of the athlete's status during and following training (i.e., at 1 month and 3 months into sports participation) is recommended to identify deterioration in rhythm resulting from the cardiovascular adaptations to chronic physical activity. Recommendations from the Bethesda Conference included consideration of the type of physical activity involved in the sport (i.e., aerobic or anaerobic). It should be remembered that an athlete's training routine for a predominantly aerobic sport frequently includes isometric activity in the weight room. It is important to remember that the young athlete is much more easily adapted to recommendations than the older one. When the possibility of future sports limitation exists because of the cardiovascular diagnosis, it is advisable to also encourage participation in nonathletic activities and in athletic activities of low physical intensity. This is suggested in order to avoid the problem of restriction of sports participation for the adolescent whose sport provides his or her sole ego reward.

TABLE 24–2
SPORTS RECOMMENDATIONS FOR THE ATHLETE WITH ARRHYTHMIA*

ARRHYTHMIA CATEGORY	RECOMMENDATION *No Restrictions*	 *No Sports*	COMMENT
Sinus/junctional bradycardia			
Normal Heart	Asymptomatic	Symptomatic	
Abnormal Heart	Asymptomatic	Symptomatic	
Second Degree AV Block			
Type I			
Normal Heart	Asymptomatic	Symptomatic	
Abnormal Heart	Asymptomatic	Symptomatic	
Type II			
Normal Heart	Asymptomatic	Symptomatic	No sports if degree of AV block increases with exercise testing
Abnormal Heart	Asymptomatic	Symptomatic	
Complete AV block			
Normal Heart		Symptomatic	No sports if ventricular arrhythmias with exercise testing
Abnormal Heart	Asymptomatic	×	
PAC, PJC			
Normal Heart	×		
Abnormal Heart	×		
PVC			
Normal Heart	×		If on treatment and can demonstrate <10 PVC/hr on Holter monitor and no ventricular arrhythmia on exercise test, then sports permitted. Parent and child should be informed of possible increased risk See also specific defect section
Abnormal Heart		×	
SVT			
Normal Heart	Asymptomatic	Symptomatic	SVT must be well controlled with medication and no episodes related to sports
Abnormal Heart	Asymptomatic	Symptomatic	
Atrial flutter/atrial fibrillation			
Normal Heart		×	If under treatment and no episodes for 6 months, sports may be permitted. Parent and child should be informed of possible increased risk
Abnormal Heart		×	
Ventricular tachycardia			
Normal Heart	Asymptomatic	Symptomatic	If patient (on or off treatment) can demonstrate no arrhythmia related to exercise, sports permitted, as long as asymptomatic
Abnormal Heart		×	
Wolff-Parkinson-White (No SVT/atrial flutter)			
Normal Heart	×		Assessment of refractory period of Kent bundle is recommended. If effective refractory period >300 ms, no restrictions. If <300 ms or is not evaluated, then parent and child should be informed of possible increased risk
Long QT (With or without ventricular arrhythmia)			
Normal or Abnormal Heart		×	

*Summarized from the 16th Bethesda Conference.

Abbreviations: AV = atrioventricular; PAC = premature atrial contractions; PJC = premature junctional contractions; PVC = premature ventricular contractions; SVT = supraventricular tachycardia.

Athletes with an apparent abnormality of sinus node function should have evaluation that includes both exercise testing and ambulatory monitoring during the athlete's sport and training routine. If the arrhythmia does not worsen with exercise, no restrictions are required if symptoms are absent. Periodic reevaluation to be certain that physiologic adaptation (i.e., training bradycardia) does not worsen the arrhythmia is important in this situation. Athletes who have syncope or light-headedness associated with this arhythmia should be held out of participation until the cause of the symptoms is adequately identified and treated. If the patient is asymptomatic for 6 months after treatment is instituted, full athletic participation may resume. However, impact or collision sports should be prohibited for the athlete with a pacemaker. Athletes with junctional escape beats or a junctional escape rhythm should be approached in the same manner as athletes with sinus node dysfunction.

Premature atrial or junctional complexes do not require limitation of sports participation in most situations. Premature supraventricular complexes in the athlete who also has symptoms suggestive of supraventricular tachycardia require further evaluation prior to sports participation.

Chronic atrial flutter or fibrillation may be well tolerated at rest because of atrioventricular conduction block but be poorly tolerated with an increase in atrioventricular conduction associated with exercise. Sports restrictions for this group of patients are recommended.

First degree atrioventricular conduction block without other abnormalities does not require sports limitations. Mobitz type I second degree atrioventricular block in asymptomatic individuals should not result in sports limitations if the degree of block improves or does not worsen with exercise. Patients who have a worsening in atrioventricular block with exercise should undergo intense evaluation before being allowed to participate. First degree atrioventricular block and Mobitz type I second degree atrioventricular block may be manifestations of the athlete's heart syndrome.

Mobitz type II second degree atrioventricular block and complete atrioventricular block are considered together for purposes of sports recommendations. Ventricular arrhythmias during exercise and syncope or presyncope are indications for atrial synchronous pacing before participation in sports with a high intensity of physical activity. Participation in sports that carry a risk of injury if syncope occurs should be restricted. Sports participation after pacemaker implant may resume, but collision sports should be avoided. Patients who have a normal heart and no symptoms may participate in sports without the need for pacemaker implantation.

Athletes with supraventricular tachycardia that is precipitated with exercise are sometimes identified by exercise testing.[92, 123] In cases with reproducible exercise-induced supraventricular tachycardia, the adequacy of therapy can be ascertained easily during exercise testing. After treatment that is adequate to prevent recurrence for a 6-month period, sports participation may be resumed. Patients with paroxysmal supraventricular tachycardia unrelated to exercise should have an attempt at treatment prior to sports participation. Exercise may increase the rate of both reentry and automatic mechanisms of supraventricular tachycardia.[123] It is helpful to know the response of tachycardia rate with exercise if sports participation is to be continued. Athletes with paroxysmal supraventricular tachycardia and a normal heart who are asymptomatic during tachycardia may participate in sports of low physical intensity or, if well controlled, participate in any sport. Patients with syncope or presyncope should not participate in sports that include a possibility of injury to themselves or others with syncope; they should not participate in competitive sports until they have been adequately treated without recurrence for at least 6 months. Association of supraventricular tachycardia with significant structural heart disease should result in limitations of athletic participation until the patient is free of recurrence for 6 months. Depending on the severity of the structural cardiac defect, other restrictions may be required as well.[124]

Wolff-Parkinson-White syndrome is rarely associated with sudden death. This risk seems to be predominantly in patients with a short antegrade refractory period of the accessory pathway. Although the athlete with Wolff-Parkinson-White syndrome who has never had symptoms may reasonably be allowed to continue to participate in sports, further investigation is desirable. Demonstration of antegrade block in the accessory connection during exercise testing can be of additional help in identifying patients with a long refractory period of the accessory connection.[51] Electrophysiologic study for measurement of the refractory period of the accessory connection may also provide important information. In some instances it is possible to do this with esophageal pacing rather than with transvenous pacing. Atrial fibrillation should be induced to identify the shortest RR interval. Because the electrophysiologic properties of the accessory connection may be altered by exercise,[125] measurement of the shortest RR interval during isoproterenol infusion or exercise should also be performed.[126, 127] Patients whose shortest RR interval during atrial fibrillation exceeds 300 ms, or whose antegrade effective refractory period of the accessory connection exceeds 220 ms during isoproterenol infusion or exercise, can be managed like other supraventricular tachycardia patients with regard to sports recommendations. While those with long refractory periods appear to do well, some patients with short refractory periods are at risk for sudden death. Untreated patients with a short refractory period should not participate in athletics. Low-intensity sports can be considered for the patient with Wolff-Parkinson-White syndrome and a short antegrade effective refractory period that can be shown to be significantly lengthened by drug therapy.

Premature ventricular contractions that disappear or do not increase in frequency during exercise testing do not require limitations in sports participation. Premature ventricular contractions that increase in frequency with exercise testing or that occur in couplets may still be relatively benign, and participation in low-intensity sports is reasonable. Participation in sports with high levels of physical intensity is not recommended for these patients without further investigation. Patients with premature ventricular contractions who are in a high-risk group (e.g., long QT interval syndrome, postoperative tetralogy of Fallot, cardiomyopathy, aortic stenosis and insufficiency, ischemic heart disease, myocarditis, and arrhythmogenic right ventricular dysplasia) should have sports participation limited.

Ventricular tachycardia may occur with exercise in young athletes and may be associated with sudden death in these individuals. Patients having ventricular tachycardia with a structurally normal heart (proven at cardiac catheterization), without any symptoms, and with monomorphic nonsustained ventricular tachycardia at a rate of 150/min or less may participate in sports. Multiform ventricular tachycardia precludes participation in sports.[26] Ventricular tachycardia patients with long QT interval syndrome and patients in the other high-risk groups previously mentioned should also be barred from sports participation. Patients with ventricular tachycardia successfully treated with no recurrence for 6 months or patients with asymptomatic tachycardia occurring at rates of 150/min or less and with an otherwise normal heart should be allowed to resume limited sports participation. Ventricular flutter or fibrillation should result in exclusion from athletics.

Asymptomatic athletes with right bundle-branch block who do not have ventricular arrhythmia or cardiac disease do not need to be restricted. Left bundle-branch block in young individuals is uncommon and may be associated with syncope. Exercise-induced left bundle-branch block is associated with structural cardiac disease.[128–131] An electrophysiology study of the young athlete with left bundle-branch block is recommended. Cases with left bundle-branch block and abnormal intracardiac atrioventricular conduction times should have pacemaker implant prior to resuming sports participation. After pacemaker implantation, collision sports should be avoided because of the pacemaker. Exercise-induced bundle-branch block has been reported with athlete's heart.[132]

Patients with hereditary prolongation of the QT interval are at risk of sudden death and should be restricted from sports participation regardless of other findings.

SPORTS AND ANTIARRHYTHMIC DRUGS

Athletes who are treated for rhythm abnormality could have special difficulty related to their drug therapy. Digitalis causes ST and T wave changes during exercise that could result in an incorrect diagnosis of ischemic heart disease.[133] Antiarrhythmic drugs that alter atrioventricular conduction have been associated with some cases of exercise-related bundle-branch block.[130, 131] Antiarrhythmic drug toxicity has been considered a contraindication to exercise testing.[134] The athlete should be closely monitored for toxicity. Evidence of toxicity certainly should be reason to interrupt athletic training and competition. Metabolic and electrolyte perturbations with extremes of athletic performance could contribute to antiarrhythmic drug toxicity.[135] β-Blocking drugs are commonly used in patients with ventricular and supraventricular arrhythmias. A slight decrease in maximal athletic performance can be noted by the athlete taking a β-blocker. Noncompliance during competition by adolescent athletes is a problem that has led us to generally avoid the use of β-blockers in these patients if possible. β-Blocking drugs are banned for international competition in several sports (such as archery and rifle shooting) in which they might result in an advantage to the athlete.

ACKNOWLEDGMENTS

Research was supported in part by grant RR-00188 from the General Clinical Research Branch, National Institutes of Health, and by the American Heart Association, Texas Affiliate Grant No. G136.

References

1. Lambert EC, Menon VA, Wagner HR, et al: Sudden unexpected death from cardiovascular disease in children. Am J Cardiol 34:89–96, 1974.
2. Garson A Jr: Sudden death in a pediatric cardiology population, 1958 to 1983: Relation to prior arrhythmias. J Am Coll Cardiol 5(suppl):138B–141B, 1985.
3. Garson A, Nihill MR, McNamara DG, et al: Status of the adult and adolescent following repair of tetralogy of Fallot. Circulation 59:1232–1240, 1979.
4. Gillette PC, Kugler JD, Garson A, et al: The mechanisms of cardiac dysrhythmias after the Mustard operation for transposition of the great arteries. Am J Cardiol 45:1225–1230, 1980.
5. Blake RS, Chung EE, Wesley H, et al: Conduction defects, ventricular arrhythmias, and late death after surgical closure of ventricular septal defect. Br Heart J 47:305–315, 1982.
6. James FW, Kaplan S, Schwartz DC, et al: Response to exercise in patients after total surgical correction of tetralogy of Fallot. Circulation 34:671–680, 1976.
7. Garson A, Gillette PC, Gutgesell HP, et al: Stress-induced ventricular arrhythmias after repair of tetralogy of Fallot. Am J Cardiol 46:1006–1012, 1980.
8. Garson A Jr, Randall DC, Gillette PC, et al: Prevention of sudden death after repair of tetralogy of Fallot: Treatment of ventricular arrhythmias. J Am Coll Cardiol 5:221–227, 1985.
9. Maron BJ, Roberts WC, McAllister HA, et al: Sudden death in young athletes. Circulation 62:218–229, 1980.
10. Maron BJ, Epstein SE, Roberts WC: Causes of sudden death in competitive athletes. J Am Coll Cardiol 7:204–214, 1986.
11. Maron BJ, Savage DD, Wolfson JK, et al: Prognostic significance of 24-hour ambulatory electrocardiographic monitoring in patients with hypertrophic cardiomyopathy: A prospective study. Am J Cardiol 48:252–257, 1981.
12. Stafford WJ, Trohman RG, Bilsker M, et al: Cardiac arrest in an adolescent with atrial fibrillation and hypertrophic cardiomyopathy. J Am Coll Cardiol 7:701–704, 1986.
13. Krikler DM, Davies MJ, Rowland E, et al: Sudden death in hypertrophic cardiomyopathy: Associated accessory atrioventricular pathways. Br Heart J 43:245–251, 1980.
14. Maron BJ, Gaffney FA, Jeresaty RM, et al: 16th Bethesda Conference. Task Force III: Hypertrophic cardiomyopathy, other myopericardial disease and mitral valve prolapse. J Am Coll Cardiol 6:1215–1217, 1985.
15. DeMaria AN, Neumann A, Lee G, et al: Alterations in ventricular mass and performance induced by exercise training in man evaluated by echocardiography. Circulation 57:237–244, 1978.
16. Longhurst JC, Kelly AR, Gonyea WJ, et al: Echocardiographic left ventricular masses in distance runners and weight lifters. J Appl Physiol 48:154–162, 1980.
17. Morganroth J, Maron BJ, Henry WL, et al: Comparative left ventricular dimensions in trained athletes. Ann Intern Med 82:521–524, 1975.
18. Underwood RH, Schwade JL: Noninvasive analysis of cardiac function of elite distance runners—echocardiography, vectorcardiography, and cardiac intervals. Ann NY Acad Sci 301:297–309, 1977.
19. Gilbert CA, Nutter DO, Feiner JM, et al: Echocardiographic study of cardiac dimensions and function in trained athletes. Am J Cardiol 40:528–533, 1977.
20. Ehsani AA, Hagberg JM, Hickson RC: Rapid changes in left ventricular dimensions and mass in response to physical conditioning and deconditioning. Am J Cardiol 42:52–56, 1978.
21. Roeske WR, O'Rourke RA, Klein A, et al: Noninvasive evaluation of ventricular hypertrophy in professional athletes. Circulation 53:286–292, 1976.
22. Geenen DL, Gilliam TB, Crowley D, et al: Echocardiographic measures in 6 to 7 year old children after an 8 month exercise program. Am J Cardiol 49:1990–1995, 1982.
23. Maron BJ, Gottdiener JS, Epstein SE: Patterns and significance of the distribution of left ventricular hypertrophy in hypertrophic cardiomyopathy: A wide-angle, two-dimensional echocardiographic study of 125 patients. Am J Cardiol 48:418–428, 1981.
24. Maron BJ: Structural features of the athlete heart as defined by echocardiography. J Am Coll Cardiol 7:190–203, 1986.
25. Cheitlin MD, DeCastro CM, McAllister HA: Sudden death as a complication of anomalous left coronary origin from the anterior sinus of Valsalva, a not so minor congenital anomaly. Circulation 50:780–787, 1974.
26. Bricker JT, Traweek MS, Smith RT, et al: Exercise

related ventricular tachycardia in children. Am Heart J 112:186–188, 1986.
27. Wiles HB, Bricker JT, McNamara DG: Treadmill exercise testing in patients with anomalous left coronary artery from the pulmonary artery. In Engle MA (ed): Abstracts of the 2nd World Congress of Pediatric Cardiology. New York, Springer-Verlag, 1985, p 117.
28. Morales AR, Romanelli R, Boucek RJ: The mural left anterior descending coronary artery, strenuous exercise and sudden death. Circulation 62:230–237, 1980.
29. Siscovick DS, Weiss NS, Fletcher RH, et al: The incidence of primary cardiac arrest during vigorous exercise. N Engl J Med 311:874–877, 1984.
30. Waller BF, Newhourse P, Pless J, et al: Exercise-related sudden death in 27 conditioned subjects aged <30 and >30 years: Coronary artery abnormalities are the culprit. J Am Coll Cardiol 3:621, 1984. Abstract.
31. Roberts WC, Maron BJ: Sudden death while playing professional football. Am Heart J 102:1061–1063, 1981.
32. McManus BM, Waller BE, Graboys TB, et al: Exercise and sudden death, part I. Curr Prob Cardiol 6:17–78, 1981.
33. Thompson PD, Funk EJ, Carleton RA, et al: Incidence of death during jogging in Rhode Island from 1975 through 1980. JAMA 247:2535–2538, 1982.
34. Nihill MR, Bricker JT, Kearney DL: Endomyocardial biopsy in infants and children. In Doyle EF, Engle MA, Gersony WM, et al (eds): Pediatric Cardiology. New York, Springer-Verlag, 1985, pp 343–347.
35. Roberts JA: Viral illnesses and sports performance. Sports Med 3(4):298–303, 1986.
36. Moss AJ, Schwartz PJ: Delayed repolarization (QT or QTU prolongation) and malignant ventricular arrhythmias. Mod Concepts Cardiovasc Dis 51:85, 1982.
37. Schwartz PJ, Periti M, Malliani A: The long Q-T syndrome. Am Heart J 89:378–390, 1975.
38. Bricker JT, Garson A Jr, Gillette PC: A family history of seizures associated with sudden cardiac deaths. Am J Dis Child 138:866–868, 1984.
39. Jeresaty RM: Mitral valve prolapse: Definition and implications in athletes. J Am Coll Cardiol 7:231–236, 1986.
40. Chesler E, King RA, Edwards JE: The myxomatous mitral valve and sudden death. Circulation 67:632–639, 1983.
41. Pocock WA, Bosman CK, Chesler E, et al: Sudden death in primary mitral valve prolapse. Am Heart J 107:378–382, 1983.
42. Bharati S, Bauernfeind R, Miller LB, et al: Sudden death in three teenagers: Conduction system studies. J Am Coll Cardiol 13:879–886, 1983.
43. Jeresaty RM: Sudden death in the mitral valve prolapse click syndrome. Am J Cardiol 37:317–319, 1976.
44. Warth DC, King ME, Cohen JM, et al: Prevalence of mitral valve prolapse in normal children. J Am Coll Cardiol 5:1173–1177, 1985.
45. McNamara DG: Idiopathic benign mitral leaflet prolapse: The pediatrician's view. Am J Dis Child 136:152–156, 1982.
46. Kavey RW, Sondheimer HM, Blackman MS: Detection of dysrhythmia in pediatric patients with mitral valve prolapse. Circulation 62:582–587, 1980.
47. Garson A Jr, Bink-Boelkens M, Hesslein PS, et al: Atrial flutter in the young: A collaborative study of 380 cases. J Am Coll Cardiol 6:871–878, 1985.
48. Braunlin EA, Dunnigan A, Mianulli M, et al: The effect of atrial flutter upon exercise capacity in adolescents following congenital heart disease surgery. Pediatr Cardiol 5:261, 1984. Abstract.
49. Gillette PC: Supraventricular arrhythmias in children. J Am Coll Cardiol 5(suppl):122B–129B, 1985.
50. Cosio FG, Benson DW Jr, Anderson RW, et al: Onset of atrial fibrillation during antidromic tachycardia: Association with sudden cardiac arrest and ventricular fibrillation in a patient with Wolff-Parkinson-White syndrome. Am J Cardiol 50:353–359, 1982.
51. Bricker JT, Porter CJ, Garson A Jr, et al: Exercise testing in children with Wolff-Parkinson-White syndrome. Am J Cardiol 55:1001–1004, 1985.
52. Olsson SB, Edvardsson N, Emanuelsson H, et al: A case of arrhythmogenic right ventricular dysplasia with ventricular fibrillation. Clin Cardiol 5:591–596, 1982.
53. Jokl E, Mackintosh RH: Sudden death of a young athlete from rupture of ascending aorta. Med Sport 5:150–152, 1971.
54. Benson DW Jr, Benditt DG, Anderson RW, et al: Cardiac arrest in young, ostensibly healthy patients: Clinical, hemodynamic, and electrophysiologic findings. Am J Cardiol 52:65–69, 1983.
55. Yasue H, Omote S, Takizawa A, et al: Circadian variation of exercise capacity in patients with Prinzemetal's variant angina: role of exercise-induced coronary arterial spasm. Circulation 59:938–948, 1979.
56. Driscoll DJ: Sudden unexpected death in children and adolescents. J Am Coll Cardiol 5(suppl):118B–121B, 1985.
57. Roberts WC, McAllister HA, Ferrans VJ: Sarcoidosis of the heart. A clinicopathologic study of 35 necropsy patients (group I) and review of 78 previously described necropsy patients (group II). Am J Med 63:86–108, 1977.
58. Thiene G, Pennelli N, Rossi L: Cardiac conduction system abnormalities as a possible cause of sudden death in young athletes. Hum Pathol 14:706–709, 1983.
59. James TN, Froggart P, Marshall TK: Sudden death in young athletes. Ann Intern Med 67:1013–1021, 1967.
60. Voigt J, Agdal N: Lipomatous infiltration of the heart. An uncommon cause of sudden, unexpected death in a young man. Arch Pathol Lab Med 106:497–498, 1982.
61. Virmani R, Robinowitz M, Clark MA, et al: Sudden death and partial absence of the right ventricular myocardium. Arch Pathol Lab Med 106:163–167, 1982.
62. Thiene G, Pennelli N, Rossi L: Cardiac conduction system abnormalities as a possible cause of sudden death in young athletes. Hum Pathol 14:704–709, 1983.
63. Isner JM, Estes M III, Thompson PD, et al: Acute cardiac events temporally related to cocaine abuse. N Engl J Med 315:1438–1443, 1986.
64. Neimann JL: Sudden death in athletes. Ann Cardiol (Paris) 34(3):145–149, 1985.
65. Baron BJ, Epstein SE, Mitchell JH: 16th Bethesda Conference: Cardiovascular abnormalities in the athlete: Recommendations regarding eligibility for

competition. Introduction. J Am Coll Cardiol 6:1189–1190, 1985.
66. Sheehan G: Electrocardiography in athletes. JAMA 224:1296, 1973.
67. Maron BJ: Structural features of the athlete heart as defined by echocardiography. J Am Coll Cardiol 7:190–203, 1986.
68. Rost R, Hollmann W: Athlete's heart—a review of its historical assessment and new aspects. Int J Sports Med 4:147–165, 1983.
69. Buytendijk FJJ, Snapper I: Ergebnisse sportarztlichen Untersuchungen bei den IX. Olympischen Spielen in Amsterdam 1928. Berlin, Springer, 1929.
70. Ikaheimo MJ, Palatsi IJ, Takkunen JT: Noninvasive evaluation of the athletic heart: Sprinters versus endurance runners. Am J Cardiol 44:24–30, 1979.
71. Palatsi IJ, Ikaheimo MJ: Runner's heart. Primary Cardiol 7(4):73–84, 1981.
72. Gibbons LW, Cooper KH, Martin RP, et al: Medical examination and electrocardiographic analysis of elite distance runners. Ann NY Acad Sci 301:283–296, 1977.
73. Cohen JL, Gupta PK, Lichstein E, et al: The heart of a dancer: Noninvasive cardiac evaluation of professional ballet dancers. Am J Cardiol 45:959–965, 1980.
74. Oakley DG, Oakley CM: Significance of abnormal electrocardiograms in highly trained athletes. Am J Cardiol 50:985–989, 1982.
75. Parker BM, Londeree BR, Cupp GV, et al: The noninvasive cardiac evaluation of long-distance runners. Chest 73:376–381, 1978.
76. Crawford MH, O'Rourke RA: The athlete's heart. Adv Intern Med 24:311–329, 1979.
77. Roeske WR, O'Rourke RA, Klein A, et al: Noninvasive evaluation of ventricular hypertrophy in professional athletes. Circulation 53:286–292, 1976.
78. Huston TP, Puffer JC, Rodney WM: The athletic heart syndrome. N Engl J Med 313:24–32, 1985.
79. Rossi F, Todaro A, Venerando A, et al: An investigation of pulmonary vascularization in endurance athletes. In Lubic T, Venerando A (eds): Sports Cardiology. Bologna, Aula Gaggi, 1980, pp 351–357.
80. Oakley DG, Oakley CM: Significance of abnormal electrocardiograms in highly trained athletes. Am J Cardiol 50:985–989, 1982.
81. Chapman JH: Profound sinus bradycardia in the athletic heart syndrome. J Sports Med Phys Fitness 22:45–48, 1982.
82. Lin Y-C, Horvath SM: Autonomic nervous control of cardiac frequency in the exercise-trained rat. J Appl Physiol 33:796–799, 1972.
83. Williams RS, Eden RS, Moll ME, et al: Autonomic mechanisms of training bradycardia: Beta-adrenergic receptors in humans. J Appl Physiol 51:1232–1237, 1981.
84. Badeer HS: Cardiovascular adaptations in the trained athlete. In Lubich T, Venerando A (eds): Sports Cardiology. Bologna, Aulo Gaggi, 1980, pp 3–12.
85. Scheuer J, Penpargkul S, Bhan AK: Experimental observations on the effects of physical training upon intrinsic cardiac physiology and biochemistry. Am J Cardiol 33:744–751, 1974.
86. Ordway GA, Charles JB, Randall DC, et al: Heart rate adaptation to exercise training in cardiac-denervated dogs. J Appl Physiol 52:1586–1590, 1982.
87. Piovano G, Caselli G, Pozzilli P: Frequency of ECG abnormalities in athletes: A study of 12,000 ECG's. In Lubich T, Venerando A (eds): Sports Cardiology. Bologna, Aulo Gaggi, 1980, pp 625–630.
88. Meytes I, Kaplinsky E, Yahini JH, et al: Wenckebach A-V block: a frequent feature following heavy physical training. Am Heart J 90:426–430, 1975.
89. Attina DA, Falorni PL, Pieri A, et al: The electrocardiogram of the middle-aged men who practice physical activity outside their normal work-time. In Lubich T, Venerando A (eds): Sports Cardiology. Bologna, Aulo Gaggi, 1980, pp 257–261.
90. Zeppilli P, Fenici R, Sassara M, et al: Wenckebach second-degree A-V block in top-ranking athletes: An old problem revisited. Am Heart J 100:281–294, 1980.
91. Han J, DeTraglia J, Millet D, et al: Incidence of ectopic beats as a function of basic rate in the ventricle. Am Heart J 72:632–639, 1966.
92. Coehlo A, Palileo E, Ashley W, et al: Tachyarrhythmias in young athletes. J Am Coll Cardiol 7:237–243, 1986.
93. Duda M: Hovik monitor aids in Cumming's diagnosis. Physician Sports Med 12:35, 1984.
94. Garson A, Williams RB, Reckless J: Long-term follow-up of patients with tetralogy of Fallot: Physical health and psychopathology. J Pediatr 85:429–433, 1974.
95. Bailey DA: The growing child and the need for physical activity. In Albinson JG, Andrew GM (eds): Sport and Physical Activity International Series on Sport Sciences, Vol 3. Baltimore, University Park Press, 1976, pp 81–93.
96. Fripp RR, Hodgson JL, Kwiterovich PO, et al: Aerobic capacity, obesity, and atherosclerotic risk factors in male adolescents. Pediatrics 75:813–818, 1985.
97. Huttenun JK, Lansimies E, Voutilainen E, et al: Effect of moderate physical exercise on serum lipoproteins. Circulation 60:1220, 1979.
98. Thorland WG, Gilliam TB: Comparison of serum lipids between habitually high and low active preadolescent males. Med Sci Sports Exer 13:316, 1981.
99. Lipson LC, Bonow RO, Schaefer EJ, et al: Effect of exercise conditioning on plasma high density lipoproteins and other lipoproteins. Atherosclerosis 37:529, 1980.
100. Dietz WH Jr, Gortmaker SL: Do we fatten our children at the television set? Obesity and television viewing in children and adolescents. Pediatrics 75:807–812, 1985.
101. Kannel WB, Sorlie P: Some health benefits of physical activity. The Framingham Study. Arch Intern Med 139:857–861, 1979.
102. Bonnano JA, Lies JE: Effects of physical training on coronary risk factors. Am J Cardiol 33:760–763, 1974.
103. Hagberg JM, Goldring D, Ehsani AA, et al: Effect of exercise training on the blood pressure and hemodynamic features of hypertensive adolescents. Am J Cardiol 52:763–768, 1983.
104. Fenici R, Caselli G, Zeppilli P, et al: High degree A-V block in 17 well-trained endurance athletes. In Lubich T, Venerando A (eds): Sports Cardiology. Bologna, Aulo Gaggi, 1980, pp 523–537.
105. Johnson ML, Burke BS, Mayer J: Relative importance of inactivity and overeating in the energy

balance of obese high school girls. Am J Clin Nutr 4:37, 1956.
106. Stunkard AJ, Pestka J: The physical activity of obese girls. Am J Dis Child 103:812, 1962.
107. Berkowitz RI, Agras WS, Korner AF, et al: Physical activity and adiposity: A longitudinal study from birth to childhood. J Pediatr 106:734, 1985.
108. Hamilton P, Andrew GM: Influence of growth and athletic training on heart and lung functions. Eur J Appl Physiol 36:27–38, 1976.
109. Pate RR, Blair SN: Exercise and the prevention of atherosclerosis: Pediatric implications. In Strong WB (ed): Atherosclerosis: Its Pediatric Aspect. New York, Grune & Stratton, 1978, chapter 13.
110. Goldberg B, Fripp RR, Lister G, et al: Effect of physical training on exercise performance of children following surgical repair of congenital heart disease. Pediatrics 68:691–699, 1981.
111. Vaccaro P, Galioto FM, Bradley LM, et al: Development of a cardiac rehabilitation programme for children. Sports Med 1:259–262, 1984.
112. Ruttenberg HD, Moller JH, Strong WB, et al: Recommended guidelines for graded exercise testing and exercise prescription for children with heart disease. J Cardiac Rehabil 4:10–16, 1984.
113. Ruttenberg HD, Adams TD, Orsmond GS, et al: Effects of exercise training on aerobic fitness in children after open heart surgery. Pediatr Cardiol 4:19–24, 1983.
114. Chen S, Fagan LF, Nouri S, et al: Ventricular dysrhythmias in children with Marfan's syndrome. Am J Dis Child 139:273–276, 1985.
115. Petren T, Sjostraud T, Sylven T: Der einfluss der trainings auf die heufigkeit der capillaren in Herz und skelettmuskulatur. Arbeitsphysiol 9:376, 1936.
116. Saltin B, Blomqvist G, Mitchell JH, et al: Response to submaximal and maximal exercise after bedrest and training. Circulation 38(suppl 7):VII-1, 1968.
117. Noakes TD, Higginson L, Opie LH: Physical training increases ventricular fibrillation thresholds of isolated rat hearts during normoxia, hypoxia and regional ischemia. Circulation 67:24–30, 1983.
118. Billman GE, Schwartz PJ, Stone HL: The effects of daily exercise on susceptibility to sudden cardiac death. Circulation 69:1182–1189, 1984.
119. Rowland TW: Aerobic response to endurance training in prepubescent children: A critical analysis. Med Sci Sports Exer 17:493–497, 1985.
120. Berg KE, LaVoie JC, Latin RW: Physiological training effects of playing youth soccer. Med Sci Sports Exer 17:656–660, 1985.
121. Zipes DP, Cobb LA Jr, Garson A, et al: Task Force VI: Arrhythmias. J Am Coll Cardiol 6:1225–1232, 1985.
122. Gutgesell HP, Gessner IH, Vetter VL, et al: Recreational and occupational recommendations for young patients with heart disease. A statement for physicians by the Committee on Congenital Cardiac Defects of the Council on Cardiovascular Disease in the Young, American Heart Association. Circulation 74:1195A, 1986.
123. Bricker JT, Traweek MS, Smith RT, et al: SVT during exercise testing in children. In: Abstracts of the 2nd World Congress of Pediatric Cardiology. New York, Springer-Verlag, 1985, p 107.
124. McNamara DG, Bricker JT, Galioto FM, et at: 16th Bethesda Conference: Cardiovascular abnormalities in the athlete: Recommendations regarding eligibility for competition. Task Force I: Congenital heart disease. J Am Coll Cardiol 6:1200–1208, 1985.
125. Frank R, Fontaine G, Tonet JL, et al: Electrophysiological studies at exercise in patients with accessory atrioventricular pathways. In Steinbach K, Glogar D, Laszkovics A, et al (eds): Cardiac Pacing. Darmstadt, Steinkopff Verlag, 1983, pp 657–662.
126. Wellens HJJ, Brugada P, Roy D, et al: Effect of isoproterenol on the anterograde refractory period of the accessory pathway in patients with the Wolff-Parkinson-White syndrome. Am J Cardiol 50:180–184, 1982.
127. Weisfogel GM, Stein RA, Fernaine A, et al: Increasing pre-excitation during exercise and isoproterenol infusion. Evidence for a catecholamine sensitive bypass tract. J Electrocardiol 12:315–320, 1979.
128. Fisch C, Zipes DP, McHenry PL: Rate dependent aberrancy. Circulation 48:714–724, 1973.
129. Bricker JT, Traweek MS, Danford DA, et al: Exercise related bundle branch block in children. Am J Cardiol 56:796–797, 1985.
130. Vasey C, O'Donnell J, Morris S, et al: Exercise induced bundle branch block and its relation to coronary artery disease. Am J Cardiol 56:892–895, 1985.
131. Wayne VS, Bishop RL, Cook L, et al: Exercise-induced bundle branch block. Am J Cardiol 52:283–286, 1983.
132. Chapman JH: Intermittent left bundle branch block in the athletic heart syndrome. Chest 71:776–779, 1977.
133. Sketch MH, Mooss AN, Butler ML, et al: Digoxin-induced positive exercise tests: Their clinical and prognostic significance. Am J Cardiol 48:655, 1981.
134. James FW, Blomqvist CG, Freed MD, et al: Standards for exercise testing in the pediatric age group. American Heart Association Council on Cardiovascular Disease in the Young, Ad Hoc Committee on Exercise Testing. Circulation 66:1378A–1397A, 1982.
135. Frizzell RT, Lang GH, Lowance DC, et al: Hyponatremia and ultramarathon running. JAMA 255:772–774, 1986.

CHAPTER 25

ARRHYTHMIAS AND SUDDEN DEATH

Arthur Garson, Jr.

Specific data on the individual arrhythmias and their likelihood to lead to sudden death are discussed in other chapters of this book. In order to provide an indication of what the pediatric cardiologist might encounter in practice, we examined the factors present in a large number of pediatric cardiology patients who had died suddenly, with specific reference to the presence of chronic arrhythmias in these patients. In the first section, data will be presented on the entire patient group. In the second and third sections, the differences between the diagnostic classes and the individual diagnoses will be discussed. Finally, each of the arrhythmias will be discussed with specific reference to this patient population and sudden death.

PATIENT DATA AND METHOD OF STUDY

The charts of all patients seen in the Pediatric Cardiology Section at Texas Children's Hospital who died in the 25-year period between 1958 and 1983 were reviewed. Patients were included in the study if the following criteria were met:

1. Patient older than 1 year at the time of death.
2. A sudden event occurred that rendered the patient unconscious, with the patient never regaining consciousness before death.
3. Occurrence of this sudden event outside the hospital.
4. Absence of acute illness in the patient shortly before sudden death.

Patients were excluded from this study if they had had cardiac catheterization or cardiac surgery within 1 month prior to death.

Certain definitions were used in the gathering of the data. The New York Heart Association criteria for clinical status were used. Cardiac catheterization hemodynamic findings were classified as excellent (normal hemodynamics), fair (unoperated or postoperative without the need for medical or surgical treatment), or poor (hemodynamics that would require eventual operative intervention, or if inoperable, subpulmonary ventricular pressure two-thirds that of systemic pressure, or end-diastolic pressures greater than 1.5 times normal), or as pulmonary hypertension (pulmonary artery systolic pressure beyond and stenoses of at least two-thirds that of systemic pressure). The presence of arrhythmias was ascertained from a review of routine resting electrocardiograms taken during two time periods: 1 week to 1 year prior to sudden death, and 1 year to 2 years before sudden death. Holter electrocardiograms were not used, because there were insufficient data on these patients to permit adequate comparison. In defining the cause of death, a "probable arrhythmia" was said to be present if indicated on an electrocardiogram obtained at the time of the sudden event, or if the event leading to sudden death had a similar history to a previous episode of a documented arrhythmia causing syncope. A "possible arrhythmia" was said to be present if a prior history of arrhythmia in a high-risk category could be obtained in a patient in whom the exact arrhythmia at the time of death was not known: for example, a patient with postoperative tetralogy of Fallot with prior ventricular arrhythmia, or a patient with prior bradyarrhythmia who had undergone Mustard repair.

RESULTS

Diagnostic Categories

Of the 981 patients seen in the Pediatric Cardiology Section at Texas Children's Hospital who died between 1958 and 1983, 101 (10.3%) died suddenly. We have divided the diagnoses of these 101 patients into five categories (Table 25–1). The largest two groups consisted of patients with unoperated congenital heart disease and patients with postoperative repair of congenital heart disease. These were followed by patients with palliated congenital heart disease, those with unoperated acquired heart disease, and those with a prolonged QT interval. Of note is the fact that no patient in this group who died suddenly had a normal heart. All of these patients, by the fact that they were seen in a pediatric cardiology clinic at least once, were thought to have heart disease. Nonetheless, no patient discharged from the clinic with a diagnosis of normal heart later died suddenly.

TABLE 25–1
DIAGNOSES IN 101 PATIENTS WHO WERE TREATED AT TEXAS CHILDREN'S HOSPITAL BETWEEN 1959 AND 1983 AND WHO SUBSEQUENTLY DIED SUDDENLY

DIAGNOSIS (TOTAL)	NUMBER OF PATIENTS
Unoperated congenital heart disease (36)	
Left-to-right shunt with pulmonary hypertension	11
Tetralogy of Fallot/pulmonary atresia + VSD	7
Cardiomyopathy	5
Aortic insufficiency	3
Hypertrophic cardiomyopathy	3
L-transposition of the great arteries	2
Aortic stenosis	2
Aortic aneurysm	1
Hypoplastic coronary arteries	1
Myxomatous mitral + tricuspid	1
Unoperated, acquired heart disease (7)	
Primary pulmonary hypertension	4
Acquired cardiomyopathy	3
Prolonged QT interval (5)	
No congenital heart disease	4
With congenital heart disease	1
Palliated congenital heart disese (17)	
Right-to-left shunt PO AP anastomosis	12
Transposition PO Blalock-Hanlon	4
Left-to-right shunt PO PA banding	1
Postoperative repair—congenital heart disease (36)	
Tetralogy of Fallot—pulmonary atresia/VSD	11
AV canal/VSD	5
Transposition—PO Mustard	5
Transposition + VSD—PO Mustard + VSD	4
Aortic valve replacement	4
Mitral valve replacement	3
Tricuspid valve replacement	1
Ostium primum ASD	1
Hypertrophic obstructive cardiomyopathy—PO myotomy	1
Patent ductus arteriosus (with CCAVB)	1

Abbreviations: AP = aorticopulmonary; ASD = atrial septal defect; AV = atrioventricular; CCAVB = congenital complete AV block; PA = pulmonary atresia; PO = postoperative; VSD = ventricular septal defect.

Clinical Information

The male:female ratio was 1.5:1 (62 male, 39 female). While this indicated a trend, it did not achieve statistical significance. Of the 101 patients, 86% had been seen in the Pediatric Cardiology Clinic within 1 year before death. The clinical status (using New York Heart Association criteria) was Class I–II in 28%, Class III in 49%, and Class IV in 23%. Therefore, 72% of the patients were thought to be in fair or poor condition at the time of their last clinic visit. On chest radiography at this last visit, 85% were found to have cardiac enlargement. Hemodynamics had been assessed at cardiac catheterization in 75 of the 101 patients. This was done an average of 2.3 years prior to the patient's death; 89% of these patients had catheterization performed less than 5 years prior to death. The hemodynamics were excellent in 6%, fair in 5%, and poor in 46%, with pulmonary hypertension in 43%. Therefore, in 89% of the patients, a severe hemodynamic abnormality was present. Overall, more than three-quarters of the patients who died suddenly in this series were either severely symptomatic, had an abnormal chest roentgenogram, or poor hemodynamics at cardiac catheterization.

Electrocardiographic Findings

ARRHYTHMIAS

A routine electrocardiogram taken between 1 week and 1 year prior to the patient's death was available in 86 patients. Of these patients, 49 (57%) had an arrhythmia, and 37 (43%) had no arrhythmia on routine electrocardiogram (Table 25–2).

The arrhythmias present on electrocardiogram 2 years before death were compared with those present within 1 year before death. In electrocardiograms taken 2 years before death, arrhythmias were present in one in 42 of the patients. Therefore, a significantly higher ($p < 0.05$) proportion of patients had arrhythmias in the year prior to their death than had arrhythmias 2 years prior to death. In six patients, the change in arrhythmia resulted from an operation that occurred in the year prior to death. It appears that in a certain number of patients, arrhythmias develop in the year before sudden death. This does not necessarily imply that the arrhythmia caused the death, only that the development of an arrhythmia was associated with later sudden death.

OTHER FINDINGS

On the electrocardiogram taken less than 1 year prior to death, nine additional patients without arrhythmias had a severe abnormality on the electrocardiogram: three had a prolonged QT interval, three had old myocardial infarction, one had left ventricular strain in hypertrophic cardiomyopathy, one had left ventricular strain after aortic valve replacement, and one had complete right bundle-branch block after a left septal myotomy for hypertrophic obstructive cardiomyopathy. If these nine patients are added to the 49 with arrhythmias prior to sudden death, then 67% of patients had an electrocardiographic abnormality other than the one that might be expected for their underlying lesion (e.g., the usual abnormality for tetralogy of Fallot is right ventricular hypertrophy; this was not included).

TABLE 25–2
ARRHYTHMIAS ON ECG 1 WEEK TO 1 YEAR BEFORE DEATH (N = 86)

ARRHYTHMIA	PERCENTAGE OF PATIENTS
PVC	20
Atrial flutter	8
Sinus bradycardia	7
Junctional rhythm	7
Complete AV block	6
Complete AV block with pacemaker	5
JR + PVC	5
CAVB + PM + PVC	2
AFL + PVC	2
SVT	1
VT	1
Total	57

Abbreviations: AFL = atrial flutter; AV = atrioventricular; CAVB = complete AV block; JR = junctional rhythm; PM = pacemaker; PVC = premature ventricular contraction; SVT = supraventricular tachycardia; VT = ventricular tachycardia. Some patients had more than one arrhythmia.

Treatment

Medical treatment had been prescribed for only a small number of these patients who died suddenly. Drug treatment at the time of death included digoxin (79%), diuretics (49%), quinidine (7%), propranolol (3%), isoproterenol (2%), mexiletine (1%), and belladonna (1%). Three patients being treated with quinidine for atrial flutter were noted at the time of their sudden episode to have a slow rate; in one, this was high grade AV block, and in the other two, slow junctional rhythm. An additional patient with junctional rhythm and premature ventricular contractions treated with quinidine was found at the time of his death to have extremely slow junctional rhythm. Propranolol had been prescribed for three patients. In one, this had been prescribed for atrial flutter and had been ineffective. The other two patients had a prolonged QT interval and were known to be noncompliant in taking their propranolol. Only one patient had been prescribed phenytoin at the time of his death. Phenytoin was effective in treating his premature ventricular contractions, but he was noncompliant. This was also the case for one patient who had been prescribed mexiletine. Therefore, four patients who died from ventricular arrhythmias were known to be noncompliant. Isoproterenol had been given to two patients with complete AV block, and belladonna had been prescribed for one patient with junctional rhythm. Three of these four patients had documented ventricular arrhythmias.

Circumstances of Death

The activity of the patient immediately preceding death was known in 46 of the 101 cases. Sudden death occurred during sports in 22% of patients, with the patient awake but not active in 50% of patients, and with the patient asleep in 28% of patients. The mean age at death was 12.4 years (range, 1 year to 30 years). In postoperative patients, sudden death occurred an average of 4.5 years after surgery (2 months to 18 years). A presumed cause of death was known in 53 of the 101 patients (Table 25–3).

Clinical Findings

DIFFERENCES AMONG DIAGNOSTIC CATEGORIES

Among the five diagnostic classes (unoperated congenital heart disease, unoperated acquired heart disease, palliated congenital heart disease, postoperative congenital heart disease, and long QT interval) the clinical findings differed in four major areas. With respect to clinical status, the unoperated patients were more limited than the palliated or postoperative congenital heart disease patients: 95% of the unoperated patients were in class III–IV, compared to 62% of those with congenital heart disease that had been palliated or repaired ($p < 0.001$).

There was a marked difference in the presence of preceding arrhythmia. An arrhythmia was present in the year prior to sudden death in 88% of those who had undergone repair of congenital heart disease compared with 35% of those in the unoperated or palliated group ($p < 0.0001$). Premature ventricular contractions in the year preceding sudden death were significantly higher in the postoperative repair group (88%) than in the unoperated or palliated group (34%) ($p < 0.01$).

The activity preceding death also varied with the group. Those patients who died during sports were in the following three groups: (1) unoperated congenital heart disease, (2) prolonged QT interval, or (3) postoperative congenital heart disease. None of the patients with palliated congenital heart disease died during sports, perhaps because these patients were not physically capable of participating in vigorous sports. Death occurred during sleep in patients in all of the groups except the prolonged QT interval group.

With respect to the cause of death, patients after repair of congenital heart disease had significantly more known or suspected arrhythmias (78%) compared with the unoperated or palliated patients (31%) ($p < 0.001$).

TABLE 25–3
KNOWN CAUSE OF DEATH (N = 53)

CAUSE	PERCENTAGE OF PATIENTS	
Arrhythmia		
Probable	32	
Possible	21	
Pacemaker	9	
Total		62
SBE		11
CVA		9
Pulmonary embolus		8
Aspiration		4
Penicillin anaphylaxis		2
Hemoptysis		2
Aortic aneurysm dissection		2
		100

Abbreviations: CVA = cerebrovascular accident; SBE = subacute bacterial endocarditis.

MOST COMMON CARDIAC DIAGNOSES

The eight most common diagnoses in these patients were, in descending order, right-to-left shunt postoperative anastomosis (12%), left-to-right shunt with pulmonary hypertension (Eisenmenger's syndrome) (11%), postoperative tetralogy of Fallot (11%), tetralogy of Fallot unoperated (7%), cardiomyopathy (5%), postoperative AV canal (5%), postoperative Mustard operation for transposition of the great arteries (5%), and prolonged QT interval (5%). These eight diagnoses made up 61% of the patients. Other diagnoses were present in 4% or less of the patients.

PRESENCE OF ARRHYTHMIAS

There were significant differences among the diagnoses with respect to the presence of arrhythmias within 1 year preceding sudden death (Table 25–4). There was a low incidence of arrhythmias (less than 25%) in the patients with left-to-right shunt and pulmonary hypertension (Eisenmenger's syndrome), and in those with unoperated or palliated tetralogy of Fallot. In all the other diagnoses, more than 50% of the patients had arrhythmias in the year prior to death. The only diagnoses in which premature ven-

TABLE 25–4
ARRHYTHMIAS PRESENT 1 WEEK TO 1 YEAR PRIOR TO DEATH

DIAGNOSIS	NUMBER OF PATIENTS	% ANY ARRHYTHMIA	% PVC	% AFL	% JR	% AVB	% COMPLEX
L-to-R shunt PH	11	14	14				
TOF	7	17				17	
CM	5	60	20	20			20
LQTS	5	75	25		50		
R-to-L Anas	12	10	10				
PO TOF	11	100	70		10	10	10
PO Canal	5	75				75	
POM	5	100		50	25		25

Abbreviations: AFL = atrial flutter; AVB = AV block; CM = cardiomyopathy; JR = junctional rhythm; LQTS = long QT syndrome; L-to-R = left to right; PH = pulmonary hypertension; PO canal = postoperative AV canal repair; POM = postoperative Mustard procedure; PO TOF = postoperative tetralogy of Fallot; PVC = premature ventricular contractions; R-to-L Anas = right-to-left shunt postoperative anastomosis; TOF = tetralogy of Fallot.

tricular contractions occurred in 25% or more of the patients were postoperative tetralogy of Fallot and long QT interval. Atrial flutter was uncommon except in postoperative Mustard patients. Sinus bradycardia and junctional rhythm occurred in less than 25% of the patients except those with a prolonged QT interval and postoperative Mustard. AV block was uncommon except in patients who had undergone repair of complete AV canal or ventricular septal defect.

CIRCUMSTANCES OF DEATH

The majority of patients died while at rest, not during sports or while asleep (Table 25–5). The only deaths that occurred during sports were in patients with a prolonged QT interval or cardiomyopathy, or in postoperative Mustard or tetralogy patients. The only patients who died during sleep were those who had unoperated tetralogy of Fallot or cardiomyopathy or were postoperative Mustard or tetralogy of Fallot patients. Either a probable arrhythmia or a possible arrhythmia was present in the majority of these diagnoses. However, an arrhythmia did not appear to be involved in patients with a left-to-right shunt and pulmonary hypertension, with unoperated tetralogy of Fallot, or with a right-to-left shunt postoperative anastomosis.

There were two groups in which patients were significantly older at the time of death than in other groups: postoperative tetralogy of Fallot and left-to-right shunt with pulmonary hypertension ($p < 0.01$). Patients who had undergone repair of AV canal died at a significantly younger age than the rest of the group. From examination of the postoperative interval, it is apparent that the postoperative AV canal patients died at a young age because they died relatively early postopera-

TABLE 25–5
CIRCUMSTANCES IN DEATH

DIAGNOSIS	NUMBER OF PATIENTS	ACTIVITY AT TIME OF DEATH: *Active* (%)	*Sleep* (%)	ARRHYTHMIA CAUSE (%)	AGE AT DEATH ± SEM (years)	PO INTERVAL ± SEM (years)
L-to-R shunt PH	11	0	0	33	15.9±2.0	—
TOF	7	0	67	25	10.6±3.4	—
CM	5	50	50	100	10.6±3.1	—
LQTS	5	67	0	100	11.4±2.5	—
R-to-L Anas	12	0	0	30	10.4±2.5	4.2±1.5
PO TOF	11	28	14	100	16.2±2.2	4.2±1.3
PO Canal	5	0	0	100	8.6±2.9	1.7±0.5
POM	5	60	40	100	11.5±3.8	7.1±2.6

Abbreviations: AFL = atrial flutter; AVB = AV block; CM = cardiomyopathy; JR = junctional rhythm; LQTS = long QT syndrome; L-to-R = left to right; PH = pulmonary hypertension; PO canal = postoperative AV canal repair; POM = postoperative Mustard procedure; PO TOF = postoperative tetralogy of Fallot; PVC = premature ventricular contractions; R-to-L Anas = right-to-left shunt postoperative anastomosis; SEM = standard error of mean; TOF = tetralogy of Fallot.

tively. The postoperative Mustard patients actually died significantly longer after surgery than did other patients, but at an earlier age than postoperative tetralogy patients. Postoperative tetralogy patients died at an older age because, presumably, reparative surgery occurred at an older age than did the Mustard operation.

Arrhythmia Findings

DIAGNOSTIC DIFFERENCES

Specific arrhythmias found in the year preceding sudden death differed among the diagnoses. Premature ventricular contractions were found in 50% or more of patients with acquired cardiomyopathy, ostium primum atrial septal defect, transposition of the great arteries, or ventricular septal defect, or following Mustard or tetralogy of Fallot repair. Atrial flutter was found in 50% or more of those with aortic insufficiency or acquired cardiomyopathy, or in those whose had undergone Mustard repair. Sinus bradycardia or junctional rhythm were found in more than 50% of patients with transposition of the great arteries, ventricular septal defect, or prolonged QT interval, or in postoperative Mustard patients. Complete AV block was found in more than 50% of patients with L-transposition of the great arteries and following patent ductus arteriosus (congenital complete AV block) surgery or tricuspid valve replacement.

The presence of arrhythmia was related to poor hemodynamics at cardiac catheterization in these patients. An arrhythmia was found in 11% of those with good hemodynamics, compared with 50% of those with poor hemodynamics ($p < 0.01$). Each of the individual arrhythmias (e.g., premature ventricular contractions) was significantly related to poor hemodynamics, with the exception of junctional rhythm. Junctional rhythm was significantly related to good hemodynamics ($p < 0.01$); good hemodynamics were found in 56% of those with junctional rhythm, compared with 5% of the patients without junctional rhythm ($p < 0.01$). This indicates that the postoperative patients with junctional rhythm (largely postoperative Mustard patients) who died suddenly had good hemodynamics.

The presumed direct cause of death was significantly related to the presence of arrhythmia in the year prior to death. However, there were some exceptions. Among the 17 patients without previous arrhythmia noted on routine electrocardiogram within 1 year prior to death, four had a probable arrhythmia at the time of death, and 13 died of other causes. Of the 28 patients with an arrhythmia in the year preceding death, only four of the 28 had another known cause for their death, leaving 24 of 28 with either a probable or possible arrhythmia responsible for their death.

HISTORICAL COMPARISON

Between 1958 and 1983, there were 23,402 patients seen in the Pediatric Cardiology Section at Texas Children's Hospital; 981 (4.2%) of these patients are known to have died. Sudden death, by our criteria, occurred in 101, nonsudden death in 730, and accidental death in 10; there was insufficient information for 140 of the patients. Since 1968, each 5-year period has seen an increase in the total number of patients seen (Table 25–6). Between 1978 and 1983, there were two major changes in arrhythmia management, with aggressive drug treatment of premature ventricular contractions and aggressive pacemaker treatment of bradydysrhythmias. During those years, none of the 18 sudden deaths occurred in patients with prior ventricular arrthythmias; however, 16 of the 69 patients who died suddenly in the previous twenty years had ventricular arrhythmias ($p < 0.05$). Since 1978, there has been one sudden death in a postoperative tetralogy patient; this was caused by a documented pacemaker failure in a patient with surgical complete AV block. Since 1977, there has been no sudden death in a patient following a Mustard procedure for transposition of the great arteries.

SUMMARY

In this study of sudden death in patients previously seen in a pediatric cardiology clinic, we attempted to identify factors that might have been associated with later sudden death. The true denominator of these factors is unknown. For example, the number of

TABLE 25–6
NUMBER OF PATIENTS SEEN AT TEXAS CHILDREN'S HOSPITAL, PEDIATRIC CARDIOLOGY SECTION, FROM 1959 TO 1983, AND FREQUENCY OF SUDDEN DEATH

	1959–1963	1964–1968	1969–1973	1974–1978	1979–1983
Number of patients	2330	1716	4668	6562	8126
Number of sudden deaths	3	27	21	37	22
Percentage of total patients	0.13	0.92	0.43	0.54	0.27

patients with these defects who have arrhythmias and do not die is not known in all cases. Further studies are planned to document the incidence of these factors in patients with similar lesions who did not die. The following conclusions can be drawn from the study:

1. More than three-quarters of the patients who died suddenly had severe limitation of activity, cardiac enlargement on chest radiograph, and poor hemodynamics at cardiac catheterization.
2. The majority of patients who died suddenly had an arrhythmia in the 12-month period preceding death. A significant number of these arrhythmias developed for the first time in the year preceding death.
3. The presence of arrhythmias was generally related to poor hemodynamics in patients who died suddenly.
4. Approximately one-quarter of the patients with arrhythmias received therapy that would currently be thought to be appropriate.
5. Most sudden deaths occurred with the patient at rest, and only approximately one-quarter occurred during sports participation.
6. Specific arrhythmias are present in association with specific conditions and appear to be correlated with the risk of sudden death in that group.
7. Conspicuously absent from the list of diagnoses are children with a normal heart and children with mitral valve prolapse.
8. With improvement in treatment practices (i.e., more aggressive drug treatment of ventricular arrhythmias and more aggressive pacemaker treatment in bradyarrhythmias), the incidence of sudden death at our institution has been reduced significantly from previous years.

Acknowledgments

Research was supported in part by grants HL24916, HL07190, and RR00188 from the National Institutes of Health, Bethesda, Maryland, and by a grant from the J. S. Abercrombie Foundation.

CHAPTER 26

FETAL DYSRHYTHMIAS

Christopher L. Case & Derek A. Fyfe

The diagnosis and treatment of dysrhythmias in the fetus has been one of the latest frontiers encountered in the field of pediatric electrophysiology. Widespread use of electronic fetal monitoring by obstetricians as well as technological advances in fetal echocardiography have been instrumental in elucidating the incidence and natural history of rhythm disturbances in the fetus. The purpose of this chapter is to summarize current concepts in the diagnosis and treatment of commonly encountered antenatal rhythm problems.

ELECTROPHYSIOLOGY AND HEMODYNAMICS OF THE NORMAL FETUS

Understanding aberrations of fetal heart function is facilitated by an appreciation of normal in utero cardiac development, electrophysiology, and hemodynamics. The conduction system of the fetal heart fully matures by the sixteenth week of gestation. The AV node and the His bundle form separately and unite at approximately the eighth week of gestation. The sinus node is structurally indistinguishable from its adult counterpart by the tenth week of gestation. By sixteen weeks, the sinus rhythm of the normal fetus can be adequately characterized by fetal echocardiography.

Studies of the normal fetal heart rate have been performed in the first, second, and third trimesters. The heart rates of 124 first trimester fetuses were determined with real-time sonography and related to gestational age. The mean embryonic heart rate increased from 100 bpm at 6 menstrual weeks, reaching a plateau at 9 menstrual weeks of 143 bpm. This study demonstrated that heart rates in the 100s are not uncommon in the early weeks of the first trimester.[1] In a different study of first trimester fetal heart rate, all pregnancies with a fetal heart rate less than 85 bpm at 5–6 menstrual weeks ended in spontaneous miscarriage.[2] Patterns of fetal heart rate during the second and third trimester as evaluated by cardiotography were described in 59 normal pregnancies.[3] These recordings showed a significant reduction in baseline heart rate as gestation advanced. The normal fetal heart rate was defined in this study as between 110 and 150 bpm. After 34 weeks of gestation, patterns of fetal heart rate seemed to be related to periods of fetal rest and activity, with rest lasting approximately 15 minutes and being characterized by a reduction in heart rate variability.

Normal fetal hemodynamics have been studied extensively in sheep and recently, with the aid of Doppler echocardiography, in humans. The ventricular compliance characteristics of the fetus are very similar to the newborn. Both right and left ventricles are less compliant than the adult counterparts.[4] Kirkpatrick et al have studied the isolated cardiac muscle mechanics of the fetus.[5] They found that there were significantly lower levels of isometric tension development in isolated fetal muscle in response to paired extra stimuli when compared to adult levels. However, like the adult, the Frank-Starling relationship has been demonstrated to be a very important determinant of fetal cardiac output.[6]

The effects of heart rate on ventricular output of the fetus is a more controversial subject. Rudolph and Heymann demonstrated that there was a direct relationship between spontaneous fetal heart rate and right and left ventricular output.[7] They also demonstrated that left and right atrial pacing produced variable degrees of augmentation of right and left ventricular output. However, experiments of Kirkpatrick and associates found that with increasing atrial pacing rates, fetal cardiac output was unchanged.[8] They did find, however, that the site of atrial pacing changed the relative contribution of the right and left ventricle to total cardiac output. The disparity that normally exists in the contribution of the left and right ventricles to total fetal cardiac output (i.e., contribution of the right greater than that of the left) was accentuated with left atrial pacing and minimized with right atrial pacing. They postulated that this difference might arise from the influence of the atrial pacing site on the direction and magnitude of flow across the patent foramen ovale, thus changing relative ventricular filling and output.

Recent experiments have attempted to clarify the conflicting results found on the effect of heart rate on fetal ventricular output. Anderson et al have demonstrated once again that variations in spontaneous heart rate correlated positively with right and left ventricular output in the fetus.[9, 10] However, with artificial right and left atrial pacing, increases in rate did not correlate positively with cardiac output, but rather correlated negatively or did not affect output at all. Thus, in summary, the effects of heart rate on fetal cardiac output are not simple. Mechanisms that cause changes in spontaneous heart rate seem to evoke corresponding changes in preload, afterload, and inotropy, which effect a corresponding positive change in cardiac output. However, with artificial atrial pacing, a consistent relationship between pacing rate and cardiac output does not seem to exist, underlying the fact that various adaptive mechanisms may be involved. These same poorly characterized mechanisms accounting for the inconsistent cardiac output effects of atrial pacing in fetal sheep may be responsible for the different pathophysiologic effects of tachycardia seen in the human fetus.

With the advent of fetal echocardiography, Doppler analysis of blood flow velocity has helped quantify normal human fetal hemodynamics.[11, 12] Allan et al demonstrated that the maximum and mean velocities of flow at each cardiac valve, expressed as a function of gestational age, showed little change throughout pregnancy. The output from the right ventricle was usually, but not always, greater than that of the left ventricle. Combined ventricular output increased from approximately 50 mL/min at 18 weeks to 1200 mL/min at term. Doppler assessment of hemodynamics in the fetus has been done and quantified using blood flow velocity waveforms obtained from the umbilical artery, umbilical vein, and descending aorta.[13–15] Some investigators have attempted to categorize abnormalities of these waveforms as predictors of perinatal mortality in the "normal fetus." Application of these methods in assessing the hemodynamics of fetal dysrhythmias has also been performed and will be discussed later.

Developmental aspects of the cellular electrophysiology in the fetus have also been recently reviewed.[16] The cardiac action potential, ionic currents responsible for various phases of that action potential, and the action potential response to pharmacologic manipulation have been studied in the chick embryo as well as in the fetal canine. Studies in the chick, rat, dog, and human have shown that action potential upstroke in utero is predominantly dependent on an inward current carried by slow channels that are calcium dependent. Later in development, inward current is carried through fast channels that are sodium dependent. Resting membrane potential has been studied in the chick embryo. As the embryo matures, the relationship between potassium concentration outside the cell and resting membrane potential is similar to that seen in the fully developed chick. However, the more immature the embryo, the greater the deviation between potassium concentration and resting membrane potential. This may reflect developmental differences in the Na^+-K^+ transport system.

Drug studies involving fetal cardiac tissues have been done in a variety of species.[17–19] Developmental aspects of drug effects on transmembrane action potential parameters seem to be species specific. Canine Purkinje fibers showed no change in sensitivity to tetrodotoxin (a sodium channel blocker) or verapamil (a calcium channel blocker) at various gestational ages. In the chick and rat myocardia, however, there appears to be a changing sensitivity of the action potential during gestation to the effects of verapamil and tetrodotoxin. Verapamil's maximum depressant effects on action potential parameters occur early in gestation, with tetrodotoxin effects becoming greater with advancing gestation. These changes in drug sensitivity are thought to reflect and parallel the changing ionic basis for the rapid depolarization phase of the action potential. Understanding the developmental aspects of fetal drug sensitivity on the cellular level may form the basis for future advances in the pharmacologic treatment of fetal dysrhythmias.

FETAL DYSRHYTHMIAS: GENERAL CONCEPTS

Fetal dysrhythmias can be defined as those aberrations of fetal heart rate or rhythm that are not associated with uterine contractions. In general, during the second and third trimester, any prolonged rate less than 110 bpm or more than 150 bpm falls beyond the range of normality.[20] However, others believe that the range of normality extends between 120 bpm and 160 bpm.[21] The predominant fetal rhythm is regular, with an undulatory pattern of variability. In a prospective study of fetal heart rate and rhythm patterns, episodes of bradycardia (defined as fewer than 100 bpm ranging from 5 to 30 seconds' duration) occurred in only 1.1% of fetuses at 30 to 35 weeks' gestation and in only 1.3% of fetuses at 36 to 41 weeks' gestation. Tachycardia (defined as episodes of more than 180 bpm ranging from 30 to 90 seconds' duration) occurred in 1.4% of the 30-to-35-week fetuses and 0.6% of the 36-to-41-week fetuses. Premature beats were also present in 1.7% of those fetuses between 36 and 41 weeks.[21] Overall the projected incidence of intrinsic fetal dysrhythmias in the third trimester seems to approach 1%.

There are three main types of fetal dysrhythmias. The first is premature beats that originate either from the atrium or ventricle; the second are tachycardias, either supraventricular (SVT) or ventricular (VT); and the third are bradycardias, either sinus or a result of some degree of AV block. Mechanisms for these dysrhythmias in the fetus have not been fully elaborated but are widely assumed to be similar to those in the neonate. For SVT, the predominant mechanism is thought to be reentry either through the AV node or an accessory atrioventricular connection. Atrial flutter, fibrillation, and chaotic atrial tachycardia have all been described in the fetus. The mechanisms of these dysrhythmias are thought to be identical to their neonatal counterparts. Ventricular dysrhythmias in the fetus may be either reentrant or the result of an automatic focus. Bradycardia unrelated to uterine contractions can be caused either by a sick sinus node or by some degree of functional or structural AV block.

The evaluation of the fetus with a suspected or documented dysrhythmia must include an investigation for associated fetal or maternal conditions that may alter dysrhythmia management. There is an increased frequency of congenital malformations in fetuses with cardiac arrhythmias.[22] Many of these congenital defects are cardiac in nature. Certainly it is well known that congenital complete AV block diagnosed in utero is associated with complex congenital heart disease, mostly atrioventricular septal defects and atrial isomerism. One series showed an 86% association between fetal heart block and structural heart disease.[23] Supraventricular tachycardia is usually not as strongly associated with congenital heart disease, though atrial flutter does seem to have a frequent association with structural abnormalities. An isolated case of fetal atrial flutter associated with X-linked dominant vitamin D–resistant rickets and cases of fetal tachycardias associated with intra-myocardial tumors have been reported.[24, 25]

There is also the well-known association between maternal rheumatologic disease, specifically systemic lupus erythematosus, and congenital complete AV block.[26] The mother may have clinical evidence of active disease during pregnancy. Commonly, however, maternal disease is manifested only by positive serum titers for autoimmune antibodies such as anti-Ro. This possibility needs to be carefully evaluated in the presence of a structurally normal heart with sustained bradycardia.

The hemodynamic consequences of fetal dysrhythmias are varied. Isolated premature contractions in a fetus with a normal structural heart generally are hemodynamically insignificant. Congestive heart failure and hydrops fetalis are a common consequence of fetal dysrhythmias. Nonimmune hydrops seems to be the common pathophysiologic expression of many fetal disease states, but its association with fetal dysrhythmias and structural heart disease is strong. In a fetus with a structurally normal heart, hydrops is a common consequence of supraventricular tachycardia. Bradycardia secondary to AV block may cause hydrops in the fetus with a normal structural heart, though cardiac compromise is more common with structural heart disease.

DIAGNOSTIC EVALUATION

On Whom?

The indications for fetal echocardiography for dysrhythmia diagnosis are still evolving. Most fetal dysrhythmia evaluations are prompted by an irregularity of the fetal heart tone noted on routine prenatal evaluation by the obstetrician. When hydrops is suspected on the basis of a routine obstetric sonogram, evaluation of the fetal rhythm should also be done because of the high association between these two entities. In the United States, generally only pregnant women with suspected fetal heart disease or whose fetuses are at high risk are examined by fetal echocardiography. In general, it is part of the routine complete fetal echocardiography exam to assess fetal heart rate and rhythm. Risk factors such as those proposed by Reed and Sahn are generally utilized as indications for fetal echocardiography.[27]

When?

The most advantageous time for fetal examination is between 16 and 32 weeks gestation. At 14 weeks the heart can be imaged but is inconsistently examinable. After 32 weeks, high quality imaging is more difficult, but examination can be performed until term.

Why?

The importance of diagnosing the cause of fetal dysrhythmias (whether they are intrinsic or extrinsic alterations of rhythm) has been well studied. Since the early 1970s, antenatal variations of the fetal heart rate in response to uterine contraction or fetal movement (stress and non-stress tests) have been used to assess fetal well-being. Obstetricians have also used fetal heart rate and variability monitored during labor to predict outcome and guide therapy. Sustained fetal tachycardia and bradycardia have been well correlated with perinatal morbidity and mortality. Fetal bradycardia coinciding with the end of uterine contraction (type 2 pattern of deceleration) has been used as a sign of fetal distress. Also, a study by Hager and Pauly has confirmed an increased risk of neonatal complications in association with intrapartum fetal tachycardia.[28]

In a study of 113 cases of intrinsic fetal bradycardias and tachycardias, Lingman et al demonstrated an increased incidence of fetal distress in labor, perinatal and neonatal mortality, and congenital malformations in the dysrhythmia group compared with the general population.[22] Fetal heart rate abnormalities are also correlated with gross congenital malformations. Biale et al noted abnormal fetal heart rates (the most common being bradycardia and variable decelerations) in 54% of fetuses with congenital malformations, versus 16% in a control group.[29] The highest rate of pathologic heart rate tracings were found in the group with multiple malformations, chromosomal aberrations, and central nervous system lesions. Therefore, when an abnormal heart rate or rhythm is diagnosed by auscultation of fetal heart tones, characterization of the dysrhythmia may be important in predicing fetal outcome and aiding in treatment planning.

By Whom?

It is important to realize that the diagnosis and treatment of fetal dysrhythmias require a team effort. Interaction between the primary obstetrician, perinatologist, pediatric cardiologist, and the neonatologist is of utmost importance to assure proper treatment planning. Many times the initial impetus for the evaluation comes from the primary care obstetrician. Many obstetric ultrasonographers are adept at performing four-chamber views of the fetal heart and beginning an initial assessment of fetal rhythm. In order to fully characterize the exact etiology and mechanism of the fetal rhythm, the pediatric cardiologist may readily provide the needed expertise. When the rhythm has been defined and the possibility of associated cardiac anomalies evaluated, interaction between the entire team is again needed to formulate treatment strategies.

How?

Electrocardiography currently is of minimal use in assessing the nature of fetal dysrhythmias. Its inability to clearly display both atrial electrical activity (P wave) and ventricular electrical activity (QRS) make electrocardiography ill suited for fetal rhythm diagnosis. For this reason, fetal echocardiography is the mainstay of evaluation. Three modes of ultrasonography (two-dimensional examination [2D], M-mode, and Doppler) are used in the assessment of fetal rhythm problems. The 2D examination is used mainly to characterize the structure of the fetal heart and associated abnormalities such as pleural or pericardial effusions seen with hydrops fetalis. Rate and rhythm can be ascertained by the 2D exam, but characterization of atrioventricular relationships is difficult.

The relationship of atrioventricular electrical events may be defined by the M-mode examination. The M-mode probe may be positioned in such a way as to image simultaneously on the same plane (1) both the atrium or the atrial septum and the ventricle, (2) an AV valve and ventricle, or (3) a semilunar valve and atrium (Fig. 26–1). Timing between atrial and ventricular electrical events and their interaction in the AV node is made by analyzing the timing of (1) atrial and ventricular contraction, (2) AV valve opening and closing, or (3) atrial contraction and semilunar valve opening (Fig. 26–2).

Doppler echocardiography is also extremely helpful in the characterization of fetal dysrhythmias (see Fig. 26–1). Pulsed Doppler echocardiography is used to define AV contraction sequences as well as atrial and ventricular rates. By using a large Doppler sample volume, which is positioned in the ventricle to simultaneously sample ventricular inflow (atrial contraction) and outflow (ventricular contraction), AV relationship can be delineated.

Hemodynamic assessment of the severity of the fetal dysrhythmia can be performed with analysis of the Doppler waveform from the fetal great arteries and veins. Analysis of umbilical vein and aortic blood flow of the fetus has been used in obstetrics to predict intrauterine growth retardation, and perinatal morbidity and mortality.[13–15, 30] Application of these techniques to quantitate the circulatory effects of fetal cardiac dysrhythmias has also been reported. Likewise, Doppler has been used to assess the hemodynamic consequences of treating fetal dysrhythmias in utero.[31–35]

SPECIFIC DYSRHYTHMIAS: TREATMENT

General Principles

Before dealing with the treatment of specific fetal dysrhythmias, it is important to review some general principles of treatment that are applicable to all rhythm disturbances. Similar to dysrhythmias that are treated after birth, fetal rhythm disturbances should be treated "in their clinical context." In other words, the mere presence of a fetal dysrhythmia may not in itself be an indication for treatment. The decision to treat should be

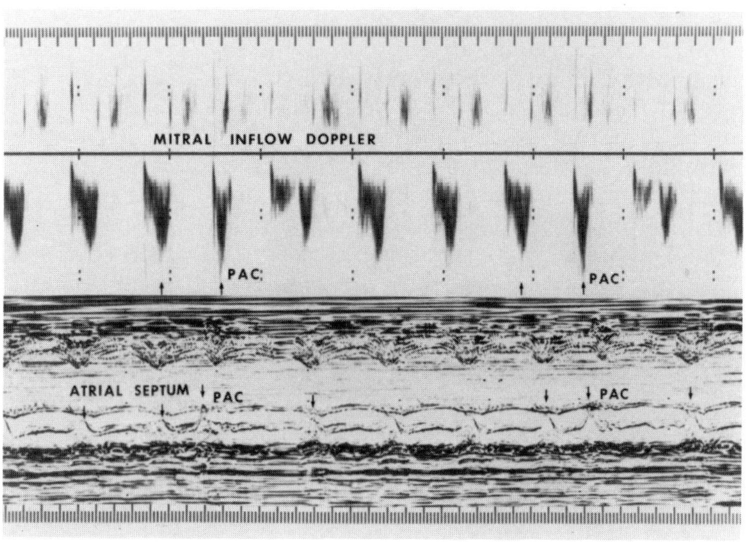

FIGURE 26–1
Upper panel: Doppler inflow signals at the mitral valve during sinus rhythm. Premature atrial contractions (PACs) are indicated and appear as early onset, higher velocity peaks of shorter duration than sinus beats. *Lower panel:* M-mode echocardiogram through the atria and atrial septum. PACs appear as early excursions of the atrial septum and free walls. A compensatory pause follows each PAC.

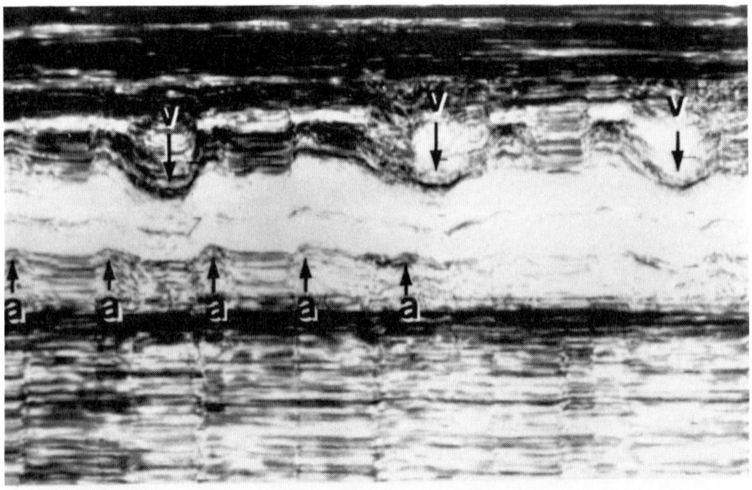

FIGURE 26–2
M-mode echocardiogram through atrial and ventricular free walls in a patient with congenital complete atrioventricular block. Note that the ventricular wall excursion (V) rate is 55 bpm and the atrial (a) rate is 160 bpm, and that no relationship exists between them.

based on the hemodynamic consequences of the dysrhythmia and its implications to fetal well-being, the gestational age of the fetus, and the possible consequences of in utero treatment to maternal health. Formulation of a risk/benefit ratio is the basis of good treatment planning. Once a specific treatment plan is established, careful follow-up in all situations is mandatory. It has been shown clinically, as well as in experimental animals, that tachycardias in the fetus can result in severe hemodynamic compromise within 48 hours.[36–38] Thus, benign dysrhythmias, such as premature contractions that are of no hemodynamic consequence at one time, within a few days may result in a severely compromised fetus should tachycardia be provoked.

When a hemodynamically significant fetal dysrhythmia is present in a near-term fetus, the treatment of choice, if possible, is delivery. Thus, fetal maturity and the possibility of perinatal morbidity and mortality due to prematurity must be weighed against the risks of treatment in utero. These decisions can be made only in conjunction with both a perinatologist and neonatologist. Clinical and laboratory assessment of fetal maturity is not exact and must be weighed against the hazards of in utero dysrhythmia therapy.

Supraventricular Tachycardia—Reentrant SVT

The diagnosis of reentrant supraventricular tachycardia requires a one-to-one relationship between arial and ventricular contractions, with a corresponding heart rate of 240 to 260 beats per minute (Fig. 26–3). This dysrhythmia is usually not associated with structural congenital heart disease; however, there is a frequent association with hydrops fetalis. During a 10-year experience with fetal dysrhythmias, Kleinman reported that out of a total of 452 patients with cardiac dysrhythmias, 34 had reentrant SVT, two of whom were subsequently noted to have Wolff-Parkinson-White syndrome after birth.[39]

Digoxin is the treatment of choice for hemodynamically significant SVT when delivery is not an option. Maternally administered digoxin may be used with intravenous loading and subsequent oral doses to keep the maternal blood level in the high therapeutic range. Usually large oral maintenance doses of 0.5–0.75 mg/d are required. Monitoring of maternal digoxin levels may be easily done, but amniocentesis with umbilical vessel sampling is required if fetal samples are to be obtained. The ratio of fetal to maternal digoxin levels may vary from 0.6 to 1. If digoxin by itself fails to control the rentrant SVT, verapamil may be added. Although the potential deleterious effects of this drug to the neonatal myocardium have been well documented, its efficacy and safety in the treatment of in utero SVT is now becoming established. Kleinman's experience has shown variable oral absorption of this agent, with steady-state levels in the fetus approximating 40% of maternal levels.[39] Digoxin may also accumulate in both mother and fetus because of impaired excretion caused by verapamil therapy. Therefore the digoxin dosage in the mother may need to be decreased by 33% to

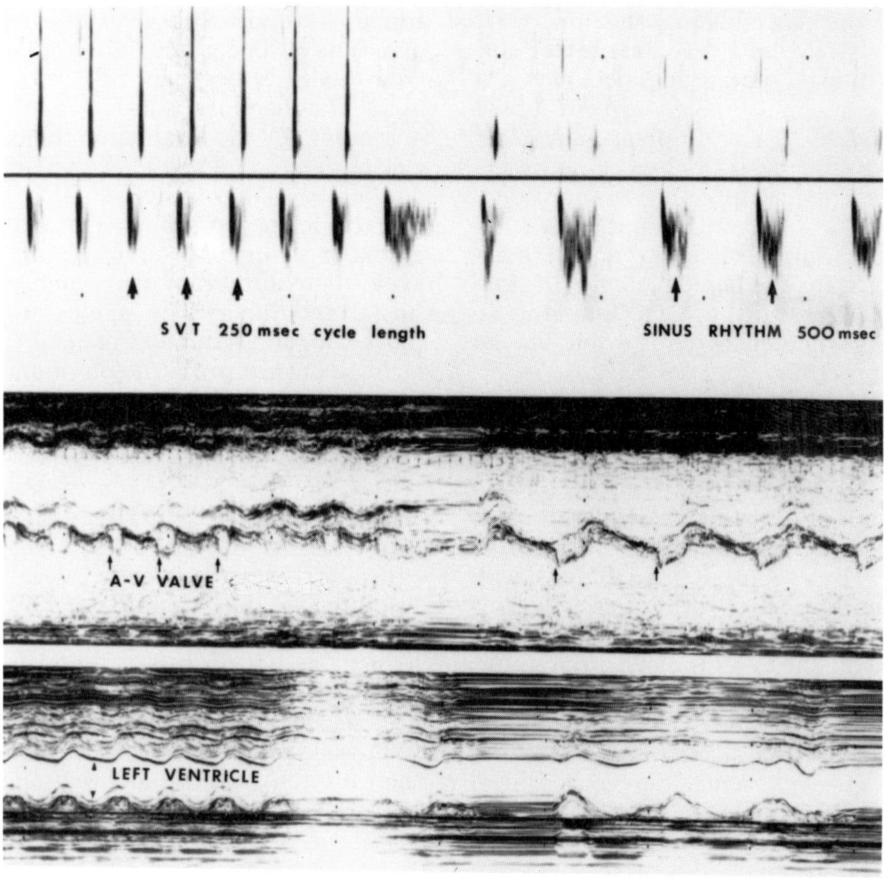

FIGURE 26–3

Upper panel shows Doppler tricuspid inflow signal during supraventricular tachycardia (SVT), 250 msec cycle length, which spontaneously converts to sinus rhythm (500 msec cycle length). Center panel shows M-mode echocardiogram recording during SVT. The atrioventricular (AV) tricuspid valve leaflets are seen to open with each atrial systole. The SVT terminates spontaneously. Lower panel shows M-mode echocardiography during SVT. The ventricles are contracting at the same rate as the atria, as established by the Doppler inflow signal and the tricuspid leaflet opening. All three panels are recorded from the same patient within a short time of each other but are not simultaneous. SVT was confirmed immediately after delivery.

50%. Although some espouse intravenous loading of the mother with 5 to 10 mg of verapamil, Kleinman prefers oral use of this medicine (80 to 120 mg every 6 to 8 hours). The use of other drugs in the treatment of in utero SVT has been described. Quinidine, procainamide, flecainide, and amiodarone have all been successfully used.[40–43] Although vagal maneuvers caused by umbilical cord or head compression have resulted in cessation of sustained SVT, such maneuvers are not recommended and provide no consistent means of preventing or terminating repeated episodes of tachycardia.

A controversial area concerning the indications for pharmacologic therapy of fetal SVT involves the patient having frequent episodes of SVT without evidence of heart failure. It is well known that fetal hemodynamic compromise from SVT may develop rapidly, that is, in less than 48 hours. This has been confirmed in the human and also in an experimental model using sheep fetus. For this reason, it is recommended that any fetus with intermittent SVT receive close follow-up. Conclusive data are lacking regarding whether to institute pharmacologic therapy prophylactically in order to deter the development of hydrops. It has been recommended that in the absence of signs of hydrops, the fetus with intermittent SVT should be treated to prevent potential hemodynamic compromise.[44]

The hemodynamic effects of in utero SVT have been quantified. Lingman and Marsal have reported the use of Doppler waveform analysis of the descending aorta flow in fetuses with dysrhythmia.[34] Despite severe cardiac arrhythmias, the aortic blood flow was within normal limits in all but one of 34 fetuses studied. Fetal Doppler waveform analysis has also been used to monitor hemodynamic changes following in utero digitalization of a fetus with supraventricular tachycardia.[35] Such techniques may be helpful in evaluating the hemodynamics of nonhydropic fetuses during SVT, and thus in determining whether the fetus would benefit from drug therapy.

Atrial Flutter/Fibrillation

Atrial flutter/fibrillation is rarer than reentrant SVT as a cause of fetal tachycardia. Kleinman[39] has reported nine fetuses with atrial flutter/fibrillation in his series, versus 34 fetuses with reentrant SVT. The echocardiographic diagnosis of in utero atrial flutter is usually made on the basis of atrial contractions at a rate of 400 to 460 beats per minute, resulting in varying degrees of ventricular response. This ventricular rate can be fixed and regular or variable and irregular. Vintzileos et al reported 22 cases of congenital atrial flutter in which the arrhythmia was detected before delivery.[24] The incidence of associated cardiac malformations in this series was 22%. Coexistent congenital heart defects worsened the prognosis. There was a 91% survival rate with appropriate in utero therapy. Eighteen of 22 fetuses responded to pharmacologic conversion with digitalis; two were not treated. Signs of congestive heart failure were present at birth in 65%. Kleinman[39] believes, that in contrast to reentrant SVT, there is a frequent association between congenital atrial flutter and structural heart disease. In his series of fetuses with atrial flutter/fibrillation, there was a high mortality rate (four out of nine, with three out of nine having associated congenital heart disease). Kleinman states that simple control of the ventricular rate is not sufficient to ameliorate the fetal hemodynamics. Actual conversion to sinus rhythm is of utmost importance.[39]

Ventricular Tachycardia

In utero ventricular tachycardia has been reported, yet its incidence is extremely low. Kleinman reported three cases in his 10-year experience. The usual rate for ventricular tachycardia is between 220 bpm and 280 bpm. The diagnosis is usually made by demonstrating AV dissociation on the basis of the lack of one-to-one relationship between atrial and ventricular contractions. It is important to exclude the possibility that a fetal tachycardia is ventricular in origin in order to avoid digoxin therapy that could exacerbate this dysrhythmia. The agents usually employed for the treatment of fetal ventricular tachycardia are propranolol, quinidine, procainamide, and phenytoin.

Sinus Bradycardia

Fetal bradycardia may be caused by a persistently low sinus rate, between 80 bpm and 100 bpm. It is important to exclude fetal hypoxia and/or distress as the primary cause for the bradycardia. A non-stress test can be used to assess heart rate variability and, thus, fetal well-being. If normal variability exists, then the fetus can be followed and delivery performed vaginally.

AV Block

Varying degrees of atrioventricular block are a common cause of fetal bradycardia (see Fig. 26–2). Experience from a number of centers has suggested that there are two large subsets of fetuses with complete heart block. The first consists of those fetuses with structurally normal hearts. This condition may be associated with maternal rheumatologic disease, particularly systemic lupus erythematosus, or serum antibodies associated with rheumatologic disorders. It has been demonstrated that the pathophysiology of this condition involves maternal antibodies that cross the placenta and initiate immune mediated destruction of the fetal AV conduction system.[45] Complete AV block in this subset of patients with structurally normal hearts is generally not associated with hydrops, though cases have been reported.[46–49] Generally, in the absence of evidence of heart failure, no intrauterine therapy for this set of patients is needed, but close follow-up is recommended. Vaginal delivery at maturity with monitoring of fetal well-being during labor using the atrial rate has been described by Kleinman.[50] In the event of hydrops developing prior to fetal maturity, the logical therapeutic option is fetal pacing. Carpenter et al have reported a successful yet short experience with fetal pacing, using a pacing catheter inserted into the fetal right ventricle through the mother's abdomen.[48] Kleinman et al believe that establishment of AV synchrony is more important than simply increasing the ventricular rate in these fetuses and thus are pessimistic about the therapeutic efficacy of ventricular pacing.

The second group of patients with fetal complete heart block consists of those with complex congenital heart disease.[23, 39, 51, 52] The association of complex congenital heart disease with AV block has a very poor prognosis in most series. The most common malformation found in these fetuses is atrioventricular septal defect and atrial isomerism. This lesion is usually fatal. In one series, there was only one survivor out of 17 fetuses with AV block, atrioventricular septal defects, and atrial isomerism.[51] If fetal pacing becomes a viable option, the fetus with complex congenital heart disease and complete heart block will benefit most from this therapy.

Blocked Atrial Bigeminy

Blocked atrial bigeminy is an important cause of fetal bradycardia that must be differentiated from congenital complete atrioventricular block. In both conditions, the heart rate may be low, but analysis of the fetal echocardiogram will help differentiate the two lesions. In blocked atrial bigeminy, there is normal AV conduction alternating with an atrial contraction that encounters a refractory AV node, and thus there is no corresponding ventricular event. Like complete AV block in a fetus with a structurally normal heart, this dysrhythmia is infrequently associated with hemodynamic compromise. In one series, Kleinman reported four fetuses with this dysrhythmia; one developed sustained SVT on the first day of life and was diagnosed as having Wolff-Parkinson-White syndrome.[50] Like neonates, if a fetus with blocked atrial bigeminy develops hemodynamic compromise in utero, digoxin is the drug of choice because of its ability to suppress premature atrial activity.

Premature Beats

Premature atrial or ventricular contractions form the bulk of diagnosed in utero dysrhythmias (see Fig. 26–1). In Kleinman's series, 385 out of 452 fetal dysrhythmia patients had only isolated extrasystoles;[39] 336 were judged to be supraventricular, while 37 were thought to be ventricular or junctional extrasystoles. Twelve patients were thought to have extrasystoles arriving from multiple sites. Most premature beats are of no hemodynamic consequence. It is important, however, to realize that premature contractions may initiate reentrant supraventricular or ventricular tachycardia. It has been recommended that such patients continue to have checks of fetal heart rate on a twice weekly basis until time of delivery. This recommendation is based on the fact that there is a 1% risk that such a patient presenting with isolated extrasystoles will later develop sustained supraventricular tachycardia.

RESEARCH AND FUTURE DEVELOPMENTS

The subject of fetal dysrhythmias is truly an evolving field. In the past 20 years, major strides have been made, not only in the recognition of significant fetal dysrhythmias, but also in their treatment. Future advances in this field most likely will rely on progress in the understanding of fetal cardiac function.

Although basic research into fetal electrophysiology and hemodynamics was started in the mid 1970s, there is still much controversy as to the relative importance of fetal heart rate, preload, and afterload in determining cardiac output in the physiologic and pathologic state. An excellent model for hydrops fetalis in the sheep, caused by rapid fetal cardiac pacing, has been developed by Stevens and further refined by Nimrod et al.[37, 38] Work with such models not only may uncover the pathophysiologic mechanism of hydrops fetalis as related to different pacing modes, but also may help explore the pathophysiology of hydrops fetalis itself.

Investigation of the cellular electrophysiology of the fetus is in its infancy. Future adances into the pharmacokinetics and pharmacodynamics of drug treatment of in utero tachycardias will be advanced by understanding the ontogeny of fetal cellular electrophysiology.

Finally, research into the more aggressive therapies for fetal bradycardias (e.g., in utero pacing) is needed to establish alternative therapeutic options. Experiments with fetal sheep and permanent pacing have been done with some success. Any therapy for in utero bradycardia caused by complete heart block must take into account the relationship between complex congenital heart disease, hydrops fetalis, and AV block. The high perinatal mortality associated with this entity makes fetal pacing a diffficult yet attractive alternative.

References

1. Hertzberg BS, Mahony BS, Bowie JD: First trimester fetal cardiac activity. Sonographic documentation of a progressive early rise in heart rate. J Ultrasound Med 7:573–575, 1988.
2. Laboda LA, Estroff JA, Benacerraf BR: First trimester bradycardia. A sign of impending fetal loss. J Ultrasound Med 8:561–563, 1989.
3. Wheeler T, Murrill A: Patterns of fetal heart rate during normal pregnancy. Br J Obstet Gynecol 85:18–27, 1978.
4. Romero T, Covell J, Friedman WF: A comparison of pressure-volume relations of the fetal, newborn and adult heart. Am J Physiol 5:1285–1290, 1972.
5. Kirkpatrick SE, Naliboff J, Pitlick PT, et al: Influence of poststimulation potentiation and heart rate on the fetal lamb heart. Am J Physiol 229:318–323, 1975.
6. Kirkpatrick SE, Pitlick PT, Naliboff J, et al: Frank-Starling relationship as an important determinant of fetal cardiac output. Am J Physiol 231:495–500, 1976.
7. Rudolph AM, Heymann MA: Cardiac output in the fetal lamb: The effects of spontaneous and induced changes of heart rate on right and left ventricular output. Am J Obstet Gynecol 124:183–192, 1976.
8. Pitlick PT, Kirkpatrick SE, Friedman WF: Distribution of fetal cardiac output: Importance of pacemaker location. Am J Physiol 231:204–208, 1976.
9. Anderson PAW, Glick KL, Killam AP, et al: The effect of heart rate on in utero left ventricular output in the fetal sheep. J Physiol 372:557–573, 1986.
10. Anderson PAW, Killam AP, Mainwaring RD, et al: In utero right ventricular output in the fetal lamb: The effect of heart rate. J Physiol 387:297–316, 1987.
11. Allan LD, Chita SK, Al-Ghazali W, et al: Doppler echocardiographic evaluation of the normal human fetal heart. Br Heart J 57:528–533, 1987.
12. Machado MVL, Chita SC, Allan DL: Acceleration time in the aorta and pulmonary artery measured by Doppler echocardiography in the midtrimester normal human fetus. Br Heart J 58:15–18, 1987.
13. Giles WB, Lingman G, Marsal K, et al: Fetal volume blood flow and umbilical artery flow velocity waveform analysis: A comparison. Br J Obstet Gynecol 93:461–465, 1986.
14. Al-Ghazali W, Chapman MG, Allan LD: Doppler assessment of the cardiac and uteroplacental circulations in normal and complicated pregnancies. Br J Obstet Gynecol 95:575–580, 1988.
15. Laurin J, Marsal K, Persson PH, et al: Ultrasound measurement of fetal blood flow in predicting fetal outcome. Br J Obstet Gynecol 94:940–948, 1987.
16. Danilo P: Electrophysiology of the fetal and neonatal heart. *In* MJ Legato (ed): Developing Heart. Boston, Martinus Nijhoff Publishing, 1984, pp 21–38.
17. Danilo P, Reder RF, Binah O, et al: Fetal canine cardiac Purkinje fibers: Electrophysiology and ultrastructure. Am J Physiol 15:H250–260, 1984.
18. Bernard C: Establishment of ionic permeabilities of myocardial membrane during embryonic development of the rat. *In* Lieberman M, Sano T (eds): Developmental and Physiological Correlates of Cardiac Muscle. New York, Raven Press, 1976, pp 169–184.
19. Shigenobu K, Sperelakis N: Development of sensitivity to terodotoxin of chick embryonic hearts with age. J Mol Cell Cardiol 3:271–286, 1971.
20. Southall DP, Richards J, Hardwick RA, et al: Prospective study of fetal heart rate and rhythm patterns. Arch Dis Child 55:506–511, 1980.
21. Kallfeiz HC: Cardiac arrhythmias in the fetus—diagnosis, significance, and prognosis. *In* Goodman MJ, Marquis RM (eds): Paediatric Cardiology. Vol 2: Heart Disease in the Newborn. Edinburgh, Churchill-Livingstone, 1979, pp 401–412.
22. Lingman G, Lundstrom NR, Marsal K, et al: Fetal cardiac arrhythmia. Clinical outcome in 113 cases. Acta Obstet Gynecol Scand 65:263–267, 1986.
23. Gembruch U, Hansmann M, Redel DA, et al: Fetal complete heart block: Antenatal diagnosis, significance and management. Eur J Obstet Gynecol Reprod Biol 31:9–22, 1989.
24. Vintzileos AM, Campbell WA, Soberman SM, et al: Fetal atrial flutter and X-linked dominant vitamin D–resistant rickets. Obstet Gynecol 65:39S–44S, 1985.
25. Birnbaum SE, McGahan JP, Janos GG, Meyers M: Fetal tachycardia and intramyocardial tumors. J Am Coll Cardiol 6:1358–1361, 1985.
26. Scott JS, Maddison PJ, Taylor PV, et al: Connective-tissue disease, antibodies to ribonucleoprotein, and congenital heart block. N Engl J Med 309:209–212, 1983.
27. Reed KL, Sahn DJ: A proposal for referral patterns for fetal cardiac studies. Semin Ultrasound CT, MR 5:249, 1984.
28. Hager DW, Pauly TH: Fetal tachycardia as an indicator of maternal and neonatal morbidity. Obstet Gynecol 66:191–194, 1985.
29. Biale Y, Brawer-Ostrosky Y, Insler V: Fetal heart rate tracings in fetuses with congenital malformations. J Reprod Med 30:43–47, 1985.
30. Laurin J, Lingman G, Marsal K, et al: Fetal blood flow in pregnancies complicated by intrauterine growth retardation. Obstet Gynecol 69:895–902, 1987.
31. Wladimiroff JW, Struyk P, Stewart PA, et al: Fetal cardiovascular dynamics during cardiac dysrhythmia. Case report. Br J Obstet Gynecol 90:573–577, 1983.
32. Tonge HM, Wladimiroff JW, Noordam MJ, et al: Fetal cardiac arrhythmias and their effect on volume

blood flow in descending aorta of human fetus. J Clin Ultrasound 14:607–612, 1986.
33. Lingman G, Dahlstrom JA, Eik-Nes SH, et al: Haemodynamic assessment of fetal heart arrhythmias. Br J Obstet Gynecol 91:647–652, 1984.
34. Lingman G, Marsal K: Circulatory effects of fetal cardiac arrhyhmias. Pediatr Cardiol 7:67–74, 1986.
35. Lingman G, Marsal K, Lundstrom NR: Intrauterine treatment of fetal heart failure monitored by combined Doppler ultrasound technique. *In* Doyle EF et al. (eds): Pediatric Cardiology. New York, Springer-Verlag, 1985, pp 52–56.
36. Kleinman CS, Copel JA, Weinstein EM, et al: In utero diagnosis and treatment of fetal supraventricular tachycardia. Semin Perinatol 9:113–129, 1985.
37. Stevens DC, Hilliard J, Schreiner RL, et al: Supraventricular tachycardia with edema, ascites, and hydrops in fetal sheep. Am J Obstet Gynecol 142:316–322, 1982.
38. Nimrod C, Davies D, Harder J, et al: Ultrasound evaluation of tachycardia-induced hydrops in the fetal lamb. Am J Obstet Gynecol 157:655–659, 1987.
39. Kleinman CS: Personal communication, Nov. 1989.
40. Spinnato JA, Shaver DC, Flinn GS, et al: Fetal supraventricular tachycardia: In utero therapy with digoxin and quinidine. Obstet Gynecol 64:730–735, 1984.
41. Dumesic DA, Silverman NH, Tobias S, et al: Transplacental cardioversion of fetal supraventricular tachycardia with procainamide. N Engl J Med 307:1128–1131, 1982.
42. Wren C, Hunter S: Maternal administration of flecainide to terminate and suppress fetal tachycardia. Br Med J (Clin Res) 296:249, 1988.
43. Arnoux P, Seyral P, Llurens M, et al: Amiodarone and digoxin for refractory fetal tachycardia. Am J Cardiol 59:166–167, 1987.
44. Maxwell DJ, Crawford DC, Curry PVM, et al: Obstetric importance, diagnosis, and management of fetal tachycardias. Br Med J 297:107–109, 1988.
45. Litsey SE, Noonan JA, O'Connor WN, et al: Maternal connective tissue disease and congenital heart block: Demonstration of immunoglobulin in cardiac tissue. N Engl J Med 312:98–100, 1985.
46. Altenburger KM, Jedziniak M, Roper WL, et al: Congenital complete heart block associated with hydrops fetalis. J Pediatr 91:618–620, 1977.
47. Martin TC, Arias F, Olander DS, et al: Successful management of congenital arioventricular block associated with hydrops fetalis. J Pediatr 112:984–986, 1988.
48. Carpenter RJ, Strasburger JF, Garson A, et al: Fetal ventricular pacing for hydrops secondary to complete atrioventricular block. J Am Coll Cardiol 8:1434–1436, 1986.
49. Moodley TR, Vaughan JE, Chuntarpursat I, et al: Congenital heart block detected in utero. A case report. S Afr Med J 70:433–434, 1986.
50. Kleinman CS, Copel JA, Hobbins JC: Combined echocardiographic and Doppler assessment of fetal congenital atrioventricular block. J Obstet Gynecol 94:967–974, 1987.
51. Machado MVL, Tynan MJ, Curry PVL, et al: Fetal complete heart block. Br Heart J 60:512–515, 1988.
52. Shenker L, Reed KL, Anderson CF, et al: Congenital heart block and cardiac anomalies in the absence of maternal connective tissue disease. Am J Obstet Gynecol 157:248–253, 1987.

CHAPTER 27

IRREGULAR HEART BEAT IN THE NORMAL CHILD

Arthur Garson, Jr.

Frequently a child has been referred to us who was found to have an irregular heart beat on routine physical examination performed by the pediatrician or general physician. It is the task of the physician caring for such children to place these arrhythmias in one of three categories: (1) those that are benign and need no further follow-up (this constitutes the vast majority of chronic arrhythmias in such children); (2) those that need not be treated but should receive continued follow-up; and (3) those that must receive treatment (the minority). In general, a child with an otherwise normal heart and an asymptomatic arrhythmia most often does not require treatment.

An electrocardiogram on the child with an irregular heart beat usually falls into one of four categories: arrhythmias usually associated with increased vagal tone, premature atrial contractions, premature ventricular contractions, and AV block. For each of these arrhythmias, a definition will be given (other chapters contain more specific information on diagnosis), as well as the clinical situations in which the arrhythmias frequently occur, an approach to diagnosis, and an approach to treatment. Children with tachyarrhythmias generally present to the physician with symptoms and are not considered in this chapter. Discussion of these arrhythmias can be found elsewhere in this book.

VAGAL ARRHYTHMIAS

The most common arrhythmias in ambulatory children are thought to be caused by the slightly enhanced vagal tone of childhood. In these arrhythmias, there is a variation throughout the atrium in the site of dominant pacemaker. In sinus arrhythmia, the P wave axis remains between 0° and +90° with a P wave preceding each QRS complex. In wandering pacemaker, the site of the P wave origin "wanders" from the high right atrium to the low right atrium (with a P wave that is negative in leads II, III, and aVF, with P waves still preceding the QRS complexes). Occasionally the rhythm wanders from low atrial to junctional, but it is unusual for a "left atrial" P wave to occur (i.e., negative in lead I).[1] In junctional rhythm, there is a normal QRS that is not preceded by a P wave. The P wave may be within or behind the QRS complex. In an adult, even an inverted P wave preceding the QRS complex may be called junctional rhythm. Electrophysiologically, it is difficult in a child for the P wave to precede the QRS complex and the origin to be above the bundle of His. Therefore, in children, a P wave preceding the QRS complex is termed low right atrial rhythm.

Clinical Situations

Most commonly, these arrhythmias present in adolescent athletes. Rarely, these arrhythmias, especially in their extreme form, may occur in any situation with heightened vagal tone, such as asthma, upper airway obstruction (in which respiratory movements are exaggerated), increased intracranial pressure, increased blood pressure, pharyngeal stimulation, or abdominal distention. It is not uncommon to encounter infants with mild to moderate sinus arrhythmia that is eliminated by decompression of the stomach after passage of a nasogastric tube. In the general population, it is rare for these arrhythmias to be a manifestation of true sick sinus syndrome.

One group of children receiving greater attention includes those who have bradycardiac spells within the first several months of life. These spells may be accompanied by apnea. These occur in full-term infants and are not manifestation of prematurity. Most of the time, the episodes of bradycardia are first noted in the newborn nursery. The heart rate and respiratory rate respond to minimal stimulation. These do not appear to be episodes of aborted sudden infant death syndrome. The etiology is unknown, although "autonomic immaturity" seems to be a reasonable choice. These spells generally disappear by 1 year of age.

Approach to Diagnosis

In vagal arrhythmias, the approach to diagnosis depends on the rhythm and symptoms of the patient. In the patient with sinus arrhythmia, wandering pacemaker or intermittent junctional rhythm while awake, no further work-up is necessary. In approximately 40% of normal children, intermittent junctional rhythm is observed during sleep on the 24-hour electrocardiogram.

If the patient has constant junctional rhythm or is symptomatic from syncope, presyncope, or light-headedness, or the patient complains of palpitations, further work-up is necessary. This should consist of an exercise test and a 24-hour electrocardiogram.

Approach to Treatment

The approach to treatment of vagal arrhythmias depends on the findings in these laboratory tests. An abnormal treadmill exercise test is defined as either depression of the maximum heart rate (the highest rate achieved during maximal exercise) or reduction of the 5-minute recovery heart rate (the patient's heart rate after 5 minutes of rest). Sinus node disease can be indicated by an inability to raise the heart rate during exercise or by a decrease in the heart rate after exercise.[2]

An abnormal 24-hour electrocardiogram is defined by the age of the child. The measurement of heart rate should be obtained over at least five beats. From the data on infants with congenital complete AV block, we know that the ventricular rate in infants needs to be above 50/min to avoid severe congestive heart failure, syncope, or even sudden death.[3] In children between 1 year of age and adolescence, a rate of less than 40/min is abnormal, as is a rate less than 30/min in a teenager. These numbers are well below the limit of normal as defined by two standard deviations below the mean.[4,5]

TREATMENT

The treatment for vagal arrhythmias depends largely on the symptoms. If a patient has recurrent syncopal episodes and has a vagal arrhythmia on routine electrocardiogram but a normal treadmill test and 24-hour electrocardiogram, then further study may be indicated. A battery of tests can be performed for autonomic dysfunction; these are discussed in chapter 23. If these tests are negative, an intracardiac electrophysiology study could be performed. This study might reveal evidence for sinus node disease. Unfortunately, even a normal electrophysiology study can be found in a patient with bradycardia. In this instance, the episodes would have to be documented by telephone transmitter. If, on any of these tests, sick sinus syndrome can be demonstrated and the patient is symptomatic, then a pacemaker should be implanted. If the patient was in a normal rhythm throughout most of the day and had only paroxysmal episodes of syncope, then a ventricular demand pacemaker should be inserted. In a patient with a vagal arrhythmia, an atrial pacemaker would not be recommended, since it is possible during these episodes that concomitant AV block could develop. Finally, if the patient has sinus bradycardia or junctional rhythm throughout the day and night, then a dual-chambered pacemaker should be inserted.

It is extremely uncommon for an asymptomatic patient with a normal heart to require a pacemaker for vagal arrhythmia. The asymptomatic patient may or may not require follow-up, depending on the rate; if the rates are extremely slow, follow-up is indicated. Usually, however, when the rate becomes extremely slow, the patient becomes symptomatic from dizzy spells or lack of energy.

Syncope is rare in these children. We do not generally recommend implantation of pacemakers in asymptomatic children with a normal heart and bradycardia. However, there must be a rate defined as "too slow," even in an asymptomatic patient. In the past 10 years, we have implanted more than 300 pacemakers in children; only two were implanted in asymptomatic children with sick sinus syndrome. Both of these children were younger than 10 years and had sleeping rates under 25/min.

Finally, we have resorted to electrophysiology study in two infants with spells of bradycardia, and found no intrinsic sinus node disease. We have not implanted pacemakers in any of these patients. However, all the patients have gone home with apnea and bradycardia monitors. The abnormalities disappeared by 18 months of age in each of the five patients that we have followed. In a group of infants reported by Simcha et al,[6] four infants had such slow rates that seizures resulted and pacemakers were implanted. In three of the four, the seizures disappeared. None of our patients have had bradycardia to this extreme degree.

PREMATURE ATRIAL CONTRACTIONS

A premature atrial contraction (PAC) is defined as a premature P wave. In this subtle form, a PAC may be demonstrated only by its deformity of the preceding T wave. This is especially important in "blocked atrial bigeminy"; in this case, the P waves occur early enough that they are not conducted to the ventricles, resulting in what appears to be regular sinus bradycardia. This occurs almost exclusively in newborns. Blocked atrial bigeminy should be suspected when "bradycardia" appears on the same rhythm strip as conduced premature atrial contractions.

In children, the presence or absence of a compensatory pause is not helpful in distinguishing a premature atrial contraction that conducts with a wide QRS complex caused by bundle-branch aberrancy from a premature ventricular contraction. The reason for this is that premature atrial contractions may occur with a fully compensatory pause, and premature ventricular contractions may occur with less than a compensatory pause. In a child with an otherwise normal heart, it is extremely rare to have both premature atrial contractions and premature ventricular contractions on the same tracing. If there are clearly premature atrial contractions, the beats with the wide QRS complexes should be examined carefully for presence of a P wave in the preceding T wave. Premature junctional contractions are recognized electrocardiographically by a premature QRS complex that has the identical morphology to the sinus QRS and is not preceded by a premature P wave. If the QRS complex is even slightly different from the sinus QRS, then this is a premature ventricular contraction. Since premature junctional contractions originate above the bifurcation of the bundle of His, it is likely that they have a similar prognosis to premature atrial contractions, and thus the following discussion applies to premature junctional contractions as well.

Clinical Situations

Premature atrial contractions usually occur in children with an otherwise completely normal heart. As much as 20% of normal children have one or more premature atrial beats on a 24-hour electrocardiogram.[5] Premature atrial beats are slightly more common than premature ventricular beats in normal patients. Rarely, premature atrial contractions can be associated with atrial enlargement, myocarditis, or hyperthyroidism, or can be a sign of overdosage in patients receiving sympathomimetic amines.

Approach to Diagnosis

The approach to the diagnosis in a patient with premature atrial contractions depends on the patient's age. In newborns with very frequent atrial contractions, occasionally a 24-hour electrocardiogram will reveal episodes of supraventricular tachycardia. Our general approach to the management of infants with premature atrial contractions is to wait 2 to 3 days and see if they diminish in frequency. If, after waiting several days, the premature atrial contractions are still relatively frequent (1 to 2 per minute), then a 24-hour electrocardiogram is obtained. In the older patient, if there are no symptoms suggestive of supraventricular tachycardia, no further work-up is obtained. If the patient has symptoms suggestive of supraventricular tachycardia, then a 24-hour electrocardiogram may be helpful to identify short bursts of supraventricular tachycardia. A telephone transmitter may be invaluable in documenting symptomatic paroxsymal arrhythmias. We usually do not obtain treadmill exercise tests in these patients unless there are exercise-related symptoms.

Approach to Treatment

We do not recommend treatment for premature atrial contractions, regardless of age. Others recommend treatment of newborns with frequent PACs. However, if supraventricular tachycardia is observed on 24-hour electrocardiogram of a newborn, or an older patient has episodes of supraventricular tachycardia documented by telephone transmitter, Holter monitor, or exercise test, then the patient should be treated for supraventricular tachycardia. The specific recommendations for treatment of supraventricular tachycardia are covered in Chapter 13.

PREMATURE VENTRICULAR CONTRACTIONS

A premature ventricular contraction (PVC) is defined as a QRS complex that has a different morphology from the sinus QRS (not necessarily a prolonged duration), that occurs before the next expected QRS complex in a regular rhythm, and that is not preceded by a premature P wave. It is not possible to distinguish, on the basis of the surface electrocardiogram, a premature junctional contraction with aberration from a premature ventricular contraction. For this reason, all beats that meet the previous definition are designated as premature ventricular contractions.

Clinical Situations

Premature ventricular contractions may occur in children with an otherwise normal heart. In studies of 24-hour electrocardiograms, approximately 5% to 10% of normal children had single uniform premature ventricular contractions.[4, 5] Approximately 10% of children with mitral valve prolapse have premature ventricular contractions on 24-hour electrocardiogram.[7] Premature ventricular contractions are also found commonly in patients with hypertrophic cardiomyopathy, congestive cardiomyopathy, arrhythmogenic right ventricular dysplasia, and myocarditis. It is important to be sure that the patient with premature ventricular contractions does not have a prolonged QT interval on the electrocardiogram. This may be hereditary and may occur with or without deafness. Any patient with premature ventricular contractions, any patient who has syncope, and probably any patient with "idiopathic seizures" should have at least one 12-lead electrocardiogram with measurement of the QT interval. Premature ventricular contractions may rarely be a sign of toxicity of psychotropic drugs.

Approach to Diagnosis

The approach to diagnosis in a patient with premature ventricular contractions begins with establishing whether the heart is normal. In addition to history and physical examination, an electrocardiogram and echocardiogram are recommended. The echocardiogram is necessary to be certain that none of the forms of cardiomyopathy are present. These may be difficult to diagnose with physical examination or chest radiograph. We also recommend a treadmill exercise test on all patients with premature ventricular contractions to be sure that the patient does not develop ventricular tachycardia on the exercise test. Exercise-induced ventricular tachycardia has a poor prognosis (see chapter 14). The characteristic response of patients with a normal heart and premature ventricular contractions is for the arrhythmia to be suppressed by exercise.[8] However, as we have performed more of these exercise tests, we have encountered children in whom the premature ventricular contractions did not disappear but instead increased with exercise. We have also encountered patients who developed multiform premature ventricular contractions or couplets with exercise. In these patients with an atypical response to exercise, we recommend the addition of a 24-hour electrocardiogram as part of the work-up. We also perform 24-hour electrocardiograms in patients found to have an abnormal heart. In newborn infants with premature ventricular contractions and a normal heart as proven by echocardiogram, we obtain a 24-hour electrocardiogram to be sure that there were not asymptomatic episodes of ventricular tachycardia.

Approach to Treatment

The approach to treatment begins with symptomatology. Any patient with premature ventricular contractions who also has syncope or presyncope should be treated. In our experience, this is limited almost entirely to patients with premature ventricular contractions and an abnormal heart. In patients with a perfectly normal heart and premature ventricular contractions, syncope is exceedingly rare. In the asymptomatic patient with single uniform premature ventricular contractions, the prognosis is entirely benign. We performed a follow-up study of 17 children with a normal heart and single uniform premature ventricular contractions on a resting electrocardiogram.[8] These patients first presented at an average age of 6.6 years. Of the 17, five had either ventricular bigeminy or trigeminy. After an average follow-up of 7.2 years, the premature ventricular contractions had disappeared in nine of the 17 patients. All of the 17, whether their premature ventricular contractions had disappeared or not, remained asymptomatic. On the basis of this study, we recommend that single uniform premature ventricular contractions in children with a normal heart not be treated, and they do not require follow-up. On the other hand, patients with premature ventricular contractions that increase with exercise or patients with multiform premature ventricular contractions or couplets need to be followed closely. If the heart is truly normal by echocardiogram, it is likely that these children do not require treatment. If any of these children become symptomatic with presyncope or syncope, treatment is recommended. The management of patients with a normal heart and ventricular tachycardia is detailed in Chapter 14, as is the management of ventricular arrhythmias in mitral valve prolapse and the various forms of cardiomyopathy.

TREATMENT

Patients with a normal heart and asymptomatic ventricular arrhythmias do not generally require treatment. The specific treatment of children with various types of abnormal heart and ventricular arrhythmias are detailed in chapter 14.

SECOND DEGREE AV BLOCK

In type I second degree AV block (also known as Wenckebach or Mobitz Type I), the PR interval lengthens progressively until a P wave is not followed by a QRS complex. In most cases, electrophysiologic studies have localized type I block to the AV node. In type II block (Mobitz type II), the PR interval is constant. In electrophysiology studies, most cases of type II second degree AV block are localized to the bundle of His or to simultaneous block in both bundle branches.

Clinical Situations

Clinical situations in which second degree AV block is found are quite varied. Type I second degree AV block occurs in approximately 3% of normal children on 24-hour electrocardiogram. Type I second degree AV block may also occur in patients with abnormally increased vagal tone. For example, patients with head trauma frequently have type I second degree AV block. Type II block does not occur in normal children in sinus rhythm. Either type I or type II second degree AV block may occur in myocarditis or cardiomyopathy.

Approach to Diagnosis

All patients with second degree AV block should have an exercise test. There are two reasons for performing the exercise test. The first is to determine the AV conduction ratio with exercise. Usually, in patients with type I second degree AV block, AV conduction improves with exercise. On the other hand, if AV conduction worsens with exercise and the ventricular rate decreases, a poor prognosis may be indicated and a pacemaker may be needed. The second reason for an exercise test is to assess exercise tolerance. Rarely, patients with advanced second degree AV block may have reduced exercise tolerance, especially if the ventricular rate does not increase appreciably with exercise.

All patients with second degree AV block on resting electrocardiogram should also have a 24-hour electrocardiogram to asssess whether there are periods of advanced AV block or even intermittent complete AV block.

Approach to Treatment

The approach to treatment of the patient with second degree AV block depends on the type of block and the presence of symptoms. The patient with syncope or presyncope and second degree AV block should probably have a pacemaker. However, in a patient with symptoms, if the AV block did not appear severe on treadmill exercise test or during 24-hour electrocardiogram, then an intracardiac electrophysiology study should be performed to be certain that a different arrhythmia can not be induced. For example, it might be possible to induce ventricular tachycardia in such a patient, and the reason for the syncope would be a tachyarrhythmia rather than a bradyarrhythmia, and a pacemaker would not be helpful.

In the asymptomatic patient with AV block, the approach to treatment depends on the type of AV block. Patients with type I second degree AV block should be followed. However, it is extremely rare for the patient with a normal heart and type I second degree AV block to progress to complete AB block, except in the first year or two of life. We have encountered several infants with type I second degree AV block in infancy that progressed to complete AV block. It is likely that these were infants with "late-appearing" congenital complete AV block. Since type I second degree AV block is generally in the AV node, even if complete AV block develops, the junctional escape rate is usually adequate to prevent serious symptoms or sudden death. Type II second degree AV block is not found in patients with normal hearts. This generally indicates abnormality of the bundle of His or bundle branches; if complete AV block developed, the escape pacemaker could be slow and irregular. For this reason, patients with presumed type II second degree AV block should have an electrophysiology study to document the site of the block. There may be rare patients in whom the site of block is in the AV node, and the concern about these patients is less than in those in whom the block is within or below the bundle of His. In a patient with type II second degree block and documented block within the bundle of His or below the bundle of His, strong consideration should be given to implanting a pacemaker.

TREATMENT

In patients requiring a pacemaker for AV block, dual-chambered pacing is usually chosen. The atrial impulses (under the normal control of the sympathetic nervous system) are sensed by the pacemaker and transmitted to the ventricles, thus allowing for a normal variation in heart rate. If the patient has only paroxysmal episodes of AV block that result in symptoms, a simple ventricular demand pacemaker can be implanted. Finally, it is possible to implant a pacemaker in the ventricle that includes a physiologic sensor (i.e., one that senses activity). This would change the rate of the pacemaker in accordance with body demand, and although this is attractive, it is preferable to have direct control of the ventricular rate by the patient's own sinus rate. Dual-chambered pacemakers are recommended in the majority of patients with AV block unless it is impossible to obtain adequate atrial sensing.

CONCLUSIONS

Management of the ambulatory child with an arrhythmia depends on whether the child is symptomatic and whether a normal heart is found on cardiac evaluation. In the child with a normal heart who is asymptomatic, the vast majority of arrhythmias can be left untreated. However, the symptomatic patient with syncope or presyncope and an abnormal heart needs urgent treatment. In patients with a normal heart and symptoms and in patients with an abnormal heart without symptoms, further testing (perhaps including intracardiac electrophysiologic study) may be helpful to demonstrate the abnormality and to choose the best method treatment.

Acknowledgments

Research was supported in part by grants HL24916, HL07190, and RR00188 from the National Institutes of Health, Bethesda, Maryland, and by a grant from the J. S. Abercrombie Foundation.

References

1. Garson A: The Electrocardiogram in Infants and Children: A Systematic Approach. Philadelphia, Lea and Febiger, 1983.
2. Kugler JD: Sinoatrial node dysfunction. *In* Gillette PC, Garson A Jr (eds): Pediatric Cardiac Dysrhythmias. New York, Grune & Stratton, 1981, pp 265–294.
3. Michaelsson M, Engle MA: Congenital complete heart block: an international study of the natural history. *In* Brest AN, Engle MA (eds): Cardiovascular Clinics. Philadelphia, FA Davis, 1972, p 85.
4. Southall DP: Study of cardiac rhythm in healthy newborn infants. Br Heart J 43:42–46, 1979.
5. Scott O, Williams GJ, Fiddler GI: Results of 24 hour ambulatory monitoring of electrocardiogram in 131 healthy boys aged 10 to 13 years. Br Heart J 44:304–308, 1980.
6. Simcha A, Rein AJJT, Uretzky G, et al: Sinus node dysfunction in infants with syncopal and apnoeic attack: Its diagnosis and treatment. *In* Doyle EF, Engle MA, Gersony WM, et al (eds): Pediatric Cardiology. Proceedings of the Second World Congress. New York, Springer-Verlag, 1985, pp 443–445.
7. Bissett GS, Schwartz DC, Meyer RA: Clinical spectrum and long-term follow-up of isolated mitral valve prolapse in 119 children. Circulation 62:423–428, 1980.
8. Jacobsen J, Garson A, Gillette PC, et al: Premature ventricular contractions in normal children. J Pediatr 92:36–38, 1978.

CHAPTER 28

UNOPERATED CONGENITAL AND ACQUIRED HEART DISEASE

Richard A. Friedman

This chapter deals with arrhythmias in children with unoperated congenital and acquired heart disease. Despite the myriad of congenital heart lesions that exist, only a few lesions have been included in studies of preoperative arrhythmias; they are discussed in this chapter. The paucity of data probably reflects the relatively recent advent of routine Holter monitoring of children and the more recent use of invasive and noninvasive electrophysiologic testing in this age group. Advances in surgery to correct or palliate congenital heart disease have altered the natural history of these diseases so that it is unusual in our experience to see arrhythmias in these patients in an unoperated state. Acquired heart disease (i.e., metabolically induced, immunologically based, or as a result of infections or other miscellaneous conditions) is examined in the second part of the chapter.

UNOPERATED CONGENITAL DISEASE

Atrial Septal Defect (ASD)

Several types of arrhythmias, predominantly supraventricular tachycardias including atrial fibrillation (AF), atrial flutter (AFl), paroxysmal supraventricular tachycardia (PSVT), and sinoatrial node dysfunction (SAND) with resultant junctional or ectopic focus atrial rhythms have been described in patients with atrial septal defects. Many of these studies have been on adult patients because of the relatively late recognition of their congenital heart disease compared with children having more complex lesions.

Hamilton et al[1] performed electrocardiograms on 384 patients (age range, 16 to 73 years) with unoperated secundum ASD. Normal sinus rhythm was present in 82%, AF or AFl was seen in 8%, minor disorders of conduction in 8%, and complete atrioventricular block in 1%. An "interventricular conduction defect" was seen in 88% of these patients on the surface electrocardiographic lead V_1. Although by history 44% complained of palpitations, only 20% had documented arrhythmias (eight patients with AF/AFl and four patients with complete right bundle-branch block [CRBBB]). The incidence of AF/AFl was correlated with increasing pulmonary resistance (Rp) at cardiac catheterization ($Rp \leq 2$ u/M^2 had 7% incidence vs 22% incidence with $Rp \geq 2$ u/M^2).

Forfang et al[2] studied 98 Norwegians (mean age, 49 years) with secundum atrial septal defect (ASD). After excluding 14 patients with concomitant lung disease or other cardiac disease, 84 patients were studied. They found a 67% incidence (56 of 84 patients) of arrhythmias prior to surgery. However, this incidence estimate was based on symptoms reported by the patients; the symptoms were ascribed to paroxysmal tachyarrhythmias, presumably of supraventricular origin. There was no difference with respect to New York Heart Association (NYHA) grading between patients complaining of a paroxysmal tachyarrhythmia and asymptomatic patients. However, those with documented AF had a worse NYHA grading than the others.

In another study of Norwegians, Rosketh and Rolf[3] surveyed the records of patients older than 40 years who had ASD. Of the 61 patients in this group, 28% had AF/AFl. This was in comparison to an additional 84 patients between 20 and 40 years of age with ASD among whom only 4% had AF/AFl.

Paolillo, Dawkins, and Miller[4] presented data on 49 unoperated patients aged 50 to 77 years. They documented 51% of their patients to have supraventricular arrhythmias. The incidence of arrhythmia was correlated with increased age (80% of patients aged 77 to 79 years had a documented arrhythmia). Unfortunately, they did not give an accurate breakdown of the specific types of arrhythmia, only noting that they included AF/AFl, supraventricular tachycardia (SVT), or premature beats (sporadic or persistent). They also commented that 73% of patients who presented in heart failure had a supraventricular arrhythmia.

Sealy et al[5] studied 108 patients with secundum ASD, 10 of whom had an associated anomalous drainage or a right pulmonary vein. Although they noted a 29% incidence of arrhythmia, documentation was present in only 19%; the remaining 10% were "positive" by history only. They also found a correlation between age and incidence of arrhythmias, with a 57% occurrence in those older than 31 years. Unlike Hamilton et al, they found no correlation between pulmonary hypertension and the presence of arrhythmia, though magnitude of shunt seemed to correlate well (11% incidence with $Qp/Qs \leq 2:1$ vs 38% incidence with $Qp/Qs \geq 3:1$). AF/AFl was most common, accounting for two-thirds of the preoperative arrhythmias, with the remainder equally divided between paroxysmal atrial tachycardia (PAT) and junctional rhythm.

Bagger et al[6] reported on nine patients (mean age, 32 years) who underwent electrophysiologic study prior to repair. Eight of the nine also had preoperative Holter monitoring, with four of the eight patients reported as normal, three patients demonstrating transient episodes of accelerated junctional rhythm, and one patient with infrequent episodes of Mobitz type II second degree AV block and episodes of sinus arrest. The preoperative ECG showed prolonged PQ segments in two patients that on intracardiac electrograms were shown to be caused by a prolonged PA (HRA-LSRA) interval in one and a prolonged AH in the other. Four other patients had CRBB on their electrocardiograms.

Benedini et al[7] examined 26 adults with unoperated ASD. Though Holter monitor results in all patients were normal, electrophysiologic catheterization studies of the sinus node sinoatrial conduction time (SACT) and sinus node recovery time (SNRT) demonstrated SAND in 17 of 26 patients. They concluded that "concealed" preoperative SAND could be a cause of postoperative "sick sinus syndrome."

There have only been a few studies in children. Clark and Kugler[8] performed 24-hour Holter monitoring and electrophysiologic catheterization on 15 patients aged 10 months to 18 years. On Holter, three patients (20%) had evidence of SAND, one had frequent premature atrial contractions (PACs), and another had paroxysmal AFl. In addition, two patients demonstrated abnormal AV node function. Electrophysiologic testing demonstrated that 10 patients (66%) had SAND, and 5 patients (33%) had abnormal AV node function. In a separate study, Clark et al[8a] demonstrated SAND in children with sinus venosus and secundum type ASDs. However, patients with the sinus venosus type had an 18% incidence, compared with a 4% incidence in patients with the secundum type. In this study, SAND was defined as documentation on surface ECG of ectopic atrial focus, absent P wave, or junctional rhythm and thus may explain the lower incidence of SAND compared with the previous study. In a similar report on children with congenital heart disease and SAND, Yabek and Jarmakani[9] found only one patient to have an operated ASD (out of a total of 30 patients).

Anderson et al[10] studied eight children aged 5 to 15 years with ASD who at cardiac catheterization had His bundle electrograms recorded. They compared this group to an age-matched control group of 16 patients with other forms of congenital heart disease. They found that the average PR interval in the ASD group was longer than that in controls (154 ms vs 135 ms) and was caused by a prolonged PA interval on the intracardiac electrogram. The AH and HV intervals were identical in the two groups. They speculated that this was a result of differences of wavefront propagation through the atrium in the ASD patients, and that the larger atria seen in patients with left-to-right shunt further slowed conduction from the sinus node to the AV node.

Ventricular Septal Defect

Two studies of patients with ventricular septal defect (VSD) who reached adulthood and did not have pulmonary hypertension found that arrhythmias were uncommon.[11, 12] In the study by Mark and Young, only 5% of 38 patients had ventricular arrhythmia, and these were felt to be secondary to digitalis therapy.[11] In the 109 patients in Otterstad, Nitter-Hauge, and Myrhe's study, only one patient had documented arrhythmia (AFl), though 37 others complained of palpitations and chest pain.[12]

Patent Ductus Arteriosus

The natural history of patients with patent ductus arteriosus (PDA) has been well studied. Marquis et al[13] studied records from 804 patients with patent ductus arteriosus from 1940 through 1979. They found that chronic atrial fibrillation was present in 11 of 13 patients whose left ventricular failure proceeded to right ventricular failure. Paroxysmal arrhythmias were uncommon in this group but included paroxysmal supraventricular tachycardia (PSVT), multiform ventricular extrasystoles, and episodes of "tachycardia of unknown origin." Of the 804 patients, one had associated syncope, and two died suddenly. McManus[14] compiled reports since 1840 that characterized 46 adults with PDA. Of 21 patients who had ECGs recorded, 15 had documented AF, and three had intermittent AF. The high incidence may be influenced by the mean age of the patients (62 years) and the fact that most had significant left-to-right shunts.

Tetralogy of Fallot

Two reports on the preoperative incidence of arrhythmias in patients with tetralogy of Fallot have concluded that ventricular arrhythmias were present in these patients preoperatively, and incidence increased with age of the patient. Sullivan et al[15] performed a Holter study on 22 patients. None of those younger than 5 years had arrhythmias, while 44% of the patients between 13 and 43 years of age had premature ventricular contractions (PVCs) (three or more per hour), couplets, or ventricular tachycardia (VT). In a related study, Deanfield et al[16] studied 145 patients and found that 20% of the uncorrected group had ventricular arrhythmia of Lown grade II (frequent uniform PVCs) or greater. The highest incidence was found in patients older than 16 years, 21% of whom had episodes of VT. Supraventricular arrhythmias were seen only in patients older than 8 years; frequent atrial extrasystoles were found in four patients, three of whom had episodes of SVT. Of 60 patients in the unoperated group, symptoms were present in only four patients (one with SVT, one with VT and syncope, and two with palpitations). The concept that a favorable milieu for the occurrence of supraventricular arrhythmias exists in patients with unoperated cyanotic congenital heart disease was studied by Dubrow et al.[17] They examined 18 acyanotic and 17 cyanotic children and found that sinoatrial conduction time and atrial refractoriness were prolonged in cyanotic children when compared with acyanotic children. Heart rate and sinus node automaticity, as determined by sinus node recovery time, were not significantly different in these two groups.

Aortic Valve Disease and Coarctation of the Aorta

Little has been written concerning preoperative arrhythmias and aortic stenosis in children. Presumably, those with severe or critical stenosis early in life receive operative intervention based on symptoms (i.e., severe congestive heart failure). Those patients with only mild aortic valve disease have been followed clinically, but rarely has routine Holter monitoring been performed. Bisset et al[18] studied 15 children with aortic valve stenosis pre- and postoperatively. Although they concluded that no conduction defects or arrhythmias were noted preoperatively, routine Holter monitoring was not performed. Other studies in children have concentrated on postoperative arrhythmias for aortic valve disease and are discussed elsewhere in this book.

Studies in unoperated adult patients have demonstrated that complex ventricular ectopy was significantly more common in patients with aortic valve disease than in age-matched controls.[19] Von Olshausen et al[20] showed that ventricular arrhythmias were common in aortic valve disease and that the state of myocardial performance was correlated with the severity of ventricular arrhythmias. Schwartz et al[21] studied syncope and sudden death in adult patients with aortic stenosis and demonstrated VT and VF with continuous electrocardiographic monitoring. Santinga et al[22] also correlated complex ventricular arrhythmias in their patients with aortic valve stenosis and depressed ventricular performance.

In a study to examine whether myocardial performance was linked to the prevalence of arrhythmias, Bush et al[23] found an "unusually high" incidence of postoperative supraventricular arrhythmias in adults after aortic valve surgery. In their study, atrial tissue was obtained from both children and adults at the time of surgery for the study of action potential characteristics. They found that in adults there was a significant disturbance of cellular action potential characteristics compared with normals and younger patients, and postulated that these disturbances could explain the observation of postoperative atrial tachycardias in adult patients. It is therefore possible to speculate that a similar evolution occurs in the ventricles of children to explain the relative lack of preoperative arrhythmias in children with aortic valve disease when compared with adults.

Coarctation of the aorta has been associated with complete atrioventricular block and Adams-Stokes disease in a few patients.[24, 25] Based on the postmortem findings of one patient, James and Jackson postulated that left ventricular hypertension during development places greater stress on the left side of the central fibrous body and influences the morphogenesis of the His bundle and AV node as well as the membranous septum. Displacement of the left part of the conduction system toward the right side would ensue, and any additional fibrosis could produce atrioventricular block. Lev et al[26] also reported on several cases of congenital atrioventricular block in patients with coexistent heart disease; one of the patients also had coarctation of the aorta. There is a report of coarctation of the aorta and Wolff-Parkinson-White syndrome (WPW).[27] This was an early report and actually documents the first known association of a congenital heart defect with WPW. The association of complete atrioventricular block or WPW and coarctation of the aorta does not appear prominent in our patient population.

Ebstein's Anomaly of the Tricuspid Valve

There have been several excellent studies of patients with Ebstein's anomaly and cardiac arrhythmias. Several have reported on the incidence and type of arrhythmia as part of a natural history study. Kumar et al[28] reviewed the natural history of 53 patients seen at Children's Hospital in Boston, Massachusetts. At their first observation, all 53 patients were noted to be in normal sinus rhythm. Subsequently, 24 patients developed an arrhythmia. PSVT was seen in 12 patients (22%) and was recurrent in seven patients. Multiple supraventricular arrhythmias (SVT, AF, junctional rhythm) were found in three more patients at different times. Wolff-Parkinson-White syndrome was seen in seven patients (13%). Long-term follow-up was available in all patients (13 patients were followed for more than 10 years). During that time, 22 patients died, two of them suddenly. One of the sudden deaths was in a patient with known SVT. Arrhythmias were noted in 38% of patients during follow-up. In another eight patients, arrhythmia occurred terminally, but in only one infant (a 4-day-old who had concomitant congestive heart failure and documented SVT that deteriorated into VT) could death be assessed as caused by arrhythmia.

Watson[29] correlated data from a large international cooperative study on 505 patients with Ebstein's anomaly. Most of the arrhythmia data came from documentation during cardiac catheterization. Of this group, 363 (72%) underwent cardiac catheterization; paroxysmal tachycardia occurred in 90 patients (25% of catheterization patients). Preexcitation was noted in 10% of patients, and an additional 28% gave a history of paroxysmal tachycardia. Arrhythmias were a frequent occurrence during catheterization; the most common arrhythmias were SVT (13%), AF or AFl (3%), SVT and VT (4.4%), multiple types of SVT (2%), VT or VF (1.4% each), and bradycardia or AV block (1% each). During cardiac catheterization, 13 patients died and an additional six patients had a cardiac arrest from which they were successfully resuscitated. Of the 13 patients who died, four developed asystole, six had rapid ventricular arrhythmias, and the other three had rapid uncontrollable SVT. In the group of six survivors, three had had asystole, and three had had a rapid ventricular arrhythmia. All 19 patients with this adverse history had been in sinus rhythm at the start of the catheterization. Preexcitation occurred in two patients (10%), and five patients (26%) had a prior history of paroxysmal tachycardia; both incidences were similar to those in the group as a whole. A history of paroxysmal tachycardia was not predictive of death or arrhythmia during catheterization nor for subsequent occurrence of sudden death.

In a large series from the Mayo Clinic, Oh et al[30] reviewed records on 52 patients seen during an 11-year period. Preoperative arrhythmias were determined to be present in 79% (either documented or by history of palpitation, near syncope or syncope). The remaining 11 patients had no symptoms or documentation of an arrhythmia. Electrocardiographic documentation was available in 34 patients [18 with SVT, 10 with AF/AFl, and 13 with ventricular arrhythmias (seven with frequent PVCs and six with nonsustained VT)]. In the 13 patients with ventricular arrhythmia, 10 also had other documented arrhythmias: five had SVT, four had AF/AFl, and one had complete AV block. Only six of the 34 (18%) were asymptomatic during their arrhythmias. Preoperative electrophysiologic assessment was performed in 14 patients whose indications were syncope (10) or WPW (four). All four patients with WPW developed sustained orthodromic reciprocating tachycardia, and three of them had sustained inducible AF or AFl. The one remaining patient had inducible nonsustained SVT. The accessory pathway was found in the right ventricular free wall in all four patients, with a second (septal) pathway in one of them. As a group, the older patients were more prone to occurrence of arrhythmia than the younger patients.

Radford, Graff, and Neilson[31] examined the natural history of 35 patients with Ebstein's anomaly. Forty percent presented as neonates, and only one patient had a serious arrhythmia (SVT at a rate faster than 300/min, associated with hydrops fetalis). Of the 10 patients who presented as infants and children, only three had SVT. Most of these patients had complete or incomplete right bundle-branch block patterns on their electrocardiograms. Of the 11 patients (31%) who presented as adolescents or adults, seven (64%) had a history of palpitation, dyspnea, or chest pain. During cardiac catheterization, "important" arrhythmias occurred in 12 patients, with cardioversion necessary in two instances. During follow-up, six of 35 patients (17%) died. Two patients died of SVT, one a 2-week-old with associated double outlet right ventricle and the other a 3-month-old infant with associated pulmonary atresia. One patient had a Kent bundle surgically divided.

In summary, arrhythmias have occurred in at least 36% of the patients described in these four studies of Ebstein's anomaly. Supraventricular tachycardia is the most frequently occurring arrhythmia, and approximately 10% of patients have WPW. Ventricular arrhythmias were also noted in at least 9% of the patients from these groups.

Transposition

d-TRANSPOSITION OF THE GREAT ARTERIES

There are two important large studies on arrhythmias in patients with unoperated complete transposition of the great arteries (d-TGA). They were performed in order to help clarify whether the atrial switch procedure was of primary importance in the genesis of postoperative arrhythmias in these patients. Southall et al[32] examined the records of 120 patients during a 7-year period. Their ages ranged from 2 weeks to 8 years; 80% had had a balloon atrial septostomy, 2% had had an atrial septectomy, and 18% had had neither. Prior to their operation, 119 of the 120 patients had normal sinus rhythm on their electrocardiograms. Holter monitoring was performed in 19 of these patients before surgery; none of the patients had a ventricular arrhythmia preoperatively. Sinus node Wenckebach and/or sinus node exit block occurred in 13 of the 19 patients. Premature atrial contractions (less than 12 per hour) occurred in four patients, and episodes of intermittent junctional rhythm occurred in seven patients. Normal sinus rhythm was seen in five patients. According to Southall et al, all these findings were essentially "normal" findings, compared with the control population. However, whether the incidence is truly identical in both populations is not clear from their data.

Martin, Radley-Smith, and Yacoub[33] performed Holter monitoring on 41 patients (mean age, 8.5 months) prior to surgery. The majority (75%) had undergone balloon atrial septostomy. Of the 41 patients, 34 (83%) had sinus rhythm only. Supraventricular arrhythmias occurred in only two patients; one had PACs and the other had paroxysmal AFl. Two patients had brief (less than 1.75 s) sinus pauses, and one patient had junctional bradycardia. In addition, six patients had ventricular arrhythmias (PVCs), but only one had Lown grade V arrhythmia; the other five patients had only Lown grade I. These investigators concluded that preoperative arrhythmias were uncommon in these patients, and when present were of similar type and frequency to those ascribed to normal children.

CORRECTED TRANSPOSITION OF THE GREAT ARTERIES

Daliento et al[34] reported on the incidence and types of arrhythmias in 17 patients with isolated corrected congenital transposition. The age range of the study group was 5 to 54 years. All the patients had surface electrocardiograms, 15 patients had Holter studies, and 10 patients underwent electrophysiologic study. On surface electrocardiogram, 10 patients had normal PR interval, two patients had first degree AV block, and five patients (29%) had complete atrioventricular block, though this finding was not present at birth. Two patients had recurrent SVT that was caused by either AV node reentry or reentry through what was thought to be a James fiber. One patient had WPW as a result of a left lateral accessory connection. Of the 15 patients who underwent Holter study, eight patients had ventricular arrhythmias. In the group with complete atrioventricular block, four of the five had Holter studies, and all had Lown grade IVa ventricular arrhythmias. One of the patients died with VT that degenerated into ventricular fibrillation (VF) 24 years after the occurrence of CAVB. In the group without complete AV block, two patients had Lown grade III, and two patients had Lown grade Ia. The authors speculated that the late onset of complete atrioventricular block was probably a result of ongoing fibrosis secondary to continued mechanical stress on the tissue, and that pacemaker implantation may be indicated even in asymptomatic patients with this disease.

Huhta et al[35] reviewed 107 patients aged 2 to 76 years with ventricular inversion. The majority of patients in this study had associated anomalies, including VSD (77%), pulmonary stenosis (53%), tricuspid valve insufficiency (34%), and dextrocardia (23%). Complete AV block was seen in 22% of these patients (four patients at birth and 19 of late onset). They found that the incidence of atrioventricular block increased with age at a rate of 2% per year after diagnosis and was not affected by surgery if atrioventricular block did not occur at the time of the operation (69 patients had at least one operation). In addition, they found that the presence of an intact ventricular septum made AV block more likely. The need for permanent pacing in some of these patients was highlighted by the occurrence of sudden death in one of their adult patients with complete AV block of late (adult) onset who had had a resting heart rate of 40 bpm.

Eisenmenger's Syndrome

If left unoperated, many types of congenital heart disease may progress to a point where fixed and elevated pulmonary vascular resistance develops. Arrhythmias may occur late in the course of the development of this syndrome. Graham[36] notes that atrial arrhythmias are more common in those Eisenmenger patients who shunt at the atrial level. Clarkson et al[37] reviewed 58 patients with Eisenmenger's syndrome and VSD. They were able to identify only one patient with an arrhythmia that was of atrial origin. Of the 17 patients who died, however, seven patients died suddenly with no previous history of a cardiac arrhythmia. Young and Mark[38] found that arrhythmias were not clinically significant in their series of 57 patients. No arrhythmias were detected in the children, though two died suddenly. The adults in their study had various arrhythmias including AFl (three), PVCs (three), premature junctional contraction (PJCs) (three), complete atrioventricular block (one), and SVT (one). Brammell et al[39] found that arrhythmias were rare in their 91 cases of Eisenmenger's syndrome. Atrial flutter was found in one patient with VSD, and 2:1 atrioventricular block was found in one patient with PDA. All remaining patients had normal sinus rhythm. In a large series of adult patients with unoperated VSDs studied in Norway by Otterstad,[12] 8% of patients developed Eisenmenger's syndrome, but arrhythmias were not a prominent feature in these patients.

Most of these studies did not include a Holter monitor on the patient. It has been our experience that late-onset atrial arrhythmias, especially symptomatic AFl, may occur in these patients and may be responsible for either syncope or severe congestive heart failure. Frequent ventricular extrasystoles, either single or in couplets, also seem to be common, but whether therapy is necessary is not resolved. Clearly a more detailed prospective study of these patients with Holter monitoring is indicated.

ACQUIRED HEART DISEASE

Connective Tissue Disease

Numerous studies have documented arrhythmias and conduction defects in the various connective tissue disorders. In 1945, Plante and Stevens[40] first described the association between congenital atrioventricular block in a fetus whose mother had systemic lupus erythematosus (SLE). The etiology of the atrioventricular block has been attributed to antibody deposition in the myocardium, with subsequent inflammation and destruction of the normal conduction tissue and replacement with fibrosis.[41–43] It has been postulated that the disease may be ongoing because of progression to complete atrioventricular block in a number of patients. In a study by McCue et al,[44] 64% of children with congenital complete atrioventricular block were born to mothers with connective tissue disease, predominantly SLE. Reed et al[42] examined 12 infants with neonatal complete AV block and found that nine of the 12 mothers had SS-A/Ro antibodies. They postulated that transplacental passage of the antibodies was responsible for the immunologic damage. They also stressed the fact that many of the mothers of these infants are asymptomatic, and thus screening the mother of an infant with congenital complete atrioventricular block for connective tissue disease should be routine. The association of infants with complete AV block and ventricular inversion and maternal connective tissue disease was noted by Litsey, Noonan, and O'Connor.[41] They speculated that this association may be explained by the possible linkage of abnormal or absent regulatory genes responsible for cardiac looping and immunoregulation.

Acute and chronic myocarditis has been noted in these infants, and ectopic atrial rhythm, AFl, and PVCs have been described.[44, 45] In addition, atrial standstill has been reported in a young adult with SLE who also had a history of SVT and bradycardia-tachycardia syndrome.[46]

Systemic sclerosis produces electrocardiographic disturbances in approximately 50% of patients with the disease.[47] Conduction system disease (left bundle-branch block, right bundle-branch block, and left anterior fascicular block) has been described and attributed to infarction and fibrosis.[48] Atrial and ventricular ectopy have been reported in 7% and 5% of patients, respectively. Patients who have systemic sclerosis with myocardial dysfunction and abnormal thallium exercise tests seem to be at greater risk of developing arrhythmias, compared with those who had normal studies. Ferri et al[48] found ventricular arrhythmias to be more common than atrial arrhythmias and included patients with multiform single PVCs and couplets as well as episodes of VT. They found that of the 23 deaths in their series of 130 patients, 43% were sudden and unexpected. Of that group, 14 had multiform and or repetitive PVCs with concomitant echocardiographic demonstration of poor left ventricular function. Thus, as in patients with congestive cardiomyopathy, the combination of these two factors may define a specific risk group for sudden death.

Other forms of connective tissue disease including ankylosing spondylitis,[49] Sjögren's syndrome,[50] and Wegener's granulomatosis[51] have been associated with complete atrioventricular block. In addition, patients with Loeffler's endomyocardial disease have been described with PACs, SVT, AF, and frequent PVCs with no evidence of complete atrioventricular block.[52] Atrial flutter, PVCs, and variable atrioventricular block have been noted in polymyositis.[53]

Neuromuscular Disorders

Supraventricular and ventricular arrhythmias as well as conduction system disturbances have been noted in patients with various neuromuscular disorders. Perloff[54] noted that in Duchenne's muscular dystrophy, the most common rhythm disturbance is inappropriate sinus tachycardia, which may either be labile or gradual in onset. The etiology is unknown but may be a result of abnormal autonomic influence on the sinus node or of infiltration of the sinus node with abnormal or scarred myocardium with resultant abnormal sinoatrial automaticity or sinus node reentry tachycardia. It is possible that this represents atrial ectopic tachycardia near the sinus node. Atrial flutter has also been described and commonly precipitates congestive heart failure in late stages of the disease.[54] Atrioventricular conduction disturbances may be seen as well. Up to 50% of patients may have a short PR interval without a delta wave and thus accelerated AV conduction similar to that seen in Pompe's disease.[54] High degree AV block in association with WPW syndrome has also been reported.[55] Premature atrial contractions and sustained atrial ectopic rhythms have been reported to be more common in these patients.[56] Ventricular arrhythmias, specifically multiform PVCs, couplets, and VT, are uncommon,[56] despite the finding that on autopsy examination, the ultrastructural changes seen in the ventricular myocardium are greater than those seen in the atrium. Fatty infiltration and fibrosis are also seen in the sinoatrial and AV node regions.[57]

Various arrhythmias are seen in other types of muscular dystrophy. Fascicular or complete AV block has been reported in slowly progressive X-linked Becker's muscular dystrophy.[54] In limb-girdle muscular dystrophy, sick sinus syndrome, AFl, bundle-branch block, first degree AV block, and complete AV block may be seen.[54] Atrial standstill, AFl, and SVT have been described in fascioscapulohumeral dystrophy[54, 58–60] and in humeroperoneal dystrophy (Emery Dreifuss disease).[54] In myotonic muscular dystrophy, some type of ECG abnormality may be seen in up to 72% of patients.[61] However, the incidence of arrhythmias is only 9% to 10%. Sinus bradycardia and atrial flutter or fibrillation have also been described.[61, 62] In addition, PACs, PVCs, (both couplets and multiform types) and SVT have been documented on Holter examinations of these patients.[62]

Kearns-Sayre syndrome (chronic, progressive external ophthalmoplegia and retinal pigmentation) is associated with complete atrioventricular block, which may progress from an interventricular conduction defect (usually CRBBB with LAD). In fact, patients with this pattern probably carry high risk of early progression to complete atrioventricular block, and elective insertion of a pacing device should be considered.[63]

In hyperkalemic periodic paralysis, ventricular arrhythmias, including PVCs (uniform and multiform), bigeminy, and bidirectional VT, are reported.[64] Although rare in children, adult patients with polio may have atrial flutter-fibrillation, multifocal atrial tachycardia, PACs, and PVCs as well as varying degrees of atrioventricular block.[54] At autopsy, these patients have degenerative changes and fibrosis in the sinus node, AV node, and His-Purkinje system. Patients with Guillain-Barré syndrome may develop sinus bradycardia and even sinus node arrest as well as complete atrioventricular block. Tachyarrhythmias (SVT and VT) have been seen in these patients, especially if mechanical ventilation is required.[54, 65–69]

Dunnigan, Pierpont, and Smith[70] described a group of patients who presented with various types of arrhythmias and who, when further investigated, were found to have skeletal muscle myopathy associated with these arrhythmias. Although the serum acyl carnitine levels were normal in nine patients, the skeletal muscle long-chain acyl carnitine was decreased in nine of 10 patients, seven had dilated and three restrictive cardiomyopathy. The arrhythmias noted were VT in six patients, SVT in two, and His-ventricular block in one. It is important to note that in none of these patients with arrhythmias was a clinically apparent muscle weakness noted.

Marfan's Syndrome

Conduction disturbances and arrhythmias are both associated with Marfan's syndrome. First degree atrioventricular block, incomplete right bundle-branch block, SVT, AFl, and multiform PVCs have been documented in two large series.[71, 72] Chen et al further stressed that the incidence of malignant ventricular arrhythmias, including multiform couplets and VT, may progress with age in these patients.[71] They noted that in Marfan patients, the combination of prolonged QTc with mitral valve prolapse is associated with a higher incidence of ventricular arrhythmias than is associated with either of these two factors alone. However, of the six patients in their study who died, all had congestive heart failure. Two had concomitant atrial flutter-fibrillation.

Infectious Agents

Many infectious agents may produce conditions of acute myocardial dysfunction with the subsequent appearance of arrhythmias. In addition, permanent or chronic damage from these agents to the myocardium may produce a milieu where arrhythmias may later develop.

Rheumatic heart disease (which has seen a slight resurgence recently) is associated with a multitude of arrhythmias. Atrial flutter-fibrillation, PACs (most frequently with mitral valve disease), multiform PVCs, VT, or VF (more common with aortic valve disease) have all been well described.[73] Acute rheumatic fever has been associated with accelerated junctional rhythm in 20% to 28% of patients.[74, 75] Sixty percent of the patients in one study developed this rhythm prior to specific evidence of carditis. However, others have found that this rhythm did not correlate with the diagnosis of carditis or affect ultimate prognosis. Atrioventricular conduction was abnormal in 84% of the patients studied by Clarke and Keith[76] and consisted primarily of first degree AV block; only 0.05% developed complete atrioventricular block. They also noted a 9.5% incidence of accelerated junctional rhythm in their patients.

Izumi, Susumo, and Akira[77] compared electrocardiograms and electrophysiologic study data in two groups of school-aged children—one with rheumatic fever and the other with proven streptococcal infection without criteria for rheumatic fever. Though present in 25% of patients with streptococcal infection, atrioventricular conduction disturbances were more common (72%) in those with rheumatic fever. Atrial fibrillation, junctional rhythm, and wandering atrial pacemaker were present in the rheumatic group only. Persistence of rhythm disturbance (greater than 5 weeks) was uncommon but was found only in the group with rheumatic carditis. In addition to supraventricular arrhythmias, VT has also been described in this disease.[78]

Rocky Mountain spotted fever, a rickettsial disease, has been associated with SVT, junctional tachycardia, and first degree atrioventricular block, though sinus tachycardia is most common.[79] Candida infections are becoming more common in the pediatric age group, especially in the immunocompromised host (i.e., newborns with indwelling catheters and cancer chemotherapy patients). Conduction alterations, tachycardias, bradycardias, and sudden death have all been described in Candida sepsis and probably represent the result of myocarditis.[80] Varicella infections, which are ubiquitous in the pediatric age group, have been associated with life-threatening ventricular arrhythmias and complete atrioventricular block.[81, 82] Chagas' disease, which is uncommon in North America but prevalent in South America, affects some 10 to 20 million people. The organism, *Trypanosoma cruzi*, can cause severe myocarditis and routinely produces CRBB; complete atrioventricular block, PVCs, nonsustained VT, and sustained, life-threatening VT may also occur.[83]

Nonspecific or presumed acute viral myocarditis is commonly associated with arrhythmias, predominantly ventricular arrhythmias (PVCs, VT) and seems to occur in those patients with compromised ventricular function.[84] Chronic myocarditis of presumed viral origin has been associated with ventricular arrhythmias in adults and children. Endomyocardial biopsy techniques have been utilized to demonstrate an inflammatory response in some patients with ventricular arrhythmias and otherwise normal hearts. Immunosuppressive therapy has been recommended to treat the presumed chronic myocarditis with some encouraging results, especially with respect to control of arrhythmias.

One of the sequelae of myocarditis may be congestive cardiomyopathy. Virtually all types of arrhythmias have been described in these patients. Previous reports have stressed the importance of ventricular arrhythmias.[85–88] However, a recent restrospective study performed at the Texas Children's Hospital demonstrated a slight predominance of atrial arrhythmias.[89] Atrial flutter was a particularly ominous finding, especially if unresponsive to therapy, as it appeared to worsen CHF. In this study, although sudden deaths occurred, none occurred in patients with a known arrhythmia, implying that more frequent Holter monitoring may be necessary.

Miscellaneous

SARCOIDOSIS

Sarcoid heart disease is more common in adults, but occasionally affects children. Malignant ventricular arrhythmias, especially VT, varying degrees of atrioventricular block (including complete AV block requiring pacing), and SVT have been reported.[90–95]

METABOLIC DISEASES

Hypothroidism is reported to be associated with sinus bradycardia (usually in patients older than 3 years),[96] QT prolongation with associated torsades de pointes,[97, 98] and atrioventricular block.[99] Thyrotoxicosis is associated with sinus node dysfunction (i.e., bradycardia-tachycardia syndrome or sinus bradycardia), SVT, and AFl.[100]

Fetal atrial flutter has been described in association with hypophosphotemic vitamin D–resistant rickets in the fetus.[101] Patients with Addison's disease may have first degree AV block, while those with pheochromocytoma may display a short PR interval as a result of enhanced AV node conduction and coexistant sinus tachycardia.[102]

OTHER DISEASES

Mesothelioma of the atrioventricular node and congenital polycystic tumor of the AV node may cause complete atrioventricular block and sudden death.[103, 104] Tumors of the ventricle have been associated with ventricular tachycardia.[105, 106] They may be visible on routine chest radiographs and easily resectable or may only be found when examined directly by the surgeon at the time of attempted resection.

References

1. Hamilton WT, Haffajee CI, Dalen JE, et al: Atrial septal defect secundum: Clinical profile and physiological correlates in children and adults. Cardiovasc Clin 10 (1):267, 1979.
2. Forfang K, Simonsen S, Andersen A, et al: Atrial septal defect of secundum type in the middle-aged. Am Heart J 94:44, 1977.
3. Rosketh R: Congenital heart disease in middle-aged adults. Acta Med Scand 183:131, 1968.
4. Paolillo V, Dawkins KD, Miller GAH: Atrial septal defect in patients over the age of 50. Int J Cardiol 9:139, 1985.
5. Sealy WC, Farmer JC, Young WG, et al: Atrial dysrhythmia and secundum defects. J Thorac Cardiovasc Surg 57:245, 1969.
6. Bagger JP, Thomsen PEB, Bjerregaard P, et al: Intracardiac electrography in patients before and after surgical repair of secundum atrial septal defect. J Electrocardiol 17:347, 1984.
7. Benedini G, Affatato A, Bellandi M, et al: Preoperative sinus node function in adult patients with atrial septal defect (ostium secundum type). Eur Heart J 6:261, 1985.
8. Clark EB, Kugler D: Preoperative secundum atrial septal defect with coexisting sinus node and atrioventricular node dysfunction. Circulation 65:976, 1982.

8a. Clark EB, Roland JMA, Varshese PJ, et al: Should the sinus venous type ASD be closed? A review of the atrial conduction defects and surgical results in 28 children. Am J Cardiol 35:127, 1975.

9. Yabek M, Jarmakani JM: Sinus node dysfunction in children, adolescents and young adults. Pediatrics 61:593, 1978.
10. Anderson PAW, Rogers MC, Canent RV, et al: Atrioventricular conduction in secundum atrial septal defects. Circulation 48:27, 1973.
11. Mark H, Young D: Congenital heart disease in the adult. Am J Cardiol 15:293, 1965.
12. Otterstad JE, Nitter-Hauge S, Myrhe E: Isolated ventricular septal defect in adults: Clinical and haemodynamic findings. Br Heart J 50:343, 1983.
13. Marquis RM, Miller HC, McCormack RJM, et al: Persistence of ductus arteriosus with left to right shunt in the older patient. Br Heart J 48:469, 1982.
14. McManus BM: Patent ductus arteriosus. In Roberts WC (ed): Adult Congenital Heart Disease. Philadelphia, FA Davis, 1987, pp 455–476.
15. Sullivan ID, Presbitero P, Gooch VM, et al: Is ventricular arrhythmia in repaired tetralogy of Fallot an effect of operation or a consequence of the course of the disease? Br Heart J 58:40, 1987.
16. Deanfield JE, McKenna WJ, Presbitero P, et al: Ventricular arrhythmia in unrepaired and repaired tetralogy of Fallot: Relation to age, timing of repair, and haemodynamic status. Br Heart J 52:77, 1984.
17. Dubrow I, Fisher E, Thanopoulos B, et al: Electrophysiologic effects of cyanosis on sinus node and atrium in children. Circulation 56 and 57 (suppl III):III-172, 1977.
18. Bisset GS, Meyer RA, Hirschfeld SS, et al: Aortic valve replacement in childhood: Evaluation of left ventricular function by electrocardiography, echocardiography and graded exercise testing. Am J Cardiol 52:568, 1983.
19. Klein RC: Ventricular arrhythmias in aortic valve disease: Analysis of 102 patients. Am J Cardiol 53:1070, 1984.
20. Von Olshausen K, Schwarz F, Apfelbach J, et al: Determinants of the incidence and severity of ventricular arrhythmias in aortic valve disease. Am J Cardiol 51:1103, 1983.
21. Schwartz LS, Goldfischer J, Sprague GJ, et al: Syncope and sudden death in aortic stenosis. Am J Cardiol 23:647, 1969.
22. Santinga JT, Kirsh MM, Brady TJ, et al: Left

ventricular function in patients with ventricular arrhythmias and aortic valve disease. Ann Thorac Surg 35:152, 1982.

23. Bush HL, Gelband H, Hoffman BF, et al: Electro physiological basis for supraventricular arrhythmias following surgical procedures for aortic stenosis. Arch Surg 103:620, 1971.
24. Clark RJ, Firminger HI: Coarctation of the aorta associated with Adams-Stokes syndrome, complete heart block and bicuspid calcareous aortic valve. N Engl J Med 24: 710, 1949.
25. James TN, Jackson DA: De subitaneis mortibus: XXVII. Histological abnormalities in the sinus node, atrioventricular node and His bundle associated with coarctation of the aorta. Circulation 56:1094, 1977.
26. Lev M, Silverman J, Fitzmaurice FM, et al: Lack of connection between the atria and the more peripheral conduction system in congenital atrioventricular block. Am J Cardiol 27:481, 1971.
27. Bodlander, JW: The Wolff-Parkinson-White syndrome in association with congenital heart disease: Coarctation of the aorta. Am Heart J 31:785, 1946.
28. Kumar AE, Fyler DC, Mietinen OS, et al: Ebstein's anomaly: Clinical profile and natural history. Am J Cardiol 28:84, 1971.
29. Watson H: Natural history of Ebstein's anomaly of tricuspid valve in childhood and adolecence: An international cooperative study of 505 cases. Br Heart J 36:417, 1974.
30. Oh JK, Holmes DR, Hayes DL, et al: Cardiac arrhythmias in patients with surgical repair of Ebstein's anomaly. J Am Coll Cardiol 6:1351, 1985.
31. Radford DJ, Graff RF, Neilson GH: Diagnosis and natural history of Ebstein's anomaly. Br Heart J 54:517, 1985.
32. Southall DP, Keeton BR, Leanage R, et al: Cardiac rhythm and conduction before and after Mustard's operation for complete transposition of the great arteries. Br Heart J 43:21, 1980.
33. Martin RP, Radley-Smith R, Yacoub MH: Arrhythmias before and after correction of transposition of the great arteries. J Am Coll Cardiol 10:200, 1987.
34. Daliento L, Corrado D, Buja G, et al: Rhythm and conduction disturbances in isolated, congenitally corrected transposition of the great arteries. Am J Cardiol 58:314, 1986.
35. Huhta JC, Maloney JD, Ritter DG, et al: Complete atrioventricular block in patients with atrioventricular discordance. Circulation 67:1374, 1983.
36. Graham TP Jr: The Eisenmenger syndrome. In Roberts WC (ed): Adult Congenital Heart Disease. Philadelphia, FA Davis Company, 1987, pp 567–581.
37. Clarkson PM, Frye RL, DuShane JW, et al: Prognosis for patients with ventricular septal defect and severe pulmonary vascular obstructive disease. Circulation 38:129, 1968.
38. Young D, Mark H: Fate of the patient with Eisenmenger syndrome. Am J Cardiol 28:658, 1971.
39. Brammell HL, Vogel JHK, Pryor R, et al: The Eisenmenger's syndrome: A clinical and physiological appraisal. Am J Cardiol 28:679, 1971.
40. Plante RK, Stevens RA: Complete AV block in a fetus: Case report. Am Heart J 13:615, 1945.
41. Litsey SE, Noonan JA, O'Connor WN: Maternal connective tissue disease and congenital heart block: Demonstration of immunoglobulin in cardiac tissue. N Engl J Med 312:98, 1985.
42. Reed BR, Lee LA, Harmon C, et al: Autoantibodies to SS-A/Ro in infants with congenital heart block. J Pediatr 103:889, 1983.
43. Chemeides L, Truex RC, Vetter V, et al: Association of maternal systemic lupus erythematosus with congenital complete heart block. N Engl J Med 297:1204, 1977.
44. McCue CM, Mantakas ME, Tingelstad JB, et al: Congenital heart block in newborns of mothers with connective tissue disease. Circulation 56:82, 1977.
45. Ansari A, Larson PH, Bates HD: Cardiovascular manifestations of systemic lupus erythematosus: Current perspective. Prog Cardiovasc Dis 27:421, 1985.
46. Hover A, Koppes GM: Atrial standstill and complete heart block in systemic lupus erythematosus. Chest 76:230, 1979.
47. Follansbee WP, Curtiss EI, Rahko PS, et al: The electrocardiogram in systemic sclerosis (scleroderma): Study of 102 consecutive cases with functional correlations and review of the literature. Am J Med 79:183, 1985.
48. Ferri C, Bernini L, Bongiorno MG, et al: Noninvasive evaluation of cardiac dysrhythmias and their relationship with multisystemic symptoms in progressive systemic sclerosis patients. Arth Rheum 28:1259, 1985.
49. Laitinen O, Kentala E, Leirisalo M; Electrocardiographic findings in patients with connective tissue disease. Scand J Rheumatol 7:193, 1978.
50. Veille JC, Sunderland C, Bennett RM: Complete heart block in a fetus associated with maternal Sjogren's syndrome. Am J Obstet Gynecol 151:660, 1985.
51. Forstot JZ, Overlie PA, Neufeld GK, et al: Cardiac complications of Wegener's granulomatosis: A case report of complete heart block and review of the literature. Semin Arth Rheum 10:148, 1980.
52. Cohen J, Davies J, Goodwin JF, et al: Arrhythmias in patients with hypereosinophilia: A comparison of patients with and without Lofflers endomyocardial disease. Postgrad Med J 56:828, 1980.
53. Singsen B, Goldreyer B, Stanton R, et al: Childhood polymyositis with cardiac conduction defects. Am J Dis Child 130:72, 1976.
54. Perloff JK: The heart in neuromuscular disease. In O'Rourke RA (ed): Current Problems in Cardiology, vol XI, no 9. Chicago, Year Book Medical Publishers, 1986.
55. Bensaid H, Marsand G, Monassier JP, et al; High degree atrioventricular block associated with Wolff-Parkinson-White syndrome during a Duchenne de Boulogne type myopathy. Ann Cardiol Angiol 24:67, 1975.
56. Perloff JK: Cardiac rhythm and conduction in Duchenne's muscular dystrophy: A prospective study of 20 patients. J Am Coll Cardiol 3:1263, 1984.
57. Nomura H, Hizawa K: Histopathological study of the conduction system of the heart in Duchenne progressive muscular dystrophy. Acta Pathol 32:1027, 1982.
58. Baldwin AJ, Talley RC, Johnson C, et al: Permanent paralysis of the atrium in a patient with fasciocapulohumeral muscular dystrophy. Am J Cardiol 31:649, 1973.
59. Bloomfield DA, Sinclair-Smith BC: Persistent atrial standstill. Am J Med 39:335, 1965.
60. Ruff P, Leier CV, Schall SF: Temporary atrial standstill. Am Heart J 98:412, 1979.
61. Moorman RJ, Coleman RE, Packer DL, et al: Cardiac involvement in myotonic muscular dystrophy. Medicine 64:6, 1985.
62. Rechavia E, Strasberg B, Agmon J: Unusual cardiac manifestations in a patient with myotonic muscular dystrophy. Int J Cardiol 11:349, 1986.
63. Charles R, Holt S, Kay JM, et al: Myocardial

ultrastructure and the development of atrioventricular block in Kearns-Sayre syndrome. Circulation 63:214, 1980.
64. Klein R, Ganelin R, Marks JF, et al: Periodic paralysis with cardiac arrhythmia. J Pediatr 62:371, 1963.
65. Emmons PR, Blume WT, Dushane JW: Cardiac monitoring and demand pacemaker in Guillain-Barré syndrome. Lancet 1:1062, 1970.
66. Narayam D, Huang MT, Matthew PK: Bradycardia and asystole requiring a pacemaker in Guillain-Barré syndrome. Am Heart J 108:426, 1983.
67. Fave H, Foex P, Guggisberg M: Use of demand pacemaker in a case of Guillain-Barré syndrome. Lancet 1:1062, 1970.
68. Stewart IM: Arrhythmias in the Guillain-Barré syndrome. Br Med J 2:665, 1973.
69. Greenland P, Griggs RC: Arrhythmic complications in the Guillain-Barré syndrome. Arch Intern Med 140:1053, 1980.
70. Dunnigan A, Pierpont ME, Smith SA: Cardiac and skeletal myopathy associated with cardiac dysrhythmias. Am J Cardiol 53:731, 1984.
71. Chen S, Fagan LF, Nouri S, et al: Ventricular dysrhythmias in children with Marfan's syndrome. Am J Dis Child 139:273, 1985.
72. Phornphutkul C, Rosenthal A, Nadas AS: Cardiac manifestations of Marfan syndrome in infancy and childhood. Circulation 47:587, 1973.
73. Taranta A (chrmn): Community resources for the management of patients with rheumatic heart disease: Rheumatic fever and rheumatic heart disease study group. Circulation 44:A-273, 1971.
74. Rodriguez-Colonel A, Miller RA: Accelerated nodal pacemaker. Pediatrics 43:430, 1969.
75. Cristal N, Stern J, Gueron M: AV dissociation in acute rheumatic fever. Br Heart J 33:12, 1971.
76. Clarke M, Keith JD: Atrioventricular conduction in acute rheumatic fever. Br Heart J 34:472,1972.
77. Izumi Y, Susumo Y, Akira S: Electrocardiographic and electrophysiological studies on arrhythmias following streptococcal infections in school children. Jpn Circ J 44:814, 1980.
78. Freed MS, Sacks P, Ellman MH: Ventricular tachycardia in acute rheumatic fever. Arch Intern Med 145:1904, 1985.
79. Marin-Garcia J, Mirvis DM: Myocardial disease in Rocky Mountain spotted fever: Clinical, functional and pathologic findings. Pediatr Cardiol 5:149, 1984.
80. Parker JC: The potentially lethal problem of cardiac candidosis. Am J Clin Pathol 73:356, 1980.
81. Woolf PK, Tae-Sun C, Stuart J, et al: Life threatening dysrhythmias in varicella myocarditis. Clin Pediatr 26:480, 1987.
82. Fiddler GI, Campbell RWF, Pottage A, et al: Varicella myocarditis presenting with unusual ventricular arrhythmias. Br Heart J 39:1150, 1977.
83. Mendoza I, Camardo J, Moleiro F, et al: Sustained ventricular tachycardia in chronic Chagasic myocarditis: Electrophysiologic and pharmacologic characteristics. Am J Cardiol 57:423, 1986.
84. Hayakawa M, Inoh T, Yokota Y, et al: Long term follow-up study of acute viral and idiopathic myocarditis. Jpn Circ J 47:1304, 1983.
85. Karjalainen J: Functional and myocarditis induced T wave abnormalities. Chest 83:6, 1983.
86. Vignola PA, Aonuma K, Swaye PS, et al: Lymphocytic myocarditis presenting as unexplained ventricular arrhythmia: Diagnosis with endomyocardial biopsy and response to immunosuppression. J Am Coll Cardiol 4:812, 1984.
87. Strain JE, et al: Results of endomyocardial biopsy in patients with spontaneous ventricular tachycardia but without apparent structural heart disease. Circulation 68:1171, 1983.
88. Taliercio CP, Seward JB, Driscoll DJ: Idiopathic dilated cardiomyopathy in the young: Clinical profile and natural history. J Am Coll Cardiol 6:1126, 1985.
89. Friedman RA, Moak JP, Garson A Jr: Idiopathic dilated cardiomyopathy in children: Arrhythmias and prognostic implications. (In press)
90. Walsh MJ: Systemic sarcoidosis with refractory ventricular tachycardia and heart failure. Br Heart J 40:931, 1978.
91. Fleming HA: Sarcoid heart disease. Br Med J 292:1095, 1986.
92. Harrison EE, Martin HM: Systemic sarcoidosis and cardiac conduction abnormalities. (Letter) Chest 80:4, 1981.
93. Fleming HA: Sarcoid heart disease: A review and an appeal. (Editorial) Thorax 35:641, 1980.
94. Johnson NM, McNicol MW, Coltart DJ: Systemic sarcoidosis with refractory ventricular tachycardia and heart failure. (Letter) Br Heart J 42:367, 1978.
95. Sewer GA, Edwards SB, Benson DW, et al: Ventricular tacharrhythmia due to cardiac sarcoidosis in a child. Pediatrics 62:322, 1978.
96. Guthrie GP, Hunsaker JC, O'Connor WN: Sudden death in hypothyroidism. (Letter) N Engl J Med 317:1291, 1987.
97. Kumar A, Bhandari AK, Rahimtoola SH: Torsades de pointes and marked QT prolongation in association with hypothyroidism. Ann Intern Med 106:712, 1987.
98. Fredlund BO, Olsson SB: Long QT interval and ventricular tachycardia of "torsade de pointes" type in hypothyroidism. Acta Med Scand 213:231, 1983.
99. Zondek H: The electrocardiogram in myxoedema. Br Heart J 26:227, 1964.
100. Talwar KK, Gupta V, Kaul U, et al: Electrophysiological studies in thyrotoxicosis with and without associated sick sinus syndrome. Clin Cardiol 10:249, 1987.
101. Vintzileos AM, Campbell WA, Soberman SM, et al: Fetal atrial flutter and X-linked dominant vitamin D-resistant rickets. Obstet Gynecol 65 (suppl):39S, 1985.
102. Huang SK, Rosenberg MJ, Denes P: Short PR interval and narrow QRS complex associated with pheochromocytoma: Electrophysiologic observations. J Am Coll Cardiol 3:872, 1985.
103. James TN, Galakhov I: De subitaneis mortibus: XXVI. Fatal electrical instability of the heart associated with benign congenital polycystic tumor of the atrioventricular node. Circulation 56:667, 1977.
104. Bharati S, Bicoff P, Fridman JL, et al: Sudden death caused by benign tumor of the atrioventricular node. Arch Intern Med 136:224, 1976.
105. Engle MA, Ebert PA, Redo SF: Recurrent ventricular tachycardia due to resectable cardiac tumor: Report of two cases in two year olds in heart failure. Circulation 59:1052, 1974.
106. Garson A, Smith RT, Moak JP, et al: Incessant ventricular tachycardia in infants: Myocardial hamartomas and surgical cure. J Am Coll Cardiol 10:619, 1987.

CHAPTER 29
CHRONIC POSTOPERATIVE ARRHYTHMIA

Arthur Garson, Jr.

The arrhythmias covered in this chapter are analyzed in detail in other chapters of this book; the purpose of this chapter is to synthesize the data concerning only arrhythmias in patients who have had repair of congenital heart disease. The overall incidence of arrhythmias and the results of electrophysiology study have been covered in detail elsewhere, and only a brief consideration to these subjects will be given. The majority of the chapter will be devoted to our current recommendations for evaluation and management of these patients. The chapter is divided into those arrhythmias primarily occurring after operations on the atria (atrial bradyarrhythmias and atrial tachyarrhythmias), followed by a discussion of those arrhythmias resulting primarily after operations on the ventricles (atrioventricular conduction disturbance and ventricular tachyarrhythmias).

CHRONIC ARRHYTHMIAS AFTER OPERATIONS ON THE ATRIA

The most striking abnormalities seem to follow both the Mustard and the Senning operation. Despite a relatively short duration of follow-up in patients after the Fontan operation, it is clear that atrial arrhythmias are also likely to be a problem in these patients. Even late after repair of a secundum atrial septal defect, sick sinus syndrome can occur.

Incidence

Approximately 5 to 10 years after the Mustard operation, between 20% and 40% of patients are in sinus rhythm, 50% have junctional rhythm or sinus bradycardia, and 10% have tachyarrhythmias, primarily atrial flutter.[1–6] With a longer duration of follow-up, there is a higher incidence of arrhythmias. On treadmill exercise testing, 83% of the patient have been reported to have a decreased maximum heart rate or a decreased heart rate after 5 minutes of recovery.[7] On 24-hour electrocardiogram, almost none of these patients are in continuous sinus rhythm. In the study by Lucet et al[5] on 123 patients who had undergone either the Mustard or the Senning operation, 20% of the patients had "severe bradycardia" with heart rates less than 30/min at night. Interestingly, the severity of the bradycardia was found to be related to the severity of coexistent tachyarrhythmias. Of those with severe bradycardia, 33% had atrial flutter, compared to an incidence of atrial flutter of 4% in the patients without severe bradycardia. In patients with no bradycardia, no episodes of atrial flutter occurred. Lucet et al found, despite a slightly increased duration of follow-up in Mustard patients, an almost identical incidence of arrhythmias after the Mustard and Senning. In this report, there were four sudden deaths (two Mustard patients, two Senning patients); three of the four had had cardiac catheterization, and all three had markedly reduced right ventricular function. Therefore, the deaths appeared to be related to poor right ventricular hemodynamics. All four of the patients had abnormal Holter electrocardiograms: two had episodes of atrial flutter (17% mortality of atrial flutter in this series); all had moderate-to-severe bradycardia in addition. None of the patients who died had normal Holter results.

In other studies,[1-4, 6] the incidence of sudden death in patients after the Mustard operation was approximately 4% to 8%. Many of these deaths have been in patients with functioning pacemakers in place. One likely conclusion is that these patients died from tachyarrhythmias rather than bradyarrhythmias. We have observed the occurrence of sudden death in four patients who were wearing Holters at the time of their death. In three, at a time of physical or emotional stress, the ventricular rate dramatically increased with 1:1 atrioventricular conduction. In two, this was followed by total asystole (without capture by pacemakers) and by ventricular fibrillation in one patient. The fourth patient had progressive increase in AV block with ventricular asystole. This patient did not have a pacemaker.

In a large collaborative study involving 380 children with atrial flutter,[1] "postoperative Mustard" was the most common diagnosis (the 6-year mortality of those with atrial flutter was 21%). An important conclusion in this study was that sudden death was four times more common in patients in whom an effective drug to treat atrial flutter could not be found, compared with those in whom an effective drug was found. In this study, a drug was only considered to be "effective" in treating atrial flutter if the episodes were entirely eliminated. Therefore a drug was not considered to be effective if episodes of atrial flutter continued, despite a "controlled" ventricular response.

Following the Fontan operation, 50% of the patients have been reported to have arrhythmias within 2 years of surgery.[8] The most common diagnosis was sinus bradycardia, followed by atrial flutter and premature ventricualr contractions. The major differences in these arrhythmias compared to those occurring after the Mustard operation is that these arrhythmias occurred within 2 months of surgery. It may also be that those with Fontan repair develop a higher incidence of late-appearing arrhythmias. One arrhythmia that we have not seen in other postoperative situations is primary atrial tachycardia, probably caused by an ectopic focus. This has developed in three of our patients after the Fontan operation.[9]

In patients who have undergone repair of ostium secundum atrial septal defect with a 20-year follow-up, 10% have serious arrhythmias, most often sinus bradycardia and atrial flutter.[10]

Routine Evaluation

In patients who have undergone the Mustard, Senning, or Fontan procedures, we recommend a 24-hour electrocardiogram before the patient leaves the hospital. A small percentage of these patients will already have severe sinus bradycardia and need to be followed more closely than the routine follow-up at 1 year. One year following surgery, we recommend a 24-hour electrocardiogram and an exercise test (if the patient is old enough). The primary reason for the treadmill test is to determine if there is objective exercise intolerance that could be associated with bradycardia. Some of these patients have fatigue and dizziness associated with a rapid decrease in heart rate immediately following exercise.

In these patients, we continue to recommend a 24-hour electrocardiogram and exercise test approximately every 2 years after surgery.

Bradyarrhythmias

MANAGEMENT BASED ON NONINVASIVE EVALUATION

The recommendations of the American Heart Association/American College of Cardiology Joint Committee on Pacing as they relate to patients after the Mustard operation[11] are to insert a pacemaker in any patient with (1) "symptomatic" bradycardia (this can include syncope or presyncope, but also exercise intolerance); (2) "extreme" bradycardia (this is not further defined in the report); and (3) any patient with a tachyarrhythmia requiring treatment with an antiarrhythmic drug other than digitalis that could suppress the sinus node (i.e., propranolol, quinidine, procainamide, verapamil, and amiodarone).

There is general agreement on the first of these recommendations. Unfortunately, it is usually quite difficult to obtain a Holter recording at the same time the patient is having symptoms. It may be possible to elicit symptoms either during or after a treadmill exercise test, in which case objective data are available. On the other hand, in a patient with a history of syncope or presyncope, if there is additional moderate bradycardia (below 60/min in an infant younger than 2 years, 50/min in children aged 2 to 10 years, or 40/min in patients older than 10 years), then we would recommend implantation of a pacemaker.

The second recommendation, to insert a pacemaker for "extreme" bradycardia, is certainly reasonable. There must be a heart rate that is "too slow" for these patients. Heart rates that have been suggested are less than 50/min in an infant younger than 1 year, less than 40/min in patients aged 1 to 10 years of age, and less than 30/min in patients older than 10 years who have had the Mustard, Senning, or Fontan operation. The concept is not unreasonable, especially since the study by Lucet et al showed that tachyarrhythmias and bradyarrhythmias were related; it may be that the long cycle length of the bradyarrhythmia predisposed to the development of the tachyarrhythmia.[5] On the other hand, it is difficult to find data proving that sudden death can be prevented by the implantation of a pacemaker in an asymptomatic patient with only sinus bradycardia. Fortunately, this situation is quite rare since the majority of patients with extremely low heart rates either have accompanying tachyarrhythmias or symptoms related to bradycardia. We recommend that implantation of a pacemaker for asymptomatic bradycardia if the "extreme bradycardia" was sustained for long periods of time and especially if the patient had extremely low rates while awake.

The third indication for pacing involved protection against bradycardia in a patient with atrial flutter being treated with antiarrhythmic drugs that could suppress the sinus node. This is also a reasonable recommendation since we and others have observed the development of progressive bradycardia in patients treated with many of these drugs (especially quinidine, procainamide, propranolol, and amiodarone). It would also seem reasonable to implant a pacemaker in such a patient to protect against the profound bradycardia that may result immediately following an episode of atrial flutter. On the other hand, it is difficult to assess the exact cause of death in patients, for example, with atrial futter being treated with digitalis and quinidine. It is possible that quinidine causes progressive sinus bradycardia, and the patients die of asystole. Alternatively, quinidine may cause bradycardia, which can then predispose to a drug-induced ventricular tachycardia that could result in ventricular fibrillation. However, these patients would also die from atrial flutter with 1:1 conduction. Implantation of a pacemaker would prevent sudden death in the first two situations, but would certainly not have any effect on the third. We continue to implant pacemakers in this situation as recommended by the Committee on Pacing, but further studies will be necessary to determine if this practice prevents sudden death.

INDICATIONS FOR ELECTROPHYSIOLOGY STUDY

We recommend electrophysiology study in a patient who has had a previous atrial operation, developed syncope or presyncope, and had an otherwise normal noninvasive evaluation. This may be an important adjunctive test, since a markedly prolonged sinus node recovery time would be helpful in assessing the reason for the syncopal episodes. Unfortunately, a negative electrophysiology study does not rule out bradycardia as a reason for syncope.[12]

We would also perform an electrophysiology study to determine the optimal type of pacemaker to implant in a patient who already had indications for pacing. Since the majority of patients generally have normal AV conduction after these operations, it has been recommended that atrial pacemakers be implanted. In the electrophysiology laboratory, if the AV conduction response to rapid atrial pacing is normal (1:1 conduction below rates of 150/min to 180/min), then it is safe to implant an atrial pacemaker. The only difficulty with this decision is that if the patient subsequently develops atrial flutter and requires treatment with drugs that could impair AV conduction (quinidine, procainamide, propranolol, or amiodarone), the atrial pacemaker will not protect against AV block. For this reason, if the patient has the slightest indication of episodes of atrial flutter, and especially if atrial flutter can be induced in the electrophysiology laboratory, we recommend implantation of a dual-chambered pacemaker. These pacemakers can now be implanted transvenously in the electrophysiology laboratory in infants weighing as little as 10 to 15 kilograms. An alternative approach is the use of an atrial antitachycardia pacemaker to avoid the need for drug treatment of atrial flutter.

At the present time, there are questions as to the necessity for performance of routine electrophysiology study after operations of this type. The reason for this is discussed in the next section.

RESULTS OF ELECTROPHYSIOLOGY STUDY

In patients who have undergone the Mustard operation, 54% have an abnormal corrected sinus node recovery time, 33% have abnormal sinoatrial conduction time, and 27% have abnormal conduction time from the high right atrium to the low lateral right atrium. However, only 5% have abnormal conduction from the high right atrium to the low septal right atrium. AV conduction was generally normal, with only 5% having a prolonged low septal right atrium–to–His conduction time, and only 2% having a prolonged HV interval.[2] While there is general correlation between the findings on the Holter and the findings on electrophysiology study, Fournier, Smith, and Garson[12] found that the electrophysiology study did not usually help in the management of the patients. There were several instances of symptomatic patients with proven sinus bradycardia on the Holter electrocardiogram and with sinus node function studies in the electrophysiology laboratory. Occasionally, however, the finding of a markedly prolonged sinus node recovery time was helpful in the management of the patient.

In the future, it will be necessary to develop better prospective tests in the electrophysiology laboratory for assessment of prognosis in the patient with possible sinus node dysfunction.

MANAGEMENT BASED ON ELECTROPHYSIOLOGY STUDY

A normal electrophysiology study is not helpful. It does not indicate the "normality" of the patient at the time of the study or offer any reassurance for the patient's future. It has been well documented that sinus node dysfunction can develop late after the Mustard operation. On the other hand, a markedly prolonged corrected sinus recovery time (greater than 2000 ms) should not, in itself, serve as an indication for pacing, but it could be "figured into the equation" in a patient with other borderline data. For example, if a patient had had dizzy spells with borderline low heart rates on the Holter, a markedly prolonged sinus node recovery time could help decide in favor of pacemaker implantation. Unfortunately, a normal sinus node recovery time in this situation is less helpful and should not be used as reassurance that the spells are benign.

Tachyarrhythmias

MANAGEMENT BASED ON NONINVASIVE TESTING

The most controversial issue in the treatment of tachyarrhythmias is whether to treat patients after the Mustard or similar operation with prophylactic digoxin. The rationale for treatment is that a patient may develop atrial flutter at any time after the operation, and if he or she is being treated with digitalis, the ventricular rate could be decreased by the digitalis, therefore resulting in better tolerance of the arrhythmia. There are data to support this practice. In the collaborative atrial flutter study of 380 children,[1] the incidence of syncope with the first episode of atrial flutter was reduced in patients taking digitalis. However, data assessing the overall practice of prophylaxis with digitalis are not available, since it is not known how many patients had sudden death with their episode of atrial flutter and whether digitalis might have prevented this. In general, it seems reasonable to use digitalis prophylactically in all patients after these operations. There are possible additional hemodynamic benefits to those Mustard/Senning patients with a systemic right ventricle or the Fontan patients with a previously dilated left ventricle. The disadvantage of chronic prophylactic treatment with digitalis is that the patient has to remember to take the drug, thus continuously reminding the patient of potential cardiac disability. We recommend prophylactic treatment of these patients with digitalis for life, but understand the reluctance of many physicians and patients to follow this recommendation.

In a patient with a known tachyarrhythmia (either discovered on Holter or suggested by the presence of rapid palpitations), it is important to make a positive diagnosis of the tachyarrhythmia. While atrial flutter is the most likely tachyarrhythmia to recur after these operations, it is possible to have AV nodal reentry, sinus node reentry, atrial ectopic tachycardia, or even ventricular tachycardia. Clearly, the treatment would be different for each of these arrhythmias. In the patient with only rapid palpitations, a telephone transmitter should be given to the patient, with encouragment to document the arrhythmia. Frequently, however, atrial flutter with 2:1 AV block is discovered in an asymptomatic patient on a routine clinic visit.

Episodes of atrial flutter must be eliminated. It is not acceptable to allow atrial flutter to continue with a "controlled" ventricular response.[1] One of our patients typifies the stories of many others. He was a 10-year-old who had previously undergone the Mustard operation and had had symptomatic sinus bradycardia early in life, followed by implantation of a ventricular demand pacemaker. He developed episodes of atrial flutter at the age of 9 years. These were not responsive to any conventional medications, and he was placed on amiodarone. He then developed shortness of breath from an episode of atrial flutter with 2:1 block. He came for an outpatient visit for shortness of breath but was reluctant to be admitted since he had had so many prior hospitalizations. We agreed to increase the amiodarone and to follow him for 1 week as an outpatient. If the atrial flutter had not converted, we would then admit him at the end of the week for cardioversion. He was told to avoid all athletics. He was on a baseball team, and his parents allowed him to go to the game but did not allow him to play. His father, the coach, thought the child was being overly rambunctious in the dugout with his friends. His father went to the dugout and scolded him loudly in front of his teammates for getting so excited. Immediately after the scolding, the patient dropped dead in front of his father. The father said his son initially had a heart rate too rapid to count and then there was no pulse. He could not be resuscitated.

This case demonstrates that atrial flutter with a "controlled ventricular rate" can suddenly accelerate, and therefore we attempt to keep these patients in sinus rhythm. We begin treatment with digitalis. If this is not effective, we implant a pacemaker and then add quinidine. If this combination is not effective, we use digoxin and amiodarone. It is possible that in the future drugs such as encainide, flecainide, or sotalol will replace amiodarone in the treatment of atrial flutter. Antitachycardia pacing is another alternative.

INDICATIONS FOR ELECTROPHYSIOLOGY STUDY

The first indication for electrophysiology study is the presence of recurrent symptomatic rapid palpitations that cannot be documented by electrocardiogram or the inability to determine the exact nature of the tachyarrhythmia from the electrocardiogram. One additional possible indication for electrophysiology study may be to attempt induction of tachyarrhythmias. The data (see following section) are not yet sufficient to recommend routine electrophysiology study in all patients, but this may be the case in the future.

RESULTS OF ELECTROPHYSIOLOGY STUDY

In two studies,[12, 13] approximately 20% of patients who had undergone the Mustard operation had a sustained tachyarrhythmia, most often atrial flutter, induced during electrophysiology study. The majority of these had evidence of a prior tachyarrhythmia. However, in the study by Vetter, Hardy, and Burton,[13] patients without preceding tachyarrhythmia who had atrial flutter induced in the electrophysiology laboratory all developed clinical atrial flutter within 1 year after the electrophysiology study. Certainly, similar to the studies for bradyarrhythmias, unsuccessful induction of atrial flutter does not imply that the patient will be free of the arrhythmia, especially as the duration from the time of surgery increases.

MANAGEMENT BASED UPON ELECTROPHYSIOLOGY STUDY

If a patient who has undergone the Mustard, Senning, or Fontan operation has sustained atrial flutter induced in the electrophysiology laboratory, even in the absence of previously documented clinical arrhythmia, then we strongly recommend prophylactic treatment with digitalis. Since there is evidence that many of the patients with induced atrial flutter will develop clinical atrial flutter,[13] it seems that these patients should certainly receive prophylactic digitalis treatment. These patients should also be followed more closely, since it is possible that a patient taking digitalis may develop atrial flutter with 2:1 block and be asymptomatic but still at risk for sudden death from 1:1 AV conduction. Therefore we recommend that a patient who has induced atrial flutter in the electrophysiology laboratory be followed every 6 months or yearly, rather than every 2 years.

If this patient then returns for a routine clinic visit, having been entirely asymptomatic while taking digoxin, and is found to have atrial flutter with a 2:1 block, the patient should have DC electrical cardioversion and be placed back on digitalis. It is possible that such patients may have only one episode. However, if the atrial flutter recurs while the patient has an adequate serum concentration of digitalis, a difficult situation presents itself. The logical step would be implantation of a pacemaker followed by initiation of either quinidine or amiodarone. However, it is extremely difficult to convince a patient who is entirely asymptomatic with atrial flutter 2:1 block that pacemaker implantation and initiation of additional drug therapy are necessary. While this is clearly likely to be the safest course of action, it may not be possible in all patients. Clearly, further therapy should be initiated and pacemaker implanted at the first sign of a symptom associated with rapid AV conduction. If the aggressive treatment strategy is not followed, the patient and parents should be informed that there is some risk of allowing atrial flutter with 2:1 block to continue.

CHRONIC ARRHYTHMIAS AFTER OPERATION ON THE VENTRICLES

Most studies of chronic arrhythmias occurring after operation on the ventricles have been done in patients who have had intracardiac repair of tetralogy of Fallot.[14–16] The findings in these patients are similar to those in patients with other defects. In general, the less serious the defect, the less serious the outcome. For example, late sudden death occurs in approximately 2% of the patients who have had ventricular septal defect repair,[17] 5% of those who have had tetralogy of Fallot repair,[14] 18% of those who have had double outlet right ventricle repair,[18] and 18% of those who have had surgery for truncus arteriosus with single pulmonary artery.[19]

Incidence

Conduction Disturbance. After repair of tetralogy of Fallot, approximately 80% of patients have complete right bundle-branch block, an additional 11% have the combination of right bundle-branch block with left axis deviation, and 3% have the combination of right bundle-branch block with left axis deviation and first degree AV block.[14] The prognosis for conduction disturbances has been controversial. The initial article by Wolff, Rowland, and Ellison[20] suggested that the combination of right bundle-branch block with left axis deviation in these patients was a predictor of later sudden death. However, in that study, all the patients who later died suddenly also had ventricular arrhythmias, and it was not possible to tell from that study which risk factor was more important. In more recent studies, it appears that the incidence of late sudden death in patients with only right bundle-branch block and left axis deviation is quite low. There has been a suggestion that this pattern, when added to the presence of transient complete AV block at the time of surgery, does form a higher risk group. We have not found that in our experience.

Ventricular Arrhythmias. In recent studies of postoperative tetralogy of Fallot, ventricular arrhythmias were evident in approximately 10% of patients on routine electrocardiogram, 40% on treadmill, and 60% on 24-hour electrocardiogram.[14, 21, 22] The presence of ventricular arrhythmias has been related to later sudden death. In one study, 38% of those with premature ventricular contractions on routine electrocardiogram died suddenly.[14] In that study, all the patients who died suddenly had the combination of a right ventricular systolic pressure greater than 70 mmHg and a right ventricular end-diastolic pressure greater than 8 mmHg.

Routine Evaluation

In the immediate postoperative period when the patient is still in the hospital, it is rare for ventricular arrhythmias to occur. However, there are a few patients with nonsustained ventricular tachycardia who should be observed more closely than the routine follow-up at 1 year; therefore a pre-discharge 24-hour electrocardiogram may be indicated, especially if the patient had ventricular arrhythmia in the recovery room. In the majority of these patients, the arrhythmias will disappear over the first month or two and are not related to the late development of arrhythmias. One year after the operation, all patients should have a 24-hour electrocardiogram and exercise test. The indications for cardiac catheterization will be discussed in the following sections. Every 2 years, patients should continue to be followed with a 24-hour electrocardiogram and exercise test.

Conduction Disturbance

MANAGEMENT BASED ON NONINVASIVE EVALUATION

The patterns of right bundle-branch block, right bundle-branch block–left axis deviation, and right bundle-branch block–left axis deviation–first degree AV block all have inconstant intracardiac correlates. In the study by Friedli and Bolens,[24] among those patients with right bundle-branch block, eight of 22 had a prolonged interval from the Q wave to the right ventricular apex. The inference was made that these eight patients had "proximal" right bundle-branch block. In only four of nine with right bundle-branch block–left axis deviation was the Q-RV apex interval prolonged. The authors made the inference that this was not true "bifascicular block," since there was left axis deviation in the presence of normal central right bundle-branch conduction. Finally, in only two of the five patients with the surface electrocardiographic pattern of "trifascicular block" was the His-ventricle interval prolonged. Therefore, since the surface electrocardiographic pattern did not always reflect the intracardiac electrophysiologic findings, the recommendation was made that the terms "bifascicular block" and "trifascicular block" should not be used when describing the surface electrocardiogram. These should only be used when there is demonstrable intracardiac correlation. "Bifascicular block" would require complete right bundle-branch block with left axis deviation and a prolonged Q-RV apex time; "trifascicular block" would require a prolonged HV interval. Since it is not possible to determine the basis for these patterns without intracardiac electrophysiologic recordings, these surface electrocardiographic patterns should not be used to determine management.

Disturbances of AV conduction that are observed with noninvasive evaluation deserve comment. The first is the presence of type I second degree AV block (Wenckebach). If the patient is asymptomatic, despite episodes of Wenckebach, then pacing is not indicated. There is no evidence that this patient is at higher risk for the development of late complete AV block. On the other hand, patients with type II second degree AV block may be at higher risk, and the American Heart Association/American College of Cardiology Committee on Pacing[11] recommends pacing for such individuals as well as for all postoperative patients who develop late complete AV block.

INDICATIONS FOR ELECTROPHYSIOLOGY STUDY

In a patient who has had an operation on the ventricles and has a normal noninvasive evaluation but also has syncope or presyncope, electrophysiology study is indicated. The cause of the syncope could be either AV block or ventricular arrhythmias, and it may be possible to determine an abnormality during intracardiac electrophysiologic study. However, similar to sinus node testing, in testing for conduction disturbances, an entirely normal intracardiac electrophysiologic study does not rule out the presence of syncope caused by paroxysmal AV block.

Routine electrophysiologic study after operations on the ventricles has not generally been recommended for assessment of AV conduction. However, the study by Friedli and Bolens[25] suggests that it may be possible to predict the development of late complete AV block by intracardiac electrophysiologic study. If these findings are reproduced in other studies, it may be that routine evaluation of the conduction system should be performed. At the present time, we are performing routine postoperative studies only under a research protocol.

RESULTS OF ELECTROPHYSIOLOGY STUDY

In our study of postoperative tetralogy,[26] 41% of patients had an abnormal corrected sinus node recovery time, 15% had an abnormal low septal right atrium–to–His bundle interval, 41% had an abnormal paced rate at the development of second degree AV block (Wenckebach rate), and 22% had a prolonged HV interval. In the study by Friedli and Bolens,[24] conduction disturbances were demonstrated in 10 of 52 patients; five had AH prolongation, four had both AH and HV prolongation, and one had only HV prolongation. In response to atrial pacing, three patients developed block below the His bundle with pacing at rates below 150/min. After a follow-up period of 5 years, two patients developed late complete AV block (2 and 5 years after electrophysiology study); both occurred in patients with previous HV prolongation in sinus rhythm and block below the His at atrial paced rates below 150/min. Therefore, in this study, late complete AV block occurred and was possibly predicted by electrophysiology study; however, the only sudden death occurred in a patient from ventricular tachycardia.

Approximately 50% of the patients have had a prolonged Q–right ventricular apex conduction time.[23, 26] This has been assumed to correlate with "central" right bundle-branch block. Those with a normal Q–right ventricular apex time are assumed to have "peripheral" bundle-branch block, which is thought to be benign. Peripheral bundle-branch block has been thought to be caused by the right ventriculotomy interrupting the distal Purkinje fibers in the right ventricular free wall.

The basis for this assumption has been brought under question in a recent study.[27] In six puppies with an otherwise normal right ventricle, a right ventriculotomy was made in the same region as that used for a repair of tetralogy of Fallot. This was performed at the age of 8 weeks, and the puppies were then allowed to recover for 1 year. None of the puppies developed right bundle-branch block. The heart was removed, and cellular electrophysiology studies were performed. There was no area of conduction delay caused by the right ventriculotomy. The impulse spread normally from inferior to superior along the margins of the ventriculotomy. While it is possible that the dog's right ventricle has a conduction system that is sufficiently different from the human structure to account for these findings, it raises the question as to whether a simple right ventriculotomy can cause the pattern of complete right bundle-branch block in humans. An alternate explanation for the human findings is that in all patients with complete right bundle-branch block, "true" right bundle-branch block exists. This could be caused either from proximal damage during repair of the ventricular septal defect or more distal damage to the right bundle branch at its junction with the moderator band. Resection of the moderator band may occur during the repair of tetralogy of Fallot. There are important implications to this hypothesis. If, in fact, the right ventriculotomy alone does not cause right bundle-branch block and if, therefore, there is "true" right bundle-branch block in all patients who have the surface electrocardiographic pattern, then in later life with the development of atherosclerotic left bundle-branch block, these patients are at risk for the development of complete AV block. Further studies should be performed in humans to examine this hypothesis.

MANAGEMENT BASED ON ELECTROPHYSIOLOGY STUDY

A pacemaker should be implanted in the patient who has syncope or presyncope, an abnormal conduction system study (either prolonged HV interval, production of block below the His at atrial paced rates below 150/min, or reduced Wenckebach cycle length), no ventricular arrhythmias. If this symptomatic patient has an abnormal conduction system study and induced ventricular arrhythmias, then therapy must be individualized; hopefully the clinical arrhythmia leading to these symptoms can be determined from the telephone transmitter. Asymptomatic patients with an abnormal conduction system study (prolonged HV interval or abnormal pacing response) should be followed closely with a 24-hour electrocardiogram and treadmill test every 6 months, but a pacemaker should not be implanted.

Ventricular Arrhythmias

MANAGEMENT BASED ON NONINVASIVE EVALUATION

We have based treatment on routine electrocardiogram and the 24-hour electrocardiogram. If any premature ventricular contractions are present on routine electrocardiogram, we recommend treatment with anti-arrhythmic drugs. Patients should be treated if premature ventricular contractions are frequent (more than one per minute) or complex (multiform PVCs, couplets, or ventricular tachycardia) as indicated on Holter monitoring. The goal of treatment in patients with frequent uniform PVCs is to eliminate ventricular arrhythmias from the Holter (i.e., less than 10 uniform PVCs per hour). While we have the same goal in patients with complex ventricular arrhythmias, we consider a drug therapy to be successful if complex ventricular arrhythmias have been eliminated and only uniform premature ventricular contractions remain. In a recent study we reported 488 patients who had had repair of tetralogy of Fallot.[23] We found no ventricular arrhythmias on routine electrocardiogram in 421 patients, and there were no sudden deaths. Of the 21 patients with ventricular arrhythmias and no treatment, 33% died. Two patients who were under treatment but did not meet the criteria for successful treatment died. Therefore, among the 23 patients with either no treatment or ineffective treatment, nine died suddenly (39% mortality). By contrast, among the 44 patients known to have ventricular arrhythmia that responded to treatment, there were no sudden deaths. Therefore, successful treatment of arrhythmias by these criteria was significantly related to management aimed at decreasing the incidence of sudden death.

INDICATIONS FOR ELECTROPHYSIOLOGY STUDY

In a patient who has had operation on the ventricles and has a normal noninvasive evaluation but also has syncope or presyncope, electrophysiology study for attempted induction of ventricular arrhythmias is indicated. Electrophysiologic testing can also provide additional information in the patient who is asymptomatic but has equivocal noninvasive data. For example, if a patient has frequent uniform premature ventricular contractions on the Holter electrocardiogram, the presence or absence of induced ventricular arrhythmias may be helpful. However, at the present time, the exact meaning of the induction, or noninduction, of ventricular arrhythmias after repair of tetralogy of Fallot has not been firmly established. For this reason, routine electrophysiology study for induction of ventricular arrhythmias after repair of tetralogy of Fallot is not recommended. We are currently performing such studies only on a research protocol.

It is important to assess the hemodynamics after repair of tetralogy of Fallot. The data are convincing that the vast majority of those patients who have had sudden death had abnormal hemodynamics. If the hemodynamics (including both the right ventricular systolic pressure and right ventricular end-diastolic pressure) can be adequately assessed by noninvasive means, then hemodynamic cardiac catheterization may not be necessary. However, if hemodynamic cardiac catheterization is necessary to provide these data, then it should be performed.

The final indication for cardiac catheterization in symptomatic patients is to perform chronic drug testing. If the patients have inducible sustained ventricular tachycardia in a drug-free state, a chronic oral medication can be given, and the patient can be returned to the electrophysiology laboratory for attempted re-induction of the arrhythmia.

RESULTS OF ELECTROPHYSIOLOGY STUDY

In our study of 26 patients, using a protocol of paired ventricular extrastimuli and burst pacing at the right ventricular apex at one cycle length, 19% had single nonbundle-branch reentry beats, 26% had nonsustained ventricular tachycardia, and 7% had sustained ventricular tachycardia.[26] In a comparison group of 77 children with an entirely normal heart, in response to the same ventricular extrastimulus protocol, no patient had even a single nonbundle-branch reentry beat induced.[28] In postoperative tetralogy patients with induced ventricular tachycardia,[26] syncope had occurred in 44%, 67% had more than 10 uniform premature ventricular contractions per hour on Holter, 56% had a right ventricular systolic pressure greater than 70 mmHg, 45% had a right ventricular ejection fraction less than 45%, and 44% had an HV interval greater than 55 ms. In those without induced arrhythmia, no patient had any of these abnormalities. Therefore, in general, the inducibility of ventricular tachycardia is correlated with clinical, electrocardiographic, and hemodynamic abnormalities. In a larger group of 309 patients, the general relationship of inducible ventricular arrhythmias to these abnormalities remained significant. Nonetheless, the interpretation of the electrophysiologic findings in an individual patient remains unsettled. Therefore, the prognosis of patients based on electrophysiologic studies still remains to be investigated with longer term follow-up.

MANAGEMENT BASED ON ELECTROPHYSIOLOGY STUDY

If the patient with syncope or presyncope and a normal noninvasive evaluation has either nonsustained or sustained ventricular tachycardia induced, and if there are no abnormalities of AV conduction, then the patient should be treated with antiarrhythmic drugs. In such a patient, since there were no arrhythmias or baseline Holter electocardiogram, the response to premature ventricular contractions cannot be used to assess treatment, and chronic electrophysiology studies with the patient receiving various antiarrhythmic agents should be used to determine the success of treatment. Kugler et al[29] studied eight patients in this way and found phenytoin to be effective in suppressing induction of ventricular tachycardia in four of eight patients and propranolol effective in four of six patients. In no patient were both drugs effective. Each patient remained on treatment with a drug found "effective." In follow-up, no patient had clinical ventricular tachycardia. Mehta et al[30] found that in two patients, phenytoin completely suppressed ventricular arrhythmias on the Holter electrocardiogram, but both patients still had inducible ventricular tachycardia in the electrophysiology laboratory when taking phenytoin. Both patients received chronic phenytoin and remained without ventricular arrhythmia in 2 years of follow-up. Dissociation between the Holter findings and the electrophysiologic results has been reported for other drugs, most notably amiodarone.[31] Phenytoin is one such drug in which it may be difficult to use electrophysiologic testing to guide therapy. Using the experience from amiodarone,[31] phenytoin is likely to be beneficial if ventricular tachycardia is not induced; however, the induction of ventricular tachycardia does not necessarily imply lack of protection by the drug against clinical episodes of ventricular tachycardia.

Treatment of asymptomatic patients based on the results of electrophysiology study awaits further confirmation. Randomized clinical trials involving treatment and nontreatment of patients with induced ventricular tachycardia should be performed. However, since the induction of this arrhythmia appears to be far beyond the range of normal, and since there is a relationship between ventricular arrhythmias and sudden death in patients who have undergone repair of tetralogy of Fallot, until further data are available, we recommend treatment of patients with induced sustained monomorphic ventricular tachycardia with antiarrhythmic drugs.

The final method of treatment for the patient who is symptomatic, has recurrent episodes of clinical ventricular tachycardia not responsive to antiarrhythmic drugs, and also has inducible sustained ventricular tachycardia is primary surgical treatment of the ventricular tachycardia. Careful endocardial mapping must be performed in the electrophysiology laboratory prior to surgery, since it is possible that the tachycardia may not be reproduced under anesthesia. We have successfully eliminated ventricular tachycardia in four out of five such patients treated surgically.

CONCLUSIONS

In the years after repair of congenital cardiac defects, numerous abnormalities of cardiac rhythm can be uncovered with diligent searching. However, the importance of some of these abnormalities is uncertain. We must infer the importance of the present data from prospective follow-up in patients who later became symptomatic or died suddenly. Since sudden death may occur without antecedent symptoms, prophylactic treatment is indicated in certain asymptomatic high risk patients. However, prophylactic treatment is justified only when the risks of treatment are small, since the risks of nontreatment (sudden death) are also relatively small.

Because treatment strategies vary throughout the world, it is important to continue an active dialogue among centers so that the true prognosis of these various abnormalities, both treated and untreated, can be determined. The eventual goal is to treat only those patients at risk for sudden death and allow the others to lead normal lives.

ACKNOWLEDGMENTS

Research was supported in part by grants HL24916, HL07190, and RR00188 from the National Institutes of Health, Bethesda, Maryland, and by a grant from the J. S. Abercrombie Foundation.

References

1. Garson A Jr, Bink-Boelkens M, Hesslein PS, et al: Atrial flutter in the young: A collaborative study of 380 cases. J Am Coll Cardiol 6:871–878, 1985.
2. Gillette PC, El-Said GM, Sivarajan N, et al: Electrophysiologic abnormalities after Mustard's operation for transposition of the great arteries. Br Heart J 36:186–191, 1974.
3. Flinn CJ: Natural history of supraventricular rhythms in 182 children following the Mustard operation. J Am Coll Cardiol 1:613–618, 1983.
4. Hayes C, Gersony WM: Arrhythmias after the Mustard operation for transposition of the great arteries: A long-term study. J Am Coll Cardiol 7:133–173, 1986.
5. Lucet V, Batisse A, Ngoc DD, et al: Troubles du rythme apres corrections atriales des transpositions des gros vaisseaus. Arch Mal Coeur 79:640–647, 1986.
6. Duster MC, Bink-Boelkens MT, Wampler D, et al: Long-term follow-up of dysrhythmias following the Mustard procedure. Am Heart J 109:1323–1326, 1985.
7. Hesslein PS, Gutgesell HP, Gillette PC: Exercise assessment of sinoatrial node function in children after Mustard's operation. Pediatr Res 14:445, 1980.
8. Battiste CE, Porter CJ, Humes RA, et al: Supraventricular tachyarrhythmias after the Fontan procedure for tricuspid atresia. Proceedings X World Congress Cardiology, Dallas, American Heart Association, 1986, p 47.
9. Ward KE, Moak JP, Garson A: Appearance and disappearance of arrhythmias after the Fontan operation. J Am Coll Cardiol 5:427, 1985.
10. Bricker JT, Gillette PC, Cooley DA, et al: Dysrhythmias after atrial septal defect repair. Pediatr Res 16:97, 1982.
11. Frye RL: Guidelines for permanent cardiac pacemaker implantation, May, 1984. Circulation 70:331A–339A, 1984.
12. Fournier A, Smith RT, Garson A: Sinus node dysfunction in children: Clinical-electrophysiologic correlation. Proceedings European Association Pediatric Cardiology, Dorchester, England, Springer International, 1986, p 7.
13. Vetter L, Hardy CE, Burton DA: Atrial endocardial mapping during basal rhythm and atrial flutter after the Mustard repair of transposition of the great arteries. Proceedings Thirteenth International Congress on Electrocardiology, 1986, p 45.
14. Garson A, Nihill MR, McNamara DG, et al: Status of the adult and adolescent following repair of tetralogy of Fallot. Circulation 59:1232–1240, 1979.
15. Kavey RE, Blackman MS, Sondheimer HM: Incidence and severity of chronic ventricular dysrhythmias after repair of tetralogy of Fallot. Am Heart J 103:342–350, 1982.
16. Fuster V, McGoon DC, Kennedy MA: Long-term evaluation (12–22 years) of open heart surgery for tetralogy of Fallot. Am J Cardiol 46:635–640, 1980.
17. Moller JH, Patton C, Varco RL, et al: Postoperative ventricular septal defect: 24–30 years follow-up of 232 patients. Proceedings Second World Congress of Pediatric Cardiology, p 20.
18. Shen WK, Holmes DR, McGoon DC, et al: Sudden death in patients after repair of double outlet right ventricle circulation. Circulation 74(suppl II):121, 1986.
19. Fyfe DA, Driscoll DJ, Danielson GK, et al: Truncus arteriosus with single pulmonary artery: Influence of pulmonary vascular obstructive disease on early and late operative results. J Am Coll Cardiol 5:1168–1172, 1985.
20. Wolff GS, Rowland TW, Ellison RC: Surgically induced right bundle branch block with left anterior hemiblock. Circulation 45:587–593, 1972.
21. Garson A, Gillette PC, Gutgesell HP, et al: Stress-induced ventricular arrhythmias after tetralogy of Fallot repair. Am J Cardiol 46:1006–1012, 1980.
22. Deanfield JE, McKenna WJ, Hallidie-Smith KA: Detection of late arrhythmia and conduction disturbance after correction of tetralogy of Fallot. Br Heart J 44:248–253, 1980.
23. Garson A, Randall DC, McVey P, et al: Prevention of sudden death after repair of tetralogy of Fallot: Treatment of ventricular arrhythmias. J Am Coll Cardiol 6:221–227, 1985.
24. Friedli B, Bolens M: Intraventricular conduction disturbances after correction of tetralogy of Fallot: Can bifascicular and trifascicular block be diagnosed from the surface ECG. Pediatr Cardiol 6:133–136, 1985.
25. Friedli B, Bolens M: Prognostic value of electrophysiological studies after tetralogy of Fallot. Proceedings Second World Congress of Pediatric Cardiology, New York, Spring-Verlag, 1985, p 100.
26. Garson A, Porter CJ, Gillette PC, et al: Induction of ventricular tachycardia during electrophysiologic study after repair of tetralogy of Fallot. J Am Coll Cardiol 1:1493–1502, 1983.
27. Nakazawa M, Okuda H, Imai Y, et al: Ventricular function in patients following external conduit repair (Rastelli procedure) for cyanotic congenital heart disease. Circulation 72(suppl III):460, 1985.
28. Garson A, Gillette PC, Porter CJ: Electrophysiologic induction of ventricular dysrhythmias in 152 children with a normal or abnormal heart. J Am Coll Cardiol 1:164, 1983.

29. Kugler JD, Cheatham JP, Gumbiner CH, et al: Results of phenytoin and propranolol drug electrophysiology studies for ventricular tachycardia in patients having repaired lesions with tetralogy of Fallot physiology. Circulation 72(suppl II):341, 1985.
30. Mehta A, Sanchez GR, O'Riordan P, et al: Phenytoin and ventricular dysrhythmias in the young. Proceedings Second World Congress of Pediatric Cardiology, New York, Springer-Verlag, 1985, p 108.
31. Waxman HL, Buxton AE, Marchlinski FE, et al: Amiodarone for sustained ventricular tachyarrhythmias: Electrophysiologic study is not predictive of clinical efficacy. Circulation 68(suppl III):382, 1983.

INDEX

Note: Page numbers in *italics* refer to illustrations; page numbers followed by (t) refer to tables.